# See Health in the Real World!

## Access to videos included with any new book.

W9-BMM-665

# REGISTER NOW!

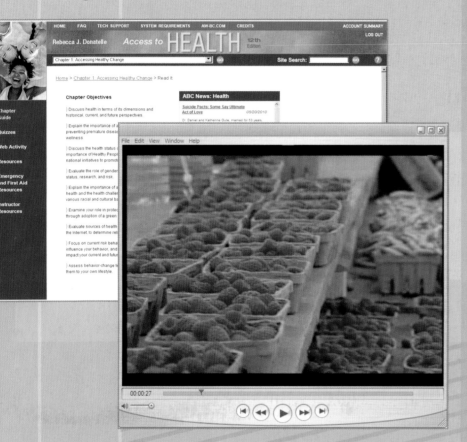

Registration will give you access to more than 30 ABC News videos and related review questions focused on health topics that matter in today's world.

# www.pearsonhighered.com/donatelle

## TO REGISTER

1. Go to www.pearsonhighered.com/donatelle
2. Pick your book cover.
3. Select any chapter from the drop-down menu and click "Go."
4. Click "See It."
5. Click "Register" and follow the on-screen instructions.

Your Access Code is:

*

## TO LOG IN

1. Go to www.pearsonhighered.com/donatelle
2. Pick your book cover.
3. Select any chapter from the drop-down menu and click "Go."
4. Click "See It."
5. Enter your login name and password under "Returning User" and click "Log In."

Hint:
Remember to bookmark the site after you log in.

Technical Support:
http://247pearsoned.custhelp.com

# BEHAVIOR CHANGE CONTRACT

Complete the Assess Yourself questionnaire. After reviewing your results and considering the various factors that influence your decisions, choose a health behavior that you would like to change, starting this quarter or semester. Sign the contract at the bottom to affirm your commitment to making a healthy change and ask a friend to witness it.

My behavior change will be:

_____

My long-term goal for this behavior change is:

_____

These are three obstacles to change (things that I am currently doing or situations that contribute to this behavior or make it harder to change):

    1. _____

    2. _____

    3. _____

The strategies I will use to overcome these obstacles are:

    1. _____

    2. _____

    3. _____

Resources I will use to help me change this behavior include:

    a friend/partner/relative: _____

    a school-based resource: _____

    a community-based resource: _____

    a book or reputable website: _____

In order to make my goal more attainable, I have devised these short-term goals:

| short-term goal | target date | reward |
|---|---|---|
| short-term goal | target date | reward |
| short-term goal | target date | reward |

When I make the long-term behavior change described above, my reward will be:

_____ target date: _____

I intend to make the behavior change described above. I will use the strategies and rewards to achieve the goals that will contribute to a healthy behavior change.

Signed: _____  Witness: _____

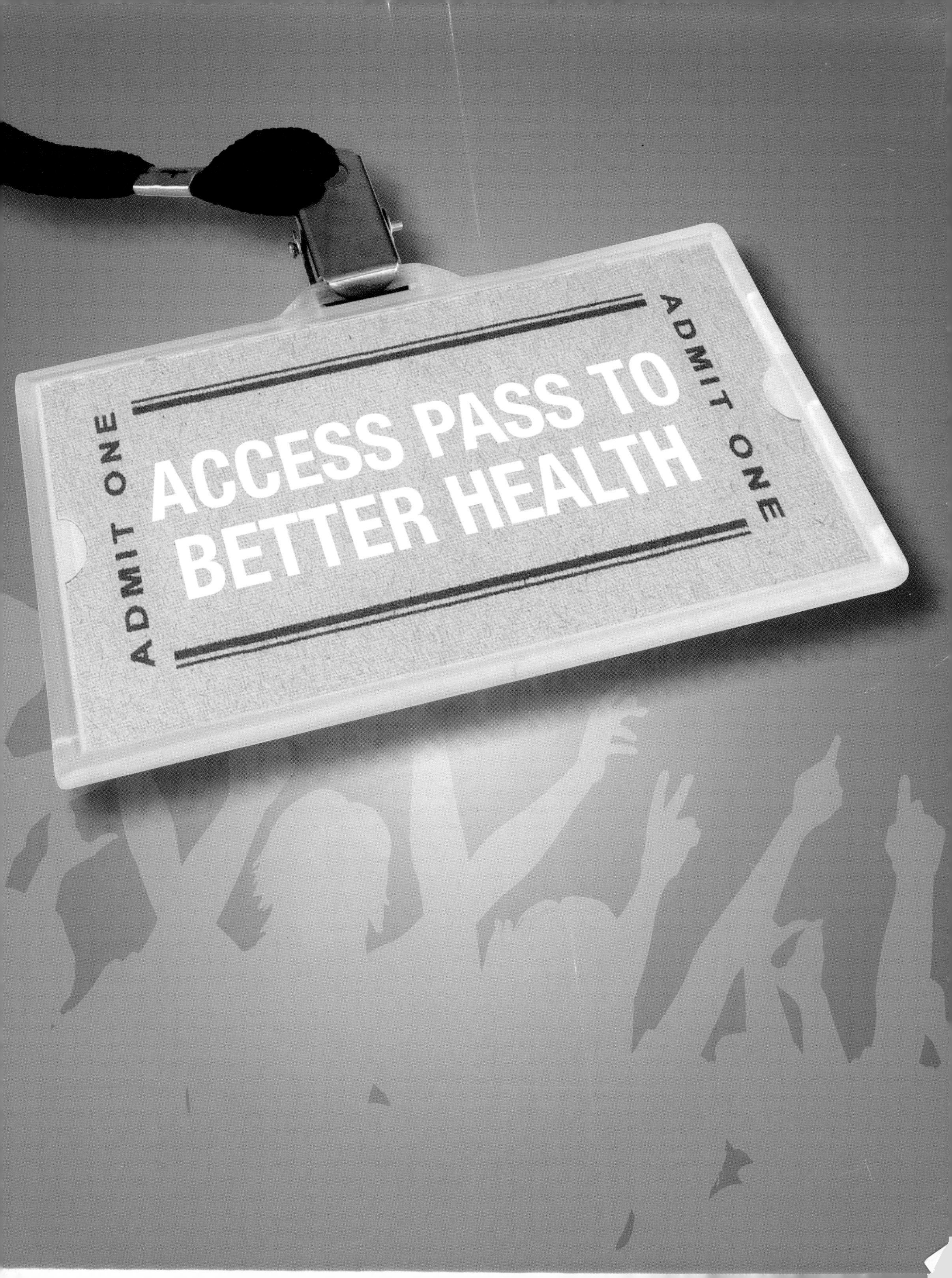
ADMIT ONE
ACCESS PASS TO
BETTER HEALTH
ADMIT ONE

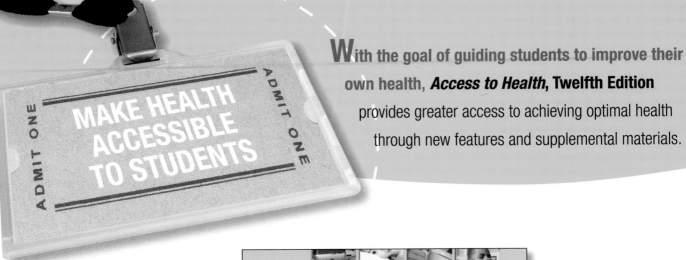

**W**ith the goal of guiding students to improve their own health, *Access to Health*, Twelfth Edition provides greater access to achieving optimal health through new features and supplemental materials.

## NEW! Focus On Chapters

These chapters address subjects that are essential to one's health and wellness, but are not usually given sufficient coverage in a personal health text. Consolidating and expanding this information and presenting it in chapter format makes it more accessible for instructors to teach and assign.

### Focus On chapters cover the following topics:

- Spiritual Health
- Sleep
- Body Image
- Health Inheritance
- Risk for Diabetes
- Risk for Unintentional Injury

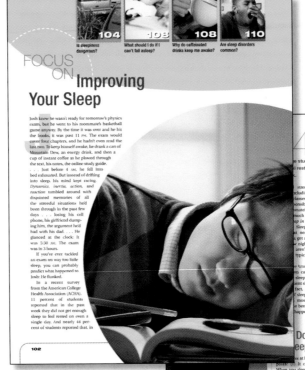

## NEW! Consumer Health Boxes

These boxes provide students with guidelines for becoming critical consumers of health products and information.

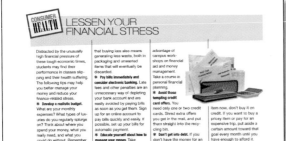

## NEW! Points of View Boxes

These boxes present controversial health issues and explain opposing viewpoints on the issues.

**Where Do You Stand?** critical thinking questions encourage students to critically evaluate the information and form their own opinions.

### POINTS OF VIEW

## Circumcision:
### RISK VERSUS BENEFIT

Circumcision, the surgical removal of the foreskin from the penis, can be a controversial issue for parents. They must balance personal, cultural, and health issues in deciding whether to circumcise a son.

Approximately 56 percent (1.1 million) of all newborn boys are circumcised in the United States each year. Here are some of the arguments against and for circumcision.

**Arguments against Circumcision**

○ It is a surgical procedure which may cause pain to the infant, and there are potential complications such as bleeding, acquiring an infection, improper healing, or cutting the foreskin too long or too short.
○ Families may feel the foreskin is needed for identity reasons, sexual pleasure reasons, or other reasons linked to religion or culture.
○ Much of the research on the relationship between circumcision and sexually transmitted infections was done in developing countries and may not be indicative of outcomes in developed nations.
○ Men lose a degree of sexual pleasure and stimulation when the foreskin is removed. Many unique nerve endings—found only in the foreskin—are lost forever.

**Arguments for Circumcision**

○ Circumcised males have a lower risk of penile cancer.
○ Circumcised males have a lower risk of urinary tract infections during their first year, easier genital hygiene, and a lower risk of foreskin infections.
○ Circumcision has been shown to have a protective effect against human immunodeficiency virus (HIV), herpes simplex virus 2 (HSV-2), and human papillomavirus (HPV) transmission in males.
○ Families may have religious or cultural reasons for wishing to circumcise their sons (in the Jewish faith, for example, circumcision is performed in a ceremony called a bris, and represents the covenant God made with the patriarch Abraham). Some people also believe a son's penis should look the same as his father's.

**Where Do You Stand?**

○ If you had a son, what decision would you make regarding circumcising him?
○ What factors—religious, cultural, aesthetic, or health-related—would have the most impact on your decision?
○ If you are male, does your circumcised or uncircumcised status affect your opinion?

**Sources:** A. A. R. Tobian, R. H. Gray, and T. C. Quinn, "Male Circumcision for the Prevention of Acquisition and Transmission of Sexually Transmitted Infections: The Case for Neonatal Circumcision," *Archives of Pediatrics & Adolescent Medicine* 164 (2010): 78–84; M. Moreno, "Advice for Patients: Male Circumcision," *Archives of Pediatrics & Adolescent Medicine* 164, no. 1 (2010): 104; Centers for Disease Control and Prevention, "Male Circumcision and Risk for HIV Transmission and Other Health Conditions: Implications for the United States," Centers for Disease Control and Prevention, Updated February 2008, www.cdc.gov/hiv/resources/factsheets/circumcision.htm; Mayo Clinic Staff, "Circumcision (Male): Why It's Done," February 2010, www.mayoclinic.com/health/circumcision/MY01023/DSECTION=why-its-done.

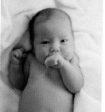

## What's Working for You?

Maybe you already are doing things to enhance your psychological health. Are any of the following true for you?

☐ I have a network of friends and advisers I can go to when I need to talk about a difficult problem.
☐ I know where to find psychological counseling on campus should I need it.
☐ I have healthy outlets for dealing with my emotions when I'm upset.
☐ I volunteer regularly in my college community, an activity that not only helps the community, but gives me a sense of purpose as well.

## NEW! What's Working for You?

These features emphasize the accessibility of healthy behaviors by calling students' attention to the little things they are already doing to improve their health.

## NEW! Why Should I Care?

This features address the relevance of health issues to students' lives by presenting information on the effects poor health habits can have on students in the here and now.

nausea, vomiting, stomach
r diarrhea. Although stress
oms, it is clearly related
of having symp-
e, people
ore sus-
rome,
ates
m.

ty
ng
on
ogy
ion-
se to
bility to
reviews of
health conse-
tress over a long period can

### "Why Should I Care?"

The evidence is compelling that stress and immune system functioning are linked. Exposure to academic stressors and self-reported stress are associated with increased upper respiratory tract infections among students. Take time to de-stress, and you might avoid being on the sidelines with a bad cold.

imp
sea
mu
as 6
sors
and
long
spo
ca
un
to im
among

**Stress**
think tha
in older pe
constant, reg
a big wrench in
life. For more inform
bido, see the **Gender & Healt**

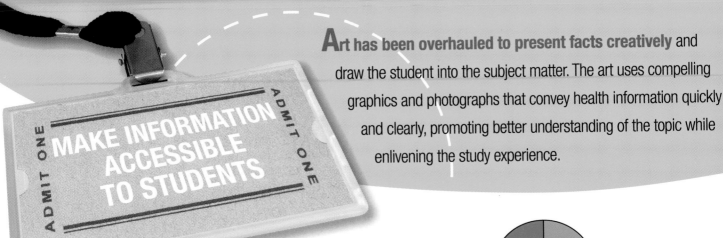

**A**rt has been overhauled to present facts creatively and draw the student into the subject matter. The art uses compelling graphics and photographs that convey health information quickly and clearly, promoting better understanding of the topic while enlivening the study experience.

Dull! ▶

# Dynamic!

Pie-charts have been made more visually appealing through innovative and informative artwork.

Other (18.4%)

Hospital (36.8%)

Prescription drugs (12.1%)

Nursing home (7.3%)

Physician services (25.4%)

**Type of expenditures**

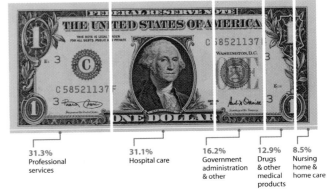

**Total expenditures = $2.2 trillion**

| 31.3% Professional services | 31.1% Hospital care | 16.2% Government administration & other | 12.9% Drugs & other medical products | 8.5% Nursing home & home care |

*Figure 18.8:* **Where do we spend our health care dollars?**

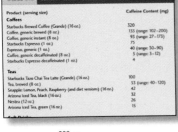

| TABLE 8.6 | Caffeine Content of Various Products |
|---|---|
| **Product (serving size)** | **Caffeine Content (mg)** |
| **Coffees** | |
| Starbucks Brewed Coffee (Grande) (16 oz.) | 320 |
| Coffee, generic brewed (8 oz.) | 135 (range: 102–200) |
| Coffee, generic instant (8 oz.) | 93 (range: 27–173) |
| Starbucks Espresso (1 oz.) | 75 |
| Espresso, generic (1 oz.) | 40 (range: 30–90) |
| Coffee, generic decaffeinated (8 oz.) | 5 (range: 3–12) |
| Starbucks Espresso decaffeinated (1 oz.) | 4 |
| | |
| **Teas** | |
| Starbucks Tazo Chai Tea Latte (Grande) (16 oz.) | 100 |
| Tea, brewed (8 oz.) | 53 (range: 40–120) |
| Snapple: Lemon, Peach, Raspberry (and diet versions) (16 oz.) | 42 |
| Arizona Iced Tea, black (16 oz.) | 32 |
| Nestea (12 oz.) | 26 |
| Arizona Iced Tea, green (16 oz.) | 15 |

◀ Flat!

# Fascinating!

Simple tables have been rendered as captivating art to more quickly convey information.

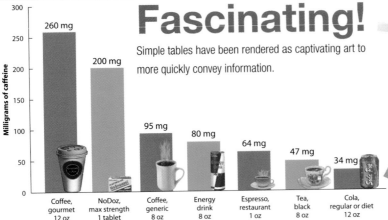

*Figure 13.5:* **Caffeine Content Comparison**

Staid! ▶

# Standout!

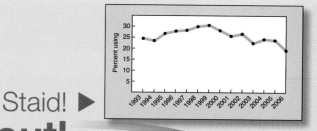

Graphs have been enhanced with eye-catching art to bring important statistics to life.

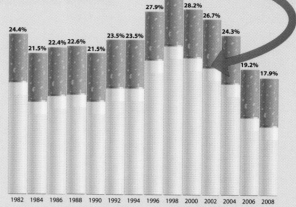

24.4% 21.5% 22.4% 22.6% 21.5% 23.5% 23.5% 27.9% 30.0% 28.2% 26.7% 24.3% 19.2% 17.9%

1982 1984 1986 1988 1990 1992 1994 1996 1998 2000 2002 2004 2006 2008

*Figure 12.1:* **Trends in Prevalence of Cigarette Smoking**

---

## Assess Yourself

### How Well Do You Communicate?

**my health lab**

Imagine that you are in each of the situations below, and indicate how confident and satisfied you are that you could communicate competently using the following scale.

1. Very dissatisfied with my ability to communicate
2. Somewhat dissatisfied with my ability to communicate
3. Not sure how effectively I could communicate
4. Somewhat satisfied that I could communicate competently
5. Very satisfied that I could communicate competently

_____ 1. Someone asks you personal questions that you feel uncomfortable answering. You'd like to tell the person that you don't want to answer.

_____ 2. You think a friend is drinking more alcohol than is healthy, and you want to bring the topic up to her.

_____ 3. Your colleague asks you to write him a letter of recommendation. You don't think he is well suited for the position to which he's applying.

_____ 4. During a heated discussion about social issues, the person with whom you are talking says, "You're not listening to anything I'm saying!"

_____ 5. A friend shares his creative writing with you. You don't think the writing is very good, but you need to respond to his request for an opinion.

_____ 6. Your roommate's bad habits are really getting on your nerves. You want to tell her you're bothered and that you'd like her to stop.

_____ 7. You arrive at a party and discover that you don't know anyone there.

_____ 8. A classmate asks you for notes for the classes he missed, but you realize he has missed half the classes and expects you to bail him out.

_____ 9. The person you have been dating declares, "I love you." You care about her, but you don't love her, at least not yet.

_____ 10. A friend comes to you with his problems, and you give him attention and advice. However, when you want to discuss your problems, he doesn't seem to have the time. You value the friendship, but you don't like feeling it's one way.

_____ TOTAL

### Interpreting Your Score

If your score indicates that you are moderately satisfied (25–39) or dissatisfied (10–24) with your communication skills, notice whether your answers are extremes (1s and 5s). Focus on improving your skills in the situations that make you uneasy.

**Source:** Based on Julia Wood and Stephanie Coopman's instructor's Resource Manual for Wood's text, *Interpersonal Communication: Everyday Encounters*, 5th ed. Copyright © 2006, Cengage Learning.

## Assess Yourself and Your Plan for Change Boxes

Using these combined features, students can assess their current health behaviors and explore specific ideas for setting goals and following through on behavior change.

Students can fill out these assessments online on the Companion Website or MyHealthLab.®

---

## YOUR PLAN FOR CHANGE

The **Assess Yourself** activity gave you the chance to look at how you communicate. Now that you have considered your responses, you can take steps toward becoming a better communicator and improving your relationships.

**Today, you can:**

○ Call a friend you haven't talked to in a while or arrange a coffee date with a new acquaintance you'd like to get to know better.

○ Start a journal in which you keep track of communication and relationship issues that arise. Look for trends and think about ways you can change your behavior to address them.

**Within the next 2 weeks, you can:**

○ Spend some time letting the people you care about know how important their relationship is to you.

○ If there is someone with whom you have a conflict, arrange a time to sit down with that person in a neutral setting away from distractions to talk about the issues.

**By the end of the semester, you can:**

○ Practice being an active listener and notice when your mind wanders while you are listening to someone.

○ Take note of your nonverbal messages. Work on maintaining good eye contact and using open body language and inviting facial expressions.

**O**rganized by learning areas and a snap to navigate, MyHealthLab® makes it easier than ever to learn about personal health and wellness.

PEARSON
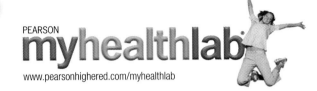
**myhealthlab**
www.pearsonhighered.com/myhealthlab

## READ IT

- Pearson eText laid out just like the book, featuring highlighting, bookmarks, and notes
- Chapter objectives, RSS feeds
- **NEW!** Pre- and post-reading quizzes that are assignable and gradable

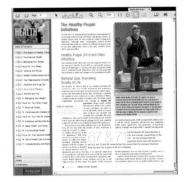
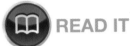

*Pearson eText*

## SEE IT

- **NEW!** More than a dozen new *ABC News* videos
- **NEW!** Assignable quizzes that speak to the gradebook

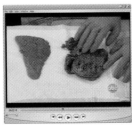

*ABC News Videos*

## HEAR IT

- MP3 Tutor Sessions for major concepts in each chapter with assignable quizzes, which speak to the gradebook
- **NEW!** Audio case studies

## DO IT

- Critical thinking questions and news quizzes
- Web links
- **NEW!** Activities based on Points of View boxes

## REVIEW IT

- Glossary with flashcards to use on mobile phones
- Practice quizzes for each chapter

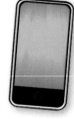

## LIVE IT

- All the Assess Yourself worksheets from the book
- **NEW!** How Healthy Are You? module
- Additional worksheets and behavior change contract, plus steps to support students through their behavior change project

## NEW! ON THE GO

More and more, students are relying on mobile devices that let them study on the go. In this section, your student will find tools to help take control of their health at any time.

- **NEW!** Tweet Your Health, a Twitter-based web application for tracking health behaviors, receiving health tips, and more!
- Mobile applications directory to help students stay on top of their health

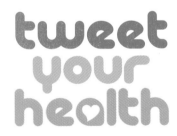

**tweet your health**

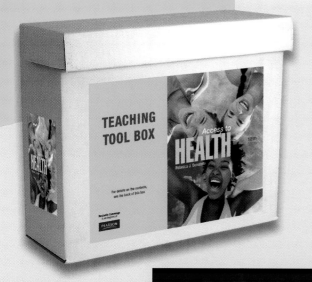

## Teaching Tool Box

Save hours of valuable planning time with one comprehensive course planning kit. In one handy box, adjunct, part-time, and full-time faculty will find a wealth of supplements and resources that reinforce key learning from the text and suit virtually any teaching style.

978-0-321-72654-4 • 0-321-72654-5

The Teaching Tool Box provides all the prepping and lecture tools an instructor needs:

- The Course-at-a-Glance Quick Reference Guide
- Instructor Resource and Support Manual
- Printed Test Bank
- An Instructor Resource DVD including PowerPoint® Lecture Outlines, PRS Clicker Questions, Quiz Show questions, *ABC News* Video Clips, Transparency Masters, and the Computerized Test Bank
- A MyHealthLab® access kit
- *Great Ideas: Active Ways to Teach Health and Wellness*
- The helpful *Eat Right! Healthy Eating in College and Beyond* student supplement
- The informative *Live Right! Beating Stress in College and Beyond* student supplement
- *Behavior Change Log Book and Wellness Journal*
- Take Charge Self-Assessment Worksheets

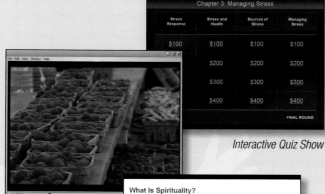

*Interactive Quiz Show*

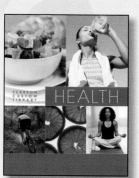

*More than a dozen new ABC News Videos*

*PowerPoint Slides*

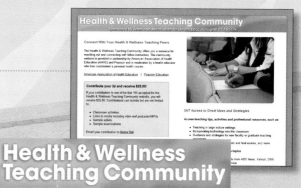

## Health & Wellness Teaching Community

www.pearsonhighered.com/healthcommunity

Connect with other health instructors! The Health & Wellness Teaching Community website, sponsored by AAHE and Pearson, serves instructors like you by offering teaching tips and ideas, and by providing a forum for you to discuss health-related issues with your peers.

## Pearson Custom Library

The Pearson Custom Library: Health and Nutrition custom publishing program gives you the freedom to create your own customized textbook for courses in health, fitness, and wellness. Select the book chapters you need, in the sequence you want. Delete chapters you don't use: Your students pay only for the material you choose. You're in control. Find out more at www.pearsoncustom.com (keyword search: health).

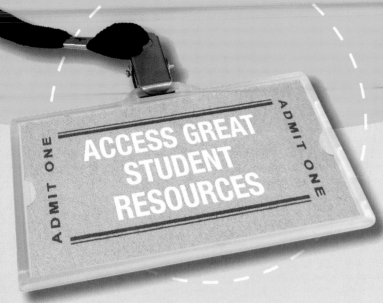

# ACCESS GREAT STUDENT RESOURCES

## Student Supplements

### Live Right! Beating Stress in College and Beyond
978-0-321-49149-7 · 0-321-49149-1

*Live Right!* gives students useful tips for coping with stressful life challenges both during college and for the rest of their lives. Topics include sleep, managing finances, time management, coping with academic pressure, and relationships.

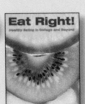

### Eat Right! Healthy Eating in College and Beyond
978-0-8053-8288-4 · 0-8053-8288-7

This handy, full-color booklet provides students with practical guidelines, tips, shopper's guides, and recipes that turn healthy eating principles into blueprints for action. Topics include healthy eating in the cafeteria, dorm room, and fast-food restaurants; planning meals on a budget; weight management; vegetarian alternatives; and how alcohol impacts health.

### Take Charge of Your Health Worksheets
978-0-321-49942-4 · 0-321-49942-5

Twelve new worksheets have been added to this edition's collection of self-assessment activities, providing a total of 50 self-assessment exercises. Worksheets are available as a gummed pad and can be packaged at no additional charge with the main text.

### Behavior Change Logbook and Wellness Journal
978-0-8053-7844-3 · 0-8053-7844-8

This assessment tool helps students track daily exercise and nutritional intake and create a long-term nutritional and fitness prescription plan. This supplement can be packaged at no additional charge with the main text.

### New Lifestyles Pedometer
978-0-321-51803-3 · 0-321-51803-9

Help students take strides to better health with this pedometer, a first step toward overall health and wellness. This pedometer measures steps, distance (miles), activity time, and calories, and provides a time clock. Available for only $8.50 when packaged with any text.

## Flexible Options

### Pearson eText Student Access Code Card
978-0-321-72657-5 · 0-321-72657-X

Pearson eText gives students access to the text whenever and wherever they can access the Internet. The eText pages look exactly like the printed text, and include powerful interactive and customization functions. This does not include the actual bound book.

### CourseSmart eTextbook
978-0-321-72658-2 · 0-321-72658-8

CourseSmart eTextbooks are an exciting new choice for students looking to save money. As an alternative to purchasing the print textbook, students can subscribe to the same content online and save up to 40% off the suggested list price of the print text. Go to www.coursesmart.com.

### Books à la Carte
978-0-321-72166-2 · 0-321-72166-7

This edition features the exact same content as **Access to Health, Twelfth Edition** in a convenient, three-hole-punched, loose-leaf version. Books à la Carte also offers a great value for your students—this format costs 35% less than a new textbook.

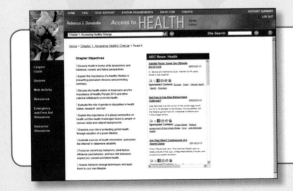

## Companion Website

www.pearsonhighered.com/donatelle

The Companion Website, organized by learning areas, includes chapter objectives, study quizzes, chapter-specific Web links, a glossary and flashcards, as well as interactive self-assessment worksheets, critical thinking activities, and health case studies.

For a complete list of supplements available with this text, please visit our Web Catalog at www.pearsonhighered.com/hk

*Access to*
# HEALTH

**12th Edition**

## Rebecca J. Donatelle
**Oregon State University**

**Benjamin Cummings**

Boston  Columbus  Indianapolis  New York  San Francisco  Upper Saddle River
Amsterdam  Cape Town  Dubai  London  Madrid  Milan  Munich  Paris  Montréal  Toronto
Delhi  Mexico City  São Paulo  Sydney  Hong Kong  Seoul  Singapore  Taipei  Tokyo

Executive Editor: Sandra Lindelof
Project Editor: Kari Hopperstead
Director of Development: Barbara Yien
Development Editor: Claire Alexander
Art Development Manager: Laura Southworth
Art Development Editor: Kari Hopperstead
Associate Editor: Brianna Paulson
Editorial Assistant: Meghan Zolnay
Associate Media Producer: Molly Crowther
Senior Managing Editor: Deborah Cogan

Senior Production Project Manager: Nancy Tabor
Production Management and Composition: Progressive
  Publishing Alternatives
Cover and Interior Designer: Hespenheide Design
Illustrators: Precision Graphics
Photo Researcher: Roman Barnes
Senior Photo Editor: Donna Kalal
Manufacturing Buyer: Jeff Sargent
Senior Marketing Manager: Neena Bali

Cover Photo Credit: Lawrence Monneret/Getty Images

Library of Congress Cataloging-in-Publication Data

Donatelle, Rebecca J., 1950–
    Access to health / Rebecca J. Donatelle. — 12th ed.
      p. cm.
    ISBN-13: 978-0-321-69908-4
    ISBN-10: 0-321-69908-4
  1. Health.    I. Title.
    RA776.D66 2012
    613—dc22
                                              2010046647

ISBN 10: 0-321-69908-4; ISBN 13: 978-0-321-69908-4 (Student edition)
ISBN 10: 0-321-72651-0; ISBN 13: 978-0-321-72651-3 (Professional copy)

1 2 3 4 5 6 7 8 9 10—DOM—14 13 12 11 10

**Benjamin Cummings**
is an imprint of

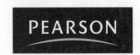

www.pearsonhighered.com

# Brief Contents

# Contents

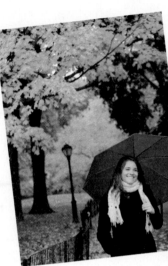
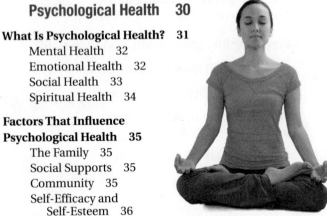

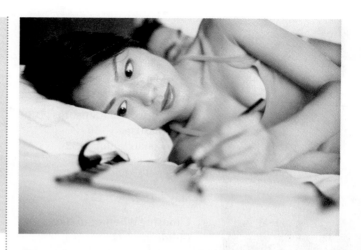

Part Two: Creating Healthy and Caring Relationships

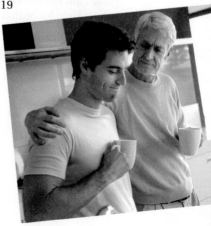

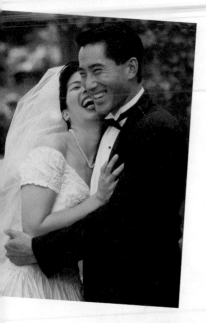

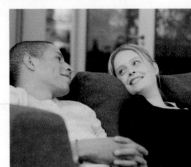
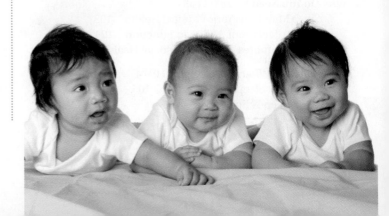

## Part Three: Building Healthly Lifestyles

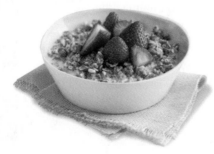

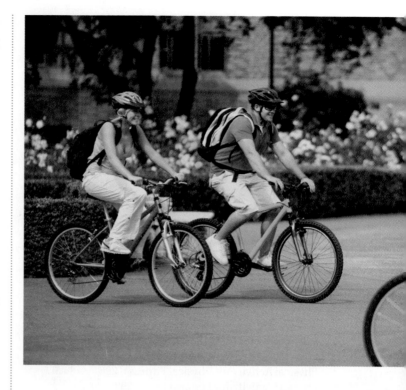

# Part Four: Avoiding Risks from Harmful Habits

## 10  Recognizing and Avoiding Addiction    328

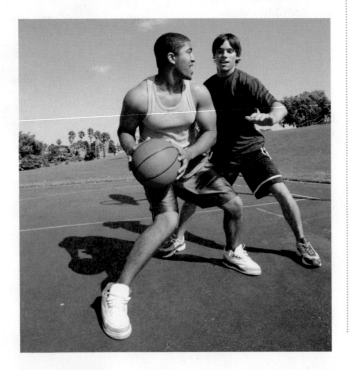

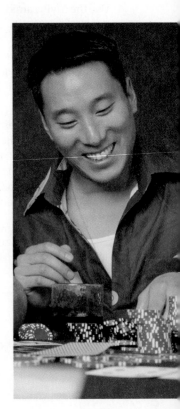

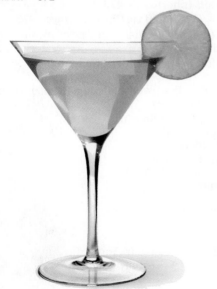

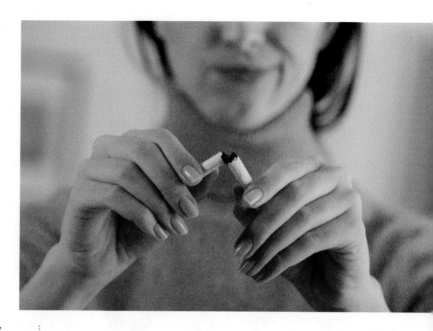

## Part Five: Preventing and Fighting Disease

## 14 Protecting against Infectious Diseases and Sexually Transmitted Infections 434

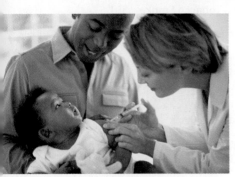

## FOCUS ON: Understanding Your Health Inheritance 472

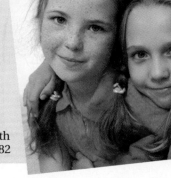

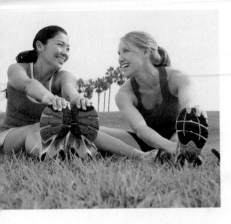

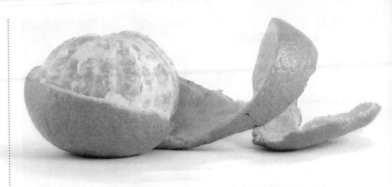

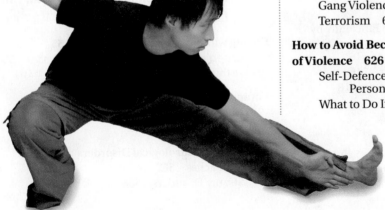

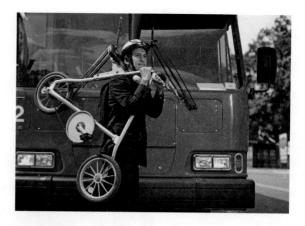

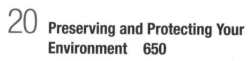

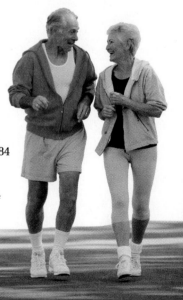

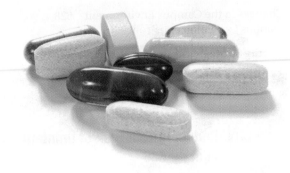

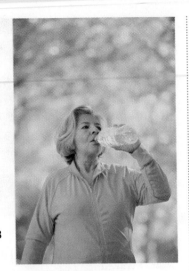

# Feature Boxes

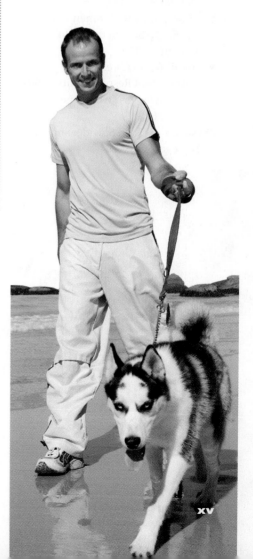

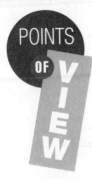

## POINTS OF VIEW

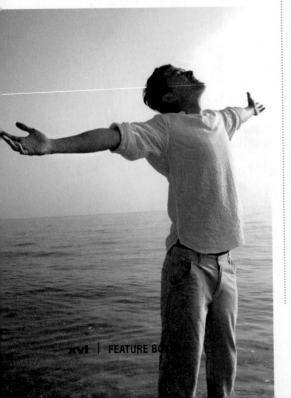

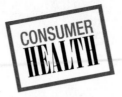

## CONSUMER HEALTH

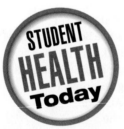

## STUDENT HEALTH Today

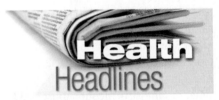

## Health Headlines

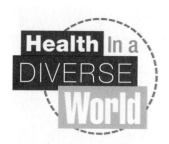

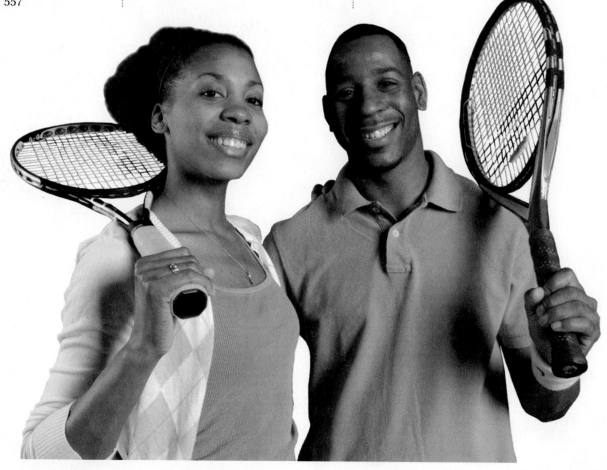

# Preface

In today's world, health is headline news. The issues and information may seem so complex and contradictory, that you may wonder how to make sense of it all. What can you do to ensure a life that is healthy and long and to help improve the health of the people around you? Getting healthy and staying healthy can be a challenge, but it is a worthwhile goal, and one that is well within reach for most of us. No matter where your health is now, you can make positive changes for a healthier future, you can help others maintain health, and you can become an agent for healthy change in your community.

My goal in writing *Access to Health*, Twelfth Edition, is to provide students with just what that title says: access to health information and to their own health potential. This book provides the most scientifically valid information available to help students be smarter in their health decision making, more positively involved in their personal health, and more active as advocates for healthy changes in their communities. Change isn't something that just happens: It takes knowledge, preparation, and effort; therefore, this book places emphasis on empowering students to identify their health risks, create plans for change, and make healthy lifestyle changes part of their daily routines.

*Access to Health* is designed to help students quickly grasp the information presented and understand its relevance to their own lives and the lives of others. Exciting revisions have been made to the art and design of the book in this new edition, with the purpose of capturing students' interest, engaging them in the subject matter, and helping them to be better prepared for whatever the future holds. In addition, six Focus On chapters have been added to delve into areas of health that are of practical importance to college students but are not always given sufficient coverage in a personal health text. These Focus On chapters spotlight spiritual health, sleep, body image, health inheritance, diabetes, and unintentional injury.

Looking back from the time when I taught my first Personal Health course as a teaching assistant in graduate school, to the completion of this, the Twelfth Edition of *Access to Health*, I am gratified by the overwhelming success that this text has enjoyed through its many revisions and changes. With each edition of the text, I have listened to the thoughtful suggestions of instructors and students using the book, as well as to the feedback from my own students in keeping the book relevant, interesting, and accessible. I hope that this edition's rich foundation of scientifically valid information, its wealth of technological tools and resources, and its thought-provoking features will stimulate you to share my enthusiasm for personal health and to become actively engaged in behaviors that will lead to better health for all.

## New to This Edition

*Access to Health*, Twelfth Edition, maintains many features that the text has become known for, while incorporating several major revisions and exciting new features. The most noteworthy changes to the text as a whole include the following:

- **New Focus On mini-chapters** address subjects that are essential to one's health and wellness, but are not usually given sufficient or consolidated coverage in a personal health text: spiritual health, sleep, body image, health inheritance, diabetes, and unintentional injuries.
- **A completely overhauled art program** presents concepts and facts creatively, with a goal of drawing the student into the subject matter. There is more art than ever before, and it uses compelling graphics and photographs to convey health information quickly and clearly, promoting better understanding of the topic while enlivening the study experience.
- **A new, innovative design** "hooks" students into the material through its vibrant, eclectic, eye-catching photos and features.
- **New Points of View boxes** present controversial health issues and explain opposing viewpoints on the issues. **Where Do You Stand?** critical thinking questions within the boxes encourage students to critically evaluate the information and form their own opinions.
- **New Why Should I Care?** features address the relevance of health issues to students' lives by presenting information on the effects poor health habits have on students in the here and now.
- **New What's Working for You?** features emphasize the accessibility of healthy behaviors by calling students' attention to the little things they are already doing to improve their health.
- **New Consumer Health** boxes provide students with guidelines for becoming critical consumers of health-related products and information.
- **Assess Yourself self-assessments** have been designed individually so that each is unique, fun, and accessible—and they encourage students to follow up on the website and course management.
- **New Pulled Statistics** draw students into the text by catching their eyes with large numerals and compelling statistics.
- **Chapter opening questions** are now tied by page number and image to a photo later in the chapter. The question is directly answered in the photo legend, making it a more visually striking and pedagogically effective tool.

- **Changes to the Companion Website include the following:**

  * **The See It** section is SMS-protected and contains *ABC News* videos with assessment questions.
  * **The Hear It** section contains new audio case studies with assessment questions.
  * **The Do It** section contains new exercises, and assessments based on the Points of View boxes in the text.
  * **The Live It** section has enhanced navigation and behavior change features, including a new How Healthy Are You? module.
  * **New On the Go** section includes Tweet Your Health, a brand new Twitter-based service that keeps students focused on behavior change.

- MyHealthLab® updates include the following:

  * **All of the same sections that appear in the Companion Website now also appear in MyHealthLab,** and the assignments all speak to the grade book. An additional set of review questions is also available for instructor assignment only.
  * **New discussion questions** about controversial health issues make creation and implementation of an online discussion forum easier and more accessible for instructors. The discussion features tie in to the Points of View boxes, *ABC News* videos, and audio case studies.
  * **New Pearson eText** is laid out just like the printed textbook. Students can create notes, highlight text in different colors, create bookmarks, zoom in and out, click hyperlinked words and phrases to view definitions, and view a video or visit a website as they read the text.

# Chapter-by-Chapter Revisions

*Access to Health,* Twelfth Edition, has been updated line by line to provide students with the most current information and references for further exploration. Portions of chapters have been reorganized to improve the flow of topics, while figures, tables, feature boxes, and photos have all been added, improved on, and updated. The following is a chapter-by-chapter listing of some of the most noteworthy changes, updates, and additions.

**Chapter 1: Accessing Your Health** This chapter has been completely rewritten to focus more on individual choices in health and the interaction between individuals and their society, as well as the personal, social, and environmental determinants influencing one's health. An expanded section on behavior change includes discussion of the social cognitive model and explores the various processes involved in behavior change at different stages of the transtheoretical model. New figures illustrate the four leading causes of preventable death and the social cognitive model. New feature boxes discuss health disparities, maintaining motivation, and changing negative self-talk.

**Chapter 2: Promoting and Preserving Your Psychological Health** New sections discuss community as a factor in psychological health, mental illness stigma, and therapy treatment models. Information has been added on borderline personality disorder. A new figure illustrates mental health concerns of college students. New feature boxes explore positive psychology, adult attention-deficit/hyperactivity disorder (ADHD), depression in different populations, nonsuicidal self-injury, and self-help books.

**Focus On: Cultivating Your Spiritual Health** ALL NEW Focus On chapter discusses the nature of spirituality and its distinction from religion, the potential benefits of focusing on spiritual health, and ways to enhance spiritual health. New figures depict the facets of spirituality and the elements of mindfulness. New feature boxes look at cultivating spirituality through service and practicing environmental mindfulness. New self-assessment evaluates spiritual IQ.

**Chapter 3: Managing Stress and Coping with Life's Challenges** New sections cover stress-related weight gain, hair loss, and digestive problems; the intellectual and psychological effects of stress; Type C and Type D personalities; procrastination; investing in loved ones; and cultivating spirituality. The revised section on personal sources of stress includes discussion of relationships and living environments. New feature boxes cover the effects of stress on libido, positive psychology approaches to stress reduction, learning to say no, and money management. New figures illustrate the acute stress response and common sources of stress among Americans.

**Focus On: Improving Your Sleep** ALL NEW Focus On chapter covers the important functions of sleep, mechanics of sleep, sleep needs, ways to improve sleep habits, and sleep disorders. The chapter includes new figures of the sleep cycle and a sleep diary, and a new table on the gender differences in sleep disorders. New feature boxes include tips for dealing with jet lag and choosing ecofriendly bedding. A new self-assessment looks at personal sleep habits.

**Chapter 4: Building Healthy Relationships and Communicating Effectively** Reorganization of the chapter pulls all of the information on successful relationships into one section. A new section discusses self-esteem and self-acceptance, and jealousy is now covered in the context of other issues confronted by couples. A revised figure on Sternberg's Triangular Theory of Love now includes components that make up companionate and passionate love, and a new figure in a revised feature box visually summarizes gender differences in communication styles. New feature boxes look at the Defense of Marriage Act and recognizing a potential abuser, and a new table presents common parenting styles.

**Chapter 5: Understanding Your Sexuality** The chapter has been reorganized to discuss anatomy and physiology first, followed by sexual identity and sexual expression. A new section discusses andropause, and a revised feature box presents opposing views on circumcision. New feature boxes discuss disorders of sexual development, sexuality and disability, and taking steps toward healthy sexuality.

## Chapter 6: Considering Your Reproductive Choices

A revised table shows the latest information on effectiveness, sexually transmitted infection (STI) protection, frequency of use, and cost of contraceptive methods. Reorganized text consistently presents the advantages and disadvantages of each contraceptive method. New sections cover choosing a method of contraception, preconception care, and infant mortality. A new figure shows proper use of a female condom. New feature boxes cover increasing men's involvement in reproductive and sexual health, fight for affordable birth control on college campuses, environmentally friendly forms of contraception, and talking about safer sex with a partner. New tables look at top-reported means of contraception among college students and types of prenatal care practitioners.

## Chapter 7: Eating for a Healthier You

A reorganized section presents guidelines on how to eat in a more healthy way. The expanded section on food allergies and intolerances includes discussion of celiac disease, and a new section looks at genetically modified crops. New feature boxes look at global nutrition, benefits of fiber, sustainable seafood, functional foods, simple rules for healthy eating, and genetically modified foods. Revised illustrated tables present water-soluble vitamins, fat-soluble vitamins, major minerals, and trace minerals separately. A new table presents common foodborne illnesses. New and revised figures illustrate trends in per capita nutrient consumption, the digestive process, anatomy of a whole grain, sustainable seafood, interpreting a food label, and the MyPyramid Plan.

## Chapter 8: Reaching and Maintaining a Healthy Weight

This chapter now begins with a discussion of factors contributing to overweight and obesity, followed by methods of determining a healthy weight. New feature boxes cover the stigma associated with obesity, the link between sedentary lifestyle and obesity, the proposed classification of obesity as a disability, and tips on making healthy eating and exercising more appealing. The body mass index figure has been revised to include more specific values and a new figure depicts potential negative effects of overweight and obesity. A new table presents recommendations for optimal body fat.

## Focus On: Enhancing Your Body Image

ALL NEW Focus On chapter discusses the nature of body image and factors that affect it, body image disorders, explanation of eating disorders and risk factors relating to them, tips for dealing with eating disorders in yourself or in friends, and exercise disorders. New figures depict the body image continuum, the eating issues continuum, factors that contribute to eating disorders, health effects of anorexia nervosa, health effects of bulimia nervosa, and the female athlete triad. A new feature box offers tips for developing a positive body image. A new self-assessment evaluates possible disordered eating.

## Chapter 9: Improving Your Physical Fitness

A completely reorganized chapter discusses motivation and guidelines for creating a fitness plan, then moves into applying the FITT principle to each component of fitness. A revised discussion of yoga, tai chi, and Pilates looks at the potential for these forms of exercise to develop multiple components of fitness, as well as core strength. New and revised figures illustrate components of physical fitness, health benefits of exercise, calories burned by different activities, how to take a pulse, and target heart rate ranges. A new table presents the 2008 Physical Activity Guidelines for Americans; another new table looks at performance-enhancing substances. Two new illustrated tables present forms of resistance training and different exercise equipment. New feature boxes discuss Title IX in athletics; physical activity for special populations; low-fat chocolate milk as a post-workout drink; and shopping for fitness facilities, equipment, and clothing. A push-up test has been added to the self-assessment.

## Chapter 10: Recognizing and Avoiding Addiction

This chapter has been reorganized to discuss the effects of addiction on family and friends earlier in the chapter. Psychological factors are now discussed in a new biopsychosocial model of addiction section. A new feature box provides tips on controlling gambling.

## Chapter 11: Drinking Alcohol Responsibly

New feature boxes include tips for drinking responsibly, discussion of changes in the legal age for drinking, review of effects of alcohol mixed with energy drinks, guidelines for dealing with an alcohol emergency, and analysis of alcohol and racial or ethnic differences. New figures illustrate a standard drink, the negative consequences of drinking among college students, the rates of alcohol use among college students, and physical and physiological effects of different blood alcohol concentration levels.

## Chapter 12: Ending Tobacco Use

New sections cover the reasons that people smoke and the use of pipes and hookahs. A new table presents symptoms to expect when quitting smoking. A new figure illustrates how trends in tobacco use correlate with lung cancer deaths. New feature boxes discuss smoking bans on college campuses, environmental tobacco smoke policies, and alternative tobacco-use cessation methods.

## Chapter 13: Avoiding Drug Misuse and Abuse

New sections have been added on the abuse of over-the-counter drugs; caffeine as a stimulant drug; and treatment and recovery from drug addiction, including treatment approaches and 12-step programs. Coverage of the nonmedical use or abuse of prescription drugs, including drugs used to treat ADHD, has been expanded. New figures show routes of drug administration, the caffeine content of various products, and college students' stated reasons for nonmedical use of ADHD drugs. New feature boxes address abuse of Vicodin and Oxy-Contin, trends in drug use among racial and ethnic minority groups, and tips for responding to an offer of drugs.

**Chapter 14: Protecting against Infectious Diseases and Sexually Transmitted Infections** A new section and new figure discuss herpes gladiatorum. Revised STI sections consistently present signs and symptoms, complications, and diagnosis and treatment of each infection. New feature boxes cover decision making about vaccinations, mandatory HIV testing and reporting, and complications of STIs in women (pelvic inflammatory disease and urinary tract infections). New and revised figures depict the "chain of infection," the body's defenses, chlamydial conjunctivitis, and the continuum of risk for various sexual behaviors. An updated feature box covers both types of the human papillomavirus vaccine, and the self-assessment has been updated and revised.

**Focus On: Understanding Your Health Inheritance** ALL NEW Focus On chapter discusses the role of inheritance in one's health. Topics include the basic makeup of genes and the role they play in inheritance, chromosomes and trait inheritance, single-gene disorders, multifactorial disorders, chromosomal disorders, genetic counseling, and the role of genes in behavior. New figures depict chromosomes, DNA, and genes; a human karyotype; the effect of dominant versus recessive alleles; inheritance patterns of single-gene disorders; and multifactorial disorders. A new feature box looks at the risks and concerns of genetic testing. A new self-assessment helps the student create a personal family health history.

**Chapter 15: Preventing Cardiovascular Disease** This chapter is reorganized to begin with an overview of the cardiovascular system. New information has been added on stents as treatment for cardiovascular disease (CVD). New feature boxes examine eating habits that affect heart health, nutritional supplements and CVD, and young adults and hypertension. New figures illustrate atherosclerosis and coronary heart disease, factors involved in metabolic syndrome, and deaths from heart disease and stroke among people of different ethnicities.

**Focus On: Minimizing Your Risk for Diabetes** ALL NEW Focus On chapter discusses the different types of diabetes and their prevalence and causes, symptoms and potential complications, treatment and management, and ways to prevent developing pre-diabetes. New and revised figures depict the prevalence of diabetes among U.S. adults, biology of diabetes, complications of diabetes, and blood glucose level tests. A new feature box offers tips for reducing diabetes risk. A self-assessment evaluates personal diabetes risk.

**Chapter 16: Reducing Your Cancer Risk** A new discussion looks at increases in lung cancer rates among those who have never smoked. New sections discuss stress and psychological factors as cancer risks, *Helicobacter pylori* and stomach cancer risk, and cancer survivorship. New feature boxes describe the controversy over mammography screening guidelines, breast awareness and self-exam (with revised art), testicular self-exam (with revised art), being a health advocate for yourself or a loved one, and new treatments for cancer.

**Chapter 17: Reducing Risks and Coping with Chronic Conditions** New sections address food allergies and inflammatory bowel disease. A new self-assessment examines potential risk for several types of chronic illness. A new feature box covers the international prevalence of chronic disease. New tables summarize types of headaches and selected modern maladies. New and revised figures show the proportion of college students with chronic conditions, the effects of asthma on the respiratory system, steps of the allergic response, and the number of days of work lost to medical conditions.

**Chapter 18: Choosing Conventional and Complementary Health Care** Both allopathic and complementary health care are now covered in one chapter. New feature boxes look at the placebo effect, the debate over national health insurance, elective surgeries, and personal advocacy in a health care crisis. New tables present information on common herbs and herbal supplements and on nonherbal dietary supplements, including benefits, research findings, and risks. New figures show the conditions that complementary and alternative medicine is most commonly used to treat, the amount of health care spending per person in different nations, and the categories of spending for each health care dollar in the United States. A revised assessment looks at health care behaviors relating to both complementary and alternative medicine.

**Chapter 19: Preventing Violence and Abuse** A revised section on violence on U.S. campuses now begins the chapter. Reorganized sections discuss gang violence and terrorism as forms of collective violence. A new section covers the impact of violence in the media. New feature boxes discuss the culture of silence surrounding sexual assault on campus, the dangers of hazing, intimate partner violence against men, and social networking safety. New figures detail crime rates in the United States, and homicide by weapon type, numbers of bias-motivated crimes, and child maltreatment rates. A new table presents homicide rates in selected nations.

**Focus On: Reducing Your Risk of Unintentional Injury** ALL NEW Focus On chapter describes common unintentional injuries and strategies for preventing them. Topics include motor vehicle safety; guidelines for recreational activities such as bicycling, skateboarding, snow sports, and boating; dangers that arise in the home, including falls and fires; effects of loud noise; and work injuries. New feature boxes discuss risk management driving techniques and hearing loss from portable music devices. New figures include the proper fit for a bicycle helmet, noise levels of various sounds, safe lifting technique, and carpal tunnel syndrome. A new self-assessment looks at personal risk for vehicular injuries.

**Chapter 20: Preserving and Protecting Your Environment** A new feature box examines the controversy over nuclear power plants as energy sources. New tables present global fertility rates and the sources and effects of selected air pollutants. New and revised figures include the Air Quality Index, world fuel consumption, sources of groundwater contamination, components of trash, and recycling rates.

## Chapter 21: Preparing for Aging, Death, and Dying

Revised and expanded text discussions include the effects of aging on the senses and rational suicide. A new table presents exercise recommendations for adults over age 65 from the American College of Sports Medicine and the American Heart Association. A new feature box looks at the controversy regarding physician-assisted suicide.

# Text Features and Learning Aids

*Access to Health*, Twelfth Edition, includes the following special features, all of which have been revised and improved upon for this edition:

- **Chapter objectives** summarize the main competencies that students will gain from each chapter and alert students to the key concepts.
- **Chapter opener questions** capture students' attention and engage them in what they will be learning. Questions are repeated and answered in photo legends within the chapter.
- **What Do You Think?** critical thinking questions within the chapter prompt students to reflect on personal and societal issues relating to the material they have just learned.
- **What's Working for You?** features (new to this edition) reinforce healthy behaviors by calling students' attention to positive things they are already doing to promote good health.
- **Why Should I Care?** features (new to this edition) lead students to recognize the relevance of health issues to their own lives in the here and now.
- **Did You Know?** figures call attention to statistics that are relevant to the lives of college students in a fun and engaging format.
- **Assess Yourself** and **Your Plan for Change** boxes are combined in each chapter. Students assess their current health behaviors and are given specific ideas for setting goals and following through on behavior change.
- **Skills for Behavior Change** boxes give students specific strategies for making lasting changes to their health behaviors.
- **Points of View** boxes (new to this edition) present viewpoints on a controversial health issue and ask students **Where Do You Stand?** questions, encouraging students to critically evaluate the information and consider their own opinions.
- **Consumer Health** boxes (new to this edition) provide students with guidelines for becoming critical consumers of health products and information.
- **Student Health Today** boxes offer current data and information about health trends specific to college students, including potential risks and safety issues that affect students' lives.

- **Health Headlines** boxes highlight new discoveries and research, as well as interesting trends in the fields of public and personal health.
- **Health in a Diverse World** boxes expand discussion of health topics to diverse groups within the United States and around the world.
- **Gender & Health** boxes help students understand unique aspects of health for both genders.
- **Be Healthy, Be Green** boxes offer information on how students can make environmentally responsible health choices.
- **A running glossary** in the margins defines terms where students first encounter them, emphasizing and supporting understanding of material.
- The sections at the ends of chapters focus on student application: **Summary** wraps up chapter content, **Pop Quiz** multiple-choice questions and **Think about It!** discussion questions encourage students to evaluate and apply new information, **Accessing Your Health on the Internet** and **References** sections offer more opportunities to explore areas of interest.
- **The appendices** at the end of the book include practical information on providing emergency care and a table of nutritive values for selected foods and fast foods.
- **A Behavior Change Contract** for students to fill out is included at the front of the book.

# Supplementary Materials

Available with *Access to Health*, Twelfth Edition, is a comprehensive set of ancillary materials designed to enhance learning and to facilitate teaching.

## Student Supplements

- **MyHealthLab** (www.pearsonhighered.com/myhealthlab). Organized by learning areas and a snap to navigate, MyHealthLab is a course management platform that makes it easier than ever to learn about personal health and wellness:

  * **Read It** contains the new Pearson eText, a full-featured electronic book that allows for note creation, highlighting, bookmarking, zooming, and linking to definitions and external sites; chapter objectives to direct student learning; and chapter-specific RSS feeds.
  * **See It** houses more than 30 *ABC News* videos about important health topics, each 5 to 10 minutes long, and followed by assignable quiz questions.
  * **Hear It** offers MP3 tutor sessions with assignable quizzes to explain the big picture concepts for each chapter, and new audio case studies with accompanying essay questions.
  * **Do It** contains activities related directly to the book's Points of View boxes, critical thinking questions, news quizzes, and Web links.
  * **Review It** provides an online glossary, flashcards available for mobile phones, and practice quizzes for each chapter.

✻ **Live It** is an electronic toolkit to help jump-start behavior change projects. With 30 assessments from the book, additional worksheets, and the new How Healthy Are You? module, it guides students through planning for change, creating a behavior change contract, journaling and logging their behaviors as they implement change, and preparing a reflection piece to aid in behavior change evaluation.

✻ **On the Go** houses tools to help students study on the go using their mobile devices, including Tweet Your Health, a brand-new Twitter application that sends students reminders about their behavior change project, and allows them to track their progress using their mobile phone.

● **Companion Website** (www.pearsonhighered.com/donatelle). Like MyHealthLab, this website is organized by learning areas. Students can study chapter objectives and follow RSS feeds (Read It), view SMS-protected *ABC News* videos on health topics (See It), listen to MP3 clips of main concepts and case studies (Hear It), learn hands-on with critical thinking activities (Do It), take practice quizzes (Review It), access the behavior-change tool kit (Live It), and utilize mobile health-tracking tools (On the Go).

● *Take Charge of Your Health!* **Worksheets.** Twelve new worksheets have been added, providing a total of 50 self-assessment exercises. Worksheets are available as a gummed pad and can be packaged at no additional charge with the main text.

● *Behavior Change Log Book and Wellness Journal.* This assessment tool helps students track daily exercise and nutritional intake and create a long-term nutrition and fitness prescription plan. It includes Behavior Change Contracts and topics for journal-based activities.

● *Eat Right! Healthy Eating in College and Beyond.* This handy, full-color booklet provides students with practical guidelines, tips, shopper's guides, and recipes that turn healthy eating principles into blueprints for action. Topics include healthy eating in the cafeteria, dorm room, and fast-food restaurants; planning meals on a budget; weight management; vegetarian alternatives; and how alcohol affects health.

● *Live Right! Beating Stress in College and Beyond.* This booklet gives students useful tips for coping with a variety of life's challenges both during college and for the rest of their lives. Topics include sleep, managing finances, time management, coping with academic pressure, relationships, and a closer look at advertised products that promise to make our lives better.

● **Digital 5-Step Pedometer.** Take strides to better health with this pedometer, which measures steps, distance (miles), activity time, and calories, and provides a time clock.

● **MyDietAnalysis** (www.mydietanalysis.com). Powered by ESHA Research, Inc., MyDietAnalysis features a database of nearly 20,000 foods and multiple reports. It allows students to track their diet and activity using up to three profiles, and to generate and submit reports electronically.

# Instructor Supplements

A full resource package accompanies *Access to Health,* Twelfth Edition, to assist the instructor with classroom preparation and presentation.

● **MyHealthLab** (www.pearsonhighered.com/myhealthlab). This course managment tool provides a one-stop spot for accessing a wealth of preloaded content and makes paper-free assigning and grading easier than ever. Instructors can electronically assign the self-assessments to students, who can complete them anonymously and still have their work reflected in the grade book. Reports on cumulative class responses allow instructors to better target certain issues in lectures. MyHealthLab contains the Pearson eText, which allows for instructor annotation to be shared with the class; includes over 30 *ABC News* videos; houses assignable chapter-specific quizzes, MP3 tutor sessions, case studies, activities, and flashcards; and provides robust electronic behavior-change tools including the How Healthy Are You? module and Tweet Your Health.

● *ABC News* **Health and Wellness Lecture Launcher Videos.** Thirty brand-new videos, each 5 to 10 minutes long, help instructors stimulate critical discussion in the classroom. Videos are provided already linked within Power-Point® lectures and are available separately in large-screen format with optional closed captioning on the Instructor Resource DVD and through MyHealthLab.

● **Instructor Resource DVD.** The Instructor Resource DVD includes 30 new *ABC News* Lecture Launcher videos; clicker questions; Quiz Show questions; PowerPoint® lecture outlines; all illustrations and tables from the text; selected photos; Transparency Masters; as well as Microsoft Word® files for the Instructor Resource and Support Manual and the Test Bank. The DVD also holds the Computerized Test Bank.

● **Teaching Tool Box.** Save hours of valuable planning time with one comprehensive course planning kit. The Teaching Tool Box provides all the prepping and lecture tools an instructor needs: the Course-at-a-Glance Quick Reference Guide; an Instructor Resource DVD including PowerPoint® Lecture Outlines, PRS Clicker Questions, Quiz Show questions, *ABC News* videos, and Transparency Masters; a MyHealthLab access kit; the Instructor Resource and Support Manual to easily find visual assets; *Great Ideas: Active Ways to Teach Health and Wellness*; Printed and Computerized Test Banks—along with helpful student supplements including the *Take Charge of Your Health!* worksheets, the *Behavior Change Log Book, Eat Right!*, and *Live Right!*—all in one convenient package!

● **Course-at-a-Glance Quick Reference Guide.** This valuable supplement acts as your road map to the Teaching Tool Box and everything it contains, with resources broken down by chapter and page number. The side for instructors provides assets that you can use when preparing for a lecture or while in class. The student side outlines where to find the resources to aid your students in their homework or in-class activities.

- **Instructor Resource and Support Manual.** Easier to use than a typical instructor's manual, this key guide provides a step-by-step visual walk-through of all the resources available to you for preparing your lectures. Also included are tips and strategies for new instructors, sample syllabi, and suggestions for integrating MyHealthLab into your classroom activities and homework assignments.
- **Test Bank.** The Test Bank incorporates Bloom's Taxonomy, or the Higher Order of Learning, to help instructors create exams that encourage students to think analytically and critically, rather than simply to regurgitate information.
- ***Great Ideas! Active Ways to Teach Health & Wellness.*** This manual provides ideas for classroom activities related to specific health and wellness topics, as well as suggestions for activities that can be adapted to various topics and class sizes.
- ***Clickers in the Classroom.*** This handbook provides detailed guidance in enhancing lectures using clicker (Classroom Response Systems) technology.
- **Course Management.** In addition to MyHealthLab, WebCT and Blackboard are available. Contact your Benjamin Cummings sales representative for details.
- **Health & Wellness Teaching Community Website** (www.pearsonhighered.com/healthcommunity). This new community website, sponsored by the American Association for Health Education (AAHE) and Pearson, serves instructors by offering teaching tips and ideas, and has a forum for peers to talk to one another about health-related issues.

# Acknowledgments

It is hard for me to believe that *Access to Health* is in its twelfth edition! Since its inception, the Personal Health textbook market has undergone remarkable changes. Whereas the text remains the foundation of information, the ability to communicate with students through the Internet and other media provides textbook authors and publishers entirely new and exciting ways of teaching, sharing information, and covering up-to-the minute health topics in every class. Each step along the way in planning, developing, and marketing a high-quality textbook and supplemental materials requires a tremendous amount of work from many dedicated professionals, and I cannot help but think how fortunate I have been to work with the gifted publishing professionals at Benjamin Cummings. From this author's perspective, the personnel personify key aspects of what it takes to be successful in the publishing world: (1) drive and motivation; (2) creativity and commitment to excellence; (3) a vibrant, youthful, and enthusiastic approach; and (4) personalities that motivate an author to continually strive to produce market-leading texts.

In particular, I am indebted to Kari Hopperstead, Project Editor *par excellence*, who has worked with me on several editions of both *Access to Health* and *Health: The Basics*. Over 12 editions of this text I have worked with several excellent editors, each of whom represented the best qualities to be found in publishing today. Without a doubt, Kari is among the best in the business! Under her leadership and guidance this text has been able to flourish, become more refined, more cutting edge, and even more accessible to students. She has wonderful instincts about student interests and needs; has been responsible for many of the improvements in art and design of the book; and goes above and beyond the call of duty to see that her books are the best available. She is truly a gem in the editorial field and a huge asset for me as an author and a credit to the publishing business.

Further praise and thanks go to the highly skilled and hardworking, creative, and charismatic Executive Editor Sandra Lindelof. Sandy keeps a steady finger on the pulse of the Personal Health market and is quick to suggest strategies to improve a text and meet the needs of instructors. She has been instrumental in the ongoing success of this text. In addition, I would like to acknowledge the contributions of Development Editor Claire Alexander. As a newcomer to the book's team, she plunged right in to the huge and complicated task of reviewing the existing text, merging content and updates with new information and ideas, and refining text revision. Overall, her exemplary work brought a fresh perspective to the text that helped us do the kind of thorough revision that was necessary.

Although these three women were key contributors to the finished work, there were many other people who worked on this revision of *Access to Health*. In particular, I would like to thank Senior Production Project Manager Nancy Tabor, who skillfully navigated production pitfalls and handled every detail, every obstacle, with patience, professionalism, and good grace. Thanks also to Linda Kern, Crystal Clifton, and the many hardworking staff at Progressive Publishing Alternatives who put everything together to make a polished finished product. Development Editor Laura Bonazzoli played a critical role in crafting the new Focus On mini-chapters and contributing to the revision of Chapter 1, while Mimi Bickel and the talented artists at Precision Graphics deserve many thanks for making our innovative new art program a reality. Gary Hespenheide and his staff at Hespenheide Design worked wonders in giving the book an exciting and fresh new look, both inside and out. Associate Editor Brianna Paulson gets major kudos for skillfully overseeing the print supplements package, and Molly Crowther, Associate Media Producer, once again pulled together an innovative and comprehensive media supplements package. Senior Project Editor Susan Malloy deserves special recognition for saving the day on more than one occasion and being ready and willing to lend a helping hand wherever needed. Additional thanks go to the rest of the team at Benjamin Cummings, especially Editorial Assistant Meghan Zolnay, Associate Project Manager Megan Power, Senior Photo Editor Donna Kalal, Senior Managing Editor Deborah Cogan, and Director of Development Barbara Yien.

The editorial and production teams are critical to a book's success, but I would be remiss without thanking another key group who ultimately help determine a book's success: the textbook representative and sales group and their leader, Senior Marketing Manager Neena Bali. Neena does a superb job of making sure that *Access to Health* gets into instructors' hands and that adopters receive the service they deserve. In keeping with my overall experiences with Benjamin Cummings, the members of the marketing and sales staff are among the best of the best. I am very lucky to have them working with me on this project and want to extend a special thanks to all of them!

# Contributors to the Twelfth Edition

Many colleagues, students, and staff members have provided the feedback, reviews, extra time, assistance, and encouragement that have helped me meet the rigorous demands of publishing this book over the years. Whether acting as reviewers, generating new ideas, providing expert commentary, or revising chapters, each of these professionals has added his or her skills to our collective endeavor.

I would like to thank specific contributors to chapters in this edition: As always, I would like to give particular thanks to Dr. Patricia Ketcham, who has helped with the *Access to Health* series since its beginnings. As Associate Director of Health Promotion in Student Health Services at Oregon State University, Dr. Ketcham provides a unique perspective on the challenges facing today's students. She contributed to Chapter 6, Considering Your Reproductive Choices; Chapter 10, Recognizing and Avoiding Addiction; Chapter 11, Drinking Alcohol Responsibly; Chapter 12, Ending Tobacco Use; Chapter 13, Avoiding Drug Misuse and Abuse; and Chapter 18, Choosing Conventional and Complementary Health Care. Dr. Peggy Pederson completed major revisions of Chapter 2, Promoting and Preserving Your Psychological Health; Chapter 4, Building Healthy Relationships and Communicating Effectively; and Chapter 5, Understanding Your Sexuality. As an Associate Professor in Community Health Education at Western Oregon State University, Dr. Pederson provided both her expertise in this area and an engaging writing style that greatly enhanced the quality and presentation of updates to this chapter. Dr. Angie Thompson, Associate Professor of Human Kinetics at St. Francis Xavier University and co-author of *Health: The Basics, Canadian Edition*, applied her wealth of teaching and research knowledge to a comprehensive update and reorganization of Chapter 9, Improving Your Physical Fitness. Dr. Karen Elliot, Assistant Professor in the Department of Public Health at Oregon State University, contributed to Focus On: Cultivating Your Spiritual Health; Focus On: Improving Your Sleep; Focus On: Enhancing Your Body Image; Focus On: Minimizing Your Risk for Diabetes; and Chapter 21, Preparing for Aging, Death, and Dying. She also provided major updates to the STI and HIV/AIDS sections of Chapter 14. Finally, a special thank you to Dr. Monica Hunsberger, R.D., Assistant Professor at Oregon Health and Sciences University, who provided a careful review and update for Chapter 7, Eating for a Healthier You, utilizing her expertise in community nutrition, healthy eating, and meal planning to add useful strategies for students interested in improving their eating behaviors.

Many thanks are also due to the talented people who contributed to the supplement package: Leslie A. Balch (Southern Connecticut State University), Elizabeth Barrington (San Diego Mesa College), Jennifer M. Jabson (Boston University), Grace Lartey (Western Kentucky University), and editor Karen Nein.

# Reviewers for the Twelfth Edition

With each new edition of *Access to Health,* we have built on the combined expertise of many colleagues throughout the country who are dedicated to the education and healthy behavioral changes of students. I thank the many reviewers of the past 11 editions of *Access to Health* who have made such valuable contributions. I want you, the instructors who have used and reviewed the book over the years, to know that I am grateful for your support and guidance. You are one of most essential resources for knowing how to best stimulate students to learn, grow, and tackle the health challenges that lie ahead of them.

For the Twelfth Edition, reviewers who have helped us continue this tradition of excellence include Gail S. Brook Arthur, MD (James Madison University), Tannah Broman, MS (Arizona State University), Elaine D. Bryan, MS (Georgia Perimeter College), Carol Cotton, PhD (University of Georgia), Deborah Stone Dailey, MS (Louisiana State University), Jennifer Dearden, EdD (Morehead State University), Nicholas DiCicco, EdD (Camden County College), Karen Edwards EdD (University of Delaware), Ping Johnson, PhD, CHES (Kennesaw State University), Erin Largo-Wight, PhD, CHES (University of North Florida), Grace Lartey, PhD (Western Kentucky University), Janis McWayne, PhD (Francis Marion University), Susie Myers, MA (Kansas City Kansas Community College), Jessica M. Poole, MS (North Georgia College and State University), Thomas E. Reed, PhD (College of DuPage), John P. Seabolt, EdD (University of Kentucky), and Cynthia Smith, MS (Central Piedmont Community College).

Many thanks to all!
Rebecca J. Donatelle, PhD

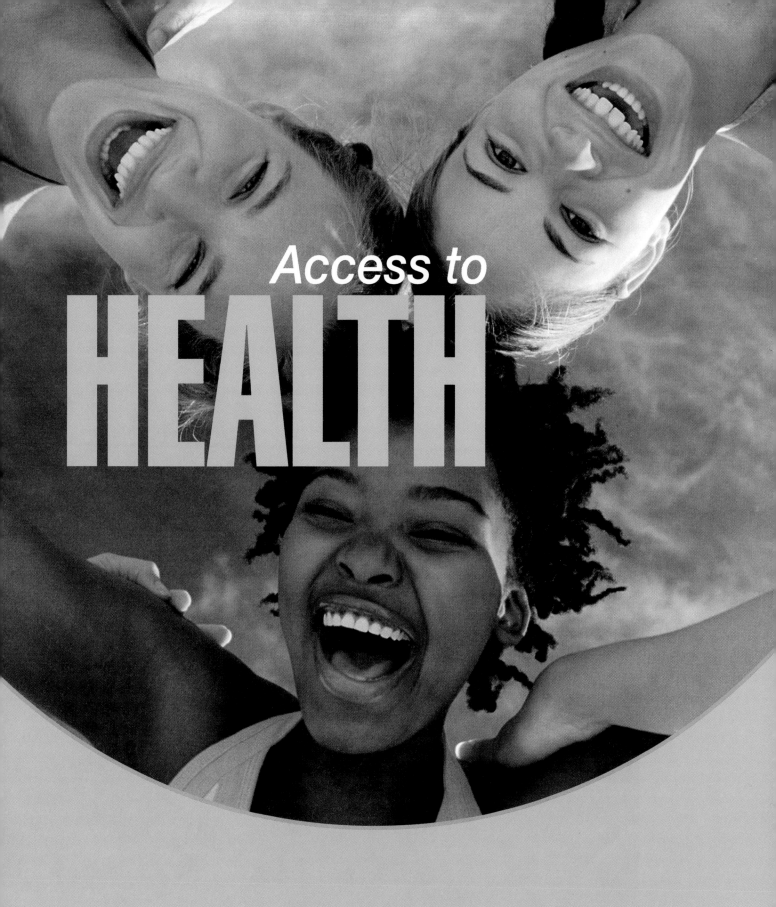

*Access to*
# HEALTH

1

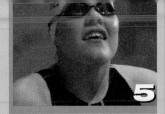

**5**

What is meant by *quality of life*?

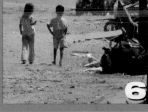

**6**

Why should I be concerned about health conditions in other places?

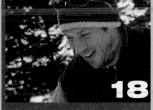

**18**

How can I stay motivated to improve my health habits?

# Accessing Your Health

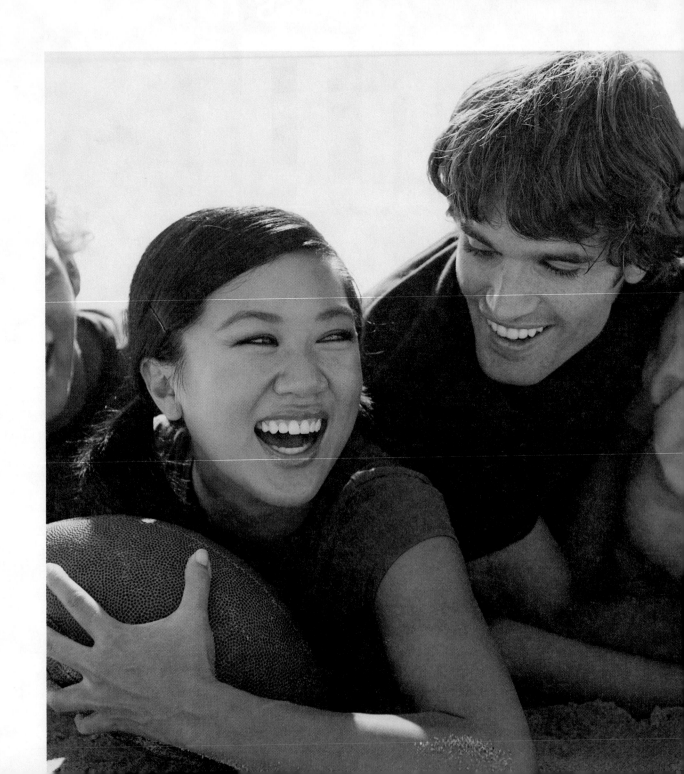

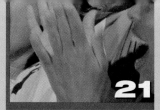

**21** How do other people influence my health behaviors?

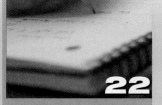

**22** What can I do to change an unhealthy habit?

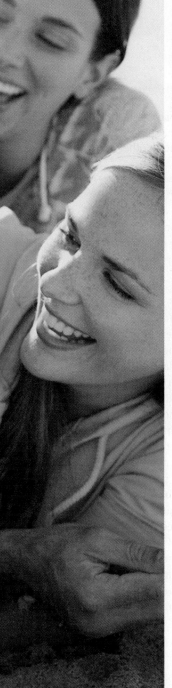

## Objectives

✳ Describe the immediate and long-term rewards of healthy behaviors and the effects that your health choices may have on others.

✳ Compare and contrast the medical model of health and the public health model, and discuss the six dimensions of health.

✳ Identify several personal factors that influence your health and classify them as modifiable or nonmodifiable.

✳ Explain how aspects of the social and physical environment influence your health.

✳ Discuss the importance of a global perspective on health, and explain how gender, racial, economic, and cultural factors influence health disparities.

✳ Compare and contrast three models of behavior change.

✳ Identify your own current risk behaviors, the factors that influence those behaviors, and the strategies you can use to change them.

*Got health?* That may sound like a simple question, but it isn't; health is a process, not something we just "get." People who are healthy in their forties, fifties, sixties, and beyond aren't just lucky or the beneficiaries of hardy genes. In most cases, those who are healthy and thriving in their later years have set the stage for good health by making it a priority in their early years. You've probably heard from your parents and grandparents that your college years will be the best years of your life. Productive careers lie ahead, special relationships are on the horizon, and the canvas is hung upon which you will paint the story of your life. Whether your story is filled with good health, happiness, and fulfillment of your life goals is largely dependent on the health choices you make—beginning right now.

## Why Health, Why Now?

We aspire to be thin and fit; we want to be more environmentally conscious; we search for relationships that are meaningful, loving, and lasting; and we want to live to a healthy, happy old age. Sound about right? In addition to our desires to improve our health, constant messages via television, the Internet, and magazines remind us of health challenges facing the world, the nation, your community, and your campus. We can't run from the health issues, we can't ignore them, and even health issues occurring in another part of the world affect us. In the twenty-first century your health is connected, not only to the people you directly interact with and the environments where you spend time, but also to people you've never met and to the well-being of the entire planet.

While the list of potential health problems is long, and it will take multiple levels of effort to improve our collective futures, individuals are at the heart of positive future health change. You can reduce your risks, improve your health status, and be a part of the solution. This chapter will help lay the foundation for good health and behavior change. *First,* you'll discover how the casual choices you make every day—from what to have for breakfast, to how much sleep you get—influence your life, your future, and the well-being of others. *Next,* you'll find out what health actually is and how it is intimately linked to—and influenced by—almost everything else in your world. *Finally,* you'll learn how to identify the health-related behaviors you'd like to change, and how to get moving toward that change.

Rather than focusing on you in some distant future, you will be honing in on what is happening in your life right now. How does what you do today influence you and those around you? Why not go for that extra helping of pizza tonight or eat the extra-large popcorn with butter at the movie theater? Why walk to your next class, when you could take the bus or drive? Why cut back on your drinking? You're healthy enough now, so why should you care? The problem with this kind of thinking is that it doesn't consider cumulative effects of poor choices on your health and the health of others. Let's take a look at how your actions and inactions matter.

# Choose Health Now for Immediate Benefits

Almost everyone knows that overeating leads to weight gain, or that drinking and driving increase the risk of motor vehicle accidents. But other, subtler choices you make every day may be influencing your well-being in ways you're not aware of. For instance, did you know that the amount of sleep you get each night could affect your body weight, your ability to ward off colds, your mood, and your driving? What's more, inadequate sleep is one of the most commonly reported impediments to academic success (Figure 1.1). Another example is smoking: It has many immediate health effects, including fatigue, throat irritation, and breathing problems. And like poor sleep, it increases your vulnerability to colds and other infections. Similarly, drinking alcohol reduces your immediate health and your academic performance. It also sharply increases your risk of unintentional injuries—not only motor vehicle accidents, but also falls, drownings, and other injuries. This is especially significant because, for people between the ages of 15 and 44, unintentional injury—whether related to alcohol use or any other factor—is the leading cause of death (Table 1.1).

It isn't an exaggeration to say that healthy choices have immediate benefits. When you're well nourished, fit, rested, and free from the influence of nicotine, alcohol, and other drugs, you're more likely to avoid illness, succeed in school, maintain supportive relationships, participate in meaningful work and community activities, and enjoy your leisure time.

**mortality** The proportion of deaths to population.
**life expectancy** Expected number of years of life remaining at a given age, such as at birth.

## Choose Health Now for Long-Term Rewards

You're probably familiar with the old proverb: "What you sow, you reap." The choices you make today are like seeds: Planting good seeds means you're more likely to enjoy the fruits of good health, including not only a longer life, but a

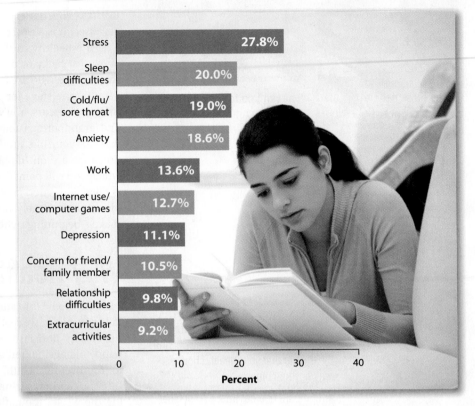

**FIGURE 1.1 Top Ten Reported Impediments to Academic Performance—Past 12 Months**
In a recent survey by the National College Health Association, students indicated that stress, poor sleep, recurrent minor illnesses, and anxiety, among other things, had prevented them from performing at their academic best.

**Source:** Data are from American College Health Association, *American College Health Association—National College Health Assessment II (ACHA-NCHA II) Reference Group Data Report, Fall 2009* (Baltimore: ACHA, 2010).

higher quality of life. In contrast, poor choices increase the likelihood of a shorter life, as well as persistent illness, addiction, and other limitations on quality of life. In other words, successful aging starts now.

## Personal Choices Influence Your Life Expectancy

According to current **mortality** statistics—which reflect the proportion of deaths within a population—the average **life expectancy** at birth in the United States is projected to be 78.3 years for a child born in 2010.[1] In other words, we can expect that American infants born today will live to an average age of over 78 years; much longer than the 47-year life expectancy for people born in the early 1900s. That's because life expectancy 100 years ago was largely determined by our susceptibility to infectious disease. In 1900, over 30 percent of all deaths occurred among children under 5 years old, and the leading cause of death was infection.[2] Even among adults, infectious diseases such as tuberculosis and pneumonia were the leading causes of death, and

## "Why Should I Care?"

Just as health problems can create impediments for your success in life, improving your health can lead to better academic performance, greater career success, more relationship satisfaction, and more joy in living overall.

| TABLE 1.1 | Leading Causes of Death in the United States, 2007, Overall and by Age Group (15 and older) | |
| --- | --- | --- |

| All Ages | Number of Deaths |
| --- | --- |
| Diseases of the heart | 616,067 |
| Malignant neoplasms | 562,875 |
| Cerebrovascular diseases | 135,952 |
| Chronic lower respiratory diseases | 127,924 |
| Accidents (unintentional injuries) | 123,706 |
| **Aged 15–24** | |
| Unintentional injuries | 15,897 |
| Homicide | 5,551 |
| Suicide | 4,140 |
| Malignant neoplasms | 1,653 |
| Diseases of the heart | 1,084 |
| **Aged 25–44** | |
| Unintentional injuries | 31,908 |
| Malignant neoplasms | 16,751 |
| Diseases of the heart | 15,062 |
| Suicide | 12,000 |
| Homicide | 7,810 |
| **Aged 45–64** | |
| Malignant neoplasms | 153,338 |
| Diseases of the heart | 102,961 |
| Unintentional injuries | 32,508 |
| Diabetes mellitus | 17,057 |
| Chronic lower respiratory diseases | 16,930 |
| **Aged 65+** | |
| Diseases of the heart | 496,095 |
| Malignant neoplasms | 389,730 |
| Cerebrovascular diseases | 115,961 |
| Chronic lower respiratory diseases | 109,562 |
| Alzheimer's disease | 73,797 |

**Source:** J. Xu et al., "Deaths: Final Data for 2007," *National Vital Statistics Reports* 58, no. 19 (Hyattsville, MD: National Center for Health Statistics, 2010).

widespread epidemics of infectious diseases such as cholera and influenza crossed national boundaries to kill millions. For example, in 1918, a worldwide influenza epidemic killed 20 million people, including half a million Americans, in less than a year.[3]

With the development of vaccines and antibiotics, life expectancy increased dramatically as premature deaths from infectious diseases decreased. As a result, the leading cause of death shifted to **chronic diseases** such as heart disease, cerebrovascular disease (which leads to strokes), cancer, and diabetes. At the same time, advances in diagnostic technologies, heart and brain surgery, radiation and other cancer treatments, as well as new medications continued the trend of increasing life expectancy into the twenty-first century.

Unfortunately, some researchers question whether this trend of increasing life expectancy will continue. In fact, a recent study projects that today's newborns will be the first generation to have a lower life expectancy than that of their parents.[4] How can this be? Clearly, our lifestyle decisions around diet, exercise, drug and alcohol consumption, smoking, and other behaviors will make a big difference. One major contributor to future reductions in life expectancy is related to obesity and sedentary lifestyle. A recent study led by researchers from the Harvard School of Public Health and the University of

**chronic disease** A disease that typically begins slowly, progresses, and persists, with a variety of signs and symptoms that can be treated but not cured by medication.

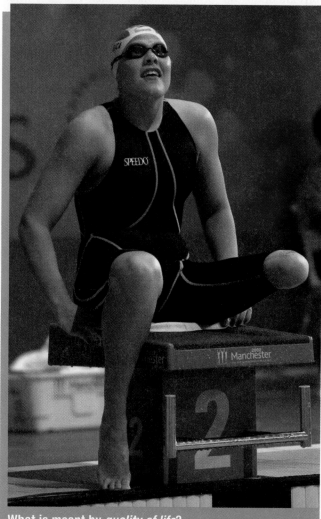

**What is meant by *quality of life*?**

Health-related *quality of life* refers to a person's or group's perceived physical and mental health over time. Just because a person has an illness or disability doesn't mean his or her quality of life is necessarily low. The South African swimmer Natalie du Toit lost her leg in a motorcycle accident at the age of 14, but that hasn't prevented her from achieving her goals and a high quality of life. In 2008, she became the first amputee to qualify for and compete in the Olympic Games.

# 67 & 71

are the *healthy* life expectancy ages of men and women, respectively, in the U.S. Note that the average total life expectancy ages of men and women in the U.S. are 75.2 and 80.4, respectively, demonstrating that many people live their last years with significant health problems that affect their quality of life.

Washington indicates that smoking, high blood pressure, elevated blood glucose, and overweight/obesity currently reduce life expectancy in the United States by 4.9 years in men and 4.1 years in women.[5]

While lifestyle may be the biggest reason for future declines in life expectancy, there are other health choices that may have an impact. For example, a growing number of persons are opting out of vaccinations for their children, while there are increasing threats from resistant pathogens and new strains of diseases. Our individual choices, whether they be to eat healthy foods, exercise, get vaccinations, pollute the environment, or take unnecessary risks are part of the life expectancy projections.

> **healthy life expectancy** Expected number of years of full health remaining at a given age, such as at birth.

**Personal Choices Influence Your *Healthy* Life Expectancy** By now you're probably beginning to see how healthful choices, such as watching what you eat, enjoying physical activity, and avoiding smoking and alcohol abuse, increase your life expectancy. But another benefit of these healthful choices is that they increase your **healthy life expectancy,** that is, the number of years of full health you enjoy, without disability, chronic pain, or significant illness. For example, if we could delay the onset of diabetes so that a person didn't develop the disease until he or she was 60 years old, rather than developing it at 30, there would be a 30-year increase in this individual's healthy life expectancy.

## Choose Health Now to Benefit Others

Our personal health choices don't affect only our own lives. They affect the lives of others, because they contribute to global health or the global burden of disease. For example, we've said that overeating and inadequate physical activity contribute to obesity. But obesity isn't a problem only for the individual. Along with its associated health problems, obesity burdens the U.S. health care system and the U.S. economy overall. *Direct* medical costs, including the costs of diagnosis and treatment, reached as high as $147 billion in 2008, and roughly half of those costs were paid by public programs (Medicaid and Medicare).[6] In addition, obesity costs the public *indirectly*. These indirect costs include, for example, reduced tax revenues because of income lost from absenteeism and premature death, increased disability payments because of an inability to remain in the workforce, and increased health insurance rates as claims rise for treatment of obesity itself as well as its associated diseases.

What's true for poor nutrition and lack of physical activity— the choices that contribute to obesity—is also true for smoking, excessive consumption of alcohol, and use of illegal drugs. All of these choices place an economic burden on our communities and our society as a whole. However, the disease burden goes beyond pure economics and includes social and emotional burdens, such as those on families left without parents or on people who lose loved ones in their prime. The burden on caregivers who must sacrifice personally to take care of those who are disabled by diseases is another part of this problem.

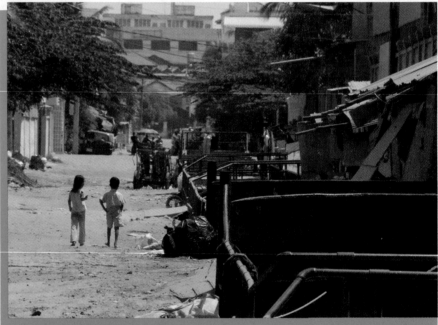

**Why should I be concerned about health conditions in other places?**

You can be affected by the health of other people—even those who live far away from you. Unhealthy conditions in one's own community, state, or country can have economic impacts on everyone living in that area through disproportionate government spending, resource allocation, or general loss in productivity. In addition, in our increasingly global society where goods, people, and information are constantly passing between nations, the pollutants, diseases, and sanitation conditions of one nation can affect the health of people in surrounding nations and around the world.

At the root of the concern that individual health choices cost society is an ethical question causing considerable debate: To what extent should the public be held accountable for an individual's unhealthy choices? Should we require individuals to somehow pay for their poor choices? Of course, in some cases, we already do. We tax cigarettes and alcohol, and a few communities are currently taxing sweetened soft drinks, which have been blamed for rising obesity rates.[7] But some people don't think such taxes go far enough: They argue that people who overeat, fail to exercise, smoke, drink in excess, or use illegal drugs should be subject to higher health insurance rates. On the other side of the argument are those who argue that smoking and drinking are addictions that require treatment, not punishment, and that obesity is a product of a society of excess in which small children learn behaviors early in life that are difficult to break. Should individuals be punished for choices that society influenced and the media promoted? Who is ultimately responsible?

Before you decide where you stand on this issue, hold on! It's not as black and white as it may first appear. That's because those seemingly personal choices that influence our health are not always entirely within our personal control. We'll explain shortly, but first, it's essential to understand what health actually is and which factors we actually may be able to control.

## what do you think?

Is obesity always a matter of willpower and lack of discipline? ● Since we tax cigarettes, is it reasonable to tax high-calorie sodas? What about taxing pre-packaged, high-fat foods? ● Who should make these decisions? ● Where would you personally draw the line?

# What Is Health?

Although we use the word **health** almost unconsciously, few people understand the broad scope of the word or how it has evolved over the years. For some, *health* simply means the antithesis of sickness. To others, it means being in good physical shape and able to resist illness. Still others use terms such as *wellness* or *well-being* to include a wide array of factors that seem to lead to positive health status. Why are there all of these variations? In part, the differences are due to an increasingly enlightened way of viewing health that has taken shape over time. In addition, as our collective understanding of illness has improved, so has our ability to understand the many nuances of health.

## Models of Health

Over the centuries, different ideals—or models—of human health have dominated. As we discuss next, our current model of health has broadened from a focus on the individual physical body to an understanding of health as a reflection not only of ourselves, but also of our communities.

## Medical Model

Prior to the twentieth century, if you made it to your fiftieth birthday, you were regarded as lucky. Survivors were believed to be of hearty, healthy stock—having what we might refer to today as "good genes." We didn't have the means to delve into factors influencing risks and as such, cleanliness, good behavior, and a bit of luck were part of the good health formula.

Throughout these years, perceptions of health were dominated by the **medical model,** in which health status focused primarily on the individual and his or her tissues and organs. The surest way to bring about improved health was to cure the individual's disease, either with medication to treat the disease-causing agent, or through surgery to remove the diseased body part. Thus, government resources focused on initiatives that led to treatment, rather than prevention, of disease.

> **health** The ever-changing process of achieving individual potential in the physical, social, emotional, mental, spiritual, and environmental dimensions.
>
> **medical model** A view of health in which health status focuses primarily on the individual and a biological or diseased organ perspective.
>
> **ecological or public health model** A view of health in which diseases and other negative health events are seen as a result of an individual's interaction with his or her social and physical environment.

## Public Health Model

Not until the early decades of the 1900s did researchers begin to recognize that entire populations of poor people, particularly those living in certain locations, were victims of environmental factors, such as polluted water, air, and food; poor housing; and unsafe work settings, over which they often had little control. As a result of this new understanding, researchers began to focus on an **ecological** or **public health model,** which views diseases and other negative health events more as a result of an individual's interaction with his or her social and physical environment.

Recognition of the public health model enabled health officials to move swiftly to control contaminants in water,

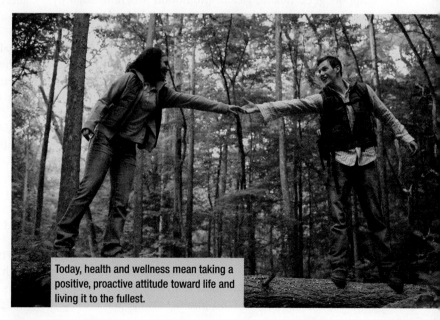

Today, health and wellness mean taking a positive, proactive attitude toward life and living it to the fullest.

for example, by building adequate sewers, and to control burning and other forms of air pollution. In the early 1900s, colleges began offering courses in health and hygiene, the predecessors of the course you are taking today, to teach students about these important factors. And over time, public health officials began to recognize and address many other forces affecting human health, including hazardous work conditions; negative influences in the home and social environment; abuse of drugs and alcohol; stress; unsafe behavior; diet; sedentary lifestyle; and cost, quality, and access to health care.

By the 1940s, progressive thinkers began calling for policies, programs, and services to improve individual health and that of the population as a whole. In other words, their focus shifted from treatment of individual illness to **disease prevention** by reducing or eliminating the factors that cause illness and injury. For example, childhood vaccination programs reduced the incidence and severity of infectious disease; installation of safety features such as seatbelts and airbags in motor vehicles reduced traffic injuries and fatalities; and laws governing occupational safety reduced injuries to and deaths of American workers.

**disease prevention** Actions or behaviors designed to keep people from getting sick.

**health promotion** The combined educational, organizational, procedural, environmental, social, and financial supports that help individuals and groups reduce negative health behaviors and promote positive change.

**risk behaviors** Actions that increase susceptibility to negative health outcomes.

**wellness** The achievement of the highest level of health possible in each of several dimensions.

In 1947 at an international conference focusing on global health issues, the World Health Organization (WHO) proposed a new definition of health: "Health is the state of complete physical, mental, and social well-being, not just the absence of disease or infirmity."[8] This new definition definitively rejected the old medical model.

Alongside prevention, the public health model began to emphasize **health promotion,** that is, policies and programs that promote behaviors known to support good health. Health-promotion programs identify healthy people who are engaging in **risk behaviors** (those that increase susceptibility to negative health outcomes) and motivate them to change their actions by changing aspects of the larger environment to increase an individual's chances of success. For instance, effective stop-smoking programs don't simply say, "Just do it." Instead, they provide information about risk behaviors and possible consequences to smokers and their secondhand-smoke victims (educational supports); they encourage smokers to participate in smoking-cessation classes and encourage employers to allow time off for worker attendance (organizational supports); they lobby for new laws governing smokers' behaviors (policy and environmental supports); and they may provide monetary incentives to motivate people to participate (financial supports).

To those of us in the field of public health, the saying "We've come a long way, baby" accurately reflects the health achievements of the past 100 years. Numerous policies, individual actions, and public services have worked

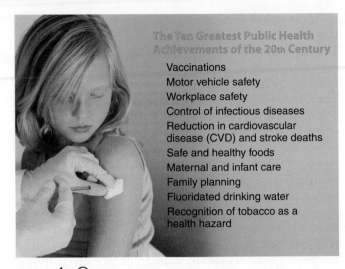

The Ten Greatest Public Health Achievements of the 20th Century

Vaccinations
Motor vehicle safety
Workplace safety
Control of infectious diseases
Reduction in cardiovascular disease (CVD) and stroke deaths
Safe and healthy foods
Maternal and infant care
Family planning
Fluoridated drinking water
Recognition of tobacco as a health hazard

FIGURE 1.2 **The Ten Greatest Public Health Achievements of the Twentieth Century**

**Source:** Adapted from Centers for Disease Control and Prevention, "Ten Great Public Health Achievements—United States, 1900–1999," *Morbidity and Mortality Weekly Report* 48, no. 12 (April 1999): 241–43.

to improve our overall health status. **Figure 1.2** lists the ten greatest public health achievements of the twentieth century.

## Wellness and the Dimensions of Health

In 1968, biologist, environmentalist, and philosopher René Dubos proposed an even broader definition of health. In his Pulitzer Prize–winning book, *So Human an Animal*, Dubos defined health as "a quality of life, involving social, emotional, mental, spiritual, and biological fitness on the part of the individual, which results from adaptations to the environment."[9] This concept of adaptability, or the ability to cope successfully with life's ups and downs, became a key element in our overall understanding of health.

Eventually the word **wellness** entered the popular vocabulary. This word further enlarged Dubos's definition of health by recognizing levels—or gradations—of health within each category. To achieve *high-level wellness*, a person must move progressively higher on a continuum of positive health indicators **(Figure 1.3)**. Those who fail to achieve these levels may move to the illness side of the continuum.

Today, the words *health* and *wellness* are often used interchangeably to mean the dynamic, ever-changing process of trying to achieve one's potential in each of six interrelated dimensions **(Figure 1.4)**, which typically include the following:

● **Physical health.** This dimension includes characteristics such as body size and shape, sensory acuity and responsiveness, susceptibility to disease and disorders, body functioning, physical fitness, and recuperative abilities. Newer

| Irreversible damage | Chronic illness | Signs of illness | Average wellness | Increased wellness | Optimal wellness |
|---|---|---|---|---|---|

**FIGURE** 1.3 **The Wellness Continuum**

definitions of physical health also include our ability to perform normal *activities of daily living (ADLs)*, or those tasks that are necessary to normal existence in society, such as getting up out of a chair, bending over to tie your shoes, or writing a check.

● **Social health.** The ability to have a broad social network and have satisfying interpersonal relationships with friends, family members, and partners is a key part of overall wellness. This implies being able to give and receive love and to be nurturing and supportive in social interactions. Successfully interacting and communicating with others, adapting to various social situations, and other daily behaviors are all part of social health.

● **Intellectual health.** The ability to think clearly, reason objectively, analyze critically, and use brainpower effectively to meet life's challenges are all part of this dimension. This includes learning from successes and mistakes and making sound, responsible decisions that consider all aspects of a situation. It also includes having a healthy curiosity about life and an interest in learning new things.

● **Emotional health.** This is the feeling component—being able to express emotions when appropriate, and to control them when not. Self-esteem, self-confidence, self-efficacy, trust, love, and many other emotional reactions and responses are all part of emotional health.

● **Environmental health.** This dimension entails understanding how the health of the environments in which you live, work, and play can positively or negatively affect you; protecting yourself from hazards in your own environment; and working to preserve, protect, and improve environmental conditions for everyone.

● **Spiritual health.** This dimension involves having a sense of meaning and purpose in your life. This may involve a belief in a supreme being or a specified way of living prescribed by a particular religion. It also may include the ability to understand and express one's purpose in life; to feel a part of a greater spectrum of existence; to experience peace, contentment, and wonder over life's experiences; and to care about and respect all living things.

Achieving wellness means attaining the optimal level of well-being for your unique limitations and strengths. For example, a physically disabled person may function at his or her optimal level of performance; enjoy satisfying interpersonal relationships; work to maintain emotional, spiritual, and intellectual health; and have a strong interest in environmental concerns. In contrast, those who spend hours lifting weights to perfect the size and shape of each muscle but pay little attention to their social or emotional health may look healthy but may not maintain a good balance in all dimensions.

Although we often consider physical attractiveness and athletic performance key measures of health, these external trappings reveal very little about a person's overall health. The perspective we need is *holistic*, emphasizing the balanced integration of mind, body, and spirit. People pursuing a goal of *mind–body health* actively work to improve other dimensions of life. Taking time to "grow yourself" intellectually, spiritually, socially, and emotionally are key aspects of mind–body work.

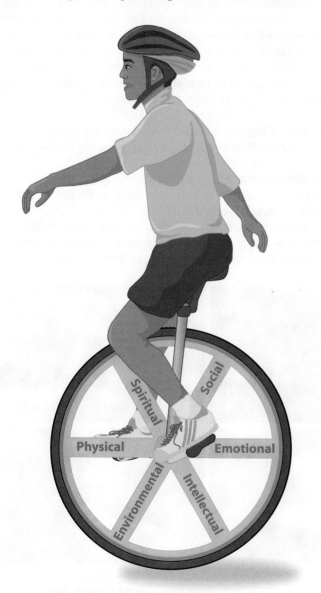

**FIGURE** 1.4 **The Dimensions of Health**
When all the dimensions are in balance and well developed, they can support your active and thriving lifestyle.

# What Influences Your Health?

If you're lucky, aspects of your world conspire to promote your health: Everyone in your family is slender and fit; your mom reminds you when it's time to see the dentist; there are fresh apples on sale at the neighborhood farmer's market; and a new bike trail opens along the river (and you have a bike!). If you're not so lucky, aspects of your world discourage health: Everyone in your family is overweight and they eat high-fat diets; your peers urge you to keep up with their drinking; there are only cigarettes, alcohol, and junk food for sale at the corner market; and you wouldn't dare walk or ride alongside the river for fear of being mugged. This variety of influences explains why we said earlier that seemingly personal choices aren't totally within an individual's control.

Public health experts refer to the factors that influence health as **determinants of health,** a term the U.S. Surgeon General defines as "the array of critical influences that determine the health of individuals and communities."[10] The Surgeon General's health promotion plan, called *Healthy People,* has been published every 10 years since 1990 with the goal of improving the quality and years of life for all Americans. *Healthy People* classifies health determinants into five large groupings: individual biology and behavior, the social environment, the physical environment, policies and interventions, and access to quality health care.[11]

**determinants of health** The array of critical influences that determine the health of individuals and communities.

## Individual Biology and Behavior

In the domain of health determinants, *biology* refers to an individual's genetics, ethnicity, age, and gender. (See the **Gender & Health** box on the next page for information on how gender influences health.) Biology also includes family history; for example, if your parents developed diabetes in their forties, that's a biological determinant for you. Your own history of illness and injury also falls within this grouping; if you suffered a serious knee injury in high school, it might influence other aspects of your health, such as your ability to participate in vigorous physical activity.

Biological determinants are things you can't change—or modify. To reinforce this idea, health experts frequently refer to these factors as *nonmodifiable determinants.* This is the term we use throughout this book.

In contrast, *behaviors* are your responses to internal and external conditions. For instance,

# 5.5 million

years of potential life are lost in the U.S. annually as a direct result of cigarette smoking.

you're feeling tense, so you go for a run. Or your roommate has just made nachos, so you have some. Possibly your parents smoke and you grow up hating the smell of smoke on your clothes and in your house, so you choose not to smoke yourself; or alternatively, your parents love high-fat foods and you learn to love them, too.

By definition, behaviors are things you can change, so health experts refer to them as *modifiable determinants.* Modifiable determinants significantly influence your risk for chronic disease. Earlier, we said that chronic diseases are the leading causes of death and disability in the United States; indeed, they are responsible for 7 out of 10 deaths.[12] Incredibly, just four modifiable determinants are responsible for most of the illness and early death related to chronic diseases (Figure 1.5). These are the following:[13]

- **Lack of physical activity.** Physical inactivity and overweight/obesity are each responsible for nearly 1 in 10 deaths in U.S. adults.
- **Poor nutrition.** High dietary salt, low dietary omega-3 fatty acids, and high dietary *trans* fatty acids are the dietary risks with the largest mortality effects.
- **Excessive alcohol consumption.** Alcohol causes 90,000 deaths in adults annually through cardiovascular disease, other medical conditions, traffic accidents, and violence.

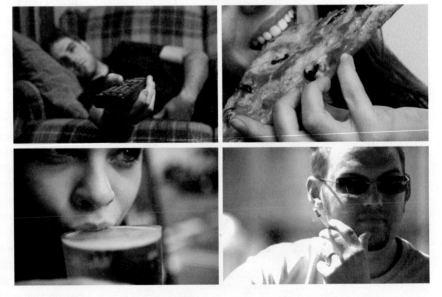

FIGURE 1.5 **Four Leading Causes of Chronic Disease in the United States** Lack of physical activity, poor nutrition, excessive alcohol consumption, and tobacco use—all modifiable health determinants—are the four most significant factors leading to chronic disease among Americans today.

# Health: His and Hers

You don't have to be a health expert to know that there are physiological differences between men and women—and these differences can extend into their health behaviors and disease risk. The following are just a few of the differences in men's and women's health:

✳ The size, structure, and function of the brain differ in women and men, particularly in areas that affect mood and behavior and in areas used to perform tasks.

✳ Bone mass in women peaks when they are in their twenties; in men, it increases gradually until age 30. At menopause, women lose bone at an accelerated rate, and 80 percent of osteoporosis cases are those of women.

✳ Women's immune systems are stronger than

men's, but women are more prone to autoimmune diseases, in which the immune system attacks the body's own cells.

✳ Men and women experience pain in different ways and may react to pain medications differently.

> Men and women may have physiological differences, but we can all benefit from a healthy, active lifestyle.

✳ When consuming the same amount of alcohol, women have a higher blood alcohol content than men, even allowing for size differences.

✳ Men smoke more than women, but women who smoke have higher rates of lung disease.

✳ Women are more likely than men to suffer a second heart attack within 1 year of their first heart attack.

✳ Women are two times more likely than men to contract a sexually transmitted infection and are ten times more likely to contract HIV when having unprotected intercourse.

✳ Depression is two to three times more common in women than it is in men, and women are more likely than men to attempt suicide; however, men are more likely to succeed at suicide.

---

● **Tobacco use.** Tobacco smoking and the high blood pressure it causes are responsible for about 1 in 5 deaths in American adults.

Other modifiable determinants include use of vitamins and other supplements, caffeine, over-the-counter medications, and illegal drugs; sexual behaviors and use of contraceptives; sleep habits; and hand washing and other simple infection-control measures. We'll explore these and many other behaviors in later chapters of this textbook.

## Social Environment

Your social environment includes your interactions with family, friends, coworkers, other students, and the people who make up your community. It also encompasses social institutions, such as your campus, other schools, places of worship, and worksites, as well as a variety of social services, such as law enforcement, public transportation, counseling services, and

senior services. A community's cultural customs and languages are also aspects of your social environment that act as health determinants, as is the level of violence in the community.[14]

Among the most powerful of all determinants of health in your social environment are economic factors: Even in affluent nations such as the United States, people who are in lower socioeconomic brackets have substantially shorter life expectancies and more illnesses than people who are wealthy.[15] Economic disadvantages exert their effects on human health within nearly all domains of life. They include the following:

● Lacking access to quality education from early childhood through adulthood
● Living in poor housing with potential exposure to asbestos, lead, dust mites, rodents and other pests, inadequate sanitation, tap water that's not safe to drink, and high levels of crime
● Being unable to pay for nourishing food, warm clothes, and sturdy shoes; heat and other utilities; medications and medical supplies; transportation; and counseling services, fitness classes, and other wellness measures
● Having insecure employment or being stuck in a low-paying job with few benefits
● Having few assets to fall back on in case of illness or injury

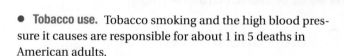

## What's Working for You?

Maybe you are already taking strides to live a more healthful life. How many of these healthy behaviors do you practice?

☐ I get a minimum of 7 hours of sleep every night.
☐ I maintain healthy eating habits and manage my weight.
☐ I regularly engage in physical activity.
☐ I practice safer sex.
☐ I limit my intake of alcohol and avoid tobacco products.
☐ I schedule regular self-exams and medical checkups.

As you can imagine, social determinants influence your health on a daily basis. Having friends who encourage you to join them at the health club and having the money for nourishing food are examples of health-promoting social determinants. On the other hand, having friends who pressure you to sniff glue and living in a dangerous neighborhood are determinants in your social environment that oppose health.

## Physical Environment

The physical environment is anything—from skyscrapers to snowfall—that you can perceive with your senses. It also includes less tangible things such as radiation and air pollution.

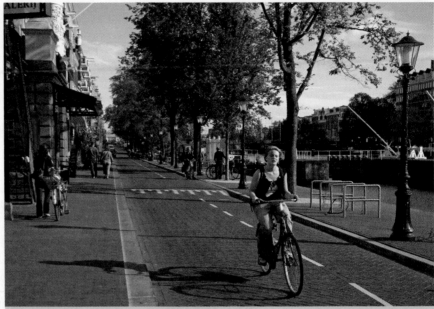

The built environment of your community can promote positive health behaviors. The bike-friendly nature of Amsterdam, Netherlands, with its wide bike paths and major thoroughfares closed to automobile traffic, encourages residents to incorporate healthy physical activity into their daily lives.

**The Built Environment** One part of the physical environment that is getting a fair amount of attention from public health officials these days is the *built environment*. As the name implies, the built environment includes anything created or modified by human beings, from buildings to roads to recreation areas and transportation systems to electric transmission lines and communications cables.

Researchers in public health have increasingly been promoting changes to the built environment that can improve the health of community members.[16] For example, Walter Willett of the Harvard School of Public Health proposes that sidewalks and bike lanes be part of every federally funded road project.[17] He asserts that, when sidewalks are built in neighborhoods and downtowns, people are more apt to start walking and slim down. Similarly, when a supermarket selling fresh produce replaces side-by-side fast-food outlets in an inner-city neighborhood, residents' dietary choices improve. Simple changes in community environments can make a difference by enabling you to make better choices.

**Pollutants and Infectious Agents** Another aspect of the physical environment is the quality of the air we breathe, our land, water, and foods. When individuals and communities are exposed to toxins, radiation, irritants, and infectious agents via their environment, they can suffer significant harm.

These effects are not necessarily limited to the local community. With the rise of global travel and commerce, the health status of one region—the pollutants it produces, or the infectious diseases it harbors—can affect the health of people around the world. Examples of such concerns include airborne pollutants from industries in Asia crossing the Pacific and harming communities along the Oregon coast; the burning of the rainforest in South America contributing to global warming; or the swift transmission of strains of severe influenza or resistant tuberculosis infecting significant portions of a population. These environmental determinants are a grim reminder of the need for a proactive international response to disease prevention and climate change (see the **Be Healthy, Be Green** box on the next page).

## Policies and Interventions

Public policies and interventions can have a powerful and positive effect on the health of individuals and communities. Examples include health promotion campaigns to prevent smoking, laws mandating child restraint and seat belt use in motor vehicles and helmets for bikes and motorcycles, vaccination programs, and public funding for mental health services.[18] For example, in 2009, the residents of Albert Lea, Minnesota, signed on to an ambitious citywide initiative to improve the health of its residents. It mandated that local restaurants make healthful changes to their menus; that schools ban eating in hallways and selling candy for fundraisers; and that neighborhoods form "walking school buses" to escort kids to school on foot. It also funded changes to the built environment, including laying new sidewalks and digging plots for community gardens. The efforts appeared to pay off with noteworthy improvements in health care claims and other behavioral improvements in less than a year.[19]

## Access to Quality Health Care

The health of individuals and communities is also determined by access to quality health care, including not only services of health care providers but also accurate and

# BE HEALTHY, BE GREEN

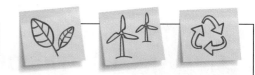

## Our Planet Needs You!

The health of our environment has always been important, but today scientists agree that global environmental conditions pose dire threats to all living things. Although debate rages over the causes and potential consequences of our environmental health concerns, it's becoming increasingly clear that the nonsustainable practices of an elite cluster of nations—including the United States—are primarily responsible for the severity of the problems we now face. Indeed, according to the Center for Environment and Population, the United States alone is responsible for 25 percent of the world's energy consumption—this in spite of the fact that the United States is home to only 5 percent of the global population.

Some of the greatest environmental challenges facing us are the following:

✱ Climate change brought about by greenhouse gas emissions from the raising of livestock for human consumption; from the burning of fossil fuels in homes and industries; and from emissions from our cars, buses, trucks, and airplanes

✱ Overreliance on fossil fuels and other nonrenewable energy sources, resulting in pollution and resource depletion

✱ Exploitation of natural resources and the endangerment of species and habitats resulting from unsustainable fishing, logging, and mining practices; urban expansion; and excess water usage

✱ Pollution of our land, water, food supply, and air by fossil-fuel emissions, medical waste, animal waste, electronic waste, toxic wastes, and nonbiodegradable trash

✱ Deforestation and desertification driven by overpopulation, poverty, nonsustainable farming techniques, and ever-increasing global demands for beef as well as wood and paper products

As more and more people become aware of these major threats to our environmental health, there has been an increasing recognition of the need to adopt environmentally responsible, or "green," practices in our homes and communities. Throughout this text, we provide useful suggestions for environmentally responsible changes that you can make as you explore different areas of your own personal health. These include ideas on how to select healthy foods that are produced sustainably, ways to reduce your environmental impact during your leisure time, and tips for locating green health care products. As with all behavior changes, small and incremental changes often reap huge rewards over time. If each of us makes the commitment today and initiates these behaviors for the rest of the term and beyond, it will help move us in the right direction.

---

# 45.4 million

**Americans do not have health insurance.**

relevant health information and products such as eyeglasses, medical supplies, and medications. This determinant can be related to economics as well as public policies and interventions related to health insurance and sponsorship of health care.

## Health Disparities

We've said that one goal of the *Healthy People* initiatives is to improve the health of Americans. In addition, in recognition of the changing demographics of the U.S. population and the vast differences in health status based on racial or ethnic background, *Healthy People 2010* included strong language about the importance of reducing these **health disparities**.[20] Publishing in late 2010, *Healthy People 2020* sets similar goals for the nation as well as trying to improve on areas that were not as successful in *Healthy People 2010*.[21] See the **Health in a**

Diverse World box on page 14 for examples of groups that often experience health disparities.

## How Can You Improve Your Health Behaviors?

We've just identified many factors critical to your health status. However, you have the most control over factors in just one category: your individual behaviors (or modifiable determinants). Clearly, change is not always easy. Your chances of successfully changing negative habits improve when you identify a behavior that you want to change and then develop a plan for gradual transformation that allows you time to unlearn negative patterns and substitute positive ones. Many experts advocate dissecting a given health behavior into smaller parts and working on them one at a time in "baby steps." In other words, to successfully change a behavior, you need to see change not as a singular *event* but instead as a *process* that

> **health disparities** Differences in the incidence, prevalence, mortality, and burden of diseases and other health conditions among specific population groups.

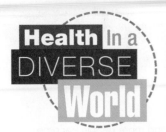

# The Challenge of Health Disparities

Among the factors that can affect an individual's ability to attain optimal health are the following:

**✳ Race and ethnicity.** Research indicates dramatic health disparities among people of certain racial and ethnic backgrounds. Socioeconomic differences, stigma based on "minority status," poor access to health care, cultural barriers and beliefs, discrimination, and limited education and employment opportunities can all affect health status.

**✳ Inadequate health insurance.** A large and growing number of people are *uninsured* or *underinsured.* Those without adequate insurance coverage may face high copayments, high deductibles, or limited care in their area.

**✳ Sex and gender.** At all ages and stages of life, men and women experience major differences in rates of disease and disability.

**✳ Economics.** One's economic status can influence one's health. For example, persistent poverty may make it difficult to buy healthy food or to afford preventive medical visits or medication.

Economics also influences access to safe, affordable exercise.

**✳ Geographic location.** Whether you live in an urban or rural area and have access to public transportation or your own vehicle can have a huge impact on what you choose to eat, the amount of physical activity you get, and your ability to visit the doctor or dentist.

**✳ Sexual orientation.** Gay, lesbian, bisexual, or transgender individuals may lack social support, are often denied health benefits due to unrecognized marital status, and face unusually high stress levels and stigmatization by other groups.

**✳ Disability.** Disproportionate numbers of disabled individuals lack access to health care services, social support, and community resources that would enhance their quality of life.

One of the ways public health officials attempt to address the problem of health disparities due to location, poverty, and lack of insurance is to organize Remote Area Medical (RAM) clinics. At a clinic like this, rural families, most with little or no insurance, wait in line for hours to receive free health care from hundreds of professional doctors, nurses, dentists, and other health workers.

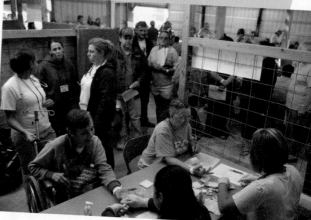

**Source:** National Institutes of Health, *National Institutes of Health (NIH) Strategic Research Plan and Budget to Reduce and Ultimately Eliminate Health Disparities: Volume 1, Fiscal Years 2002–2006* (Bethesda, MD: National Institutes of Health, May 12, 2006).

---

requires preparation, has several steps or stages, and takes time to succeed.

# Models of Behavior Change

Over the years, social scientists and public health researchers have developed a variety of models to reflect this multifaceted process of behavior change. We explore three of those here.

**Health Belief Model** We often assume that when rational people realize their behaviors put them at risk, they will change those behaviors and reduce that risk. However, it doesn't work that way for many of us. Consider the number of health professionals who smoke, consume junk food, and act in other unhealthy ways. They surely know better, but their "knowing" is disconnected from their "doing." One classic model of behavior change proposes that our beliefs may help to explain why this occurs.

A **belief** is an appraisal of the relationship between some object, action, or idea (e.g., smoking) and some attribute of that

**Did you Know?**

According to an annual survey conducted by Franklin Covey, 35% of people who make New Year's resolutions break them by the end of January!

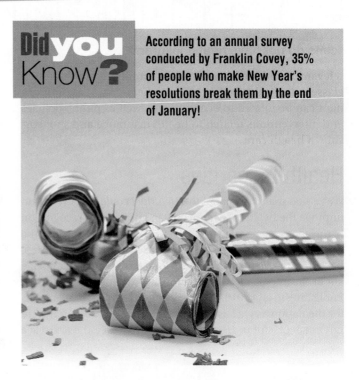

object, action, or idea (e.g., "Smoking is expensive, dirty, and causes cancer"—or, "Smoking is sociable and relaxing"). Psychologists studying the relationship between beliefs and health behaviors have determined that although beliefs may subtly influence behavior, they may or may not cause people to behave differently. In 1966, psychologist I. Rosenstock developed a classic theory, the **health belief model (HBM),** to show when beliefs affect behavior change.[22] The HBM holds that several factors must support a belief before change is likely:

● **Perceived seriousness of the health problem.** How severe would the medical and social consequences be if the health problem were to develop or be left untreated? The more serious the perceived effects are, the more likely that action will be taken.
● **Perceived susceptibility to the health problem.** What is the likelihood of developing the health problem? People who perceive themselves at high risk are more likely to take preventive action.
● **Cues to action.** A person who is reminded or alerted about a potential health problem is more likely to take action.

People follow the HBM many times every day. Take, for example, smokers. Older smokers are likely to know other smokers who have developed serious heart or lung problems. They are thus more likely to perceive tobacco as a threat to their health than are teenagers who have just begun smoking. The greater the perceived threat of health problems caused by smoking, the greater the chance a person will quit.

However, many chronic smokers know the risks yet continue to smoke. Why do they miss these cues to action? According to Rosenstock, some people do not believe they are susceptible to a severe problem—they act as though they are immune to it—and are unlikely to change their behavior. They also may feel that the immediate pleasure outweighs the long-range cost.

## Social Cognitive Model
The **social cognitive model** developed from the work of several researchers over the past several decades, but is most closely associated with the work of psychologist Albert Bandura. Fundamentally, the model proposes that three factors interact in a reciprocal fashion to promote and motivate change. These are the social environment in which we live, our thoughts or cognition (including our values, perceptions, beliefs, expectations, and sense of self-efficacy), and our behaviors (Figure 1.6). We change our behavior in part by observing models in our environments—from childhood to the present moment—reflecting on our observations, and regulating ourselves accordingly.

For instance, if as a child we observed our mother successfully quitting smoking, we are more apt to believe we can do it, too. In addition, when we succeed in changing ourselves, we change our thoughts about ourselves, and this in turn may promote further behavior change: After we've successfully quit smoking, we may feel empowered to increase our level of physical activity. Moreover, as we change

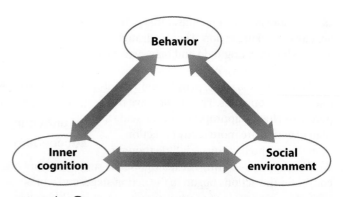

FIGURE 1.6 **Social Cognitive Model**
We are constantly changing our behavior in response to factors in our social environment and our inner world (our thoughts and feelings). In a reciprocal fashion, our behaviors change our environments as well as our thoughts and feelings—including our sense of our ability to make positive change.

ourselves, we change our world; in our example, we become a model of successful smoking cessation for others to observe. Thus, we are not just products of our environments, but producers.

## Transtheoretical Model
Why do so many New Year's resolutions fail before Valentine's Day? According to Drs. James Prochaska and Carlos DiClemente, it's because we are going about things in the wrong way; fewer than 20 percent of us are really prepared to take action. After considerable research, Prochaska and DiClemente have concluded that behavior changes usually do not succeed if they start with the change itself. Instead, we must go through a series of stages to adequately prepare ourselves for that eventual change.[23] According to Prochaska and DiClemente's **transtheoretical model** of behavior change (also called the *stages of change model*), our chances of keeping those New Year's resolutions will be greatly enhanced if we have proper reinforcement and help during each of the following stages:

**belief** Appraisal of the relationship between some object, action, or idea and some attribute of that object, action, or idea.
**health belief model (HBM)** Model for explaining how beliefs may influence behaviors.
**social cognitive model** Model of behavior change emphasizing the role of social factors and thought processes (cognition) in behavior change.
**transtheoretical model** Model of behavior change that identifies six distinct stages people go through in altering behavior patterns; also called the *stages of change model*.

**1. Precontemplation.** People in the precontemplation stage have no current intention of changing. They may have tried to change a behavior before and given up, or they may be in denial and unaware of any problem.
**2. Contemplation.** In this phase, people recognize that they have a problem and begin to contemplate the need to change. Despite this acknowledgment, people can languish in this stage for years, realizing that they have a problem but lacking the time or energy to make the change.

**3. Preparation.** Most people at this point are close to taking action. They've thought about what they might do and may even have come up with a plan.

**4. Action.** In this stage, people begin to follow their action plans. Those who have prepared for change appropriately and made a plan of action are more ready for action than those who have given it little thought.

**5. Maintenance.** During the maintainance stage a person continues the actions begun in the action stage, and works toward making these changes a permanent part of his or her life. In this stage, it is important to be aware of the potential for relapses and to develop strategies for dealing with such challenges.

**6. Termination.** By this point, the behavior is so ingrained that constant vigilance may be unnecessary. The new behavior has become an essential part of daily living.

We don't necessarily go through these stages sequentially. They may overlap, or we may shuttle back and forth from one to another—say, contemplation to preparation, then back to contemplation—for a while before we become truly committed to making the change. Still, it's useful to recognize "where we're at" with a change, so that we can consider the appropriate strategies to move us forward.

## Step One: Increase Your Awareness

Before you can decide what you might want to change, you need to learn what researchers know about the behaviors that contribute to and detract from your health. Each chapter in this book provides a foundation of information focused on these factors. Check out the Table of Contents at the front of the book to locate chapters with the information you're looking for.

This is also a good time to take stock of the health determinants in your life: What aspects of your biology and behavior support your health, and which are obstacles to overcome? What elements of your social and physical environment could you tap into to help you change, and what elements might hold you back? Does your campus have policies that support student health, and interventions such as a health clinic and counseling services? Making a list of all of the health determinants that affect you—both positively and negatively—should greatly increase your understanding of what you might want to change, and what you might need to do to make that change happen.

## Step Two: Contemplate Change

Now that you've increased your awareness of the behaviors that contribute to wellness in populations, and the specific health determinants affecting you, you may find yourself contemplating change. In this stage, the following strategies may be helpful.

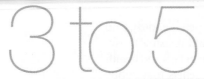

**is the number of times most people will attempt to change an unhealthy behavior before succeeding.**

**Examine Your Current Health Habits and Patterns** To help you zero in on a behavior you might want to change, examine your current habits and behavior patterns. Do you routinely stop at Dunkin' Donuts for breakfast? Smoke when you're feeling stressed? Party too much on the weekends? Get to bed way past 2 AM? When considering such habits and patterns, ask yourself the following:

- How long has this been going on?
- How often does it happen?
- How serious are the consequences of the habit or pattern?
- What are some of your reasons for continuing this problematic behavior?
- What kinds of situations trigger the behavior?
- Are other people involved in this behavior? If so, in what way?

As we've explored throughout this chapter, health behaviors involve elements of personal choice, but are also influenced by other determinants that make them more or less likely. Some are *predisposing factors*—for instance, if your parents smoke, you're 90 percent more likely to start smoking than someone whose parents don't smoke. Some are *enabling factors*—for example, if your peers smoke, you are 80 percent more likely to smoke. Identifying the factors that may encourage or discourage the habit you're exploring is part of contemplating behavior change.

Various *reinforcing factors* can also contribute to your current habits. If you decide to stop smoking but your family and friends all smoke, you may lose your resolve. In such cases, it can be helpful to employ the social cognitive model and deliberately change aspects of your social environment. For instance, you could spend more time with nonsmoking friends to give yourself a chance to observe people modeling the positive behavior you want to emulate.

**Identify a Target Behavior** To clarify your thinking about the various behaviors you might like to target, ask yourself these questions:

- **What do I want?** What is your ultimate goal? To lose weight? Exercise more? Reduce stress? Have a lasting relationship? Whatever it is, you need a clear picture of your target outcome.
- **Which change is the greatest priority at this time?** People often decide to change several things at once. Suppose you are gaining unwanted weight. Rather than saying, "I need to eat less and start exercising," identify one specific behavior that contributes significantly to your greatest problem, and tackle that first.
- **Why is this important to me?** Think through why you want to change. Are you doing it because of your health? To improve your academic performance? To look better? To win

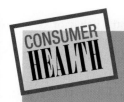
# SURFING FOR THE LATEST IN HEALTH

The Internet can be a wonderful resource for quickly finding answers to your questions, but it can also be a source of much *misinformation.* If you're not careful, you could end up feeling frazzled, confused, and— worst of all—misinformed. To ensure that the sites you visit are reliable and trustworthy, follow these tips:

✱ Look for websites sponsored by an official government agency, a university or college, or a hospital/medical center. Government sites are easily identified by their *.gov* extensions (e.g., the National Institute of Mental Health's website is www.nimh.nih.gov). College and university sites typically have *.edu* extensions (e.g., Johns Hopkins University's website is www.jhu.edu). Hospitals often have an extension of *.org* (e.g., the Mayo Clinic's website is www.mayoclinic.org). Major philanthropic foundations, such as the Robert Wood Johnson Foundation, the Kellogg Foundation, and others, often provide informa-

tion about selected health topics. In addition, national nonprofit organizations, such as the American Heart Association and the American Cancer Society, are often good, authoritative sources of information. Foundations and nonprofits usually have URLs ending with a *.org* extension.

✱ Search for well-established, professionally peer-reviewed journals such as the *New England Journal of Medicine* (http://content.nejm.org) or the *Journal of the American Medical Association (JAMA;* http://jama.ama-assn.org). Although some of these sites require a fee for access, you can often locate concise abstracts and information, such as a weekly table of contents, that can help you conduct a search. Other times, you can pay a basic fee for a certain number of hours of unlimited searching. Your college may have Internet access to these journals that they make available to students for no cost.

✱ Consult the Centers for Disease Control and Prevention (www.cdc.gov) for consumer news, updates, and alerts.

✱ For a global perspective on health issues, visit the World Health Organization (www.who.int/en).

✱ There are many government- and education-based sites that are independently sponsored and reliable. The following is just a sample. We provide more in each chapter as we cover specific topics:

**1.** Aetna Intelihealth: www.intelihealth.com

**2.** FamilyDoctor.org: http://familydoctor.org

**3.** MedlinePlus: www.nlm.nih.gov/medlineplus

**4.** Go Ask Alice!: www.goaskalice.columbia.edu

**5.** WebMD health: http://my.webmd.com

✱ The nonprofit health care accrediting organization Utilization Accreditation Review Commission (URAC; www.urac.org) has devised

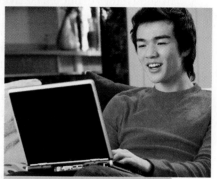
Find reliable health information at your fingertips!

more than 50 criteria that health sites must satisfy to display its seal. Look for the "URAC Accredited Health Web Site" seal on websites you visit.

✱ And, finally, don't believe everything you read. Cross-check information against reliable sources to see whether facts and figures are consistent. Be especially wary of websites that try to sell you something. When in doubt, check with your own health care provider, health education professor, or state health division website.

---

someone else's approval? It's best to target a behavior because it's right for you rather than because you think it will help you win others' approval.

Another aspect of targeting is filling in the details. All too often we berate ourselves by using generalities: "I'm lousy to my friends; I need to be a better person." Identifying the specific behavior you would like to change—in contrast to the general problem—will allow you to set clear goals. How are you a lousy friend? Are you gossiping or lying about your friends? Have you been a taker rather than a giver? Or are you really a good friend most of the time?

**Learn More about the Target Behavior** Once you've clarified exactly what behavior you'd like to change, you're ready to learn more about that behavior. Again, the information in this

textbook will help. In addition, this is a great time to learn how to gain access to accurate and reliable health information on the Internet (see the **Consumer Health** box above).

As you conduct your research, don't limit your focus to the behavior and its effects. Also think about what aspects of your world might pose obstacles to your success, and learn all you can about those. For instance, let's say you decide you want to meditate for 15 minutes a day. You face a big ramp-up just in learning what meditation is, how it's practiced, and what benefits you might expect from it. But in addition, what might pose an obstacle to meditation? Do you think of yourself as hyper? Do you live in a super-noisy dorm? Are you afraid your friends might think meditating is weird? In short, learn everything you can—positive and negative—about your target behavior now, and you'll be better prepared for change.

## Assess Your Motivation and Your Readiness to Change

On any given morning, many of us get out of bed and resolve to change a given behavior that day. Whether it be losing weight, drinking less, exercising more, being nicer to others, managing time better, or some other change, we start out with enthusiasm and high expectations. However, most of us soon return to our old behavior patterns.

Wanting to change is an essential prerequisite of the change process, but to achieve change, you need more than desire. You need real **motivation,** which isn't just a feeling, but a social and cognitive force that directs your behavior. To understand what goes into motivation, let's return for a moment to two models of change discussed earlier: the health belief model and the social cognitive model.

**motivation** A social, cognitive, and emotional force that directs human behavior.

**self-efficacy** Belief in one's ability to perform a task successfully.

Remember that, according to the HBM, your beliefs affect your ability to change. For example, when reaching for another cigarette, smokers sometimes tell themselves, "I'll stop tomorrow," or "They'll have a cure for lung cancer before I get it." These beliefs allow them to continue what they're doing. To put it another way, they dampen motivation. So as you contemplate change, take some time to think about your beliefs and consider whether they are likely to motivate you to achieve lasting change. Ask yourself the following:

• Do you believe that your current pattern could lead you to a serious problem? The more severe the consequences are, the more motivated you'll be to change the behavior. For example, smoking can cause cancer, emphysema, and other deadly diseases. The fear of developing those diseases can help you stop smoking. But what if cancer and emphysema were just words to you? In that case, you could study up on these disorders and the tissue destruction, pain, loss of function, and emotional suffering they cause. Doing so might increase your motivation: In Canada, a recent law requires that graphic images of gangrenous limbs, diseased organs, and chests sawed open for autopsy cover at least half of cigarette packages. The year after the law took effect, 38 percent of smokers who tried to quit cited the images as a motivating factor.[24]

• Do you believe that you are personally likely to experience the consequences of your behavior? For example, losing a loved one to lung cancer could motivate you to work harder to stop smoking. If you really couldn't convince yourself that your behavior will affect you personally, you might ask your health care provider to give you an honest assessment of your risk.

Let's say you're still struggling to perceive the behavior as serious or the consequences as personal. If that's true, try employing the social cognitive model to help change those beliefs. For instance, you could interview people struggling with the consequences of the behavior you want to change. Ask them what their life is like, and if, when they were engaging in the behavior, they believed that it would harm them. Your health care provider may be able to put you in touch with patients who would be happy to support your behavior change plan in this way. And don't ignore the motivating potential of positive role models. Do you know people who have successfully lost weight, stopped drinking, or quit smoking? Hang out with them! Finding ways to stay motivated is a key purpose behind many of the behavior change steps and processes we have been describing throughout this section. The **Skills for Behavior Change** box on the next page summarizes some of these tips for maintaining motivation.

Even though motivation is powerful, by itself it's not enough to achieve change. Motivation has to be combined with common sense, commitment, and a realistic understanding of how best to move from point A to point B. *Readiness* is the state of being that precedes behavior change. People who are ready to change possess the knowledge, skills, and external and internal resources that make change possible.[25]

## Develop Self-Efficacy

**Self-efficacy**—an individual's belief that he or she is capable of achieving certain goals or of performing at a level that may influence events in life—is one

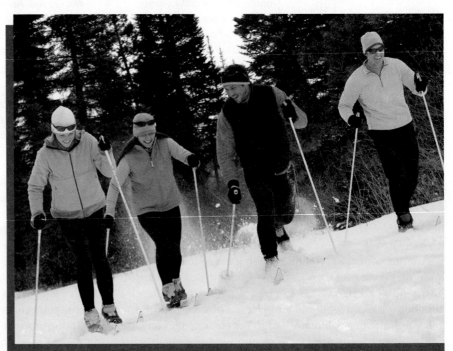

**How can I stay motivated to improve my health habits?**

Many people find it easiest to keep themselves motivated by planning small incremental changes, working toward a goal, and rewarding themselves along the way. Your friends can also help you stay motivated by modeling healthy behaviors, offering support, joining you in your change efforts, and providing reinforcement.

of the most important factors that influences our health status. Prior success in academics, athletics, or social interactions will lead to expectations of success in the future. In general, people who exhibit high self-efficacy are confident that they can succeed, and they approach challenges with a positive attitude. In turn, they may be more motivated to change and more likely to succeed.

Conversely, someone with low self-efficacy or with self-doubts about what they can and cannot do may give up easily or never even try to change a behavior. These people tend to shy away from difficult challenges. They may have failed before, and when the going gets tough, they are more likely to give up or revert to old patterns of behavior.

If you suspect your have low self-efficacy, the contemplation stage is a great time to get to work developing it! A technique of cognitive-behavioral therapy called *cognitive restructuring* (see Chapter 3) can help. Find out more by visiting your campus student counseling services.

**Cultivate an Internal Locus of Control** The conviction that you have the power and ability to change is a powerful motivator. Individuals who feel that they have limited control over their lives often find it more difficult to initiate positive changes.[26] If they believe that someone or something else controls a situation or that they dare not act in a particular way because of peer repercussions, they may become easily frustrated and give up. People with these characteristics have an *external* **locus of control.** In contrast, people who have a stronger *internal* locus of control believe that they have power over their own actions. They are more driven by their own thoughts and are more likely to state their opinions and be true to their own beliefs.

Having an internal or external locus of control can vary according to circumstance. For instance, someone who finds out that diabetes runs in his family may resign himself to facing the disease one day, instead of taking an active role in modifying his lifestyle to minimize his risk of developing diabetes. On this front, he would be demonstrating an external locus of control. However, the same individual might exhibit an internal locus of control when being pressured by friends to smoke. He knows that he does not want to smoke and does not want to risk the potential consequences of the habit, so he takes charge and resists the pressure. Developing and maintaining an internal locus of control can help you take charge of your health behaviors.

# what do you think?

In general, do you have an internal or an external locus of control? ● Can you think of some good friends whom you'd describe as more internally controlled? Externally controlled? ● How have you seen these demonstrated?

## Step Three: Prepare for Change

You've contemplated change for long enough! Now it's time to set a realistic goal, anticipate barriers, reach out to others, and commit. Here's how.

**Skills for Behavior Change**

## Maintain Your Motivation

✱ **Pick one specific behavior you want to change.** Trying to change too many things at once can be overwhelming and cause you to lose motivation.

✱ **Assess the one behavior you wish to change.** Figure out why it is important to you to change. If it doesn't feel important to you, then you'll have a hard time finding motivation, and it probably isn't a behavior you should address at this time.

✱ **Set achievable and incremental goals.** By developing both short- and long-term goals, and by taking baby steps, you improve your chances of accomplishing those goals and staying motivated to move forward.

✱ **Give yourself rewards.** Create a list of things you would find rewarding and plan for giving yourself specific ones once you reach specific goals. Having something to look forward to can help you stay focused and motivated.

✱ **Avoid or anticipate barriers and temptation.** By controlling or eliminating the environmental cues that provoke the behavior you want to change you'll make it easier for yourself to succeed at lasting change.

✱ **Remind yourself why you are trying to change.** Prepare a list of benefits you'll realize from making this change, both now and down the road. You can also prepare a list of the risks you face if you don't make this change. Post the lists where you will see them daily.

✱ **Enlist the help and support of others.** Other people can be major motivators for positive change—either as role models, a cheering squad, or partners in change. Let the people you care about know about your plans for change and ask them for help.

✱ **Don't be discouraged by lapses.** Everyone experiences temporary setbacks, no matter how committed they are. A brief lapse doesn't mean the entire cause is lost. Reexamine your plan, look for new strategies to motivate you, set some new short-term goals, and get right back on the horse.

**Set a Realistic Goal** A realistic goal is one that you truly can achieve—not some day, when other things in your life change, but within the circumstances of your life right now. Knowing that your goal is attainable increases your motivation. This, in turn, leads to a better chance of success and to a greater sense of self-efficacy—which can motivate you to succeed even more. To set realistic goals, use the SMART system, and employ shaping.

**locus of control** The location, *external* (outside oneself) or *internal* (within oneself), that an individual perceives as the source and underlying cause of events in his or her life.

**Use the SMART System** Unsuccessful goals are vague and open-ended; for instance, "Get into shape by exercising more." In contrast, successful goals are SMART:

- **S**pecific. A specific goal would be, "Attend the Tuesday/Thursday aerobics class at the YMCA."
- **M**easurable. A measurable goal would be, "Reduce my alcohol intake on Saturday nights from three drinks to two."
- **A**ction-oriented. An action-oriented goal would be, "Volunteer at the animal shelter on Friday afternoons."
- **R**ealistic. A realistic goal would be, "Increase my daily walk from 15 to 20 minutes."
- **T**ime-oriented. A time-oriented goal would be, "Stay in my strength-training class for the full 10-week session, then reassess."

**Use Shaping Shaping** is a stepwise process of making a series of small changes. Suppose you want to start jogging 3 miles every other day, but right now you get tired and winded after half a mile. Shaping would dictate a process of slow, progressive steps such as walking 1 hour every other day at a slow, relaxed pace for the first week; walking for an hour every other day but at a faster pace that covers more distance the second week; and speeding up to a slow run the third week.

**shaping** Using a series of small steps to gradually achieve a particular goal.

**modeling** Learning specific behaviors by watching others perform them.

Regardless of the change you plan, remember that current habits didn't develop overnight, and they won't change overnight, either. Prepare your goals and your plan of action with these shaping points in mind:

- Start slowly to avoid hurting yourself or causing undue stress.
- Keep the steps of your program small and achievable.
- Be flexible and ready to change your original plan if it proves to be uncomfortable.
- Master one step before moving on to the next.

## Anticipate Barriers to Change

Anticipating *barriers to change,* or possible stumbling blocks, will help you prepare fully and adequately for change. For example, if you want to lose weight, you may face several barriers to change, including social determinants (your family members and friends are overweight), aspects of the built environment (the only food vendors on or near your campus are convenience stores and fast-food outlets), or lack of adequate health care (you have an inexpensive health insurance policy that doesn't cover treatment for weight loss). In addition to negative determinants, the following are a few general barriers to change:

- **Overambitious goals.** Remember the advice to set realistic goals? Even with the strongest motivation, overambitious goals can derail change. Most people cannot lose weight, stop smoking, and begin running 3 miles a day all at the same time. Wanting to achieve dramatic change within unrealistically short time frames—such as losing 20 pounds in 1 month—tends to be equally unsuccessful. Habits are best changed one small step at a time.
- **Self-defeating beliefs and attitudes.** As the health belief model explains, believing you're too young or fit or lucky to have to worry about the consequences of your behavior can keep you from making a solid commitment to change. Likewise, thinking you are helpless to change your eating, smoking, or other habits can also undermine your efforts. Greater self-efficacy and more positive expectations may help.
- **Failing to accurately assess your current state of wellness.** You might assume that you will be able to walk the 2 miles to campus each morning, for example, only to discover that you're aching and winded after only a mile. Failing to make sure that the planned change is realistic for *you* can be a barrier that leaves you with weakened motivation and commitment.
- **Lack of support and guidance.** If you want to cut down on your drinking, peers who drink heavily may be powerful barriers to that change. To succeed, you need to recognize the people in your life who can't support, or might even actively oppose, your decision to change, and limit your interactions with them.
- **Emotions that sabotage your efforts and sap your will.** Sometimes the best laid plans go awry because you're having a bad day or are fighting with someone you care about. Emotional reactions to life's challenges aren't inherently bad. However, they can sabotage your efforts to change by distracting you and draining your reserves. Seek help for more severe psychological problems, and recognize that you may need to focus on those before you can effect significant change in other aspects of your health.

**Enlist Others as Change Agents** The social cognitive model recognizes the importance of our social contacts in successful change. Most of us are highly influenced by the approval or disapproval (real or imagined) of close friends, family members, and the social and cultural group to which we belong. In addition, watching others successfully change their behavior can give you ideas and encouragement for your own change. This **modeling,** or learning from role models, is a key component of the social cognitive model of change. Observing a friend who is a good conversationalist, for example, can help you improve your communication skills. Or find someone to share your plan for change! For instance, get your roommate

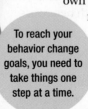

To reach your behavior change goals, you need to take things one step at a time.

to commit to a daily walk with you, or sign a contract with a friend stipulating that you will never let each other drink and drive.

**Family Members** From the time of your birth, your parents and other family members have given you strong cues about which actions are and are not socially acceptable. Your family also influenced your food choices, your religious beliefs, your political beliefs, and many of your other values and actions. Strong and positive family units provide care, trust, and protection; are dedicated to the healthful development of all family members; and work to reduce problems.

When the loving family unit does not exist or when it does not provide for basic human needs, it becomes difficult for a child to learn positive health behaviors. Healthy families provide the foundation for a clear and necessary understanding of what is right and wrong, what is positive and negative. Without this fundamental grounding, many young people have great difficulties.

**Friends** Just as your family influences your actions during your childhood, your friends and significant others influence your behaviors as you grow older. Most of us desire to fit the "norm" and avoid hassles in our daily interactions with others. If you deviate from the actions expected in your hometown or among your friends, you may suffer ostracism, strange looks, and other negative social consequences. But if your friends offer encouragement, or even express interest in joining with you in the behavior change, you are more likely to remain motivated. Thus, cultivating and maintaining close friends who share your personal values can greatly affect your behaviors.

**Professionals** Sometimes the change you seek requires more than the help of well-meaning family members and friends. Depending on the type and severity of the problem, you may want to enlist support from professionals such as your health instructor, PE instructor, coach, health care provider, academic adviser, or minister. As appropriate, consider the counseling services offered on campus, as well as community services such as smoking cessation programs, Alcoholics Anonymous support groups, and your local YMCA.

**Sign a Contract** It's time to get it in writing! A formal *behavior change contract* serves many powerful purposes. It functions as a promise to yourself; as a public declaration of intent; as an organized plan that lays out start and end dates and daily actions; as a listing of barriers you may encounter; as a place to brainstorm strategies to overcome barriers; as a list of sources of support; and as a reminder of the benefits of sticking with the program. Writing a behavior change contract will help you clarify your goals and make a commitment to change. Fill out the Behavior Change Contract at the beginning of this book to help you set a goal, anticipate obstacles, and create strategies to overcome those obstacles. Figure 1.7 on page 22 shows an example of a completed contract.

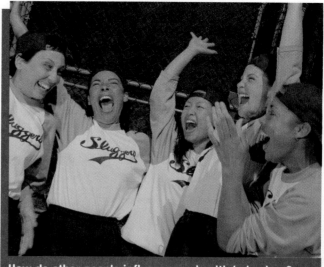

**How do other people influence my health behaviors?**

The people in your life—including family, friends, neighbors, coworkers, and society in general—can play a huge role—both positive and negative—in the health choices you make. The behaviors of those around you can predispose you to certain health habits, at the same time enabling and reinforcing them. Seeking out the support and encouragement of friends who have similar goals and interests will strengthen your commitment to develop and maintain positive health behaviors.

## Step Four: Take Action to Change

It's time to put your plan into action! Behavior change strategies include visualization, countering, controlling the situation, changing your self-talk, rewarding yourself, and journaling. The options don't stop here, but these are a good place to start.

**Visualize New Behavior** Mental practice can transform unhealthy behaviors into healthy ones. Athletes and others often use a technique known as **imagined rehearsal** to reach their goals. By visualizing their planned action ahead of time, they will be prepared when they put themselves to the test. Careful mental and verbal rehearsal of how you intend to act will help you anticipate problems and greatly improve the likelihood of success.

> **imagined rehearsal** Practicing, through mental imagery, to become better able to perform an event in actuality.
> **countering** Substituting a desired behavior for an undesirable one.

**Learn to "Counter"** **Countering** means substituting a desired behavior for an undesirable one. You may want to stop eating junk food, for example, but "cold turkey" just isn't realistic—unless the turkey's on a sandwich! Instead, compile a list of substitute foods and places to get them and have this ready before your mouth starts to water at the smell of a burger and fries.

**Control the Situation** Sometimes, the right setting or the right group of people will positively influence your behaviors. Any behavior has both antecedents and consequences.

**Behavior Change Contract**

My behavior change will be:
To snack less on junk food and more on healthy foods.

My long-term goal for this behavior change is:
Eat junk food snacks no more than once a week

These are three obstacles to change (things that I am currently doing or situations that contribute to this behavior or make it harder to change):
1. The grocery store is closed by the time I come home from school.
2. I get hungry between classes, and the vending machines only carry candy bars.
3. It's easier to order pizza or other snacks than to make a snack at home.

The strategies I will use to overcome these obstacles are:
1. I'll leave early for school once a week so I can stock up on healthy snacks in the morning.
2. I'll bring a piece of fruit or other healthy snack to eat between classes.
3. I'll learn some easy recipes for snacks to make at home.

Resources I will use to help me change this behavior include:
a friend/partner/relative: my roommates: I'll ask them to buy healthier snacks instead of chips when they do the shopping.
a school-based resource: The dining hall: I'll ask the manager to provide healthy foods we can take to eat between classes.
a community-based resource: The library: I'll check out some cookbooks to find easy snack ideas
a book or reputable website: The USDA nutrient database at www.ars.usda.gov: I'll use this site to make sure the foods I select are healthy choices.

In order to make my goal more attainable, I have devised these short-term goals:
short-term goal Eat a healthy snack 3 times per week    target date September 15    reward new CD
short-term goal Learn to make a healthy snack    target date October 15    reward concert tickets
short-term goal Eat a healthy snack 5 times per week    target date November 15    reward new shoes

When I make the long-term behavior change described above, my reward will be:
ski lift tickets for winter break    target date: December 15

I intend to make the behavior change described above. I will use the strategies and rewards to achieve the goals that will contribute to a healthy behavior change.

Signed: Elizabeth King    Witness: Susan Bauer

FIGURE 1.7 **Example of a Completed Behavior Change Contract**

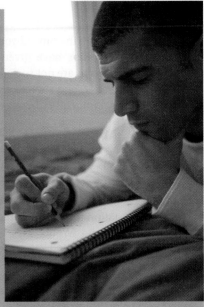

**What can I do to change an unhealthy habit?**

One of the best tools for helping you change your habits is journaling. Keeping track of your goals, behaviors, feelings, accomplishments, and setbacks can reinforce the healthy changes you are trying to make and provide motivation to continue. Other useful tools include shaping, enlisting support, visualization, countering, controlling the situation, changing your self-talk, and rewarding yourself.

*Antecedents* are the events or aspects of the situation that come beforehand; these cue or stimulate a person to act in certain ways. Antecedents can be physical events, thoughts, emotions, or the actions of other people. *Consequences*—the results of behavior—affect whether a person will repeat that action. Consequences can also consist of physical events, thoughts, emotions, or the actions of other people. A diary noting your undesirable behaviors and identifying the settings in which they occur can be useful in helping you determine the antecedents and consequences involved. Once you have recognized the antecedents of a given behavior, you can employ **situational inducement** to modify those that are working against you. By carefully considering which settings will help and which will hurt your effort to change, and by seeking the first and avoiding the second, you will improve your chances for change. Similarly, identifying substitute antecedents that can support a more positive result gives you a strategy for controlling the situation.

**situational inducement** Attempt to influence a behavior through situations and occasions that are structured to exert control over that behavior.

**self-talk** The customary manner of thinking and talking to yourself, which can affect your self-image.

**Change Your Self-Talk** **Self-talk,** or the way you think to yourself, can also play a role in modifying health-related behaviors. Self-talk can reflect your feelings of *self-efficacy*, discussed earlier in this chapter. When we don't feel self-efficacious, it's tempting to engage in negative self-talk, which can sabotage our best intentions. Following and in the **Skills for Behavior Change** box on the next page are some suggested strategies for changing self-talk.

**Use Rational, Positive Statements** The rational-emotive form of cognitive therapy, or self-directed behavior change, is based on the premise that there is a close connection between what people say to themselves and how they feel. According to psychologist Albert Ellis, most emotional problems and related behaviors stem from irrational statements that people make to themselves when events in their lives are different from what they would like them to be.[27]

For example, suppose that after doing poorly on a test you say to yourself, "I can't believe I flunked that easy exam. I'm so stupid." By changing this irrational, "catastrophic" self-talk into rational, positive statements about what is really going on, you can increase the likelihood that you will make a positive behavior change. Positive self-talk might be phrased as follows: "I really didn't study enough for that exam. I'm certainly not stupid, I just need to prepare better for the next test." Such self-talk will help you recover quickly from disappointment and take positive steps to correct the situation.

**Practice Blocking and Stopping** By purposefully blocking or stopping negative thoughts, a person can concentrate on taking positive steps toward behavior change. For example, suppose you are preoccupied with your ex-partner, who has recently left you for someone else. By refusing to dwell on negative images and forcing yourself to focus elsewhere, you can avoid wasting energy, time, and emotional resources and move on to positive change.

**Reward Yourself** Another way to promote positive behavior change is to reward yourself for it. This is called **positive reinforcement.** Each of us is motivated by different reinforcers.

Most positive reinforcers can be classified under five headings: consumable, activity, manipulative, possessional, and social:

- *Consumable reinforcers* are edible items that you enjoy, such as your favorite fruit or snack mix.
- *Activity reinforcers* are opportunities to do something enjoyable, such as going on a hike or taking a trip.
- *Manipulative reinforcers* are incentives such as getting a lower rent in exchange for mowing the lawn or the promise of a better grade for doing an extra-credit project.
- *Possessional reinforcers* are tangible rewards such as a new electronic gadget or sports car.
- *Social reinforcers* are signs of appreciation, approval, or love, such as loving looks, affectionate hugs, and praise.

The difficulty with employing positive reinforcment often lies in determining which incentive will be most effective. Your reinforcers may initially come from others (extrinsic rewards), but as you see positive changes in yourself, you will begin to reward and reinforce yourself (intrinsic rewards). Keep in mind that reinforcers should immediately follow a behavior, but beware of overkill. If you reward yourself with a movie every time you go jogging, this reinforcer will soon lose its power. It would be better to give yourself this reward after, say, a full week of adherence to your jogging program.

**what do you think?**

What type of reinforcers would most likely get you to change a behavior? Money? Praise or recognition from someone in particular? ● Why would you find this reinforcer motivating? ● Can you think of some healthy options for reinforcing your own behavior changes?

## Challenge the Thoughts That Sabotage Change

Are any of the following thought patterns and beliefs holding you back? If so, try the strategies that follow them.

✳ **"I don't have enough time!"** Chart your hourly activities for 1 day. What are your highest priorities? What can you eliminate? Plan to make some time for a healthy change next week.

✳ **"I'm too stressed!"** Assess your major stressors right now. List those you can control and those you can change or avoid. Then identify two things you enjoy that can help you reduce stress now.

✳ **"I'm worried about what others may think."** Ask yourself how much others influence your decisions about drinking, sex, eating habits, and the like. What is most important to you? What actions can you take to act in line with these values?

✳ **"I don't think I can do it."** Just because you haven't done something before doesn't mean you can't do it now. To develop some confidence, take baby steps and break tasks into small segments of time.

✳ **"I can't break this habit!"** Habits are difficult to break, but not impossible. What triggers your behavior? List ways you can avoid these triggers. Ask for support from friends and family.

**Journal** Journaling, or writing personal experiences, interpretations, and results in a journal, notebook, or a journal file on your laptop, is an important skill for behavior change. Your journal can be the place where you log your daily activities, monitor your progress, record how you feel about it, and note ideas for improvement.

**positive reinforcement** Presenting something positive following a behavior that is being reinforced.

## Let's Get Started!

After you acquire the skills to support successful behavior change, you're ready to apply those skills to your target behavior. Create a behavior change contract incorporating the goals and skills we've discussed, and place it where you will see it every day and where you can refer to it as you work through the chapters in this text. Consider it a visual reminder that change doesn't "just happen." Reviewing your contract helps you to stay alert to potential problems, to be aware of your alternatives, to maintain a firm sense of your values, and to stick to your goals under pressure.

# How Healthy Are You?

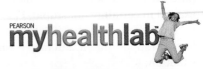

Although we all recognize the importance of being healthy, it can be a challenge to sort out which behaviors are most likely to cause problems or which ones pose the greatest risk. *Before* you decide where to start, it is important to look at your current health status.

By completing the following assessment, you will have a clearer picture of health areas in which you excel and those that could use some work. Taking this assessment will also help you to reflect on components of health that you may not have thought about.

Answer each question, then total your score for each section and fill it in on the Personal Checklist at the end of the assessment for a general sense of your health profile. Think about the behaviors that influenced your score in each category. Would you like to change any of them? Choose the area that you'd like to improve, and then complete the Behavior Change Contract at the front of your book. Use the contract to

Fill out this assessment online at www.pearsonhighered.com/myhealthlab or www.pearsonhighered.com/donatelle.

think through and implement a behavior change over the course of this class.

Each of the categories in this questionnaire is an important aspect of the total dimensions of health, but this is not a substitute for the advice of a qualified health care provider. Consider scheduling a thorough physical examination by a licensed physician or setting up an appointment with a mental health counselor at your school if you need help making a behavior change.

For each of the following, indicate how often you think the statements describe you.

## 1 Physical Health

| | Never | Rarely | Some of the Time | Usually or Always |
|---|---|---|---|---|
| 1. I am happy with my body size and weight. | 1 | 2 | 3 | 4 |
| 2. I engage in vigorous exercises such as brisk walking, jogging, swimming, or running for at least 30 minutes per day, three to four times per week. | 1 | 2 | 3 | 4 |
| 3. I get at least 7 to 8 hours of sleep each night. | 1 | 2 | 3 | 4 |
| 4. My immune system is strong, and my body heals itself quickly when I get sick or injured. | 1 | 2 | 3 | 4 |
| 5. I listen to my body; when there is something wrong, I try to make adjustments to heal it or seek professional advice. | 1 | 2 | 3 | 4 |

Total score for this section: _____

## 2 Social Health

| | Never | Rarely | Some of the Time | Usually or Always |
|---|---|---|---|---|
| 1. I am open, honest, and get along well with others. | 1 | 2 | 3 | 4 |
| 2. I participate in a wide variety of social activities and enjoy being with people who are different from me. | 1 | 2 | 3 | 4 |
| 3. I try to be a "better person" and decrease behaviors that have caused problems in my interactions with others. | 1 | 2 | 3 | 4 |
| 4. I am open and accessible to a loving and responsible relationship. | 1 | 2 | 3 | 4 |
| 5. I try to see the good in my friends and do whatever I can to support them and help them feel good about themselves. | 1 | 2 | 3 | 4 |

Total score for this section: _____

## 3 Emotional Health

| | Never | Rarely | Some of the Time | Usually or Always |
|---|---|---|---|---|
| 1. I find it easy to laugh, cry, and show emotions like love, fear, and anger, and try to express these in positive, constructive ways. | 1 | 2 | 3 | 4 |
| 2. I avoid using alcohol or other drugs as a means of helping me forget my problems. | 1 | 2 | 3 | 4 |
| 3. I recognize when I am stressed and take steps to relax through exercise, quiet time, or other calming activities. | 1 | 2 | 3 | 4 |
| 4. I try not to be too critical or judgmental of others and try to understand differences or quirks that I note in others. | 1 | 2 | 3 | 4 |
| 5. I am flexible and adapt or adjust to change in a positive way. | 1 | 2 | 3 | 4 |

Total score for this section: _____

## 4 Environmental Health

| | Never | Rarely | Some of the Time | Usually or Always |
|---|---|---|---|---|
| 1. I buy recycled paper and purchase biodegradable detergents and cleaning agents, or make my own cleaning products, whenever possible. | 1 | 2 | 3 | 4 |
| 2. I recycle paper, plastic, and metals; purchase refillable containers when possible; and try to minimize the amount of paper and plastics that I use. | 1 | 2 | 3 | 4 |
| 3. I try to wear my clothes for longer periods between washing to reduce water consumption and the amount of detergents in our water sources. | 1 | 2 | 3 | 4 |
| 4. I vote for pro-environment candidates in elections. | 1 | 2 | 3 | 4 |
| 5. I minimize the amount of time that I run the faucet when I brush my teeth, shave, or shower. | 1 | 2 | 3 | 4 |

Total score for this section: _____

## 5 Spiritual Health

| | Never | Rarely | Some of the Time | Usually or Always |
|---|---|---|---|---|
| 1. I take time alone to think about what's important in life—who I am, what I value, where I fit in, and where I'm going. | 1 | 2 | 3 | 4 |
| 2. I have faith in a greater power, be it a supreme being, nature, or the connectedness of all living things. | 1 | 2 | 3 | 4 |
| 3. I engage in acts of caring and goodwill without expecting something in return. | 1 | 2 | 3 | 4 |
| 4. I sympathize and empathize with those who are suffering and try to help them through difficult times. | 1 | 2 | 3 | 4 |
| 5. I go for the gusto and experience life to the fullest. | 1 | 2 | 3 | 4 |

Total score for this section: _____

## 6 Intellectual Health

| | Never | Rarely | Some of the Time | Usually or Always |
|---|---|---|---|---|
| 1. I carefully consider my options and possible consequences as I make choices in life. | 1 | 2 | 3 | 4 |
| 2. I learn from my mistakes and try to act differently the next time. | 1 | 2 | 3 | 4 |
| 3. I have at least one hobby, learning activity, or personal growth activity that I make time for each week, something that improves me as a person. | 1 | 2 | 3 | 4 |
| 4. I manage my time well rather than let time manage me. | 1 | 2 | 3 | 4 |
| 5. My friends and family trust my judgment. | 1 | 2 | 3 | 4 |

Total score for this section: _____

Although each of these six aspects of health is important, there are some factors that don't readily fit in one category. As college students, you face some unique risks that others may not have. For this reason, we have added a section to this self-assessment that focuses on personal health promotion and disease prevention. Answer these questions and add your results to the Personal Checklist in the following section.

## 7 Personal Health Promotion/ Disease Prevention

| | Never | Rarely | Some of the Time | Usually or Always |
|---|---|---|---|---|
| 1. If I were to be sexually active, I would use protection such as latex condoms, dental dams, and other means of reducing my risk of sexually transmitted infections. | 1 | 2 | 3 | 4 |
| 2. I can have a good time at parties or during happy hours without binge drinking. | 1 | 2 | 3 | 4 |
| 3. I have eaten too much in the last month and have forced myself to vomit to avoid gaining weight. | 4 | 3 | 2 | 1 |
| 4. If I were to get a tattoo or piercing, I would go to a reputable person who follows strict standards of sterilization and precautions against bloodborne disease transmission. | 1 | 2 | 3 | 4 |
| 5. I engage in extreme sports and find that I enjoy the highs that come with risking bodily harm through physical performance. | 4 | 3 | 2 | 1 |

Total score for this section: _____

## Personal Checklist

Now, total your scores for each section on the next page and compare them to what would be considered optimal scores. Are you surprised by your scores in any areas? Which areas do you need to work on?

| | Ideal Score | Your Score |
|---|---|---|
| Physical health | 20 | _____ |
| Social health | 20 | _____ |
| Emotional health | 20 | _____ |
| Environmental health | 20 | _____ |
| Spiritual health | 20 | _____ |
| Intellectual health | 20 | _____ |
| Personal health promotion/ disease prevention | 20 | _____ |

## What Your Scores in Each Category Mean

### Scores of 15–20:

Outstanding! Your answers show that you are aware of the importance of these behaviors in your overall health. More important, you are putting your knowledge to work by

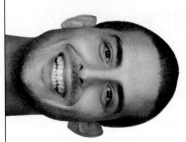

practicing good health habits that should reduce your overall risks. Although you received a very high score on this part of the test, you may want to consider areas in which your scores could be improved.

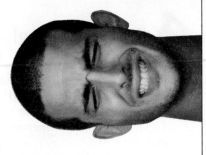

### Scores of 10–14:

Your health risks are showing! Find information about the risks you are facing and why it is important to change these behaviors. Perhaps you need help in deciding how to make the changes you desire. Assistance is available from this book, your professor, and student health services at your school.

### Scores below 10:

You may be taking unnecessary risks with your health. Perhaps you are not aware of the risks and what to do about them. Identify each risk area and make a mental note as you read the associated chapter in the book. Whenever possible, seek additional resources, either on your campus or through your

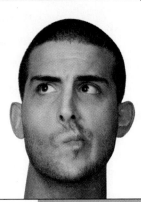

local community health resources, and make a serious commitment to behavior change. If any area is causing you to be less than functional in your class work or personal life, seek professional help. In this book you will find the information you need to help you improve your scores and your health. Remember that these scores are only indicators, not diagnostic tools.

# YOUR PLAN FOR CHANGE

The **Assessyourself** activity gave you the chance to look at the status of your health in several dimensions. Now that you have considered these results, you can take steps toward changing certain behaviors that may be detrimental to your health.

### Today, you can:

◯ Evaluate your behavior and identify patterns and specific things you are doing.

◯ Select one pattern of behavior that you want to change.

◯ Fill out the Behavior Change Contract at the front of your book. Be sure to include your long- and short-term goals for change, the rewards you'll give yourself for reaching these goals, the potential obstacles along the way, and the

strategies for overcoming these obstacles. For each goal, list the small steps and specific actions that you will take.

### Within the next 2 weeks, you can:

◯ Start a journal and begin charting your progress toward your behavior change goal.

◯ Tell a friend or family member about your behavior change goal, and ask them to support you along the way.

◯ Reward yourself for reaching your short-term goals, and reevaluate your plan if you find they are too ambitious.

### By the end of the semester, you can:

◯ Review your journal entries and consider how successful you have been in following your plan. What helped you be successful? What made change more difficult? What will you do differently next week?

◯ Revise your plan as needed: Are the goals attainable? Are the rewards satisfying? Do you have enough support and motivation?

# Summary

* Choosing good health has immediate benefits, such as reducing the risk of injury and illnesses, and improving academic performance; long-term rewards, such as disease prevention, longevity, and improved quality of life; and societal and global benefits, such as reducing the global disease burden.
* For the U.S. population as a whole, the leading causes of death are heart disease, cancer, and stroke. In the 15- to 24-year-old age group, the leading causes are unintentional injuries, homicide, and suicide.
* The average life expectancy at birth in the United States is 78.3 years. This has increased greatly over the past century; however, unhealthy behaviors related to chronic disease may prevent further increases in total life expectancy and cause a reduction in *healthy* life expectancy.
* The definition of *health* has changed over time. The medical model focused on treating disease, whereas the current ecological or public health model focuses on factors contributing to health, disease prevention, and health promotion.
* Health can be seen as existing on a continuum and encompassing the dynamic process of fulfilling one's potential in the physical, social, emotional, spiritual, intellectual, and environmental dimensions of life. Wellness means achieving the highest level of health possible in several dimensions.
* Health is influenced by factors called *determinants*. The Surgeon General's health promotion plan, *Healthy People*, classifies determinants as individual biology and behavior, the social environment, the physical environment, policies and interventions, and access to quality health care. Disparities in health among different groups contribute to increased risks.
* Models of behavior change include the health belief model, the social cognitive model, and the transtheoretical (stages of change) model. A person can increase the chance of successfully changing a health-related behavior by viewing change as a process containing several steps and components.
* When contemplating a behavior change, it is helpful to examine current habits, learn about a target behavior, and assess motivation and readiness to change. When preparing to change, it is helpful to set realistic and incremental goals that employ shaping, anticipate barriers to change, enlist the help and support of others, and sign a behavior change contract. When taking action to change, it is helpful to visualize new behavior, practice countering, control the situation, change self-talk, reward oneself, and keep a log or journal.

# Pop Quiz

1. Our ability to perform everyday tasks, such as walking up the stairs or tying your shoes, is an example of
   a. improved quality of life.
   b. physical health.
   c. health promotion.
   d. activities of daily living.

2. Janice describes herself as confident and trusting, and she displays both high self-esteem and high self-efficacy. The dimension of health this relates to is the
   a. social dimension.
   b. emotional dimension.
   c. spiritual dimension.
   d. intellectual dimension.

3. What statistic is used to describe the number of deaths from heart disease this year?
   a. Morbidity
   b. Mortality
   c. Incidence
   d. Prevalence

4. Because Craig's parents smoked, he is 90 percent more likely to start smoking than someone whose parents didn't. This is an example of what factor influencing behavior change?
   a. Circumstantial factor
   b. Enabling factor
   c. Reinforcing factor
   d. Predisposing factor

5. Suppose you want to lose 20 pounds. To reach your goal, you take small steps. You start by joining a support group and counting calories. After 2 weeks, you begin an exercise program and gradually build up to your desired fitness level. What behavior change strategy are you using?
   a. Shaping
   b. Visualization
   c. Modeling
   d. Reinforcement

6. After Kirk and Tammy pay their bills, they reward themselves by watching TV together. The type of positive reinforcement that motivates them to pay their bills is a(n)
   a. activity reinforcer.
   b. consumable reinforcer.
   c. manipulative reinforcer.
   d. possessional reinforcer.

7. Jake is exhibiting *self-efficacy* when he
   a. believes that he can and will be able to bench-press 125 pounds in his specified time frame.
   b. is doubtful that his bad shoulder will heal enough to bench-press the weight he is hoping for.
   c. claims he is not good enough to do any physical exercise that will ever allow him to bench-press 125 pounds.
   d. does not possess personal control over this situation.

8. The setting events for a behavior that cue or stimulate a person to act in certain ways are called
   a. antecedents.
   b. frequency of events.
   c. consequences.
   d. cues to action.

9. What strategy for change is advised for an individual in the preparation stage of change?
   a. Seeking out recommended readings
   b. Finding creative ways to maintain positive behaviors
   c. Setting realistic goals
   d. Publicly stating the desire for change

10. Spiritual health is
    a. exclusive to religiosity.
    b. optional for achieving wellness.
    c. related to one's purpose in life.
    d. finding fulfilling relationships.

*Answers to these questions can be found on page A-1.*

# Think about It!

1. How are the words *health* and *wellness* similar? What, if any, are important distinctions between these terms? What is health promotion? Disease prevention?

2. How healthy is the U.S. population today? Are we doing better or worse in terms of health status than we have done previously? What factors influence today's disparities in health?

3. What are some of the health disparities existing in the United States today? Why do you think these differences exist? What policies do you think would most effectively address or eliminate health disparities?

4. What is the health belief model? How may this model be working when a young woman decides to smoke her first cigarette? Her last cigarette?

5. Using the transtheoretical model, discuss what you might do (in stages) to help a friend stop smoking. Why is it important that a person be ready to change before trying to change?

# Accessing Your Health on the Internet

The following websites explore further topics and issues related to personal health. For links to the websites below, visit the Companion Website for *Access to Health,* 12th Edition, at www.pearsonhighered.com/donatelle.

1. *CDC Wonder.* This is a clearinghouse for comprehensive information from the Centers for Disease Control and Prevention (CDC), including special reports, guidelines, and access to national health data. http://wonder.cdc.gov

2. *MayoClinic.com.* This reputable resource for specific information about health topics, diseases, and treatment options is provided by the staff of the Mayo Clinic. It is easy to navigate and is consumer friendly. www.mayoclinic.com

3. *National Center for Health Statistics.* This is an outstanding place to start for information about health status in the United States. It contains links to key reports; national survey information; and information on mortality by age, race, gender, geographic location, and other important data. www.cdc.gov/nchs

4. *National Health Information Center.* This is an excellent resource for consumer information about health. www.health.gov/nhic

5. *World Health Organization.* This resource for global health information provides information on the current state of health around the world, such as illness and disease statistics, trends, and illness outbreak alerts. www.who.int/en

# References

1. U.S. Census Bureau, *The 2010 Statistical Abstract of the United States: Births, Deaths, Marriages, and Divorces,* "Table 102 Expectations of Life at Birth, 1970 to 2006, and Projections 2010 and 2020," 2010, Available at www.census.gov/compendia/statab/cats/births_deaths_marriages_divorces.html.

2. Centers for Disease Control and Prevention, "Achievements in Public Health, 1900–1999: Control of Infectious Diseases," *MMWR* 48, no. 29 (1999): 621–29, Available at www.cdc.gov/mmwr/preview/mmwrhtml/mm4829a1.htm.

3. Ibid.

4. S. J. Olshansky et al., "A Potential Decline in Life Expectancy in the United States in the 21st Century," *New England Journal of Medicine* 352, no. 11 (2005): 1138–45.

5. G. Danaei et al., "The Promise of Prevention: The Effects of Four Preventable Risk Factors on National Life Expectancy and Life Expectancy Disparities by Race and County in the United States," *PLoS Medicine* 7, no. 3 (2010): e1000248, Available at www.plosmedicine.org/article/info%3Adoi%2F10.1371%2Fjournal.pmed.1000248.

6. E. A. Finkelstein et al., "Annual Medical Spending Attributable to Obesity: Payer- and Service-Specific Estimates," *Health Affairs* 28, no. 5 (2009): w822–31.

7. M. Bittman, "Soda: A Sin We Sip Instead of Smoke?" *New York Times*, February 12, 2010, Available at www.nytimes.com/2010/02/14/weekinreview/14bittman.html.

8. World Health Organization (WHO), "Constitution of the World Health Organization," *Chronicles of the World Health Organization* (Geneva: WHO, 1947), Available at www.who.int/governance/eb/constitution/en/index.html.

9. R. Dubos, *So Human an Animal: How We Are Shaped by Surroundings and Events* (New York: Scribner, 1968), 15.

10. U.S. Department of Health and Human Services, *Healthy People 2010* (Washington, DC: U.S. Government Printing Office, 2000).

11. Ibid.

12. Centers for Disease Control and Prevention, Chronic Disease and Health Promotion, *Chronic Disease Overview*, December 17, 2009, Available at www.cdc.gov/chronicdisease/overview/index.htm#2.

13. G. Danaei et al., "The Preventable Causes of Death in the United States: Comparative Risk Assessment of Dietary, Lifestyle, and Metabolic Risk Factors," *PLoS Medicine* 6,

no. 4 (2009): e1000058, Available at www.plosmedicine.org/article/info:doi/10.1371/journal.pmed.1000058; Centers for Disease Control and Prevention, *Chronic Disease Overview*, 2009.

14. U.S. Department of Health and Human Services, *Healthy People 2010*, 2000.

15. R. Wilkinson and M. Marmot, eds., *Social Determinants of Health: The Solid Facts*, 2nd ed. (Geneva: World Health Organization, 2003), Available at www.euro.who.int/en/what-we-publish/abstracts/social-determinants-of-health.-the-solid-facts.

16. Prevention Institute, *The Built Environment and Health: 11 Profiles of Neighborhood Transformation*, July 2004, Available at www.preventioninstitute.org/index.php?option=com_jlibrary&view=article&id=114&Itemid=127.

17. W. C. Willett and A. Underwood, "Crimes of the Heart," *Newsweek*, February 5, 2010, Available at www.newsweek.com/id/233006.

18. U.S. Department of Health and Human Services, *Healthy People 2010*, 2000.

19. W. C. Willett and A. Underwood, "Crimes of the Heart," 2010.

20. National Institutes of Health, *National Institutes of Health (NIH) Strategic Research Plan and Budget to Reduce and Ultimately Eliminate Health Disparities: Volume 1, Fiscal Years 2002–2006* (Bethesda, MD: National Institutes of Health, May 12, 2006), Available at http://ncmhd.nih.gov/our_programs/strategic/pubs/VolumeI_031003EDrev.pdf.

21. U.S. Department of Health and Human Services, "*Healthy People 2020*: The Road Ahead," Revised 2009, www.healthypeople.gov/HP2020.

22. I. Rosenstock, "Historical Origins of the Health Belief Model," *Health Education Monographs* 2, no. 4 (1974): 328–35.

23. J. O. Prochaska and C. C. DiClemente, "Stages and Processes of Self-Change of Smoking: Toward an Integrative Model of Change," *Journal of Consulting and Clinical Psychology* 51 (1983): 390–95.

24. W. C. Willett and A. Underwood, "Crimes of the Heart," 2010.

25. M. Hesse, "The Readiness Ruler as a Measure of Readiness to Change Polydrug Use in Drug Abusers," *Journal of Harm Reduction* 3, no. 3 (2006): 1477–81; M. Cismaru, "Using Protection Motivation Theory to Increase the Persuasiveness of Public Service Communications," The Saskatchewan Institute of Public Policy, Public Policy Series paper no. 40 (February 2006); E. A. Fallon, S. Wilcox, and M. Laken, "Health Care Provider Advice for African American Adults Not Meeting Health Behavior Recommendations," *Preventing Chronic Disease* 3, no. 2 (2006): A45; M. R. Chacko et al., "New Sexual Partners and Readiness to Seek Screening for Chlamydia and Gonorrhea: Predictors among Minority Young Women," *Sexually Transmitted Infections* 82 (2006): 75–79.

26. J. M. Twenge, Z. Liqing, and C. Im, "It's Beyond My Control: A Cross-Temporal Meta-Analysis of Increasing Externality in Locus of Control, 1960–2002," *Personality and Social Psychology Review* 8 (2004): 308–20.

27. A. Ellis and M. Benard, *Clinical Application of Rational Emotive Therapy* (New York: Plenum, 1985).

2

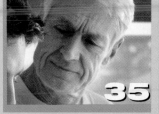
35
How do others influence my psychological well-being?

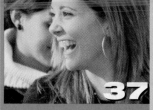
37
Is laughter really the best medicine?

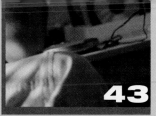
43
What are the symptoms of depression?

# Promoting and Preserving Your Psychological Health

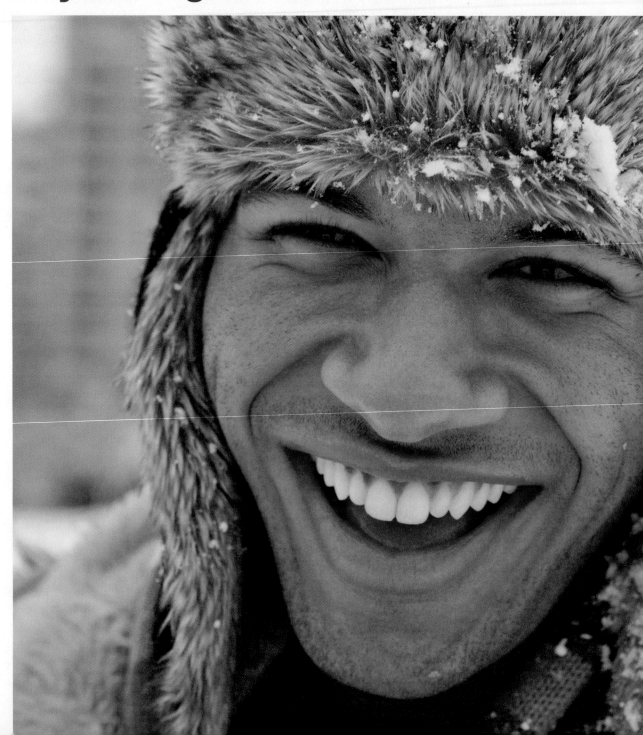

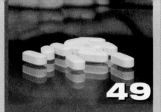

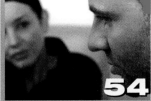

**49**

**What should I do if someone I know is suicidal?**

**54**

**How can I choose the right therapist for me?**

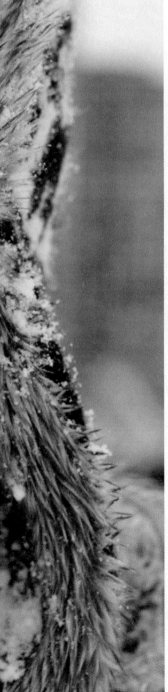

## Objectives

✳ Define each of the four components of psychological health, and identify the basic traits shared by psychologically healthy people.

✳ Learn what factors affect your psychological health; discuss the positive steps you can take to enhance psychological well-being.

✳ Identify psychological disorders, such as mood disorders, anxiety disorders, personality disorders, and schizophrenia, and explain their causes and treatments.

✳ Discuss warning signs of suicide and actions that can be taken to help a suicidal individual.

✳ Explain the different types of treatments and mental health professionals, and examine how they can play a role in managing mental health disorders.

Although the vast majority of college students describe their college years as among the best of their lives, many find the pressure of grades, financial concerns, relationship problems, and the struggle to find themselves to be extraordinarily difficult. Psychological distress caused by relationship issues, family issues, academic competition, and adjusting to life as a college student is rampant on college campuses today. Experts believe that the anxiety-inducing campus environment is a major contributor to poor health decisions such as high levels of alcohol consumption and, in turn, to health problems that ultimately affect academic success and success in life.

Fortunately, even though we often face seemingly insurmountable pressures, human beings possess a resiliency that enables us to cope, adapt, and thrive, regardless of life's challenges. How we feel and think about ourselves, those around us, and our environment can tell us a lot about our psychological health and whether we are healthy emotionally, socially, spiritually, and mentally.

# What Is Psychological Health?

Psychological health is the sum of how we think, feel, relate, and exist in our day-to-day lives. Our thoughts, perceptions, emotions, motivations, interpersonal relationships, and behaviors are a product of our experiences and the skills we have developed along the way to meet life's challenges. **Psychological health** includes mental, emotional, social, and spiritual dimensions (Figure 2.1).

**psychological health** The mental, emotional, social, and spiritual dimensions of health.

Most experts identify several basic elements shared by psychologically healthy people:

● **They feel good about themselves.** They are not typically overwhelmed by fear, love, anger, jealousy, guilt, or worry. They know who they are, have a realistic sense of their capabilities, and respect themselves even though they realize they aren't perfect.

● **They feel comfortable with other people and express respect and compassion toward others.** They enjoy satisfying and lasting personal relationships and do not take advantage of others, or allow others to take advantage of them. They recognize that there are others whose needs are greater than their own and take responsibility for their fellow human beings. They can give love, consider others' interests, take time to help others, and respect personal differences.

● **They control tension and anxiety.** They recognize the underlying causes and symptoms of stress and anxiety in their lives and consciously avoid irrational thoughts, hostility, excessive excuse making, and blaming others for their problems. They use resources and learn skills to control reactions to stressful situations.

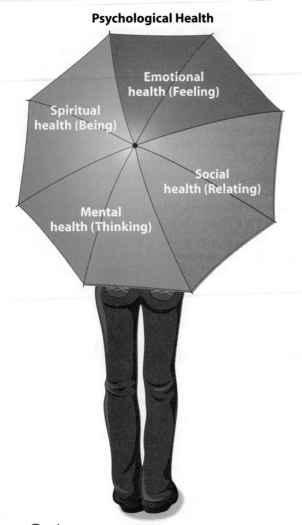

**Psychological Health**

Emotional health (Feeling)

Spiritual health (Being)

Social health (Relating)

Mental health (Thinking)

FIGURE 2.1 **Psychological Health**
Psychological health is a complex interaction of the mental, emotional, social, and spiritual dimensions of health. Possessing strength and resiliency in these dimensions can maintain your overall well-being and help you weather the storms of life.

● **They meet the demands of life.** They try to solve problems as they arise, accept responsibility, and plan ahead. They set realistic goals, think for themselves, and make independent decisions. Acknowledging that change is inevitable, they welcome new experiences.

**mental health** The thinking part of psychosocial health; includes your values, attitudes, and beliefs.
**emotional health** The feeling part of psychosocial health; includes your emotional reactions to life.
**emotions** Intensified feelings or complex patterns of feelings we constantly experience.

● **They curb hate and guilt.** They acknowledge and combat tendencies to respond with anger, thoughtlessness, selfishness, vengefulness, or feelings of inadequacy. They do not try to knock others aside to get ahead, but rather reach out to help others.

● **They maintain a positive outlook.** They approach each day with a presumption that things will go well. They look to the future with enthusiasm rather than dread. Fun and making time for themselves are integral parts of their lives.

● **They value diversity.** They do not feel threatened by those of a different race, gender, religion, sexual orientation, ethnicity, or political party. They are nonjudgmental and do not force their beliefs and values on others.
● **They appreciate and respect nature.** They take time to enjoy their surroundings, are conscious of their place in the universe, and act responsibly to preserve their environment.

Psychologists have long argued that before we can achieve any of the above characteristics of psychologically healthy people, we must have certain basic needs met in our lives. In the 1960s, human theorist Abraham Maslow developed a *hierarchy of needs* to describe this idea (Figure 2.2): At the bottom of his hierarchy are basic *survival needs,* such as food, sleep, and water; at the next level are *security needs,* such as shelter and safety; at the third level—*social needs*—is a sense of belonging and affection; at the fourth level are *esteem needs,* self-respect and respect for others; and at the top are needs for *self-actualization* and self-transcendence.

According to Maslow's theory, a person's needs must be met at each of these levels before that person can ever truly be healthy. Failure to meet one of the lower levels of needs will interfere with a person's ability to address the upper-level ones. For example, someone who is homeless or worried about threats from violence will be unable to focus on fulfilling social, esteem, or actualization needs. Maslow believed that people are more likely to behave badly if they are frustrated by a lack of need fulfillment.[1]

In sum, psychologically healthy people are emotionally, mentally, socially, and spiritually resilient. They usually respond to challenges and frustrations in appropriate ways, despite occasional slips (see Figure 2.3 on page 34). When they do slip, they recognize it and take action to rectify the situation.

Attaining psychological well-being involves many complex processes. This chapter will help you understand not only what it means to be psychologically well, but also why we may run into problems in our psychological health. Learning how to assess your own health and take action to help yourself are important aspects of psychological health.

## Mental Health

The term **mental health** is used to describe the "thinking" or "rational" dimension of our health. A mentally healthy person perceives life in realistic ways, can adapt to change, can develop rational strategies to solve problems, and can carry out personal and professional responsibilities. In addition, a mentally healthy person has the intellectual ability to sort through information, messages, and life events; attach meaning to these events; and respond appropriately. This is often referred to as *intellectual health,* a subset of mental health.[2]

## Emotional Health

The term **emotional health** refers to the feeling, or subjective, side of psychological health. **Emotions** are intensified feelings or complex patterns of feelings that we experience

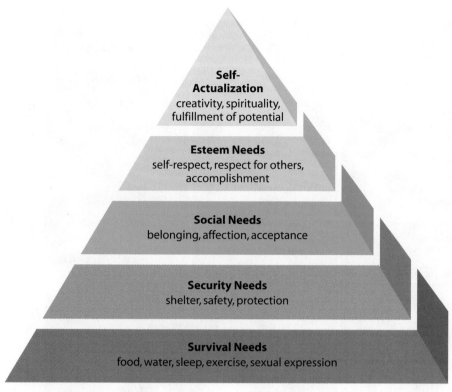

FIGURE 2.2 **Maslow's Hierarchy of Needs**

on a regular basis, including love, hate, frustration, anxiety, and joy, just to name a few. Typically, emotions are described as the interplay of four components: physiological arousal, feelings, cognitive (thought) processes, and behavioral reactions. As rational beings, we are responsible for evaluating our individual emotional responses, the environment that is causing them, and the appropriateness of our actions.

Emotionally healthy people usually respond appropriately to upsetting events. Rather than reacting in an extreme fashion or behaving inconsistently or offensively, they can express their feelings, communicate with others, and show emotions in appropriate ways. Emotionally unhealthy people are much more likely to let their feelings overpower them. They may be highly volatile and prone to unpredictable emotional responses, which may be followed by inappropriate communication or actions.

Emotional health also affects social and intellectual health. Someone feeling hostile, withdrawn, or moody may become socially isolated.[3] Because they are not much fun to be around, their friends may avoid them at the very time they are most in need of emotional support. For students, a more immediate concern is the impact of emotional trauma on academic performance. Have you ever tried to study for an exam after a fight with a close friend or family member? Emotional turmoil may seriously affect your ability to think, reason, and act rationally.

## Social Health

**Social health** includes your interactions with others on an individual and group basis, your ability to use social resources and support in times of need, and your ability to adapt to a variety of social situations. Socially healthy individuals enjoy a wide range of interactions with family, friends, and acquaintances and are able to have healthy interactions with an intimate partner. Typically, socially healthy individuals can listen, express themselves, form healthy attachments, act in socially acceptable and responsible ways, and find the best fit for themselves in society. Numerous studies have documented the importance of positive relationships with family members, friends, and significant others in overall well-being and longevity.[4]

**Social bonds** reflect the level of closeness and attachment that we develop with individuals and are the very foundation of human life. They provide intimacy, feelings of belonging, opportunities for giving and receiving nurturance, reassurance of one's worth, assistance and guidance, and advice. Although you may have many friends, the ones you share your deepest thoughts with, those you seek out when you are in trouble, and those you miss the most when they are away reflect your degree of bonding. Social bonds take multiple forms, the most common of which are social support and community engagements.

The concept of **social support** is more complex than many people realize. In general, it refers to

**social health** Aspect of psychosocial health that includes interactions with others, ability to use social supports, and ability to adapt to various situations.
**social bonds** Degree and nature of interpersonal contacts.
**social support** Network of people and services with whom you share ties and from whom you get support.

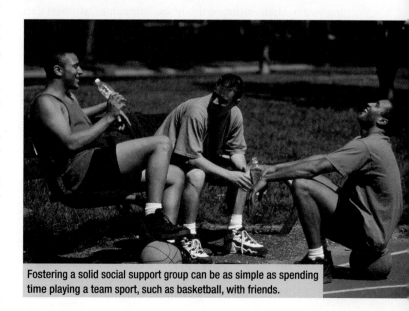

Fostering a solid social support group can be as simple as spending time playing a team sport, such as basketball, with friends.

| | | | |
|---|---|---|---|
| No zest for life; pessimistic/cynical most of the time; spiritually down | Shows poorer coping than most, often overwhelmed by circumstances | Works to improve in all areas, recognizes strengths and weaknesses | Possesses zest for life; spiritually healthy and intellectually thriving |
| Laughs, but usually at others, has little fun | Has regular relationship problems, finds that others often disappoint | Healthy relationships with family and friends, capable of giving and receiving love and affection | High energy, resilient, enjoys challenges, focused |
| Has serious bouts of depression, "down" and tired much of time; has suicidal thoughts | Tends to be cynical/critical of others; tends to have negative/critical friends | Has strong social support, may need to work on improving social skills but usually no major problems | Realistic sense of self and others, sound coping skills, open minded |
| A "challenge" to be around, socially isolated | Lacks focus much of the time, hard to keep intellectual acuity sharp | Has occasional emotional "dips" but overall good mental/emotional adaptors | Adapts to change easily, sensitive to others and environment |
| Experiences many illnesses, headaches, aches/pains, gets colds/infections easily | Quick to anger, sense of humor and fun evident less often | | Has strong social support and healthy relationships with family and friends |

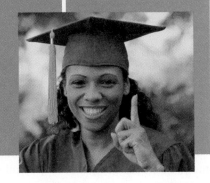

FIGURE 2.3 **Characteristics of Psychologically Healthy and Unhealthy People**
Where do you fall on this continuum?

the networks of people and services with whom and which we interact and share social connections. These ties can provide *tangible support,* such as babysitting services or money to help pay the bills, or *intangible support,* such as encouraging you to share intimate thoughts. Sometimes, support can be felt as perceiving that someone would be there for us in a crisis. Generally, the closer and the higher the quality of the social bond, the more likely a person is to ask for and receive social support. For example, if your car broke down on a dark country road in the middle of the night, whom could you call for help and know that the person would do everything possible to get there? Common descriptions of strong social support include the following:[5]

● Being cared for and loved, with shared intimacy
● Being esteemed and valued; having a sense of self-worth
● Sharing companionship, communication, and mutual obligations with others; having a sense of belonging
● Having "informational" support—access to information, advice, community services, and guidance from others

**spiritual health** The aspect of psychosocial health that relates to having a sense of meaning and purpose to one's life, as well as a feeling of connection with others and with nature.

Social health also reflects the way we react to others. Look for more information about interpersonal relationships in Chapter 4.

## Spiritual Health

It is possible to be mentally, emotionally, and socially healthy and still not achieve optimal psychological well-being. What is missing? For many people, the difficult-to-describe element that gives purpose to life is the spiritual dimension.

According to the National Center for Complementary and Alternative Medicine (NCCAM), *spirituality* is broader in meaning than religion and is defined as an individual's sense of purpose and meaning in life; it goes beyond material values.[6] Spirituality may be practiced in many ways, including through religion; however, religion does not have to be part of a spiritual person's life. **Spiritual health** refers to the sense of belonging to something greater than the purely physical or personal dimensions of existence. For some, this unifying force is nature; for others, it is a feeling of connection to other people; for still others, the unifying force is a god or other higher power.

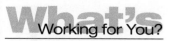
Maybe you already are doing things to enhance your psychological health. Are any of the following true for you?

☐ I have a network of friends and advisers I can go to when I need to talk about a difficult problem.

☐ I know where to find psychological counseling on campus should I need it.

☐ I have healthy outlets for dealing with my emotions when I'm upset.

☐ I volunteer regularly in my college community, an activity that not only helps the community, but gives me a sense of purpose as well.

**Focus On: Cultivating Your Spiritual Health** beginning on page 60 will help you explore your spiritual health in more detail and better understand the role spirituality plays in your overall psychological health.

# Factors That Influence Psychological Health

Our psychological health is the product of many influences throughout our lives. In this section, we first discuss how your psychological health can be influenced by multiple environmental factors, including your family, your social supports, and the community in which you live. Then we show how your psychological health is shaped by your sense of self-efficacy and self-esteem, your personality, and your life span development.

## The Family

Families have a significant influence on psychological development. Healthy families model and help develop the cognitive and social skills necessary to solve problems, communicate emotions in socially acceptable ways, manage stressors, and develop both a sense of self-worth and purpose in life. Consistent love and nurturing from family members develop our capacity to value ourselves and to relate to others in respectful and caring ways. Children raised in healthy, nurturing homes are more likely to become well-adjusted, productive adults. In adulthood, family support is one of the best predictors of health and happiness.[7] Children brought up in **dysfunctional families**—in which there is violence; distrust; anger; dietary deprivation; drug abuse; parental discord; or sexual, physical, or emotional abuse—may have a harder time adapting to life and may run an increased risk of psychological problems. In dysfunctional families, love, security, and unconditional trust may be so lacking that children become psychologically damaged. Yet not all people raised in dysfunctional families become psychologically unhealthy, and not all people from healthy environments become well adjusted.

**dysfunctional families** Families in which there is violence; physical, emotional, or sexual abuse; parental discord; or other negative family interactions.

## Social Supports

Our initial social support may be provided by family members, but as we grow and develop the support of peers and friends becomes more and more important. We rely on

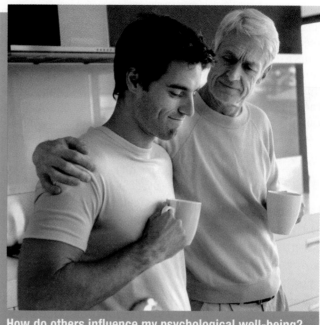

**How do others influence my psychological well-being?**

Your outlook on life is determined in part by your social and cultural surroundings, and your general sense of well-being can be strongly affected by the positive or negative nature of your social bonds. In particular, your family members shape your psychological health. As you were growing up, they modeled behaviors and skills that helped you develop cognitively and socially. Their love and support can give you a sense of self-worth and encourage you to treat others with compassion and care.

friends to help us figure out who we are and what we want to do with our lives. A recent study involving college students clearly demonstrated that the availability of a social network (a sense of belonging) predicted health.[8] Think about some of the questions you may be asking yourself now, like "What should I choose as a major? How can I keep my student loans in check? Should I take my relationship with Chris to the next level?" or "How can I cut back on my partying, because it is starting to affect my grades?" These challenges require us to make a realistic consideration of our goals and values, recognize our emotional responses, think through our options, and make decisions. We often check in with friends to bounce ideas off them and see if they think we are being logical or smart or practical or fair. Having people in our lives that we can trust and rely on is important to our psychological health.

## Community

The communities we live in can have a positive impact on our psychological health through collective actions. Neighbors who work together to create a functioning, informal network of people who show concern for one another and their community create a collective efficacy.[9] A *collective efficacy* occurs when a group has an expectation that its members can successfully achieve an intended goal through collective action. For example, neighbors may join together to get rid of trash on the street, participate in a neighborhood watch to keep children safe, help each other with home repairs, or initiate a community picnic. Religious institutions, schools, clinics, and retail stores can also enhance collective efficacy through policies and practices that demonstrate support and caring for community members. Likewise, you are a part of a campus community. That community may support and care for your psychological health by creating a safe environment to explore and develop your mental, emotional, social, and spiritual dimensions. Your participation in athletics, recreational sports, academic support and advising services, a fraternity or sorority, campus religious organizations, student health services, campus counseling services, student government, performing arts groups, or campus cultural centers may be a part of the collective efficacy of your campus community.

## what do you think?

What are some ways in which people in your community work together in a form of "collective efficacy?" ● What type of groundwork must be established before this type of working together can occur? ● What factors can get in the way of having a community where collective efficacy exists?

## Self-Efficacy and Self-Esteem

During our formative years, successes and failures in school, athletics, friendships, intimate relationships, our jobs, and every other aspect of life subtly shape our beliefs about our personal worth and abilities. These beliefs in turn become internal influences on our psychosocial health.

As we defined in Chapter 1, *self-efficacy* describes a person's belief about whether he or she can successfully engage in and execute a specific behavior. *Self-esteem* refers to one's sense of self-respect or self-worth. People with high levels of self-efficacy and self-esteem tend to express a positive outlook on life.

Our self-esteem is a result of the relationships we have with our parents and family during our formative years; with our friends as we grow older; with our significant others as we form intimate relationships; and with our teachers, coworkers, and others throughout our lives. How can you build up your self-esteem? The Skills for Behavior Change box at right suggests small things you can do every day that can significantly affect the way you feel about yourself.

### Learned Helplessness versus Learned Optimism

Psychologist Martin Seligman has proposed that people who continually experience failure may develop a pattern of responding known as **learned helplessness** in which they give up and fail to take any action to help themselves. Seligman ascribes this response in part to society's tendency toward *victimology*—blaming one's problems on other people and circumstances.[10] Although viewing ourselves as victims may make us feel better temporarily, it does not address the underlying causes of a problem. Ultimately, it can

**learned helplessness** Pattern of responding to situations by giving up because of repeated failure in the past.
**learned optimism** Teaching oneself to think positively.

### Build Your Self-Efficacy and Self-Esteem

* Pay attention to your own needs and wants. Listen to what your body, mind, and heart are telling you.
* Make a list of things that make you happy and do something from that list every day.
* Do things you are good at and enjoy the satisfaction in a job well done.
* Do something that you have been putting off, such as cleaning out your closet or paying a bill that you've been ignoring, to give yourself a sense of accomplishment.
* Acknowledge that you are a great person by rewarding yourself regularly.
* Don't engage in self put downs or self-criticism.
* Write down the good things about yourself and practice positive affirmations.
* Spend time with people who make you feel good about yourself. Avoid people who treat you poorly or make you feel bad about yourself.
* Display or keep close by items that you like and take time to reflect on your achievements, your friends, or special times.
* Take advantage of any opportunity to learn something new.
* Do something nice for another person. There is no greater way to feel better about yourself than to help someone in need.

erode self-efficacy by making us feel that we cannot do anything to improve the situation.

Today, many people have developed self-help programs that use elements of Seligman's principle of **learned optimism.** The basis for these programs is the thought that just as we learn to be helpless, so we can teach ourselves to be optimistic. By changing our self-talk, examining our reactions, and blocking negative thoughts, we can "unlearn" negative thought processes that have become habitual. Some programs practice "positive affirmations" with clients, teaching them the sometimes difficult task of learning to acknowledge positive things about themselves. Often we are our own worst critics, and learning to be kinder to ourselves is difficult.

## Personality

Your personality is the unique mix of characteristics that distinguishes you from others. Heredity, environment, culture, and experience influence how each person develops. Personality determines how we react to the challenges of life, interpret our feelings, and resolve conflicts.

Most recent schools of psychological theory promote the idea that we have the power to understand our behavior and to change it, thus molding our own personalities. Although

**75%** of the general U.S. population is estimated to be extroverted, as measured by the Myers–Briggs Type Indicator personality test.

this is more difficult if social environments are inhospitable, there may be opportunities for making positive changes. One way to examine personality is by looking at traits that are associated with psychological health. In general, the following personality traits are often related to psychological well-being:[11]

● **Extroversion**—the ability to adapt to a social situation and demonstrate assertiveness as well as power or interpersonal involvement
● **Agreeableness**—the ability to conform, be likable, and demonstrate friendly compliance and love
● **Openness to experience**—the willingness to demonstrate curiosity and independence (also referred to as inquiring intellect)
● **Emotional stability**—the ability to maintain emotional control
● **Conscientiousness**—the qualities of being dependable and demonstrating self-control, discipline, and a need to achieve
● **Resiliency**—the ability to adapt to change and stressful events in healthy and flexible ways

## Life Span and Maturity

Our temperaments change as we grow, which is illustrated by the extreme emotions that children and many young teens experience. Most of us learn to control our emotions as we advance toward adulthood. The college years mark a critical transition period for young adults as they move away from families and establish themselves as independent adults. This transition will be easier for those who have successfully accomplished earlier developmental tasks such as learning how to solve problems, make and evaluate decisions, define and adhere to personal values, and establish both casual and intimate relationships. People who have not fulfilled these earlier tasks may find their lives interrupted by recurrent crises left over from earlier stages. For example, if they did not learn to trust others in childhood, they may have difficulty establishing intimate relationships as adults.

## The Mind–Body Connection

Can negative emotions make us physically ill? Can positive emotions help us stay well? Researchers are

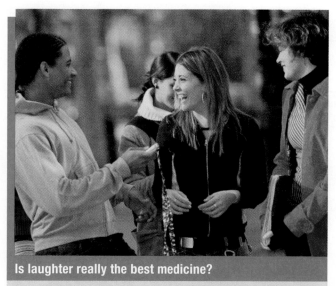

**Is laughter really the best medicine?**

Research is inconclusive regarding whether the act of laughing actually improves your health, but we've all experienced the sense of well-being that a good laugh can bring. Regardless of whether it actually increases blood flow, boosts immune response, lowers blood sugar levels, or facilitates better sleep, there is no doubting that sharing laughter and fun with others can strengthen social ties and bring joy to your everyday life.

exploring the interaction between emotions and health, especially in conditions of uncontrolled, persistent stress. In fact, the NCCAM and other organizations are investing more and more dollars in large research projects designed to explore the link between mind and body. At the core of the mind–body connection is the study of **psychoneuroimmunology (PNI),** or how the brain and behavior affect the body's immune system.

One area of study that appears to be particularly promising in enhancing physical health is *happiness*— a collective term for several positive states in which individuals actively embrace the world around them.[12] In examining the characteristics of happy people, scientists have found that this emotion can have a profound impact on the body. Happiness, or related mental states such as hopefulness, optimism, and contentment, appears to reduce the risk or limit the severity of cardiovascular disease, pulmonary disease, diabetes, hypertension, colds, and other infections. Laughter can promote increases in heart and respiration rates and can reduce levels of stress hormones in much the same way as light exercise can. For this reason, it

**psychoneuroimmunology (PNI)** The science that examines the relationship between the brain and behavior and how this affects the body's immune system.

Calming your mind may help heal your body.

has been promoted as a possible risk reducer for people with hypertension and other forms of cardiovascular disease.[13]

**Subjective well-being** is that uplifting feeling of inner peace or an overall "feel-good" state, which includes happiness. Subjective well-being is defined by three central components: satisfaction with present life, relative presence of positive emotions, and relative absence of negative emotions.[14] You do not have to be happy all the time to achieve overall subjective well-being. Everyone experiences disappointments, unhappiness, and times when life seems unfair. However, people with a high level of subjective well-being are typically resilient, are able to look on the positive side and get back on track fairly quickly, and are less likely to fall into despair over setbacks.

**subjective well-being** An uplifting feeling of inner peace.

Scientists suggest that some people may be biologically predisposed to happiness. Psychologist Richard Davidson has proposed that happiness and other emotions may, in part, be related to actual differences in brain physiology—that neurotransmitters, the chemicals that transfer messages between neurons, may function more efficiently in happy people.[15] Other psychologists suggest that we can develop happiness by practicing positive psychological actions.[16] The **Skills for Behavior Change** box at left provides some suggestions for things you can do to incorporate positive psychology principles into your own life.

# Strategies to Enhance Psychological Health

As we have seen, psychological health involves four dimensions. Attaining self-fulfillment is a lifelong, conscious process that involves enhancing each of these components. Strategies include building self-efficacy and self-esteem, understanding and controlling emotions, maintaining support networks, and learning to solve problems and make decisions. In addition to the advice in this chapter, see Chapter 3 for tips on effective stress reduction, relaxation techniques, and other tools for enhancing your psychological health.

- **Find a support group.** The best way to promote self-esteem is through a support group—peers who share your values. A support group can make you feel good about yourself and force you to take an honest look at your actions and choices. Keeping in contact with old friends and important family members can provide a foundation of unconditional love that will help you through life transitions.
- **Complete required tasks.** A good way to boost your sense of self-efficacy is to learn new skills and develop a history of success. Most college campuses provide study groups and learning centers that can help you manage time, develop study skills, and prepare for tests. Poor grades, or grades that do not meet expectations, are major contributors to emotional distress among college students.
- **Form realistic expectations.** If you expect perfect grades, a steady stream of Saturday-night dates, and the perfect job, you may be setting yourself up for failure. Assess your current resources and the direction in which you are heading. Set small, incremental goals that you can actually meet.
- **Make time for you.** Taking time to enjoy yourself is another way to boost your self-esteem and psychosocial health. View a new activity as something to look forward to and an opportunity to have fun. Anticipate and focus on the fun things that you have to look forward to each day.
- **Maintain physical health.** Regular exercise fosters a sense of well-being. More and more research supports the role of exercise in improved mental health. Nourishing meals can help

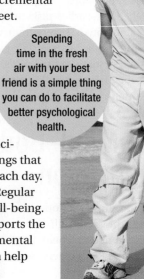

Spending time in the fresh air with your best friend is a simple thing you can do to facilitate better psychological health.

you stay well and avoid the weight gain and related depression many college students experience.

● **Examine problems and seek help when necessary.** Knowing when to seek help from friends, support groups, family, or professionals is an important factor in boosting self-esteem. Sometimes you can handle life's problems alone; at other times, you need assistance. Get help before you feel overwhelmed.

● **Get adequate sleep.** Getting enough sleep on a daily basis is a key factor in physical and psychological health. Not only do our bodies need to rest to conserve energy for our daily activities, but we also need to restore supplies of many of the neurotransmitters that we use up during our waking hours. For more information on the importance of sleep, see **Focus On: Improving Your Sleep** beginning on page 102.

## When Psychological Health Deteriorates

Sometimes circumstances overwhelm us to such a degree that we need help to get back on track to healthful living. Stress, abusive relationships, anxiety, loneliness, financial upheavals, and other traumatic events can derail our coping resources, causing us to turn inward or to act in ways that are outside of what might be considered normal. Chemical imbalances, drug interactions, trauma, neurological disruptions, and other physical problems also may contribute to these behaviors. **Mental illnesses** are disorders that disrupt thinking, feeling, moods, and behaviors, and cause varying degrees of impaired functioning in daily living. They are believed to be caused by a variety of biochemical, genetic, and environmental factors.[17] Risk factors for developing or triggering mental illness include the following: having other biological relatives with a mental illness; malnutrition or exposure to viruses while in the womb; stressful life situations, such as financial problems, a loved one's death, or a divorce; chronic medical conditions, such as cancer; combat; taking psychoactive drugs during adolescence; childhood abuse or neglect; and lack of friendships or healthy relationships.[18] As with physical disease, mental illnesses can range from mild to severe and can exact a heavy toll on quality of life, both for people with the illnesses and those who come in contact with them.

Mental disorders are common in the United States and worldwide. The basis for diagnosing mental disorders in the United States is the *Diagnostic and Statistical Manual of Mental Disorders,* Fourth Edition, Text Revision (*DSM-IV-TR*). An estimated 26.2 percent of Americans aged 18 and older—about 1 in 4 adults—suffer from a diagnosable mental disorder in a given year and nearly half of them have more than one mental illness

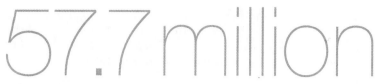

# 57.7 million

**U.S. adults suffer from a diagnosable mental disorder in any given year.**

at the same time.[19] This translates to 57.7 million people. Out of these, about 6 percent, or 1 in 17, suffer from a serious mental illness requiring close monitoring, residential care in many instances, and medication.

Mental disorders are the leading cause of disability in the United States and Canada for people aged 15 to 44.[20]

> **mental illnesses** Disorders that disrupt thinking, feeling, moods, and behaviors, and that impair daily functioning.

## Mental Health Threats to College Students

Mental health problems are common among college students and they appear to be increasing in number and severity.[21] The most recent National College Health Assessment survey found that nearly 1 in 3 undergraduates reported "feeling so depressed it was difficult to function" at least once in the past year. Just over 6 percent of students reported "seriously considering attempting suicide" in the past year.[22] **Figure 2.4** on page 40 shows more results from this survey. In another study based on a nationally representative sample, almost half of college students met the *DSM-IV-TR* criteria for at least one mental disorder in the previous year.[23] Although these data may appear alarming, it is important to note that increases in help-seeking behavior rather than actual increases in overall prevalence of disorders may be contributing to these trends. More effective psychotropic medications, combined with young people having more access to effective treatments during adolescence that allow them to function well enough to attend college, may lead to more persons with mental disorders attending college.[24]

Although there are many types of mental illnesses, we will focus here on those disorders that are most common among college students: mood disorders, anxiety disorders, personality disorders, and schizophrenia (see the **Health Headlines** box on page 41 for information on another growing mental health concern among young adults, attention-deficit/hyperactivity disorder). For information about other disorders, consult the Accessing Your Health on the Internet section at the end of this chapter or ask your instructor for local resources.

**"Why Should I Care?"**

Mental health problems can affect people of any age and have a huge impact on the kind of life you lead—including your success in academics, career, and relationships, as well as your general ability to function and enjoy life. Also, mental health concerns are so prevalent among college students that it is possible your roommate or a friend could have a problem, and may need your help and support.

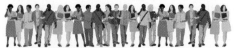

**Felt overwhelmed by all they needed to do 84.6%**

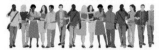

**Thought things were hopeless 45.9%**

**Had difficulty functioning because of depression 29.6%**

**Seriously considered suicide 6.1%**

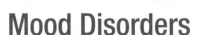

**Intentionally injured themselves 5.2%**

**Attempted suicide 1.3%**

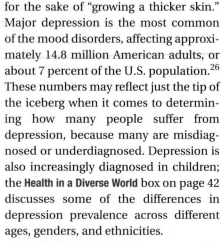

= 2%

FIGURE 2.4 **Mental Health Concerns of American College Students, Past 12 Months**

Source: Data are from American College Health Association, *American College Health Association–National College Health Assessment II (ACHA-NCHA II) Reference Group Data Report Fall 2009* (Baltimore: ACHA, 2010).

# Mood Disorders

**Chronic mood disorders** are disorders that affect how you feel, such as persistent sadness or feelings of euphoria. They include major depression, dysthymic disorder, bipolar disorder, and seasonal affective disorder. In any given year, approximately 10 percent of Americans aged 18 or older—or 20.9 million people—suffer from a mood disorder.[25]

## Major Depression

Sometimes life throws us down the proverbial stairs. We experience loss, pain, disappointment, or frustration, and we can be left feeling beaten and bruised. How do we know if these emotions are really signs of a **major depression**? Major or clinical depression is not the same as having a bad day or feeling down after a negative experience. It is also not something that can be willed or wished away, or ignored

**chronic mood disorder** Experience of persistent emotional states, such as sadness, despair, and hopelessness.
**major depression** Severe depressive disorder that entails chronic mood disorder, physical effects such as sleep disturbance and exhaustion, and mental effects such as the inability to concentrate; also called *clinical depression*.

for the sake of "growing a thicker skin." Major depression is the most common of the mood disorders, affecting approximately 14.8 million American adults, or about 7 percent of the U.S. population.[26] These numbers may reflect just the tip of the iceberg when it comes to determining how many people suffer from depression, because many are misdiagnosed or underdiagnosed. Depression is also increasingly diagnosed in children; the **Health in a Diverse World** box on page 42 discusses some of the differences in depression prevalence across different ages, genders, and ethnicities.

Major depression is characterized by a combination of symptoms that interfere with work, study, sleep, appetite, relationships, and enjoyment of life. Symptoms can last for weeks, months, or years and vary in intensity.[27] Sadness and despair are the main symptoms of depression. Other common signs include the following:

- Loss of motivation or interest in pleasurable activities
- Preoccupation with failures and inadequacies; concern over what others are thinking
- Difficulty concentrating; indecisiveness; memory lapses
- Loss of sex drive or interest in close interactions with others
- Fatigue and loss of energy; slow reactions
- Sleeping too much or too little; insomnia
- Feeling agitated, worthless, or hopeless
- Withdrawal from friends and family
- Diminished or increased appetite
- Significant weight loss or weight gain
- Recurring thoughts that life isn't worth living; thoughts of death or suicide

**Depression in College Students** Mental health problems, particularly depression, have gained increased recognition as major obstacles to success and healthy adjustment on campuses throughout the country. Students who have weak communication skills; who find that college isn't what they expected; or who find that people they've known seem different often have difficulties. Stressors such as anxiety over relationships, pressure to get good grades and win social acceptance, abuse of alcohol and other drugs, poor diet, and lack of sleep can create a toxic cocktail that can overwhelm even the most resilient students. In its most recent survey, the American College Health Association found that the number of students who reported "having been diagnosed with depression" was 11.1 percent.[28]

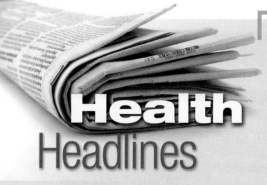

# Health Headlines

## WHEN ADULTS HAVE ADHD

Attention-deficit/hyperactivity disorder (ADHD) is a common neurobehavioral disorder that affects 5 to 8 percent of school-aged children. In as many as 60 percent of cases, symptoms persist into adulthood. In any given year, 4.1 percent of adults are identified as having ADHD.

People with ADHD are hyperactive or distracted most of the time. Even when they try to concentrate, they find it hard to pay attention. They have a hard time organizing things, listening to instructions, remembering details, and controlling their behavior. As a result, people with ADHD often have problems getting along with other people at home, at school, or at work.

### ADULT ADHD MYTHS AND FACTS

**Myth:** ADHD is just a lack of willpower. Persons with ADHD focus well on things that interest them; they could focus on any other tasks if they really wanted to.
**Fact:** ADHD looks very much like a willpower problem, but it isn't. It's essentially a chemical problem in the management systems of the brain.

**Myth:** Everybody has the symptoms of ADHD, and anyone with adequate intelligence can overcome these difficulties.
**Fact:** ADHD affects persons of all levels of intelligence. Although everyone sometimes is prone to distraction or impulsivity, only those with chronic impairments from ADHD symptoms warrant an ADHD diagnosis.

**Myth:** Someone can't have ADHD and also have depression, anxiety, or other psychiatric problems.
**Fact:** A person with ADHD is six times more likely to have another psychiatric

or learning disorder than most other people. Attention-deficit/hyperactivity disorder usually overlaps with other disorders.

**Myth:** Unless you have been diagnosed with ADHD as a child, you can't have it as an adult.
**Fact:** Many adults struggle all their lives with unrecognized ADHD impairments. They haven't received help because they assumed that their chronic difficulties, like depression or anxiety, were caused by other impairments that did not respond to usual treatment.

### EFFECTS OF ADULT ADHD

Left untreated, ADHD can disrupt everything from your career to your relationships and financial stability. Although most of us sometimes have challenges in these areas, the persistent chaos and disorganization of ADHD can make managing the problems worse and worse. Some key areas of disruption might include the following:

* **Health.** Impulsivity and trouble with organization can lead to problems with health, such as compulsive eating, alcohol and drug abuse, or forgetting to take medication for a chronic condition.
* **Work and finances.** Difficulty concentrating, completing tasks, listening, and relating to others can lead to trouble at work. Managing finances also may be a concern. You may find yourself struggling to pay your bills, losing paperwork, missing deadlines, or spending impulsively, resulting in debt.
* **Relationships.** You might wonder why loved ones constantly nag you to tidy up, get organized, and take care of business. Or if your loved one has ADHD, you might be hurt that your loved one doesn't seem to listen to you, blurts out hurtful things, and leaves you with the bulk of organizing and planning.

### GET EDUCATED ABOUT ADHD

If you suspect you or someone close to you has ADHD, learn as much as you can about adult ADHD and treatment options.

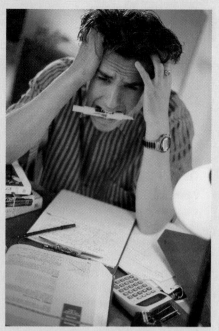

Disorder and chaos can be headaches for us all, but ADHD sufferers may find them insurmountable obstacles.

The organization Children and Adults with Attention-Deficit Hyperactivity Disorder (CHADD) is a good source of information and support (www.chadd.org). Adult ADHD can be a challenge to diagnose, as there is no simple test for it and it often occurs concurrently with other conditions, such as depression or anxiety disorders. To ensure that you have the best treatment plan, secure a diagnosis and treatment plan from a qualified professional with experience in ADHD.

**Sources:** Centers for Disease Control and Prevention, "Attention-Deficit Hyperactivity Disorder," www.cdc.gov/ncbddd/adhd, Updated October 2009; Helpguide.org, "Adult ADD/ADHD: Signs, Symptoms, Effects, and Treatment," Reviewed November 2010, www.helpguide.org/mental/adhd_add_adult_symptoms.htm; National Institute of Mental Health, "The Numbers Count," www.nimh.nih.gov/health/publications/the-numbers-count-mental-disorders-in-america/index.shtml, 2008; H. R. Searight, J. M. Burke, and F. Rottnek, "Adult ADHD: Evaluation and Treatment in Family Medicine," *American Family Physician* 62, no. 9 (2000): 2091–92; T. Brown, *Attention Deficit Disorder: The Unfocused Mind in Children and Adults* (New Haven, CT: Yale University Press, 2005).

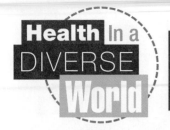
# Depression across Gender, Age, and Ethnicity

Although depression may affect persons of every age, gender, and ethnicity, it does not always manifest itself in the same way across all populations.

## DEPRESSION AND GENDER

Women are almost twice as likely to experience depression as men are. Hormonal changes may be factors in this increased rate. Women also face various stressors in their lives related to multiple responsibilities—work, child rearing, single parenthood, household work, and caring for elderly parents—at rates that are higher than those of men. Researchers have observed gender differences in coping strategies (responses to certain events or stimuli) and have proposed that some women's strategies make them more vulnerable to depression. Typically, men try to distract themselves from a depressed mood, whereas women focus on it. If focusing obsessively on negative feelings intensifies these feelings, women who do this may predispose themselves to depression.

Depression in men is often masked by alcohol or drug abuse, or by the socially acceptable habit of working excessively long hours. Typically, depressed men present not as hopeless and helpless, but as irritable, angry, and discouraged— often personifying a "tough guy" image. Men are less likely to admit they are depressed, and doctors are less likely to suspect it, based on what men report during doctor's visits.

Depression can affect men's physical health in a different way than it can women's health. Although depression is associated with an increased risk of coronary heart disease in both men and women, it is also associated with a higher risk of death by heart disease in men. Men are also more likely to act on suicidal feelings than are women, and they are usually more successful at suicide as well; suicide rates among

depressed men are four times those among depressed women.

## DEPRESSION AND AGE

Today, depression in children is increasingly reported, with 1 in 10 children between ages 6 and 12 experiencing persistent feelings of sadness, the hallmark of depression. Depressed children may pretend to be sick, refuse to go to school or have a sudden drop in school performance, sleep incessantly, engage in self-mutilation, abuse drugs or alcohol, feel misunderstood, and attempt suicide.

Before adolescence, girls and boys experience depression at about the same rate, but by adolescence and young adulthood, girls experience depression more than boys do. This may be due to biological and hormonal changes; girls' struggles with self-esteem and perceptions of success and approval; and an increase in girls' exposure to traumas that may contribute to depression, such as childhood sexual abuse and poverty.

As adults reach their middle and older years, most are emotionally stable and lead active and satisfying lives. However, when depression does occur, it is often undiagnosed or untreated, particularly in people in lower income groups or who do not have access to community resources and supports or medications. Depression is considered the most common mental disorder of people aged 65 and older. Older adults may be less likely to discuss feelings of sadness, loss, help-lessness, or other symptoms, or they

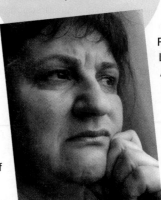

Regardless of gender, age or ethnicity, none of us is immune of depression.

may attribute their depression to aging.

## DEPRESSION AND RACE/ETHNICITY

Rates of depression among Latino, African American, and Asian American/Pacific Islander populations are difficult to determine, as members of these groups may have diffi-culty accessing mental health services because of economic barriers, social and cultural differences, language barriers, and lack of cultur-ally competent providers. Data from the 2008 U.S. National Health and Wellness Survey indicated that when whites report depression symptoms to a health care provider, they are much more likely to be officially diagnosed with depression. Seventy-six percent of whites with reported depressive symptoms were officially diagnosed versus 58.7 percent of African Americans, 62.7 percent of Latinos, and 47.4 percent of Asian Americans.

**Sources:** National Institute of Mental Health (NIMH), *Women and Depression: Discovering Hope,* NIH Publication no. 09-4779, revised 2009, Available at www.nimh.nih.gov/health/publications/women-and-depression-discovering-hope/index.shtml; NIMH, "Real Men. Real Depression." NIH Publication no. 03-5300, March 2003, Available at www.nimh.nih.gov/health/publications/real-men-real-depression-easy-to-read/index.shtml; American Psychiatric Association (APA), Healthy Minds. Healthy Lives, "Children," 2010, www.healthyminds.org/More-Info-For/Children.aspx; APA, Healthy Minds. Healthy Lives, "Seniors," 2010, www.healthyminds.org/More-Info-For/Seniors.aspx; H. Kannan, S. Bolge, and S. Wagner, "Depression: Ethnic Differences in Prevalence, Diagnosis, and Symptoms" (Princeton, NJ: Consumer Health Sciences, 2009), Poster presented at the International Society of Pharmacoeconomics and Outcomes Research (ISPOR) 14th Annual International Meeting, May 2009, Available at www.chsinternational.com/Resources/2009_05_20_ISPOR_Poster_no3_Depression-Ethnicity.pdf.

# 30 years old is the median age of onset for mood disorders.

Being far from home without the security of family and friends can exacerbate problems and make coping difficult; international students are particularly vulnerable to depression and other mental health concerns. Most campuses have counseling centers, cultural centers, and other services available; however, many students do not use them because of persistent stigma about going to a counselor. The **Student Health Today** box on page 44 discusses some of the strategies colleges are adopting to address mental health concerns on campuses.

## Dysthymic Disorder

Many people suffer from **dysthymic disorder (dysthymia),** a less severe syndrome of chronic, mild depression. Dysthymia can be harder to recognize than major depression. Dysthymic individuals may appear to function all right, but they may lack energy or may fatigue easily; be short-tempered, overly pessimistic, and ornery; or just not feel quite up to par without having any significant, overt symptoms. People with dysthymia may cycle into major depression over time. For a diagnosis, symptoms must persist for at least 2 years in adults (1 year in children). This disorder affects approximately 1.5 percent of the U.S. population aged 18 and older in a given year, or about 3.3 million American adults.[29]

## Bipolar Disorder

Another type of depressive mood disorder is **bipolar disorder,** also called *manic depression.* People with bipolar disorder often have severe mood swings, ranging from extreme highs (mania) to extreme lows (depression). Sometimes these swings are dramatic and rapid; other times they are slow and gradual. When in the manic phase, people may be overactive, talkative, and have tons of energy; in the depressed phase, they may experience some or all of the typical symptoms of major depression.

Although the exact cause of bipolar disorder is unknown, biological, genetic, and environmental factors, such as drug abuse and stressful or psychologically traumatic events, seem to be involved in triggering episodes of the illness. Once diagnosed, persons with bipolar disorder have several counseling and pharmaceutical options, and most will be able to live a healthy, functional life while being treated. Bipolar dis-

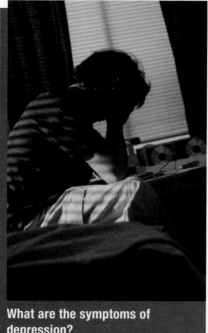

**What are the symptoms of depression?**

There is more to depression than simply feeling blue. When a person is clinically depressed, he finds it difficult to function, sometimes struggling just to get out of bed in the morning or to follow a conversation.

order affects 5.7 million adults in the United States, or approximately 2.6 percent of the population.[30]

## Seasonal Affective Disorder

Another form of depression, **seasonal affective disorder (SAD),** strikes during the winter months and is associated with reduced exposure to sunlight. People with SAD suffer from irritability, apathy, carbohydrate craving and weight gain, increased sleep time, and general sadness. Several factors are implicated in SAD development, including disruption in the body's natural circadian rhythms and changes in levels of the hormone melatonin and the brain chemical serotonin.[31]

The most beneficial treatment for SAD is light therapy, in which patients are exposed to lamps that simulate sunlight. Eighty percent of patients experience relief from their symptoms within 4 days. Other treatments for SAD include diet change (such as eating more complex carbohydrates), increased exercise, stress-management techniques, sleep restriction (limiting the number of hours slept in a 24-hour period), psychotherapy, and prescription medications.

## Causes of Mood Disorders

Mood disorders are caused by the interaction between multiple factors including biological differences, hormones, inherited traits, life events, and early childhood trauma.[32] The biology of mood disorders is related to individual levels of brain chemicals called *neurotransmitters.* Several types of depression, including bipolar disorder, appear to have a genetic component. Depression can also be triggered by a serious loss, difficult relationships, financial problems, and pressure to succeed. Early childhood trauma, such as loss of a parent, may cause permanent changes in the brain, making one more prone to depression. In recent years, researchers have shown that changes in the body's physical health can be accompanied by mental changes, particularly depression. Stroke, heart attack, cancer, Parkinson's disease, problems with chronic pain, type 2 diabetes, certain medications, alcohol, hormonal disorders, and a wide range of afflictions can cause

**dysthymic disorder (dysthymia)** A type of depression that is milder and harder to recognize than major depression; chronic; and often characterized by fatigue, pessimism, or a short temper.

**bipolar disorder** A form of mood disorder characterized by alternating mania and depression; also called *manic depression.*

**seasonal affective disorder (SAD)** A type of depression that occurs in the winter months, when sunlight levels are low.

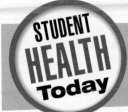
## Mental Health Problems on Campus: Universities Respond

According to the latest National College Health Assessment Survey, nearly 32 percent of female students and 26 percent of male students on campuses throughout the country reported that they had felt too depressed to function at least once during the past year. At the same time, 50 percent of college women and 39 percent of college men felt hopeless one or more times, and another 6 percent of college women and 6 percent of college men had seriously considered suicide. Universities are enacting a range of policies to help these students, including the following:

✳ Student leave is a growing trend on campuses. For example, New York University, Texas A&M, and Cornell University have established various forms of a mandatory 6-month or 1-year leave of absence for students who seem to be at highest risk for mental health problems.
✳ Some institutions, such as the University of Illinois at Urbana-Champaign, mandate counseling for students who are suicidal, requiring a minimum of four therapy sessions following a suicide attempt.
✳ Increasing numbers of institutions offer time-management workshops; massage

and destressing sessions during examinations; and workshops on relationships, coping with loss and grief, and other challenges throughout the academic year.
✳ Classes on stress management, coping, relaxation, meditation, yoga, and other mental health strategies are increasingly common on campuses, either as electives or as part of a professional curriculum.
✳ Most on-campus health services now include counseling centers with easy 24/7 access. Students are encouraged to use them, and increased advertising in new-student orientation sessions lets students know what kind of help is available.
✳ Many universities offer extensive first-year orientations at the beginning of each academic year. Students engage in group activities, such as camping trips and special seminars, to get to know one another in social settings. Professors; sophomores, juniors, and seniors; and others offer special assistance and lead discussion groups to help incoming students cope with adjusting to life away from home and to foster awareness of the wide range of

First-year orientation programs are one strategy universities have adopted to help students transition into college life and to address potential mental health concerns.

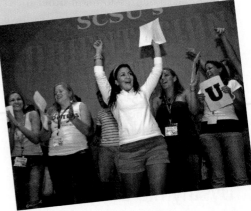

student resources available when students can't handle multiple pressures.

**Sources:** J. Feirman, "The New College Drop-Out," *Psychology Today* 38, no. 3 (2005): 38–39; American College Health Association, *American College Health Association–National College Health Assessment II (ACHA–NCHA II): Reference Group Data Report Fall 2009* (Baltimore: American College Health Association, 2010).

---

you to become depressed, frustrated, and angry. When this happens, recovery is often more difficult. A person who feels exhausted and defeated may lack the will to fight illness and do what is necessary to optimize recovery.

## Anxiety Disorders

**Anxiety disorders** include generalized anxiety disorder, panic disorders, phobic disorders, obsessive-compulsive disorder, and post-traumatic stress disorder. They are characterized by persistent feelings of threat and worry. Consider John Madden, former head coach of the Oakland Raiders and a true "man's man," who outfitted his own bus and, for many years, drove every weekend across the country to serve as commentator for NFL football games. What was the reason behind this exhausting driving schedule? Madden is terrified of getting on a plane.

**anxiety disorders** Mental illnesses characterized by persistent feelings of threat and worry in coping with everyday problems.

**generalized anxiety disorder (GAD)** A constant sense of worry that may cause restlessness, difficulty in concentrating, tension, and other symptoms.

Anxiety disorders are the number one mental health problem in the United States, affecting more than 40 million people ages 18 and older each year, or about 18 percent of all adults.[33] Anxiety is also a leading mental health problem among adolescents, affecting 13 million Americans aged 9 to 17. Among U.S undergraduates, 9.4 percent report being diagnosed with or treated for anxiety in the past year.[34] Costs associated with an overly anxious populace are growing rapidly; conservative estimates cite nearly $50 billion a year spent in doctors' bills and workplace losses in America.[35]

## Generalized Anxiety Disorder

One common form of anxiety disorder, **generalized anxiety disorder (GAD),** is severe enough to interfere significantly with daily life. Generally, the person with GAD is a consummate worrier who develops a debilitating level of anxiety. To be diagnosed with GAD, one must exhibit at least three of the following symptoms for more days than not during a 6-month period: restlessness or feeling keyed up or on edge; being easily fatigued; difficulty concentrating or mind going blank; irritability; muscle tension; sleep disturbances.[36] Generalized anxiety disorder often runs in families and is readily treatable.

## Panic Disorders

Panic disorders are characterized by the occurrence of **panic attacks,** a form of acute anxiety reaction that brings on an intense physical reaction. You may dismiss the feelings as the jitters from too much stress, or the reaction may be so severe that you fear you will have a heart attack and die. Approximately 6 million Americans aged 18 and older experience panic attacks each year, usually in early adulthood.[37] Panic attacks and disorders are increasing in incidence, particularly among young women.

Although highly treatable, panic attacks may become debilitating and destructive, particularly if they happen often and cause the person to avoid going out in public or interacting with others. A panic attack typically starts abruptly, peaks within 10 minutes, lasts about 30 minutes, and leaves the person tired and drained.[38] Symptoms include increased respiration, chills, hot flashes, shortness of breath, stomach cramps, chest pain, difficulty swallowing, and a sense of doom or impending death.

Although researchers aren't sure what causes panic attacks, heredity, stress, and certain biochemical factors may play a role. Your chances of having a panic attack increase if a close relative has them. Some researchers believe that people who suffer panic attacks are experiencing an overreactive fight-or-flight physical response (see Chapter 3).

Many people are uneasy around spiders, but if your fear of them is irrational, it may be a phobia.

## Phobic Disorders

**Phobias,** or phobic disorders, involve a persistent and irrational fear of a specific object, activity, or situation, often out of proportion to the circumstances. Phobias result in a compelling desire to avoid the source of the fear. About 9 percent of American adults suffer from specific phobias, such as fear of spiders, snakes, or public speaking.[39]

Another 7 percent of American adults suffer from **social phobia,** also called social anxiety disorder.[40] Social phobia is an anxiety disorder characterized by the persistent fear and avoidance of social situations. Essentially, the person dreads these situations for fear of being humiliated, embarrassed, or even looked at. These disorders vary in scope. Some cause difficulty only in specific situations, such as getting up in front of the class to give a report. In more extreme cases, a person avoids all contact with others.

## Obsessive-Compulsive Disorder

People who feel compelled to perform rituals over and over again; who are fearful of dirt or contamination; who have an unnatural concern about order, symmetry, and exactness; or who have persistent intrusive thoughts that they can't shake may be suffering from **obsessive-compulsive disorder (OCD).** Approximately 2 million Americans aged 18 and over have OCD.[41] Not to be confused with being a perfectionist, a person with OCD often knows the behaviors are irrational and senseless, yet is powerless to stop them. According to the *DSM-IV-TR,* for a person to be diagnosed with OCD, the obsessions must consume more than 1 hour per day and interfere with normal social or life activities. Although the exact cause is unknown, genetics, biological abnormalities, learned behaviors, and environmental factors have all been considered. Obsessive-compulsive disorder usually begins in adolescence or early adulthood; the median age of onset is 19.

**panic attack** Severe anxiety reaction in which a particular situation, often for unknown reasons, causes terror.

**phobia** A deep and persistent fear of a specific object, activity, or situation that results in a compelling desire to avoid the source of the fear.

**social phobia** A phobia characterized by fear and avoidance of social situations; also called *social anxiety disorder.*

**obsessive-compulsive disorder (OCD)** A form of anxiety disorder characterized by recurrent, unwanted thoughts and repetitive behaviors.

**post-traumatic stress disorder (PTSD)** A collection of symptoms that may occur as a delayed response to a serious trauma.

## Post-Traumatic Stress Disorder

People who have experienced or witnessed a natural disaster, serious accident, violent assault, terrorist incident, or other traumatic life event may develop **post-traumatic stress disorder (PTSD).** Often PTSD affects soldiers returning home from war, particularly those who have seen friends killed or

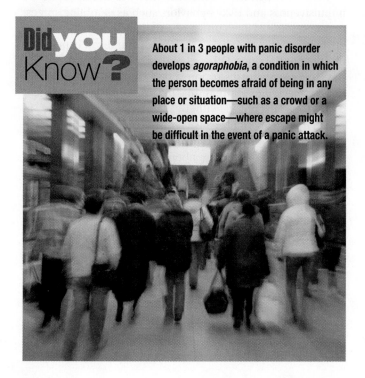

**Did you Know?**

About 1 in 3 people with panic disorder develops *agoraphobia*, a condition in which the person becomes afraid of being in any place or situation—such as a crowd or a wide-open space—where escape might be difficult in the event of a panic attack.

maimed or who have themselves received terrible wounds. Responses from a survey given to a sample of service personnel deployed to Iraq indicated that 90 percent had been shot at and a high percentage reported knowing someone who was injured or had been killed, or had killed an enemy combatant. This study of armed services members found that 1 in 8 reported symptoms of PTSD.[42] Unfortunately, less than half of those with problems sought help, fearing stigma and damage to their careers.

Symptoms of PTSD include the following:

- Dissociation, or perceived detachment of the mind from the emotional state or even the body
- Intrusive recollections of the traumatic event, such as flashbacks, nightmares, and recurrent thoughts or visual images
- Acute anxiety or nervousness, in which the person is hyperaroused, may cry easily, or experience mood swings
- Insomnia and difficulty concentrating
- Intense physiological reactions, such as shaking or nausea, when something reminds the person of the traumatic event

**personality disorders** A class of mental disorders that are characterized by inflexible patterns of thought and beliefs that lead to socially distressing behavior.

**self-injury** Intentionally causing injury to one's own body in an attempt to cope with overwhelming negative emotions; also called *self-mutilation, self-harm,* or *nonsuicidal self-injury* (NSSI).

Although these symptoms may be appropriate as initial responses to traumatic events, PTSD may be diagnosed if a person experiences them for at least 1 month following the traumatic event. In some cases, symptoms don't appear until months or even years after the event.

## Causes of Anxiety and Phobic Disorders

Because anxiety disorders vary in complexity and degree, scientists have yet to find clear reasons why one person develops them and another doesn't. The following factors are often cited as possible causes:[43]

- **Biology.** Some scientists trace the origin of anxiety to the brain and its functioning. Using sophisticated positron-emission tomography (PET) scans, scientists can analyze areas of the brain that react during anxiety-producing events. Families appear to display similar brain and physiological reactivity, so we may inherit tendencies toward anxiety disorders.
- **Environment.** Anxiety can be a learned response. Although genetic tendencies may exist, experiencing a repeated pattern of reaction to certain situations programs the brain to respond in a certain way. For example, if your mother or father screamed whenever a large spider crept into view, or if other anxiety-raising events occurred frequently, you might be predisposed to react with anxiety to similar events later in your life.

- **Social and cultural roles.** Cultural and social roles also may be a factor in risks for anxiety. Because men and women are taught to assume different roles in society (such as man as protector, woman as victim), women may find it more acceptable to scream, shake, pass out, and otherwise express extreme anxiety. Men, in contrast, may have learned to repress such anxieties rather than act on them.

# Personality Disorders

According to the *DSM-IV-TR,* a **personality disorder** is an "enduring pattern of inner experience and behavior that deviates markedly from the expectation of the individual's culture and is pervasive and inflexible."[44] Researchers at the National Institute of Mental Health have found that about 9 percent of adults in the United States have some form of personality disorder as defined by the *DSM-IV-TR.*[45] People who live, work, or are in relationships with individuals suffering from personality disorders often find interactions with them to be very challenging and destructive.

One common type of personality disorder is *paranoid personality disorder,* which involves pervasive, unfounded suspicion and mistrust of other people, irrational jealousy, and secretiveness. Persons with this illness have delusions of being persecuted by everyone, from their family members and loved ones to the government. *Narcissistic personality disorders* involve an exaggerated sense of self-importance and self-absorption. Persons with narcissistic personalities are fascinated with themselves and are preoccupied with fantasies of how wonderful they are. Typically they are overly needy and demanding and believe that they are "entitled" to nothing but the best.

*Borderline personality disorder (BPD)* is characterized by impulsiveness and risky behaviors such as gambling sprees, unsafe sex, use of illicit drugs, and daredevil driving.[46] Sufferers have trouble stabilizing their moods and can experience erratic mood swings. Other characteristics of this mental illness include reality distortion and the tendency to see things in only black-and-white terms. In addition, 70 to 80 percent of persons diagnosed with BPD engage in **self-injury,** in which they deliberately cause harm to their own body—such as by cutting or burning themselves—as a way to cope with their emotions.[47] For more about self-injury, see the **Student Health Today** box at right.

# Schizophrenia

Perhaps the most frightening of all psychological disorders is **schizophrenia,** which affects about 1 percent of the U.S. population.[48] Schizophrenia is characterized by alterations of the senses (including auditory and visual hallucinations); the inability to sort out incoming stimuli and make appropriate responses; an altered sense of self; and radical changes in emotions, movements, and behaviors. Typical symptoms of

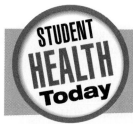
When some people are unable to deal with the pain, pressure, or stress they experience in everyday life, they may resort to self-harm in an effort to cope. *Self-injury*, also termed *self-mutilation, self-harm,* or *nonsuicidal self-injury* (NSSI), is the act of deliberately harming one's body in an attempt to cope with overwhelming negative emotions. Self-injury is an attempt at coping; it is not an attempt at suicide.

The most common method of self-harm is cutting (with razors, glass, knives, or other sharp objects). Other methods include burning, bruising, excessive nail biting, breaking bones, pulling out hair, and embedding sharp objects under the skin. Seventy-five percent of those who harm themselves do so in more than one way.

Researchers estimate that between 2 and 8 million Americans have engaged in self-harm at some point in their lives and the prevalence of NSSI in college students is reported between 17 and 38 percent. Many people who inflict self-harm suffer from larger mental health conditions and have experienced sexual, physical, or emotional abuse as children or adults. Self-harm is also commonly associated with mental illnesses such as borderline personality disorder, depression, anxiety disorders, substance abuse disorders, post-traumatic stress disorder, and eating disorders.

Signs of self-injury include multiple scars, current cuts and abrasions, and implausible explanations for wounds and ongoing injuries. A self-injurer may attempt to conceal scars and injuries by wearing long sleeves and pants. Other symptoms can include difficulty handling anger, social withdrawal, sensitivity to rejection, or body alienation. If you or someone you know is engaging in self-injury, seek professional help. Treatment is challenging; not only must the self-injurious behavior be stopped, but the sufferer must also learn to recognize and manage the feelings that triggered the behavior.

If you are a recovering cutter, some of the following steps may be part of your treatment:

**1.** Start by being aware of feelings and situations that trigger your urge to cut.
**2.** Identify a plan of what you can do instead of cutting when you feel the urge.
**3.** Create a list of alternatives, including:
  * Things that might distract you
  * Things that might soothe and calm you
  * Things that might help you express the pain and deep emotion
  * Things that might help release physical tension and distress
  * Things that might help you feel supported and connected
  * Things that might substitute for the cutting sensation

For more information, try these resources: American Self-Harm Information Clearinghouse, www.selfinjury.org; S.A.F.E. Alternatives, www.selfinjury.com; and Self-Injury Support, www.sisupport.org.

Previously, self-injury was thought to be more common in females, but recent research indicates that rates are generally the same for men and women.

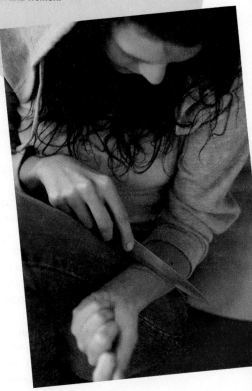

**Sources:** J. Bennett, "Why She Cuts," *Newsweek* Web Exclusive, December 29, 2008, www .newsweek.com/id/177135; M. J. Prinstein, "Introduction to the Special Section on Suicide and Nonsuicidal Self-Injury: A Review of Unique Challenges and Important Directions for Self-Injury Science," *Journal of Consulting and Clinical Psychology* 76, no. 1 (2008): 1–8; Mayo Clinic Staff, MayoClinic.com, "Self-Injury/Cutting," August 2008, www.mayoclinic.com/health/self-injury/DS00775.

---

schizophrenia include fluctuating courses of delusional behavior, hallucinations, incoherent and rambling speech, inability to think logically, erratic movement and odd gesturing, and difficulty with normal activities of daily living.[49] The net effect is that such individuals are often regarded by society at large as being odd; viewed that way, they have difficulties in social interactions and may withdraw.

For decades, scientists believed that schizophrenia was an environmentally provoked form of madness. They blamed abnormal family interactions or early childhood traumas.

Since the mid-1980s, however, when magnetic resonance imaging (MRI) and PET scans began allowing us to study brain function more closely, scientists have recognized that schizophrenia is a biological disease of the brain. The brain damage occurs early in life, possibly as early as the second trimester of fetal development. Fetal exposure to toxic substances, infections, or medications has been studied as a possible risk. In

**schizophrenia** A mental illness with biological origins that is characterized by irrational behavior, severe alterations of the senses, and often an inability to function in society.

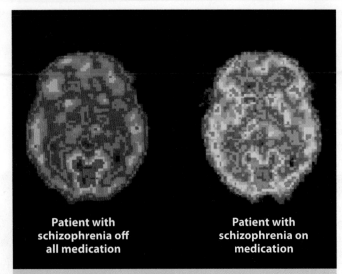

**Patient with schizophrenia off all medication**

**Patient with schizophrenia on medication**

These brain images reveal a significant reduction in brain activity in a person with untreated schizophrenia. Yellow and red identify areas of greatest activity, and blue signifies reduced activity.

addition, possible hereditary links are being explored. Symptoms usually appear in men in their late teens and twenties and in women in their late twenties and early thirties.[50]

Even though environmental theories of the causes of schizophrenia have been discarded in favor of biological ones, a stigma remains attached to the disease. Families of people with schizophrenia frequently experience anger and guilt. They often need information, family counseling, and advice on how to meet the schizophrenic person's needs for shelter, medical care, vocational training, and social interaction.

At present, schizophrenia is treatable but not curable. Treatments usually include some combination of hospitalization, medication, and supportive psychotherapy. Supportive psychotherapy, as opposed to psychoanalysis, can help the patient acquire skills for living in society. With proper medication, public understanding, support of loved ones, and access to therapy, many schizophrenics lead normal lives. In the absence of these forms of assistance and treatment, they may have great difficulty.

# Suicide: Giving Up on Life

Each year there are more than 33,000 reported suicides in the United States.[51] Experts estimate that there may actually be closer to 100,000 cases; the discrepancy is due to the difficulty in determining the causes of many suspicious deaths. More lives are lost to suicide than to any other cause except cancer and cardiovascular disease. It is the third leading cause of death for 15- to 24-year-olds and the fourth leading cause of death for 10- to 14-year-olds.[52]

College students are more likely than the general population to attempt suicide; it's the second leading cause of death on college campuses. The pressures, joys, disappointments, challenges, and changes of the college environment are believed to be partially responsible for the emotional turmoil that can lead a young person to contemplate suicide. However, young adults who choose not to go to college but who are searching for direction in careers, relationships, and other life goals are also at risk. Specific risk factors include a family history of suicide, previous suicide attempts, excessive drug and alcohol use, prolonged depression, financial difficulties, serious illness in oneself or a loved one, and loss of a loved one through death or rejection.

Recent studies indicate that suicide is the eighth leading cause of death for men and the sixteenth leading cause of death for women.[53] Whether they are more likely to attempt suicide or are more often successful in their attempts, nearly four times as many men die by suicide than women. Overall, firearms, suffocation, and poison are by far the most common methods of suicide. However, men are almost twice as likely as women to commit suicide with firearms, whereas women are almost three times as likely as men to commit suicide by poisoning.[54]

## Warning Signs of Suicide

In most cases, suicide does not occur unpredictably. In fact, 75 to 80 percent of people who commit suicide give an indication of their intentions, though the warnings are not always recognized as such by the people around them.[55] Anyone who expresses a desire to kill himself or herself or who has made an attempt is at risk. Common signs that a person may be contemplating suicide include the following:[56]

**90%** of people who kill themselves have a diagnosable mental disorder, most commonly a depressive disorder or a substance abuse disorder.

- Recent loss and a seeming inability to let go of grief
- A history of depression
- Change in personality, such as sadness, withdrawal, irritability, anxiety, tiredness, indecisiveness, apathy
- Change in behavior, such as inability to concentrate, loss of interest in classes or work, unexplained demonstration of happiness following a period of depression
- Sexual dysfunction (such as impotence) or diminished sexual interest
- Expressions of self-hatred and excessive risk-taking, or an "I don't care what happens to me" attitude
- Change in sleep patterns and/or eating habits
- A direct statement about committing suicide, such as "I might as well end it all"
- An indirect statement, such as "You won't have to worry about me anymore"
- Final preparations such as writing a will, giving away prized possessions, or writing revealing letters

- A preoccupation with themes of death
- Marked changes in personal appearance

## Preventing Suicide

Most people who attempt suicide really want to live but see death as the only way out of an intolerable situation. Crisis counselors and suicide hotlines may help temporarily, but the best way to prevent suicide is to get rid of conditions and substances that may precipitate attempts, including alcohol, drugs, loneliness, isolation, and access to guns.

If someone you know threatens suicide or displays warning signs of doing so, get involved—ask questions and seek help. Specific actions you can take include the following:[57]

- **Monitor the warning signals.** Keep an eye on the person or see that there is someone around the person as often as possible. Don't leave him or her alone.
- **Take threats seriously.** Don't brush them off as "just talk."
- **Let the person know how much you care about him or her.** State that you are there to help.
- **Listen.** Try not to discredit or be shocked by what the person says. Empathize, sympathize, and keep the person talking.
- **Ask directly,** "Are you thinking of hurting or killing yourself?"
- **Do not belittle the person's feelings.** Don't tell the person that he or she doesn't really mean it or couldn't succeed at suicide. To some people, these comments offer the challenge of proving you wrong.
- **Help the person think about alternatives to suicide.** Offer to go for help along with the person. Call your local suicide hotline, and use all available community and campus resources.
- **Tell your friend's spouse, partner, parents, siblings, or counselor.** Do not keep your suspicions to yourself. Don't let a suicidal friend talk you into keeping your discussions confidential. If your friend succeeds in a suicide attempt, you may find that others will question your decision, and you may blame yourself.

## Seeking Professional Help

A physical ailment will readily send most of us to the nearest health professional, but many people view seeking professional help for psychological problems as an admission of

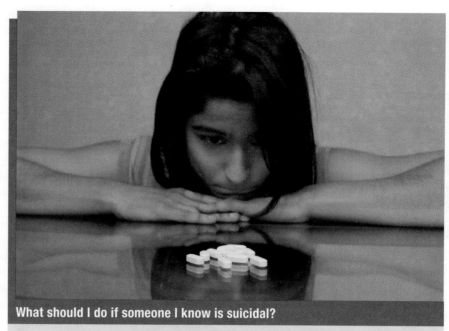

**What should I do if someone I know is suicidal?**

If you notice warning signs of suicide in someone you know, it is imperative that you take action. Suicidal people urgently need professional assistance; your willingness to talk to the person about depression and suicide in a nonjudgmental way can be the encouragement he or she needs to seek help. Remember: Always take thoughts of or plans for suicide seriously; a life may depend on it.

personal failure. However, increasing numbers of Americans are turning to mental health professionals, and nearly 1 in 5 seeks such help. Researchers view breakdowns in support systems, high societal expectations, and dysfunctional families as three major reasons that more people are asking for assistance than ever before.

Consider seeking help if any of the following occurs:

- You feel that you need help.
- You experience wild mood swings or inappropriate emotional responses to normal stimuli.
- Your fears or feelings of guilt frequently distract your attention.
- You begin to withdraw from others.
- You have hallucinations.
- You feel inadequate or worthless or feel that life is not worth living.
- Your daily life seems to be nothing but a series of repeated crises.
- You are considering suicide.
- You turn to drugs or alcohol to escape your problems.
- You feel out of control.

In addition to seeking professional help, there are other positive steps you can take now to help pull yourself out of negative thoughts and feelings; the **Skills for Behavior Change** box on page 50 presents some of these. You may find some books helpful, as well, but be cautious when turning to self-help books (see the **Points of View** box on page 51).

## Dealing with and Defeating Depression

The first step in defeating depression is recognizing it. If you feel you have depression symptoms, set up an appointment with a counselor. Depression is often a biological condition that you can't just "get over" on your own. You may need talk therapy, sometimes combined with antidepressant medication, to help you reach a place where you are able to play a greater role in getting well. Once you've started along a path of therapy and healing, the following strategies may help you feel better faster.

* Set realistic goals in light of the depression and assume a reasonable amount of responsibility.
* Break large tasks into small ones, set some priorities, and do what you can as you can.
* Try to be with other people and to confide in someone.
* Mild exercise, going to a movie or a ballgame, or participating in religious or social activities may help.
* Take a course in meditation, yoga, tai chi, or some other mind–body practice. These disciplines can help you connect with your inner feelings, release tension, and empty your mind to make room for positive thoughts.
* Expect your mood to improve gradually, not immediately. Feeling better takes time.
* Consider postponing important decisions until the depression has lifted. Before deciding to make a significant transition, change jobs, or get married or divorced, discuss it with others who know you well and have a more objective view of your situation.
* Let your family and friends help you.
* Continue working with your counselor. If he or she isn't helpful, look for another one.

## Mental Illness Stigma

Mental health advocates have stated that the last great stigma of the twentieth century was the stigma of mental illness. **Stigmas** are negative stereotypes about people. Common stigmas about people with mental illness are that they are dangerous, irresponsible, childlike and requiring constant care, or that they "just need to get over it." Derogatory terms such as *nut job, wacko, crazy, insane, madman, bonkers,* and *demented* are still commonly heard in our society to describe persons with mental illness. The reality is that very few people who suffer with a mental illness are dangerous to society. Most live independ-

**stigmas** Negative stereotypes about groups of people.

ently, go to school, hold jobs, and are productive members of society. A mental illness is like any other chronic disease. You can't decide just to "get over it."

The stigma of mental illness often leads to feelings of shame, guilt, loss of self-esteem, and a sense of isolation and hopelessness. Many people who have successfully managed their mental illness report that the stigma they faced was more disabling at times than the illness itself.[58] One very significant consequence of mental illness stigma is that people who are struggling with a mental illness may delay seeking treatment or avoid care that could dramatically alter their symptoms and improve their quality of life.

In 2001, college student Alison Malmon founded the group Active Minds after her older brother, Brian, committed suicide. Brian had suffered from mental illness for several years, but had concealed his symptoms from everyone close to him. Today there are almost 250 Active Mind chapters on college campuses across the country, working to end the stigma of mental illness and to encourage those at risk to seek help and quality care.[59]

### what do you think?

Do you notice social stigma against mental illness in your community? ● How often do you hear terms like "crazy" or "wacko" used to describe people who appear to have a mental health problem? Why are those words harmful to others? ● What could you do to combat mental illness stigma?

## Getting Evaluated for Treatment

If you are considering treatment for a psychological problem, schedule a complete evaluation first. Consult a credentialed health professional for a thorough examination, which should include three parts:

**1.** *A physical checkup,* which will rule out thyroid disorders, viral infections, and anemia—all of which can result in depressive-like symptoms—and a neurological check of coordination, reflexes, and balance to rule out brain disorders

**2.** *A psychiatric history,* which will attempt to trace the course of the apparent disorder, genetic or family factors, and any past treatments

**3.** *A mental status examination,* which will assess thoughts, speaking processes, and memory, and will include an in-depth interview with tests for other psychiatric symptoms

Once physical factors have been ruled out, you may decide to consult a professional who specializes in psychological health.

## Mental Health Professionals

Several types of mental health professionals are available to help you; Table 2.1 on page 52 compares several of the most common. When choosing a therapist, the most important criterion is not how many degrees this person has, but whether you feel you can work with him or her. A qualified mental health professional should be willing to answer all

# Self-Help Books:
## BENEFICIAL OR BALONEY?

These days, self-help books abound, and they cover everything from losing weight to having a better sex life to improving your golf swing to managing your finances. These books, and the programs, seminars, DVDs, and other products that support them, offer accessible, relatively inexpensive guidance to individuals hoping to bring about positive change in their lives. But are these books really helpful, or are they a marketing scam, taking money from innocent consumers without providing any real service?

### Arguments in favor of Self-help Books

○ Self-help books can provide another perspective on a problem, helping the reader become "unstuck."
○ Some self-help books are directive and practical enough to help people change their lives for the better.
○ Self-help books can provide useful information and can point people to concrete resources.
○ Self-help books provide a private way for people to find information about problems that they may have difficulty discussing.
○ Using a self-help book to read up on a condition or disease may help a person empathize more with another struggling person.
○ Self-help books are generally inexpensive compared with many other kinds of help, such as psychological counseling.

### Arguments against Self-help Books

○ Books can't make you change—real change has to come from within an individual.
○ These books often make claims of an outcome that seems just too good to be true.
○ Merely reading a self-help book may give a person a false sense of solving a problem, when doing so is really in the actual work of tackling that problem.
○ Self-help books encourage self-diagnosis of health problems, which carries many risks.
○ Anyone can write a self-help book—you don't have to be a professional to be published and the book doesn't have to be based on scientific evidence of effectiveness.
○ When it comes to your health, it's worth it to find qualified health care providers who can help you, even if doing so costs more than buying a book.

### Where Do You stand?

○ Do you think self-help books tend to be more helpful or harmful? In which situations do you think a self-help book is most likely to be valuable?
○ Would you use a self-help book if you felt you had a problem?

If so, how would you determine what book to use?
○ Do you know anyone who has used one? Did it help? How?
○ Suppose your cousin were looking to buy a self-help book. What advice would you give her?

---

your questions during an initial consultation. Questions to ask the therapist and yourself include the following:

● **Can you interview the therapist before starting treatment?** An initial meeting will help you determine whether this person will be a good fit for you.
● **Do you like the therapist as a person?** Can you talk to him or her comfortably?
● **Is the therapist watching the clock or easily distracted?** You should be the main focus of the session.

● **Does the therapist demonstrate professionalism?** Be concerned if your therapist is frequently late or breaks appointments, suggests social interactions outside your therapy sessions, talks inappropriately about himself or herself, has questionable billing practices, or resists releasing you from therapy.
● **Will the therapist help you set your own goals and timetables?** A good professional should evaluate your general situation and help you set small goals to work on between sessions.

| What Are They Called? | What Kind of Training Do They Have? | What Kind of Therapy Do They Do? | Professional Association |
|---|---|---|---|
| Psychiatrist | Medical doctor (MD) degree, followed by 4 years of specialized mental health training | As a licensed MD, a psychiatrist can prescribe medications and may have admitting privileges at a local hospital. | American Psychiatric Association www.psych.org |
| Psychologist | Doctoral (PhD) degree in counseling or clinical psychology, followed by several years of supervised practice to earn license | Psychologists are trained in various types of therapy, including behavior and insight therapy. They may be trained in certain specialties, such as family counseling or sexual counseling. | American Psychological Association www.apa.org |
| Clinical/psychiatric social worker | Master's degree in social work (MSW) followed by 2 years of experience in a clinical setting to earn license | Social workers may be trained in certain specialties, such as substance abuse counseling or child counseling. | National Association of Social Workers www.socialworkers.org |
| Counselor | Master's degree in counseling, psychology, educational psychology, or related human service; generally must complete at least 2 years of supervised practice before obtaining a license | Many counselors are trained to provide individual and group therapy. They often specialize in one type of counseling, such as family, marital, relationship, children, or drug. | American Counseling Association www.counseling.org |
| Psychoanalyst | Postgraduate degree in psychology or psychiatry (PhD or MD), followed by 8 to 10 years of training in psychoanalysis, which includes undergoing analysis themselves | Psychoanalysis is based on the theories of Freud and his successors. It focuses on patterns of thinking and behavior and the recall of early traumas that have blocked personal growth. Treatment is intensive, lasting 5 to 10 years, with 3 or 4 sessions per week. | American Psychoanalytic Association www.apsa.org |
| Licensed marriage and family therapist (LMFT) | Master's or doctoral degree in psychology, social work, or counseling, specializing in family and interpersonal dynamics; generally must complete at least 2 years of supervised practice before obtaining a license | LMFTs treat individuals or families in the context of family relationships. Treatment is typically brief (20 sessions or fewer) and focused on finding solutions to specific relational problems. | American Association for Marriage and Family Therapy www.aamft.org |

Remember, in most states, the use of the title *therapist* or *counselor* is unregulated. Make your choice carefully.

## Pharmacological Treatment

Drug therapy can be an important adjunct in the treatment of many psychological disorders and new generations of medications are continually being developed. Table 2.2 includes information about the major classes of medications used to treat the most common mental illnesses. These drugs require a doctor's prescription and have been approved by the U.S. Food and Drug Administration (FDA). These medications are not, however, without side effects and contraindications for use. Recently the FDA proposed new warnings about suicidal thinking and behavior in young adults who take antidepressant medications, including a labeling change that warns about increased risks of suicidal thinking and behavior in young adults aged 18 to 24 during initial treatment.[60]

Potency, dosage, and side effects of drugs within medication categories can vary greatly. It is very imporant that you talk to your health care provider so that you completely understand the risks and benefits of any medication you may be prescribed. Likewise, your doctor needs to be aware as soon as possible of any adverse effects you may experience. With some drug therapies, such as antidepressants, you may not feel the therapeutic effects for several weeks, so patience is important. Finally, compliance with your doctor's recommendations for beginning or ending a course of any medication is very important.

TABLE
2.2

## Types of Medications Used to Treat Mental Illness

| Antidepressants | Used to treat depression, panic disorders, anxiety disorders | |
|---|---|---|
| Selective serotonin-reuptake inhibitors (SSRIs) | *Examples:* fluoxetine (Prozac), paroxetine (Paxil, Seroxat), escitalopram (Lexapro, Esipram), citalopram (Celexa), and sertraline (Zoloft) | The current standard drug treatment for depression; also frequently prescribed for anxiety disorders |
| Noradrenergic and specific serotonergic antidepressants (NaSSAs) | *Examples:* mirtazapine (Avanza, Zispin, Remeron) | Reportedly has fewer sexual dysfunction side effects than do SSRIs |
| Serotonin-norepinephrine reuptake inhibitors (SNRIs) | *Examples:* venlafaxine (Effexor), duloxetine (Cymbalta) | Also sometimes prescribed for ADHD |
| Norepinephrine-dopamine reuptake inhibitors (NDRIs) | *Examples:* bupropion (Wellbutrin, Zyban) | Also used in smoking cessation; fewer weight gain or sexual dysfunction side effects than SSRIs |
| Tricyclic antidepressants (TCAs) | *Examples:* imipramine, amitriptyline, nortriptyline, and desipramine | Negative side effects; usually used as a 2nd or 3rd line of treatment when other medications prove ineffective |
| Monoamine oxidase inhibitors (MAOIs) | *Examples:* phenelzine (Nardil), tranylcypromine (Parnate), and isocarboxazid (Marplan) | Dangerous interactions with many other drugs and substances in food; generally no longer prescribed |
| **Anxiolytics (antianxiety drugs)** | **Used to treat anxiety disorders including OCD, GAD, panic disorders, phobias, PTSD** | |
| Benzodiazepines | *Examples:* lorazepam (Ativan), clonazepam (Klonopin), alprazolam (Xanax), diazepam (Valium) | Short-term relief, sometimes taken on an as-needed basis; dangerous interactions with alcohol; possible to develop tolerance or dependence |
| Serotonin 1A agonists | *Examples:* buspirone (BuSpar) | Longer-term relief; must be taken for at least 2 weeks to achieve antianxiety effects |
| **Mood stabilizers** | **Used to treat bipolar disorder, schizophrenia** | |
| Lithium | *Examples:* lithium carbonate | Drug most commonly used to treat bipolar disorder; blood levels must be closely monitored to determine proper dosage and avoid toxic effects |
| Anticonvulsants | *Examples:* valproic acid (Depakene), divalproex sodium (Depakote), sodium valproate (Depacon) | Used more frequently for acute mania than for long-term maintenance of bipolar disorder |
| **Antipsychotics (neuroleptics)** | **Used to treat schizophrenia, mania, bipolar disorder** | |
| Atypical antipsychotics | *Examples:* clozapine (Clozaril), risperidone (Risperdal) | First line of treatment for schizophrenia; fewer adverse effects than earlier antipsychotics |
| First-generation antipsychotics | *Examples:* haloperidol (Haldol), chlorpromazine (Thorazine) | Earliest forms of antipsychotics; unpleasant side effects such as tremor and muscle stiffness |
| **Stimulants** | **Used to treat ADHD, narcolepsy** | |
| Methylphenidate | *Brand names:* Ritalin, Metadate, Concerta | Can lead to tolerance and dependence; frequently abused for both performance enhancement and recreational use |
| Amphetamines | *Examples:* amphetamine (Adderall), dextroamphetamine (Dexedrine, Dextrostat), pemoline (Cylert) | Can lead to tolerance and dependence; frequently abused for both performance enhancement and recreational use |

**Source:** Data from National Institute of Mental Health.

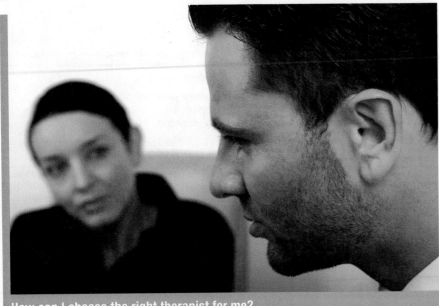

**How can I choose the right therapist for me?**

The choice of therapist is very individual—when you begin seeing a mental health professional you enter into a relationship with that person, and, just as in any relationship, there will be some therapists with whom you connect more than others. Depending on your mental health concerns, you may need to find someone with a particular specialty or degree, but regardless, you'll want to be comfortable with the person you choose. Schedule an initial interview with more than one therapist and ask a lot of questions. If one person doesn't "feel right" to you, trust your instincts and look for someone else. Remember that your mental health is important; you deserve to find the best possible help and support.

## What to Expect in Therapy

The first trip to a therapist can be extremely difficult. Most of us have misconceptions about what therapy is and what it can do. That first visit is a verbal and mental sizing up between you and the therapist. If you decide that this professional is not for you, you will at least have learned how to present your problem and what qualities you need in a therapist.

Before meeting, briefly explain your needs. Ask what the fee is. Arrive on time, wear comfortable clothing, and expect your visit to last about an hour. The therapist will want to take down your history and details about the problems that have brought you to therapy. Answer as honestly as possible. Do not be embarrassed to acknowledge your feelings. It is critical to the success of your treatment that you trust this person enough to be open and honest.

Do not expect the therapist to tell you what to do or how to behave. The responsibility for improved behavior lies with you. If after your first visit (or even after several visits), you feel you cannot work with this person, say so. You have the right to find a therapist with whom you feel comfortable.

**Treatment Models** Many different types of counseling exist, including individual therapy, which involves one-on-one work between therapist and client, and group therapy, in which two or more clients meet with a therapist to discuss problems. Treatment for mental disorders can include various cognitive-behavioral therapies. *Cognitive therapy* focuses on the impact of thoughts and ideas on our feelings and behavior. It helps a person to look at life rationally and correct habitually pessimistic or faulty thinking patterns. *Behavioral therapy*, as the name implies, focuses on what we do. Behavior therapy uses the concepts of stimulus, response, and reinforcement to alter behavior patterns. It is not uncommon for psychotherapeutic treatment to combine cognitive-behavioral therapies with drug therapies.

# How Psychologically Healthy Are You?

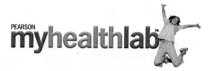

Fill out this assessment online at www.pearsonhighered.com/myhealthlab or www.pearsonhighered.com/donatelle.

Being psychologically healthy requires both introspection and the willingness to work on areas that need improvement. Begin by completing the following assessment scale. Use it to determine how well each statement describes you. When you're finished, ask someone who is very close to you to take the same test and respond with his or her own perceptions of you.

Carefully assess areas in which your responses differ from those of your friend or family member. Which areas need some work? Which are in good shape?

| | Never | Rarely | Fairly Frequently | Most of the Time | All of the Time |
|---|---|---|---|---|---|
| 1. My actions and interactions indicate that I am confident in my abilities. | 1 | 2 | 3 | 4 | 5 |
| 2. I am quick to blame others for things that go wrong in my life. | 1 | 2 | 3 | 4 | 5 |
| 3. I am spontaneous and like to have fun with others. | 1 | 2 | 3 | 4 | 5 |
| 4. I am able to give love and affection to others and show my feelings. | 1 | 2 | 3 | 4 | 5 |
| 5. I am able to receive love and signs of affection from others without feeling uneasy. | 1 | 2 | 3 | 4 | 5 |
| 6. I am generally positive and upbeat about things in my life. | 1 | 2 | 3 | 4 | 5 |
| 7. I am cynical and tend to be critical of others. | 1 | 2 | 3 | 4 | 5 |
| 8. I have a large group of people whom I consider to be good friends. | 1 | 2 | 3 | 4 | 5 |
| 9. I make time for others in my life. | 1 | 2 | 3 | 4 | 5 |
| 10. I take time each day for myself for quiet introspection, having fun, or just doing nothing. | 1 | 2 | 3 | 4 | 5 |
| 11. I am compulsive and competitive in my actions. | 1 | 2 | 3 | 4 | 5 |
| 12. I handle stress well and am seldom upset or stressed out by others. | 1 | 2 | 3 | 4 | 5 |

| | Never | Rarely | Fairly Frequently | Most of the Time | All of the Time |
|---|---|---|---|---|---|
| 13. I try to look for the good in everyone and every situation before finding fault. | 1 | 2 | 3 | 4 | 5 |
| 14. I am comfortable meeting new people and interact well in social settings. | 1 | 2 | 3 | 4 | 5 |
| 15. I would rather stay in and watch TV or read than go out with friends or interact with others. | 1 | 2 | 3 | 4 | 5 |
| 16. I am flexible and can adapt to most situations, even if I don't like them. | 1 | 2 | 3 | 4 | 5 |
| 17. Nature, the environment, and other living things are important aspects of my life. | 1 | 2 | 3 | 4 | 5 |
| 18. I think before responding to my emotions. | 1 | 2 | 3 | 4 | 5 |
| 19. I tend to think of my own needs before those of others. | 1 | 2 | 3 | 4 | 5 |
| 20. I am consciously trying to be a better person. | 1 | 2 | 3 | 4 | 5 |
| 21. I like to plan ahead and set realistic goals for myself. | 1 | 2 | 3 | 4 | 5 |
| 22. I accept others for who they are. | 1 | 2 | 3 | 4 | 5 |
| 23. I value diversity and respect others' rights, regardless of culture, race, sexual orientation, religion, or other differences. | 1 | 2 | 3 | 4 | 5 |

| | Never | Rarely | Fairly Frequently | Most of the Time | All of the Time |
|---|---|---|---|---|---|
| **24.** I try to live each day as if it might be my last. | ① | ② | ③ | ④ | ⑤ |
| **25.** I have a great deal of energy and appreciate the little things in life. | ① | ② | ③ | ④ | ⑤ |
| **26.** I cope with stress in appropriate ways. | ① | ② | ③ | ④ | ⑤ |
| **27.** I get enough sleep each day and seldom feel tired. | ① | ② | ③ | ④ | ⑤ |
| **28.** I have healthy relationships with my family. | ① | ② | ③ | ④ | ⑤ |

| | Never | Rarely | Fairly Frequently | Most of the Time | All of the Time |
|---|---|---|---|---|---|
| **29.** I am confident that I can do most things if I put my mind to them. | ① | ② | ③ | ④ | ⑤ |
| **30.** I respect others' opinions and believe that others should be free to express their opinions, even when they differ from my own. | ① | ② | ③ | ④ | ⑤ |

## Interpreting Your Scores

Look at items 2, 7, 11, 15, and 19. Add up your score for these five items and divide by 5. Is your average for these items above or below 3? Did you score a 5 on any of these items? Do you need to work on any of these areas? Now look at your scores for the remaining items (there should be 25 items). Total these scores and divide by 25. Is your average above or below 3? On which items did you score a 5? Obviously you're doing well in these areas. Now remove these items from this grouping of 25 (scores of 5), and add up your scores for the remaining items. Then divide your total by the number of items included. Now what is your average?

Do the same for the scores completed by your friend or family member. Which scores, if any, are different, and how do they differ? Which areas do you need to work on? What actions can you take now to improve your ratings in these areas?

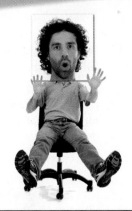

# YOUR PLAN FOR CHANGE

The **Assessyourself** activity gave you the chance to look at various aspects of your psychological health and compare your self-assessment with a friend's perceptions. Now that you have considered these results, you can take steps to change behaviors that may be detrimental to your psychological health.

### Today, you can:

◯ Evaluate your behavior and identify patterns and specific things you are doing that negatively affect your psychological health. What can you change now? What can you change in the near future?

◯ Start a journal and note changes in your mood. Look for trends and think about ways you can change your behavior to address them.

◯ Make a list of the things that bring you joy—friends, family, activities, entertainment, nature. Commit yourself to making more room for these joy-givers in your life.

### Within the next 2 weeks, you can:

◯ Visit your campus health center and find out about the counseling services they offer. If you are feeling overwhelmed, depressed, or anxious, make an appointment with a counselor.

◯ Pay attention to the negative thoughts that pop up throughout the day. Note times when you find yourself devaluing or undermining your abilities, and notice when you project negative attitudes on others. Bringing your awareness to these thoughts gives you an opportunity to stop and reevaluate them.

### By the end of the semester, you can:

◯ Make a commitment to an ongoing therapeutic practice aimed at improving your psychological health. Depending on your current situation, this could mean anything from seeing a counselor or joining a support group to practicing meditation or attending religious services.

◯ Volunteer regularly with a local organization you care about. Focus your energy and gain satisfaction by helping to improve others' lives or the environment.

## Summary

* Psychological health is a complex phenomenon involving mental, emotional, social, and spiritual dimensions.
* Many factors influence psychological health, including life experiences, family, the environment, other people, self-esteem, self-efficacy, and personality.
* The mind–body connection is an important link in overall health and well-being. Positive psychology emphasizes happiness as a key factor in determining overall reaction to life's challenges.
* Developing self-esteem and self-efficacy, making healthy connections, having a positive outlook on life, and maintaining physical health are key to enhancing psychological health.
* College life is a high-risk time for developing mental disorders such as depression or anxiety disorders because of high stress levels, pressures for grades, and financial problems, among others.
* Mood disorders include major depression, dysthymic disorder, bipolar disorder, and seasonal affective disorder. Anxiety disorders include generalized anxiety disorder, panic disorders, phobic disorders, obsessive-compulsive disorder, and post-traumatic stress disorder. Personality disorders include paranoid, narcissistic, and borderline personality disorders.
* Schizophrenia is a disorder once believed to be the result of environmental causes. Now brain function studies have shown that it is instead a biological disease of the brain.
* Suicide is a result of negative psychosocial reactions to life. People intending to commit suicide often give warning signs of their intentions. Such people can often be helped.
* Mental health professionals include psychiatrists, psychoanalysts, psychologists, social workers, and counselors. Many therapy methods exist, including group and individual, cognitive, and behavioral therapies.

## Pop Quiz

1. A person with high self-esteem
   a. possesses feelings of self-respect and self-worth.
   b. believes he or she can successfully engage in a specific behavior.
   c. believes external influences shape one's psychosocial health.
   d. has a high altruistic capacity.

2. All of the following traits have been identified as characterizing psychologically healthy people *except*
   a. conscientiousness.
   b. introversion.
   c. openness to experience.
   d. agreeableness.

3. Subjective well-being includes all of the following components *except*
   a. psychological hardiness.
   b. satisfaction with present life.
   c. relative presence of positive emotions.
   d. relative absence of negative emotions.

4. People who have experienced repeated failures at the same task may eventually give up and quit trying altogether. This pattern of behavior is termed
   a. post-traumatic stress disorder.
   b. learned helplessness.
   c. self-efficacy.
   d. introversion.

5. The term that most accurately refers to the feeling or subjective side of psychological health is
   a. social health.
   b. mental health.
   c. emotional health.
   d. spiritual health.

6. Which statement below is *false*?
   a. One in four adults in the United States suffers from a diagnosable mental disorder in a given year.
   b. Mental disorders are the leading cause of disability in the United States.
   c. Dysthymia is an example of an anxiety disorder.
   d. Bipolar disorder can also be referred to as manic depression.

7. This disorder is characterized by a need to perform rituals over and over again; fear of dirt or contamination; or an unnatural concern with order, symmetry, and exactness.
   a. personality disorder
   b. obsessive-compulsive disorder
   c. phobic disorder
   d. post-traumatic stress disorder

8. What is the number one mental health problem in the United States?
   a. Depression
   b. Anxiety disorders
   c. Alcohol dependence
   d. Schizophrenia

9. Every winter, Stan suffers from irritability, apathy, weight gain, and sadness. He most likely has
   a. panic disorder.
   b. generalized anxiety disorder.
   c. seasonal affective disorder.
   d. chronic mood disorder.

10. A person with a PhD in counseling psychology and training in various types of therapy is a
    a. psychiatrist.
    b. psychologist.
    c. social worker.
    d. psychoanalyst.

*Answers to these questions can be found on page A-1.*

## Think about It!

1. What is psychological health? What indicates that you are or are not psychologically healthy? Why might the college environment provide a challenge to psychological health?
2. Discuss the factors that influence your overall level of psychological health. Which factors can you change? Which ones may be more difficult to change?
3. What psychological dimensions do you need to work on? Which are most important to you, and why? What actions can you take today?
4. What are the warning signs of suicide? Of depression? Why are some groups more vulnerable to suicide and depression than others? What would you do if you heard a friend in the cafeteria say to no one in particular that he was going to "do the world a favor and end it all"?
5. Discuss the different types of health professionals and therapies. If you felt depressed about breaking off a long-term relationship, which professional and which therapy do you think would be most beneficial to you?

## Accessing Your Health on the Internet

The following websites explore further topics and issues related to personal health. For links to the websites below, visit the Companion Website for *Access to Health*, 12th Edition, at www.pearsonhighered.com/donatelle.

1. *American Foundation for Suicide Prevention.* This group provides resources for suicide prevention and support for family and friends of those who have committed suicide. www.afsp.org
2. *American Psychological Association Help Center.* This site includes infor-

mation on psychology at work, the mind–body connection, psychological responses to war, and other topics. http://apahelpcenter.org
3. *National Alliance on Mental Illness.* This group is a support and advocacy organization of families and friends of people with severe mental illnesses. www.nami.org
4. *National Institute of Mental Health (NIMH).* The NIMH provides an overview of mental health information and new research relating to mental health. www.nimh.nih.gov
5. *Mental Health America.* This organization works to promote mental health through advocacy, education, research, and services. www.nmha.org
6. *Helpguide.* You can find resources here for improving mental and emotional health as well as specific information on topics such as self-injury, sleep, depressive disorders, and anxiety disorders. www.helpguide.org
7. *Active Minds.* This campus education and advocacy organization was formed to combat the stigma of mental illness, encourage students who need help to seek it early, and prevent tragedies related to untreated mental illness.
www.activeminds.org

## References

1. A. H. Maslow, *Motivation and Personality,* 2nd ed. (New York: Harper and Row, 1970).
2. U.S. Department of Health and Human Services, *Mental Health: A Report of the Surgeon General—Executive Summary* (Rockville, MD: U.S. Department of Health and Human Services, Substance Abuse and Mental Health Services Administration, National Institute of Mental Health, 1999), Available at www.surgeongeneral .gov/library/mentalhealth/summary.html.
3. T. M. Chaplin, "Anger, Happiness, and Sadness: Association with Depressive Symptoms in Late Adolescence," *Journal of Youth and Adolescence* 35, no. 6 (2006): 977–86.
4. A. F. Jorm, "Social Networks and Health: It's Time for an Intervention Trial," *Journal of Epidemiology and Community Health* 59 (2005): 537–39; C. Huang, "Elderly Social Support System and Health Status in the

Urban and Rural Areas," Paper presented at the American Public Health Association Annual Meeting (New Orleans, LA, 2005); C. Alarie, *Impact of Social Support on Women's Health: A Literature Review* (Winnipeg, MB: Women's Center of Excellence, 1998), Available at www.pwhce.ca/ limpactDuSupport.htm; A. Sherman, J. Lansford, and B. Volling, "Sibling Relationships and Best Friendships in Young Adulthood: Warmth, Conflict and Well-Being," *Personal Relationships* 13, no. 2 (2006): 151–65; N. Stevens, "Marriage, Social Integration, and Loneliness in the Second Half of Life," *Research on Aging* 28, no. 2 (2006): 713–29.
5. K. Karren et al., *Mind/Body Health,* 4th ed. (San Francisco: Benjamin Cummings, 2010).
6. National Center for Complementary and Alternative Medicine (NCCAM), "Prayer and Spirituality in Health: Ancient Practices, Modern Science," *CAM at the NIH: Focus on Complementary and Alternative Medicine* 12, no. 1 (2005), Updated October 2007, Available at http://nccam.nih .gov/news/newsletter/archive.htm.
7. W. Schneider and L. Davidson, "Physical Health and Adult Well-Being," in *Well-Being: Positive Development across the Life Course,* eds. M. H. Bornstein, L. Davidson, and C. Keyes (Mahwah, NJ: Lawrence Erlbaum Associates, 2003), 407–23.
8. C. Hale, J. Hannum, and D. Espelage, "Social Support and Physical Health: The Importance of Belonging," *Journal of American College Health* 53, no. 6 (2005): 276–84.
9. K. S. Berger, *The Developing Person through the Life Span,* 6th ed. (New York: Worth, 2005), 9–10.
10. M. Seligman and C. Peterson, "Learned Helplessness," in *International Encyclopedia for the Social and Behavioral Sciences,* vol. 13, ed. N. Smelser (New York: Elsevier, 2002), 8583–866.
11. M. Seligman, *Learned Optimism: How to Change Your Mind and Your Life* (New York: Free Press, 1998); J. H. Martin, "Motivation Processes and Performance: The Role of Global and Facet Personality," PhD dissertation, University of North Carolina at Chapel Hill, 2002.
12. M. Lemonick, "The Biology of Joy," *Time* (January 17, 2005): A12–A14; P. Herschberger, "Prescribing Happiness: Positive Psychology and Family Medicine," *Family Medicine* 37, no. 9 (2005): 630–34.
13. J. Kluger, "The Funny Thing about Laughter," *Time* (January 17, 2005): A25–A29; M. Miller and W. F. Fry, "The Effect of Mirthful Laughter on the Human Cardiovascular System," *Medical Hypotheses* 73, no. 5 (2009): 636–39; S. Horowitz, "The Effect of

Positive Emotions on Health: Hope and Humor," *Alternative and Complementary Therapies* 15, no. 4 (2009): 196–202.

14. J. Kluger, "The Funny Thing about Laughter," 2005.

15. R. Davidson et al., "The Privileged Status of Emotion in the Brain," *Proceedings of the National Academy of Sciences of the United States of America* 101, no. 33 (2004).

16. E. Diener and M. E. P. Seligman, "Beyond Money: Toward an Economy of Well-Being," *Psychological Science in the Public Interest* 5 (2004): 1–31; C. Peterson and M. Seligman, *Character Strengths and Virtues* (London: Oxford University Press, 2004).

17. Mayo Clinic Staff, MayoClinic.com, "Mental Illness: Causes," 2008, www.mayoclinic.com/health/mental-illness/DS01104/DSECTION=causes.

18. Ibid.

19. National Institute of Mental Health, "The Numbers Count: Mental Disorders in America," Reviewed September 2010, www.nimh.nih.gov/health/publications/the-numbers-count-mental-disorders-in-america.shtml.

20. Ibid.

21. J. Hunt and D. Eisenberg, "Mental Health Problems and Help-Seeking Behavior among College Students," *Journal of Adolescent Health* 46, no. 1 (2010): 3–10.

22. American College Health Association, *American College Health Association–National College Health Assessment II (ACHA–NCHA II): Reference Group Data Report Fall 2009* (Baltimore: American College Health Association, 2010), Available at www.acha-ncha.org/reports_ACHA-NCHAII.html.

23. C. Blanco et al., "Mental Health of College Students and Their Non-College Attending Peers: Results from the National Epidemiologic Study on Alcohol and Related Conditions," *Archives of General Psychiatry* 65, 12 (2008): 1429–37.

24. J. Hunt and D. Eisenberg, "Mental Health Problems and Help-Seeking Behavior among College Students," 2010.

25. National Institute of Mental Health, "The Numbers Count," 2009.

26. Ibid.

27. National Institute of Mental Health, "Depression," 2009, www.nimh.nih.gov/publicat/depression.cfm.

28. American College Health Association, *ACHA–NCHA II: Reference Group Data Report Fall 2009*, 2010.

29. National Institute of Mental Health, "The Numbers Count," 2009.

30. Ibid.

31. American Psychiatric Association, Healthy Minds. Healthy Lives., "Seasonal Affective Disorder," 2010, www.healthyminds.org/Main-Topic/Seasonal-Affective-Disorder.aspx.

32. Mayo Clinic Staff, MayoClinic.com, "Depression: Causes," 2010, www.mayoclinic.com/health/depression/DS00175/DSECTION=causes.

33. National Institute of Mental Health, "The Numbers Count," 2009.

34. American College Health Association, *ACHA–NCHA II: Reference Group Data Report Fall 2009*, 2010.

35. M. Jacofsky et al., MentalHelp.net, "Understanding Anxiety and Anxiety Disorders Introduction," Updated June 2010, www.mentalhelp.net/poc/view_doc.php?type=doc&id=38463&cn=1.

36. National Institute of Mental Health, "Generalized Anxiety Disorder, GAD," Reviewed July 7, 2009, www.nimh.nih.gov/health/publications/anxiety-disorders/generalized-anxiety-disorder-gad.shtml.

37. National Institute of Mental Health, "The Numbers Count," 2009.

38. Mayo Clinic Staff, MayoClinic.com, "Panic Attacks and Panic Disorder: Symptoms," 2010, www.mayoclinic.com/health/panic-attacks/DS00338/DSECTION=symptoms.

39. National Institute of Mental Health, "The Numbers Count," 2009.

40. Ibid.

41. Ibid.

42. C. W. Hoge et al., "Combat Duty in Iraq and Afghanistan, Mental Health Problems, and Barriers to Care," *New England Journal of Medicine* 351 (2004): 13–22.

43. National Institute of Mental Health, "Generalized Anxiety Disorder, GAD," 2009.

44. W. T. O'Donohue, K. A. Fowler, and S. O. Lilienfeld, *Personality Disorders: Toward the DSM-V* (Thousand Oaks, CA: Sage Publications, 2007).

45. National Institute of Mental Health, "National Survey Tracks Prevalence of Personality Disorders in U.S. Population," October 18, 2007, www.nimh.nih.gov/science-news/2007/national-survey-tracks-prevalence-of-personality-disorders-in-us-population.shtml.

46. Mayo Clinic Staff, MayoClinic.com, "Borderline Personality Disorder," 2010, www.mayoclinic.com/health/borderline-personality-disorder/DS00442.

47. J. Cole, "Facts," BPDWORLD, 2010, www.bpdworld.org/demo-category/106-facts.

48. National Institute of Mental Health, "The Numbers Count," 2009.

49. National Institute of Mental Health, "Schizophrenia," Reviewed March 2010, www.nimh.nih.gov/health/topics/schizophrenia/index.shtml.

50. Ibid.

51. National Institute of Mental Health, "Suicide in the U.S.: Statistics and Prevention," NIH Publication no. 06-4594, Reviewed September 2010, www.nimh.nih.gov/health/publications/suicide-in-the-us-statistics-and-prevention/index.shtml.

52. J. Xu et al., "Deaths: Final Data for 2007," *National Vital Statistics Reports* 58, no. 19 (Hyattsville, MD: National Center for Health Statistics, 2010).

53. National Institute of Mental Health, "Suicide in the U.S.: Statistics and Prevention," 2009.

54. Ibid.

55. Crisis Link, "Suicide Myths (Adult)," 2009, www.crisislink.org/resources/suicide/suicide_myths_adult.html.

56. National Institute of Mental Health, "Suicide in the U.S.: Statistics and Prevention," 2009.

57. American Association of Suicidology, "Understanding and Helping the Suicidal Individual," Accessed March 2010, www.suicidology.org/web/guest/how-can-you-help.

58. Mayo Clinic Staff, MayoClinic.com, "Mental Health: Overcoming the Stigma of Mental Illness," 2009, www.mayoclinic.com/health/mental-health/MH00076; P. Corrigan and R. Lundin, *Don't Call Me Nuts: Coping with the Stigma of Mental Illness* (Tinley Park, IL: Recovery Press, 2001).

59. Active Minds: Changing the Conversation about Mental Health, "About Us: FAQ," Accessed March 2010, www.activeminds.org/index.php?option=com_content&task=view&id=40&Itemid=109.

60. U.S. Food and Drug Administration, "New Warnings Proposed for Antidepressants," May 2007, www.fda.gov/ForConsumers/ConsumerUpdates/ucm048950.htm.

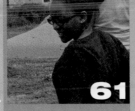
How many college students focus on their spiritual health?

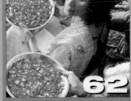
Is spirituality the same as religion?

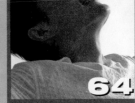
Does spirituality influence health?

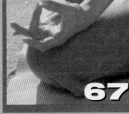
Is meditation boring?

# FOCUS ON Cultivating Your Spiritual Health

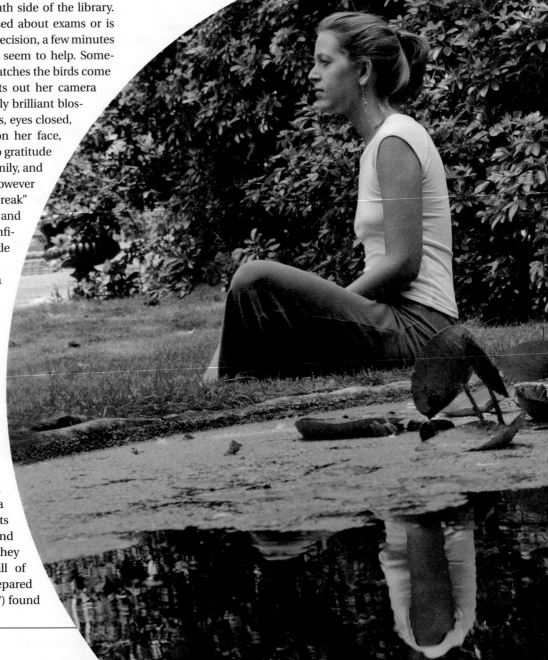

Lia's favorite spot on campus is the secluded Japanese garden on the south side of the library. Whether she's feeling stressed about exams or is mulling over an important decision, a few minutes alone in the garden always seem to help. Sometimes she sits quietly and watches the birds come and go. Sometimes she gets out her camera and photographs particularly brilliant blossoms. Often she simply rests, eyes closed, feeling the sun's warmth on her face, and lets her thoughts turn to gratitude for her health, her loving family, and her opportunity to study. However she spends it, her "garden break" leaves Lia feeling refreshed and refocused, with greater confidence in her ability to tackle the challenges of her day.

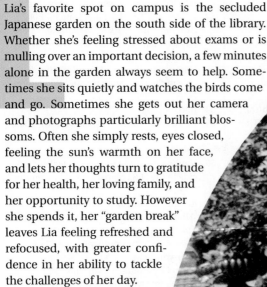

Lia's desire to find a sense of purpose, meaning, and harmony in her life is shared by a majority of American college students. According to UCLA's Higher Education Research Institute, (HERI) although undergraduates' religious attendance declines during the college years, they show significant growth in a wide spectrum of spiritual and ethical considerations.[1] Data from nearly 15,000 students at more than 136 colleges and universities (taken as they entered college in the fall of 2004 and again as they prepared for their senior year in 2007) found that interest in the following goals increased by more than 10 percent during the college years, to levels representing more than half of all students surveyed:

- Attaining inner harmony
- Developing a meaningful philosophy of life
- Seeking beauty in life
- Becoming a more loving person

Also, researchers found that, compared with college first-year students, juniors and seniors were more desirous of reducing pain and suffering in the world, were more thankful for all that had happened to them, and expressed higher levels of ecumenical worldviews—that is, views

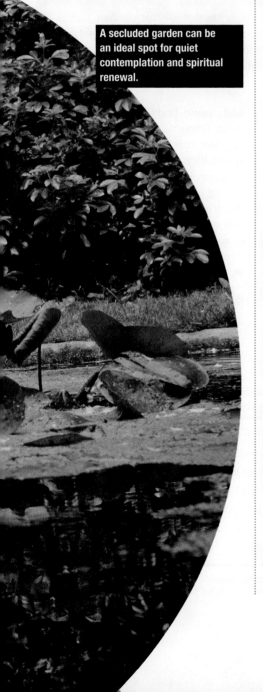

A secluded garden can be an ideal spot for quiet contemplation and spiritual renewal.

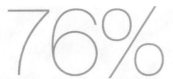

**of college students say they are "searching for meaning and purpose in life."**

expressing tolerance and respect for other religions and philosophies—and a commitment to understanding other countries and cultures.

Back in Chapter 1, we identified spiritual health as one of six key dimensions of health (see Figure 1.4 on page 9). Lia's sense of wonder and respect for the natural world, her gratitude for the good things in her life, and her belief in a "universal spirit" suggest that spiritual health is an important focus of her daily life, bringing her greater awareness and serenity. If you're feeling as if you could use a little more of these qualities in your own life, read on: This chapter will help you explore ways to sharpen your spiritual focus.

# What Is Spirituality?

From one day to the next, many of us attempt to satisfy our needs for belonging and self-esteem by acquiring material possessions. But at some point we come to realize that new gadgets, clothes, or concert tickets don't necessarily make us happy or improve our sense of self-worth. That's when many of us begin to contemplate another side of ourselves: our spirituality.

But what is spirituality? It isn't easy to define. Although part of the universal human experience, it's highly personal, and involves feelings and senses that are often intangible. As such, it tends to defy the boundaries that strict definitions would impose. Let's begin by exploring its root, *spirit*, which in many cultures refers to *breath*, or the force that animates life. When you're "inspired," your energy flows. You're not held back by doubts about the purpose or meaning of your work and life. Indeed, many definitions of spirituality

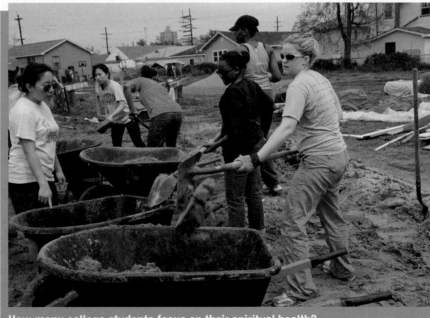

**How many college students focus on their spiritual health?**

Spiritual and ethical concerns are important to a majority of American college students. For example, more than 80 percent of college seniors desire to become a more loving person. One of the ways college students express their spirituality is by working to reduce suffering in the world; many contribute their time and skills to volunteer organizations, as these students are doing by working to build homes for Habitat for Humanity.

incorporate this sense of transcendence. For example, the National Center for Complementary and Alternative Medicine (NCCAM) defines **spirituality** as an individual's sense of purpose and meaning in life, beyond material values.[2] Similarly, Harold G. Koenig, MD, one of the foremost researchers of spirituality and health, defines *spirituality* as the personal quest for understanding answers to ultimate questions about life, about meaning, and about our relationship with the sacred or transcendent.[3] The sacred or transcendent could be a higher power or it could relate to our relationship with nature or forces we cannot explain.

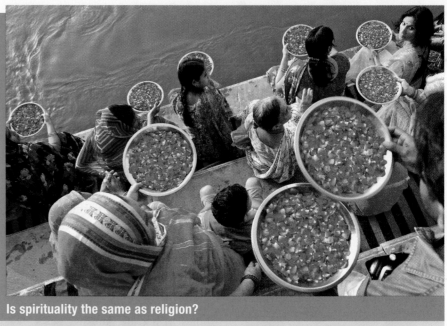

**Is spirituality the same as religion?**

Spirituality and religion are not the same. Many people find that religious practices, such as attending services or making offerings—such as the flowers these Hindus are preparing to place in the sacred Ganges River—help them to focus on their spirituality. However, religion does not have to be part of a spiritual person's life.

## Religion and Spirituality Are Distinct Concepts

Spirituality may or may not lead to participation in organized **religion,** that is, a system of beliefs, practices, rituals, and symbols designed to facilitate closeness to the sacred or transcendent.[4] In other words, although spirituality and religion do share some common elements, they are not the same thing. Most Americans consider spirituality to be important in their lives, but not necessarily in the form of religion: A recent national survey of more than 35,000 Americans revealed that 92 percent believe in some kind of "higher power," but not all of these respondents identified themselves as being affiliated with a particular religion.[5] Thus, it's clear that religion does not have to be part of a spiritual person's life. Table 1 identifies some characteristics that can help you distinguish between religion and spirituality.

Another finding of the same survey was that 70 percent of Americans affiliated with a religious tradition agreed that other religions are also valid.[6] Perhaps this is because all major religions express a belief in a unifying spiritual concept, a oneness with a greater power. It seems that a majority of Americans recognize and respect this underlying unity of spiritual ideas, expressed in different religious and spiritual practices.

## Spirituality Integrates Three Facets

Brian Luke Seaward, a professor at the University of Northern Colorado and author of several books on spirituality and mind–body healing, identifies three facets of human existence that together constitute the core of human spirituality: relationships, values, and purpose in life (Figure 1).[7] Questions arising in these three domains prompt many of us to look for spiritual answers. At the same time, spiritual well-being is characterized by healthy relationships, strong personal values, and a sense that we have a meaningful purpose in life.

**Relationships** Have you ever wondered if someone you were attracted to

**spirituality** An individual's sense of purpose and meaning in life, beyond material values.
**religion** A system of beliefs, practices, rituals, and symbols designed to facilitate closeness to the sacred or transcendent.

| TABLE 1 | Characteristics Distinguishing Religion and Spirituality | |
|---|---|---|
| **Religion** | | **Spirituality** |
| Community focused | | Individualistic |
| Observable, measurable, objective | | Less measurable, more subjective |
| Formal, orthodox, organized | | Less formal, less orthodox, less systematic |
| Behavior oriented, outward practices | | Emotionally oriented, inwardly directed |
| Authoritarian in terms of behaviors | | Not authoritarian, little accountability |
| Doctrine separating good from evil | | Unifying, not doctrine oriented |

**Source:** National Center for Complementary and Alternative Medicine (NCCAM), "Prayer and Spirituality in Health: Ancient Practices, Modern Science," *CAM at the NIH* 12, no. 1 (2005): 1–4.

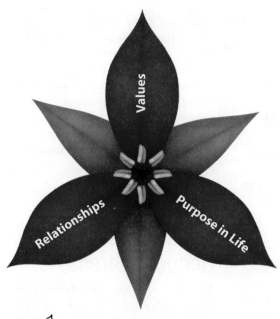

**FIGURE 1** **Three Facets of Spirituality**
Most of us are prompted to explore our spirituality because of questions relating to our relationships, values, and purpose in life. At the same time, these three facets together constitute spiritual well-being.

is really right for you? Or, conversely, if you should break off a long-term relationship? Have you ever wished you had more friends, or that you were a better friend to yourself? Have you ever tried to make a connection with some sort of Presence or Higher Self? For many people, such questions and yearnings are natural triggers for spiritual growth: As we contemplate whom we should choose as a life partner or how to mend a quarrel with a friend, we begin to foster our own inner wisdom. At the same time, healthy relationships are a sign of spiritual well-being. When we treat ourselves and others with respect, honesty, integrity, and love, we are manifesting our spiritual health.

**Values** Our personal **values** are our principles—not only the things we say we care about, but also the things that cause us to behave the way we do. For instance, if you value honesty, then you are not likely to call in sick for work when you intend to spend the day at the beach. In other words, our value system is the set of fundamental rules by which we conduct our lives. It's what we stand for. When we attempt to clarify our values, and then to live

according to those values, we're engaging in spiritual work. Spiritual health is characterized by a strong personal value system.

**Meaningful Purpose in Life** What career do you plan to pursue after you graduate? Do you hope to marry? Do you plan to have or adopt children? What things will make you happy and feel "complete"? How do these choices reflect what you hold as your purpose in life? At the end of your days, what things would you want people to say about how you've lived your life and what your life has meant to others? Contemplating these questions fosters spiritual growth. People who are spiritually healthy are able to articulate their purpose, and to make choices that manifest that purpose. In thinking about your own purpose, avoid the temptation to get too ambitious, as in, "I'm here to eradicate world hunger!" Instead, try to articulate just what you see as your unique contribution to the world—something you can actually do, starting now.

## Spiritual Intelligence Is an Inner Wisdom

Our relationships, values, and sense of purpose together contribute to our overall **spiritual intelligence (SI).** This term was introduced by physicist and philosopher Danah Zohar, who defined it as "the intelligence that makes us whole, that gives us our integrity. It is the soul's intelligence, the intelligence of the deep self."[8] Zohar includes qualities such as self-awareness, spontaneity, and compassion in her definition of *spiritual intelligence,* explaining that SI helps us use adversity in a positive way and live according to our values and our vision.

Since Zohar's introduction of SI, dozens of clerics, psychologists, and

even business consultants have expanded on the definition. For example, Rabbi Yaacov Kravitz of the Center for Spiritual Intelligence explains that SI helps us find a moral and ethical path to help guide us through life. Similarly, psychologist Robert Emmons emphasizes the ability of people with a high level of SI to solve problems and attain goals.[9] Would you like to find out your own spiritual IQ? See the **Assess Yourself** box on page 70.

## How Is It Beneficial to Focus on Your Spiritual Health?

The importance of people's spirituality to their wellness and health has been widely acknowledged and is based on hundreds of published studies.[10]

## Spiritual Health Contributes to Physical Health

The emerging science of mind–body medicine is a research focus of the NCCAM. One area under study is the association between spiritual health and general health and longevity. The NCCAM cites evidence of a positive influence of spirituality on health, and suggests that the connection may be due to improved immune function, cardiovascular function, and/or other physiological changes.[11] Evidence from a variety of other studies also supports this association. For example, several recent studies have found that Americans who attend religious services regularly, particularly those whose religious tenets

---

**values** Principles that influence our thoughts and emotions, and guide the choices we make in our lives.
**spiritual intelligence (SI)** The intelligence of the deep self; a capacity to live in alignment with our inner wisdom, values, and vision.

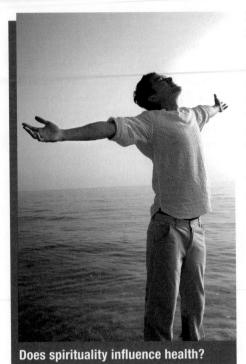

**Does spirituality influence health?**

Spirituality is widely acknowledged to have a positive impact on health and wellness. The benefits range from reductions in overall morbidity and mortality to improved abilities to cope with illness and stress.

restrict smoking, alcohol use, and engaging in other risk behaviors, live longer—on average—than those who do not. Although religious attendance is often cited as being related to good health, it really isn't attendance per se that is the key.[12] Other factors, such as living a life reflective of spirituality, including such things as kindness, balance, harmony, selflessness, and respect for others, are probably the most important contributors to these positive outcomes.

Some researchers believe that a key to understanding the improved health and longer life in spiritually healthy people is their greater self-control. That is, people who are more spiritually healthy may have an increased capacity to restrain themselves from overeating, smoking, and abusing alcohol and other drugs. They may also be more disciplined about getting adequate exercise and sleep.[13]

When we do get sick, the National Cancer Institute (NCI) contends that spiritual or religious well-being may

help restore health and improve quality of life in the following ways:[14]

- By decreasing anxiety, depression, anger, discomfort, and feelings of isolation
- By decreasing alcohol and drug abuse
- By decreasing blood pressure and the risk of heart disease
- By increasing the person's ability to cope with the effects of illness and with medical treatments
- By increasing feelings of hope and optimism, freedom from regret, satisfaction with life, and inner peace

Several studies show an association between spiritual health and a person's ability to cope with any of a variety of physical illnesses in addition to cancer.[15] For example, a study of people living with chronic pain and fatigue showed a benefit of spiritual health.[16] Another study of people with HIV showed a slower disease progression over a period of 4 years in people who become more spiritually focused after their diagnosis.[17]

## Spiritual Health Contributes to Psychosocial Health

Current research also suggests that spiritual health contributes to psychosocial health. For instance, the NCI and independent studies have found a benefit of spirituality in reducing levels of anxiety and depression.[18] And certain spiritual practices, such as yoga, deep meditation, and prayer, can positively affect brain chemistry in much the same way that conventional antianxiety and antidepressant medications do.[19]

People who have found a spiritual community also benefit from increased social support among members. For instance, participation in religious services, charitable organizations, and social gatherings can help members avoid isolation. At such gatherings, clerics and other members

may offer spiritual support on challenges that participants may be facing. Or a community may have retired members who offer child care for harried parents, meals for members with disabilities, or transportation to those needing to get to medical appointments. All such measures can contribute to members' overall feelings of security and belonging.

## Spiritual Health Contributes to Reduced Stress

Both the NCCAM and the NCI cite stress reduction as one probable mechanism among spiritually healthy people for improved health and longevity, and for better coping with illness.[20] In addition, several small studies support the contention that positive religious coping supports effective stress management.[21] And a recent study suggests that increasing mindfulness through meditation reduces stress levels not only in people with physical and mental disorders, but in healthy people as well.[22]

## What Can You Do to Focus on Your Spiritual Health?

Cultivating your spiritual side takes just as much work as becoming physically fit or improving your diet. Here, we introduce some ways to develop your spiritual health by training your body, expanding your mind, tuning in, and reaching out.

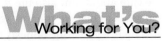

**What's Working for You?**

Maybe you're already focusing on enhancing your spiritual health. Do you incorporate any of the following behaviors into your daily life?

☐ I practice yoga.
☐ I meditate.
☐ I do volunteer work.
☐ I maintain healthy relationships.

## Train Your Body

For thousands of years, in regions throughout the world, seekers have cultivated transcendence through physical means. One of the foremost examples is the practice of various forms of **yoga.** Although in the West we think of yoga as involving controlled breathing and physical postures, traditional forms also emphasize meditation, chanting, and other practices that are believed to cultivate unity with the *Atman,* or Absolute.

If you are interested in exploring yoga, sign up for a class on campus, at your local YMCA, or at a dedicated yoga center. Make sure you choose a form that seems right to you: Some, such as *hatha yoga,* focus on developing flexibility, deep breathing, and tranquility, whereas others, such as *ashtanga yoga,* are fast-paced and demanding, and thus more appropriate for developing physical fitness than spiritual health. (See Chapter 3 and Chapter 9 for more about individual styles of yoga.) For your first class, dress comfortably in relaxed fabrics that are somewhat close fitting so that, when you bend at the waist or lift your leg, you won't feel constricted or exposed. No shoes or socks are worn. At the beginning of the class, the instructor will likely lead you through some gentle warm-up poses, and then add more challenging poses with coordinated inhalations and exhalations to align, stretch, and invigorate each region of your body. Most classes provide yoga mats to cushion your joints as you work through the postures. Your class will probably conclude with several minutes of relaxation and deep breathing.

Training your body to improve your spiritual health doesn't necessarily require you to engage in a formal practice such as yoga. By energizing your body and sharpening your mental focus, jogging, biking, aerobics, or any other exercise you do every day can contribute to your spiritual health. To transform an exercise session into a spiritual workout, begin by acknowledging gratitude for your body's strength and speed, then, throughout the session, try to maintain mindfulness of your breathing. We'll say more about mindful breathing in the discussion of meditation below.

You can also cultivate spirituality through fully engaging your body's senses. In fact, you can think of vision, hearing, taste, smell, and touch as five portals to spiritual health. Viewing an engaging piece of artwork or listening to beautiful music can calm the mind and soothe the spirit. A key reason that Lia, in our opening story, finds sustenance in nature is that she fully

**yoga** A system of physical and mental training involving controlled breathing, physical postures *(asanas)*, meditation, chanting, and other practices that are believed to cultivate unity with the *Atman,* or Absolute.

eyes and sitting in silence removes the distraction of visual and auditory stimuli, helping you to focus within. To take advantage of silence, turn off your cell phone and take a long, solitary walk. You might even spend a weekend at one of the many retreat centers throughout the United States. To find one, see the state-by-state listing at www.SpiritSite.com.

## Expand Your Mind

For many people, psychological counseling is a first step toward improving their spiritual health. Therapy helps you let go of the hurts of the past, accept your limitations, manage stress and anger, reduce anxiety and depression, and take control of your life—all of which are also steps toward spiritual growth. If you've never engaged in therapy, making the first appointment can feel daunting. Your campus health department can usually help by providing a referral.

Another practical way to expand your mind is to study the sacred texts of the world's major religions and spiritual practices. Many seekers find guidance in the writings of great spiritual teachers. Libraries and bookstores are filled with volumes that explore the diverse approaches humans take to achieve spiritual fulfillment.

Finally, you can expand your awareness of different spiritual practices by exploring on-campus meditation groups, taking classes in spirituality or comparative religions, attending meetings of student organizations where different religious tenets are explored, going to different churches in your local area and noting what spiritual elements they hold in common, attending public lectures and critically evaluating whether the speakers demonstrate a spiritual bent or

## 15.8 million

U.S. adults practice yoga, according to a recent survey by *Yoga Journal.*

engages her senses—smelling the freshly cut grass, listening to the birds, and photographing the flowers.

The flip side of cultivating your senses is depriving them! Closing your

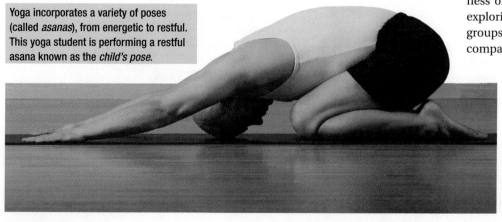

Yoga incorporates a variety of poses (called *asanas*), from energetic to restful. This yoga student is performing a restful asana known as the *child's pose.*

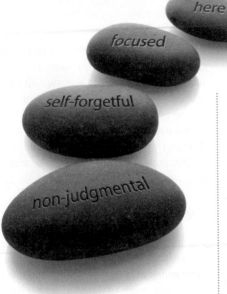

**FIGURE 2** Qualities of Mindfulness

---

**contemplation** A practice of concentrating the mind on a spiritual or ethical question or subject, a view of the natural world, or an icon or other image representative of divinity.
**mindfulness** A practice of purposeful, nonjudgmental observation in which we are fully present in the moment.
**meditation** A practice of emptying the mind of thought.

---

reflect bias or exclusion in their lectures, and checking out the official websites of various spiritual and religious organizations.

# Tune in to Yourself and Your Surroundings

Focusing on your spiritual health has been likened to tuning in on a radio: Inner wisdom is perpetually available to us, but if we fail to tune our "receiver," we won't be able to hear it for all the "static" of daily life. Fortunately, four ancient practices still used throughout the world can help you tune in. These are contemplation, mindfulness, meditation, and prayer, which you can think of as studying, observing, emptying, and communing with the Divine.

## Contemplation

If you were to look up the word *contemplation* in a dictionary, you'd find that it means a study of something—whether a candle flame or a theory of quantum mechanics. In the domain of spirituality, **contemplation** usually refers to a practice of concentrating the mind on a spiritual or ethical question or subject, a view of the natural world, or an icon or other image representative of divinity. For instance, a Zen Buddhist might contemplate a riddle, called a *koan,* such as, what is the sound of one hand clapping? A Sufi might contemplate the 99 names of God. A Roman Catholic might contemplate an image of the Virgin Mary. Spiritual people with no religious affiliation might contemplate the natural world, a favorite poem, or an ethical question such as, what is the origin of evil? In addition, most religious and spiritual traditions advocate engaging in the contemplation of gratitude, forgiveness, and unconditional love.

When practicing contemplation, it can be helpful to keep a journal to record any insights that arise. In addition, journaling itself can be a form of contemplation. For example, you might want to make a list of 20 things in your life that you are grateful for or write a poem of forgiveness for yourself or a loved one. You might also use your journal to record inspirational quotations that you encounter in your readings.

**Mindfulness** A practice of focused, nonjudgmental observation, **mindfulness** is the ability to be fully present in the moment (Figure 2). If you have ever "forgotten yourself" while watching the sun set over a mountain, or listening to a great pianist playing Bach, or even while performing a challenging calculation in math, then you have experienced a moment of mindfulness. In other words, mindfulness is an awareness of present-moment reality—a holistic sensation of being totally involved in the moment rather than focused on some past worry or future event.[23]

So how do you practice mindfulness? The range of opportunities is as infinite as the moments of our everyday lives. According to molecular biologist and guru of mindfulness Jon Kabat-Zinn, living mindfully means "making more of your ordinary moments notable and noteworthy by taking note of them."[24] For instance, the next time you get ready to eat an orange, pay attention! What does it feel like to pierce the skin with your thumbnail? Do you smell the fragrance of the orange as you peel it? What does the rind really look like? How do the drops of juice splatter as you separate the orange into segments? And finally, what does it taste like, and how does the taste change from the first bite to the last?

Pursuing almost any endeavor that requires close concentration can help you develop mindfulness. For instance, think of physical and mental challenges, such as a competitive diver leaping from the board, or a physician attempting a difficult diagnosis. Or consider creative and performing arts such as sculpting, painting, writing, dancing, or playing a musical instrument. Even household

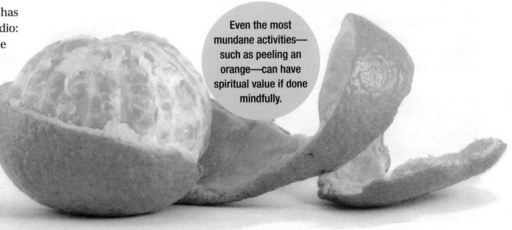

Even the most mundane activities—such as peeling an orange—can have spiritual value if done mindfully.

# BE HEALTHY, BE GREEN

## Developing Environmental Mindfulness

In her recent book, *Mindfully Green*, environmentalist Stephanie Kaza emphasizes the connection between mindfulness and environmental consciousness. Kaza argues that more people need "to bring their best ethical and spiritual attention to environmental concerns." We need to base our decisions on "compassion, restraint, and acceptance of universal responsibility for the well-being of the earth."

To be mindfully green, Kaza claims, requires us to contemplate a wide variety of troubling questions, to answer them for ourselves, and to commit to taking the right actions that result from our reflection. These questions include, but are not limited to, the following:

✳ How can I investigate the nature of desire?

✳ How can I challenge its allure for me, as a consumer?

✳ What do I actually need?

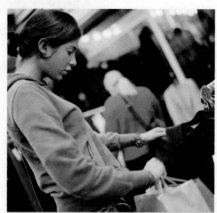

To be mindfully green requires us to ask ourselves some tough questions, such as, what is my fair share? and how much do I really need?

✳ What is my fair share?

✳ How do my choices influence the resources available to others?

✳ Can I both practice restraint and cultivate contentment?

✳ Am I willing to witness suffering?

✳ How can I recognize, evaluate, and work to reduce environmental harm?

✳ How can I cultivate kindness toward birds, trees, waters, and lands?

✳ Can I acknowledge my responsibility to inflict no unnecessary harm?

✳ How shall I respond to the harm inflicted by others?

✳ How can I more fully recognize my interdependence with all living organisms and with all elements of the natural world?

In short, Kaza explains that being mindfully green is "about staying present, one action at a time, always asking, What is the kind thing to do now?"

**Source:** From *Mindfully Green,* by Stephanie Kaza, © 2008 by Stephanie Kaza. Reprinted by arrangement with Shambhala Publications Inc., Boston, MA. www.shambhala.com.

---

activities such as cooking or cleaning can foster mindfulness—as long as you pay attention while you do them!

In this era of global environmental concerns, we can also cultivate mindfulness by paying attention to how our choices affect our world. This doesn't only mean mindfulness about recycling our soda cans and taking the subway instead of our car. Those are the easy examples. Instead, mindfulness of our environment calls on us to examine our values and behaviors as we share our Earth every moment of each day. The **Be Healthy, Be Green** box will help you begin.

## what do you think?

Why do you think mindfulness practices are gaining more recognition? ● What are the benefits of mindfulness? ● In today's fast-paced, multitasking world, do you think it is challenging to practice mindfulness on a regular basis?

**Meditation** **Meditation** is a practice of emptying the mind, of cultivating stillness. Although the precise details vary with different schools of meditation, the fundamental task is the same: to quiet the mind's noise (variously referred to as "chatter," "static," or "monkey mind").

## 39%
### of Americans meditate at least once a week.

Why would you want to cultivate the stillness of meditation? For thousands of years, human beings of different cultures and traditions have found that achieving periods of meditative stillness each day enhances their spiritual health. Today, researchers are beginning to

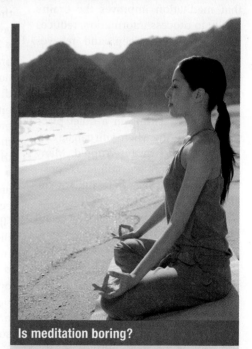

**Is meditation boring?**

Once you get the hang of it, meditation is anything but boring. As expert Jon Kabat-Zinn notes, "[When] you pay attention to boredom, it gets unbelievably interesting."

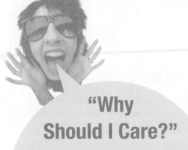

discover why. The NCCAM reports that by using brain-scanning techniques, researchers have found that experienced meditators show a significantly increased level of *empathy,* the ability to understand and share another person's experience.[25] Similarly, another recent study found that meditation increased the capacity for forgiveness among college students.[26] And there are other benefits, too. Studies suggest that meditation improves the brain's ability to process information, reduces stress, improves sleep, and relieves chronic pain.[27]

So how do you meditate? Detailed instructions are beyond the scope of this text, but most teachers advise beginning by sitting in a quiet place with low lighting where you can be certain you won't be interrupted. Many advocate assuming a "full lotus" position, with both legs bent fully at the knees, and each ankle over the opposite knee. However, this position can be painful for beginners, people with poor flexibility, and people with joint pain. Thus, you may want to assume a modified lotus position, in which your legs are simply crossed in front of you. Lying down is not recommended because you may fall asleep. Rest your hands palm upward on your knees. This position uncrosses the two bones of the forearm. Your eyes can be

---

**prayer** Communication with a transcendent Presence.

open, half-open, or closed, but if you are a beginner, you may find it easier to meditate with your eyes closed.

Once you're in a position conducive to meditation, it's time to start emptying your mind. Different schools of meditation teach different methods to achieve this. For example:

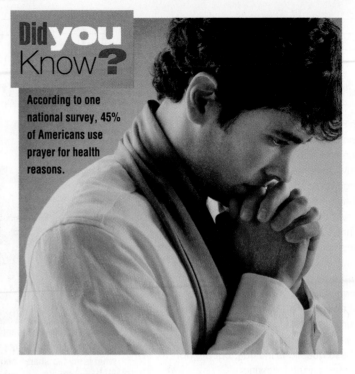

● **Mantra meditation.** Focus on a *mantra,* a single word such as *Om, Amen, Love,* or *God.* Keep repeating this word silently to yourself. When a distracting thought arises, simply set it aside. It may help to imagine the thought as a leaf, and mentally place it on a gently flowing stream that carries it away. Do not fault yourself for becoming distracted. Simply notice the thought, release it, and return to your mantra.

● **Breath meditation.** Count each breath: Pay attention to each inhalation, the brief pause that follows, and the exhalation. Together, these equal one breath. When you have counted ten breaths, return to one. As with mantra meditation, as distractions arise, release them and return to the breath.

● **Color meditation.** When your eyes are closed, you may perceive a field of color, such as a deep blue "pearl" or "flame." Focus on this color. Treat distractions as for other forms of meditation.

● **Object meditation.** With your eyes open, focus on an object, such as a picture of a religious symbol or figure, or a flower or stone. Allow your eyes to soften as you meditate on this object. Treat distractions as for other forms of meditation.

After several minutes of meditation, and with practice, you may come to experience a sensation sometimes described as "dropping down," in which you feel yourself release into the meditation. In this state, which can be likened to a wakeful sleep, distracting thoughts are far less likely to arise, and yet you may suddenly receive surprising insights.

When you're just starting out, try meditating for just 10 to 20 minutes a session, once or twice a day. In time, you can increase your sessions to 30 minutes or more. As you meditate for longer periods, you will likely find yourself feeling more rested and less stressed throughout your day, and you may begin to experience the increased levels of empathy recorded among expert meditators.

**Prayer** In **prayer,** rather than emptying the mind, an individual focuses the mind in communication with a transcendent Presence. Spiritual traditions throughout the world distinguish several forms that this communication can take. For many, prayer offers a sense of comfort; a sense that we are not alone; and an avenue for expressing concern for others, for admission of transgressions, for seeking forgiveness, and for renewing hope and purpose. Focusing on the things we can be grateful for in life can move people to look to the future

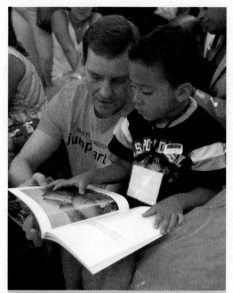

Volunteering can be a fun and fulfilling way to broaden your experience, connect with your community, and focus on your spiritual health.

## Finding Your Spiritual Side through Service

Recognizing that we are all part of a greater system and that we have responsibilities to and for others is a key part of spiritual growth and development. Volunteering your time and energy is a great way to connect with others and help make the world a better place while improving your own health. Here are some ways you can go about this:

✳ Offer to help elderly neighbors by providing lawn care, hauling away trash and debris, or making their homes energy efficient for the winter.
✳ Volunteer for Meals on Wheels, Senior Companions, a local soup kitchen, a food bank, or another program to help neighbors with low food security levels.
✳ Organize or participate in an after-school or summertime activity for neighborhood children.
✳ Participate in a highway, beach, or neighborhood cleanup; restoration of park trails and rivers; or other environmental preservation projects.
✳ Volunteer at the local humane society walking dogs, grooming cats, cleaning, fostering pets, or raising money for spaying and neutering.
✳ Join a Big Brother or Big Sister program and work to instill self-esteem in those who may face significant challenges or have poor role models.
✳ Join a student organization working on a cause such as global warming or hunger, or start one yourself. Think that's impossible? Check out these inspiring examples: Students Against Global Apathy (SAGA) was founded by a University of Alberta student to confront global poverty and injustice; Students for the Environment (S4E) was founded by students at the University of Delaware to focus on local, national, and global environmental issues. And the National Student Campaign Against Hunger and Homelessness is a project of student-level Public Interest Research Groups.
✳ Spend your vacation volunteering in a neighborhood challenged by poverty, low literacy levels, or a natural disaster. Or volunteer with an organization such as Habitat for Humanity to build homes or provide other aid to developing communities.

with hope and give them the strength to get through the most challenging times.

## Reach Out to Others

**Altruism,** the giving of oneself out of genuine concern for others, is a key aspect of a spiritually healthy lifestyle. Volunteering to help others, choosing to work for a not-for-profit organization, donating money or other resources to a food bank or other program—even spending an afternoon picking up litter in your neighborhood—all of these are ways to serve others and simultaneously enhance your own spiritual health. Most colleges and universities offer opportunities for community practicums and service that can also facilitate future career opportunities.

Community service can also take the form of **environmental stewardship,** which the Environmental Protection Agency (EPA) defines as the responsibility for environmental quality shared by all those whose actions

affect the environment.[28] Responsibility manifests in action. At home, simple actions such as reducing and recycling packaging, turning off the lights, making sure the heat or air-conditioning maintains an ecofriendly room temperature, replacing old lightbulbs with energy-efficient varieties, and taking shorter showers are all part of environmental stewardship.

For more strategies to enhance your spiritual health by reaching out to others, refer to the **Skills for Behavior Change** box.

---

**altruism** The giving of oneself out of genuine concern for others.
**environmental stewardship** A responsibility for environmental quality shared by all those whose actions affect the environment.

# Assess yourself

## What's Your Spiritual IQ?

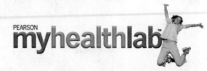

At least a dozen tools are now available for assessing your spiritual intelligence. Although each differs significantly according to its target audience (therapy clients, business executives, church members, and so on), most share certain underlying principles, reflected in the questionnaire below. Answer each question as follows:

0 = not at all true for me
1 = somewhat true for me
2 = very true for me

_____ 1. I frequently feel gratitude for the many blessings of my life.

_____ 2. I am often moved by the beauty of Earth, music, poetry, or other aspects of my daily life.

_____ 3. I readily express forgiveness toward those whose missteps have affected me.

_____ 4. I recognize in others qualities that are more important than their appearance and behaviors.

_____ 5. When I do poorly on an exam, lose an important game, or am rejected in a relationship, I am able to know that the experience does not define who I am.

_____ 6. When fear arises, I am able to know that I am eternally safe and loved.

_____ 7. I meditate or pray daily.

_____ 8. I frequently and fearlessly ponder the possibility of an afterlife.

_____ 9. I accept total responsibility for the choices that I have made in building my life.

_____ 10. I feel that I am on Earth for a unique and sacred reason.

### Scoring

The higher your score on this quiz means the higher your spiritual intelligence. To improve your score, apply the suggestions for spiritual practices from this chapter.

---

# YOUR PLAN FOR CHANGE

The **Assess yourself** activity gave you the chance to evaluate your own spiritual intelligence, and the chapter introduced you to some practices used successfully by millions of people over many generations to enhance their spiritual health. If you are interested in cultivating your own spirituality further, consider taking some of the small but significant steps listed below to start you on your journey.

### Today, you can:

◯ Find a quiet spot; turn off your cell phone; close your eyes; and contemplate, meditate, or pray for 10 minutes. Or spend 10 minutes in quiet mindfulness of your surroundings.

◯ In a journal or on your computer, begin compiling a numbered list of things you are grateful for. Today, list at least ten things. Include people, pets, talents and abilities, achievements, favorite places, foods . . . whatever comes to mind!

### Within the next 2 weeks, you can:

◯ Explore the options on campus for beginning psychotherapy, joining a spiritual or religious student group, or volunteering with a student organization working for positive change.

◯ Think of a person in your life with whom you have experienced conflict. Spend a few minutes contemplating forgiveness toward

this person and then write him or her an e-mail or letter apologizing for any offense you may have given and offering your forgiveness in return. Wait for a day or two before deciding whether you are truly ready to send the message.

### By the end of the semester, you can:

◯ Develop a list of several spiritual texts that you would like to read during your break.

◯ Begin exploring options for volunteer work next summer.

# References

1. Higher Education Research Institute, "Press Release: Students Experience Spiritual Growth During College: UCLA Study Reveals Significant Changes in Undergraduates' Values and Beliefs," December 18, 2007, Available at http://spirituality.ucla.edu/publications/news.
2. National Center for Complementary and Alternative Medicine (NCCAM), "Prayer and Spirituality in Health: Ancient Practices, Modern Science," *CAM at the NIH* 12, no. 1 (2005): 1–4, Available at http://nccam.nih.gov/news/newsletter/archive.htm.
3. H. G. Koenig, M. McCullough, and D. B. Larson, *Handbook of Religion and Health: A Century of Research Reviewed* (New York: Oxford University Press, 2001).
4. Ibid.
5. Pew Forum on Religion & Public Life, *U.S. Religious Landscape Survey Religious Beliefs and Practices: Diverse and Politically Relevant* (Washington, DC: Pew Research Center, 2008), Available at http://religions.pewforum.org/reports.
6. Ibid.
7. B. L. Seaward, *Health of the Human Spirit: Spiritual Dimensions for Personal Health* (Boston: Allyn & Bacon, 2001), 85–90; B. L. Seaward, *Managing Stress: Principles and Strategies for Health and Well Being*, 6th ed. (Sudbury, MA: Jones and Bartlett, 2009).
8. D. Zohar, *ReWiring the Corporate Brain: Using the New Science to Rethink How We Structure and Lead Organizations* (San Francisco: Berrett Koehler, 1997).
9. R. A. Emmons, *The Psychology of Ultimate Concerns: Motivation and Personality in Spirituality* (New York: Guilford Press, 2003).
10. A. Moreira-Almeida and H. G. Koenig, "Retaining the Meaning of the Words Religiousness and Spirituality," *Social Science and Medicine* 63, no. 4 (2006): 843–45.
11. NCCAM, "Prayer and Spirituality in Health," 2005.
12. A. J. Weaver and H. G. Koenig, "Religion, Spirituality, and Their Relevance to Medicine: An Update," *American Family Physician* 73, no. 8 (2006): 1336–37; R. F. Gillum, D. E. King, T. O. Obisesan, and H. G. Koenig, "Frequency of Attendance at Religious Services and Mortality in a U.S. National Cohort," *Annals of Epidemiology* 18, no. 2 (2008): 124–29.
13. M. E. McCullough and B. L. B. Willoughby, "Religion, Self-Regulation, and Self-Control: Associations, Explanations, and Implications," *Psychological Bulletin* 135, no. 1 (2009): 69–93.
14. National Cancer Institute (NCI), "Spirituality in Cancer Care," Modified March 6, 2009, www.cancer.gov/cancertopics/pdq/supportivecare/spirituality/patient.
15. F. A. Curlin, S. A. Sellergren, J. D. Lantos, and M. H. Chin, "Physicians' Observations and Interpretations of the Influence of Religion and Spirituality on Health," *Archives of Internal Medicine* 167, no. 7 (2007): 649–54.
16. M. Baetz and R. Bowen, "Chronic Pain and Fatigue: Associations with Religion and Spirituality," *Pain Research & Management* 13, no. 5 (2008): 383–88.
17. G. Ironson, R. Stuetzle, and M. A. Fletcher, "An Increase in Religiousness/Spirituality Occurs after HIV Diagnosis and Predicts Slower Disease Progression over 4 Years in People with HIV," *Journal of General Internal Medicine* 21, no. 5 (2006): S62–S68.
18. A. Moreira-Almeida and H. G. Koenig, "Religiousness and Spirituality in Fibromyalgia and Chronic Pain Patients," *Current Pain and Headache Reports* 12, no. 5 (2008): 327–32; B. R. Doolittle and M. Farrell, "The Association between Spirituality and Depression in an Urban Clinic," *Primary Care Companion to the Journal of Clinical Psychiatry* 6, no. 3 (2004): 114–18; NCI, "Spirituality in Cancer Care," 2009.
19. M. Javnbakht, R. Hejazi Kenari, and M. Ghasemi, "Effects of Yoga on Depression and Anxiety of Women," *Complementary Therapies in Clinical Practice* 15, no. 2 (2009): 102–04; A. Woolery, H. Myers, B. Sternlieb, and L. Zeltzer, "A Yoga Intervention for Young Adults with Elevated Symptoms of Depression," *Alternative Therapies in Health and Medicine* 10, no. 2 (2004): 60–63.
20. NCCAM, "Prayer and Spirituality in Health," 2005; NCI, "Spirituality in Cancer Care," 2009.
21. G. G. Ano and E. B. Vasconcelles, "Religious Coping and Psychological Adjustment to Stress: A Meta-Analysis," *Journal of Clinical Psychology* 61, no. 4 (2005): 461–80; U. Winter, D. Hauri, S. Huber, J. Jenewein, U. Schnyder, and B. Kraemer, "The Psychological Outcome of Religious Coping with Stressful Life Events in a Swiss Sample of Church Attendees," *Psychotherapy and Psychosomatics* 78, no. 4 (2009): 240–44.
22. A. Chiesa and A. Serretti, "Mindfulness-Based Stress Reduction for Stress Management in Healthy People: A Review and Meta-Analysis," *Journal of Alternative and Complementary Medicine* 15, no. (2009): 593–600.
23. J. A. Astin, S. L. Shapiro, D. M. Eisenberg, and K. L. Forys, "Mind-Body Medicine: State of the Science, Implications for Practice," *Journal of the American Board of Family Practice* 16, no. 2 (2003): 131–47; J. Bishop et al., "Mindfulness: A Proposed Operational Definition," *Clinical Psychology: Science and Practice* 11 (2004): 230–41.
24. J. Kabat-Zinn, *Coming to Our Senses: Healing Ourselves and the World through Mindfulness* (New York: Hyperion, 2005).
25. National Center for Complementary and Alternative Medicine (NCCAM), "Research Spotlight: Meditation May Increase Empathy," Modified October 2009, http://nccam.nih.gov/research/results/spotlight/060608.htm.
26. D. Oman, S. Shapiro, C. Thoreson, T. Plante, and T. Flinders, "Meditation Lowers Stress and Supports Forgiveness among College Students: A Randomized Controlled Trial," *Journal of American College Health* 56, no. 5 (2008): 425–31.
27. National Center for Complementary and Alternative Medicine (NCCAM), "Research Spotlight: Meditation May Make Information Processing in the Brain More Efficient," Modified October 2009, http://nccam.nih.gov/research/results/spotlight/082307.htm; A. Chiesa and A. Serretti, "Mindfulness-Based Stress Reduction for Stress Management in Healthy People," 2009; N. Y. Winbush, C. R. Gross, and M. J. Kreitzer, "The Effects of Mindfulness-Based Stress Reduction on Sleep Disturbance: A Systematic Review. *EXPLORE: The Journal of Science and Healing* 3, no. 6 (2007): 585–91; N. E. Morone, C. S. Lynch, C. M. Greco, H. A. Tindle, and D. K. Weiner, "'I Felt Like a New Person.' The Effects of Mindfulness Meditation on Older Adults with Chronic Pain: Qualitative Narrative Analysis of Diary Entries," *Journal of Pain*, no. 9 (2008): 841–48.
28. Environmental Protection Agency (EPA), "Environmental Stewardship," Updated January 6, 2010, www.epa.gov/stewardship.

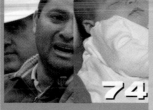
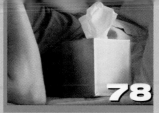
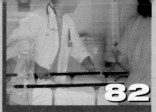

**74** Isn't some stress healthy?

**78** Why do I always get sick during finals week?

**82** Who is most prone to stress?

# Managing Stress and Coping with Life's Challenges

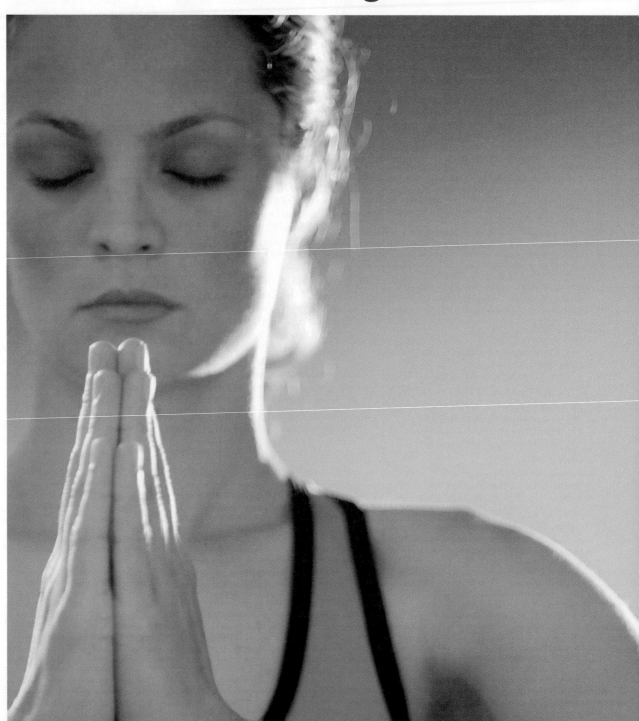

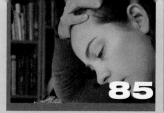

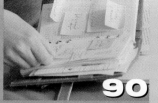

**85**

Are college students more stressed out than other groups?

**90**

How can I manage my time more effectively?

Rising tuition, roommates who bug you, dating anxiety, pressure to get good grades, money, and future career worries—they all lead up to STRESS! In today's fast-paced, 24/7 connected world, stress can cause us to feel overwhelmed. It can also cause us to push ourselves to improve performance, bring excitement and a "rush" into an otherwise humdrum life, and leave us exhilarated. While we work, play, socialize, and sleep, stress affects us in myriad ways, many of which we may not even notice.

**9%**

of college students report experiencing "tremendous stress" over the past 12 months.

According to a recent American Psychological Association poll, 75 percent of American adults reported experiencing moderate to high levels of stress in the past month. Nearly half of American adults (45%) believe that their stress has increased over the past 5 years, affecting their personal and professional lives.[1] The exact toll stress exerts on us during a lifetime of overload is unknown, but we know stress is a significant health hazard. It can rob the body of needed nutrients, damage the cardiovascular system, raise blood pressure, increase our risks for cancer and diabetes, and dampen the immune system's defenses. In addition, it can drain our emotional reserves; contribute to depression, anxiety, fatigue, and irritability; and punctuate social interactions with hostility and anger.

Is too much stress an inevitable negative part of life? Fortunately, the answer is no. To make stress more a friend than an enemy, we can learn to anticipate and recognize our personal stressors and develop skills to reduce or better manage those stressors we cannot avoid or control. First, we must understand what stress is and what effects it has on the body.

## Objectives

✳ Define stress and examine its potential impact on health, relationships, and success in college.

✳ Explain the phases of the general adaptation syndrome and the physiological changes that occur during them.

✳ Examine the physical, emotional, and social health risks that may occur with chronic stress.

✳ Discuss sources of stress and examine the unique stressors that affect college students.

✳ Explore stress-management techniques and ways to enrich your life with positive experiences and attitudes.

## What Is Stress?

Most current definitions state that **stress** is the mental and physical response and adaptation by our bodies to the real or perceived changes and challenges in our lives. A **stressor** is any real or perceived physical, social, or psychological event or stimulus that causes our bodies to react or respond.[2] Several factors influence one's response to stressors including *characteristics of the stressor* (Can you control it? Is it predictable? Does it occur often?); *biological factors* (e.g., your age or gender); and *past experiences* (e.g., things that have happened to you, their consequences, and how you responded). Stressors may be tangible, such as a failing grade on a test, or intangible, such as the angst associated with meeting your significant other's parents for the first time. Importantly, stress is in the eye of

**stress** A series of physiological responses and adaptations in response to a real or imagined threat to one's well-being.

**stressor** A physical, social, or psychological event or condition that upsets homeostasis and produces a stress response.

the beholder: Each person's unique combination of heredity, life experiences, personality, and ability to cope influences how the person perceives an event and what meaning he or she attaches to it. What "stresses out" one person may not even bother the next person.

Stress can be associated with most daily activities. Generally, positive stress is called **eustress.** Eustress presents the opportunity for personal growth and satisfaction and can actually improve health. It can energize you, motivate you, and raise you up when you are down. Getting married or winning a major competition can give rise to the pleasurable rush associated with eustress. **Distress,** or negative stress, is caused by events that result in debilitative tension and strain, such as financial problems, the death of a loved one, academic difficulties, and the breakup of a relationship. There are two kinds of distress: **Acute stress** is typically intense, flares quickly, and disappears

quickly. If you view a TV program in which a knife-wielding murderer lurks in a bedroom closet and watches a sleeping victim, your stress response might zoom into overdrive for a short time, only to be relieved when the CSI team swoops in and intervenes. **Chronic stress** may not appear as intense but it can linger indefinitely and wreak silent havoc on your body systems. Losing your mother after her long battle with breast cancer can cause prolonged stress responses in your body. For months after her death, you may struggle to balance the need to process emotions such as anger, grief, loneliness, and guilt, while focusing to stay caught up in classes and with your life.[3]

# Your Body's Response to Stress

From the beginning of human life on Earth, when the need to respond quickly to danger was a matter of life or death, the body's physiological responses evolved to protect humans from harm. If you didn't respond by fighting or fleeing, you might have been eaten by a saber-toothed tiger or killed by a marauding enemy clan. Today, although we sometimes face real or perceived tigers in angry friends, vicious verbal attacks, or more insidious insults, these same, very real, physiological responses must be contained or repressed. Continually having to "stuff" our reactions rather than letting our physiological responses run their course can harm our health over time.

## The General Adaptation Syndrome

When stress levels are low, the body is often in a state of **homeostasis:** All body systems are operating smoothly to maintain equilibrium. Stressors trigger a "crisis-mode" physiological response, after which the body attempts to return to homeostasis by means of an **adaptive response.** First characterized by Hans Selye in 1936, the internal fight to restore homeostasis in the face of a stressor is known as the **general adaptation syndrome (GAS)** (Figure 3.1). The GAS has three distinct phases: alarm, resistance, and exhaustion.[4] It's important to note that regardless of whether positive or negative events cause your eustress or distress, similar physiological changes will occur in your body.

**Alarm Phase** Suppose you are walking to your residence hall after a night class on a dimly lit campus. As you pass a particularly dark area, you hear someone

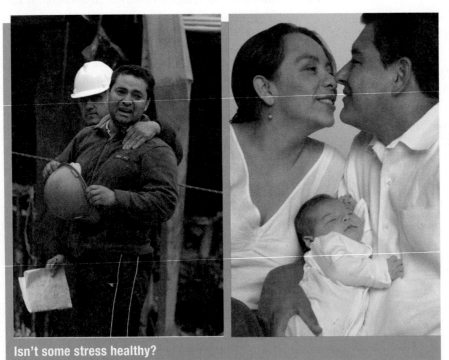

**Isn't some stress healthy?**

Absolutely! Stress isn't necessarily bad for you: Although events that cause prolonged *distress,* such as a natural disaster, can undermine your health, events that cause *eustress,* such as the birth of a child, can have positive effects on your growth and well-being. In general, people perform at their best and live their lives to the fullest when they experience a moderate level of stress—just enough to keep them challenged and motivated—and deal with that stress in a productive manner. Just as too much stress can be detrimental to your health, too little stress leaves you stagnant and unfulfilled.

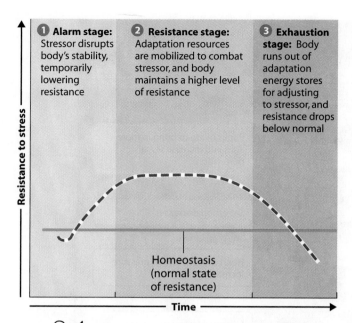

**FIGURE 3.1 The General Adaptation Syndrome (GAS)**
The GAS describes the body's method of coping with prolonged stress.

cough behind you, and you sense someone approaching rapidly. You walk faster, only to hear the quickened footsteps of the other person. Your senses become increasingly alert, your breathing quickens, your heart races, and you begin to perspire. In desperation you stop, rip off your backpack, and prepare to fling it at your attacker to defend yourself. You turn around quickly and let out a blood-curdling yell. To your surprise, the only person you see is a classmate: She has been trying to stay close to you out of her own anxiety about walking alone in the dark. She screams and backs off the sidewalk into the bushes, and you both stare at each other in startled embarrassment. You have just experienced the alarm phase of the GAS. Also known as the **fight-or-flight response,** this physiological reaction is one of our most basic, innate survival instincts.[5]

How does this work, exactly? When the mind perceives a real or imaginary stressor, the cerebral cortex, the region of the brain that interprets the nature of an event, triggers an **autonomic nervous system (ANS)** response that prepares the body for action. The ANS is the portion of the central nervous system regulating body functions that we do not normally consciously control, such as heart and glandular functions and breathing.

The ANS has two branches: sympathetic and parasympathetic. The **sympathetic nervous system** energizes the body for fight or flight by signaling the release of several stress hormones. The **parasympathetic nervous system** functions to slow all the systems stimulated by the stress response—in effect, it counteracts the actions of the sympathetic branch.

The responses of the sympathetic nervous system to stress involve a series of biochemical exchanges between different parts of the body. The **hypothalamus,** a structure in the brain, functions as the control center of the sympathetic nervous system and determines the overall reaction to stressors. When the hypothalamus perceives that extra energy is needed to fight a stressor, it stimulates the adrenal glands, located near the top of the kidneys, to release the hormone **epinephrine,** also called *adrenaline.* Epinephrine causes more blood to be pumped with each beat of the heart, dilates the airways in the lungs to increase oxygen intake, increases the breathing rate, stimulates the liver to release more glucose (which fuels muscular exertion), and dilates the pupils to improve visual sensitivity (see **Figure 3.2** on page 76). The body is then poised to act immediately.

In addition to the fight-or-flight response, the alarm phase can also trigger a longer-term reaction to stress. The hypothalamus uses chemical messages to trigger the pituitary gland within the brain to release a powerful hormone, *adrenocorticotropic hormone (ACTH).* ACTH signals the adrenal glands to release **cortisol,** a hormone that makes stored nutrients more readily available to meet energy demands. Finally, other parts of the brain and body release endorphins, which relieve pain that a stressor may cause.

**Resistance Phase** In the resistance phase of the GAS, the body tries to return to homeostasis by resisting the alarm responses. However, because some perceived stressor still exists, the body does not achieve complete calm or rest. Instead, the body stays activated or aroused at a level that causes a higher metabolic rate in some organ tissues. For example, if a loved one develops an aggressive form of cancer, you may be wild with grief or anxiety after hearing the diagnosis and all of your systems may respond in the alarm phase. As you get used to the diagnosis, you calm down somewhat, but your body does not return completely to rest. The organs and systems of resistance are working overtime.

**Exhaustion Phase** A prolonged effort to adapt to the stress response leads to **allostatic load,** or exhaustive wear and tear on the body.[6] In the exhaustion phase of the GAS, the physical and emotional energy used to fight a stressor has been depleted. As the body adjusts to chronic unresolved stress, the adrenal glands continue to release cortisol, which remains in the bloodstream for longer periods of time as a result of slower metabolic responsiveness. Over time, cortisol can reduce **immunocompetence,** or the ability of the immune system to respond to attack. Blood

**fight-or-flight response**
Physiological arousal response in which the body prepares to combat or escape a real or perceived threat.
**autonomic nervous system (ANS)**
The portion of the central nervous system regulating body functions that a person does not normally consciously control.
**sympathetic nervous system**
Branch of the autonomic nervous system responsible for stress arousal.
**parasympathetic nervous system**
Branch of the autonomic nervous system responsible for slowing systems stimulated by the stress response.
**hypothalamus** A structure in the brain that controls the sympathetic nervous system and directs the stress response.
**epinephrine** Also called *adrenaline,* a hormone that stimulates body systems in response to stress.
**cortisol** Hormone released by the adrenal glands that makes stored nutrients more readily available to meet energy demands.
**allostatic load** Wear and tear on the body caused by prolonged or excessive stress responses.
**immunocompetence** The ability of the immune system to respond to attack.

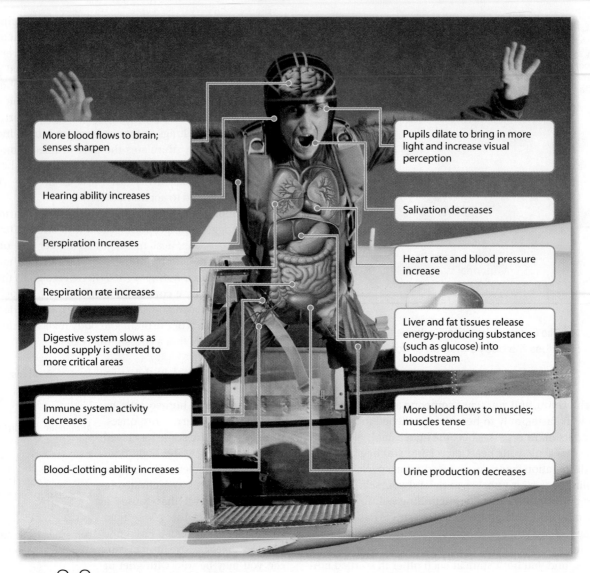

FIGURE 3.2 **The Body's Acute Stress Response**
Exposure to stress of any kind causes a complex series of involuntary physiological responses.

Labels in figure:
- More blood flows to brain; senses sharpen
- Hearing ability increases
- Perspiration increases
- Respiration rate increases
- Digestive system slows as blood supply is diverted to more critical areas
- Immune system activity decreases
- Blood-clotting ability increases
- Pupils dilate to bring in more light and increase visual perception
- Salivation decreases
- Heart rate and blood pressure increase
- Liver and fat tissues release energy-producing substances (such as glucose) into bloodstream
- More blood flows to muscles; muscles tense
- Urine production decreases

pressure can remain dangerously elevated, you may catch colds more easily, or your body's ability to control blood glucose levels can be affected.

## Effects of Stress on Your Life

Much has been written about the negative effects of stress, but researchers have only recently begun to untangle the complex web of physiological and emotional responses that can take a toll on a person's physical, intellectual, and emotional well-being. Stress is often described as a "disease of prolonged arousal" that leads to a cascade of negative health effects. The longer you are chronically stressed, the more likely will be the negative health effects.

# 40%

**of deaths in the United States are related wholly or in part to stress.**

Nearly all body systems become potential targets, and the long-term effects may be devastating. Some warning symptoms of prolonged stress are shown in Figure 3.3.

## Physical Effects of Stress

Studies show that 40 percent of deaths and 70 percent of diseases in the United States are related, in whole or in part, to stress.[7] The list of ailments related to chronic stress includes heart disease, diabetes, cancer, headaches, ulcers, low back pain, depression, and the common cold. Increases in rates of suicide, homicide, and domestic violence across the United States are additional symptoms of a nation under stress.

**Stress and Cardiovascular Disease** Perhaps the most studied and documented health consequence of unresolved

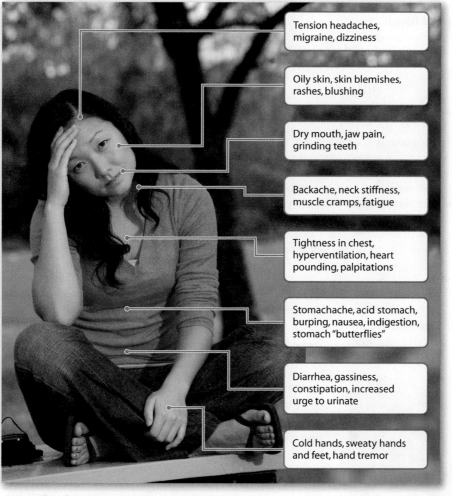

FIGURE 3.3 **Common Physical Symptoms of Stress**
Sometimes you may not even notice how stressed you are until your body starts sending you signals. Do you frequently experience any of these physical symptoms of stress?

Tension headaches, migraine, dizziness

Oily skin, skin blemishes, rashes, blushing

Dry mouth, jaw pain, grinding teeth

Backache, neck stiffness, muscle cramps, fatigue

Tightness in chest, hyperventilation, heart pounding, palpitations

Stomachache, acid stomach, burping, nausea, indigestion, stomach "butterflies"

Diarrhea, gassiness, constipation, increased urge to urinate

Cold hands, sweaty hands and feet, hand tremor

stress is cardiovascular disease (CVD). Research on this topic demonstrates the impact of chronic stress on heart rate, blood pressure, heart attack, and stroke.[8] The largest epidemiological study to date, the INTERHEART Study with almost 30,000 participants in 52 countries, identified stress as one of the key modifiable risk factors for heart attack.[9]

Historically, the increased risk of CVD from chronic stress has been linked to increased arterial plaque buildup due to elevated cholesterol, hardening of the arteries, alterations in heart rhythm, increased and fluctuating blood pressures, and difficulties in cardiovascular responsiveness due to all of the above.[10] In the past two decades, research into the relationship between stress and CVD contributors has shown direct links between the incidence and progression of CVD and stressors such as job strain, caregiving,

bereavement, and natural disasters.[11] For more information about CVD, see Chapter 15.

**Stress and Weight Gain** If you have a nagging suspicion that when you are extremely stressed, you tend to eat more and gain more weight, guess what? You didn't imagine it. Higher stress levels may increase cortisol levels in the bloodstream. Because cortisol contributes to increased hunger and seems to activate fat-storing enzymes, people who are stressed may get a double whammy of risks from higher-circulating cortisol levels. Animal and human studies seem to support the theory that cortisol plays a role in laying down extra belly fat and increasing eating behaviors.[12]

**Stress and Hair Loss** Too much stress can lead to thinning hair, and even baldness, in men and women. The most common type of stress-induced hair loss is *telogen effluvium*. Often seen in individuals who have suffered a death in the family, had a difficult pregnancy, or experienced severe weight loss, this condition pushes colonies of hair to go into a resting phase. Over time (usually a few months), simply washing or combing the hair may cause clumps of it to fall out. A similar stress-related condition known as *alopecia areata* occurs when stress triggers white blood cells to attack and destroy hair follicles, usually in patches. If stress is prolonged, varying degrees of baldness may occur.[13]

**Stress and Diabetes** Controlling stress levels is critical for preventing development of type 2 diabetes, as well as for successful short- and long-term diabetes management.[14] People under lots of stress often don't get enough sleep, don't eat well, and may drink or take other drugs to help them get through a stressful time. All of these behaviors can alter blood sugar levels and promote development of diabetes. For full information on diabetes, see Focus On: Minimizing Your Risk for Diabetes beginning on page 514.

Losing hair? Maybe you need to de-stress!

**Stress and Digestive Problems** Digestive disorders are physical conditions whose causes are often unknown. It is widely assumed that an underlying illness, pathogen, injury, or inflammation is already present when stress triggers nausea, vomiting, stomach cramps and related gut pain, or diarrhea. Although stress doesn't directly cause these symptoms, it is clearly related and may actually make your risk of having symptoms even worse.[15] For example, people with depression or anxiety are more susceptible to irritable bowel syndrome, probably because stress stimulates colon spasms via the nervous system.

## Stress and Impaired Immunity

As discussed in Chapter 2, a growing area of scientific investigation known as *psychoneuroimmunology (PNI)* analyzes the intricate relationship between the mind's response to stress and the immune system's ability to function effectively. Several recent reviews of research linking stress to adverse health consequences suggest that too much stress over a long period can negatively affect various aspects of the cellular immune response.[16] How long do you have to be stressed to suffer from

### "Why Should I Care?"

The evidence is compelling that stress and immune system functioning are linked. Exposure to academic stressors and self-reported stress are associated with increased upper respiratory tract infections among students. Take time to de-stress, and you might avoid being on the sidelines with a bad cold.

impaired immunity? A look at the research yields evidence of impaired immunity from the initial stress to as long as 6 months later following acute stressors such as arguments, public speaking, and academic examinations.[17] More prolonged stressors such as the loss of a spouse, exposure to a natural disaster, caregiving, living with a handicap, and unemployment also have been shown to impair the natural immune response among various populations over time.[18]

**Stress and Libido** Although we might think that a lack of interest in sex occurs only in older people and that young people enjoy constant, regular sex, too much stress can throw a big wrench in your sex life at any age and stage of life. For more information on stress and its impact on libido, see the **Gender & Health** box on the next page.

# Intellectual Effects of Stress

In a recent national survey of college students, more than half of the respondents said that they had felt overwhelmed by all that they had to do within the past 2 weeks. Forty percent of students felt they had been under more than average stress in the past 12 months, whereas 9.8 percent reported being under tremendous stress during that same time period. Not surprisingly, these same students rated stress as their number one impediment to academic performance,

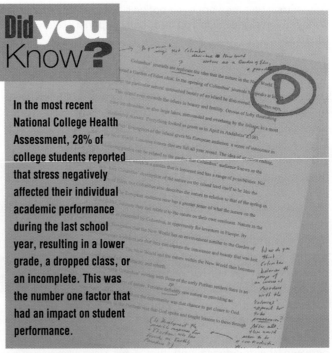

**Why do I always get sick during finals week?**

Prolonged stress can compromise your immune system, leaving you vulnerable to infection. If you spend exam week in a state of high stress—sleeping too little, studying too hard, and worrying a lot—chances are you'll reduce your body's ability to fight off any cold or flu bugs you may encounter.

## Did you Know?

In the most recent National College Health Assessment, 28% of college students reported that stress negatively affected their individual academic performance during the last school year, resulting in a lower grade, a dropped class, or an incomplete. This was the number one factor that had an impact on student performance.

**Source:** Data are from American College Health Association, *American College Health Association—National College Health Assessment II (ACHA-NCHA II) Reference Group Data Report Fall 2009* (Baltimore: ACHA, 2010).

# Stress and Your Sex Drive

Sexual drive, or *libido,* is complex and can be influenced by several psychological and physiological factors. Time pressures, concerns over appearance, anxiety over performance, exhaustion from work, lack of sleep, and the multiple demands of classes and social life can wreak havoc on the libidos of both men and women.

In men, high stress levels can lead to declines in hormone production and low levels of testosterone. A man who is feeling anxious may have trouble having an erection. Even if a male achieves an erection, worries that he should be studying, hasn't started his homework, or can't afford tuition can shut down the erection right in the middle of intercourse. If a male is also prone to erectile dysfunction from other causes (medications, injury, etc.), stress may knock out erections even more quickly.

In women, fluctuating reproductive hormones and irregular menstrual cycles can cause major emotional swings. Stress can disrupt virtually all of the reproductive hormones, causing changes in mood, increased anxiety, and other emotional issues. This stress and hormonal roller coaster can become a vicious cycle, making women particularly vulnerable to stress-related changes in libido. When women are physically and emotionally exhausted or suffering from stress-related insomnia, sex drive is likely to wane. Virtually any extreme stressor on the body, be it the major assault of starvation from anorexia nervosa, exposure to prolonged environmental conditions such as heat and drought, or intense pain and grief, can trigger declines in sexual desire.

Too much stress can have a negative impact on all aspects of your life— including your love life!

**Sources:** V. Bitsika, C. Sharpley, and R. Bell, "The Contribution of Anxiety and Depression to Fatigue among a Sample of Australian University Students: Suggestions for University Counselors," *Counseling Psychology Quarterly* 22, no. 2 (2009): 243–53; A. Katz, "'Not Tonight, Dear': The Elusive Female Libido," *AJN, American Journal of Nursing* 107, no. 12 (2007): 32–34.

followed by lack of sleep.[19] Stress can play a huge role in whether students stay in school, get good grades, and succeed on their career path. It can also wreak havoc on students' ability to concentrate, remember key information for exams, and understand and retain complex information.

**Stress, Memory, and Concentration** Although the exact reasons stress can affect grades are complex, the mystery of how and why stress affects memory and concentration in humans is slowly unraveling. Animal studies have provided compelling indicators of how glucocorticoids—stress hormones released from the adrenal cortex—are believed to affect memory. In humans, acute stress has been shown to impair short-term memory, particularly verbal memory.[20] Exciting new studies have linked prolonged exposure to cortisol (a key stress hormone) to actual shrinking of the hippocampus, the brain's major memory center. In rats that were chronically stressed, the decision-making regions of the brain actually shriveled, whereas brain sectors responsible for habitual behaviors that didn't rely on memory increased.[21]

## Psychological Effects of Stress

Stress may be one of the single greatest contributors to mental disability and emotional dysfunction in industrialized nations. Studies have shown that the rates of mental disorders, particularly depression and anxiety, are associated with various environmental stressors, including divorce, marital conflict, economic hardship, and other stressful life events.[22] In particular, stressful life events and inadequate sources of

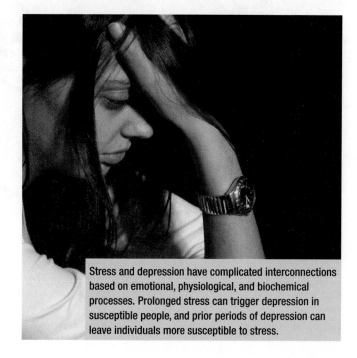

Stress and depression have complicated interconnections based on emotional, physiological, and biochemical processes. Prolonged stress can trigger depression in susceptible people, and prior periods of depression can leave individuals more susceptible to stress.

social support can contribute to mental disorders among people aged 15 to 24 more than among other age groups. Researchers suggest that as individuals move from adolescence into adulthood, they face increased stressors of all kinds, from school to employment to relationships, that may challenge their mental health.[23] The high incidence of suicide among college students is assumed to indicate high personal and societal stress in the lives of young people.[24]

# What Causes Stress?

On any given day, we all experience eustress and distress, usually from a wide range of obvious and not-so-obvious sources. Several studies in recent years have examined sources of stress among various populations in the United States and globally. One of the most comprehensive is conducted annually by the American Psychological Association; the 2009 survey found that concerns over money, work, family, and housing were major sources of stress among American adults (Figure 3.4).[25] College students, in particular, face stressors that come from internal sources, as well as external pressures to succeed in a competitive environment that is often geographically far from the support of family and lifelong friends. Awareness of the sources of stress can do much to help you develop a plan to avoid, prevent, and control the things that cause you stress.

## Psychosocial Stressors

*Psychosocial stressors* refer to the factors in our daily routines and in our social and physical environments that cause us to experience stress. Key psychosocial stressors include adjustment to change, hassles, interpersonal relationships, academic and career pressures, frustrations and conflicts, overload, and stressful environments.

**Adjustment to Change** Any time change occurs in your normal routine, whether good or bad, you experience stress. The more changes you experience and the more adjustments you must make, the greater the chances are that stress will have an impact on your health. Unfortunately, although your first days on campus can be exciting, they can also be among the most stressful you will face in your life. Moving away from home, trying to fit in and make new friends from diverse backgrounds, adjusting to a new schedule, learning to live with strangers in housing that is often lacking in the comforts of home: All of these things can cause sleeplessness and anxiety and keep your body in a continual fight-or-flight mode.

**Hassles: The Little Things That Bug You** Some psychologists have proposed that little stressors, frustrations, and petty annoyances, known collectively as *hassles*, can be just as stressful as the major life changes.[26] Listening to classmates who talk too much during lecture, having to hear someone airing their dirty laundry on a loud cell phone call, not finding parking on campus, and a host of other bothersome situations can push your buttons and result in frustration, anger, and fight-or-flight responses.[27] For many people, the fast pace of technology creates new hassles and adds to their stress. See the **Student Health Today** box on the next page for more on technostress.

**The Toll of Relationships** Let's face it, relationships can trigger some of the biggest fight-or-flight reactions of all time. Remember that wild, exhilarating feeling of new love? You couldn't focus, you couldn't sleep, and

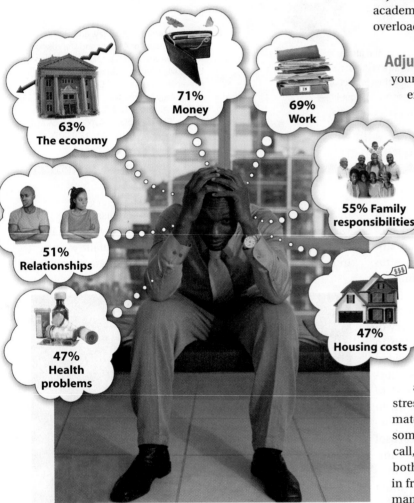

FIGURE 3.4 **What Stresses Us?**
Not surprisingly, over the past few years, the annual *Stress in America* survey has indicated that American adults are increasingly experiencing money, work, and housing concerns as major sources of stress in their lives.

**Source:** Data are from the American Psychological Association, *Stress in America 2009, Executive Summary,* 2009, www.apa.org/news/press/releases/stress/index.aspx.

# Taming Technostress

Are you "twittered out"? Is all that texting causing your thumbs to seize up in protest? If so, you're not alone. Like millions of others, you may find that all of the pressure for contact is stressing you out! Known as *technostress,* this bombardment is defined as stress created by a dependence on technology and the constant state of connection, which can include a perceived obligation to respond, chat, or tweet.

There is much good that comes from all that technological wizardry. For some folks, however, technomania can become obsessive—when people would rather hang out online talking to strangers, than study, talk to friends, socialize in person, or generally connect in the real world. Although technology can allow us to multitask, work on the go, and communicate in new and different ways, there are some clear downsides to all of that "virtual" interaction.

✳ **Distracted driving.** The National Safety Council estimates at least 28 percent of all traffic crashes—or at least 1.6 million crashes each year—are caused by drivers talking on cell phones or texting. A recent survey conducted by Zogby International, a public opinion research group, indicated that as many as 66 percent of young adults aged 18 to 24 are sending text messages while driving, whereas another survey showed that 83 percent of respondents thought the practice should be banned. Right now, more than 19 states have laws banning texting while driving for all drivers.

✳ **BlackBerry thumb.** If you are one of a growing number of persons who have this malady, you already know that it refers to a problem experienced by too much thumb use on today's personal digital assistant (PDA) devices. It causes pain, swelling, or numbness of the thumb. There are exercises to strengthen thumb muscles and help stretch tight muscles and tendons, pain relievers, and more drastic treatments involving injections or surgery, but the best advice is to avoid the malady by stretching thumb muscles before texting and keeping messaging to a minimum.

✳ **Other repetitive stress injuries.** Sitting in front of a computer screen set at the wrong height, or working hunched over a laptop for hours can result in back pain, neck cramps, and carpal tunnel syndrome. Keeping sessions short, stretching muscles frequently, and getting an ergonomic check of your workstation can all help prevent repetitive stress injuries.

✳ **Social distress.** Authors Michell Weil and Larry Rosen describe *technosis,* a very real syndrome in which people become so immersed in technology that they risk losing their own identity. Worrying about checking your voice mail, constantly switching to e-mail or Facebook to see who has left a message or is online, perpetually posting to Twitter, and so on can keep you distracted and take important minutes or hours from your day.

To avoid technosis and to prevent technostress, set time limits on your technology usage, and make sure that you devote at least as much time to face-to-face interactions with people you care about as a means of cultivating and nurturing your relationships. Screen your contacts, especially when you are in public or engaged in face-to-face communication with someone. You don't always need to answer your phone or respond to a text or e-mail immediately.

Leave your devices at home or turn them off when you are out with others or on vacation. If you can't leave your PDA, laptop, or cell phone at home—or turned off—when you are out with others, or on vacation, then there is a problem. Tune in to your surroundings, your loved ones and friends, your job, and your classes by shutting off your devices.

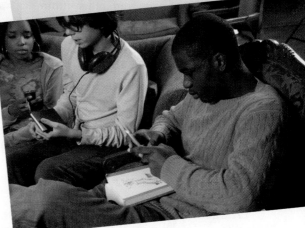

Technology may keep you in touch, but it can also add to your stress and take you away from real-world interactions.

**Sources:** National Safety Council, "National Safety Council Estimates That at Least 1.6 Million Crashes Are Caused Each Year by Drivers Using Cell Phones and Texting," Press Release, January 12, 2010, www.nsc.org/Pages/NSCestimates16million crashescausedbydriversusingcellphonesandtexting .aspx; Governors Highway Safety Association, "Cell Phone and Texting Laws," 2010, www.ghsa.org/ html/stateinfo/laws/cellphone_laws.html; Zogby International, "Text Messaging While Driving Ban in Effect Today," October 2009, www.zogby.com/ SOUNDBITES/ReadClips.cfm?ID=19087; M. Weil and L. Rosen, "Technostress: Are You a Victim?" 2007, www.technostress.com.

you didn't get much work done while thinking about your *new* love interest. Likewise, remember when you ultimately broke up with someone you thought you were deeply in love with, or they broke up with you? You couldn't focus, you couldn't sleep, and you didn't get much done while thinking about your *former* love interest. Love relationships are the ones we often think of first, but friends, family members, and coworkers can be the sources of overwhelming struggles, just as they can be sources of strength and support. These relationships can make us strive to be the best that we can be and give us hope for the future, or they can diminish our self-esteem and leave us reeling from a destructive interaction.

## Academic and Financial Pressure

It isn't surprising that putting a group of top high school graduates into today's colleges and universities and telling them to compete for grades, athletic positions, and jobs and other future goals can cause mind-boggling amounts of pressure. Challenging classes can be tough enough, but many students also work at least part-time to pay the bills. Even in times of economic prosperity, students often have a tough time meeting all of their costs and obligations. Today's economic downturn can have major effects on college students and make distant dreams even harder to realize.

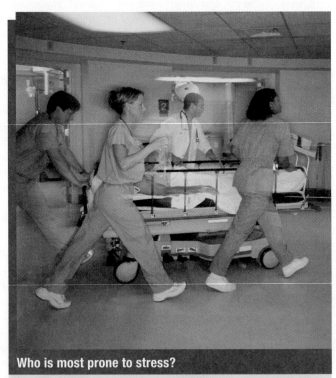

Traffic jams and noise pollution are examples of the daily hassles and frustrations that can add up and jeopardize our health.

**Frustrations and Conflicts** Whenever there is a disparity between our goals (what we hope to obtain in life) and our behaviors (actions that may or may not lead to these goals), frustration can occur. For example, you realize that you must get good grades in college to enter graduate school, which is your ultimate goal. If you know you should be getting good grades, but are having too much fun with friends when you should be studying, these inconsistencies between your goals and your behavior can cause significant stress.

Conflicts occur when we are forced to decide among competing motives, impulses, desires, and behaviors, or when we are forced to face pressures of demands that are incompatible with our own values and sense of importance. College students who are away from their families for the first time may face a variety of conflicts among parental values, their own beliefs, and the beliefs of others who are very different from themselves.

**Overload** We've all experienced times in our lives when the demands of work, responsibilities, deadlines, and relationships all seem to be pulling us underwater with a 200-pound weight tied to our feet. **Overload** occurs when, try as we might, there are not nearly enough hours in the day to do what we are required to do and our physical, mental, and emotional reserves are not sufficient to deal with all we have on our plate. Students suffering from overload may experience depression, sleeplessness, mood swings, frustration, anxiety, or a host of other symptoms. Binge drinking; high consumption of junk foods; and fighting with friends, family, and coworkers can all add fuel to the overload fire.[28] Unrelenting stress and overload can lead

**overload** A condition in which a person feels overly pressured by demands.
**background distressors** Environmental stressors of which people are often unaware.

to a state of physical and mental exhaustion known as *burnout*.

**Stressful Environments** For many students, where they live and the environment around them cause significant levels of stress. Many students cannot afford quality housing, and unscrupulous landlords have been known to exploit students by leasing them substandard, even unhealthy, apartments. Roommates can cause major environmental stress by not cleaning up after themselves, creating excessive clutter, invading your privacy, damaging your property, and being inconsiderate in many other ways.

Although rare, natural disasters can wreak havoc on our lives, causing environmental stress. Flooding, earthquakes, hurricanes, blizzards, and tornadoes can all disrupt students' ability to attend class and conduct their daily lives. Often as damaging as one-time disasters are **background distressors** in the environment, such as noise, air, and water pollution; allergy-aggravating pollen and dust; or

### Who is most prone to stress?

Everyone experiences stress in his or her life, but some people have personalities and attitudes that leave them more susceptible, whereas others have careers or life circumstances that impose greater external pressures on them. Individuals such as doctors and nurses face long work hours and a high-stakes work environment, making them especially prone to stress, overload, and burnout.

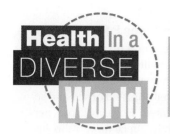

# Health In a DIVERSE World

## International Student Stress

International students experience unique adjustment issues related to language barriers, cultural barriers, and a lack of social support, among other challenges. Academic stress may pose a particular problem for the more than 670,000 international students who have left support networks of family and friends in their native countries to study in the United States. Accumulating evidence suggests that seeking emotional support from others is among the most effective ways to cope with stressful and upsetting situations. Yet, many international students refrain from doing so because of cultural norms, feelings of shame, and the belief that seeking support is a sign of weakness that calls inappropriate attention to both the individual and the respective ethnic group. This reluctance, coupled with the language barriers, cultural conflicts, and other stressors, can lead international students to suffer significantly more stress-related

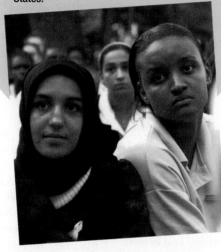

Language barriers, cultural conflicts, racial prejudices, and a reluctance to seek social support all contribute to a significantly higher rate of stress-related illnesses among international students studying in the United States.

illnesses than their American counterparts. Even if we can't solve the many

problems international students encounter, there are things we can do to make one person's life (or maybe two or three persons' lives) a little less stressful: Share companionship and communication, and lend a helping hand. To paraphrase a popular Hindu proverb: "Help thy neighbor's boat across and thine own boat will also reach the shore."

**Sources:** S. Sumer, "International Students' Psychological and Sociocultural Adaptation in the United States," Georgia State University, Doctoral Dissertation, 2009, http://digitalarchive.gsu.edu/cps_diss/34; Institute of International Education, "Record Numbers of International Students in U.S. Higher Education," Press Release, November 16, 2009, http://opendoors.iienetwork.org/?p=150649; S. T. Mortenson, "Cultural Differences and Similarities in Seeking Social Support as a Response to Academic Failure: A Comparison of American and Chinese College Students," *Communication Education* 55 no. 2 (2006): 127–46.

## what do you think?

Do you get stressed out by things in your home or school environment? ● Which environmental stressors bug you the most? ● When you encounter these environmental stressors, what actions do you take, if any?

environmental tobacco smoke. As with other challenges, our bodies respond to environmental distressors with the GAS. People who cannot escape background distressors may exist in a constant resistance phase.

### Bias and Discrimination

Racial and ethnic diversity of students, faculty members, and staff enriches everyone's educational experience on campus. It also challenges us to examine our personal attitudes, beliefs, and biases. Students come to campus from vastly different backgrounds and with very different life experiences. Often, those perceived as dissimilar may become victims of subtle and not-so-subtle forms of bigotry, insensitivity, harassment, or hostility, or they may simply be ignored. Race, ethnicity, religious affiliation, age, sexual orientation, or other "differences"—whether in viewpoints, appearance, behaviors, or backgrounds—may hang like a

dark cloud over these students.[29] See the **Health in a Diverse World** box above for more on stress and international students.

Evidence of the health effects of excessive stress in minority groups abounds. For example, African Americans suffer higher rates of hypertension, CVD, and most cancers than do whites.[30] Although poverty and socioeconomic status have been blamed for much of the spike in hypertension rates for African Americans and other marginalized groups, this chronic, physically debilitating stress may reflect real and perceived effects of harassment in society more than it reflects actual poverty.[31]

## Internal Stressors

Although stress can come from the environment and other external sources, it can result from internal factors as well. Internal stressors such as negative appraisal, low self-esteem, and low self-efficacy can cause unsettling thoughts or feelings, and can ultimately affect your health.[32] It is important to address and manage these internal stressors.

**Appraisal and Stress** Throughout life, we encounter many different types of demands and potential stressors—some biological, some psychological, and others sociological. In any case, it is our appraisal of these demands, not the demands themselves, that results in our experiencing stress. **Appraisal** is defined as the interpretation and evaluation of information provided to the brain by the senses. Appraisal is not a conscious activity, but rather a natural process that the brain constantly performs. As new information becomes available, appraisal helps us recognize stressors, evaluate them on the basis of past experiences and emotions, and decide how to cope with them. When you perceive that your coping resources are sufficient to meet life's demands, you experience little or no stress. By contrast, when you perceive that life's demands exceed your coping resources, you are likely to feel strain and distress.

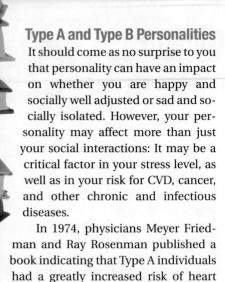

How daunting that pile of books and homework is all depends on your own appraisal of it.

**Self-Esteem and Self-Efficacy** As we learned in Chapters 1 and 2, *self-esteem* refers to how you feel about yourself. Self-esteem varies; it can and does continually change.[33] When you feel good about yourself, you are less likely to respond to or interpret an event as stressful. Conversely, if you place little or no value on yourself and believe you have inadequate coping skills, you become susceptible to stress and strain.[34] Of particular concern, research with high school and college students has found that low self-esteem and stressful life events significantly predict **suicidal ideation,** a desire to die and thoughts about suicide. On a more positive note, research has also indicated that it is possible to increase an individual's ability to cope with stress by increasing self-esteem.[35] In Chapter 2 we discussed several ways to develop and maintain self-esteem.

*Self-efficacy,* also introduced in earlier chapters, is another important factor in the ability to cope with life's challenges. Self-efficacy refers to belief or confidence in one's skills and performance abilities.[36] Self-efficacy is considered one of the most important personality traits that influences psychological and physiological stress responses and has been found to predict a number of health behaviors in college students.[37] Developing self-efficacy is also vital to coping with and overcoming academic pressures and worries. For example, by learning to handle anxiety around testing situations, you improve your chances of performing well; the more you feel yourself capable to handle testing situations, the greater will be your sense of academic self-efficacy. For tips on how to deal with test-taking anxiety and build your testing self-efficacy, see the **Skills for Behavior Change** box on the next page.

**appraisal** The interpretation and evaluation of information provided to the brain by the senses.

**suicidal ideation** A desire to die and thoughts about suicide.

**hostility** The cognitive, affective, and behavioral tendencies toward anger and cynicism.

**psychological hardiness** A personality trait characterized by control, commitment, and the embrace of challenge.

**Type A and Type B Personalities** It should come as no surprise to you that personality can have an impact on whether you are happy and socially well adjusted or sad and socially isolated. However, your personality may affect more than just your social interactions: It may be a critical factor in your stress level, as well as in your risk for CVD, cancer, and other chronic and infectious diseases.

In 1974, physicians Meyer Friedman and Ray Rosenman published a book indicating that Type A individuals had a greatly increased risk of heart disease.[38] *Type A* personalities are defined as hard-driving, competitive, time-driven perfectionists. In contrast, *Type B* personalities are described as being relaxed, noncompetitive, and more tolerant of others.

Today, most researchers recognize that none of us will be wholly Type A or Type B all of the time. We might exhibit either type as we respond to the various challenges of our daily lives. In addition, recent research indicates that not all Type A people experience negative health consequences; in fact, some hard-driving individuals seem to thrive on their supercharged lifestyles. Only those Type A individuals who exhibit a "toxic core"; have disproportionate amounts of anger; are distrustful of others; and have a cynical, glass-half-empty approach to life—a set of characteristics referred to as **hostility**—are at increased risk for heart disease.[39]

**Type C and Type D Personalities** In addition to CVD risks, personality types have been linked to increased risk for a variety of illnesses, ranging from asthma to cancer. *Type C* personality is one such type. Typically, Type C people are stoic and tend to deny feelings. They have a tendency to conform to the wishes of others (or to be "pleasers"), a lack of assertiveness, and an inclination toward feelings of helplessness or hopelessness. Possibly as a result of these characteristics, research indicates they are more susceptible to illnesses such as asthma, multiple sclerosis, autoimmune disorders, and cancer.[40] They are the "nice" guys and gals who really do finish last when it comes to their health.

A more recently identified personality type is *Type D* (distressed), which is characterized by a tendency toward excessive negative worry, irritability, gloom, and social inhibition. Several recent studies have shown that Type D people may be up to eight times more likely to die of a heart attack or sudden cardiac death.[41]

**Psychological Hardiness** According to psychologist Susanne Kobasa, **psychological hardiness** may negate self-imposed stress associated with Type A behavior. Psychologically

## Overcoming Test-Taking Anxiety

Testing well is a skill needed in college and beyond. Try these helpful hints on your next exam.

### BEFORE THE EXAM

✴ Manage your study time. Start studying a week before your test to reduce anxiety. Do a limited review the night before, get a good night's sleep, and arrive for the exam early.

✴ Build your test-taking self-esteem. On an index card, write down three reasons you will pass the exam. Keep the card with you and review it whenever you study. When you get the test, write your three reasons on the test or on a piece of scrap paper.

✴ Eat a balanced meal before the exam. Avoid sugar and rich or heavy foods, as well as foods that might upset your stomach. You want to feel your best.

✴ If you feel that you are a slow reader and need more time, discuss this in advance with your teacher or test administrator.

### DURING THE TEST

✴ Manage your time during the test. Decide how much time you need to take the test, review your answers, and go back over questions you might be stuck on. Hold to this schedule.

✴ Slow down and pay attention. When you open your test book, always write "RTFQ" (Read the Full Question) at the top. Make sure you understand the question before answering.

✴ Stay on track. If you begin to get anxious, reread your three reasons for success.

hardy people are characterized by control, commitment, and willingness to embrace challenge.[42] People with a sense of control are able to accept responsibility for their behaviors and change those that they discover to be debilitating. People with a sense of commitment have good self-esteem and understand their purpose in life. Those who embrace challenge see change as a stimulating opportunity for personal growth. The concept of hardiness has been studied extensively, and many researchers believe it is the foundation of an individual's ability to cope with stress and remain healthy.[43]

# Managing Stress in College

College students thrive under a certain amount of stress, but excessive stress can leave them overwhelmed and less than enthusiastic about their classes and social interactions. In fact, two 2009 studies by the Higher Education Research Institute found that 40 percent of first-year students and 35 percent of seniors were overwhelmed much of the time.[44] Relationships, school events, safety, and feeling deviant from school norms are particularly distressful. In addition, studies have indicated that first-year students report not only more problems with these issues, but also more emotional reactivity in the form of anger, hostility, frustration, and a greater sense of being out of control.[45] Sophomores and juniors reported fewer problems with these issues, and seniors reported the fewest problems. This may indicate students' progressive emotional growth through experience, maturity, increased awareness of support services, and more social connections.

Students generally report using health-enhancing methods to combat stress, but research has found that students sometimes resort to health-compromising activities to escape the stress and anxiety of college.[46] Numerous researchers have found stress among college students to be correlated to unhealthy behaviors such as substance abuse, lack of physical activity, poor psychological and physical health, lack of social problem solving, and infrequent use of social support networks.[47]

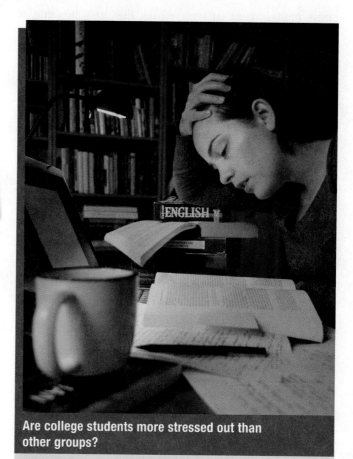

**Are college students more stressed out than other groups?**

Studies suggest that college students are indeed more stressed out than many other groups of people. The combination of a new environment; peer and parental pressure; and the many demands of course work, campus activities, and social life likely contributes to this higher-than-usual stress.

Being on your own in college may pose challenges; but it also lets you take control of and responsibility for your life, evaluate your unique situation, and take steps that fit your schedule and lifestyle to reduce negative stressors in your life.

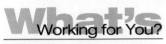
Although you can't eliminate all life stressors, you can train yourself to recognize the events that cause stress and to anticipate your reactions to them. **Coping** is the act of managing events or conditions to lessen the physical or psychological effects of excess stress.[48] One of the most effective ways to combat stressors is to build coping strategies and skills, known collectively as *stress-management techniques,* such as the ones discussed in the following sections.

## Practicing Mental Work to Reduce Stress

Stress management isn't something that just happens. It calls for getting a handle on what is going on in your life, taking a careful look at yourself, and coming up with a personal plan of action. Because your perceptions are often part of the problem, assessing your "self-talk," beliefs, and actions are good first steps. Why are you so stressed? How much of it is due to perception rather than reality? What's a realistic plan of action for you? Think about your situation and map out a strategy for change. The tools in this section will help you.

**Assess Your Stressors and Solve Problems** Assessing what is really going on in your life is an important first step to solving problems and reducing your stress. Here's how:

- Make a list of the major things that you are worried about right now.
- Examine the causes of the problems and worries.
- Consider how big each problem is. What are the consequences of doing nothing? Of taking action?
- List your options, including ones that you may not like very much.
- Outline an action plan, and then act. Remember that even little things can sometimes make a big difference and that you shouldn't expect immediate results.
- After you act, evaluate. How did you do? Do you need to change your actions to achieve a better outcome next time? How?

One useful way of coping with your stressors, once you have identified them, is to consciously

coping Managing events or conditions to lessen the physical or psychological effects of excess stress.
stress inoculation Stress-management technique in which a person consciously tries to prepare ahead of time for potential stressors.
cognitive restructuring The modification of thoughts, ideas, and beliefs that contribute to stress.

anticipate and prepare for specific stressors, a technique known as **stress inoculation.** For example, suppose speaking in front of a class scares you. Practice in front of friends or in front of a video camera to banish panic and prevent your freezing up on the day of the presentation. The assumption is that by dealing with smaller fears, you develop resistance, so that larger fears do not seem so overwhelming.

**Change the Way You Think and Talk to Yourself** As noted earlier, our appraisal of people and situations is what makes these things stressful, not the people or situations themselves. Several types of negative self-talk exist, but among the most common are *pessimism,* or focusing on the negative; *perfectionism,* or expecting superhuman standards; *"should-ing,"* or reprimanding yourself for items that you should have done; *blaming* yourself or others for circumstances and events; and *dichotomous thinking,* in which everything is either black or white (good or bad) instead of gradated.[49] To combat negative self-talk, we must first become aware of it, then stop it, and finally replace the negative thoughts with positive ones—a process referred to as **cognitive restructuring.** Once you realize that some of your thoughts may be irrational or overreactive, interrupt this self-talk by saying, "Stop" (under your breath or out loud), and make a conscious effort to think positively. If you can learn to view stressors in a positive light, you can reduce your stress levels without having to remove the stressors. See the **Skills for Behavior Change** box on the next page for other suggestions of ways to rethink your thinking habits.

## Developing a Support Network

As you plan a stress-management program, remember the importance of social networks and social bonds. Friendships are an important aspect of inoculating yourself against harmful stressors. Studies of college students have demonstrated the importance of social support in buffering individuals from the effects of stress.[50] It isn't necessary to have a large number of friends. However, different friends often serve different needs, so having more than one is usually beneficial.

Family members and friends are often a steady base of support when the pressures of life seem overwhelming. But if friends or family are unavailable, most colleges and universities offer counseling services at no cost for short-term crises. Clergy, instructors, and residence hall supervisors also may be excellent resources. If university services are unavailable, or if you are concerned about confidentiality, most communities offer low-cost counseling through mental health clinics.

**Invest in Your Loved Ones** Imagine if you had absolutely no one you could call when you were in financial trouble or if a loved one died and no one called you. Many people find that they've spent so much of their time pushing ahead in careers or self-improvement that they are alone at the worst times of their lives. As our lives get busy and obligations become over-

## Rethink Your Thinking Habits

✳ **Reframe a distressing event from a positive perspective.** Reframing is a stress-management technique that helps you change your perspective on a situation to a more positive vantage point.

✳ **Worry less.** Don't waste time and energy worrying about things you can't change or events that may never happen. Listen to your self-talk. Tell yourself to *stop*.

✳ **Look at life as being fluid.** If you accept that change is a natural part of living and growing, it will be easier to take.

✳ **Consider alternatives.** There is seldom only one appropriate action. Thinking about your options will help you adjust quickly.

✳ **Moderate your expectations.** Be realistic about your circumstances and motivation.

✳ **Weed out trivia.** Cardiologist Robert Eliot offers two rules for coping with life's challenges: "Don't sweat the small stuff," and remember, "It's all small stuff."

✳ **Don't rush into action.** Think before you act. Consider possible consequences to yourself and others.

✳ **Tolerate mistakes by yourself and others.** Rather than getting upset by mishaps, evaluate what happened and learn from them.

✳ **Live simply.** Eliminate unnecessary things and obligations. Learn to say no. Prioritize. Make commitments only to things you want or have to do.

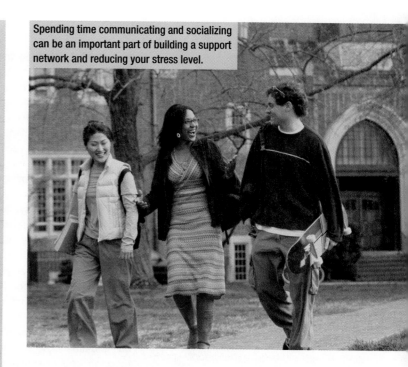

Spending time communicating and socializing can be an important part of building a support network and reducing your stress level.

whelming, we often don't make time for the very people who are most important to us: our friends, family, and other loved ones. In order to have a healthy social support network, we have to invest time and energy. Cultivate and nurture the relationships that matter: those built on trust, mutual acceptance and understanding, honesty, and genuine caring. In addition, treating others empathically provides them with a measure of emotional security and reduces *their* anxiety. If you want others to be there for you to help you cope with life's stressors, you need to be there for them.

### Cultivate Your Spiritual Side

One of the most important factors in reducing overall stress in your life is taking the time and making the commitment to cultivate your spiritual side: finding your purpose in life and living your days more fully. Spiritual health and spiritual practices can be vital components of your support system, often linking you to a community of like-minded individuals and giving you perspective on the things that truly matter in your life. For specific information on the various aspects of spirituality and how it can affect your overall health, see Focus On: Cultivating Your Spiritual Health beginning on page 60.

## Managing Emotional Responses

Have you ever gotten all worked up about something only to find that your perceptions were totally wrong? We often get upset not by realities, but by our faulty perceptions. For example, suppose you found out that everyone except you is invited to a party. You might begin to wonder why you were excluded. Does someone dislike you? Have you offended someone? Such thoughts are typical. However, the reality of the situation may have absolutely nothing to do with your being liked or disliked. Perhaps party organizers didn't have your correct e-mail address, a spam filter blocked the invitation, or it was a simple oversight.

Stress management requires that you examine your emotional responses to interactions with others. With any emotional response to a stressor, you are responsible for the emotion and the resulting behaviors. Learning to tell the difference between normal emotions and emotions based on irrational beliefs or expressed and interpreted in an over-the-top manner can help you stop the emotion or express it in a healthy and appropriate way.

**Learn to Laugh, Be Joyful, and Cry** Have you ever noticed that you feel better after a belly laugh or a good cry? Adages such as "laughter is the best medicine" and "smile and the world smiles with you" didn't just evolve out of the blue. Humans have long recognized that smiling, laughing, singing, dancing, and other actions can elevate our moods, relieve stress, make us feel good, and help us improve our relationships. Crying can have similar positive physiological effects in relieving tension. Several research articles have indicated that laughter and joy may increase endorphin levels, increase oxygen levels in the blood, decrease stress levels, relieve pain, enhance productivity, and reduce risks of chronic disease;

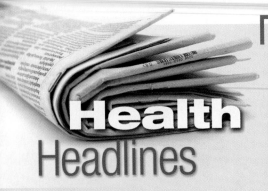

# Health
## Headlines

## FIND HAPPINESS AND REDUCE STRESS

Don't we all just want to be happy? In the past few decades, a field of research called *positive psychology* has emerged to study the truth of that idea. Psychologists in this field believe that people *want* to lead meaningful and fulfilling lives; to cultivate what is best within themselves; and to enhance their life experiences in love, at work, and at play. In studying people's attitudes and choices, and evaluating the outcomes, some positive psychologists found that people who are generally more optimistic or happier have fewer mental and physical health problems. If happiness and optimism are keys to health and stress reduction, how can *you* find them? Experts have a range of opinions on how to achieve the glass-half-full attitude.

✳ **Set realistic goals.** In her best-selling book, *Be Happy without Being Perfect,* psychologist Alice Donner says that striving for a 100 percent dose of contentment and perfection is unrealistic. She suggests that managing your *expectations* is a key. Decide what is realistic for you and work to get to a realistic place in your social structure, your classes, your relationships, and your career.

✳ **Remember that money doesn't buy happiness.** In fact, too much focus on the acquisition of things rather than on relationships and connections may be a major cause of discontent. Also, people who have to pay for a lot of material things tend to work longer hours, vacation less, and in general not take time for themselves.

✳ **Lose yourself in the moment.** According to Mihaly Csikszentmihalyi, a leading expert on positive psychology, finding your flow, a state of effortless concentration and enjoyment, should be a daily goal. What is it that energizes you, makes time fly by, and causes you to concentrate fully on the present? The more often you find and follow that, the happier you'll be.

✳ **Count your blessings.** Although we all can find time to be critical and complain, focusing on our many positive attributes and being thankful for all the good things in our lives should become a daily ritual. For some, this might include daily journaling, a time when they can contemplate all of the good things about their day. Telling your parents how much you appreciate them, telling your friends that they enrich your life, and bringing a smile to someone's face—even if you don't know them—are all important.

✳ **Make changes and reinvigorate.** If you find that your life is ho hum, try new things. For example, try new recipes, find new ways of exercising, plan a fun outing with someone you enjoy once a month, find a new place on campus to study, plan a trip somewhere different in the next 6 months, learn a new skill, or help someone by volunteering your time.

✳ **Forgive and forget.** Rather than ruminating over some slight or indiscretion, try to understand what may have caused someone to act toward you in a hurtful manner, and then move on.

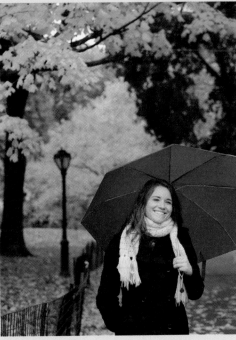

Don't forget to make time for joy and beauty in your life.

✳ **Remember you are worth the time and energy.** Rather than letting yourself succumb to stress, force yourself to prioritize *you*. Your own happiness is as important as that of others in your life. Limit the time you spend with people who bring you down. Instead, find time for breaks, fun interludes, and time alone.

**Sources:** M. Csikszentmihalyi, *Flow: The Psychology of Optimal Experience* (New York: Harper & Row, 1990); The Positive Psychology Center at the University of Pennsylvania, "Frequently Asked Questions," 2007, www.ppc.sas .upenn.edu/faqs.htm; M. E. P. Seligman, *Authentic Happiness: Using the New Positive Psychology to Realize Your Potential for Lasting Fulfillment* (New York: Free Press/Simon & Schuster, 2002); A. Donner, *Be Happy without Being Perfect: How to Break Free from the Perfection Deception* (New York: Random House, 2008).

---

however, the evidence for *long-term* effects on immune functioning and protective effects for chronic diseases is only just starting to be understood.[51] For ideas on how to find more joy and laughter in your daily life, see the **Health Headlines** box above.

**Fight the Anger Urge** Anger usually results when we feel we have lost control of a situation or are frustrated by a situation that we can do little about. Major sources of anger include (1) perceived *threats* to self or others we care about;

(2) *reactions to injustice* such as unfair actions, policies, or behaviors; (3) *fear,* which leads to negative responses; (4) *faulty emotional reasoning,* or misinterpretation of normal events; (5) *low frustration tolerance,* often fueled by stress, drugs, lack of sleep, and other factors; (6) *unreasonable expectations* about ourselves and others; and (7) *people rating,* or applying derogatory ratings to others.

Each of us likely has learned by this point in our lives that there are three main approaches to dealing with anger:

expressing it, suppressing it, or calming it. You may be surprised to find out that expressing your anger is probably the healthiest thing to do in the long run, if you express anger in an assertive rather than an aggressive way. However, it's a natural reaction to want to respond aggressively, and that is what we must learn to keep at bay. To accomplish this, there are several strategies you can use:[52]

- **Identify your anger style.** Do you express anger passively or actively? Do you hold anger in, or do you explode? Do you throw the phone, smash things, or scream at others?
- **Learn to recognize patterns in your anger responses and how to de-escalate them.** For 1 week, keep track of everything that angers you or keeps you stewing. What thoughts or feelings lead up to your boiling point? Keep a journal and listen to your anger. Try to change your self-talk. Explore how you can interrupt patterns of anger, such as counting to 10, getting a drink of water, or taking some deep breaths.
- **Find the right words to de-escalate conflict.** Recent research has shown that when couples are angry and fight, using words that suggest thoughtfulness can reduce conflict.[53] Words such as *think, because, reason, why* demonstrate more consideration for your partner and the issues under fire, as well as a more rational approach.
- **Plan ahead.** Explore options to minimize your exposure to anger-provoking situations such as traffic jams.
- **Develop a support system.** Find a few close friends whom you can confide in or vent your frustration to. Allow them to listen and perhaps provide insight or another perspective that your anger has blinded you to. Don't wear down your supporter with continual rants.
- **Develop realistic expectations of yourself and others.** Anger is often the result of unmet expectations, frustrations, resentments, and impatience. Are your expectations of yourself and others realistic? Try talking with those involved about your feelings at a time when you are calm.
- **Turn complaints into requests.** When frustrated or angry with someone, try reworking the problem into a request. Instead of screaming and pounding on the wall because your neighbors' blaring music woke you up at 2 AM, talk with them. Try to reach an agreement that works for everyone.
- **Leave past anger in the past.** Learn to resolve issues that have caused pain, frustration, or stress. If necessary, seek the counsel of a professional to make that happen.

## Taking Physical Action

Physical activities can complement the emotional and mental strategies of stress management. Key to this is finding some form of exercise that you really enjoy and doing it regularly as something to look forward to, something that helps fuel your inner energy.

**Exercise Regularly** It is important to remember that the human stress response is intended to end in physical activity. The outpouring of glucose into the bloodstream is meant to feed the muscles and brain as part of the fight-or-flight

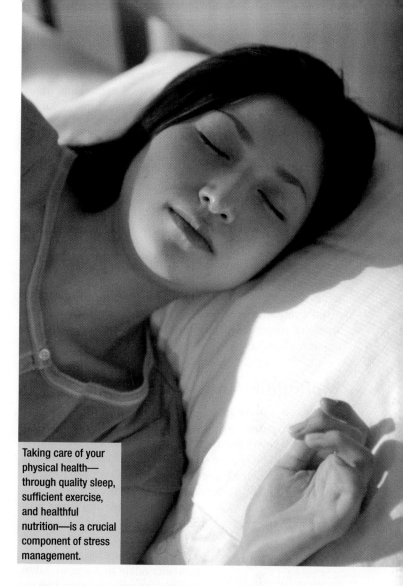

Taking care of your physical health—through quality sleep, sufficient exercise, and healthful nutrition—is a crucial component of stress management.

response. If the threat persists, hormones are released into the bloodstream to maintain the response. Although most threats induce a physical response, we usually aren't able to fight or flee. Typically, we have to wait until such time as we can move and use up those products of the stress response. Exercise "burns off" existing stress hormones by directing them toward their intended metabolic function.[54] Exercise can also help combat stress by raising levels of endorphins—mood-elevating, painkilling hormones—in the bloodstream, increasing energy, reducing hostility, and improving mental alertness. For more information on the beneficial effects of exercise, see Chapter 9.

**Get Enough Sleep** Increasingly, sleep is being recognized as one of the single greatest remedies for a host of threats to health. Adequate amounts of sleep allow you to refresh your vital energy, cope with multiple stressors more effectively, and be productive when you need to be. In fact, sleep is one of the biggest stress busters of them all. These benefits and others are discussed in much more depth in Focus On: Improving Your Sleep beginning on page 102.

**Learn to Relax** Like exercise, relaxation can help you cope with stressful feelings, preserve your energy, and refocus your energies. Once you have learned simple relaxation techniques, you can use them at any time—before a difficult exam, for example. As your body relaxes, your heart rate slows, your blood pressure and metabolic rate decrease, and many other body-calming effects occur, all of which allow you to channel energy appropriately. We discuss specific relaxation techniques later in the chapter.

**Eat Healthfully** Whether foods can calm us and nourish our psyches is a controversial question. High-potency supplements that are supposed to boost resistance against stress-related ailments are nothing more than gimmicks. However, it is clear that eating a balanced, healthy diet will help provide the stamina you need to get through problems and will stress-proof you in ways that are not fully understood. It is also known that undereating, overeating, and eating the wrong kinds of foods can create distress in the body. In particular, avoid **sympathomimetics,** foods that produce (or mimic) stresslike responses, such as caffeine. For more information about the benefits of sound nutrition, see Chapter 7.

## Managing Your Time

Ever go to a party when an exam was looming over your head? Ever put off writing a paper until the night before it was due? If you're like 15 to 20 percent of all adults and up to 95 percent of all college students, you **procrastinate,** or voluntarily delay doing some task despite expecting to be worse off for the delay.[55] These delays can result in academic difficulties, financial problems, relationship problems, and a multitude of stress-related ailments.[56] For some, the reasons for procrastination may relate to a fear of failure or a wish to avoid being put on the spot. For others, distractions can send them off in pursuit of fun and excitement, rather than the steady course of studying. When the consequences of their dalliances hit, stress levels increase, and in a last-ditch attempt to finish projects that should have been started weeks before, sleep goes by the wayside, coffee intake increases, and emotions flare.

How can you avoid the procrastination bug? According to psychologist Shane Owens and his colleagues at Hofstra University, one key is setting clear "implementation intentions."[57] For example, you could specify that you will do work on your paper from 6 PM to 7 PM each night for the next week, as a way of ensuring that you'll stay on task. By making a clear plan of action with set deadlines and rewarding yourself for meeting these deadlines, you can motivate yourself toward project completion. Another strategy is to get started early and set a personal end date that is well ahead of the class due date.

Learning to manage your time better overall is key to reducing stress. Keep a journal for 1 week to become aware of how you spend your time. Write down your activities every day—everything from going to class to doing your laundry to texting your friends—and the amount of time you spend doing each (see **Figure 3.5** for a sample journal format). Once

**sympathomimetics** Food substances that can produce stresslike physiological responses.
**procrastinate** To intentionally put off doing something.

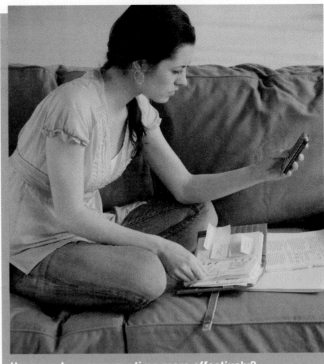

**How can I manage my time more effectively?**

Learning to manage your time means recognizing that there are only 24 hours in a day and you can't do everything. Instead, you need to prioritize your "to do's" and set realistic time limits. You also need to identify the things that cause you to waste time, and find ways to avoid them. Establishing routines and using a calendar or other planning device to keep track of schedules and tasks can help you implement an effective time-management plan.

you have kept track for several days, you can assess your activities. Are you completing the tasks you need to do on a daily basis? Are there any activities you can stop doing or that you would like to do more frequently? Use the following time-management tips in your stress-management program:

- **Do one thing at a time.** Don't try to watch television, wash clothes, and write your term paper all at once. Stay focused.
- **Clean off your desk.** Go through the things on your desk, toss unnecessary papers, and put into folders the papers for tasks that you must do. Read your mail, recycle what you don't need, and file what you will need later.
- **Prioritize your tasks.** Make a daily "to do" list and stick to it. Categorize the things you must do today, the things that you must do but not immediately, and the things that it would be nice to do. Consider the "nice to do" items only if you finish the others or if they include something fun.
- **Find a clean, comfortable place to work, and avoid interruptions.** When you have a project that requires total concentration, schedule uninterrupted time. Don't answer the phone; close your door and post a "Do Not Disturb" sign; or go to a quiet room in the library or student union where no one will find you.
- **Reward yourself for work completed.** Did you finish a task on your list? Then do something nice for yourself. Rest

| Activity | Monday | Tuesday | Wednesday | Thursday | Friday | Saturday | Sunday | Total Hours |
|---|---|---|---|---|---|---|---|---|
| Getting ready | | | | | | | | |
| On the road | | | | | | | | |
| In class | | | | | | | | |
| Working for pay | | | | | | | | |
| Exercising | | | | | | | | |
| Eating (meals & snacks) | | | | | | | | |
| Studying | | | | | | | | |
| Watching TV, videos | | | | | | | | |
| Using computer (school-related) | | | | | | | | |
| Using computer (recreational) | | | | | | | | |
| Spending time with friends | | | | | | | | |
| Leisure activities | | | | | | | | |
| Other (specify) | | | | | | | | |
| Other (specify) | | | | | | | | |
| Total Hours | | | | | | | | |

FIGURE 3.5 **How Do You Spend Your Time?**
Use this schedule to keep track of where your time goes for 1 week. Each day, fill in the amount of time you spend on different activities. Once you have kept track for a week, total the hours for each activity and assess how you spend your time. Are there any activities you can stop doing or that you would like to do more frequently?

breaks give you time to yourself to help you recharge and refresh your energy levels.
● **Work when you're at your best.** If you're a morning person, study and write papers in the morning, and take breaks when you start to slow down.
● **Break overwhelming tasks into small pieces, and allocate a certain amount of time to each.** If you are floundering on a task, move on and come back to it when you're refreshed.
● **Remember that time is precious.** Many people learn to value their time only when they face a terminal illness. Try to value each day. Time spent not enjoying life is a tremendous waste! If you have trouble saying no to people and projects that steal your time, see the **Skills for Behavior Change** box on page 92 for some suggestions.

## Managing Your Finances

Higher education can impose a huge financial burden on parents, students, and communities. In recent studies, nearly two-thirds of students have indicated that they have "some" or "major" concerns regarding their ability to pay for their education.[58] The economic downturn of the past few years is likely pushing already financially stressed students further toward the breaking point.

**35%** of college students report that their finances have been very difficult to handle during the past 12 months.

Several factors are converging to increase today's students' financial woes. First, a recession has caused many parents to lose their jobs. Faced with dwindling resources at home, many students are being forced to look for part-time or even full-time work. These students may encounter increasing competition for even the lowest-paying jobs as displaced workers take these jobs to remain financially afloat. Already known to carry a disproportionate level of credit card debt, students are resorting to using plastic to pay for essentials, leading to more debt and higher stress. The **Consumer Health** box on page 93 offers tips on how to deal with financial woes in these tough times.

## Learn to Say No and Mean It!

Is your calendar always so full you barely have time to breathe? Are you unable to say no to other people? For overachievers, a bulging calendar can be a misplaced badge of honor. Ditch the idea that a jammed calendar is a good thing, that you're indespensible, or that you're superhuman. When you're asked to do something you don't really want to do, practice the following tips to avoid overcommitment:

✳ **Be sympathetic, but firm.** Explain that although you think it's a great cause or idea, you just can't take on one more project right now. If they persist in pressuring you, tell them it was nice talking, but you have to run.

✳ **Don't say you want to think about it and will get back to them.** This only leads to more forceful requests later. Say, "not this time," and reiterate that you are overwhelmed and can't take on any more obligations.

✳ **Don't give in to guilt.** Stick to your guns. Remember you don't owe anyone your time.

✳ **Even if something sounds good, avoid spontaneous "yes" responses to new projects.** Make a rule that you will take at least a day to think about committing your time. If you still think it might be a good idea after 24 hours, decide what you can take *off* your plate in order to do this thing.

✳ **Schedule time for yourself first.** If you don't have time for the things you love to do, stop and prioritize your activities. Keep two or three of the "must do's" on your list each day. Cross off the "I don't have to, but I said yes to" events. Be honest, admit you overcommitted, and bow out of the event. Add one or two, "I really want to do" things.

✳ **Remember that there are only 24 hours in every day and you need at least 8 for sleeping.** Consider how each thing you add to your list will help you grow personally, professionally, or will help contribute to society. Choose wisely.

## Consider Downshifting

Today's lifestyles are hectic and pressure packed, and stress often comes from trying to keep up. Many people are questioning whether "having it all" is worth it, and they are taking a step back and simplifying their lives. This trend has been labeled *downshifting,* or *voluntary simplicity*. Moving from a large urban area to a smaller town, leaving a high-paying and high-stress job for one that makes you happy, and a host of other changes in lifestyle typify downshifting.

Downshifting involves a fundamental alteration in values and honest introspection about what is important in life. It means cutting down on shopping habits, buying only what you need to get by, and living within modest means. When you contemplate any form of downshift or perhaps even start your career this way, it's important to move slowly and consider the following:

● **Plan for health care costs.** Make sure that you budget for health insurance and basic preventive health services if you're not covered under your parents' plan. Understand your coverage. This should be a top priority.

● **Determine your ultimate goal.** What is most important to you, and what will you need to reach that goal? What can you do without?

● **Make both short- and long-term plans for simplifying your life.** Set up your plans in doable steps, and work slowly toward each step.

● **Complete a financial inventory.** How much money will you need to do the things you want to do? Will you live alone or share costs with roommates? Do you need a car, or can you rely on public transportation? Pay off your debt, and get used to paying with cash. If you don't have the cash, don't buy.

● **Select the right career.** Look for work that you enjoy and that isn't necessarily driven by salary. Can you be happy taking a lower-paying job if it is less stressful?

● **Consider options for saving money.** Downshifting doesn't mean you renounce money; it means you choose not to let money dictate your life. Saving is still important. If you're just getting started, you need to prepare for emergencies and for future plans.

### what do you think?

Who are the role models in your life? ● Are they constantly "on the go" or more relaxed? ● Would you characterize them as stressed out? ● Could you follow their lead without becoming stressed out yourself?

## Relaxation Techniques for Stress Management

Relaxation techniques to reduce stress have been practiced for centuries, and there is a wide selection from which to choose. Some common techniques include yoga, qigong, tai chi, deep breathing, meditation, visualization, progressive muscle relaxation, massage therapy, biofeedback, and hypnosis.

**Yoga** Yoga is an ancient practice that combines meditation, stretching, and breathing exercises designed to relax, refresh, and rejuvenate. It began about 5,000 years ago in India and has been evolving ever since. Some 20 million adults practice many versions in the United States today.

*Classical yoga* is the ancestor of nearly all modern forms of yoga. Breathing, poses, and verbal mantras are often part of classical yoga. Of the many branches of classical yoga, *Hatha yoga* is the most well known because it is the most

# LESSEN YOUR FINANCIAL STRESS

Distracted by the unusually high financial pressure of these tough economic times, students may find their performance in classes slipping and their health suffering. The following tips may help you better manage your money and reduce your finance-related stress.

* **Develop a realistic budget.** What are your monthly expenses? What types of luxuries do you regularly splurge on? Think about where you spend your money, what you really need, and what you could do without. Remember that buying less also means generating less waste, both in packaging and unwanted items that will eventually be discarded.

* **Pay bills immediately and consider electronic banking.** Late fees and other penalties are an unnecessary way of depleting your bank account and are easily avoided by paying bills as soon as you get them. Sign up for an online account to pay bills quickly and easily. If possible, set up your bills for automatic payment.

* **Educate yourself about how to manage your money.** Take advantage of campus workshops on financial aid and money management. Take a course in personal financial planning.

* **Avoid those tempting credit card offers.** You need only one or two credit cards. Shred extra offers you get in the mail, and put them straight into the recycling bin.

* **Don't get into debt.** If you don't have the money for an item now, don't buy it on credit. If you want to buy a pricey item or pay for an expensive trip, put aside a certain amount toward that goal every month until you have enough to afford it.

---

body focused. This style of yoga involves the practice of breath control and *asanas*—held postures and choreographed movements that enhance strength and flexibility. Several other, more athletic, forms of yoga are discussed in Chapter 9.

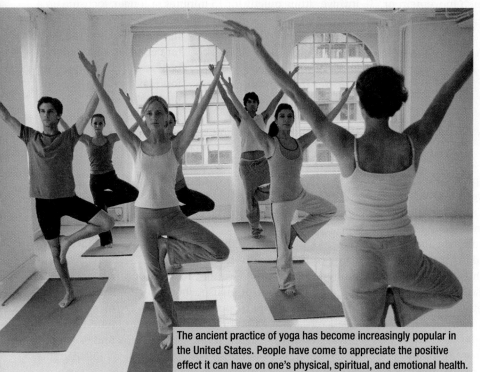

The ancient practice of yoga has become increasingly popular in the United States. People have come to appreciate the positive effect it can have on one's physical, spiritual, and emotional health.

**Qigong** *Qigong* (pronounced "chee-kong") is one of the fastest-growing and most widely accepted forms of mind–body health exercises. Even some of the country's largest health care organizations, such as Kaiser Permanente, include this relaxation technique in their system, particularly for people suffering from chronic pain or stress. Qigong is an ancient Chinese practice that involves becoming aware of and learning to control *qi* (or *chi*, pronounced "chee") or vital energy in your body. According to Chinese medicine, a complex system of internal pathways called *meridians* carry *qi* throughout your body. If your *qi* becomes stagnant or blocked, you'll feel sluggish or powerless. Qigong incorporates a series of flowing movements, breath techniques, mental visualization exercises, and vocalizations of healing sounds designed to restore balance and integrate and refresh the mind and body.

**Tai Chi** *Tai chi* (pronounced "ty-chee") is sometimes described as "meditation in motion." Originally developed in China as a form of self-defense, this graceful form of exercise has existed for about 2,000 years. Tai chi is noncompetitive and self-paced. To do tai chi, you perform a defined series of postures or

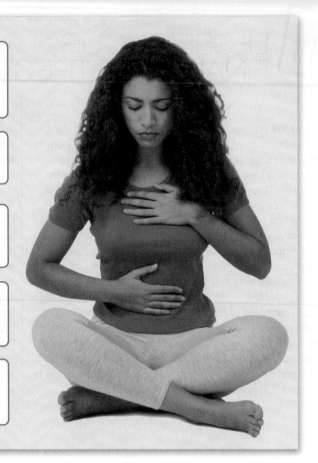

1. Assume a natural, comfortable position either sitting up straight with your head, neck, and shoulders relaxed, or lying on your back with your knees bent and your head supported. Close your eyes and loosen binding clothes.

2. In order to feel your abdomen moving as you breathe, place one hand on your upper chest and the other just below your rib cage.

3. Breathe in slowly and deeply through your nose. Feel your stomach expanding into your hand. The hand on your chest should move as little as possible.

4. Exhale slowly through your mouth. Feel the fall of your stomach away from your hand. Again, the hand on your chest should move as little as possible.

5. Concentrate on the act of breathing. Shut out external noise. Focus on inhaling and exhaling, the route the air is following, and the rise and fall of your stomach.

FIGURE 3.6 **Diaphragmatic Breathing**
This exercise will help you learn to breathe deeply as a way to relieve stress. Practice this for 5 to 10 minutes several times a day, and soon diaphragmatic breathing will become natural for you.

movements in a slow, graceful manner. Each movement or posture flows into the next without pause. Tai chi has been widely practiced in China for centuries and is now becoming increasingly popular around the world, both as a basic exercise program and as a complement to other health care methods. Health benefits include stress reduction, greater balance, and increased flexibility.

**9.4%**

**Diaphragmatic or Deep Breathing** Typically, we breathe using only the upper chest and thoracic region rather than involving the abdominal region. Simply stated, diaphragmatic breathing is deep breathing that maximally fills the lungs by involving the movement of the diaphragm and lower abdomen. This technique is commonly used in yoga exercises and in other meditative practices. Try the diaphragmatic breathing exercise in Figure 3.6 right now and see whether you feel more relaxed!

**meditation** A relaxation technique that involves deep breathing and concentration.
**visualization** The creation of mental images to promote relaxation.

**Meditation** There are many different forms of **meditation.** Most

**of American adults report having practiced some form of meditation in the past 12 months.**

involve sitting quietly for 15 minutes or longer, focusing on a particular word or symbol, and controlling breathing. Practiced by Eastern religions for centuries, meditation is believed to be an important form of introspection and personal renewal. In stress management, it can calm the body and quiet the mind, creating a sense of peace. Meditation and other aspects of spiritual health are discussed in detail in Focus On: Cultivating Your Spiritual Health beginning on page 60.

**Visualization** Often it is our own thoughts and imagination that provoke distress by conjuring up worst-case scenarios. Our imagination, however, can also be tapped to reduce stress. In **visualization,** you create mental scenes using your imagination. The choice of mental images is unlimited, but natural settings such as ocean beaches and mountain lakes are often used, because they simulate vacation locations where people typically go to escape the stress of the home, school, or work environment. Recalling physical senses of sight, sound, smell, taste, and touch can replace stressful stimuli with peaceful or pleasurable thoughts.

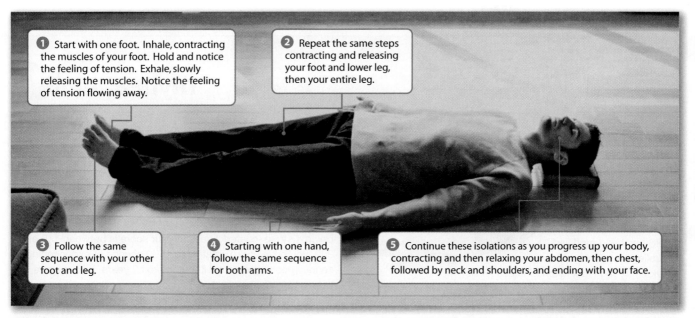

1 Start with one foot. Inhale, contracting the muscles of your foot. Hold and notice the feeling of tension. Exhale, slowly releasing the muscles. Notice the feeling of tension flowing away.

2 Repeat the same steps contracting and releasing your foot and lower leg, then your entire leg.

3 Follow the same sequence with your other foot and leg.

4 Starting with one hand, follow the same sequence for both arms.

5 Continue these isolations as you progress up your body, contracting and then relaxing your abdomen, then chest, followed by neck and shoulders, and ending with your face.

FIGURE 3.7 **Progressive Muscle Relaxation**
Sit or lie down in a comfortable position and follow the steps described to increase your awareness of tension in your body.

**Progressive Muscle Relaxation** Progressive muscle relaxation involves systematically contracting and relaxing different muscle groups in your body. The standard pattern is to begin with the feet and work your way up your body, contracting and releasing as you go (Figure 3.7). The process is designed to teach awareness of the different feelings of muscle tension and muscle release. With practice, you can quickly identify tension in your body when you are facing stressful situations and consciously release that tension to calm yourself.

**Massage Therapy** If you have ever had someone massage your stiff neck or aching feet, you know that massage is an excellent way to relax. Techniques vary from deep-tissue massage to the gentler acupressure. Chapter 18 provides more information about the benefits of massage as well as other body-based methods such as acupressure and shiatsu.

**Biofeedback** Biofeedback involves monitoring your physical responses to stress via machine. The machine records perspiration, heart rate, respiration rate, blood pressure, surface body temperature, muscle tension, and other stress responses. You use various relaxation techniques while hooked up to a biofeedback machine, and through trial and error and signals from the machine, you learn to lower the stress response. Eventually, you develop the ability to recognize and lower stress responses without using the machine.

**biofeedback** A technique using a machine to self-monitor physical responses to stress.
**hypnosis** A trancelike state that allows people to become unusually responsive to suggestion.

**Hypnosis** Hypnosis requires a person to focus on one thought, object, or voice, thereby freeing the right hemisphere of the brain to become more active. The person then becomes unusually responsive to suggestion. Whether self-induced or induced by someone else, hypnosis can reduce certain types of stress.

## What's Your Stress Level?

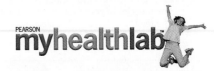

Fill out this assessment online at www.pearsonhighered.com/myhealthlab or www.pearsonhighered.com/donatelle.

# 1 The Student Stress Scale

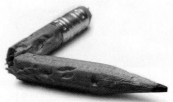

The Student Stress Scale represents an adaptation of Holmes and Rahe's Social Readjustment Rating Scale (SRRS). The SRRS has been modified for college students and provides a rough indication of stress levels and health consequences. In the scale, each event is given a score that represents the amount of readjustment a person must make as a result of the life change. To determine your stress score, check each event that you have experienced in the past 12 months, and then sum the number of points corresponding to each event.

| | | | |
|---|---|---|---|
| 1. | Death of a close family member | _____ | 100 |
| 2. | Death of a close friend | _____ | 73 |
| 3. | Divorce between parents | _____ | 65 |
| 4. | Jail term | _____ | 63 |
| 5. | Major personal injury or illness | _____ | 63 |
| 6. | Marriage | _____ | 58 |
| 7. | Firing from a job | _____ | 50 |
| 8. | Failure in an important course | _____ | 47 |
| 9. | Change in health of a family member | _____ | 45 |
| 10. | Pregnancy | _____ | 45 |
| 11. | Sex problems | _____ | 44 |
| 12. | Serious argument with close friend | _____ | 40 |
| 13. | Change in financial status | _____ | 39 |
| 14. | Change of major | _____ | 39 |
| 15. | Trouble with parents | _____ | 39 |
| 16. | New girlfriend or boyfriend | _____ | 37 |
| 17. | Increase in workload at school | _____ | 37 |
| 18. | Outstanding personal achievement | _____ | 36 |
| 19. | First quarter/semester in school | _____ | 36 |
| 20. | Change in living conditions | _____ | 31 |
| 21. | Serious argument with an instructor | _____ | 30 |
| 22. | Lower grades than expected | _____ | 29 |
| 23. | Change in sleeping habits | _____ | 29 |
| 24. | Change in social activities | _____ | 29 |
| 25. | Change in eating habits | _____ | 28 |
| 26. | Chronic car trouble | _____ | 26 |
| 27. | Change in number of family gatherings | _____ | 26 |
| 28. | Too many missed classes | _____ | 25 |
| 29. | Change of college | _____ | 24 |
| 30. | Dropping of more than one class | _____ | 23 |
| 31. | Minor traffic violations | _____ | 20 |

Total: _____

## Scoring Part 1

If your score is 300 or higher, you may be at high risk for developing a stress-related illness. If your score is between 150 and 300, you have approximately a 50-50 chance of experiencing a serious health problem within the next 2 years. If your score is below 150, you have a 1 in 3 chance of experiencing a serious health change in the next few years.

**Source:** Adapted from T. Holmes and R. H. Rahe, "The Social Readjustment Rating Scale," *Journal of Psychosomatic Research* 11, no. 8 (1967): 213–18. Copyright © 1967 Elsevier, Inc. Used with permission.

# 2 How Do You Respond to Stress?

Read the following scenarios and choose the response that you would most likely have to these stressful events.

1. You've been waiting 20 minutes for a table in a crowded restaurant, and the hostess seats a group that arrived after you.

   a. You yell, "Hey! I was here first" in an irritated voice to the hostess.

   b. You say, "Excuse me" in a polite voice and inform the other group or the hostess that you were there first.

   c. You walk out of the restaurant in disgust. Obviously the hostess was willfully ignoring you.

2. You come home to find the kitchen looking like a disaster area and your spouse/roommate lounging in front of the TV.

   a. You pick a fight about how your spouse/roommate never does anything and always expects you to clean up after him or her.

   b. You sit down next to your spouse/roommate and ask if he or she would take a 5-minute break from the TV show to help you clean.

   c. You don't say anything but instead tense up and angrily start cleaning the kitchen, making as much noise as possible.

3. You have to present a paper in front of your class, and you are anxious about doing a good job.

   a. You get flustered during the presentation and snap at your fellow classmates when they ask questions about your topic.

b. You ask a friend to help you practice the presentation ahead of time so you can feel confident going in to class.

c. You lose sleep worrying about the presentation, and afterward you spend the rest of the day reliving all the mistakes you made.

4. Your partner is seen out with another person and appears to be acting quite close to the person.

a. You immediately assume your partner is cheating on you. Infuriated, you launch into a stream of accusations the next time you are together.

b. The next time you see your partner, you calmly mention your concerns and describe your feelings, giving him or her a chance to explain the situation.

c. You decide your partner no longer cares about you and spend the evening reproaching yourself for being so unlovable.

5. You aren't able to study as much as you'd like for an exam, and when you get it back, you find that you did horribly.

a. You angrily bad-mouth your professor to your friends and anyone else who will listen.

b. You make an appointment to talk with the professor and determine what you can do to improve on the next exam.

c. You decide you're just crummy at the subject and don't even bother studying at all the next time.

## Analyzing Part 2

If you chose mostly "a" responses, you are probably a hot reactor who responds to mildly stressful situations with a fight-or-flight adrenaline rush. Before you honk or make obscene gestures at the guy who cuts you off in traffic, remember that the only thing you'll hasten by reacting is a decline in health. Look at ways to change your perceptions and cope more effectively.

If you chose mostly "b" responses, you are probably a cool reactor who tends to roll with the punches when a situation becomes stressful. This usually indicates a good level of coping; overall, you will suffer fewer health consequences when stressed. The key here is that you really are not stressed, and you really are calm and unworried about the situation—not just behaving as though you were.

If you chose mostly "c" responses, you have intense reactions to stress that you are prone to directing inward. This can negatively affect your health just as much as being explosive. To change your approach to stress, work on ways of building your senses of self-efficacy and self-esteem. Changing the way you think about yourself and others can help you approach stress in a more balanced and productive way.

# YOUR PLAN FOR CHANGE

The **Assessyourself** activity gave you the chance to look at your stress responses and identify particular situations in your life that cause stress. Now that you are aware of these patterns, you can change behaviors that lead to increased stress.

### Today, you can:

○ Practice one new stress-management technique. For example, you could spend 10 minutes doing a deep-breathing exercise or find a good spot on campus to meditate.

○ Buy a journal and write down stressful events or symptoms of stress that you experience. Try to focus on intense emotional experiences and explore how they affect you.

### Within the next 2 weeks, you can:

○ Attend a class or workshop in yoga, tai chi, qigong, meditation, or some other stress-relieving activity. Look for beginner classes offered on campus or in your community.

○ Make a list of the papers, projects, and tests that you have over the coming semester and create a schedule for them. Break projects and term papers into small, manageable tasks, and try to be realistic about how much time you'll need to get these tasks done.

### By the end of the semester, you can:

○ Keep track of the money you spend and where it goes. Establish a budget and follow it for at least a month.

○ Find some form of exercise you can do regularly. You may consider joining a gym or just arranging regular "walk dates" or pickup basketball games with your friends. Try to exercise at least 30 minutes every day. See Chapter 9 for more information about physical fitness.

## Summary

* Stress is an inevitable part of our lives. *Eustress* refers to stress associated with positive events; *distress* refers to stress associated with negative events.
* The alarm, resistance, and exhaustion phases of the general adaptation syndrome (GAS) involve physiological responses to both real and imagined stressors and cause a complex cascade of hormones to rush through the body. Prolonged arousal may be detrimental to health.
* Undue stress for extended periods of time can compromise the immune system and result in serious health consequences. Stress has been linked to numerous health problems, including cardiovascular disease (CVD), weight gain, hair loss, diabetes, digestive problems, increased susceptibility to infectious diseases, and diminished libido. Psychoneuroimmunology is the science that analyzes the relationship between the mind's reaction to stress and the function of the immune system.
* Stress can have negative impacts on your intellectual and psychological health, including impairing memory and concentration, and contributing to depression, anxiety, and other mental health disorders.
* Multiple factors contribute to stress and the stress response. Psychosocial factors include change, hassles, relationships, pressure, conflict, overload, and environmental stressors. Persons subjected to discrimination or bias may face unusually high levels of stress. Some sources of stress are internal and are related to appraisal, self-esteem, self-efficacy, personality, and psychological hardiness.
* College can be especially stressful. Recognizing the signs of stress is the first step toward better health. Managing stress begins with learning coping skills. Finding out what works best for you—probably some combination of managing emotional responses, taking mental or physical action, downshifting, learning time management, managing finances, or learning relaxation techniques—will help you better cope with stress in the long run.

## Pop Quiz

1. Even though Andre experienced stress when he graduated from college and moved to a new city, he viewed these changes as an opportunity for growth. What is Andre's stress called?
   a. Strain
   b. Distress
   c. Eustress
   d. Adaptive response

2. The branch of the autonomic nervous system that is responsible for energizing the body for either fight or flight and for triggering many other stress responses is the
   a. central nervous system.
   b. parasympathetic nervous system.
   c. sympathetic nervous system.
   d. endocrine system.

3. During what phase of the general adaptation syndrome has the physical and psychological energy used to fight the stressor been depleted?
   a. Alarm phase
   b. Resistance phase
   c. Endurance phase
   d. Exhaustion phase

4. A state of physical and mental exhaustion caused by excessive stress is called
   a. conflict.
   b. overload.
   c. hassles.
   d. burnout.

5. Losing your keys is an example of what psychosocial source of stress?
   a. Pressure
   b. Inconsistent behaviors
   c. Hassles
   d. Conflict

6. After 5 years of 70-hour workweeks, Tom decided to leave his high-paying, high-stress law firm and lead a simpler lifestyle. What is this trend called?
   a. Adaptation
   b. Conflict resolution
   c. Burnout reduction
   d. Downshifting

7. Which of the following test-taking techniques is *not* recommended to reduce test-taking stress?
   a. Plan ahead and study over a period of time for the test.
   b. Take regular breaks to refresh the overstimulated brain.
   c. Do all your studying the night before the exam so it is fresh in your mind.
   d. Practice by testing yourself with other classmates' sample test questions.

8. Which of the following is *not* an example of a time-management technique?
   a. Scheduling one's time with a calendar or day planner
   b. Identifying time robbers
   c. Practicing procrastination in completing homework assignments
   d. Developing a game plan

9. Which of the following is an example of a chronic stressor?
   a. Giving a talk in public
   b. Meeting a deadline for a big project
   c. Dealing with a permanent disability
   d. Dealing with the death of a family member or close friend

10. In which stage of the general adaptation syndrome does the fight-or-flight response occur?
    a. Exhaustion stage
    b. Alarm stage
    c. Resistance stage
    d. Response stage

*Answers to these questions can be found on page A-1.*

1. Describe the alarm, resistance, and exhaustion phases of the general adaptation syndrome and the body's physiological response to stress. Does stress lead to more irritability or emotionality, or does emotionality lead to stress? Provide examples to support your case.
2. What are some of the health risks that result from chronic stress? How does the study of psychoneuroimmunology link stress and illness?
3. Why are the college years often high-stress years for many? What factors increase stress risks? What actions can you take to manage your stressors?
4. How does anger affect the body? Discuss the steps you can take to manage your own anger and help your friends control theirs.
5. How much of a procrastinator are you? What can you do to reduce procrastination?

## Accessing Your Health on the Internet

The following websites explore further topics and issues related to personal health. For links to the websites below, visit the Companion Website for *Access to Health*, 12th Edition, at www.pearsonhighered.com/donatelle.

1. *American College Counseling Association.* The website of the professional organization for college counselors offers useful links and articles. www.collegecounseling.org
2. *American College Health Association.* This site provides information and data from the National College Health Assessment survey. www.acha.org
3. *American Psychological Association.* Here you can find current information and research on stress and stress-related conditions. www.apa.org/topics/stress

4. *Higher Education Research Institute.* This organization provides annual surveys of first-year and senior college students that cover academic, financial, and health-related issues and problems. www.heri.ucla.edu
5. *National Institute of Occupational Safety and Health, Stress at Work.* This site is an excellent source for information and resources on workplace stress. www.cdc.gov/niosh/topics/stress
6. *National Institute of Mental Health.* This comprehensive site from the National Institutes of Health is a resource for information on all aspects of mental health, including the effects of stress. www.nimh.nih.gov

## References

1. American Psychological Association, *Stress in America 2009, Executive Summary.* 2009, Available at www.apa.org/news/press/releases/stress.
2. K. Glanz and M. Schwartz, "Stress, Coping and Health Behavior," in *Health Behavior and Health Education: Theory, Research and Practice*, 4th ed., eds. K. Glanz, B. Rimer, and K. Viswanath (San Francisco: Jossey Bass, 2002), 210–36.
3. B. L. Seaward, *Managing Stress: Principles and Strategies for Health and Well-Being,* 6th ed. (Sudbury, MA: Jones and Bartlett, 2009), 8.
4. H. Selye, *Stress without Distress* (New York: Lippincott, 1974), 28–29.
5. W. B. Cannon, *The Wisdom of the Body* (New York: Norton, 1932).
6. B. S. McEwen, "Mood Disorders and Allostatic Load," *Biological Psychiatry* 54 (2003): 200–07.
7. A. Mokdad et al., "Actual Causes of Death in the United States, 2000," *Journal of the American Medical Association* 291 (2004): 1238–45.
8. S. Cohen, D. Janicki-Deverts, and G. Miller, "Psychological Stress and Cardiovascular Disease," *Journal of the American Medical Association* 298, no. 14 (2007): 1685–87; A. Väänänen et al., "Lack of Predictability at Work and Risk of Acute Myocardial Infarction: An 18-Year Prospective Study of Industrial Employees," *American Journal of Public Health* 98, no. 12 (2008): 2264–71; J. Bremner et al., *Stress and Health: Effects of a Cognitive Stress Challenge on Myocardial Perfusion and Plasma Cortisol in Coronary Heart Disease Patients with Depression* (San Francisco: John Wiley & Sons, 2009); A. Sgoifo, N. Montano, C. Shively, J. Thayer, and A. Steptoe, "The Inevitable Link between Heart and Behavior: New Insights from Biomedical Research and Implications for Practice," *Neuroscience and Biobehavioral Reviews* 33, no. 2 (2008): 61–67; K. Monyeki and H. Kemper, "The Risk Factors for Elevated Blood Pressure and How to Address Cardiovascular Risk Factors: A Review in Pediatric Populations," *Journal of Human Hypertension* 22 (2008): 450–59; F. Sparrenberger et al., "Does Psychological Stress Cause Hypertension? A Systematic Review of Observational Studies," *Journal of Human Hypertension* 23 (2009): 12–19; M. Hamer, G. Molloy, and E. Stamatakis, "Psychological Distress as a Risk Factor for Cardiovascular Events," *Journal of the American College of Cardiology* 52 (2008): 2156–62.
9. S. Yusef et al., "Effect of Potentially Modifiable Risk Factors Associated with Myocardial Infarction in 52 Countries (The INTERHEART Study): Case-Control Study," *Lancet* 364, no. 9438 (2004): 937–52.
10. J. Dimsdale, "Psychological Stress and Cardiovascular Disease," *Journal of the American College of Cardiology* 51 (2008): 1237–46.
11. B. Aggarwart, M. Liao, A. Christian, and L. Mosca, "Influence of Care-Giving on Lifestyle and Psychosocial Risk Factors among Family Members of Patients Hospitalized with Cardiovascular Disease," *Journal of General Internal Medicine* 24, no. 1 (2009): 1497–1525; F. Sparrenberger et al., "Does Psychological Stress Cause Hypertension?" 2009; M. Kivimäki et al., "Socioeconomic Position, Psychosocial Work Environment, and Cerebrovascular Disease among Women: The Finnish Public Sector Study," *International Journal of Epidemiology* (January 20, 2009); A. Väänänen et al., "Lack of Predictability at Work and Risk of Acute Myocardial Infarction," 2008; A. Miller and B. Arquilla, "Chronic Disease and Natural Hazards: Impact of Disasters on Diabetes, Renal and Cardiac Patients," *Prehospital Disaster Medicine* 23, no. 2 (2008): 185–94; I. Weissbecker, S. Sephton, M. Martin, and D. Simpson, "Psychological and Physiological Correlates of Stress in Children Exposed to Disaster: Current Research and Recommendations for Intervention," *Children, Youth and Environments* 18, no. 1 (2008): 30–70.
12. V. Vicennati et al., "Stress-Related Development of Obesity and Cortisol in Women," *Obesity* 17, no. 19 (2009): 1678–83; C. Shively, T. Register, and T. Clarkson, "Social Stress, Visceral Obesity and Coronary Atherosclerosis in Female Primates,"

*Obesity* 17, no. 8 (2009): 1513–20; L. Brydon et al., "Stress-Induced Cytokine Responses and Central Adiposity in Young Women," *International Journal of Obesity* 32, no. 3 (2008): 443–50; R. Pasquali et al., "Sex Dependent Role of Glucocorticoids and Androgens in the Pathophysiology of Human Obesity," *International Journal of Obesity* 32 (2008): 1764–79.

13. D. K. Hall-Flavin, "Stress and Hair Loss: Are They Related?" Mayo Clinic.com, 2008, www.mayoclinic.com/health/stress-and-hair-loss/AN01442.

14. M. Scollan-Koliopoulos, "Managing Stress Response to Control Hypertension in Type 2 Diabetes," *Nurse Practitioner* 30, no. 2 (2005): 46–49.

15. University of Maryland Medical Center, "Digestive Disorders: Irritable Bowel Syndrome," March 2009, www.umm.edu/digest/ibs.htm; National Digestive Diseases Information Clearinghouse (NDDIC), "Irritable Bowel Syndrome," NIH Publication no. 07-693, September 2007; Johns Hopkins Health Alerts, "Four Relaxation Techniques to Soothe Your Digestive Discomfort," 2008, www.johnshopkinshealthalerts.com/reports/digestive_health/2683-1.html?ty.

16. S. Lightman, "Chronic Stress Can Significantly Damage Health," *Discover Health* (2008), http://health.discovery.com/centers/stress/interviews/liteman_int.html; J. Walburn et al., "Psychological Stress and Wound Healing in Humans: A Systematic Review and Meta-Analysis," *Journal of Psychosomatic Research* 67, no. 3 (2009): 253–71; T. Denson, M. Spanovic, and N. Miller, "Cognitive Appraisals and Emotions Predict Cortisol and Immune Responses: A Meta-Analysis of Acute Laboratory Social Stressors and Emotion Inductions," *Psychological Bulletin* 135, no. 6 (2009): 823–53; S. Seagerstrom and G. Miller, "Psychological Stress and the Human Immune System: A Meta-Analytic Study of 30 Years of Inquiry," *Psychological Bulletin* 130, no. 4 (2004) 601–30; E. R. Volkmann and N. Y. Weekes, "Basal SigA and Cortisol Levels Predict Stress-Related Health Outcomes," *Stress and Health* 22 (2006): 11–23.

17. G. Miller, N. Rohleder, and S. Cole, "Chronic Interpersonal Stress Predicts Activation of Pro- and Anti-Inflammatory Signaling 6 Months Later," *Psychosomatic Medicine* 71, no. 1 (2009): 57–62.

18. R. Ader, *Psychoneuroimmunology*, 2007; S. Seagerstrom and G. Miller, "Psychological Stress and the Human Immune System: A Meta-Analytic Study of 30 Years of Inquiry," Psychological *Bulletin* 130, no. 4 (2004) 601–30.

19. American College Health Association (ACHA), *American College Health Association—National College Health Assessment II (ACHA-NCHA II) Reference Group Data Report Fall 2009,* (Baltimore: ACHA, 2010), Available at www.acha-ncha.org/reports_ACHA-NCHAII.html.

20. L. Schwabe, T. Wolf, and M. Oitzi. "Memory Formation under Stress: Quantity and Quality," *Neuroscience and Biobehavioral Reviews* 34, no. 4 (2009): 584–91.

21. E. Dias-Ferreira et al., "Chronic Stress Causes Frontostriatal Reorganization and Affects Decision-Making," *Science* 325, no. 5940 (2009): 621–25; D. de Quervan et al., "Glucocorticoids and the Regulation of Memory in Health and Disease," *Frontiers in Neuroendocrinology* 30, no. 3 (2009): 358–70.

22. D. A. Katerndahl and M. Parchman, "The Ability of the Stress Process Model to Explain Mental Health Outcomes," *Comprehensive Psychiatry* 43 (2002): 351–60; R. C. Kessler et al., "The Epidemiology of Major Depressive Disorder," *Journal of the American Medical Association* 289 (2003): 3095–105.

23. R. L. Turner and D. A. Lloyd, "Stress Burden and the Lifetime Incidence of Psychiatric Disorder in Young Adults: Racial and Ethnic Contrasts," *Archives of General Psychiatry* 61 (2004): 481–88; A. Väänänen et al., "Sources of Social Support as Determinants of Psychiatric Morbidity after Severe Life Events: Prospective Cohort Study of Female Employees," *Journal of Psychosomatic Research* 58 (2005): 459–67.

24. V. R. Wilburn and D. E. Smith, "Stress, Self-Esteem, and Suicidal Ideation in Late Adolescence," *Adolescence* 40 (2005): 33–46.

25. American Psychological Association, *Stress in America 2009, Executive Summary,* 2009.

26. R. Lazarus, "The Trivialization of Distress," in *Preventing Health Risk Behaviors and Promoting Coping with Illness,* eds. J. Rosen and L. Solomon (Hanover, NH: University Press of New England, 1985), 279–98.

27. D. J. Maybery and D. Graham, "Hassles and Uplifts: Including Interpersonal Events," *Stress and Health* 17 (2001): 91–104; R. Blonna, *Coping with Stress in a Changing World,* 4th ed. (New York: McGraw-Hill, 2006).

28. C. L. Park, S. Armeli, and H. Tennen, "The Daily Stress and Coping Process and Alcohol Use among College Students," *Journal of Studies on Alcohol* 65, no. 1 (2004): 126–30; B. E. Miller et al., "Alcohol Misuse among College Athletes: Self-Medication for Psychiatric Symptoms?" *Journal of Drug Education* 32 (2002): 41–52.

29. S. Sumer, "International Students' Psychological and Sociocultural Adaptation in the United States," Georgia State University, Doctoral Dissertation, 2009, http://digitalarchive.gsu.edu/cps_diss/34; L. Johnson and D. Sandhu, "Isolation, Adjustment and Acculturation Issues of International Students: Intervention Strategies for Counselors," in *A Handbook for Counseling International Students in the U.S.,* eds. S. Singaravelu and M. Pope (Alexandria, VA: American Counseling Association, 2007), 13–36.

30. Z. Djuric et al., "Biomarkers of Psychological Stress in Health Disparities Research," *The Open Biomarkers Journal* 1 (2008): 7–19; J. Watson, H. Logan, and S. Tomar, "The Influence of Active Coping and Perceived Stress on Health Disparities in a Multi-Ethnic Low Income Sample," *BMC Public Health* 8 (2008): 41; C. M. Arthur, "A Little Bit of Rain Each Day: Psychological Stress and Health Disparities," *California Journal of Health Promotion* 5, Special Edition (2007): 58–67.

31. N. Buchanan et al., "Unique and Joint Effects of Sexual and Racial Harassment on College Students' Well-Being," Basic and *Applied Social Psychology* 31, no. 3 (2009): 267–85.

32. D. Stang, "Calming Down: An Introduction to Stress and Stress Solutions," HealthVideo.com, Accessed November 2010, www.healthvideo.com/article.php?id=1174.

33. K. Karren et al., *Mind/Body Health: The Effects of Attitudes, Emotions, and Relationships,* 3rd ed. (San Francisco: Benjamin Cummings, 2006).

34. K. Karren et al., *Mind/Body Health,* 2006; B. L. Seaward, *Managing Stress,* 2009; V. R. Wilburn and D. E. Smith, "Stress, Self-Esteem, and Suicidal Ideation," 2005.

35. V. R. Wilburn and D. E. Smith, "Stress, Self-Esteem, and Suicidal Ideation," 2005; D. Robotham and C. Julian, "Stress and the Higher Education Student: A Critical Review of the Literature," *Journal of Further and Higher Education* 30, no. 2 (2006): 107–17.

36. K. Glanz, B. Rimer, and F. Levis, eds., *Health Behavior and Health Education: Theory, Research, and Practice,* 3rd ed. (San Francisco: Jossey-Bass, 2002).

37. A. D. Von et al., "Predictors of Health Behaviors in College Students," *Journal of Advanced Nursing* 48, no. 5 (2004): 463–74.

38. M. Friedman and R. H. Rosenman, *Type A Behavior and Your Heart* (New York: Knopf, 1974).

39. K. Karren et al., *Mind/Body Health,* 2006; R. Niaura et al., "Hostility, Metabolic Syndrome, and Incident Coronary Heart Disease," *Health Psychology* 21, no. 6 (2002): 588–93.

40. M. Jawer and M. Micozzi, *The Spiritual Anatomy of Emotion: How Feelings Link the Brain, the Body, and the Sixth Sense* (Rochester, VT: Park Street Press, 2009).

41. J. Denollet, "Prognostic Value of Type D Personality Compared with Depressive Symptoms," *Archives of Internal Medicine* 168, no. 4 (2008): 431–35; N. Kupper and J. Denollet, "Type D Personalities as a Prognostic Factor in Heart Disease: Assessment and Mediating Mechanisms," *Journal of Personality Assessment* 89, no. 3 (2007): 265–66; L. Williams et al., "Type D Personality Mechanisms of Effect: The Role of Health-Related Behavior and Social Support," *Journal of Psychosomatic Research* 64, no. 1 (2008): 63–68.

42. S. Kobasa, "Stressful Life Events, Personality, and Health: An Inquiry into Hardiness," *Journal of Personality and Social Psychology* 37 (1979): 1–11.

43. B. J. Crowley, B. Hayslip, and J. Hobdy, "Psychological Hardiness and Adjustment to Life Events in Adulthood," *Journal of Adult Development* 10 (2003): 237–48; S. R. Maddi, "The Story of Hardiness: Twenty Years of Theorizing, Research, and Practice," *Consulting Psychology Journal: Practice and Research* 54 (2002): 173–86.

44. S. Ruiz et al., *Findings from the 2009 Administration of the Your First College Year (YFCY): National Aggregates* (Los Angeles: Cooperative Institutional Research Program at the Higher Education Research Institute at UCLA, 2010), Available at www.heri.ucla.edu/publications-brp.php; R. Franke et al., *Findings from the 2008 Administration of the College Senior Survey (CSS): National Aggregates* (Los Angeles: Cooperative Institutional Research Program at the Higher Education Research Institute at UCLA, 2009), Available at www.heri.ucla.edu/publications-brp.php.

45. J. H. Pryor et al., *The American Freshman: National Norms Fall 2009* (Los Angeles: Higher Education Research Institute, 2010), Available at www.heri.ucla.edu/publications-brp.php.

46. M. E. Pritchard and G. S. Wilson, "Do Coping Styles Change during the First Semester of College?" *Journal of Social Psychology* 146, no. 1 (2006): 125–27; C. L. Broman, "Stress, Race, and Substance Use in College," *College Student Journal* 39, no. 2 (2005): 340–52; D. Kariv, D. Heilman, and T. Heilman, "Task-Oriented versus Emotion-Oriented Coping Strategies: The Case of College Students," *College Student Journal* 39, no. 1 (2005): 72–84; K. M. Kiefer et al., "Test and Study Worry and Emotionality in the Prediction of College Students' Reasons for Drinking: An Exploratory Investigation," *Journal of Alcohol and Drug Education* 50, no. 1 (2006): 57–81.

47. P. A. Bovier, E. Chamot, and T. V. Perneger, "Perceived Stress, Internal Resources, and Social Support as Determinants of Mental Health among Young Adults," *Quality of Life Research* 13, no. 1 (2004): 161–70; E. Largo-Wright, P. M. Peterson, and W. W. Chen, "Perceived Problem Solving, Stress, and Health among College Students," *American Journal of Health Behavior* 29, no. 4 (2005): 360–70; C. L. Park et al., "The Daily Stress and Coping Process and Alcohol Use among College Students," 2004, 126–35.

48. K. Glanz and M. Schwartz, "Stress, Coping and Health Behavior," in *Health Behavior and Health Education: Theory, Research and Practice*, 4th ed., eds. K. Glanz, B. Rimer, and K. Viswanath (San Francisco: Jossey-Bass, 2002), 210–36.

49. B. L. Seaward, *Managing Stress*, 2009.

50. P. A. Bovier, E. Chamot, and T. V. Perneger, "Perceived Stress, Internal Resources, and Social Support as Determinants of Mental Health among Young Adults," 2004; E. Largo-Wright, P. M. Peterson, and W. W. Chen, "Perceived Problem Solving, Stress, and Health among College Students," 2005; C. L. Park, S. Armeli, and H. Tennen, "The Daily Stress and Coping Process and Alcohol Use among College Students," 2004; A. M. McLaughlin, L. Doane, A.

Costiuc, and N. Feeny, *Determinants of Minority Mental Health and Wellness* (New York: Springer, 2009); L. Crockett et al., "Acculturative Stress, Social Support and Coping: Relations to Psychological Adjustment among Mexican American College Students," *Cultural Diversity and Ethnic Minority Psychology* 13, no. 4 (2007): 347–55; M. Neely et al., "Self Kindness When Facing Stress: The Role of Compassion, Self Regulation and Support in College Students' Well Being," *Motivation and Emotion* 33 (2009): 88–97; J. Ruthig et al., "Perceived Academic Control: Mediating the Effects of Optimism and Social Support on College Students' Psychological Health," *Social Psychology of Education* 12, no. 7 (2009): 233–49.

51. M. Bennett and C. Lengacher, "Humor and Laughter May Influence Health IV: Humor and Immune Function," *Evidence-Based Complementary and Alternative Medicine* 6, no. 2 (2009): 159–64.

52. P. Holmes, "Managing Anger," 2004; B. L. Seaward, *Managing Stress*, 2009.

53. J. Graham et al., "Cognitive Word Use during Marital Conflict and Increases in Proinflammatory Cytokines," *Health Psychology* 28, no. 5 (2009): 621–30.

54. D. A. Girdano, D. E. Dusek, and G. S. Everly, *Controlling Stress and Tension*, 8th ed. (San Francisco: Benjamin Cummings, 2009), 375.

55. P. Steel, "The Nature of Procrastination: A Meta-Analytic and Theoretical Review of Quintessential Self-Regulatory Failure," *Psychological Review* 133, no. 1 (2007): 65–94.

56. T. Gura, "Procrastinating Again? How to Kick the Habit," *Scientific American Mind,* December 2008, www.sciam.com/article.cfm?id=procrastinating-again.

57. Ibid.

58. J. H. Pryor et al., *The American Freshman: National Norms Fall 2009*, 2010.

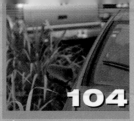

**104**

Is sleepiness dangerous?

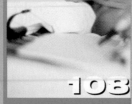

**108**

What should I do if I can't fall asleep?

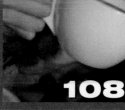

**108**

Why do caffeinated drinks keep me awake?

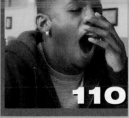

**110**

Are sleep disorders common?

FOCUS ON

# Improving Your Sleep

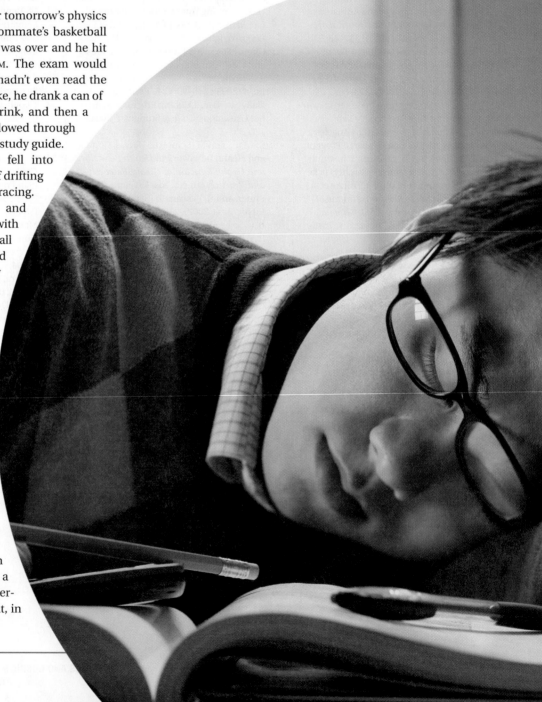

Josh knew he wasn't ready for tomorrow's physics exam, but he went to his roommate's basketball game anyway. By the time it was over and he hit the books, it was past 11 PM. The exam would cover four chapters, and he hadn't even read the last two. To keep himself awake, he drank a can of Mountain Dew, an energy drink, and then a cup of instant coffee as he plowed through the text, his notes, the online study guide. . . . Just before 4 AM, he fell into bed exhausted. But instead of drifting into sleep, his mind kept racing. *Dynamics, inertia, action,* and *reaction* tumbled around with disjointed memories of all the stressful situations he'd been through in the past few days . . . losing his cell phone, his girlfriend dumping him, the argument he'd had with his dad. . . . He glanced at the clock: It was 5:30 AM. The exam was in 3 hours.

If you've ever tackled an exam on way too little sleep, you can probably predict what happened to Josh: He flunked.

In a recent survey from the American College Health Association (ACHA), 11 percent of students reported that in the past week they did not get enough sleep to feel rested on even a single day. And nearly 44 per- cent of students reported that, in the past week, they'd felt rested on fewer than 3 days.[1] It's widely acknowledged that college students are among the most sleep-deprived age group in the United States.[2] Today's students are going to bed an average of 1 to 2 hours later and sleeping 1 to 1.6 fewer hours than students of their parents' generation did.[3]

One factor commonly implicated in reduced sleep time among college students is the Internet and its 24-hour access to online games, social networking sites, videos, and news. Other things keeping students awake include academic pressures, an underlying sleep disorder, chronic pain and other disease symptoms, anxiety or depression, the use of drugs (including alco-

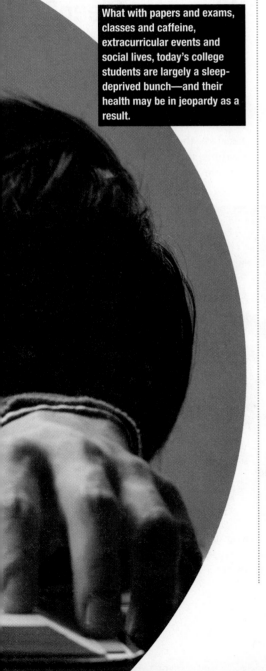

What with papers and exams, classes and caffeine, extracurricular events and social lives, today's college students are largely a sleep-deprived bunch—and their health may be in jeopardy as a result.

# 44%

of college students say they don't feel rested most days of the week.

hol), and stress from a variety of sources, including the stress of juggling finances, classes, and homework with a job or responsibilities at home.

Unfortunately, the statistics don't improve much for working adults. A recent *Sleep in America* poll from the National Sleep Foundation (NSF) found that nearly a third (32%) of Americans get a good night's sleep on only a few nights per month.[4] When there just aren't enough hours in the day, what typically gets shortchanged is sleep.

Because Americans are managing to function on campus and on the job with less sleep, you might conclude that sufficient sleep isn't all that necessary. In fact, getting an adequate amount of sleep is much more important than most people realize. Let's look at the benefits of sleep, and find out what happens when you don't get enough.

# Why Do You Need to Sleep?

Sleep serves at least two biological purposes: (1) It conserves body energy. When you sleep, your core body temperature and the rate at which you burn calories drop. This leaves you with more energy to perform activities throughout your waking hours. (2) It restores you both physically and mentally. For example, certain reparative chemicals are released while you sleep. And there is some evidence, discussed shortly, that during sleep the brain is cleared of daily minutiae, learning is synthesized, and memories are consolidated. In short, getting enough sleep to feel ready to meet daily challenges is essential.

# Sleep Maintains Your Physical Health

Sleep has beneficial effects on most body systems. That's why, when you consistently don't get a good night's rest, your body doesn't function as well, and you become more vulnerable to a wide variety of health problems.[5] Researchers are only just beginning to explore the physical benefits of sleep. The following is a brief summary of what we've learned so far.

● **Sleep helps maintain your immune system.** The common cold, strep throat, the flu, mononucleosis, cold sores, and a variety of other ailments are more common when your immune system is depressed. And that's more likely to happen if you're not getting enough sleep. For instance, one recent study found that poor sleep quality and shorter sleep duration increased susceptibility to the common cold.[6]

● **Sleep helps reduce your risk for cardiovascular disease.** A study of more than 5,000 adults suggested that high blood pressure is more common in people who get fewer than 7 hours of sleep a night.[7] In addition, two separate studies found that poor sleep quality or reduced sleep time increased the prevalence of high levels in the blood of a substance called C-reactive protein (CRP), which is a risk factor for heart disease.[8] Sleep also seems to influence the risk of stroke (a blockage affecting a blood vessel in the brain): A study of more than 93,000 women suggested that sleep duration of 6 or fewer hours a night increases the risk of stroke.[9]

● **Sleep contributes to a healthy metabolism and body weight.** Every moment of your life your body's cells are participating in chemical reactions, many of which involve the breakdown of food and the synthesis of new compounds that the body needs. The sum of all these reactions is called *metabolism*. Several recent studies suggest that sleep contributes to healthy metabolism and thus helps you maintain a healthy body weight. In contrast, inadequate sleep may play a role in our population's increased prevalence of

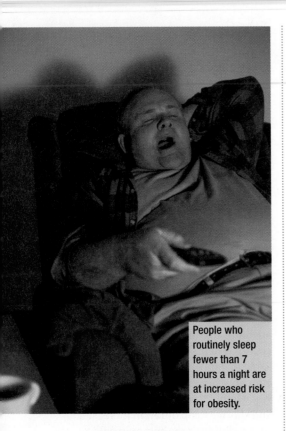

People who routinely sleep fewer than 7 hours a night are at increased risk for obesity.

*type 2 diabetes*, a disorder of glucose metabolism, as well as obesity.[10]

## Sleep Affects Your Ability to Function

If you routinely shortchange yourself on sleep, you could be sabotaging your grades and, if you drive while drowsy, endangering your life. Let's look at what the research reveals about how sleep helps you to function.

● **Sleep contributes to neurological functioning.** Restricting sleep can cause a wide range of neurological problems, including lapses of attention, slowed or poor memory, reduced cognitive ability, and a tendency for your thinking to get "stuck in a rut."[11] Your ability not only to remember facts but also to integrate those facts, make meaningful generalizations about them, and consolidate what you've learned into lasting memories requires adequate sleep time.[12] Studies have shown that college students who pull all-nighters, as well as students who are short sleepers, have significantly lower overall grade-point averages compared with classmates who get adequate sleep.[13]

● **Sleep improves motor tasks.** Sleep also has a restorative effect on motor function, that is, the ability to perform tasks such as shooting a basket, playing a musical instrument, or driving a car.[14] It's one thing to mess up on a Schubert sonata, but the consequences are potentially fatal when sleep deprivation makes you mess up behind the wheel. Some sleep researchers contend that a night without sleep impairs your motor skills and reaction time as much as if you were driving drunk.[15] As Americans have become more and more sleep-deprived, the incidence of drowsy driving and so-called fall-asleep crashes has become a national concern. The NSF reports that 37 percent of Americans admit to having fallen asleep at the wheel in the past year, and more than 1,500 Americans die in fatigue-related crashes annually.[16]

## Sleep Promotes Your Psychosocial Health

Research suggests that certain brain regions, including the cerebral cortex (your "master mind"), can achieve some form of essential rest only during sleep.[17] So if your roommate says you're grouchy after you've gone for a few nights without enough sleep, don't take it too personally: Your irritability is actually just a sign of brain fatigue.

In addition, you're more likely to feel stressed-out, worried, or sad when you're sleep-deprived. The relationship between sleep and stress is highly complex: Stress can cause or contribute to sleep problems, and sleep problems can cause or increase your level of stress! The same is true of clinical psychiatric conditions such as depression and anxiety disorders: Reduced or poor quality sleep can trigger these disorders, but it's also a common symptom resulting from them.[18]

## What Goes on When You Sleep?

If you've ever taken a flight that crossed two or more time zones, you've probably experienced *jet lag*, a feeling that your body's "internal clock" is out of sync with the hours of daylight and darkness at your destination. Jet lag happens because the new day/night pattern disrupts the 24-hour cycle by which you are accustomed to going to sleep,

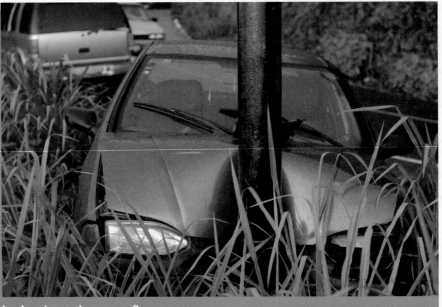

**Is sleepiness dangerous?**

Lack of sleep impairs your reflexes, cognitive functioning, and motor skills, all of which you need to ride a bike or operate a car safely. The National Sleep Foundation estimates that 100,000 sleep-related auto accidents, resulting in 1,500 deaths, occur in the United States every year.

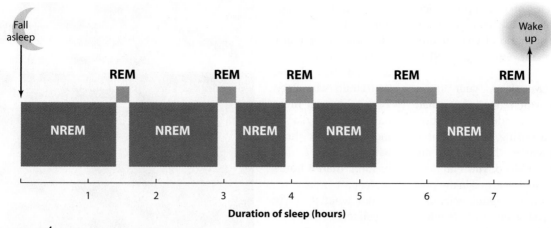

FIGURE 1 **The Nightly Sleep Cycle**
As the number of hours you sleep increases, your brain spends more and more time in REM sleep.
Thus, sleeping for too few hours could mean you're depriving yourself primarily of needed REM sleep.

waking up, and performing habitual behaviors throughout your day. This cycle, known as your **circadian rhythm,** is regulated in part by a tiny gland in your brain called the *pineal body:* It releases a **hormone** called *melatonin* that induces drowsiness.

You can fight the effects of melatonin for hours—even days!—especially if, like Josh in our opening story, you load up on caffeine. But like all human beings, and in fact all mammals, you will eventually succumb to **sleep,** which is clinically defined as a readily reversible state of reduced responsiveness to, and interaction with, the environment.[19] Sleep researchers generally distinguish between two primary sleep states: a state that is not characterized by rapid eye movement, called **non-REM (NREM) sleep,** and a state in which rapid eye movement does occur, called **REM sleep.** During the night, you slide through the stages of NREM sleep, then into REM, then back through NREM again, repeating one full cycle about once every 90 minutes.[20] Overall, you spend about 75 percent of each night in NREM sleep, and 25 percent in REM (Figure 1).

## Non-REM Sleep Is Restorative

During non-REM sleep the body rests. Movement can occur, for instance, to shift your position in bed, but muscle tension is reduced. Both your body temperature and your energy use drop; sensation is dulled; and your brain waves, heart rate, and breathing slow. In contrast, digestive processes speed up, and your body stores nutrients. During NREM sleep, you do not typically dream. Four distinct stages of NREM sleep have been distinguished by their characteristic brain-wave patterns.

**Stage 1.** Your eyes may be open or closed, but essentially, you're drifting off. Stage 1 lasts only a few minutes, and is the lightest stage of sleep from which you are most easily awakened.

**Stage 2.** This stage is slightly deeper than stage 1 and lasts from 5 to 15 minutes. Your eyes are closed, eye and body movements gradually cease, and you disengage from your environment.

**Stage 3.** NREM sleep is also called *slow-wave sleep,* because during stages 3 and 4, a sleeper's brain generates slow, large-amplitude delta waves as shown on an electroencephalogram (EEG). Your blood pressure drops, your heart rate and respiration slow considerably, and you enter deep sleep.

**Stage 4.** This is the deepest stage of sleep. Human growth hormone is released and signals your body to repair worn tissues. Speech and movement are rare during this stage, but can and do sometimes occur. For example, sleepwalking typically occurs during the first stage 4 period of the night. You've probably heard that it's difficult to awaken a sleepwalker, and that's true of anyone in stage 4 sleep.

## REM Sleep Is Energizing

Dreaming takes place primarily during REM sleep. On an EEG, a REM sleeper's brain-wave activity is almost indistinguishable from that of someone who is wide awake, and the brain's energy use is higher than that of a person who is performing a difficult math problem![21] Your muscles are paralyzed during REM sleep: You may dream that you're rock climbing, but your body is incapable of movement. Almost the only exceptions are your respiratory muscles, which allow you to breathe, and

---

**circadian rhythm** The 24-hour cycle by which you are accustomed to going to sleep, waking up, and performing habitual behaviors.

**hormone** A "chemical messenger" that is released from one of the body's endocrine glands and travels in the bloodstream to another site where it helps to regulate body functions.

**sleep** A readily reversible state of reduced responsiveness to, and interaction with, the environment.

**non-REM (NREM) sleep** A period of restful sleep dominated by slow brain waves; during non-REM sleep, rapid eye movement is rare.

**REM sleep** A period of sleep characterized by brain-wave activity similar to that seen in wakefulness; rapid eye movement and dreaming occur during REM sleep.

the tiny muscles of your eyes, which move your eyes rapidly as if you were following the scenario of your dream. This rapid eye movement gives REM sleep its name.

During REM sleep, your brain processes the experiences you've had and consolidates the information you've learned during the day. Some researchers theorize that, if you are deprived of REM sleep, you may lose information or skills learned in the previous 24 to 48 hours. Other scientists believe that REM sleep has little effect on memory.[22] As the night progresses, the duration of NREM sleep declines and you spend more and more time in REM. That's why a full night's sleep is important for getting as much REM sleep as you need.

## How Much Sleep Do You Need?

Given the importance of adequate sleep, especially REM sleep, you're probably asking yourself how much you really need. Unfortunately, there's no magic number. Let's find out why.

## Sleep Need Includes Baseline Plus Debt

The short answer to how much sleep you need is about 7 to 8 hours. This recommendation is used by researchers as the standard for "average" sleep

# 7 to 8

**hours is the sleep duration period associated with optimal health and functioning.**

**sleep debt** The difference between the number of hours of sleep an individual needed in a given time period and the number of hours he or she actually slept.
**sleep inertia** A state characterized by cognitive impairment, grogginess, and disorientation that is experienced upon rising from short sleep or an overly long nap.

time, and is supported by a variety of studies over many years.[23] For instance, research has shown that adults who sleep 7 to 8 hours a night have a lower risk of mortality than those who get fewer than 7 or more than 8 hours of sleep.[24]

But what if you're absolutely certain that you get by just fine on 5 or 6 hours a night? Then you might be interested in the results of another study in which young people who claimed they needed less sleep were found to need the average 7 to 8 hours when monitored in a sleep lab![25]

Still, sleep is not a "one size fits all" proposition. Individual variations do occur according to age (kids need more sleep), gender (women need more sleep), and many other factors. In addition, when trying to figure out your sleep needs, you have to consider two aspects: your body's physiological need plus your current **sleep debt.** That's the total number of hours of missed sleep you're carrying around with you, either because you got up before your body was fully rested, or because your sleep was interrupted. Let's say that last week you managed just 5 hours of sleep a night Monday through Thursday. Even if you get 7 to 8 hours a night Friday through Sunday, that unresolved sleep debt of 8 to 12 hours will still leave you feeling tired and groggy when you start the week again. That means you need *more than* 8 hours a night for the next several nights to "catch up."

The good news is that you *can* catch up if you go about it sensibly. Getting 5 hours of sleep a night all semester long, then sleeping 48 hours the first weekend you're home on break won't restore your functioning, and it's likely to disrupt your circadian rhythm. Instead, whittle away at

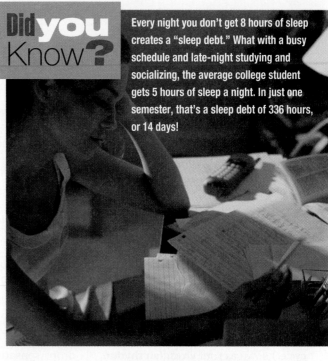

*Every night you don't get 8 hours of sleep creates a "sleep debt." What with a busy schedule and late-night studying and socializing, the average college student gets 5 hours of sleep a night. In just one semester, that's a sleep debt of 336 hours, or 14 days!*

that sleep debt by sleeping 9 hours a night throughout your break—then start the new term resolved to sleep 7 to 8 hours a night.

## what do you think?

Do you find it difficult to get 7 or 8 hours of sleep each night? ● Do you think you are able to catch up on sleep you miss? ● Have you noticed any negative consequences in your own life when you get too little sleep?

## Do Naps Count?

Speaking of catching up, do naps count? Although naps can't entirely cancel out a significant sleep debt, they can help to improve your mood, alertness, and performance.[26] It's best to nap in the early to mid-afternoon, when the pineal body in your brain releases a small amount of melatonin and your body experiences a natural dip in its circadian rhythm. Never nap in the late afternoon, as it could interfere with your ability to fall asleep that night. Keep your naps short, because a nap of more than 30 minutes can leave you in a state of **sleep inertia,** which is characterized by cognitive impairment, grogginess, and a disoriented feeling.

# BE HEALTHY, BE GREEN

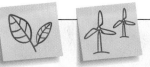

## Bedding Down in Green

We may not lie awake thinking about our bed's impact on the environment, but we can still make healthier and environmentally sound choices through the bedding products we buy. To begin with, ecofriendly and organic versions of most textile products—including sheets and blankets—have become widely available.

During the production of conventional cotton, or nonorganic cotton, synthetic pesticides and other environmentally harmful chemicals are used. The conventional cotton industry also uses a large number of chemicals after harvest, including bleach and petroleum-based dyes. Conversely, organic cotton is grown using organic farming techniques, such as crop rotation and biological pest control, aimed at producing crops without exhausting the soil or polluting the environment. In addition, organic cotton products are typically processed without bleach and use natural dyes.

Another textile fiber with environmental benefits is bamboo, which offers a soft fabric from a rapidly renewable resource. Bamboo is actually a type of grass that can grow extremely fast, up to several feet per day! Further, bamboo does not require replanting and helps offset greenhouse gases by absorbing $CO_2$ from the atmosphere. This plant is naturally resistant to pests and infection, so no pesticides are used in its cultivation, and its natural antibacterial and antifungal properties are an added bonus of using bamboo bedding.

For most people, a mattress is an extremely important purchase: The bed you choose can affect the quality of your rest and your overall health for years. Your choice of mattress can affect the planet's health, too. Synthetic materials used in conventional mattresses, such as polyurethane foam, can emit volatile organic compounds that have been associated with poor respiratory function. Moreover, conventional mattresses are often treated with synthetic chemicals that are known to "off-gas," affecting indoor air quality.

More healthful and environmentally responsible mattress materials include organic cotton, wool, and natural latex. Some ecofriendly mattresses combine organic cotton with wool, a natural fire retardant. Wool is also nonabsorbent and, consequently, is less hospitable to microorganisms, meaning no antimicrobial chemicals are necessary on wool products. Similarly, mattresses and pillows made of natural latex, derived from the resin of the rubber tree, are hypoallergenic, mold and mildew resistant, and breathable. They are also biodegradable and are produced from a renewable resource—rubber trees are not killed or damaged by the process of tapping them for their resin, so they can continue producing resin and contributing to counterbalancing greenhouse gases for years.

With ecofriendly beds and bedding, you can sleep more easily knowing that your choices are healthier for you and for the environment, both inside and outside your home.

---

# How Can You Get a Good Night's Sleep?

Do you need a jolt of caffeine to get you jump-started in the morning? Do you find it hard to stay awake in class? Have you ever nodded off behind the wheel? These are all signs of inadequate or poor quality sleep. To find out whether you're sleep-deprived, take the **Assess Yourself** questionnaire on page 114.

## To Promote Restful Sleep, Try These Tips

The following tips can help you get a longer and more restful night's sleep.

- **Let there be light.** Throughout the day, stay in sync with your circadian rhythm by spending time in the sunlight. If you live in an area where the sun seldom shines for weeks at a time, invest in special light-emitting diode (LED) lighting designed to mimic the sun's rays. Exposure to natural light outdoors is most beneficial, but opening the shades indoors and, on overcast days, turning on room lights can also help keep you alert.
- **Stay active.** It's hard to feel sleepy if you've been sedentary all day, so make sure you get plenty of physical activity during the day. Resist the temptation to postpone exercise until you're sleeping better. Start gently, but start now, because regular exercise may help you maintain regular sleep habits.

- **Sleep tight.** Don't let a pancake pillow, scratchy or pilled sheets, or a threadbare blanket keep you from sleeping soundly. If your mattress is uncomfortable and you can't replace it, try putting a foam mattress overlay on top of it. For information about ecofriendly bedding, see the **Be Healthy, Be Green** box.
- **Create a sleep "cave."** Take a lesson from bats, bears, and burrowing animals! As bedtime approaches, keep your bedroom quiet, cool, and dark. Start by turning off your computer and cell phone. If you live in an apartment or dorm where there's noise outside or in the halls, wear ear plugs or get an electronic device that produces "white noise" such as the sound of gentle rain. Turn down the thermostat or, on hot nights, run a quiet electric

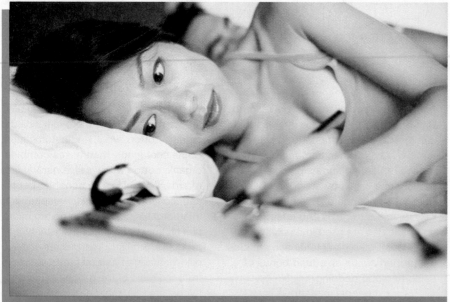

**What should I do if I can't fall asleep?**

If you have difficulty falling asleep, it may be that noises, lights, interruptions, or persistent worries are keeping you awake. Use ear plugs or a white noise machine to block out noise, wear an eye shade to block out light, and turn off your phone and computer to prevent interruptions. If a worry keeps you awake, jot it down in a journal. You'll be better prepared to handle it in the morning after you've had a good night's sleep.

fan. Install room-darkening shades or curtains or wear an eye mask if necessary to block out any light from the street.

- **Condition yourself into better sleep.** Go to bed and get up at the same time each day. Establish a bedtime ritual that signals to your body that it's time for sleep. For instance, sit by your bed and listen to a quiet song, meditate, write in a journal, take a warm bath or shower, or read something that lets you quietly wind down.
- **Breathe.** Do it deeply, as soon as your head hits the pillow. Inhale through your nose slowly, filling your lungs completely, then exhale slowly through slightly pursed lips. Repeat several times. Giving your body the oxygen it needs, deep breathing can also decrease anxiety and tension that sometimes make it difficult to fall asleep.
- **Don't toss and turn.** If you're not asleep after 20 minutes, get up. Turn on a low light, and read something relaxing, not stimulating, or listen to some gentle music. Once you feel sleepy, go back to bed.

## To Prevent Sleep Problems, Avoid These Behaviors

Maybe you're already doing most of the actions suggested above, and you still can't sleep. If so, perhaps it's time to learn what *not* to do:

- Don't nap in the late afternoon or evening, and don't nap for longer than 30 minutes.
- Don't engage in strenuous exercise within several hours of bedtime. Activity speeds up your metabolism and makes it harder to fall asleep.
- Don't read, study, watch TV, use your laptop, talk on the phone, eat, or smoke in bed. In fact, don't smoke at all: Besides promoting cancer and heart disease, smoking is known to disturb your sleep.
- Don't try to sleep if you're starving or stuffed. Allow at least 3 hours between your evening meal and bedtime and, if you feel hungry before bed, have a light snack.
- Don't drink coffee, energy drinks, or anything else that contains caffeine

within several hours of bedtime. Once you consume caffeine, which is a powerful stimulant, it takes your body about 6 hours to clear just *half* of it from your system.[27]

- Don't drink alcohol within several hours of bedtime. Although initially it can make you drowsy, it interferes with your natural sleep stages and can cause you to awaken in the middle of the night, unable to get back to sleep.
- Don't drink large amounts of any liquid before bed, to prevent having to get up in the night to use the bathroom.
- Don't take sleeping pills or nighttime pain medications unless they have been prescribed by your health care provider. Casual use of over-the-counter sleeping aids can interfere

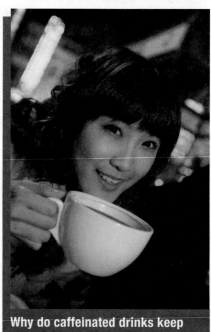

**Why do caffeinated drinks keep me awake?**

After-dinner coffee? Not unless it's decaf. Caffeine promotes alertness by blocking the neurotransmitter adenosine in your brain—a useful thing when you are studying, but a potential problem when you are trying to sleep. Your body needs 6 hours to process half of the caffeine you drink (and another 6 to process half of what remains, and so on). So coffee at 8 PM means you won't be sleeping soundly until well after midnight.

with your brain's natural progression through the healthy stages of sleep. You may also experience "payback" later when you try to stop using the drug and your sleep challenges return, at a level worse than they were before you started using the medication.

● Don't get triggered. Remember the earlier advice about turning off your cell phone as you begin to prepare for bed? One reason is to avoid those late-night phone calls that can end up in arguments, disappointments, and other emotional stressors. If something—or someone—does trigger you shortly before bed, journal about it briefly, then promise yourself that you'll make time the next day to explore your feelings more deeply.

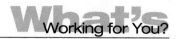

### Working for You?

Maybe you're already practicing ways to get a better night's sleep. Which of the following sleep-promoting behaviors are you already incorporating into your life?

☐ I exercise regularly.
☐ I turn off my computer at night.
☐ I drink only beverages that are caffeine free late in the day.
☐ I make sure not to nap late in the day.

# What If You're Not Sleeping Well?

If you're following the advice in this chapter and you still aren't sleeping well, then it's time to see your health care provider, as you may be one of the estimated 50 to 70 million Americans who have a clinical sleep disorder.[28] To aid in diagnosis, you will probably be asked to keep a sleep diary like the one in Figure 2, and you may be referred to a sleep disorders center for an overnight stay. This type of evaluation is known as a clinical **sleep study.** While you are asleep in the sleep center, sensors and electrodes record data that will be reviewed by a sleep specialist who will help your primary health care provider determine the precise nature of your sleep problem.

The American Academy of Sleep Medicine identifies more than 80 specific sleep disorders. The most common

---

**sleep study** A clinical assessment of sleep in which the patient is monitored while spending the night in a sleep disorders center.

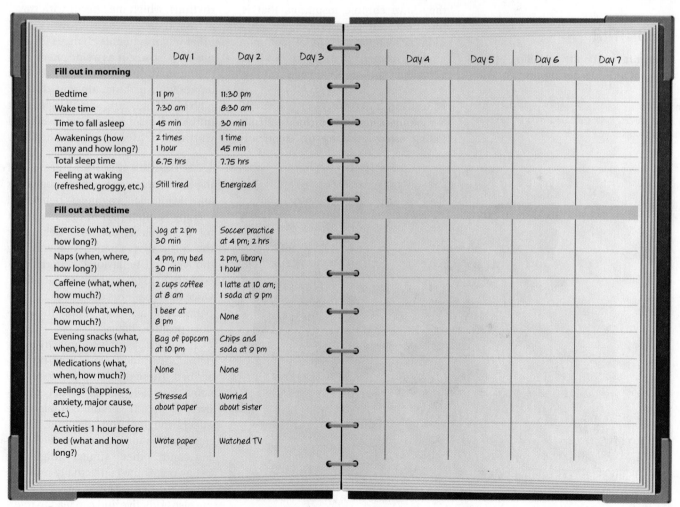

| | Day 1 | Day 2 | Day 3 | Day 4 | Day 5 | Day 6 | Day 7 |
|---|---|---|---|---|---|---|---|
| **Fill out in morning** | | | | | | | |
| Bedtime | 11 pm | 11:30 pm | | | | | |
| Wake time | 7:30 am | 8:30 am | | | | | |
| Time to fall asleep | 45 min | 30 min | | | | | |
| Awakenings (how many and how long?) | 2 times 1 hour | 1 time 45 min | | | | | |
| Total sleep time | 6.75 hrs | 7.75 hrs | | | | | |
| Feeling at waking (refreshed, groggy, etc.) | Still tired | Energized | | | | | |
| **Fill out at bedtime** | | | | | | | |
| Exercise (what, when, how long?) | Jog at 2 pm 30 min | Soccer practice at 4 pm; 2 hrs | | | | | |
| Naps (when, where, how long?) | 4 pm, my bed 30 min | 2 pm, library 1 hour | | | | | |
| Caffeine (what, when, how much?) | 2 cups coffee at 8 am | 1 latte at 10 am; 1 soda at 9 pm | | | | | |
| Alcohol (what, when, how much?) | 1 beer at 8 pm | None | | | | | |
| Evening snacks (what, when, how much?) | Bag of popcorn at 10 pm | Chips and soda at 9 pm | | | | | |
| Medications (what, when, how much?) | None | None | | | | | |
| Feelings (happiness, anxiety, major cause, etc.) | Stressed about paper | Worried about sister | | | | | |
| Activities 1 hour before bed (what and how long?) | Wrote paper | Watched TV | | | | | |

FIGURE 2 **Sample Sleep Diary**
Using a sleep diary such as this one can help you and your health care provider discover any behavioral factors that might be contributing to your sleep problem.

### Sleep Disorder Prevalence by Gender and Ethnicity

| Sleep Disorders | White | | Black | | Asian | | Hispanic | |
|---|---|---|---|---|---|---|---|---|
| | Men | Women | Men | Women | Men | Women | Men | Women |
| Any | 22% | 19% | 24% | 16% | 10% | 9% | 17% | 20% |
| Insomnia | 9% | 10% | 2% | 5% | 3% | 5% | 7% | 7% |
| Sleep apnea | 10% | 2% | 20% | 10% | 5% | 4% | 9% | 7% |
| Restless legs syndrome | 4% | 8% | <1% | 1% | 3% | – | 3% | 4% |

**Source:** National Sleep Foundation, *2010 Sleep in America Poll Summary of Findings* (Washington, DC: National Sleep Foundation, 2010), 51, Used with permission of the National Sleep Foundation. For further information, please visit www.sleepfoundation.org.

disorders in adults are insomnia, sleep apnea, and restless legs syndrome. **Table 1** compares the prevalence of these disorders among men and women across different ethnicities. Other common sleep disorders include narcolepsy and a group of disorders called parasomnias.

## Insomnia

**Insomnia**—difficulty in falling asleep, frequent arousals during sleep, or early

> **insomnia** A disorder characterized by difficulty in falling asleep quickly, frequent arousals during sleep, or early morning awakening.

morning awakening—is the most common sleep complaint. Annual *Sleep in America* polls dating back at least 10 years reveal that more than 50 percent of Americans experience insomnia at least a few nights a week.[29] About 10 to 15 percent of Americans report that they have chronic insomnia, that is, insomnia that persists longer than a month. Insomnia is more common among women than men, and its prevalence increases with age.

### Insomnia Symptoms and Causes

Symptoms of insomnia include difficulty falling asleep, waking up frequently during the night, difficulty returning to sleep, waking up too early in the morning, unrefreshing sleep, daytime sleepiness, and irritability. Sometimes insomnia is related to stress and worry. In other cases it may be related to disruptions to the body's circadian rhythms, which may occur with travel across time zones, shift work, and other major schedule changes. Insomnia can also occur as a side effect from taking medications for heart disease, depression, asthma, thyroid disease, high blood pressure, and allergies. Left untreated, insomnia can be associated with an increased illness or morbidity.

**Treatment for Insomnia** Because of the close connection between behavior and insomnia, cognitive behavioral therapy is often part of any treatment for insomnia. A cognitive behavioral therapist assists a patient in identifying thought and behavioral patterns that contribute to the inability to fall asleep. Once these patterns are recognized, the patient practices new habits that produce positive change.

In some cases of insomnia, *hypnotic* or *sedative* medications may be prescribed. These drugs induce sleep, and some may help relieve anxiety. However, some have undesirable side effects ranging from daytime sleepiness and hallucinations to sleepwalking and other strange nighttime behaviors. Some can actually promote anxiety or depression. Many sedatives are also addictive and can lead to tolerance and dependence. Antidepressants are also commonly prescribed for insomnia.

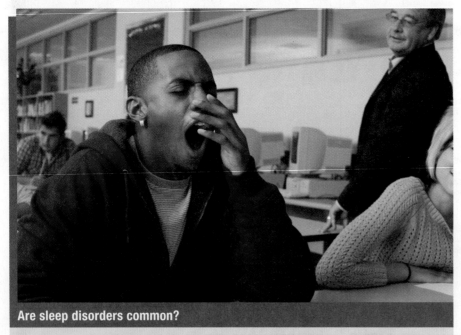

**Are sleep disorders common?**

From insomnia to sleepwalking to narcolepsy, sleep disorders are more common than you might think. There are more than 80 different clinical sleep disorders, and it is estimated that between 50 and 70 million Americans—children and adults—suffer from one. Many aren't even aware of their disorder, and many others never seek treatment.

## Beat Jet Lag

Insomnia, fatigue, stomachache, and headache: These are symptoms of jet lag and not a great way to spend a spring break vacation. In general, the more time zones you cross, the worse the jet lag will be. There are ways to avoid or reduce jet lag. Here's how:

* Begin the trip rested (preexisting sleep deprivation intensifies jet lag).
* Schedule a daytime flight.
* Reset your watch as soon as you depart.
* Avoid alcohol, caffeine, and nicotine.
* Eat small meals at the appropriate mealtime for your destination.
* Several days before going west, go to bed and wake up 1 hour later each day.
* Once in the west, seek morning light and avoid afternoon light.
* Several days before going east, go to bed and wake up 1 hour earlier each day.
* Once in the east, seek evening light and avoid morning light.
* If you take an overnight flight, avoid sleeping too much on the day of your arrival. You'll find it hard to fight the fatigue, but sleeping during the day will make it harder for you to adjust to your new time zone's schedule.

Relaxation techniques, including yoga and meditation, can be especially helpful in preparing the body to sleep. Exercise, done early in the day, can also be helpful in reducing stress and promoting deeper sleep. The **Skills for Behavior Change** box presents some specific tips for preventing insomnia related to jet lag and other schedule disruptions.

## Sleep Apnea

**Sleep apnea** is a disorder in which breathing is briefly and repeatedly interrupted during sleep.[30] *Apnea* refers to a breathing pause that lasts at least 10 seconds. During that time, the chest may rise and fall, but little or no air may be exchanged, or the person may actually not breathe until the brain triggers a gasping inhalation. Sleep apnea affects more than 18 million Americans, or 1 in every 15 people.[31]

**Causes of Sleep Apnea** There are two major types of sleep apnea: central and obstructive. *Central sleep apnea* occurs when the brain fails to tell the respiratory muscles to initiate breathing. This condition often occurs in people who have other medical conditions involving the brain, such as stroke or neurodegenerative diseases. Consumption of alcohol, certain illegal drugs, and certain medications can also lead to central sleep apnea.

*Obstructive sleep apnea (OSA)*, which is the more common form, occurs when air cannot move in and out of a person's nose or mouth, even though the body tries to breathe. Typically, OSA occurs when a person's throat muscles and tongue relax during sleep and block the airways. This condition can occur in people of any age and either sex, but certain factors are associated with increased risk: having a small upper airway, being overweight or obese, having a recessed chin or small jaw, large neck size, and smoking and alcohol use.[32] Prevalence is greater in people over age 40 and of African-American, Pacific-Islander, or Hispanic ethnicity. Obstructive sleep apnea also may have a genetic link, as it appears to run in families.

**Symptoms of Sleep Apnea** People with OSA are prone to heavy snoring, snorting, and gasping. These sounds occur because, as oxygen saturation levels in the blood fall, the body's autonomic nervous system is stimulated to trigger inhalation, often via a sudden gasp of breath. This response may wake the person, preventing deep sleep and causing the person to wake up in the morning feeling tired and unwell.

People with sleep apnea tend to be sleep-deprived, and may suffer from sleeplessness and a wide range of other symptoms that include difficulty concentrating; depression; irritability; sexual dysfunction; learning and memory difficulties; and falling asleep while at work, on the phone, or driving. Left untreated, symptoms of sleep apnea can lead to further complications including high blood pressure, heart attack, congestive heart failure, cardiac arrhythmia, stroke, or depression.

**Treatment of Sleep Apnea** The most commonly prescribed therapy for OSA is use of a continuous positive airway pressure (CPAP) device, which consists of an airflow device, long tube, and mask (see **Figure 3** on page 112). People with sleep apnea wear this mask during sleep, and air is forced into the nose to keep the airway open.

Other methods for treating OSA include dental appliances, which reposition the lower jaw and tongue, and upper airway surgery to remove tissue in the airway. In general, these approaches are most helpful for mild disease or heavy

**sleep apnea** A disorder in which breathing is briefly and repeatedly interrupted during sleep.

### "Why Should I Care?"

If you experience persistent trouble sleeping, it's worth your time to see a doctor. Not only can sleep disorders by themselves be threatening to your health, but the fact that they deprive you of quality sleep can also lead to a host of other problems including academic difficulties, weight gain, high blood pressure, and chronic stress.

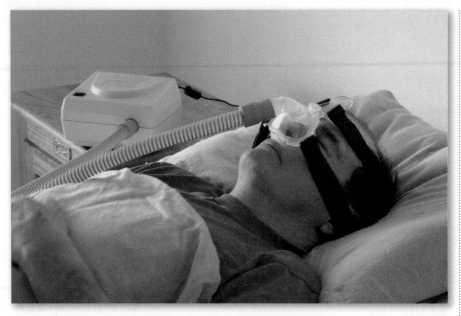

## Narcolepsy

**Narcolepsy** is a neurological disorder caused by the brain's inability to properly regulate sleep–wake cycles. The result of this disorder is excessive, intrusive sleepiness and daytime sleep attacks. Narcolepsy occurs in about 1 of every 2,000 people, and affects men and women equally.[34]

**Symptoms and Causes of Narcolepsy** Narcolepsy is characterized by overwhelming and uncontrollable sleepiness during the day. Narcoleptics are prone to falling asleep at inappropriate times and places—in class, at work, while driving or eating, or even mid-conversation. These sleep attacks can last from a few seconds to several minutes. Other symptoms of narcolepsy include *cataplexy* (the sudden loss of voluntary muscle tone, often triggered by emotional stimuli), hallucinations during sleep onset or upon awakening, and brief episodes of paralysis during sleep–wake transitions.

In most cases narcolepsy appears to be caused by a deficiency in the brain of hypocretin, a chemical that plays a role in sleep regulation. The reason for this chemical deficiency is still being studied, but there appears to be a genetic basis for the disorder.[35] Other factors can contribute to the development of narcolepsy, including having another sleep disorder, using certain medications, or having a mental disorder or substance abuse disorder.

**Treatment for Narcolepsy** The most common way to treat narcolepsy is by medication. Various stimulants are often prescribed to improve alertness, and antidepressants may be prescribed to treat cataplexy, hallucinations, and sleep paralysis. Behavioral therapy can also be effective in helping narcoleptics cope with their condition. Some lifestyle changes, such as scheduling brief naps during the day or not eating heavy meals, may also be helpful.

## Parasomnias

A **parasomnia** is a disorder in which undesired events occur while a person

snoring. Lifestyle changes, which may include losing weight, avoiding alcohol, and quitting smoking, are often effective ways of reducing symptoms of OSA.

## Restless Legs Syndrome

**Restless legs syndrome (RLS)** is a neurological disorder characterized by unpleasant sensations in the legs when at rest combined by an uncontrollable urge to move in an effort to relieve these feelings. These sensations range in severity from uncomfortable to irritating to painful. Some researchers estimate that RLS affects as many as 12 million Americans, whereas others think it may be even more common but is underdiagnosed or misdiagnosed.[33]

**Symptoms and Causes of RLS** Restless legs syndrome sensations are often described as burning, creeping, or tugging, or like insects crawling inside the legs. Moving the legs relieves the discomfort, so people with RLS often keep their legs in motion. In general, the symptoms are more pronounced in the evening or at night. Lying down or trying to relax activates the symptoms, so people with RLS often have difficulty falling and staying asleep.

In most cases, the cause of RLS is unknown. A family history of the condition is seen in approximately 50 percent of such cases, suggesting a genetic form of the disorder. People with familial RLS tend to be younger when symptoms start and have a slower progression of the condition. In other cases, RLS appears to be related to other conditions including Parkinson's disease, diabetes, and anemia.

**Treatment of RLS** If there is an underlying condition, treatment of that condition may provide relief. Other treatment options include use of prescribed medication, decreasing tobacco and alcohol use, and applying heat to the legs. For some people practicing relaxation techniques or performing stretching exercises can help alleviate symptoms.

**restless legs syndrome (RLS)** A neurological disorder characterized by an overwhelming urge to move the legs when they are at rest.
**narcolepsy** Excessive, intrusive sleepiness.
**parasomnia** A disorder characterized by the occurrence of undesirable events while a person is sleeping.

is sleeping. Two common parasomnias are REM sleep behavior disorder (RBD) and sleepwalking.

### REM Sleep Behavior Disorder (RBD)
REM sleep behavior disorder (RBD) occurs when a person acts out vivid dreams during REM sleep. The activity involved may be mild, such as moving the hands, or violent, such as tackling an imaginary attacker. People with RBD do not have their eyes open and rarely get up and walk, but they may shout, punch, jump, or kick. The episodes may begin in the first cycle of REM sleep and continue to occur during subsequent REM stages until the sleeper awakes in the morning.

RBD occurs most commonly in adult men, often after age 50.[36] RBD often occurs as the result of another medical condition, and it has been associated with other sleep disorders including sleep apnea and narcolepsy. RBD has also been associated with use of certain medications, sleep deprivation, and alcohol withdrawal. RBD is usually treated with medications. In addition to medication, people with RBD may need to "injury-proof" their bedrooms or take other precautions to prevent hurting themselves or others during an episode.

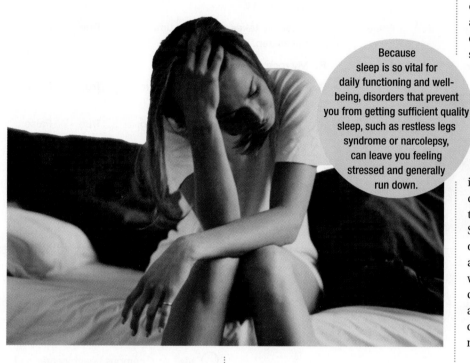

Because sleep is so vital for daily functioning and well-being, disorders that prevent you from getting sufficient quality sleep, such as restless legs syndrome or narcolepsy, can leave you feeling stressed and generally run down.

### Sleepwalking
Sleepwalking is another type of parasomnia in which a sleeper gets up and walks around, typically with eyes open, all while entirely asleep. Unlike RBD, it typically occurs during stage 3 or 4 of NREM sleep. The sleepwalker may eat, perform a chore, urinate, or even get in a car and drive. Sleepwalking is more common in children, but up to 4 percent of adults sleepwalk.[37]

In children, sleepwalking usually goes away on its own as they enter the teen years. Causes of sleepwalking in adults can include alcohol use, sleep deprivation, use of certain medications, and physical or emotional stress. Sleepwalking can also occur as a result of obstructive sleep apnea. If OSA is also being treated, symptoms of sleepwalking often improve. A doctor's visit can assess whether a medication for another health condition may be the cause, and switching prescriptions may be necessary.

# Assess yourself

## Are You Sleeping Well?

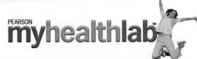

Read each statement below, then circle True or False according to whether or not it applies to you in the current school term.

Fill out this assessment online at
www.pearsonhighered.com/myhealthlab or
www.pearsonhighered.com/donatelle.

1. I sometimes doze off in my morning classes.    True    False

2. I sometimes doze off in my last class of the day.    True    False

3. I go through most of the day feeling tired.    True    False

4. I feel drowsy when I'm a passenger in a bus or car.    True    False

5. I often fall asleep while reading or studying.    True    False

6. I often fall asleep at the computer or watching TV.    True    False

7. It usually takes me a long time to fall asleep.    True    False

8. My roommate tells me I snore.    True    False

9. I wake up frequently throughout the night.    True    False

10. I have fallen asleep while driving.    True    False

If you answer True more than once, you may be sleep-deprived. Try the strategies in this chapter for getting more or better quality sleep, but if you still experience sleepiness, see your health care provider.

# YOUR PLAN FOR CHANGE

The **Assess yourself** activity gave you the chance to determine whether you are sleep-deprived. Now that you have considered your answers, you can take steps to improve your sleep, starting tonight.

### Today, you can:

○ Evaluate your behaviors and identify things you're doing that get in the way of a good night's sleep. Develop a plan. What can you do differently starting today?

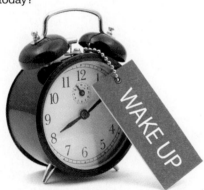

○ Write a list of personal Dos and Don'ts. For instance: Do turn off your cell phone after 11 PM. Don't drink anything with caffeine after 3 PM.

### Within the next 2 weeks, you can:

○ Keep a sleep diary, noting not only how many hours of sleep you get each night, but also how you feel and how you function the next day.

○ Arrange your room to promote restful sleep. Remember the "cave": Keep it quiet, cool, and dark, and replace any uncomfortable bedding.

○ Visit your campus health center and ask for more information about getting a good night's sleep.

### By the end of the semester, you can:

○ Establish a regular sleep schedule. Get in the habit of going to bed and waking up at the same time, even on weekends.

○ Create a ritual, such as stretching, meditation, reading something light, or listening to music, that you follow each night to help your body ease from the activity of the day into restful sleep.

○ If you are still having difficulty sleeping and feel you may have a sleep disorder or an underlying health problem disrupting your sleep, contact your health care provider.

# References

1. American College Health Association, *American College Health Association–National College Health Assessment II (ACHA–NCHA II): Reference Group Data Report Fall 2009* (Baltimore: American College Health Association, 2010), Available at www.achancha.org/reports _ACHA-NCHAII.html.

2. Central Michigan University, "College Student Sleep Patterns Could Be Detrimental," *ScienceDaily* (May 13, 2008), www.sciencedaily.com/releases/2008/ 05/080512145824.htm, Accessed March 18, 2009.

3. D. Law, "Exhaustion in University Students and the Effect of Coursework Involvement," *Journal of American College Health* 55, no. 4 (2007): 239–45.

4. National Sleep Foundation, *Longer Work Days Leave Americans Nodding Off on the Job*, Press Release (March 3, 2008), www .sleepfoundation.org/article/press -release/longer-work-days-leave -americans-nodding-the-job.

5. S. Banks and D. F. Dinges, "Behavioral and Physiological Consequences of Sleep Restriction," *Journal of Clinical Sleep Medicine* 3, no. 5 (2007): 519–28.

6. S. Cohen et al., "Sleep Habits and Susceptibility to the Common Cold," *Archives of Internal Medicine* 169, no. 1 (2009): 62–67.

7. D. J. Gottlieb et al., "Association of Usual Sleep Duration with Hypertension: The Sleep Heart Health Study," *Sleep* 29, no. 8 (2006): 1009–14.

8. S. R. Patel et al., "Sleep Duration and Biomarkers of Inflammation," *Sleep* 32, no. 2 (2009): 200–04; M. L. Okun, M. Coussons-Read, and M. Hall, "Disturbed Sleep Is Associated with Increased C-Reactive Protein in Young Women," *Brain, Behavior, and Immunity* 23, no. 3 (2009): 351–54.

9. J-C. Chen et al., "Sleep Duration and Risk of Ischemic Stroke in Postmenopausal Women," *Stroke* 30, no. 12 (2008): 3185–92.

10. K. L. Knutson et al., "The Metabolic Consequences of Sleep Deprivation," *Sleep Medicine Reviews* 11, no. 3 (2007): 163–78; National Sleep Foundation, "Obesity and Sleep," 2009, www.sleepfoundation.org/ article/sleep-topics/obesity-and-sleep.

11. S. Banks and D. F. Dinges, "Behavioral and Physiological Consequences of Sleep Restriction," *Journal of Clinical Sleep Medicine* 3, no. 5 (2007): 519–28.

12. H. Eichenbaum, "To Sleep, Perchance to Integrate," *Proceedings of the National Academy of Sciences of the United States of America* 104, no. 18 (2007): 7317–18; J. M. Ellenbogen, P. T. Hu, D. Titone, and M. P. Walker, "Human Relational Memory Requires Time and Sleep," *Proceedings of the National Academy of Sciences of the United States of America* 104, no. 18 (2007): 7723–28; J. M. Ellenbogen, J. C. Hulbert, Y. Jiang, and R. Stickgold, "The Sleeping Brain's Influence on Verbal Memory: Boosting Resistance to Interference," *PLoS ONE* 4, no. 1 (2009): e4117.

13. P. V. Thatcher, "University Students and the 'All-Nighter': Correlates and Patterns of Students' Engagement in a Single Night of Total Sleep Deprivation," *Behavioral Sleep Medicine* 6, no. 1 (2008): 16–31.

14. B. R. Sheth, D. Janvelyan, and M. Khan, "Practice Makes Imperfect: Restorative Effects of Sleep on Motor Learning," *PLoS ONE* 3, no. 9 (2008): e3190.

15. T. Jan, "Colleges Calling Sleep a Success Prerequisite," *Boston Globe* (September 30, 2008), www.boston.com/news/ education/higher/articles/2008/09/30/ colleges_calling_sleep_a_success _prerequisite.

16. National Sleep Foundation, *State of the States Report on Drowsy Driving: Summary of Findings* (Washington, DC: National Sleep Foundation, 2008) Executive Summary, p. 2, Available at http://drowsydriving.org/resources/ 2008-state-of-the-states-report-on -drowsy-driving.

17. M. F. Bear, B.W. Connors, and M. A. Paradiso, *Neuroscience: Exploring the Brain*, 3d ed. (Baltimore: Lippincott Williams & Wilkins, 2007), 600.

18. National Sleep Foundation, "Depression and Sleep," www.sleepfoundation.org/ article/sleep-topics/depression-and- sleep, Accessed March 2009; T. Roth, "Expert Column-Stress, Anxiety, and Insomnia: What Every PCP Should Know," *Current Perspectives in Insomnia* 4 (2004), Available at http://cme.med- scape.com; A. Gregory et al., "The Direction of Longitudinal Associations between Sleep Problems and Depression Symptoms: A Study of Twins Aged 8 and 10 Years," *Sleep* 32, no. 2 (2009): 189–99.

19. M. F. Bear, B.W. Connors, and M. A. Paradiso, *Neuroscience*, 2007, 594.

20. Ibid., 596.

21. Ibid.

22. L. Genzel et al., "Slow Wave Sleep and REM Sleep Awakenings Do Not Affect Sleep Dependent Memory Consolidation," *Sleep* 32, no 3. (2009): 302–10.

23. J. Ferrie et al., "A Prospective Study of Change in Sleep Duration: Associations with Mortality in the Whitehall II Cohort," *Sleep* 30, no. 12 (2007): 1659–66; C. Hublin et al., "Sleep and Mortality: A Population-Based 22-Year Follow-Up Study," *Sleep* 30, no. 12 (2007): 1614–15.

24. C. Hublin et al., "Sleep and Mortality: A Population-Based 22-Year Follow-Up Study," *Sleep* 30, no. 10 (2007): 1245–53; D. L. Wingard and L. F. Berkman, "Mortality Risk Associated with Sleeping Patterns among Adults," *Sleep* 6, no. 2 (1983): 102–07.

25. E. B. Klerman and D. Dijk, "Interindividual Variation in Sleep Duration and Its Association with Sleep Debt in Young Adults," *Sleep* 28, no. 10 (2005): 1253–59.

26. National Sleep Foundation, "Napping," 2009, www.sleepfoundation.org/article/ sleep-topics/napping.

27. National Sleep Foundation, "Caffeine and Sleep," 2009, www.sleepfoundation.org/ article/sleep-topics/caffeine-and-sleep.

28. American Academy of Sleep Medicine, "A Sleep Study May Be Your Best Investment for Long-Term Health," 2008, www .sleepeducation.com/Article.aspx?id =1083.

29. National Sleep Foundation, "Can't Sleep? What to Know about Insomnia," 2009, www.sleepfoundation.org/article/sleep- related-problems/insomnia-and-sleep.

30. National Sleep Foundation, "Sleep Apnea and Sleep," 2009, www.sleepfoundation .org/article/sleep-related-problems/ obstructive-sleep-apnea-and-sleep.

31. Sleep Disorders Guide, "Sleep Apnea Statistics," 2009, www.sleepdisordersguide .com/sleepapnea/sleep-apnea-statistics .html.

32. National Sleep Foundation, "Sleep Apnea and Sleep," 2009; American Sleep Apnea Association, "Sleep Apnea Information," 2008, www.sleepapnea.org/info/index .html.

33. National Institute of Neurological Disorders and Stroke, "Restless Legs Syndrome Fact Sheet," Updated March 2010, www .ninds.nih.gov/disorders/restless_legs/ detail_restless_legs.htm.

34. National Institute of Neurological Disorders and Stroke, "Narcolepsy Fact Sheet," Updated October 2009, www.ninds.nih .gov/disorders/narcolepsy/detail _narcolepsy.htm.

35. Ibid.

36. American Academy of Sleep Medicine, "REM Sleep Behavior Disorder," Updated October 21, 2005, www.sleepeducation .com/Disorder.aspx?id=29.

37. American Academy of Sleep Medicine, "Sleepwalking," Updated August 31, 2007, www.sleepeducation.com/Disorder.aspx? id=14.

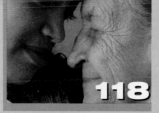
**118**
Does an intimate relationship have to be sexual?

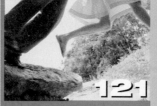
**121**
What are the most important characteristics of a healthy relationship?

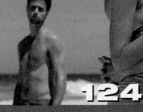
**124**
Is it normal to be jealous?

# Building Healthy Relationships and Communicating Effectively

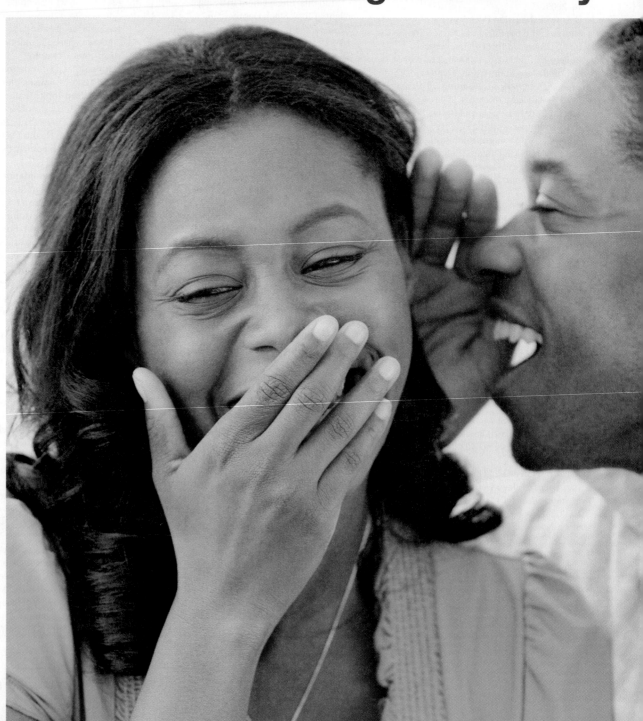

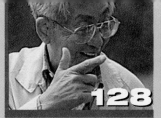
**128**

How can I communicate better?

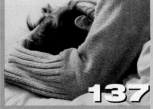
**137**

How do I cope with a bad breakup?

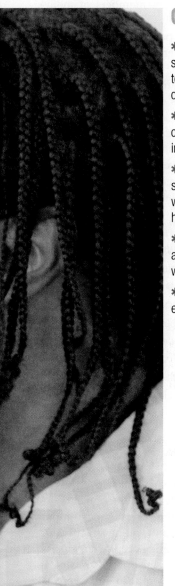

## Objectives

* Identify the characteristics of successful relationships, including how to maintain them and overcome common obstacles.

* Discuss ways to improve communication skills and interpersonal interactions.

* Examine what determines the success of an intimate relationship, and where to get help when a relationship has problems.

* Examine relationship factors that affect life decisions, for example, whether to have children.

* Discuss when and why relationships end, and how to cope when they do.

Humans are social animals—we have a basic need to belong and to feel loved, appreciated, and wanted. We can't live without interacting with others in some way. The ability to relate well with people, as well as to give and receive love and support throughout your life, are essential components of ensuring a productive and healthy future. We build "social capital" or networks of supportive friends, significant others, family members, and others who play important roles in helping us meet life's challenges. Numerous studies have shown that having supportive interpersonal relationships is beneficial to health.[1]

In spite of their potential to improve quality of life, all relationships involve a degree of risk. However, only by taking these risks can we grow and truly experience all that life has to offer. In this chapter, we examine healthy relationships and the communication skills necessary to create and maintain them. Why is communication so important? For one thing, the way we communicate influences whether we are accepted by others. For another, most of us sincerely want to express ourselves clearly and honestly in our relationships. Clear communication can help us bridge our differences, and it can also affect health. Expressing ourselves well and knowing how to understand what others are saying are both vitally important skills. These abilities lay the groundwork for healthy relationships, which are significant factors in overall health.

# Characteristics and Types of Intimate Relationships

Experts in the field of interpersonal relationships define **intimate relationships** in terms of four characteristics: *behavioral interdependence, need fulfillment, emotional attachment,* and *emotional availability.* Each of these characteristics may be related to interactions with family, close friends, and romantic partners.

*Behavioral interdependence* refers to the mutual impact that people have on each other as their lives and daily activities intertwine. What one person does influences what the other person wants to and can do. Behavioral interdependence may become stronger over time, to the point that each person would feel a great void if the other were gone.

> **intimate relationships** Relationships with family members, friends, and romantic partners, characterized by behavioral interdependence, need fulfillment, emotional attachment, and emotional availability.

Intimate relationships also fulfill psychological needs and are therefore a means of *need fulfillment.* Through relationships with others, we fulfill our needs for the following:

● **Intimacy**—someone with whom we can share our feelings freely
● **Social integration**—someone with whom we can share worries and concerns
● **Nurturance**—someone we can take care of and who will take care of us

- **Assistance**—someone to help us in times of need
- **Affirmation**—someone who will reassure us of our own worth and tell us that we matter

In mutually rewarding intimate relationships, partners and friends meet each other's needs. They disclose feelings, share confidences, and provide support and reassurance. Each person comes away feeling better for the interaction and validated by the other person.

In addition to behavioral interdependence and need fulfillment, intimate relationships involve strong bonds of *emotional attachment,* or feelings of love. When we hear the word *intimacy,* we often think of a sexual relationship. Although sex can play an important role in emotional attachment, a relationship can be very intimate and yet not sexual. Two people can be emotionally intimate (share feelings) or spiritually intimate (share spiritual beliefs and meanings), or they can be intimate friends.

*Emotional availability,* the ability to give to and receive from others emotionally without fear of being hurt or rejected, is the fourth characteristic of intimate relationships. At times, all of us may limit our emotional availability—for example, after a painful breakup, we may decide not to jump into another relationship immediately, or we may decide not to talk about it with every friend. Holding back can offer time for introspection and healing, as well as for considering the lessons learned. However, some people who have experienced intense trauma find it difficult ever to be fully available emotionally. This limits their ability to experience intimate relationships.

**family of origin** People present in the household during a child's first years of life—usually parents and siblings.

In the early years of people's lives, families provide the most significant relationships. Gradually, the circle widens to include friends, coworkers, and acquaintances. Ultimately, most of us develop romantic or sexual relationships with a significant other. Each of these relationships plays a significant role in psychological, social, spiritual, and physical health.

## Family Relationships

A family is a recognizable group of people with roles, tasks, boundaries, and personalities whose central focus is to protect, care for, love, and socialize with one another. Because the family is a dynamic institution that changes as society changes, the definition of *family,* and those individuals believed to constitute family membership, changes over time as well. Who are members of today's families? Historically, most families have been made up of people related by blood, marriage or long-term committed relationships, or adoption. Yet today, many other groups of people are being recognized and are functioning as family units. Although there is no "best" family type, we do know that a healthy family's key roles and tasks are to nurture and support. Healthy families foster a sense of security and feelings of belonging that are central to growth and development. It is from our **family of origin,** the people present in our household during our first years of life, that we initially learn about feelings, problem solving, love, intimacy, and gender roles. We learn to negotiate relationships and have opportunities to communicate effectively, develop attitudes and values, and explore spiritual belief systems. It is not uncommon when we establish relationships outside the family to rely on these initial experiences and on skills modeled by our family of origin.

# 58%
**of Americans live in a nuclear family (husband and wife plus biological offspring).**

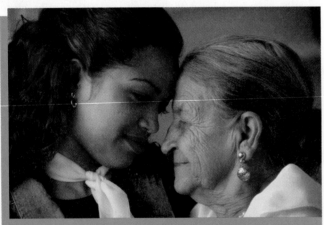

**Does an intimate relationship have to be sexual?**

We may be accustomed to hearing *intimacy* used to describe romantic or sexual relationships, but intimate relationships can take many forms. The emotional bonds that characterize intimate relationships often span the generations and help individuals gain insight and understanding into each other's worlds.

**what do you think?**

What values about relationships did you learn from your family?
● Did your family foster open, honest, and caring communication? ● Were they demonstrative in showing their love and feelings for others? ● How do you think they influenced you in your relationships today?

## Relating to Yourself

You have probably heard the idea that you must love and care for yourself before you can honestly love someone else. The truth behind this saying is that, ultimately, the most important relationship in your life is the one you have with yourself. But how do you learn to value and accept who you are? Most of us begin to develop a healthy sense of self growing up with our families. Parents provide assurance and appreciation for our talents and skills. We develop a sense of being loved, of being able to reach out to others, and of being able to accomplish our goals. That positive sense of self grows as we enter high school and college and as we are accepted by others and excel in classes, athletics, or other venues. Forming loving relationships is a natural part of that growth and development experience for many. People with high self-esteem show respect for themselves by remaining true to their values and beliefs. They feel worthy of success in love and relationships and are well positioned for successful relationships.

Two personal qualities that are especially important to any good relationship are *accountability* and *self-nurturance*. **Accountability** entails recognizing that you are responsible for your own decisions, choices, and actions. Having a sense of accountability means you don't hold your relationship partners responsible for positive or negative experiences and you don't buy into the "blame game." **Self-nurturance,** which goes hand in hand with accountability, means developing individual potential through a balanced and realistic appreciation of self-worth and ability. To make good choices in life, a person must balance many physical and emotional needs, including sleeping, eating, exercising, working, relaxing, and socializing. When the balance is disrupted, as it will inevitably be, self-nurturing people are patient with themselves and try to put things back on course. It is a lifelong process to learn to live in a balanced and healthy way. Individuals who are on a path of accountability and self-nurturance have a much better chance of maintaining a satisfying relationship with others.

**Self-Esteem and Self-Acceptance** Important factors that affect your ability to nurture yourself and maintain healthy relationships with others include the way you define yourself (*self-concept*) and the way you evaluate yourself (*self-esteem*). How you define yourself is your self-concept. Are you an athlete, a mother, an honor student, an activist, a pianist? Your self-concept is like a mental mirror that reflects how you view your physical features, emotional states, talents, likes and dislikes, values, and roles. How you feel about yourself or evaluate yourself constitutes your self-esteem. You might consider yourself an excellent student, a horrible singer, a great lover, or a "10" in terms of appearance—such judgments indicate your level of self-esteem or self-evaluation.

Your perception and acceptance of yourself influences your relationship choices. If you feel unattractive, uncomfortable, or inferior to others, you may choose not to interact with them or to avoid social events. Or you may unconsciously seek out individuals who confirm your negative view of yourself by treating you poorly. Conversely, if you are secure about your unique characteristics and talents, that positive self-concept will make it easier to form relationships with people who support and nurture you, and to interact with a variety of people in a healthy, balanced way.

## Friendships

Unlike most of the other relationships in our lives, friendship is uniquely voluntary. Our relatives are designated by blood or legal ties and our neighbors by proximity, but

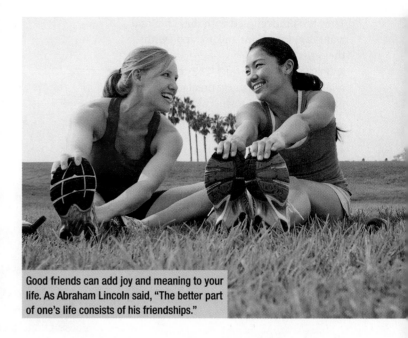

Good friends can add joy and meaning to your life. As Abraham Lincoln said, "The better part of one's life consists of his friendships."

friends are selected. Friendships are often the first relationships we form outside of our immediate families and they can be some of our lives' most stable and enduring relationships. Being able to establish and maintain strong friendships may be a good predictor of your success in establishing love relationships, as each requires shared interests and values, mutual acceptance, trust, understanding, respect, and levels of confiding.

**accountability** Accepting responsibility for personal decisions, choices, and actions.
**self-nurturance** Developing individual potential through a balanced and realistic appreciation of self-worth and ability.

Investing in friendships is important because friends provide emotional stability throughout our lives. Getting to know someone well requires time, effort, and commitment. And the effort is worth it: A good friend can be an honest and trustworthy companion, someone who honors and respects your strengths as well as your weaknesses, someone who can share your joys as well as your sorrows, and someone you can count on for support.

**what do you think?**
Take a few minutes to examine one of your current friendships. What characteristics in that relationship keep your friendship intact? ● What do you gain from your friendship? ● What does your friend gain?

## Romantic Relationships

Most people choose at some point to enter into an intimate romantic and sexual relationship with another person. Romantic relationships typically include all the characteristics of friendship as well as the following characteristics related to passion and caring:

● **Fascination.** Lovers tend to pay attention to the other person even when they should be involved in other activities.

They are preoccupied with the other and want to think about, talk to, or be with the other.

- **Exclusiveness.** Lovers have a special relationship that usually precludes having the same relationship with a third party. The love relationship often takes priority over all others.
- **Sexual desire.** Lovers desire physical intimacy and want to touch, hold, and engage in sexual activities with the other.
- **Giving the utmost.** Lovers care enough to give the utmost when the other is in need, sometimes to the point of extreme sacrifice.
- **Being a champion or advocate.** Lovers actively champion each other's interests and attempt to ensure that the other succeeds.

## Theories of Love
What is love? This four-letter word has been written about and engraved on walls; it has been the theme of countless novels, movies, and plays. There is no single definition of *love*, and the word may mean different things to different people, depending on cultural values, age, gender, and situation. Although we may not know how to put our feelings into words, we all know it when the "lightning bolt" of love strikes.

Many social scientists maintain that love may be of two kinds: *companionate* and *passionate*. Companionate love is a secure, affectionate, and trusting attachment, similar to what we may feel for family members or close friends. In companionate love, two people are attracted, have much in common, care about each other's well-being, and express reciprocal liking and respect. *Passionate love* is an intense state of wanting to bond with another person. It has three components: cognitive, emotional, and behavioral. In the cognitive component, someone has a preoccupation with another person, he or she idealizes that person, and has an intense desire to know that person. The emotional component includes strong feelings about another person, physiological arousal and attraction, including sexual attraction, and a desire for sexual intimacy with the other person. The behavioral component encompasses actions to know the other person's feelings and to maintain physical closeness and be helpful to the other person.[2]

Several other theories have been proposed to help provide insight into how and why love develops. In his classic Triangular Theory of Love, psychologist Robert Sternberg proposes the following three key components to loving relationships (Figure 4.1):[3]

- **Intimacy.** The emotional component, which involves closeness, sharing, and mutual support

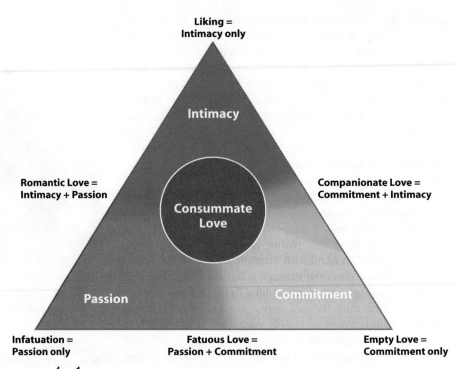

FIGURE 4.1 **Sternberg's Triangular Theory of Love**
According to Sternberg's model, three elements—intimacy, passion, and commitment—existing alone or in combination form different types of love. The most complete, ideal type of love in the model is consummate love, which combines balanced amounts of all three elements.

- **Passion.** The motivational component, which includes lust, attraction, sexual arousal, and sharing
- **Commitment.** The cognitive component, which includes the decision to be open to love in the short term and the commitment to the relationship in the long term

The quality of love relationships is reflected by the level of intimacy, passion, and commitment each person brings to the relationship over time. Sternberg believes that relationships that include two or more of the above are more likely to endure than those that include only one. He uses the term *consummate love* to describe a combination of intimacy, passion, and commitment—an ideal and deep form of love that is, unfortunately, all too rare.

An alternate theory of love and attraction, based on brain circuitry and chemistry, is quite different from that of Sternberg. Anthropologist Helen Fisher, among others, has hypothesized that attraction and falling in love follow a fairly predictable pattern based on the following: (1) *imprinting*, in which our evolutionary patterns, genetic predispositions, and past experiences trigger a romantic reaction; (2) *attraction*, in which neurochemicals produce feelings of euphoria and elation; (3) *attachment*, in which endorphins—natural opiates—cause lovers to feel peaceful, secure, and calm; and (4) *production of a cuddle chemical*, in which the brain secretes the hormone oxytocin, thereby stimulating sensations during lovemaking and eliciting feelings of satisfaction and attachment.[4]

According to Fisher's theory, lovers who claim that they are swept away by passion may not be far from the truth. Why? The love-smitten person's endocrine system secretes chemical substances such as dopamine, norepinephrine, and phenylethylamine (PEA), which are chemical cousins of amphetamines.[5] Although attraction may in fact be a "natural high," this passion loses effectiveness over time as the body builds up a tolerance. Many people may become attraction junkies, seeking the intoxication of love much as the drug user seeks a chemical high. Fisher speculates that PEA levels drop significantly over a 3- to 4-year period, leading to the "4-year itch" that manifests in the peaking fourth-year divorce rates present in over 60 cultures. Romances that last beyond the 4-year mark are influenced by endorphins that give lovers a sense of security, peace, and calm. In her recent work, Fisher has focused on how we develop attractions to specific individuals based on body chemistry, learned influences from family and friends, and our unique personalities.[6]

# Strategies for Success in Relationships

Our definition of success in a relationship tends to be based on whether a couple stays together or a friendship remains close over the years. Learning to communicate, respecting each other, and sharing a genuine fondness are crucial to relationship success. Many social scientists agree that the happiest committed relationships are flexible enough to allow the partners to grow throughout their lives.

How can you ensure that your relationships with family, friends, or a romantic partner succeed? In this section we talk about what a healthy relationship looks like and make suggestions for nurturing your existing relationships. Most relationships start with great optimism and true love or caring. So why do so many run into trouble? One contributing factor is the message (or myth) that many of us grew up with about romantic relationships: the idea that if we found the right person, we would live "happily ever after." What is missing from that message is that healthy relationships don't just happen; they require psychosocial skills and continued effort.

# Characteristics of Healthy Relationships

Satisfying and stable relationships share certain identifiable traits, such as good communication, intimacy, friendship, and other factors. A key ingredient is trust, the degree of confidence each person feels in a relationship. Without trust, intimacy will not develop, and the relationship will likely fail. Trust includes three fundamental elements:

**1.** *Predictability* means that you can predict your partner's behavior, based on the knowledge that he or she acts in consistently positive ways.

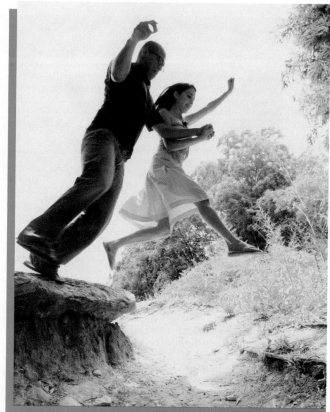

**What are the most important characteristics of a healthy relationship?**

Healthy relationships can come in all shapes and sizes but they do have some characteristics in common, including communication, caring, respect, and support. One of the most important components of a strong relationship is trust, which is made up of predictability, dependability, and faith.

**2.** *Dependability* means that you can rely on your partner to give support in all situations, particularly those in which you feel threatened with hurt or rejection.

**3.** *Faith* means that you feel absolutely certain about your partner's intentions and behavior.

Trust can develop even when it is initially lacking. This requires opening yourself to others, which carries the risk of hurt or rejection.

How do you know if you are in a healthy relationship? Some of the characteristics of healthy and unhealthy relationships are contrasted in Figure 4.2. Answering some basic questions can help you determine if your relationships are working.

- Do you love and care for yourself while in the relationship to the same extent that you did before the relationship? Do you feel that you can be yourself in the relationship?
- Do you share interests, values, and opinions? Is there mutual respect for differences and civil discussion of differences?
- Is there mutual encouragement and emotional support? Do you trust each other?

| In an unhealthy relationship... | In a healthy relationship... |
| --- | --- |
| You care for and focus on another person only and neglect yourself or you focus only on yourself and neglect the other person. | You both love and take care of yourselves before and while in a relationship |
| One of you feels pressure to change to meet the other person's standards and is afraid to disagree or voice ideas. | You respect each other's individuality, embrace your differences, and allow each other to "be yourselves." |
| One of you has to justify what you do, where you go, and whom you see. | You both do things with friends and family and have activities independent of each other. |
| One of you makes all the decisions and controls everything without listening to the other's input. | You discuss things with each other, allow for differences of opinion, and compromise equally. |
| One of you feels unheard and is unable to communicate what you want. | You express and listen to each other's feelings, needs, and desires. |
| You lie to each other and find yourself making excuses for the other person. | You both trust and are honest with yourselves and with each other. |
| You don't have any personal space and have to share everything with the other person. | You respect each other's need for privacy. |
| Your partner keeps his or her sexual history a secret or hides a sexually transmitted infection from you, or you do not disclose your history to your partner. | You share sexual histories and information about sexual health with each other. |
| One of you is scared of asking the other to use protection or has refused the other's requests for safer sex. | You both practice safer sex methods. |
| One of you has forced or coerced the other to have sex. | You both respect sexual boundaries and are able to say no to sex. |
| One of you yells and hits, shoves, or throws things at the other in an argument. | You resolve conflicts in a rational, peaceful, and mutually agreed upon way. |
| You feel stifled, trapped, and stagnant. You are unable to escape the pressures of the relationship. | You both have room for positive growth, and you both learn more about each other as you develop and mature. |

FIGURE 4.2 **Healthy versus Unhealthy Relationships**

**Source:** Advocates for Youth, Washington, DC, 20036, www.advocatesforyouth.org. Copyright © 2000. Used with permission.

● Are you honest with each other? Can you comfortably express your feelings, your needs, or your desires? Do you talk about things that you know may cause disagreement?
● Is there genuine caring and goodwill? Are you there for each other and do you support each other unconditionally?
● Is there room in your relationship for growth as you both evolve and mature?

Relationships are nurtured by consistent communication, actions, and self-reflection. Poor communication can weaken bonds and create mistrust. We all need to take the time periodically to reflect on how we have been relating to others in our lives through words and actions. Have we been honest, direct, fair, and open in our conversations? Have we really listened to others' thoughts, wants, and needs? Have we behaved in ways consistent with our words, values, and beliefs?

## Choosing a Romantic Partner

The choice of a relationship partner is influenced by more than just the chemical and psychological processes described in researchers' theories of love. One important factor is *proximity*, or being in the same place at the same time. The more often that you see a person in your hometown, at social gatherings, or at work, the more likely that interaction will occur. Thus, if you live in New York, you'll probably end up with another New Yorker. (With the advent of the Internet, however, geographic proximity has become less important. See the **Consumer Health** box on the next page for some guidelines on meeting and dating online friends.)

You also choose a partner based on *similarities* (in attitudes, values, intellect, interests, education, and socioeconomic status); the old adage that "opposites attract"

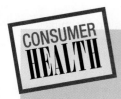
# MEETING PEOPLE ONLINE

The Internet has revolutionized our access to information and the way we communicate. Literally thousands of websites specialize in helping people meet one another. Sites such as Facebook, MySpace, and Friendster allow people to network not only in their own community, but also around the world, finding others who share their taste in music, movies, politics, popular culture, and much more.

Sites such as Match.com and eHarmony.com provide dating services, which help people find others who match particular profiles. Websites that provide these services may be free, or they may charge fees for access. Dating service sites usually explicitly restrict participation to people over 18 years old, but most of them rely on a credit card to authenticate age, and there isn't much they can do if teenagers or younger children have

access to credit card numbers.

Social networking sites may have fewer restrictions and a younger audience than dating sites, but they also have less policing. Sites such as Facebook and MySpace have policies that allow for reporting and removal of illegal, offensive, or pornographic material. In an effort to protect young teens from sexual predators, these sites are not open to individuals under the age of 13 (Facebook) or 14 (MySpace), and the sites encourage parents to talk to their children about online safety and to monitor their profiles.

In addition to creating casual friendships, matchmaking, or simply communicating with others, Internet users can also get involved in *cybersex*. People chatting online can describe themselves or each other in sexual situations or interactions that are age inappropriate and may be

disturbing for some. Many divorces have resulted from cybersex, when one spouse gets upset about the other's intimacy with a stranger, even via the Internet.

## PRACTICAL GUIDELINES FOR SOCIAL NETWORKERS OF ALL AGES

✱ As you are getting to know someone online, ask questions about lots of things you are interested in, such as hobbies, politics, religion, education, birth date, family background, and marital history and status. Keep the answers you receive and beware of contradictions.

✱ Be suspicious of anyone who seems too good to be true, such as someone who agrees with your taste on every single preference or interest. Trying too hard to please may mark a manipulative and potentially dangerous personality.

✱ Be honest about yourself; state your own interests and

characteristics fairly, including things you think might be less attractive than stereotypes and cultural norms dictate.

✱ If you get to the point of exchanging pictures, be sure that you see photos of the person in a wide variety of situations and with other people, to ensure they aren't sending you pictures of someone else.

✱ If you decide to arrange a meeting, plan something brief and in public, preferably during daylight hours. Set up a double date or group date if possible. Meet in a well-lit, busy public place such as a coffee shop. Do not meet with anyone who wants to keep the location and time a secret.

✱ Tell a friend or family member the details of where and when you are going to meet, and provide that person with any information you have about the person you are meeting. Make sure to plan your own way of getting home.

---

usually isn't true. If your potential partner expresses interest or liking, you may react with mutual regard known as *reciprocity*. The more you express interest, the safer it is for someone else to return the regard, and the cycle spirals onward.

## what do you think?

What factors do you consider most important in a potential partner? ● Which factors are absolute musts? ● Are there any differences between what you believe to be important in a relationship and the things your parents feel are important?

A final factor that plays a significant role in selecting a partner is *physical attraction*. Whether such attraction is caused by a chemical reaction or a socially learned behavior, men and women appear to have different attraction criteria. This attraction is complex and influenced by social, biological, and cultural factors.[7]

## Confronting Couple Issues

Couples seeking a long-term relationship must confront several issues that can either enhance or diminish their chances of success. Some of these issues involve gender roles, power sharing, and open communication about unmet expectations.

**Jealousy** Jealousy has been described as an aversive reaction evoked by a real or imagined relationship involving one's partner and a third person. As one psychologist put it, "Jealousy is like a San Andreas fault running beneath the surface of an intimate relationship. Most of the time, its eruptive potential lies hidden. But when it begins to rumble, the destruction can be enormous."[8] Contrary to what many of us believe, jealousy is not a sign of intense devotion.

**jealousy** An aversive reaction evoked by a real or imagined relationship involving a person's partner and a third person.

Instead, jealousy often indicates underlying problems, such as insecurity or possessiveness, that may prove to be a significant barrier to a healthy intimate relationship. Often, jealousy is rooted in a past relationship in which an individual experienced deception and loss. Other causes of jealousy typically include the following:

- **Overdependence on the relationship.** People who have few social ties and who rely exclusively on their significant other tend to be fearful of losing them.
- **Severity of the threat.** People may feel uneasy if someone with stunning good looks and a great personality appears interested in their partner.
- **High value on sexual exclusivity.** People who believe that sexual exclusivity is a crucial indicator of love are more likely to become jealous.
- **Low self-esteem.** People who think poorly of themselves are more likely to feel unworthy or fear that someone is going to snatch their partner away.
- **Fear of losing control.** Some people need to feel in control of every situation. Feeling that they may be losing the attachment of or control over a partner can cause jealousy.

In both sexes, jealousy is related to believing it would be difficult to find another relationship if the current one ends. For men, jealousy is positively correlated with the degree to which the man's self-esteem is affected by his partner's judgments. Although a certain amount of jealousy can be expected in any loving relationship, it doesn't have to threaten a relationship as long as partners communicate openly about it.[9]

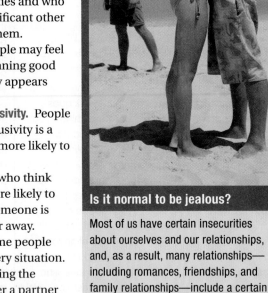

**Is it normal to be jealous?**

Most of us have certain insecurities about ourselves and our relationships, and, as a result, many relationships—including romances, friendships, and family relationships—include a certain amount of jealousy. As long as you communicate about the issue, your relationship shouldn't suffer, and you can move past the jealousy. However, if jealousy is ignored or becomes extreme, it can undermine and threaten a relationship.

# what do you think?

Have you ever experienced jealousy in a relationship? ● Do you think that jealousy indicates "love" for a partner, or "disrespect" for them? ● Are there ever times when jealousy is justified?

## Changing Gender Roles

Throughout history, women and men have taken on various roles in their relationships. In colonial America, gender roles were determined by tradition, and each task within a family unit held equal importance. Our modern society has very few gender-specific roles. Women and men alike drive cars, care for children, operate computers, manage finances, and perform equally well in the tasks of daily living. Rather than taking on traditional female and male roles, many couples find it makes more sense to divide tasks on the basis of schedule, convenience, and preference. However, it rarely works out that the division is equal. Even when women work full-time, they tend to bear heavy family and household responsibilities. Today's working woman, living in a dual-career family and coping with the responsibilities of being a partner, a mother, and a professional, is often stressed and frustrated. Men, who may have expected a more traditional role for their partners, may experience difficulties. Over time, if couples are unable to communicate how they feel about performing certain tasks, the relationship may suffer.

**Sharing Power** **Power** can be defined as the ability to make and implement decisions. There are many ways to exercise power, but powerful people are those who know what they want and have the ability to attain it. In traditional relationships, men were the wage earners and consequently had decision-making power. Women exerted much influence, but in the final analysis they needed a man's income for survival. As women have become wage earners in increasing numbers and have begun enjoying their own financial resources, the power dynamics between women and men have shifted considerably. Part of the increase in the divorce rate in the past century undoubtedly reflects the recognition by working women that they are financially independent and can support themselves by choice rather than remaining in relationships that don't work.

In general, successful couples have relationships that are more equal, with each sharing responsibilities, power, and control. Even when both members of a couple are financially equal, power in other areas may be an issue. If one partner always has the final say in deciding social plans, for example, the unequal distribution of power may affect the quality of the relationship.

All couples have conflicts. Learning to handle them maturely is vital to relationship success.

**Unmet Expectations** We all have expectations of ourselves and our partners—how we will spend our time, how we will spend our money, how and how often we will express love and intimacy, and

**power** The ability to make and implement decisions.

how we will grow together as a couple. Expectations are an extension of our values, beliefs, hopes, and dreams for the future. When communicated and agreed on, these help relationships thrive. If we are unable to communicate our expectations, we set ourselves up for disappointment and hurt. Partners in healthy relationships can communicate wants and needs and have honest discussions when things aren't going as expected or as planned.

# Communicating: A Key to Good Relationships

From the moment of birth, we struggle to be understood. We flail our arms, cry, scream, smile, frown, and make sounds and gestures to get a reaction from someone we care about or to have someone understand what we want or need from him or her. By the time we enter adulthood, each of us has developed a unique way of communicating to others with gestures, words, expressions, and body language. No two people communicate in the exact same way or have the same need for connecting with others. Some of us are outgoing and quick to express our emotions and thoughts. Others are quiet, reluctant to talk about feelings, and may prefer to spend time alone rather than with others.

Different cultures have unique languages and dialects, as well as different ways of expressing feelings and using body language. Some cultures gesture broadly; others maintain a closed and rigid means of speaking. Some are offended by direct eye contact; others welcome a steady gaze. Men and women also tend to have different styles of communication, which are largely dictated by culture and socialization (see the **Gender & Health** box on page 126).

Although people differ in the way they communicate, this doesn't mean that one sex, culture, or group is better at it than another. We have to be willing to accept differences and work to keep communication lines open and fluid. Remaining interested, actively engaged in the interaction, and open and willing to exchange ideas and thoughts are all things that we typically learn with practice and hard work.

When two people begin a relationship, they bring their past communication styles with them. How often have you heard someone say, "We just can't communicate" or "You're sending me mixed messages"? These exchanges occur regularly as people start relationships or work through ongoing communication problems in an existing relationship. Because communication is a process, our every action, word, facial expression, gesture, or body posture becomes part of our shared experience and part of the evolving impression we make on others. If we are angry in our responses, others will be reluctant to interact with us. If we bring "baggage" from past bad interactions to new relationships, we may be cynical, distrustful, and guarded in our exchanges

with others. If we are positive, happy, and share openly with others, they will be more likely to communicate openly with us. This ability to communicate assertively is an important skill in relationships. Assertive communicators are in touch with their feelings and values and can communicate their needs directly and honestly to defend choices in a positive manner.

All of us can learn to be better communicators. By understanding how to deliver and interpret information, we can enhance our relationships. Three aspects of strong communications skills are sharing information through self-disclosure, becoming a better listener, and understanding nonverbal communication.

## Learning Appropriate Self-Disclosure

Sharing personal information with others is called **self-disclosure.** If you are willing to share personal information with others, they will likely share personal information with you. In other words, if you want to learn more about someone, you have to be willing to share parts of your personal self with that person. Self-disclosure is not storytelling or sharing secrets; rather, it is revealing how you are reacting to the present situation and giving any information about the past that is relevant to the other person's understanding of your current reactions.

**self-disclosure** Sharing personal feelings or information with others.

Self-disclosure can be a double-edged sword, for there is risk in divulging personal insights and feelings. If you sense that sharing feelings and personal thoughts will result in a closer relationship, you will likely take such a risk. But if you believe that the disclosure may result in rejection or alienation, you may not open up so easily. If the confidentiality of previously shared information has been violated, you may hesitate to disclose yourself in the future.

However, the risk in not disclosing yourself to others is that you will lack intimacy in relationships. Noted psychologist Carl Rogers stressed the importance of understanding yourself and others through self-disclosure. Rogers believed that weak relationships were characterized by inhibited self-disclosure.[10]

If self-disclosure is such a key element in creating healthy

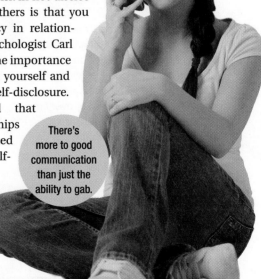

There's more to good communication than just the ability to gab.

# He Says/She Says

## Women

**FACIAL EXPRESSIONS**
- Smile and nod more often
- Maintain better eye contact

**SPEECH PATTERNS**
- Higher pitched, softer voices
- Use approximately 5 speech tones
- May sound more emotional
- Make more tentative statements
- Interrupt less often

**BODY LANGUAGE**
- Take up less space
- Gesture toward the body
- Lean forward when listening
- More gentle when touching others
- More feedback via body language

**BEHAVIORAL DIFFERENCES**
- More emotional approach
- Express intimate feelings more readily
- Tendency to hold grudges
- Give more compliments
- Gossip more
- More likely to ask for help
- Tend to take rejection more personally
- Apologize more frequently
- Talk is primarily a means of rapport, establishing connections, and negotiating relationships

## Men

**FACIAL EXPRESSIONS**
- Frown more often
- Often avoid eye contact

**SPEECH PATTERNS**
- Lower pitched, louder voices
- Use approximately 3 speech tones
- May sound more abrupt
- Make more direct statements
- More likely to interrupt

**BODY LANGUAGE**
- Occupy more space
- Gesture away from the body
- Lean back when listening
- More forceful gestures
- Less feedback via body language

**BEHAVIORAL DIFFERENCES**
- More inclined to be analytical
- Have more difficulty in expressing intimate feelings
- Hold fewer grudges
- Give fewer compliments
- Gossip less
- Less likely to ask for help
- Tend to take rejection less personally
- Apologize less often
- Talk is primarily a means of preserving independence and negotiating and maintaining status

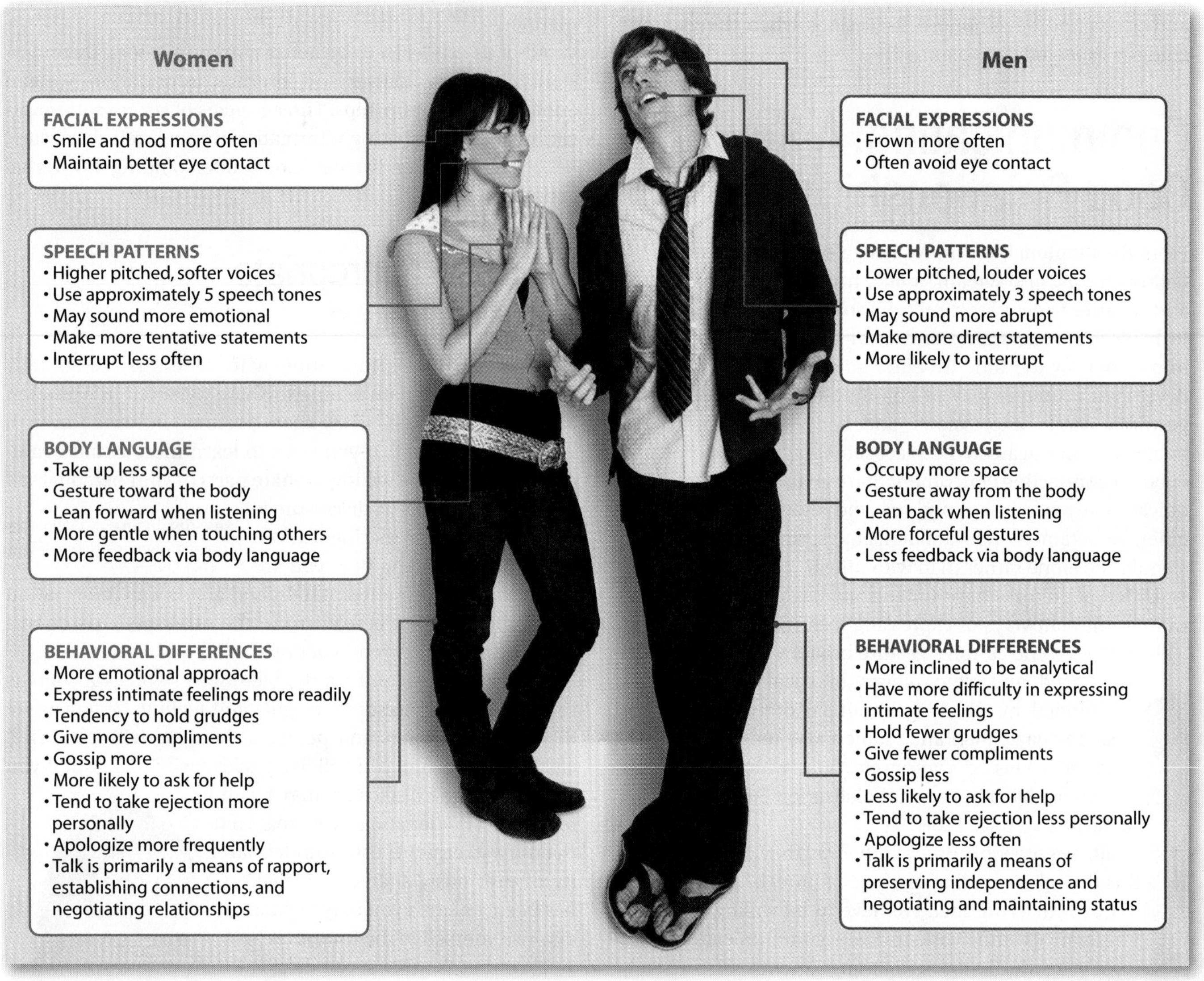

Although men and women may make decisions differently, act differently in terms of their sexual and partnering behaviors, and respond in ways that are somewhat distinctive to their genders, these lines have begun to blur over time. Books, such as *Men Are from Mars, Women Are from Venus,* that focus on these differences capture media attention, but they also have their critics.

According to Dr. Cynthia Burggraf Torppa at Ohio State University, differences in communication between men and women are really quite minor. What is most important, she says, is the way in which men and women interpret or process the same message. She indicates that studies support the idea that women, to a greater extent than men, are sensitive to the interpersonal meanings that lie between the lines in the messages they exchange with their mates. This is because societal expectations often make women responsible for regulating intimacy. Men, on the other hand, are more sensitive than women to subtle messages about status. For them, societal expectations dictate that they negotiate hierarchy, or who's the captain and who's the crew.

Within our society and in light of these general trends, there are some gender-specific communication patterns and behaviors that are obvious to the casual observer (see the figure above). Recognizing these differences and how they make us unique is a good first step in avoiding unnecessary frustrations and irritations.

**Sources:** C. Burggraf Torppa, Family and Consumer Sciences, Ohio State University Extension, "Gender Issues: Communication Differences in Interpersonal Relationships," 2010, http://ohioline.osu.edu/flm02/pdf/fs04.pdf. J. Wood, *Gendered Lives: Communication, Gender, and Culture,* 8th ed. (Belmont, CA: Cengage, 2010); M. L. Knapp and A. L. Vangelisti, *Interpersonal Communication and Human Relationships,* 5th ed. (Boston: Allyn & Bacon, 2004).

communication, but fear is a barrier to that process, what can we do? The following suggestions can help:

● **Get to know yourself.** Remember that your self includes your feelings, beliefs, thoughts, and concerns. The more you know about yourself, the more likely you will be able to communicate with others about yourself.

● **Become more accepting of yourself.** No one is perfect or has to be.

● **Be willing to discuss your sexual history.** In a culture that puts many taboos on discussions of sex in everyday conversation, it's no wonder we find it hard to disclose our sexual feelings to those with whom we are intimate. However, with the soaring rate of sexually transmitted infections and the ever-looming threat of AIDS, there has never been a more important time to disclose sexual feelings and history. The life-altering effects of an unwanted pregnancy or contracting HIV underscore the need to communicate about sex before you become intimate.

● **Choose a safe context for self-disclosure.** When and where you make such disclosures and to whom may greatly influence the response. Choose a setting in which you feel safe to let yourself be known.

## Becoming a Better Listener

Listening is a vital part of interpersonal communication; it allows us to share feelings, express concerns, communicate wants and needs, and let our thoughts and opinions be known. We must do the necessary work to improve both our speaking and listening skills, which will enhance our relationships, improve our grasp of information, and allow us to interpret more effectively what others say. We listen best when (1) we believe that the message is somehow important and relevant to us; (2) the speaker holds our attention through humor, dramatic effect, use of the media, or other techniques; and (3) we are in the mood to listen (free of distractions and worries).

When we really listen effectively, we try to understand what people are thinking and feeling from their perspective. We hear the words, and we try to understand what is really being said. How many times have you been caught pretending to be listening when you were not? After several moments of nodding and saying "uh-huh," your friend finally asks you a question, and you haven't a clue what she has been saying. Sometimes tuning out is due to lacking sleep, being overly stressed, being preoccupied, having too much to drink, or being under the influence of drugs. Other times it's because you perceive the speaker as a "motor mouth" who talks for the sake of talking, or because you find them or what they are talking about boring. Some of the most common listening difficulties are things that we can work to improve. See the **Skills for Behavior Change** box at right for suggestions on improving your listening skills.

**The Three Basic Listening Modes** There are three main ways in which we listen. Knowing when to use each of these

Skills for Behavior Change

### Learning to Really Listen

To become a better listener, try practicing the following skills and consciously using them on a daily basis:

✳ Be present in the moment. Good listeners participate and acknowledge what the other person is saying through nonverbal cues such as nodding, smiling, saying "yes" or "uh-huh," and asking questions at appropriate times.

✳ Show empathy and sympathy.

✳ Ask for clarification. If you aren't sure what the speaker means, indicate that you're not sure you understand, or paraphrase what you think you heard.

✳ Control that deadly desire to interrupt. Try taking a deep breath for 2 seconds, then hold your breath for another second and really listen to what is being said as you slowly exhale.

✳ Avoid snap judgments based on what other people look like or are saying.

✳ Resist the temptation to "set the other person straight."

✳ Focus on the speaker. Hold back the temptation to launch into a story about your own experience in a similar situation.

will enhance the way in which you listen and improve the outcome:

**1.** **Competitive, or combative, listening** happens when we are more interested in promoting our own point of view than in understanding or exploring someone else's. We listen either for openings to take the floor or for flaws and weak points that we can attack. Looking at your watch, sighing, nodding vigorously, and staring into space are meant to discourage speakers or make them relinquish the floor.

**2.** **Passive, or attentive, listening** occurs when we are genuinely interested in hearing and understanding the other person's point of view. By being attentive and passively listening, we encourage further discussion. We assume that we heard and understand correctly, but we stay passive and don't verify it.

**3.** **Active, or reflective, listening** is the single most useful and important listening skill. In active listening, we are genuinely interested in understanding what the other person is thinking, feeling, and wanting, and we are interested in what the message means. We are active in confirming our understanding before we respond with our own new message by restating or paraphrasing what we think the other person means, reflecting it back to the sender for verification. This verification or feedback process is what distinguishes active listening and makes it effective.

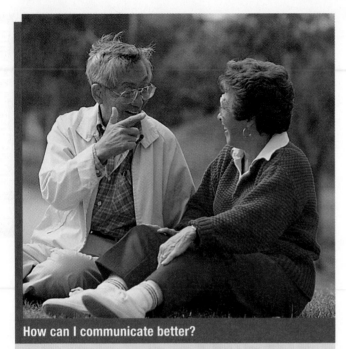

**How can I communicate better?**

One way to communicate better is to pay attention to your body language. Researchers have found that 93% of communication effectiveness is determined by nonverbal cues. Laughing, smiling, and gesturing all help convey meaning and assure your partner you are actively engaged in communicating.

Nonverbal communication can include the following:[12]

- **Touch.** This can be a handshake, a warm hug, a hand on the shoulder, or a kiss on the cheek.
- **Gestures.** These can include physical mannerisms that replace words, such as a thumbs-up or a wave hello or good-bye, or movements that augment verbal communication, such as fanning your face when you are hot or indicating with your hands how big the fish was that got away. Gestures can also be rude, such as glancing at one's watch and rolling one's eyes.
- **Interpersonal space.** This is the amount of physical space that separates two people. Getting "in someone's face" or too close when your presence isn't wanted is offensive.
- **Facial expressions.** These can signal moods and emotions and often have universal meaning. Frowning, smiling, and grimacing all signal various responses.
- **Body language.** This includes things such as folding your arms across your chest, crossing your legs, leaning forward in your chair, and shaking your head no.
- **Tone of voice.** This refers not to what you say, but how you say it—the elements of speaking that color the use of words, such as pitch, volume, and speed.

To communicate as effectively as possible, it is important to recognize and use nonverbal cues that support and help clarify your verbal messages. Awareness and practice of your verbal and nonverbal communication will also enhance your skills in interpreting others' messages.

## Using Nonverbal Communication

Understanding what someone is saying often involves much more than listening and speaking. Often, what is not actually said may speak louder than any words. Smiling, looking away rather than maintaining eye contact, making body movements and hand gestures—all these nonverbal clues influence the way our conversational partners interpret our messages. **Nonverbal communication** includes all unwritten and unspoken messages, both intentional and unintentional. Ideally, our nonverbal communication matches and supports our verbal communication. This is not always the case. Research shows that when verbal and nonverbal communications don't match, we are more likely to believe the nonverbal cues.[11] This is one reason it is important to be aware of all the nonverbal cues we use regularly and to understand how others might interpret them.

**nonverbal communication** All unwritten and unspoken messages, both intentional and unintentional.
**conflict** An emotional state that arises when the behavior of one person interferes with the behavior of another.
**conflict resolution** A concerted effort by all parties to constructively resolve points of contention.

**"Why Should I Care?"**

Learning how to communicate effectively isn't just some touchy-feely notion—it's actually vital to your current and future success in life. Unless you decide to be a hermit, there is hardly a career or life path you might choose that won't require communicating and cooperating with others. Develop good communication skills now, and you'll be poised for success in your post-college life.

**What's Working for You?**

Maybe you already communicate well. Below is a list of some things you can do to improve communication. Which of these are you already incorporating into your life?
- ☐ I listen actively—I actively try to understand what my friend or partner is saying.
- ☐ I let people finish what they are saying before I cut in with my thoughts
- ☐ I tell my friends when I am upset, and work problems out with them.
- ☐ When the right time comes, I discuss my intimate thoughts and feelings with my partner.

## Managing Conflict through Communication

A **conflict** is an emotional state that arises when the behavior of one person interferes with that of another. Conflict is inevitable whenever people live or work together. Not all conflict is bad; in fact, airing feelings and coming to some form of resolution over differences can sometimes strengthen relationships. **Conflict resolution** and successful conflict management form a systematic approach to resolving differences fairly and constructively, rather than allowing them to fester. The goal of conflict resolution is to solve differences peacefully and creatively.

Most conflicts revolve around two message components: content and relationship. *Content* is usually easy to discern, as it is the subject of the participants' sentences. It deals with the issues on the surface. *Relationship* is more difficult to discern, because it embodies the interactions between the people concerned and usually involves issues that are much more deeply rooted. Because of the double-pronged nature of messages, many arguments arise out of seemingly innocuous situations. For instance, a housemate comes home from the library, walks into the kitchen, and asks, "What's for dinner?" The other responds, "Whatever you make! When are you going to take care of yourself for once?" On the surface, the conflict may be about dinner. From a relationship standpoint, however, one roommate feels used and underappreciated.

Prolonged conflict can destroy relationships unless the parties agree to resolve points of contention constructively. As two people learn to negotiate and compromise on their differences, the number and intensity of conflicts should diminish. Conflict resolution can therefore be a growth process as people learn to recognize problems and solutions based on past experience.

During a heated conflict, try to pause for a moment before responding, consider the possible impact of your comments or actions, and speak slowly and state your point positively and constructively. You can also dismiss yourself from the situation and walk away by saying something like, "I can see we aren't going to resolve this right now. Let's save it for a time when we've both cooled off and can discuss this more calmly."

E-mail messages are easily misunderstood because we can't see or hear the person talking. Was that last comment meant to be snippy and mean, or did I misinterpret what they were saying? In general, when you read something on e-mail and find that you are ready to flip back a nasty response, stop. If you must, write the message and have a 24-hour rule—don't hit Send until the next day, if you still want to. Usually, you'll find that by the next day, it's better to hit the Delete button and move on.

Rude or inconsiderate behavior usually develops in situations in which a person fails to recognize the feelings or rights of another. To avoid this type of behavior, try to see the other person's point of view, listen actively, avoid interrupting, and avoid making gestures that indicate disagreement, such as head-shaking or finger-pointing. A key element of successfully managing conflict is to validate others' opinions and treat them as you would like to be treated. Maintain respect and concern for others' welfare at all times.

Here are some strategies for conflict resolution.

**1. Identify the problem or issues.** Talk with each other to clarify exactly what the conflict or problem is. Try to understand both sides of the problem. In this first stage, you must say what you want and listen to what the other person wants. Focus on using "I" messages and avoid using any blaming "you" messages. Be an active listener—repeat what the other person has said and ask questions for clarification or additional information. The **Skills for Behavior Change** box at right suggests some ways to express difficult feelings.

**2. Generate several possible solutions.** Brainstorm options for addressing and solving the problem. Base your search for solutions on the goals and interests identified in the first step. Come up with several different alternatives, and avoid evaluating any of them until you have finished brainstorming.

**3. Evaluate the alternative solutions.** Review the various suggested solutions. Discard any that are unacceptable to either of you, and keep narrowing down the solutions to one or two that seem to work for both parties. Be honest with each other about a solution that you feel is unsatisfactory, but also be open to compromise. Focus on finding a solution that you both feel is satisfactory.

**4. Decide on the best solution.** Choose an alternative that is acceptable to both parties. You both need to be committed to the decision in order for this solution to be effective.

**5. Implement the solution.** Discuss how the decision will be carried out. Establish who is responsible to do what and when. The solution stands a better chance of working if you agree on the plans for implementing it.

**what do you think?**

How well do you manage conflict in your personal relationships?
● Do you think you fight fairly?
● What could you improve about the way you resolve conflict in your relationships?

**6. Follow up.** Evaluate whether the solution is working. Check in with your partner to see how he or she feels about it. Check in with yourself to see if you are satisfied with the way the solution is working out. If something is not working as planned, or if circumstances have changed, discuss revising the plan. Remember that both parties must agree to any changes to the plan, as they did the original idea.

# Committed Relationships

Commitment in a relationship means that there is an intent to act over time in a way that perpetuates the well-being of the other person, oneself, and the relationship. The majority of people strive to develop loving, committed relationships and expect their love interest to reciprocate. These commitments can take several forms, including marriage, cohabitation, and gay and lesbian partnerships.

## Marriage

In many societies around the world, traditional committed relationships take the form of marriage. In the United States, marriage means entering into a legal agreement that includes shared financial plans, property, and responsibility for raising children. Many Americans also view marriage as a religious sacrament that emphasizes certain rights and obligations for each spouse.

Historically, close to 90 percent of Americans marry at least once during their lifetime, and at any given time, close to 60 percent of U.S. adults are married (Figure 4.3). However, in recent years Americans have become less likely to marry; since 1960, annual marriages of adult men and women have steadily declined.[13] This decrease may be due to several factors, including delay of first marriages, increase in cohabitation, and a small decrease in the number of divorced persons who remarry. In 1960, the median age for first marriage was 23 years for men and 20 years for women; by 2009, the median age of first marriage had risen to 28.1 years for men and 25.9 years for women.[14]

**monogamy** Exclusive sexual involvement with one partner.
**serial monogamy** A series of monogamous sexual relationships.
**open relationship** A relationship in which partners agree that sexual involvement can occur outside the relationship.

Many Americans believe that marriage involves **monogamy,** or exclusive sexual involvement with one partner. In fact, the lifetime pattern for many Americans appears to be **serial monogamy,** which means that a person has a monogamous sexual relationship with one partner before moving on to another monogamous relationship. However, some people prefer an **open relationship,** or open marriage, in which both partners agree that each person may be sexually involved with others outside their relationship.

Marriage is socially sanctioned and highly celebrated in our culture, so there are numerous incentives for couples to formalize their relationship in this manner. A healthy marriage provides emotional support by combining the benefits

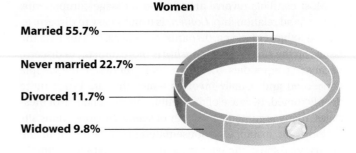

**Women**

Married 55.7%
Never married 22.7%
Divorced 11.7%
Widowed 9.8%

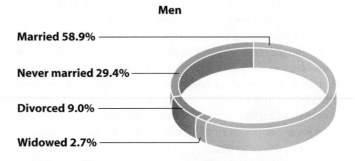

**Men**

Married 58.9%
Never married 29.4%
Divorced 9.0%
Widowed 2.7%

FIGURE 4.3 **Marital Status of the U.S. Population by Sex**

**Source:** U.S. Census Bureau, *The 2010 Statistical Abstract*, table 57, "Marital Status of the Population by Sex and Age: 2008," 2010, Available at www.census.gov/compendia/statab.

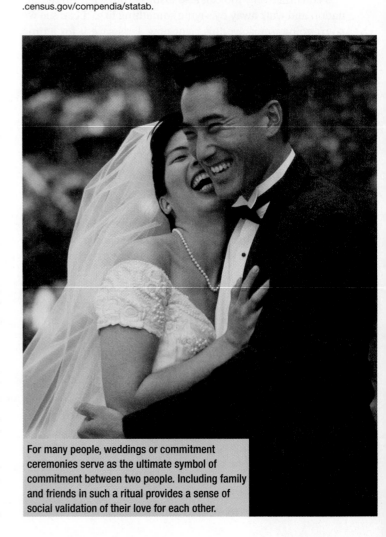

For many people, weddings or commitment ceremonies serve as the ultimate symbol of commitment between two people. Including family and friends in such a ritual provides a sense of social validation of their love for each other.

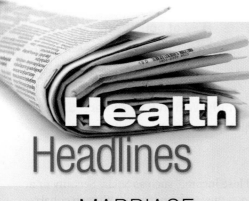

# Health Headlines

## MARRIAGE DEMYSTIFIED

What does marriage mean to you? It is the great unknown for many young people, and you may wonder when Mr. or Ms. Right will come along, where you'll find your lifetime partner, or if there is such a thing as the "perfect" marriage. The National Marriage Project studies the state of marriage in the United States and worldwide and educates the public on marital status and child well-being. The following facts and myths are from the National Marriage Project's research findings:

**FACT**— *The most likely way to find a future marriage partner is through an introduction by family, friends, or acquaintances.* Despite the romantic notion that people meet and fall in love through chance or fate, the evidence suggests that social networks are important in bringing together individuals of similar interests and backgrounds, especially when it comes to selecting a marriage partner.

**FACT**— *The more similar people are in their values, backgrounds, and life goals, the more likely they are to have a successful marriage.* Opposites may attract but they may not live together harmoniously as married couples. People who share common backgrounds and similar social networks are better suited as marriage partners than people who are very different in their backgrounds and networks.

**FACT**— *For large segments of the population, the risk of divorce is far below 50 percent.* Although the overall divorce rate in America remains close to 50 percent of all marriages, it has been dropping gradually over the past two decades. Also, the risk of divorce is far below 50 percent for educated people marrying for the first time, and lower still for people who wait to marry until at least their mid-twenties, who haven't lived with many different partners prior to marriage, or who are strongly religious and marry someone of the same faith.

**MYTH**— *Having a child together will help a couple improve their marital satisfaction and prevent a divorce.*
**FACT**— *Many studies have shown that the most stressful time in a marriage is after the first child is born.* Couples who have children together have a slightly decreased risk of divorce compared to couples without children, but the decreased risk is far less than it used to be when parents with marital problems were more likely to stay together "for the sake of the children."

**MYTH**— *Married people have less satisfying sex lives, and less sex, than single people.*
**FACT**— *Contrary to the popular belief that married sex is boring and infrequent, married people report higher levels of sexual satisfaction than both sexually active singles and cohabiting couples.* The higher level of commitment in marriage is probably the reason for the high level of reported sexual satisfaction; marital commitment contributes to a greater sense of trust and security, less drug- and alcohol-infused sex, and more mutual communication.

**MYTH**— *The keys to long-term marital success are good luck and romantic love.*

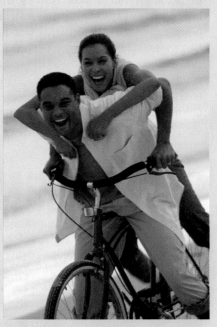

Sharing common interests and taking pleasure in each other's company are two keys to marital success.

**FACT**— *Rather than luck and love, the most common reasons that couples give for their long-term marital success are commitment and companionship.* They define their marriage as a creation that has taken hard work, dedication, and commitment (to each other and to the institution of marriage). The happiest couples are friends who share lives and have compatible interests and values.

**Sources:** D. Popenoe, "Top Ten Myths of Marriage," 2002, Copyright © 2002 by the National Marriage Project at Rutgers University; D. Popenoe, "Top Ten Myths of Divorce," 2001, Copyright © 2001 by the National Marriage Project at Rutgers University; and D. Popenoe and B. D. Whitehead, "Ten Important Research Findings on Marriage and Choosing a Marriage Partner," 2004, Copyright © 2004 by the National Marriage Project at Rutgers University. Reprinted by permission of the National Marriage Project, all available at www.virginia.edu/marriageproject/tenthingsseries.html. E O. Laumann et. al, *The Social Organization of Sexuality* (Chicago: University of Chicago Press, 1994), 234–35.

of friendship and a loving committed relationship. A happy marriage also provides stability for both the couple and for those involved in their lives. It is important to note, however, that traditional marriage does not work for everyone, and it is not the only path to a successful committed relationship. See the **Health Headlines** box above for some common misperceptions about marriage.

Considerable research indicates that married people live longer, feel happier, remain mentally alert longer, and suffer fewer physical and mental health problems.[15] Couples in healthy marriages have less stress, which in turn contributes to better overall health. Healthy marriage contributes to lower levels of stress in three important ways: financial stability, expanded support networks, and improved personal behaviors. According to the Centers for Disease Control and Prevention, married adults are about half as likely to be smokers as single, divorced, or separated adults.[16] They are also less likely to be heavy drinkers or to engage in risky sexual behavior. The one negative health indicator for married people is body weight. Married adults, particularly men, weigh more than do single adults.

## Cohabitation

**Cohabitation** is defined as a relationship in which two unmarried people with an intimate connection live together in the same household. For a variety of reasons, increasing numbers of Americans are choosing cohabitation. In some states, cohabitation that lasts a designated number of years (usually 7) legally constitutes a **common-law marriage** for purposes of purchasing real estate and sharing other financial obligations.

---

**cohabitation** Living together without being married.
**common-law marriage** Cohabitation lasting a designated period of time (usually 7 years) that is considered legally binding in some states.

---

Cohabitation can offer many of the same benefits as marriage: love, sex, companionship, and the ongoing opportunity to know a partner better over time. In addition to enjoying emotional and physical benefits, some people may cohabit for practical reasons such as the opportunity to share bills and housing costs. Over the past 20 years, there has been a large increase in the number of persons who have ever cohabited. In fact, cohabitation is increasingly the first coresidential partnership formed by young adults.[17]

Until recently, many people thought that cohabitation before marriage was likely to lead to the ultimate breakup of the marriage. However, the long-term outcomes or implications of living together may be related more to who chooses to cohabit, when, and why, rather than the experience of cohabitation itself. According to a report from the National Center for Health Statistics, cohabitation isn't a clear predictor of marriage success or failure. In a group of 13,000 men and women aged 15 to 44, 71 percent of men who were already engaged when they moved in with their fiancée were still married to her after 10 years.[18] For men who didn't cohabit before getting married, the success rate dropped slightly, to 69 percent. Sixty-five percent of cohabiting engaged women made it to 10 years, compared to 66 percent of women who waited until the marriage was official to move in with their husband.

Cohabitation can serve as a prelude to marriage, but for some people, it is an alternative to marriage. It is more common among those of lower socioeconomic status, those who are less religious, those who have been divorced, and those who have experienced parental divorce or high levels of parental conflict during childhood. Many cohabitants are young, but some older adults also choose this lifestyle

**46%** of couples living together in a given year are doing so as a precursor to marriage, according to one study. Within 5 to 7 years, 52% of those couples will have actually married and 31% will have split up.

because they would lose income, such as Social Security or a late spouse's pension, if they were to marry. Although cohabitation has its advantages, it also has some drawbacks. Perhaps the greatest disadvantage is the lack of societal validation for the relationship, especially if the couple subsequently has children. Many cohabitants must deal with pressures or disapproval from parents and friends, difficulties in obtaining insurance and tax benefits, and legal issues over property.

## Gay and Lesbian Partnerships

Whether they are gay or straight, men or women, most adults want intimate, committed relationships. Lesbians and gay men seek the same things in primary relationships that heterosexual partners do: love, friendship, communication, validation, companionship, and a sense of stability. The 2008 American Community Survey identified an estimated 564,743 same-sex couples in the United States. Those states with some

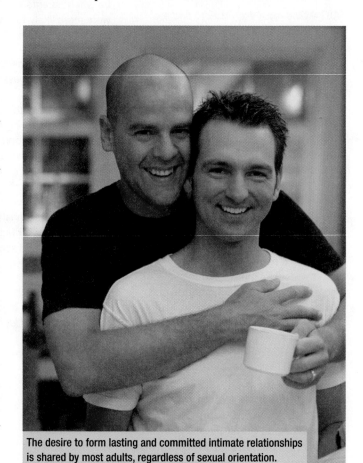

The desire to form lasting and committed intimate relationships is shared by most adults, regardless of sexual orientation.

# The Defense of Marriage Act:
## FOR BETTER OR FOR WORSE?

The federal Defense of Marriage Act (DOMA) is a U.S. law requiring that no state can treat a relationship between persons of the same sex as a marriage, even if the relationship is considered a marriage in another state. DOMA states that the federal government defines *marriage* as a legal union exclusively between one man and one woman. Thus, DOMA denies gay couples the federal protections and benefits that apply to heterosexual couples. In addition, DOMA allows a state to refuse to recognize the civil marriage of a same-sex couple that was performed legally in another state. It also states that federal statutes, regulations, and rulings applicable to married heterosexual people do not apply to married people of the same sex.

Before DOMA was enacted, federal law deferred to states in defining marriage. At the time DOMA was enacted, same-sex couples were not allowed to marry in any U.S. state. Since then, eight states and the District of Columbia have recognized equal marriage rights for same-sex couples, and thousands of couples have married. Three of those state laws were later overturned, but the states still honor the marriages that took place while the law was in effect. However, because of DOMA, the federal government does not recognize or provide federal legal protections for any of these same-sex marriages. Should DOMA be repealed? Here are some of the arguments for and against the law.

### Arguments to Keep DOMA

○ Marriage is largely a religious institution, and most religious organizations are opposed to the idea of same-sex marriage.

○ Civil unions and domestic partnerships offer same-sex couples many of the same protections and rights as marriage, so allowing same-sex couples to marry is unnecessary.

○ Allowing same-sex couples to marry would undermine the institution of marriage itself.

### Arguments to Repeal DOMA

○ The U.S. Constitution is supposed to guarantee equal rights for all U.S. citizens. Having unequal marriage rights is a form of discrimination.

○ Civil unions and domestic partnerships do not offer all of the benefits of marriage, and they vary greatly from state to state.

○ The U.S. Constitution requires each state to give "full faith and credit" to the laws of other states, including states' obligations to honor marriages validated in other states and districts.

### Where Do You Stand?

○ Do you think all legally married couples should be treated equally under the law? Do you think states should be able to make their own determinations about who can legally marry?

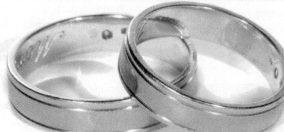

○ Are you aware of what rights, responsibilities, and protections are granted to married couples at the federal level?

○ Who or what institution do you think should define marriage?

○ Do you think DOMA should be repealed? Why or why not?

---

form of legal relationship recognition for same-sex couples report the most same-sex couples: District of Columbia, Maine, Massachusetts, Oregon, and Washington.[19]

Challenges to successful lesbian and gay relationships often stem from discrimination and difficulties dealing with social, legal, and religious doctrines. For lesbian and gay couples, obtaining the same level of "marriage benefits," such as tax deductions, power-of-attorney rights, partner health insurance, child custody rights, and other rights, continues to be a challenge. In 1996, the U.S. Congress reaffirmed tax advantages for married couples and effectively blocked

cohabiting couples—both homosexual and heterosexual—from these benefits through the Defense of Marriage Act (DOMA). The purpose of DOMA was to normalize heterosexual marriage on a federal level and to permit each state to decide whether or not to recognize same-sex unions. See the **Points of View** box above for more on the two sides to this issue.

At the time of this writing in 2010, Massachusetts, Connecticut, Iowa, New Hampshire, Vermont, and the District of Columbia are the only states or districts to grant same-sex couples marriage equality. Five other states currently have broad relationship-recognition laws that extend to same-sex couples all, or nearly all, the state rights and responsibilities of married heterosexual couples, whether labeled "civil unions" or "domestic partnerships." More limited rights and protections for same-sex couples are legislated in five additional states.[20] Worldwide, the number of countries that have legalized same-sex marriages or who approve civil unions or registered domestic partnerships for same-sex couples continues to grow.

## Staying Single

Increasing numbers of adults of all ages are electing to marry later or to remain single altogether. According to data from 2008, 52.8 percent of women aged 20 to 34 have never been married. Likewise, men in this age group postponed marriage in increasing numbers, with 62.8 percent remaining unmarried in 2008.[21]

Today, large numbers of people choose to remain single or to delay marriage. Singles clubs, social outings arranged by communities and religious groups, extended family environments, and many social services support the single lifestyle. Many singles live rich, rewarding lives and maintain a large network of close friends and families. Although sexual intimacy may or may not be present, the intimacy achieved through other interactions with loved ones is a key aspect of the single lifestyle.

## Choosing Whether to Have Children

If you decide to raise children, your relationship with your partner will change. Resources of time, energy, and money are split many ways, and you will no longer be able to give each other undivided attention. Babies and young children do not time their requests for food, sleep, and care for the

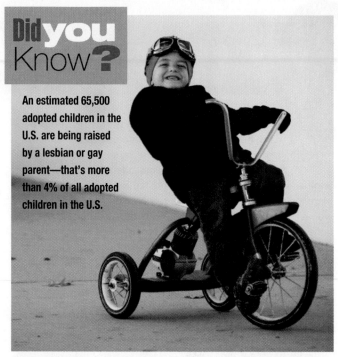

**Source:** Data are from G. Gates, L. M. V. Badgett, J. E. Macomber, and K. Chambers, *Adoption and Foster Care by Gay and Lesbian Parents in the United States,* The Urban Institute and the Charles R. Williams Institute on Sexual Orientation Law and Public Policy, March 2007.

convenience of adults. Therefore, if your own basic needs for security, love, and purpose are already met, you will be better parents. Any stresses existing in your relationship will be further accentuated when parenting is added to your responsibilities. Having a child does not save a bad relationship—in fact, it seems only to compound the problems that already exist. A child cannot and should not be expected to provide the parents with self-esteem and security.

Changing patterns in family life affect the way children are raised. In modern society, it is not always clear which partner will adjust his or her work schedule to provide the primary care of children. Nearly half a million children each year become part of a blended family when their parents remarry; remarriage creates a new family of stepparents and stepsiblings.[22] In addition, you might be among the increasing numbers of individuals choosing to have children in a family structure other than a heterosexual marriage. Single women or lesbian couples can choose adoption or alternative insemination as a way to create a family. Single men or gay couples can choose to adopt or obtain the services of a surrogate mother. According to the U.S. Census Bureau, in 2009 over 26 percent of all children under age 18 were living in families headed by a man or woman raising a child alone, reflecting a growing trend in America and in the international community.[23] Regardless of the structure of the family, certain factors remain important to the well-being of the unit: consistency, communication, affection, and mutual respect. Good parenting does not necessarily come naturally. Many people parent as they were parented (see Table 4.1). This strategy may or may not follow sound child-rearing principles.

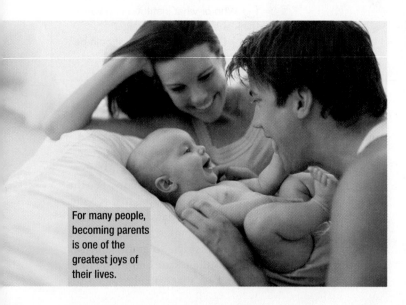

For many people, becoming parents is one of the greatest joys of their lives.

| Authoritarian "giving orders" | Parents use a set of rules that are clear and unbending. Obedience is highly valued and rewarded. Misbehavior is punished. Children may behave for a reward or out of fear of punishment. Children are not encouraged to think for themselves or to question those in authority. |
|---|---|
| Permissive "giving in" | Parents take a hands-off approach. Children are allowed great freedom with few boundaries, minimal guidance, and little discipline. Without limits and expectations, children often struggle with impulse control, poor choices, and insecurity, and have trouble taking responsibility for their actions. |
| Assertive–Democratic "giving choices" | Parents have clear expectations for children, clarify issues, and give reasons for limits. Children are given lots of practice in making choices and are guided to see the consequences of their decisions. Encouragement and acknowledgment of good behavior form the focal point of this style. Misbehavior is handled with an appropriate consequence or by problem solving with the child. |

**Source:** Adapted from Sue Dinwiddie, *Effective Parenting Styles: Why Yesterday's Models Won't Work Today.* Copyright © Sue Dinwiddie. Retrieved January 12, 2009, from www.kidsource.com/better.world.press/parenting.html. Used with permission.

Establishing a positive, respectful parenting style sets the stage for healthy family growth and development.

Finally, as a potential parent you must consider the financial implications of deciding to have a child. It is estimated that a family that had a child in 2009 will spend between $200,000 and $475,000 for food, clothing, shelter, education, and other necessities for the child over the next 17 years. Keep in mind that these numbers do not include the cost of childbearing or the major expense that all of you are struggling with right now: the costs of a college education![24] Compared to 1975, when only 39 percent of women with children under the age of 5 worked outside the home, nearly 64 percent of mothers with children under the age of 5 work outside the home today.[25] Day care workers, family members, friends, grandparents, neighbors, and nannies "mind the kids." Some employers offer family leave arrangements that allow parents more latitude in taking time away from work.

Some people become parents without a lot of forethought. Some children are born into a relationship that was supposed to last and didn't. This does not mean it is too late to do a good job of parenting. Children are amazingly resilient and forgiving if parents show respect and communicate about household activities that affect their lives. Even children who grew up in a household of conflict can feel loved and respected if the parents treat them fairly. This means that parents must take responsibility for their own emotions and make it clear to children that they are not the reason for the conflict.

# When Relationships Falter

Breakdowns in relationships usually begin with a change in communication, however subtle. Either partner may stop listening and cease to be emotionally present for the other. In turn, the other feels ignored, unappreciated, or unwanted.

Unresolved conflicts increase, and unresolved anger can cause problems in sexual relations.

When a couple who previously enjoyed spending time together find themselves continually in the company of others, spending time apart, or preferring to stay home alone, it may be a sign that the relationship is in trouble. Of course, the need for individual privacy is not a cause for worry—it's essential to health. If, however, a partner decides to change the amount and quality of time spent together without the input or understanding of the other, it may be a sign of hidden problems.

College students, particularly those who are socially isolated and far from family and hometown friends, may be particularly vulnerable to staying in unhealthy relationships. They may become emotionally dependent on a partner for everything from sharing meals to spending recreational time. Mutual obligations, such as shared rental arrangements, transportation, and child care, can make it tough to leave. It's also easy to mistake sexual advances for physical attraction or love. Without a network of friends and supporters to talk with, to obtain validation for feelings, or to share concerns, a student may feel stuck in a relationship that is headed nowhere.

**48%** of U.S. marriages undertaken by women under the age of 18 end within 10 years.

Honesty and verbal affection are usually positive aspects of a relationship. In a troubled relationship, however, they can be used to cover up irresponsible or hurtful behavior. "At least I was honest" is not an acceptable substitute for acting in a trustworthy way. "But I really do love you" is not a license for being inconsiderate or rude. Relationships that are lacking in mutual respect and consideration can become physically or emotionally abusive; see the **Student Health Today** box on page 136 describing some warning signs.

## Recognizing a Potential Abuser

Is that new "item" in your life really what he or she appears to be? Your new love interest may seem like the perfect catch in the beginning. He or she appears sensitive, gentle, caring, respectful, considerate—all the things you've been looking for. It can be hard to tell what someone is really like early on, as that person tries to make a good impression on you. To avoid getting into a long-term relationship with an abuser, watch carefully and trust your instincts. Ask others about the person and find out about his or her relationship history with partners, friends, and family. All are important indicators of an emotionally and socially healthy person. When you are beginning a relationship, be immediately wary if your partner demonstrates any of the following red flags:

✻ Gets extremely angry and swears at you or others.
✻ Hurts you by making fun of you or putting you down.

✻ Takes too much control. In a healthy relationship, partners share decision making.
✻ Displays excessive jealousy. Someone who is constantly jealous may lack the self-esteem to have a healthy relationship.
✻ Tries to shut out people you want to see, and wants to spend more and more time alone with you.
✻ Expresses continual negativity. Sulks, angers easily, throws tantrums when things don't go his or her way.
✻ Pushes you verbally or physically to have unwanted sex or intimacy.
✻ Damages your property in fits of anger.
✻ Threatens you.
✻ Verbally or physically hurts children or animals.
✻ Is always in trouble or fighting with someone.

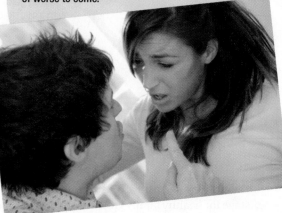

Verbal and physical threats are never part of a healthy relationship — and they may be signs of worse to come.

The list above is not exhaustive, and there are degrees of seriousness for each. However, if someone you have known only for a short time displays any sign of physical anger or pushes, shoves, slaps, restrains, or threatens you early on, it's time to walk.

## When and Why Relationships End

Often we hear in the news that 50 percent of American marriages end in divorce. This number is based on the annual marriage rate compared with the annual divorce rate. This is misleading, because in any given year, the people who are divorcing are not the same as those who are marrying. The preferred method to determine the divorce rate is to calculate how many people who have ever married subsequently divorce. Using this calculation, the divorce rate in the United States has never exceeded 41 percent.[26] Although this number is still high, the divorce rate in this country has declined from previous decades. This decrease may be related to an increase in the age at which persons first marry and also a higher level of education among those who are marrying—both contribute to marital stability.[27]

The divorce rate represents only a portion of the actual number of failed relationships. Many people never go through a legal divorce process; as a result, they are not counted in these statistics. Cohabitants and unmarried partners who raise children, own homes together, and exhibit all the outward appearances of marriage without the license are also not included.

Why do relationships end? There are many reasons, including illness, financial concerns, and career problems. Other breakups arise from unmet expectations. Many people enter a relationship with certain expectations about how they and their partner will behave. Failure to communicate these beliefs can lead to resentment and disappointment. Differences in sexual needs may also contribute to the demise of a relationship. Under stress, communication and cooperation between partners can break down. Conflict, negative interactions, and a general lack of respect between partners can erode even the most loving relationship.

### what do you think?

What factors do you think contribute most to divorce?
● What factors contribute most to couples staying together?
● How do societal attitudes about marriage and divorce affect relationships in the United States?
● Do you feel as if divorce is sometimes the best resort when a marriage experiences difficulties? If not, how would you avoid the possibility in your own marriage?

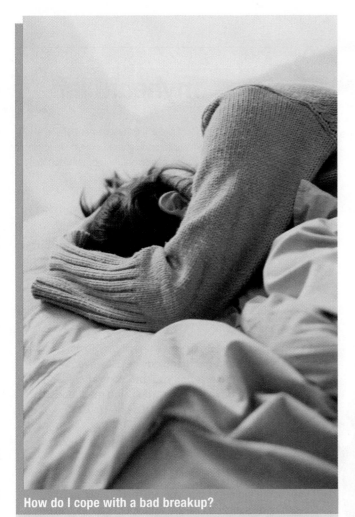

**How do I cope with a bad breakup?**

It may feel as if there is no end to the sorrow, anger, and guilt that often attend a difficult breakup, but time is a miraculous healer. Acknowledging your feelings, finding healthful ways to express them, spending time with friends, and allowing yourself to take as much time as you need to recover are all helpful strategies for dealing with the end of a romantic relationship.

# Coping with Failed Relationships

No relationship comes with a guarantee, no matter how many promises partners make to be together forever. Losing a love is as much a part of life as falling in love. That being said, the uncoupling process can be very painful (see the **Skills for Behavior Change** box at right for advice on approaching this difficult process). Whenever we risk getting close to another, we also risk being hurt if things don't work out. Remember that knowing, understanding, and feeling good about oneself before entering the relationship is very important. Consider these tips for coping with a failed relationship:

## How Do You End It?

Relationship endings are just as important as their beginnings. Healthy closure affords both parties the opportunity to move on without wondering or worrying about what went wrong and whose fault it was. If you need to end a relationship, do so in a manner that preserves and respects the dignity of both partners. If you are the person "breaking up," you have probably had time to think about the process and may be at a different stage from your partner.

Here are some tips for ending a relationship in a respectful and caring way:

✳ Arrange a time and quiet place where you can talk without interruption.
✳ Say in advance that there is something important you want to discuss.
✳ Accept that your partner may express strong feelings and be prepared to listen quietly.
✳ Consider in advance if you might also become upset and what support you might need.
✳ Communicate honestly using "I" messages and without personal attacks. Explain your reasons as much as you can without being cruel or insensitive.
✳ Don't let things escalate into a fight, even if you have very strong feelings.
✳ Provide another opportunity to talk about the end of the relationship when you both have had time to reflect.

● **Recognize and acknowledge your feelings.** These may include grief, loneliness, rejection, anger, guilt, relief, or sadness. Seek professional help and support as needed.
● **Find healthful ways to express your emotions, rather than turning them inward.** Go for a walk, talk to friends, listen to music, work out at the gym, volunteer with a community organization, or write in a journal.
● **Spend time with current friends, or reconnect with old friends.** Get reacquainted with yourself, what you enjoy doing, and the people whose company you enjoy.
● **Don't rush into a "rebound" relationship.** You need time to resolve your past experience rather than escape from it. You can't be trusting and intimate in a new relationship if you are still working on getting over a past relationship.

## How Well Do You Communicate?

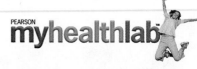

PEARSON
myhealthlab

Fill out this assessment online at www.pearsonhighered.com/myhealthlab or www.pearsonhighered.com/donatelle.

Imagine that you are in each of the situations below, and indicate how confident and satisfied you are that you could communicate competently using the following scale.

1. Very dissatisfied with my ability to communicate
2. Somewhat dissatisfied with my ability to communicate
3. Not sure how effectively I could communicate
4. Somewhat satisfied that I could communicate competently
5. Very satisfied that I could communicate competently

_____ **1.** Someone asks you personal questions that you feel uncomfortable answering. You'd like to tell the person that you don't want to answer.

_____ **2.** You think a friend is drinking more alcohol than is healthy, and you want to bring the topic up to her.

_____ **3.** Your colleague asks you to write him a letter of recommendation. You don't think he is well suited for the position to which he's applying.

_____ **4.** During a heated discussion about social issues, the person with whom you are talking says, "You're not listening to anything I'm saying!"

_____ **5.** A friend shares his creative writing with you. You don't think the writing is very good, but you need to respond to his request for an opinion.

_____ **6.** Your roommate's bad habits are really getting on your nerves. You want to tell her you're bothered and that you'd like her to stop.

_____ **7.** You arrive at a party and discover that you don't know anyone there.

_____ **8.** A classmate asks you for notes for the classes he missed, but you realize he has missed half the classes and expects you to bail him out.

_____ **9.** The person you have been dating declares, "I love you." You care about her, but you don't love her, at least not yet.

_____ **10.** A friend comes to you with his problems, and you give him attention and advice. However, when you want to discuss your problems, he doesn't seem to have the time. You value the friendship, but you don't like feeling it's one way.

_____ TOTAL

## Interpreting Your Score

If your score indicates that you are moderately satisfied (25–39) or dissatisfied (10–24) with your communication skills, notice whether your answers are extremes (1s and 5s). Focus on improving your skills in the situations that make you uneasy.

**Source:** Based on Julia Wood and Stephanie Coopman's Instructor's Resource Manual for Wood's text, *Interpersonal Communication: Everyday Encounters,* 5th ed. Copyright © 2006, Cengage Learning.

# YOUR PLAN FOR CHANGE

The **Assess yourself** activity gave you the chance to look at how you communicate. Now that you have considered your responses, you can take steps toward becoming a better communicator and improving your relationships.

**Today, you can:**

○ Call a friend you haven't talked to in a while or arrange a coffee date with a new acquaintance you'd like to get to know better.

○ Start a journal in which you keep track of communication and relationship issues that arise. Look for trends and think about ways you can change your behavior to address them.

**Within the next 2 weeks, you can:**

○ Spend some time letting the people you care about know how important their relationship is to you.

○ If there is someone with whom you have a conflict, arrange a time to sit down with that person in a neutral setting away from distractions to talk about the issues.

**By the end of the semester, you can:**

○ Practice being an active listener and notice when your mind wanders while you are listening to someone.

○ Take note of your nonverbal messages. Work on maintaining good eye contact and using open body language and inviting facial expressions.

# Summary

* Characteristics of intimate relationships include behavioral interdependence, need fulfillment, emotional attachment, and emotional availability. These influence how we interact with others and the types of intimate relationships we form. Family, friends, and partners or lovers provide the most common opportunities for intimacy. Each relationship may include healthy and unhealthy characteristics that may affect daily functioning. Self-esteem and self-acceptance are important factors in the success and failure of relationships.

* There are many strategies for building better relationships. Examining one's own behaviors to determine what to change and how to change it is an important ingredient of success. Characteristics of satisfying and successful relationships include good communication, intimacy, friendship, and trust. Issues that can cause problems in relationships include jealousy, differences over gender roles, power struggles, and unmet expectations.

* To improve our ability to communicate with others, we need to address several factors, including learning how to use self-disclosure, listening effectively, conveying and interpreting nonverbal communication, establishing a proper climate for communicating, and managing and resolving conflicts.

* For most people, commitment is an important ingredient in successful relationships. The major types of committed relationships include marriage, cohabitation, and gay and lesbian partnerships (which may involve either marriage or cohabitation). Success in committed relationships requires understanding the elements of a good relationship.

* Life decisions such as whether to marry or have children require serious consideration. Remaining single is more common than ever before. Most single people lead healthy, happy, and well-adjusted lives. Those who decide to have or not have children can also lead rewarding, productive lives as long as they have given this decision the utmost thought, weighing the pros and cons of each alternative in the context of their lifestyles.

* Before relationships fail, many warning signs often appear. By recognizing these signs and taking action to change behaviors, partners may save and enhance their relationship.

# Pop Quiz

1. Intimate relationships fulfill our psychological need for someone to listen to our worries and concerns. This is known as our need for
   a. dependence.
   b. social integration.
   c. enjoyment.
   d. spontaneity.

2. Lovers tend to pay attention to the other person even when they should be involved in other activities. This is called
   a. inclusion.
   b. exclusivity.
   c. fascination.
   d. authentic intimacy.

3. All of the following are typical causes of jealousy EXCEPT
   a. overdependence on the relationship.
   b. low self-esteem.
   c. a past relationship that involved deception.
   d. belief that relationships can easily be replaced.

4. According to anthropologist Helen Fisher, attraction and falling in love follow a pattern based on
   a. lust, attraction, and attachment.
   b. intimacy, passion, and commitment.
   c. imprinting, attraction, attachment, and the production of a cuddle chemical.
   d. fascination, exclusiveness, sexual desire, giving the utmost, and being a champion.

5. The goal of conflict resolution is to
   a. constructively resolve points of contention.
   b. declare a winner and a loser.
   c. ensure that couples argue as little as possible.
   d. set a time limit on discussion of difficult issues.

6. Terms such as *behavioral interdependence, need fulfillment,* and *emotional availability* describe which type of relationship?
   a. Dysfunctional
   b. Sexual
   c. Intimate
   d. Behavioral

7. Predictability, dependability, and faith are three fundamental elements of
   a. trust.
   b. friendship.
   c. attraction.
   d. attachment.

8. *Competitive listening* refers to
   a. attentive listening to what the other person is saying.
   b. paraphrasing what the other person is communicating to you.
   c. arguing or debating without listening to what the other person is trying to express.
   d. promoting your own point of view.

9. One of the most important ways to express difficult feelings with another person is to
   a. be specific rather than general about how you feel.
   b. express anger and resentment so the other person feels your heartache.

c. point your finger at the other person.

d. blame the other person for the difficulty you are experiencing.

10. One important factor in choosing a partner is *proximity*, which refers to
    a. mutual regard.
    b. attitudes and values.
    c. physical attraction.
    d. being in the same place at the same time.

*Answers to these questions can be found on page A-1.*

# Think about It!

1. What are the characteristics of intimate relationships? What are behavioral interdependence, need fulfillment, emotional attachment, and emotional availability, and why is each important in relationship development?

2. What problems can form barriers to intimacy? What actions can you take to reduce or remove these barriers?

3. What are common elements of good relationships? Warning signs of trouble? What actions can you take to improve your own interpersonal relationships?

4. What is nonverbal communication, and why is it important to develop skills in this area? Give examples of some things that you do to communicate without words.

5. How can you tell the difference between a love relationship and one that is based primarily on attraction? What characteristics do love relationships share?

6. Name some common misconceptions about people who choose to remain single and about couples who choose not to have children. Do you want to have children? Why or why not? What characteristics show that a couple is ready to have children?

# Accessing Your Health on the Internet

The following websites explore further topics and issues related to personal health. For links to the websites below, visit the Companion Website for *Access to Health*, 12th Edition, at www.pearsonhighered.com/donatelle.

1. *Gay and Lesbian Couples National Network.* This is a link into a network for same-sex couples and singles, with resources about gay and lesbian issues. http://couples-national.org

2. *The Gottman Institute.* This organization helps couples directly and provides training to therapists. The website includes research information, self-help tips for relationship building, and a relationship quiz. www.gottman.com

3. *National Center for Health Statistics.* This division of the Centers for Disease Control and Prevention has up-to-date statistics on trends in marriage, divorce, and cohabitation. www.cdc.gov/nchs

4. *Relationship Growth Online.* This site provides information, quizzes, games, advice, and links to more information on how to build better relationships. www.relationshipweb.com

5. *The Conflict Resolution Information Source.* This site provides information, news, research, and links to resources for resolving conflicts in interpersonal relationships, marriages, families, organizations, and more. www.crinfo.org

# References

1. J. Snelgrove, P. Hynek, and M. Stafford, "A Multi-Level Analysis of Social Capital and Self-Rated Health: Evidence from the British Household Panel Survey," *Social Science and Medicine* 68, no. 11 (2009): 1993–2001; C. J. Hale, J. W. Hannum, and D. L. Espelage, "Social Support and Physical Health: The Importance of Belonging," *Journal of American College Health*, 53 (2005): 276–84; S. Braithwaite, R. Delevi, and F. Fincham, "Romantic Relationships and the Physical and Mental Health of College Students," *Personal Relationships* 17, no. 1 (2010): 1–12; E. Cornwell and L. Waite, "Social Disconnectedness, Perceived Isolation, and Health among Older Adults" *Journal of Health and Social Behavior*, 50, no.11 (2009): 31–48.

2. E. Hatfield, J. T. Pillemer, M. U. O'Brien, and Y. L. Le, "The Endurance of Love: Passionate and Companionate Love in Newlywed and Long-Term Marriages," *Interpersona: An International Journal of Personal Relationships* 2 (June 2008): 35–64; E. Hatfield and R. L. Rapson, *Love, Sex, and Intimacy: Their Psychology, Biology, and History* (New York: Harper Collins, 1993).

3. R. Sternberg, "Construct Validation of a Triangular Love Scale," *European Journal of Social Psychology* 27 (1997): 313–35.

4. H. Fisher, *Why We Love* (New York: Henry Holt, 2004); H. Fisher, A. Aron, D. Mashek, H. Li, and L. L. Brown, "Defining the Brain System of Lust, Romantic Attraction, and Attachment," *Archives of Sexual Behavior* 31, no. 5 (2002): 413–19.

5. Ibid.

6. H. Fisher, *Why Him? Why Her? How to Find and Keep a Lasting Love* (New York: Henry Holt, 2009).

7. Ibid.

8. S. Brehm et al., *Intimate Relationships*, 3rd ed. (New York: McGraw-Hill, 2002), 263.

9. M. Gatzeva and A. Paik, "Emotional and Physical Satisfaction in Noncohabiting, Cohabiting, and Marital Relationships: The Importance of Jealous Conflict," *Journal of Sex Research* 25 (2009): 1–14; D. Nannini and L. Mayers, "Jealousy in Sexual and Emotional Infidelity: An Alternative to the Evolutionary Explanation," *Journal of Sex Research* 37, no. 2 (2000): 117–22.

10. C. R. Rogers, "Interpersonal Relationship: The Core of Guidance" in *Person to Person: The Problem of Being Human*, eds. C. R. Rogers and B. Stevens (Lafayette, CA: Real People Press, 1967).

11. J. Wood, *Interpersonal Communication: Everyday Encounters* (Belmont, CA: Cengage, 2010); J. K. Burgoon, C. Segrin, and N. E. Dunbar, "Nonverbal Communication and Social Influence," in *Persuasion: Developments in Theory and Practice*, eds. J. P. Dillard and M. Pfau (Thousand Oaks, CA: Sage, 2002), 445–76.

12. R. S. Miller, D. Perlman, and S. S. Brehm, *Intimate Relationships*, 4th ed. (New York: McGraw-Hill, 2007), 150–56.

13. The National Marriage Project, University of Virginia, *The State of Our Unions: Marriage in America, 2009: Money & Marriage* (Charlottesville, VA: National Marriage Project and the Institute for

American Values, 2009), Available at www.stateofourunions.org.

14. U.S. Census Bureau News, "Press Release: March 2009 Current Population Survey: Census Bureau Reports Families with Children Increasingly Face Unemployment," January 15, 2010, www.census.gov/newsroom/releases/archives/families_households/cb10-08.html.

15. K. McCoy, "Can Marriage Help You Live Longer?" HealthLibrary, EBSCO Publishing, Updated April 2010, http://healthlibrary.epnet.com/GetContent.aspx?token=af362d97-4f80-4453-a175-02cc6220a387&chunkiid=43793.

16. C. A. Schoenborn, "Marital Status and Health: United States, 1999–2002," *Advance Data from Vital and Health Statistics,* no. 351, DHHS Publication No. 2005-1250 (Hyattsville, MD: National Center for Health Statistics, 2004), Available at www.cdc.gov/nchs/products/ad.htm.

17. P. Y. Goodwin, W. D. Mosher, and A. Chandra, "Marriage and Cohabitation in the United States: A Statistical Portrait Based on Cycle 6 (2002) of the National Survey of Family Growth, National Center for Health Statistics," *Vital Health Statistics* 23, no. 28 (2010), Available at www.cdc.gov/nchs/nsfg/nsfg_products.htm.

18. Ibid.

19. G. J. Gates, "Same-Sex Spouses and Unmarried Partners in the American Community Survey, 2008" (Los Angeles: The Williams Institute, UCLA School of Law, 2009), Available at www.law.ucla.edu/williamsinstitute/publications/Policy-Census-index.html.

20. National Gay and Lesbian Task Force, "Relationship Recognition Map for Same-Sex Couples in the U.S.," September 2010, www.thetaskforce.org/reports_and_research/relationship_recognition.

21. U.S. Census Bureau, "2008 American Community Survey, Marital Status," table S1210, 2008, http://factfinder.census.gov/servlet/DatasetMainPageServlet?_program=ACS&_submenuId=datasets_3&_lang=en&_ts=.

22. U.S. Census Bureau, Housing and Household Economic Statistics Division, Fertility & Family Statistics Branch, "America's Families and Living Arrangements: 2009," 2010, www.census.gov/population/www/socdemo/hh-fam/cps2009.html.

23. Ibid.

24. M. Lino, *Expenditures on Children by Families, 2009* (Alexandria, VA: U.S. Department of Agriculture, Center for Nutrition Policy and Promotion, 2010), Available at www.cnpp.usda.gov/ExpendituresonChildrenbyFamilies.htm.

25. U.S. Bureau of Labor Statistics, "Women in the Labor Force: A Databook 2009 Edition," 2009, http://data.bls.gov/cgi-bin/print.pl/cps/wlf-databook2009.htm.

26. D. Hurley, "Divorce Rate: It's Not as High as You Think," *New York Times,* April 19, 2005.

27. The National Marriage Project, University of Virginia, *The State of Our Unions: Marriage in America, 2009: Money & Marriage,* 2009.

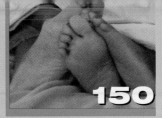
**147**
Do all women get PMS?

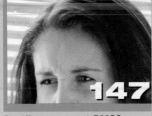
**150**
How does aging affect one's libido?

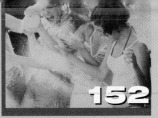
**152**
What influences sexual identity besides biology?

# 5

# Understanding Your Sexuality

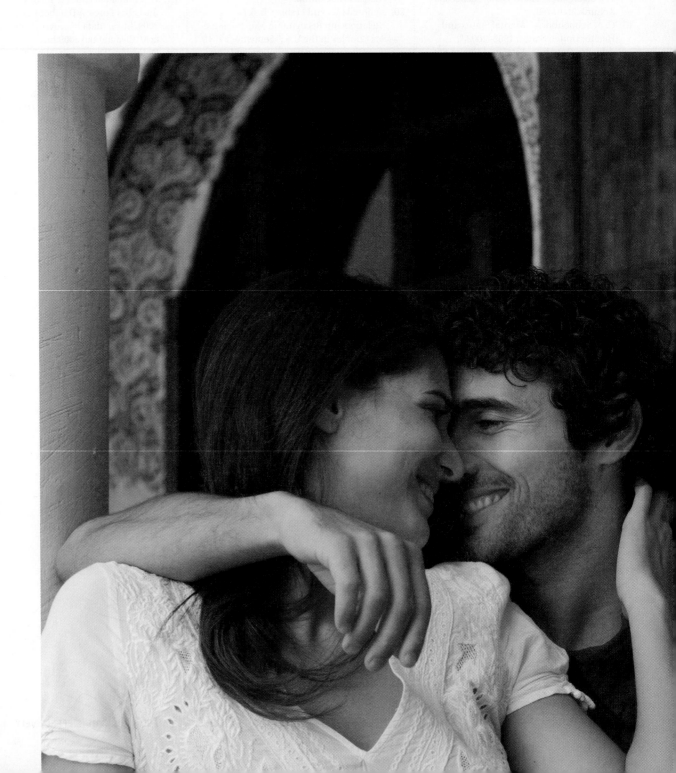

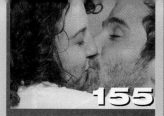

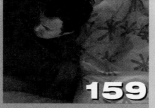

**155**

What is "normal" sexual behavior?

**159**

Are sexual disorders more physical or more psychological?

## Objectives

✶ Identify major features and functions of male and female sexual anatomy and physiology.

✶ Discuss the stages of the human sexual response and what factors may influence these during your life.

✶ Define *sexual identity,* and discuss its major components, including biology, gender identity, gender roles, and sexual orientation.

✶ Discuss the options available for the expression of one's sexuality.

✶ Classify sexual dysfunctions, and describe major disorders.

✶ Examine the effects of various drugs on sexual behavior.

How do you see yourself as a sexual person? Do you identify as transgendered? Gay? Straight? Are the sexual behaviors you engage in similar to those of other students? Are you "comfortable in your own skin"? Do you know enough about sexual anatomy and physiology to maximize your sexual pleasure or control your fertility? All these questions relate directly to your sexuality. Sexuality begins with our biological sex, gender, sexual anatomy and physiology, and sexual functions, but it also encompasses values, beliefs, and attitudes about how we see ourselves as a sexual being and how we relate to others.

Human sexuality can be fascinating, complex, contradictory, and sometimes frustrating. It presents challenges in the areas of personal values, interpersonal relationships, cultural traditions, social norms, new technologies, current research findings, and changing political agendas. **Sexuality** is much more than sexual feelings or intercourse. Rather, it includes all the thoughts, feelings, and behaviors associated with being male or female, experiencing attraction, being in love, and being in relationships that include sexual intimacy and activity. These interwoven elements of sexuality include the following:

● **Sensuality.** Awareness and feelings about your body and other people's bodies, especially that of your sexual partner. Sensuality enables us to feel good about how our bodies look and feel and to enjoy the pleasure they can give to us and others.
● **Intimacy.** The ability to be close to another human being emotionally and to accept closeness in return.
● **Sexual identity.** A person's understanding of who she or he is sexually, including one's sense of maleness or femaleness.
● **Sexual health and reproduction.** A person's attitudes and behaviors related to producing children, care and maintenance of the sex and reproductive organs, and health consequences of sexual behavior.
● **Sexualization.** The use of sexuality to influence, control, or manipulate others, in ways that may be harmful or exploitative.

Because our sexuality is central to who we are, many of these topics are discussed throughout this text. In this chapter, we will focus primarily on sexual identity, aspects of sexual health and reproduction, and sensuality. In the end, having a comprehensive understanding of your sexuality will help you prepare to make healthful, responsible, and satisfying decisions about your life and your interpersonal relationships. Let's start exploring our sexuality by reviewing sexual anatomy and physiology.

**sexuality** All the thoughts, feelings, and behaviors associated with being male or female, experiencing attraction, being in love, and being in relationships that include sexual intimacy and activity.

# Sexual Anatomy and Physiology

Understanding the functions of the male and female reproductive systems will help you derive pleasure and satisfaction from your sexual relationships, be sensitive to your partner's wants and needs, and make responsible choices regarding your own sexual health.

## Female Sexual Anatomy and Physiology

The female reproductive system includes two major groups of structures, the external genitals and the internal organs (Figure 5.1). The external female genitals are collectively known as the **vulva** and include the structures that are outwardly visible, specifically the mons pubis, the labia minora and majora, the clitoris, and the urethral and vaginal openings. The **mons pubis** is a pad of fatty tissue covering and protecting the pubic bone; after the onset of puberty, it becomes covered with coarse hair. The **labia majora** are folds of skin and erectile tissue that enclose the urethral and vaginal openings; the **labia minora,** or inner lips, are folds of mucous membrane found just inside the labia majora.

The **clitoris** is located at the upper end of the labia minora and beneath the mons pubis, and its only known function is to provide sexual pleasure. Directly below the clitoris is the **urethral opening** through which urine is expelled from the body. Below the urethral opening is the vaginal opening. In some women, the vaginal opening is covered by a thin membrane called the **hymen.** It is a myth that an intact hymen is proof of virginity, as the hymen can be stretched or torn by physical activity, and is not present in all women to begin with.

The **perineum** is the area of smooth tissue found between the vulva and the anus. Although not technically part of the external genitalia, the tissue in this area has many nerve endings and is sensitive to touch; it can play a part in sexual excitement.

The internal female genitals include the vagina, uterus, fallopian tubes, and ovaries. The **vagina** is a tubular organ that serves as a passageway from the uterus to the outside of the body. This passage allows menstrual flow to exit from the uterus during a woman's monthly cycle, receives the penis during intercourse, and serves as the birth canal during childbirth. The **uterus (womb)** is a hollow, muscular, pear-shaped organ. Hormones acting on the inner lining of the uterus (the **endometrium**), either prepare the uterus for implantation and development of a fertilized egg or signal that no fertilization has taken place, in which case the endometrium deteriorates and becomes menstrual flow.

The lower end of the uterus, the **cervix,** extends down into the vagina. Its actual opening is refered to as the *cervical os.* The **ovaries,** almond-sized organs suspended on either side of the uterus, produce the hormones estrogen and progesterone and are also the reservoir for immature eggs. All the eggs a woman will ever have are present in her ovaries at birth. Eggs mature and are released from the ovaries in response to hormone levels. Extending from the upper end of the uterus are two thin, flexible tubes called the **fallopian tubes** (also known as **oviducts**). The fallopian tubes, which do not actually touch the ovaries, capture eggs as they are released from the ovaries during ovulation, and they are the site where sperm and egg meet and fertilization takes place. The fallopian tubes then serve as the passageway to the uterus, where the fertilized egg becomes implanted and development continues.

### The Onset of Puberty and the Menstrual Cycle
With the onset of puberty, the female reproductive system matures, and the development of **secondary sex characteristics,** including the development of breasts, the widening of hips, and the growth of underarm and pubic hair, signals the transition of young girls into young women. The first sign of puberty is the beginning of breast development, which generally occurs around age 11. The **pituitary gland,** the **hypothalamus,** and the ovaries all secrete hormones that act as chemical messengers among them. Working in a feedback system, hormonal levels in the bloodstream act as the trigger mechanism for release of more or different hormones.

Around the time a girl reaches 9½ to 11½ years old, the hypothalamus receives the message to begin secreting *gonadotropin-releasing hormone (GnRH).* The release of GnRH in turn signals the pituitary gland to release hormones called *gonadotropins.* Two specific gonadotropins, *follicle-stimulating hormone (FSH)* and *luteinizing hormone (LH),* signal the ovaries to start producing **estrogens** and **progesterone.** Estrogens regulate the menstrual cycle, and increased estrogen levels assist in the development of female secondary sex characteristics. Progesterone helps the endometrium to develop in preparation for nourishing a fertilized egg and helps maintain pregnancy. The normal age range for the onset of the

**vulva** Collective term for the external female genitalia.

**mons pubis** Fatty tissue covering the pubic bone in females; in physically mature women, the mons is covered with coarse hair.

**labia majora** "Outer lips," or folds of tissue covering the female sexual organs.

**labia minora** "Inner lips," or folds of tissue just inside the labia majora.

**clitoris** A pea-sized nodule of tissue located at the top of the labia minora; central to sexual arousal in women.

**urethral opening** The opening through which urine is expelled.

**hymen** Thin tissue covering the vaginal opening in some women.

**perineum** Tissue that forms the "floor" of the pelvic region in both men and women.

**vagina** The passage in females leading from the vulva into the uterus.

**uterus (womb)** Hollow, pear-shaped muscular organ whose function is to contain the developing fetus.

**endometrium** Soft, spongy matter that makes up the uterine lining.

## "Why Should I Care?"

It is more difficult to please a partner sexually or to descibe to a partner how to please you if you don't really know and understand basic sexual anatomy. For example, the clitoris in females is very responsive to touch and when stimulated often leads to orgasm. The urethral opening located nearby is not.

## External Anatomy

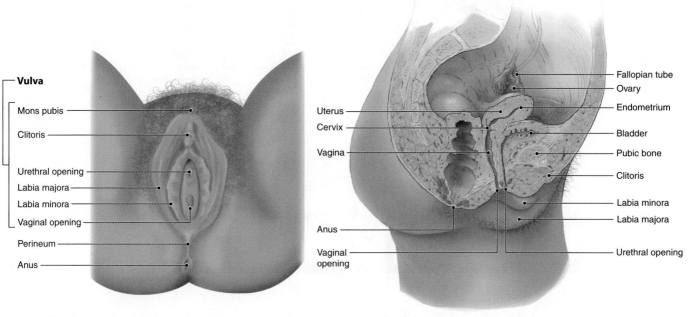

**Vulva**
- Mons pubis
- Clitoris
- Urethral opening
- Labia majora
- Labia minora
- Vaginal opening
- Perineum
- Anus

## Internal Organs

- Fallopian tube
- Ovary
- Endometrium
- Bladder
- Pubic bone
- Clitoris
- Labia minora
- Labia majora
- Urethral opening
- Uterus
- Cervix
- Vagina
- Anus
- Vaginal opening

FIGURE 5.1 **Female Reproductive System**

first menstrual period, or **menarche,** is 9 to 17 years, with the average age being 11 to 13 years. Body fat heavily influences the onset of puberty, and increasing rates of obesity in children may account for the fact that girls here and in other countries seem to be reaching puberty much earlier than they used to.[1] Very thin girls, such as young athletes, tend to start menstruating later.

The average menstrual cycle lasts 28 days and consists of three phases: the proliferative phase, the secretory phase, and the menstrual phase **(Figure 5.2)**. The *proliferative phase*

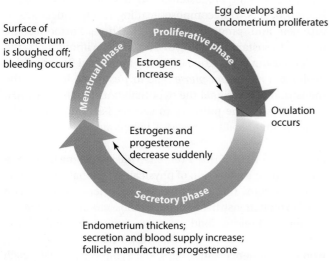

Surface of endometrium is sloughed off; bleeding occurs

Egg develops and endometrium proliferates

Proliferative phase

Estrogens increase

Ovulation occurs

Menstrual phase

Estrogens and progesterone decrease suddenly

Secretory phase

Endometrium thickens; secretion and blood supply increase; follicle manufactures progesterone

FIGURE 5.2 **The Three Phases of the Menstrual Cycle**

**Source:** Rathus, et al., *Human Sexuality in a World of Diversity* Figure "The Three Phases of the Menstrual Cycle," © 2005 Allyn & Bacon. Reproduced with permission of Pearson Education, Inc.

begins with the end of menstruation. During this time, the endometrium develops, or "proliferates." How does this process work? By the end of menstruation, the hypothalamus senses very low levels of estrogen and progesterone in the blood. In response, it increases its secretions of GnRH, which in turn triggers the pituitary gland to release FSH. When FSH reaches the ovaries, it signals several **ovarian follicles** to begin maturing. Normally, only one of the follicles, the **graafian follicle,** reaches full maturity in the days preceding ovulation. While the follicles mature, they begin producing estrogen, which in turn signals the endometrial lining of the uterus to proliferate. If fertilization occurs, the endometrium will become a nesting place for the developing embryo. High estrogen levels signal the pituitary to slow down FSH production and increase release of LH. Under the influence of LH, the graafian follicle ruptures and releases a mature **ovum** (plural: *ova*), a single mature egg cell, near a fallopian tube. This event, which usually occurs around

**cervix** Lower end of the uterus that opens into the vagina.
**ovaries** Almond-sized organs that house developing eggs and produce hormones.
**fallopian tubes (oviducts)** Tubes that extend from near the ovaries to the uterus; site of fertilization and passageway for fertilized eggs.
**secondary sex characteristics** Characteristics associated with sex but not directly related to reproduction, such as vocal pitch, degree of body hair, and location of fat deposits.
**pituitary gland** The endocrine gland controlling the release of hormones from the gonads.
**hypothalamus** An area of the brain located near the pituitary gland; works in conjunction with the pituitary gland to control reproductive functions.
**estrogens** Hormones secreted by the ovaries that control the menstrual cycle.
**progesterone** Hormone secreted by the ovaries; helps the endometrium develop and helps maintain pregnancy.
**menarche** The first menstrual period.
**ovarian follicles** Areas within the ovary in which individual eggs develop.
**graafian follicle** Mature ovarian follicle that contains a fully developed ovum, or egg.
**ovum** A single mature egg cell.

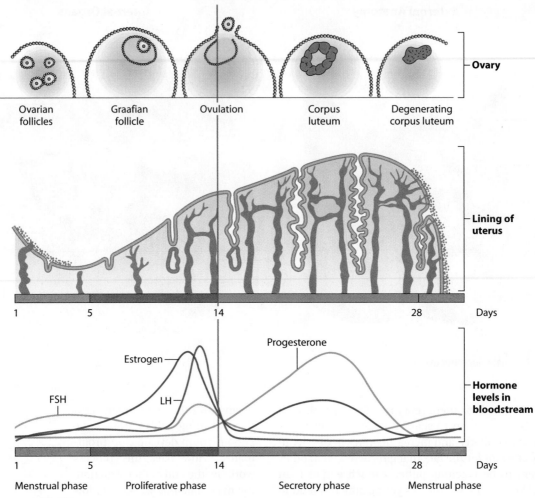

Ovary

Ovarian follicles | Graafian follicle | Ovulation | Corpus luteum | Degenerating corpus luteum

Lining of uterus

1   5   14   28   Days

Progesterone

Estrogen

FSH   LH

Hormone levels in bloodstream

1   5   14   28   Days

Menstrual phase | Proliferative phase | Secretory phase | Menstrual phase

FIGURE 5.3 **Hormonal Control and Phases of the Menstrual Cycle**

day 14 of the cycle, is referred to as **ovulation.** The other ripening follicles degenerate and are reabsorbed by the body. Occasionally, two ova mature and are released during ovulation. If both are fertilized, fraternal (nonidentical) twins develop. Identical twins develop when one fertilized ovum (called a *zygote*) divides into two separate zygotes.

The phase following ovulation is called the *secretory phase.* The ruptured graafian follicle, which has remained in the ovary, is transformed into the **corpus luteum** and begins secreting large amounts of estrogen and progesterone. These hormone secretions peak around the twentieth or twenty-first days of the average cycle and cause the endometrium to thicken. If fertilization and implantation take place, cells surrounding the developing embryo release a hormone called *human chorionic gonadotropin* (*HCG*), increasing estrogen and progesterone secretions that maintain the endometrium and signal the pituitary not to start a new menstrual cycle. If no implantation occurs, the hypothalamus responds by signaling the pituitary to stop producing FSH and LH, thus peaking the levels of progesterone in the blood. The corpus luteum begins to decompose, leading to rapid declines in estrogen and progesterone levels. These hormones are needed to sustain the lining of the uterus. Without them, the endometrium is sloughed off in the menstrual flow, and this begins the *menstrual phase.* The low estrogen levels of the menstrual phase signal the hypothalamus to release GnRH, which acts on the pituitary to secrete FSH, and the cycle, depicted graphically in **Figure 5.3**, begins again.

**Menstrual Problems** **Premenstrual syndrome (PMS)** is a term used for a collection of physical, emotional, and behavioral symptoms that many women experience 7 to 14 days prior to their menstrual period. The most common symptoms are tender breasts, food cravings, fatigue, irritability, and depression. It is estimated that 75 percent of menstruating women experience some signs and symptoms of PMS each month. For the majority of women, these disappear as their period begins, but for a small subset of women (3–5%), their symptoms are severe enough to affect their daily routines and activities to the point of being disabling. This severe form of

**ovulation** The point of the menstrual cycle at which a mature egg ruptures through the ovarian wall.

**corpus luteum** A body of cells that forms from the remains of the graafian follicle following ovulation; it secretes estrogen and progesterone during the second half of the menstrual cycle.

**premenstrual syndrome (PMS)** Comprises the mood changes and physical symptoms that occur in some women during the 1 or 2 weeks prior to menstruation.

PMS has its own psychiatric designation, **premenstrual dysphoric disorder (PMDD)**, with symptoms that include severe depression, hopelessness, anger, anxiety, low self-esteem, difficulty concentrating, irritability, and tension.

There are several natural approaches to managing PMS that can also help PMDD. These strategies include eating more carbohydrates (grains, fruits, and vegetables), reducing caffeine and salt intake, exercising regularly, and taking measures to reduce stress. Recent investigation into methods of controlling severe emotional swings has led to the use of antidepressants for treating PMDD, primarily selective serotonin reuptake inhibitors (SSRIs; e.g., Prozac, Paxil, and Zoloft).

**Dysmenorrhea** is a medical term for menstrual cramps, the pain or discomfort in the lower abdomen that many women experience just before or after menstruation. Along with cramps, some women can experience nausea and vomiting, loose stools, sweating, and dizziness. Menstrual cramps can be classified as primary or secondary dysmenorrhea. Primary dysmenorrhea doesn't involve any physical abnormality and usually begins 6 months to a year after a woman's first period, whereas secondary dysmenorrhea has an underlying physical cause such as endometriosis or uterine fibroids.[2] If you experience primary dysmenorrhea, you can reduce your discomfort by using over-the-counter nonsteroidal anti-inflammatory drugs (NSAIDs) such as aspirin, ibuprofen (Advil or Motrin), or naproxen (Aleve). Other self-care strategies such as soaking in a hot bath or using a heating pad on your abdomen may also ease your cramps. For severe cramping, your health care provider may recommend a low-dose oral contraceptive to prevent ovulation, which in turn may reduce the production of prostaglandins and therefore the severity of your cramps. Managing secondary dysmenorrhea involves treating the underlying cause.

*Toxic shock syndrome (TSS)*, although rare today, is still something women should be aware of. It is caused by a bacterial infection facilitated by tampon or diaphragm use (see Chapter 6). Symptoms, which occur during one's period or a few days afterward, are sometimes hard to recognize because they mimic the flu and include sudden high fever, vomiting, diarrhea, dizziness, fainting, or a rash that looks like sunburn. Proper treatment usually assures recovery in 2 to 3 weeks.

**Menopause** Just as menarche signals the beginning of a woman's potential reproductive years, **menopause**—the permanent cessation of menstruation—signals the end. Generally occurring between the ages of 40 and 60, and at age 51 on

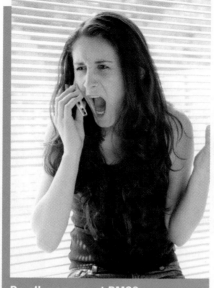

**Do all women get PMS?**

About 75% of menstruating women experience some PMS symptoms every month, but for most women these symptoms are mild and short lived. Stress reduction, regular exercise, and a healthy diet are all good strategies for coping with PMS symptoms, which can include irritability and moodiness, fatigue, breast tenderness, and food cravings.

**51** is the average age of onset for menopause among American women.

average in the United States, menopause results in decreased estrogen levels, which may produce troublesome symptoms in some women. Decreased vaginal lubrication, hot flashes, headaches, dizziness, and joint pain have been associated with the onset of menopause. In some women, menopause and the physical symptoms related to it can lead to a decline in **libido,** or sex drive.

Hormones, such as estrogen and progesterone, have long been prescribed as **hormone replacement therapy** to relieve menopausal symptoms and reduce the risk of heart disease and osteoporosis. (The National Institutes of Health prefers the term **menopausal hormone therapy,** because hormone therapy is not a replacement and does not restore the physiology of youth.) However, recent studies, including results from the Women's Health Initiative (WHI), suggest that hormone therapy may actually do more harm than good. In fact, the WHI terminated its research into the effects of hormone therapy ahead of schedule due to concerns about participants' increased risk of breast cancer, heart attack, stroke, blood clots, and other health problems.[3] All women need to discuss the risks and benefits of menopausal hormone therapy with their health care provider to make an informed decision. Adopting a healthy lifestyle, which includes regular exercise, a balanced diet, and adequate calcium intake, can also help protect postmenopausal women from heart disease and osteoporosis.

## Male Sexual Anatomy and Physiology

The structures of the male reproductive system are divided into external and internal genitals (Figure 5.4). The external genitals are the penis and the scrotum. The internal male genitals include the testes, epididymides, vasa deferentia, ejaculatory ducts, urethra, and three other structures—the seminal vesicles, the prostate gland,

**premenstrual dysphoric disorder (PMDD)** Collective name for a group of negative symptoms similar to but more severe than PMS, including severe mood disturbances.
**dysmenorrhea** Condition of pain or discomfort in the lower abdomen just before or after menstruation.
**menopause** The permanent cessation of menstruation, generally between the ages of 40 and 60.
**libido** Sexual drive or desire.
**hormone replacement therapy** or **menopausal hormone therapy** Use of synthetic or animal estrogens and progesterone to compensate for decreases in estrogens in a woman's body during menopause.

## External Anatomy

## Internal Organs

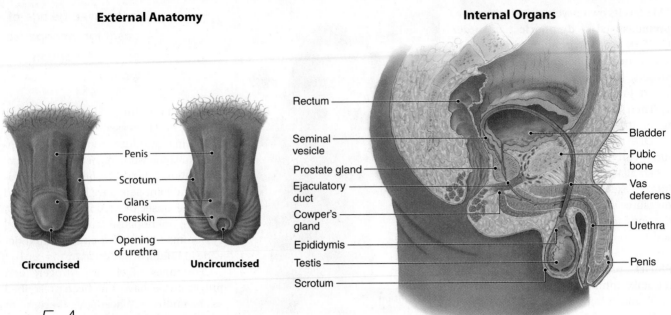

FIGURE 5.4 **Male Reproductive System**

and the Cowper's glands—that secrete components that, with sperm, make up semen. These three structures are sometimes referred to as the *accessory glands.*

The **penis** is the organ that deposits sperm in the vagina during intercourse. The urethra, which passes through the center of the penis, acts as the passageway for both semen and urine to exit the body. During sexual arousal, the spongy tissue in the penis becomes filled with blood, making the organ stiff (erect). Further sexual excitement leads to **ejaculation,** a series of rapid, spasmodic contractions that propels semen out of the penis.

Debate continues over the practice of *circumcision,* the surgical removal of a fold of skin covering the end of the penis known as the *foreskin.* Most circumcisions are performed for religious or cultural reasons or because of hygiene concerns. However, recent research supports the claim that circumcision yields medical benefits, including decreased risk of urinary tract infections in the first year, decreased risk of penile cancer (although cancer of the penis is very rare to begin with), and decreased risk of sexual transmission of human papillomavirus (HPV) and human immunodeficiency virus (HIV).[4] See the **Points of View** box on the next page for further discussion of the controversy surrounding circumcision.

Situated behind the penis and also outside the body is a sac called the **scrotum.** The scrotum encases the testes, pro-

**penis** Male sexual organ that releases sperm into the vagina.
**ejaculation** The propulsion of semen from the penis.
**scrotum** External sac of tissue that encloses the testes.
**testes** Male sex organs that manufacture sperm and produce hormones.
**testosterone** The male sex hormone manufactured in the testes.
**spermatogenesis** The development of sperm.
**epididymis** The duct system atop the testis where sperm mature.
**vas deferens** Tube that transports sperm from the epididymis to the ejaculatory duct.
**seminal vesicles** Glandular ducts that secrete nutrients for the semen.
**semen** Fluid containing sperm and nutrients that increase sperm viability and neutralize vaginal acid.

tecting them and helping control their internal temperature, which is vital to proper sperm production. The **testes** (singular: *testis*) manufacture sperm and **testosterone,** the hormone responsible for the development of male secondary sex characteristics, including deepening of the voice and growth of facial, body, and pubic hair.

The development of sperm is referred to as **spermatogenesis.** Like the maturation of eggs in the female, this process is governed by the pituitary gland. Follicle-stimulating hormone (FSH) is secreted into the bloodstream to stimulate the testes to manufacture sperm. Immature sperm are released into a comma-shaped structure on the back of each testis called the **epididymis** (plural: *epididymides*), where they ripen and reach full maturity.

Each epididymis contains coiled tubules that gradually "unwind" and straighten out to become the **vas deferens.** The two vasa deferentia, as they are called in the plural, make up the tubular transportation system whose sole function is to store and move sperm. Along the way, the **seminal vesicles** provide sperm with nutrients and other fluids that compose **semen.**

The vasa deferentia eventually connect each epididymis to the **ejaculatory ducts,** which pass through the prostate gland and empty into the urethra. The **prostate gland** contributes more fluids to the semen, including chemicals that help the sperm fertilize an ovum and neutralize the acidic environment of the vagina to make it more conducive to sperm motility and potency. Just below the prostate gland are two pea-shaped nodules called the **Cowper's glands.** The Cowper's glands secrete a fluid that lubricates the urethra and neutralizes any acid that may remain in the urethra after urination. Urine and semen do not come into contact with each other. During ejaculation of semen, a small valve closes off the tube to the urinary bladder.

# Circumcision:
## RISK VERSUS BENEFIT

Circumcision, the surgical removal of the foreskin from the penis, can be a controversial issue for parents. They must balance personal, cultural, and health issues in deciding whether to circumcise a son.

Approximately 56 percent (1.1 million) of all newborn boys are circumcised in the United States each year. Here are some of the arguments against and for circumcision.

### Arguments against Circumcision

○ It is a surgical procedure which may cause pain to the infant, and there are potential complications such as bleeding, acquiring an infection, improper healing, or cutting the foreskin too long or too short.

○ Families may feel the foreskin is needed for identity reasons, sexual pleasure reasons, or other reasons linked to religion or culture.

○ Much of the research on the relationship between circumcision and sexually transmitted infections was done in developing countries and may not be indicative of outcomes in developed nations.

○ Men lose a degree of sexual pleasure and stimulation when the foreskin is removed. Many unique nerve endings—found only in the foreskin—are lost forever.

### Arguments for Circumcision

○ Circumcised males have a lower risk of penile cancer.

○ Circumcised males have a lower risk of urinary tract infections during their first year, easier genital hygiene, and a lower risk of foreskin infections.

○ Circumcision has been shown to have a protective effect against human immunodeficiency virus (HIV), herpes simplex virus 2 (HSV-2), and human papillomavirus (HPV) transmission in males.

○ Families may have religious or cultural reasons for wishing to circumcise their sons (in the Jewish faith, for example, circumsicion is performed in a ceremony called a bris, and represents the covenant God made with the patriarch Abraham). Some people also believe a son's penis should look the same as his father's.

### Where Do You Stand?

○ If you had a son, what decision would you make regarding circumcising him?

○ What factors—religious, cultural, aesthetic, or health-related—would have the most impact on your decision?

○ If you are male, does your circumcised or uncircumcised status affect your opinion?

**Sources:** A. A. R. Tobian, R. H. Gray, and T. C. Quinn, "Male Circumcision for the Prevention of Acquisition and Transmission of Sexually

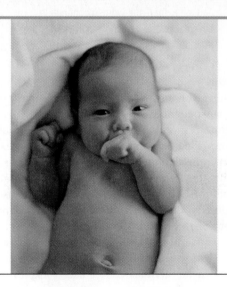

Transmitted Infections: The Case for Neonatal Circumcision," *Archives of Pediatrics & Adolescent Medicine* 164 (2010): 78–84; M. Moreno, "Advice for Patients: Male Circumcision," *Archives of Pediatrics & Adolescent Medicine* 164, no. 1 (2010): 104; Centers for Disease Control and Prevention, "Male Circumcision and Risk for HIV Transmission and Other Health Conditions: Implications for the United States, Centers for Disease Control and Prevention," Updated February 2008, www.cdc.gov/hiv/resources/factsheets/circumcision.htm; Mayo Clinic Staff, "Circumcision (Male): Why It's Done," February 2010, www.mayoclinic.com/health/circumcision/MY01023/DSECTION=why-its-done.

---

**Andropause** Testosterone levels in men vary greatly and in general, older men have lower testosterone levels than do younger men. Men, however, do not experience a rapid hormone decline in middle age that directly affects their reproductive capacity as women do during menopause. Instead, men typically experience a gradual decline in testosterone levels throughout adulthood, about 1 percent a year on average after the age of 30.[5] Many doctors use the term *andropause* to describe age-related hormone changes in men. Some men with lower testosterone levels do not

experience signs and symptoms. Those who do may experience the following:

● **Changes in sexual function.** These may include reduced sexual desire, fewer spontaneous erections—such as during sleep—and infertility. Testes may become smaller as well.

**ejaculatory duct** Tube formed by the junction of the seminal vesicle and the vas deferens that carries semen to the urethra.

**prostate gland** Gland that secretes nutrients and neutralizing fluids into the semen.

**Cowper's glands** Glands that secrete a fluid that lubricates the urethra and neutralizes any acid remaining in the urethra after urination.

- **Changes in sleep patterns.** Sometimes low testosterone causes insomnia or other sleep disturbances.
- **Physical changes.** Various physical changes are possible, including increased body fat, reduced muscle bulk and strength, and decreased bone density. Swollen or tender breasts (gynecomastia) and hair loss are possible.
- **Emotional changes.** Low testosterone levels may contribute to a decrease in motivation or self-confidence, cause sadness or depression, or interfere with concentrating or remembering things.[6]

Treatment is available for age-related low testosterone levels, but it is not without controversy. For some men, testosterone therapy relieves their bothersome signs and symptoms. For others, especially older men, the benefits aren't clear. There are risks for testosterone therapy as well. Testosterone therapy may increase the risk of prostate cancer or other health problems. It is important to discuss the pros and cons of testosterone treatment in detail with your doctor to decide if it is right for you.

# Human Sexual Response

Psychological traits greatly influence sexual response and sexual desire. Thus, we may find relationships with one partner vastly different from those we might experience with another. For both men and women, sexual response is a physiological process that generally follows a pattern that can be divided into four stages: excitement/arousal, plateau, orgasm, and resolution (Figure 5.5). Researchers agree that each individual has a personal response pattern that may or may not conform to these phases. Regardless of the type of sexual activity (stimulation by a partner or self-stimulation), the response stages are the same.

During the first stage, *excitement/arousal,* **vasocongestion** (increased blood flow that causes swelling in the genitals) stimulates male and female genital responses. The vagina begins to lubricate in preparation for penile penetration, and the penis becomes partially erect. Both sexes may exhibit a "sex flush," or a light blush all over their bodies. Excitement/arousal can be generated through fantasy or by touching, kissing, viewing films or videos, or reading erotic literature.

During the *plateau phase,* the initial responses intensify. Voluntary and involuntary muscle tensions increase. The woman's nipples and the man's penis become erect. The

**vasocongestion** The engorgement of the genital organs with blood.

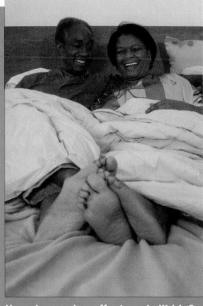

**How does aging affect one's libido?**

Both men and women frequently experience a decline in libido, or sex drive, as they grow older—particularly after menopause in women and andropause in men, when lower sex drive can result from reduced sex hormone production. However, the desire for physical contact and intimacy does not decrease with age, and many men and women continue to have active and fulfilling sex lives well into their golden years.

penis secretes a few drops of preejaculatory fluid, which may contain sperm.

During the *orgasmic phase,* vasocongestion and muscle tension reach their peak, and rhythmic contractions occur through the genital regions. In women, these contractions are centered in the uterus, outer vagina, and anal sphincter. In men, the contractions occur in two stages. First, contractions within the prostate gland begin propelling semen through the urethra. In the second stage, the muscles of the pelvic floor, urethra, and anal sphincter contract. Semen usually, but not always, is ejaculated from the penis. In both sexes, spasms in other major muscle groups also occur, particularly in the buttocks and abdomen. Feet and hands may also contract, and facial features often contort.

Muscle tension and congested blood subside in the *resolution phase* as the genital organs return to their pre-arousal states. Both sexes usually experience deep feelings of well-being and profound relaxation. Following orgasm and resolution, many women can become aroused again and experience additional orgasms. However, most men experience a refractory period, during which their systems are incapable of subsequent arousal. This refractory period may last from a few minutes to several hours and tends to lengthen with age.

Although men and women experience the same stages in the sexual response cycle, the length of time spent in any one stage varies. Thus, one partner may be in the plateau phase while the other is in the excitement/arousal or orgasmic phase. Such variations in response rates are entirely normal. Some couples believe that simultaneous orgasm is desirable for sexual satisfaction. Although simultaneous orgasm is pleasant, it may be difficult to achieve because of differences in arousal and response.

Sexual pleasure and satisfaction are also possible without orgasm or even intercourse. Expressing sexual feelings for another person involves many pleasurable activities, of which intercourse and orgasm may be only a part.

## what do you think?

Why do we place so much importance on orgasm? ● Can sexual pleasure and satisfaction be achieved without orgasm? ● What is the role of desire in sexual response?

## Sexual Responses among Older Adults

Older adults are commonly stereotyped as being incapable of or uninterested in sexual relations. The truth is, though we do

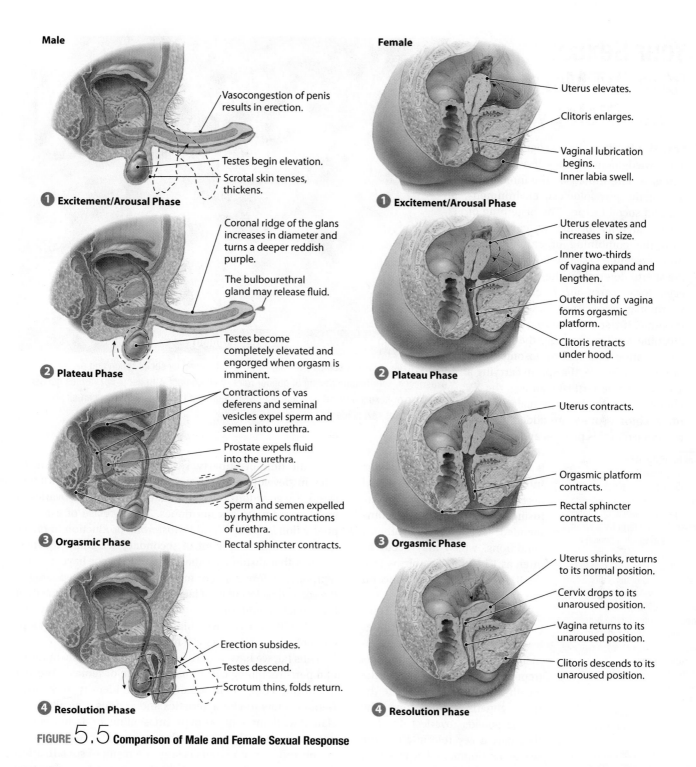

**Male**

**1** Excitement/Arousal Phase
- Vasocongestion of penis results in erection.
- Testes begin elevation.
- Scrotal skin tenses, thickens.

**2** Plateau Phase
- Coronal ridge of the glans increases in diameter and turns a deeper reddish purple.
- The bulbourethral gland may release fluid.
- Testes become completely elevated and engorged when orgasm is imminent.

**3** Orgasmic Phase
- Contractions of vas deferens and seminal vesicles expel sperm and semen into urethra.
- Prostate expels fluid into the urethra.
- Sperm and semen expelled by rhythmic contractions of urethra.
- Rectal sphincter contracts.

**4** Resolution Phase
- Erection subsides.
- Testes descend.
- Scrotum thins, folds return.

**Female**

**1** Excitement/Arousal Phase
- Uterus elevates.
- Clitoris enlarges.
- Vaginal lubrication begins.
- Inner labia swell.

**2** Plateau Phase
- Uterus elevates and increases in size.
- Inner two-thirds of vagina expand and lengthen.
- Outer third of vagina forms orgasmic platform.
- Clitoris retracts under hood.

**3** Orgasmic Phase
- Uterus contracts.
- Orgasmic platform contracts.
- Rectal sphincter contracts.

**4** Resolution Phase
- Uterus shrinks, returns to its normal position.
- Cervix drops to its unaroused position.
- Vagina returns to its unaroused position.
- Clitoris descends to its unaroused position.

FIGURE 5.5 **Comparison of Male and Female Sexual Response**

experience some physical changes as we age, they generally do not cause us to stop enjoying sex.

In women, the most significant physical changes follow menopause. Skin becomes less elastic; most internal sexual organs, including the uterus and cervix, shrink somewhat; the vaginal walls become thinner; and vaginal lubrication during sexual arousal may decrease. The resulting increased friction during penetration can be painful; the use of artificial lubricants usually resolves this problem. Women who remain sexually active as they age report fewer problems with age-related changes in sexual functioning.

Although men do not experience menopause, their bodies also change as a result of the aging process. They require more direct and prolonged stimulation to achieve an erection, and erections become less firm. They are slower to obtain a full erection and to reach orgasm, and their refractory periods are longer. Older men also experience a decrease in the intensity of ejaculation. Semen seeps out during ejaculation rather than being forcefully expelled as is typical in younger men. However, the majority of healthy older men, like healthy older women, enjoy a regular and satisfying sex life.

# Your Sexual Identity: More Than Biology

**Sexual identity,** the recognition and acknowledgment of oneself as a sexual being, is determined by the interaction of genetic, physiological, environmental, and social factors. The beginning of sexual identity occurs at conception with the combining of chromosomes that determine sex. The father's fertilizing sperm determines the child's sex. All eggs (ova) carry an X chromosome; sperm may carry either an X or a Y chromosome. If a sperm carrying an X chromosome fertilizes an egg, the resulting combination of sex chromosomes (XX) produces a female. If a sperm carrying a Y chromosome fertilizes an egg, the XY combination produces a male. Sometimes chromosomes are added, lost, or rearranged in this process and the sex of the offspring

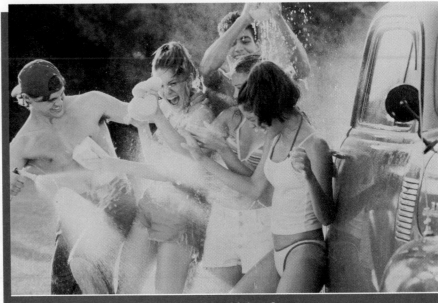

**What influences sexual identity besides biology?**

How you perceive yourself as a sexual being is influenced by socialization and personal experience. Your understanding of gender roles, your contact with people of various gender identities or sexual orientations, and your own degree of emotional maturity can all affect your sense of sexual identity.

is not clear, a condition known as **intersex.** *Disorders of sexual development (DSDs)* is a less confusing term that has been recommended to refer to intersex conditions, which may occur as often as 1 in 1,500 live births (see the **Health in a Diverse World** box on the next page).[7]

The genetic instructions included in the sex chromosomes lead to the differential development of male and female **gonads** (reproductive organs) at about the eighth week of fetal life. Once the male gonads (testes) and the female gonads (ovaries) develop, they play a key role in all future sexual development, because they are responsible for the production of sex hormones. As previously discussed, the primary female sex hormones are estrogen and progesterone. The primary male sex hormone is testosterone. The release of testosterone in a maturing fetus signals the development of a penis and other male genitals. If no testosterone is produced, female genitals form.

At the time of **puberty,** sex hormones again play major roles in development. Hormones released by the pituitary gland, the gonadotropins, stimulate the testes and ovaries to make appropriate sex hormones. The increase of estrogen production in females and testosterone production in males leads to the development of secondary sex characteristics, features that distinguish the sexes but do not have a direct reproductive function. For males these include deepening of the voice, development of facial and body hair, and growth of the skeleton and musculature. For females they include growth of the breasts, widening of the hips, and the development of pubic and underarm hair.

Thus far, we have described sexual identity only in terms of a person's biological status as a male or female. Another important component of our sexual identity is gender. **Gender** refers to characteristics and actions typically associated with men or women (masculine or feminine) as defined by the culture in which one lives. Our sense of masculine and feminine traits is largely a result of **socialization** during our childhood. **Gender roles** are the behaviors and activities we use to express our maleness or femaleness in ways that conform to society's expectations. For example, you may learn to play with dolls, or play with trucks and guns, based on how your parents influence your actions. For some, gender roles can be very confining when they lead to stereotyping. Bounds established by **gender-role stereotypes** can make it difficult to express one's true sexual identity. Men are traditionally expected to be independent, aggressive, logical, and always in control of their emotions. Women are traditionally expected to be passive, nurturing,

**sexual identity** Recognition of oneself as a sexual being; a composite of biological sex characteristics, gender identity, gender roles, and sexual orientation.

**intersex** General term for a variety of conditions in which a person is born with reproductive or sexual anatomy that doesn't seem to fit the typical definitions of female or male. Also termed *disorders of sexual development (DSDs).*

**gonads** The reproductive organs in a male (testes) or female (ovaries) that produce sperm (male), eggs (female), and sex hormones.

**puberty** The period of sexual maturation.

**gender** The psychological condition of being feminine or masculine as defined by the society in which one lives.

**socialization** Process by which a society communicates behavioral expectations to its individual members.

**gender roles** Expressions of maleness or femaleness in everyday life.

**gender-role stereotypes** Generalizations concerning how men and women should express themselves and the characteristics each possesses.

**androgyny** High levels of traditional masculine and feminine traits in a single person.

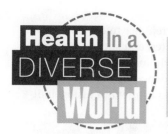

## Health In a DIVERSE World

## Disorders of Sexual Development

The South African middle-distance runner Caster Semenya is one of the fastest women around today. But after she won the gold medal in the 800-meter race at the 2009 World Championships, she was required to undergo gender testing and was subsequently barred from competition. Officials at the International Association of Athletics Federations (IAAF) wanted to determine whether Semenya has a disorder of sexual development (DSD; also called intersex) resulting in testosterone levels that give her an unfair athletic advantage over other women competitors. After 11 months, in July 2010, the IAAF announced that Semenya was again eligible to compete against other women, following the conclusions of a panel of medical experts.

The details of Semenya's test results and whether she received medical treatment in order to regain her eligibility remain confidential; however, Semenya's case highlights the challenges facing athletes and other people with both male and female characteristics. People with DSDs are born with various levels of male and female biological characteristics, ranging from different chromosomal arrangements to altered hormone produc-

tion to variation in primary and secondary sex characteristics. Whereas most people are born with either XX or XY chromosomes, some are born with XXY or XO chromosomes (where O signifies a missing or damaged chromosome). In some people, gonads do not develop fully into ovaries or testicles, although there may be no external signs to indicate this, and in others, external genitalia may be ambiguous.

Many, but not all, DSDs require some degree of medical intervention, whether hormonal or surgical, to ensure a person's physical health. It is also necessary to "assign" a gender to all children as early as possible to ensure their psychological health. If this assignment is later found to be inconsistent with the child's own sense of personal gender, he or she may choose to adopt a different gender identity. Most people born with DSDs today are allowed to grow up, establish their own gender identity, and choose as adults whether to have additional surgeries to alter any sexual tissues they feel that are incongruent with their gender. To find out more about DSDs, visit the website of Accord Alliance at www.accordalliance.org.

Many people considered it an invasion of privacy when World Champion runner Caster Semenya was required to submit to gender testing before being allowed to return to competition.

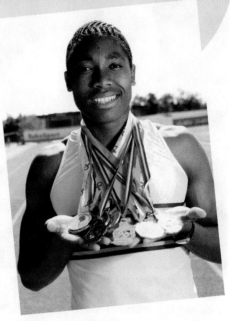

**Sources:** A. Kessel, "Caster Semenya May Return to Track This Month after IAAF Clearance," *The Guardian,* July 6, 2010, www.guardian.co.uk/sport/2010/jul/06/caster-semenya-iaaf-clearance; "Consensus Statement on Management of Intersex Disorders," *Pediatrics* 118 (2006): e488–e500.

---

intuitive, sensitive, and emotional. **Androgyny** refers to the combination of traditional masculine and feminine traits in a single person. Androgynous people do not always follow traditional sex roles but instead choose behaviors based on the given situation.

Whereas gender roles are an expression of cultural expectations for behavior, **gender identity** refers to the personal sense or awareness of being masculine or feminine, a male or a female. A person's gender identity does not always match his or her biological sex: This is called being **transgendered.** There is a broad spectrum of expression among transgendered persons that reflects the degree of dissatisfaction they have with their sexual anatomy. Some transgendered persons are very comfortable with their bodies and are content simply to dress and live as the other gender. At the other end of the spectrum are

**transsexuals,** who feel extremely trapped in their bodies and may opt for therapeutic interventions, such as sex reassignment surgery.

## Sexual Orientation

**Sexual orientation** refers to a person's enduring emotional, romantic, sexual, or affectionate attraction to other persons. You may be primarily attracted to members of the opposite sex **(heterosexual),** the same sex **(homosexual),** or both sexes

**gender identity** Personal sense or awareness of being masculine or feminine, a male or a female.
**transgendered** Having a gender identity that does not match one's biological sex.
**transsexual** A person who is psychologically of one sex but physically of the other.
**sexual orientation** A person's enduring emotional, romantic, sexual, or affectionate attraction to other persons.
**heterosexual** Experiencing primary attraction to and preference for sexual activity with people of the opposite sex.
**homosexual** Experiencing primary attraction to and preference for sexual activity with people of the same sex.

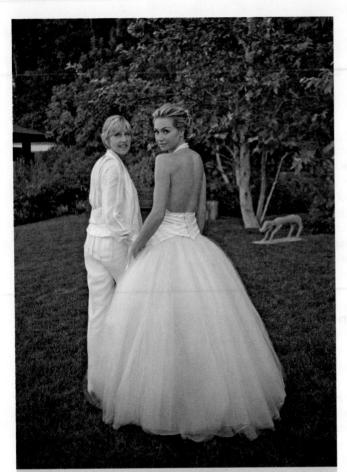

The presence of gay and lesbian celebrities in the media contributes to the increasing acceptance of gay relationships in everyday life. Talk show host Ellen DeGeneres and actress Portia de Rossi are an openly gay couple who married in 2008.

sexual prejudice (or *sexual bias*). Prejudice refers to negative attitudes and hostile actions directed at a social group and its members. Hate crimes, discrimination, and hostility toward sexual minorities are evidence of ongoing sexual prejudice. Recent data from the Department of Justice indicated that bias regarding sexual orientation was the motivation for approximately 17.6 percent of all hate crimes reported.[8]

Sexual orientation is often viewed as a concept based entirely on whom one has sex with, but this is an inaccurate and overly simplistic idea. Researcher Fritz Klein developed a questionnaire that not only looks at who you are sexually attracted to, fantasize about, and actually have sex with, but also considers factors such as those individuals you feel close to emotionally and like to socialize with, and in which "community" you feel most comfortable. You can find this questionnaire in the **Assess Yourself** box on page 164. After completing it, you may realize that there are not just two (homosexual, heterosexual) or three (homosexual, heterosexual, bisexual) orientations, but indeed a whole range of complex, interacting, and fluid factors influencing your sexuality over time.

**(bisexual).** Many homosexuals prefer the terms **gay,** queer, or **lesbian** to describe their sexual orientation. *Gay* and *queer* can apply to both men and women, but *lesbian* refers specifically to women.

Researchers today agree that sexual orientation is best understood using a model that incorporates biological, psychological, and socioenvironmental factors. Biological explanations focus on research into genetics, hormones, and differences in brain anatomy, whereas psychological and socioenvironmental explanations examine parent–child interactions, sex roles, and early sexual and interpersonal interactions. Collectively, this growing body of research suggests that the origins of homosexuality, like heterosexuality, are complex. To diminish the complexity of sexual orientation to "a choice" is a clear misrepresentation of current research. Homosexuals do not "choose" their sexual orientation any more than heterosexuals do.

Gay, lesbian, and bisexual persons are often the targets of

**bisexual** Experiencing attraction to and preference for sexual activity with people of both sexes.
**gay** Sexual orientation involving primary attraction to people of the same sex.
**lesbian** Sexual orientation involving attraction of women to other women.
**sexual prejudice** Negative attitudes and hostile actions directed at sexually identified social groups; also referred to as *sexual bias.*

# Expressing Your Sexuality

Finding healthy ways to express your sexuality is an important part of developing sexual maturity. Many avenues of sexual expression are available.

## Sexual Behavior: What Is "Normal"?

Most of us want to fit in and be identified as normal, but how do we know which sexual behaviors are considered normal? What or whose criteria should we use? These are not easy questions.

Every society sets standards and attempts to regulate sexual behavior. Boundaries arise that distinguish good from bad, acceptable from unacceptable, and result in criteria used to establish what is viewed as normal or abnormal. Some of the common sociocultural standards for sexual behavior in Western culture today include the following:[9]

- **The coital standard.** Penile–vaginal intercourse (coitus) is viewed as the ultimate sex act.

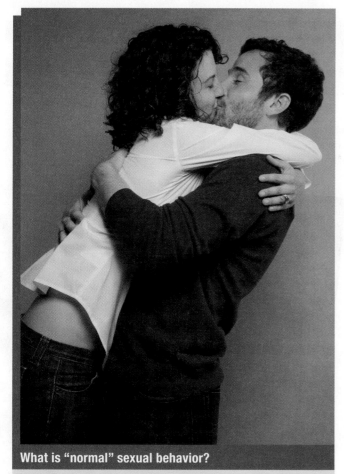

**What is "normal" sexual behavior?**

As with any other human behavior, the idea of "normal" sexual behavior varies from person to person and from society to society, usually along a spectrum of perceived acceptability or appropriateness. For example, in most modern cultures kissing is a common way to express affection; however, societies have different standards—and individuals have different comfort levels—for the circumstances in which a full-on smack is considered appropriate.

- **The orgasmic standard.** Sexual interaction should lead to orgasm.
- **The two-person standard.** Sex is an activity to be experienced by two people.
- **The romantic standard.** Sex should be related to love.
- **The safer-sex standard.** If we choose to be sexually active, we should act to prevent unintended pregnancy or disease transmission.

These are not laws or rules but are rather social scripts that have been adopted over time. Sexual standards often shift through the years, and many people choose not to follow them. Rather than making blanket judgments about normal versus abnormal, we might ask the following questions:[10]

- Is a sexual behavior healthy and fulfilling for a particular person?
- Is it safe?
- Does it involve the exploitation of others?
- Does it take place between responsible, consenting adults?

In this way, we can view behavior along a continuum that takes into account many individual factors. As you read about the options for sexual expression in the pages ahead, use these questions to explore your feelings about what is normal for you.

## Options for Sexual Expression

The range of human sexual expression is virtually infinite. What you find enjoyable may not be an option for someone else—everything from cultural norms to upbringing, to personal comfort level to physical limitations can influence how you express your sexuality (see the **Health in a Diverse World** box on page 156 for a discussion of sexuality and disability). The ways you choose to meet your sexual needs today may be very different from what they were 2 weeks ago or will be 2 years from now. Accepting yourself as a sexual person with individual desires and preferences is the first step in achieving sexual satisfaction. Are you curious about your college peers' sexual behavior? Then check out the **Student Health Today** box on page 157.

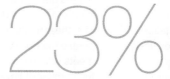

**23%** of college students report having had more than one sex partner in the past 12 months.

**Celibacy** **Celibacy** is avoidance of or abstention from sexual activities with others. Some people choose celibacy for religious or moral reasons. Others may be celibate for a period of time due to illness, the breakup of a long-term relationship, or lack of an acceptable partner. For some, celibacy is a lonely, agonizing state, but others find it an opportunity for introspection, values assessment, and personal growth.

**Autoerotic Behaviors** **Autoerotic behaviors** involve sexual self-stimulation. The two most common are sexual fantasy and masturbation.

**Sexual fantasies** are sexually arousing thoughts and dreams. Fantasies may reflect real-life experiences, forbidden desires, or the opportunity to practice new or anticipated sexual experiences. The fact that you fantasize about a particular sexual experience does not necessarily mean that you want to, or have to, act that experience out. Sexual fantasies are just that—fantasy.

**Masturbation,** or self-stimulation of the genitals, is one of the most common ways that humans seek sexual pleasure throughout their lives. It is a valuable and important means for all people to explore sexual feelings and responsiveness. In

**celibacy** State of abstaining from sexual activity.
**autoerotic behaviors** Sexual self-stimulation.
**sexual fantasies** Sexually arousing thoughts and dreams.
**masturbation** Self-stimulation of genitals.

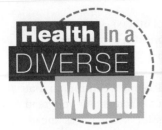

# Sexuality and Disability

Many of us tend to think of disabled people as asexual. It may be difficult to understand what sex would be like as or with a disabled person, but disabled people are not asexual as a rule, and it is possible for a disabled person to have a sex life. A major challenge for disabled people is meeting others who are interested in a romantic or sexual relationship. There are many hurdles to overcome, including our society's cultural standards of beauty and perfection, and our preconceptions about what disabled people can and can't do sexually.

Disabled people may be born with their disability; they may have become disabled as a young child, or, through disease or accident, become disabled later in their lives. These distinctions are significant; for people who became disabled after they became sexually active, there may be the expectation of performing sexually the way they used to. Coming to terms with a change in sexual performance due to disability can be a difficult process.

The challenges a disabled person faces with respect to having a satisfying sexual relationship include both physical and psychological difficulties. Being disabled, or "incapacitated by illness or injury," means that a person is in some way unable to function physically. That can mean many things, and the disability may or may not directly affect sexual function. For example, someone who is deaf is legally disabled, but sexually functional. A person living with polio, paralyzed from the neck down, may be able to have an orgasm, in spite of being unable to move.

Some people have disabilities that have minimal direct impact on their ability to pursue social connections. A person who has lost a limb, for example, is often still able to take part in everyday social—and perhaps athletic—activities to the same extent as most able-bodied people. Other disabilities can even foster certain

social connections—for example, many deaf individuals consider themselves part of a vibrant Deaf culture that provides rich social interaction and support.

On the other hand, some disabilities can be very socially isolating. For example, a person who is paralyzed has obstacles to overcome in finding a romantic or sexual partner. Just consider the physical hurdles: This person must have help getting out of the house to go on a date. The sheer number of people the person meets will be limited by the number of times he or she can get out socially. He or she may need help making a phone call. He or she may not be able to get undressed or lie down on a bed without aid. He or she may not be able to move to touch and arouse a partner. The psychological challenges for disabled people in finding a romantic or sexual partner can also be significant, and may include overcoming anger about the situation, dealing with the feeling that their sexual drives are illegitimate, and overcoming feelings that they don't measure up in the estimation of other people.

For anyone with a disability, counseling or therapy to deal with sexuality issues can help. Cognitive therapy and sex therapy—the treatment of sexual dysfunction, such as premature ejaculation or erectile dysfunction, low libido, sexual addiction, painful sex, or lack of sexual confidence, and other sexual problems—may help, or the person may want to see a certified sex surrogate. Surrogates offer therapeutic exercises

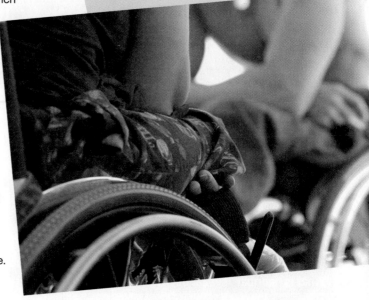

Whether able-bodied or disabled, we are all sexual beings deserving of intimacy and fulfilling sexual relationships.

to help the patient. These may include relaxation techniques, intimate communication, social skills, and sexual touching. One or a combination of these methods may help disabled people who want to explore the sexual side of their life. In addition, resources such as the National Sexuality Resource Center (http://nsrc.sfsu.edu/issues/sex-and-disability) can help those who want more information about sexuality and disability.

Whether a person is born with a disability or acquires it, each disabled person is unique, and it's important to consider that unique person's challenges, problems, and feelings as he or she comes to grips with his or her sexuality. There is no hard and fast rule about who can and can't have sex or a sensual relationship. Even if a person has lost sensation in his or her genitals, he or she may still be able to become aroused and have an orgasm. A disabled person can certainly benefit from and enjoy physical touch, whether sexual or not.

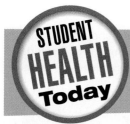
## MISPERCEPTIONS ABOUT SEX ON CAMPUS

College students often think everyone is having more sex than they are and with numerous partners. These perceptions may cause them to feel self-conscious about their own lack of sexual activity or encourage increased promiscuity in order to "measure up." In reality, college students' opinions about sex, relationships, and contraception and their attitudes toward sexual activity vary greatly. Results from a recent survey answered by college students nationwide might help you sort through some of these misperceptions:

✱ Approximately 76 percent of college students reported having had 0 to 1 sexual (oral, anal, or vaginal) partners within the past school year. However, 83 percent thought the typical student at their school had had *more* than one sexual partner in the past school year.

✱ Forty-four percent of students reported having had oral sex one or more times in the past 30 days, but 93 percent thought the typical student had oral sex at least once during that time.

✱ Forty-nine percent of students reported having had vaginal intercourse one or

more times in the past 30 days, yet 95 percent thought the typical student had vaginal intercourse at least once during that time.

✱ Five percent of students reported having anal intercourse one or more times in the past 30 days, whereas 57 percent thought the typical student had anal sex at least once during that time.

✱ Two percent of college females who had vaginal intercourse within the past school year reported experiencing an unintentional pregnancy and 2.1 percent of males who had had vaginal intercourse in the past year reported having gotten someone pregnant unintentionally.

**Source:** American College Health Association, *American College Health Association—National College Health Assessment: Reference Group Data Report Spring 2008* (Baltimore: American College Health Association, 2009), Available at www.acha-ncha .org/reports_ACHA-NCHAoriginal.html.

Are you the only one on your campus not living the life of the typical reality TV hottie? Probably not. You may think everyone else is having more sex with more partners than you are, but generally speaking, the actual numbers don't measure up to college students' perceptions.

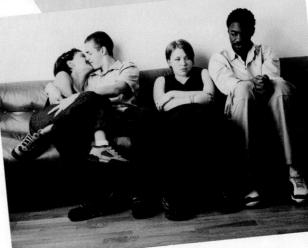

---

one survey of college students, 48 percent of women and 92 percent of men reported that they have masturbated.[11]

**Kissing and Erotic Touching** Kissing and erotic touching are two very common forms of nonverbal sexual communication. Both men and women have **erogenous zones,** areas of the body that lead to sexual arousal when touched. These may include genital as well as nongenital areas, such as the earlobes, mouth, breasts, and inner thighs. Almost any area of the body can be conditioned to respond erotically to touch. Spending time with your partner to explore and learn about his or her erogenous areas is another pleasurable, safe, and satisfying means of sexual expression.

**Manual Stimulation** Both men and women can be sexually aroused and achieve orgasm through manual stimulation of the genitals by a partner. For many women, orgasm is more likely to be achieved through manual stimulation than through intercourse. *Sex toys* include a wide variety of objects that can be used for sexual stimulation alone or with a partner. Vibrators and dildos are two common types of toys

and can be found in a variety of shapes, styles, and sizes. These toys can add zest to sexual experiences and, for women who may not reach orgasm by intercourse, can provide another option for satisfaction. Toys must be cleaned after each use.

**Oral–Genital Stimulation** Cunnilingus refers to oral stimulation of a woman's genitals and **fellatio** to oral stimulation of a man's genitals. Many partners find oral stimulation intensely pleasurable. In the most recent National College Health Assessment (NCHA), 40 percent of college students reported having oral sex in the past month.[12] For some people, oral sex is not an option because of moral, religious, or aesthetic beliefs. Note that HIV and other sexually transmitted infections (STIs) can be transmitted via unprotected oral–genital sex just as they can through intercourse. Use of an appropriate barrier device is strongly recommended if either partner's health status is in question.

**erogenous zones** Areas of the body that, when touched, lead to sexual arousal.

**cunnilingus** Oral stimulation of a woman's genitals.

**fellatio** Oral stimulation of a man's genitals.

# 52.4%
of college students report using a contraceptive the last time they had vaginal intercourse.

**Vaginal Intercourse** The term *intercourse* generally refers to **vaginal intercourse** (*coitus,* or insertion of the penis into the vagina), which is the most frequently practiced form of sexual expression. In the latest NCHA survey, more than 46 percent of college students reported having vaginal intercourse in the past month.[13] Coitus can involve a variety of positions, including missionary (man on top facing the woman), woman on top, side by side, or man behind (rear entry). Many partners enjoy experimenting with different positions. Knowledge of yourself and your body, along with your ability to communicate effectively, will play a large part in determining the enjoyment and meaning of intercourse for you and your partner. Whatever your circumstances, you should practice safer sex to avoid disease and unintended pregnancy.

> **vaginal intercourse** The insertion of the penis into the vagina.
> **anal intercourse** The insertion of the penis into the anus.
> **variant sexual behavior** A sexual behavior that is not practiced by most people.

**Anal Intercourse** The anal area is highly sensitive to touch, and some couples find pleasure in stimulation there. **Anal intercourse** is insertion of the penis into the anus. Research indicates that over 21 percent of college-aged men and women have had anal sex.[14] Stimulation of the anus by the mouth, fingers, or sex toys is also practiced. As with all forms of sexual expression, anal stimulation or intercourse is not for everyone. If you do enjoy this form of sexual expression, remember to use condoms and/or dental dams to avoid transmitting disease. Also,

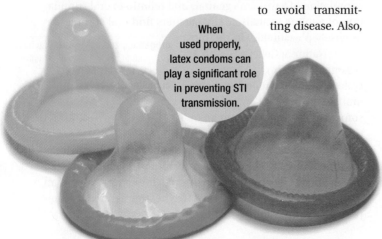

When used properly, latex condoms can play a significant role in preventing STI transmission.

anything inserted into the anus should not then be directly inserted into the vagina, as bacteria commonly found in the anus can cause vaginal infections.

## Variant Sexual Behavior

Although attitudes toward sexuality have changed substantially over time, some people still believe that any sexual behavior other than heterosexual intercourse is abnormal or perverted. People who study sexuality prefer to use the neutral term **variant sexual behavior** to describe sexual behaviors that most people do not engage in, for example:

● **Group sex.** Sexual activity involving more than two people. Participants in group sex run a higher risk of exposure to HIV and other STIs.
● **Transvestism.** Wearing the clothing of the opposite sex. Most transvestites are male, heterosexual, and married.
● **Fetishism.** Sexual arousal achieved by looking at or touching inanimate objects, such as underclothing or shoes.

Some variant sexual behaviors can be harmful to the individual, to others, or to both. Many of the following activities are illegal in at least some states:

● **Exhibitionism.** Exposing one's genitals to strangers in public places. Most exhibitionists are seeking a reaction of shock or fear from their victims. Exhibitionism is a minor felony in most states.
● **Voyeurism.** Observing other people for sexual gratification. Most voyeurs are men who attempt to watch women undressing or bathing. Voyeurism is an invasion of privacy and is illegal in most states.
● **Sadomasochism.** Sexual activities in which gratification is received by inflicting pain (verbal or physical abuse) on a partner or by being the object of such infliction. A sadist is a person who enjoys inflicting pain, and a masochist enjoys experiencing pain.
● **Pedophilia.** Sexual activity or attraction between an adult and a child. Any sexual activity involving a minor, including possession of child pornography, is illegal.
● **Autoerotic asphyxiation.** The practice of reducing or eliminating oxygen to the brain, usually by tying a cord around one's neck while masturbating to orgasm. Tragically, some individuals accidentally strangle themselves.

## Sexual Dysfunction

Research indicates that **sexual dysfunction,** the term used to describe problems that can hinder sexual functioning, is quite common. Don't feel embarrassed if you experience sexual dysfunction at some point in your life. The sexual part of you does not come with a lifetime warranty. You can have breakdowns involving your sexual function just as in any other body system. Sexual dysfunction can be divided into

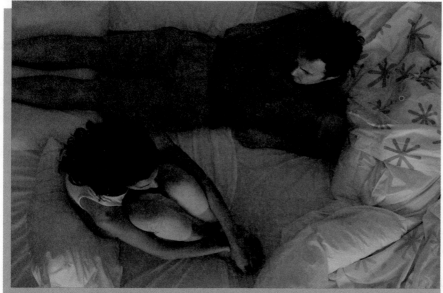

**Are sexual disorders more physical or more psychological?**

Sexual disorders can have both physical and psychological roots. Sexual desire disorders, orgasmic disorders, and sexual performace disorders often arise as a result of stress, fatigue, depression, or anxiety, but they frequently have physiological bases, such as medication or substance use, as well. Sexual arousal disorders and sexual pain disorders, on the other hand, often are strongly related to physical conditions and risk factors, but they may be exacerbated by stress and mental health problems. Interpersonal problems, including lack of trust and communication between partners, are also significant contributors to the development of sexual dysfunctions.

# 50%

of the 30 million American men with erectile dysfunction are under age 65.

every man experiences erectile dysfunction. Risk factors that can contribute to erectile dysfunction include medical conditions, using tobacco, being overweight, certain medical treatments, injuries, medications, psychological conditions, drug and alcohol use, and prolonged bicycling.[17] Some 30 million men in the United States, half of them under age 65, suffer from ED. The condition generally becomes more of a problem as men age, affecting 1 in 4 men over the age of 65.[18] The U.S. Food and Drug Administration has approved several drugs, such as Viagra (sildenafil citrate), Levitra (vardenafil hydrochloride), and Cialis (tadalafil) to treat ED. These drugs work by relaxing the smooth muscle cells in the penis, allowing for increased blood flow to the erectile tissues. Additional oral medicines are being tested for safety and effectiveness. The best prevention for ED is to take care of your general mental and physical health.

five major classes: disorders of sexual desire, sexual arousal, orgasm, sexual performance, and sexual pain. All of them can be treated successfully.

## Sexual Desire Disorders

The most frequent reason people seek out a sex therapist is **inhibited sexual desire.**[15] Inhibited sexual desire is the lack of a sexual appetite or simply a lack of interest and pleasure in sexual activity. A low sex drive (decreased libido) may be caused by a drop in normal production of estrogen in women or in testosterone in both men and women. Fatigue, stress, and common medical conditions such as depression and anxiety can cause a decrease in libido. Antidepressant medications (e.g., Prozac, Zoloft, Paxil) are well known for reducing sexual desire in both men and women.[16] **Sexual aversion disorder** is another type of desire dysfunction, characterized by sexual phobias (unreasonable fears) and anxiety about sexual contact. The psychological stress of a punitive upbringing, a rigid religious background, or a history of physical or sexual abuse may be sources of these desire disorders.

## Sexual Arousal Disorders

The most common sexual arousal disorder is **erectile dysfunction (ED)**—difficulty in achieving or maintaining a penile erection sufficient for intercourse. At some time in his life,

## Orgasmic Disorders

**Premature ejaculation**—ejaculation that occurs prior to or very soon after the insertion of the penis into the vagina—affects up to 50 percent of men at some time in their lives. Treatment for premature ejaculation first involves a physical examination to rule out organic causes. If the cause of the problem is not physiological, therapy is available to help a man learn how to control the timing of his ejaculation. Fatigue, stress, performance pressure, and alcohol use can all contribute to orgasmic disorders in men.

In a woman, the inability to achieve orgasm is called **female orgasmic disorder.** A woman with this disorder often blames herself and learns to fake orgasm to avoid embarrassment or to preserve her partner's ego. Contributing to this response are the messages women

**sexual dysfunction** Problems associated with achieving sexual satisfaction.

**inhibited sexual desire** Lack of sexual appetite or simply a lack of interest and pleasure in sexual activity.

**sexual aversion disorder** Desire dysfunction characterized by sexual phobias and anxiety about sexual contact.

**erectile dysfunction (ED)** Difficulty in achieving or maintaining a penile erection sufficient for intercourse.

**premature ejaculation** Ejaculation that occurs prior to or almost immediately following penile penetration of the vagina.

**female orgasmic disorder** A woman's inability to achieve orgasm.

have historically been given about sex as a duty rather than a pleasurable act. As with men who experience orgasmic disorders, the first step in treatment is a physical exam to rule out organic causes. However, the problem is often solved by simple self-exploration to learn more about what forms of stimulation are arousing enough to produce orgasm. Through masturbation, a woman can learn how her body responds sexually to various types of touch. Once she has become orgasmic through masturbation, she learns to communicate her needs to her partner.

## Sexual Performance Disorders

Both men and women can experience **sexual performance anxiety** when they anticipate some sort of problem in the sex act. A man may become anxious and unable to maintain an erection, or he may experience premature ejaculation. A woman may be unable to achieve orgasm or to allow penetration because of the involuntary contraction of vaginal muscles. Both can overcome performance anxiety by learning to focus on immediate sensations and pleasures rather than on orgasm.

**sexual performance anxiety** A condition of sexual difficulties caused by anticipating some sort of problem with the sex act.
**dyspareunia** Pain experienced by women during intercourse.
**vaginismus** A state in which the vaginal muscles contract so forcefully that penetration cannot occur.

## Sexual Pain Disorders

Two common disorders in this category are dyspareunia and vaginismus. **Dyspareunia** is pain experienced by a woman during intercourse that may be caused by diseases such as endometriosis, uterine tumors, chlamydia, gonorrhea, or urinary tract infections. Damage to tissues during childbirth and insufficient lubrication during intercourse may also cause discomfort. Dyspareunia can also be psychological in origin. As with other sexual problems, dyspareunia can be treated, with good results.

**Vaginismus** is the involuntary contraction of vaginal muscles, making penile insertion painful or impossible. Most cases of vaginismus are related to fear of intercourse or to unresolved sexual conflicts. Treatment involves teaching a woman to achieve orgasm through nonvaginal stimulation.

## Seeking Help for Sexual Dysfunction

Sexual dysfunctions are most common in the early adult years, with the majority of people seeking care for these conditions during their late twenties and into their thirties. The incidence of dysfunction increases again during perimenopause and postmenopause years in women and in older age for both men and women.[19] Many theories and treatment models can help people with sexual dysfunction. It is important not to be afraid to talk to a counselor or medical professional. Most colleges and universities have medical and counseling services available on campus that would be a good place to start if you are seeking advice. If you are looking for a qualified sex therapist or counselor outside of your university setting, the American Association of Sex Educators, Counselors, and Therapists (AASECT) can help. AASECT has been in the forefront of establishing criteria for certifying sex therapists. These criteria include appropriate degree(s) in the helping professions, specialized coursework in human sexuality, and sufficient hours of practical therapy work under the direct supervision of a certified sex therapist. Lists of certified counselors, sex therapists, and clinics that treat sexual dysfunctions can be obtained by visiting the AASECT website: www.aasect.org.

## Drugs and Sex

Because psychoactive drugs affect the body's entire physiological functioning, it is only logical that they affect sexual behavior. Promises of increased pleasure make drugs very tempting to people seeking greater sexual satisfaction. Too often, however, drugs become central to sexual activities and damage the relationship. Drug use can also lead to undesired sexual activity, as well as a tendency to blame the drug for negative behavior or unsafe sexual activities. "I can't help what I did last night because I was drunk" is a statement that demonstrates sexual immaturity. A sexually mature person carefully examines risks and benefits and makes decisions accordingly. If drugs are necessary to increase erotic feelings, it is likely that the partners are being dishonest about their feelings for each other. Good sex should not depend on chemical substances.

Alcohol is notorious for reducing inhibitions and promoting feelings of well-being and desirability. At the same time, alcohol inhibits sexual response; thus, the mind may be willing, but not the body. In addition to alcohol use, an increasing number of young men have begun experimenting with the recreational use of drugs intended to treat erectile dysfunction, including Viagra, Cialis, and Levitra. Young men who take this type of medication are hoping to increase their sexual stam-

## what do you think?

Why do we find it so difficult to discuss sexual dysfunction?
● Do you think it is more difficult for men than for women to talk about dysfunction? Or vice versa?
● Have you ever used alcohol or some other drug to enhance your sexual performance or reduce sexual inhibitions?

### "Why Should I Care?"

Generally, we don't talk about sexual dysfunction in our society. When problems occur, it can be easy to assume we are alone if we experience them. If you or your partner ever experiences a problem, knowing you're not alone, and understanding sexual dysfunction, can help get you started finding the resources to solve the problem.

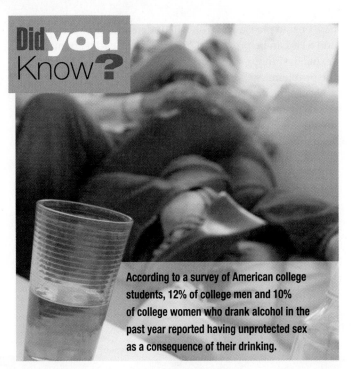
ina, or counteract sexual performance anxiety or the effects of alcohol or other drugs. However, these drugs probably have only a placebo effect in men with normal erections, and combining them with other drugs, such as cocaine, MDMA (Ecstasy), amyl nitrate ("poppers"), and methamphetamine, can lead to potentially fatal drug interactions. In particular, when combined with amyl nitrate these drugs can lead to a sudden drop in blood pressure, and possible cardiac arrest.[20]

"Date rape" drugs have been a growing concern in recent decades. They have become prevalent on college campuses, where they are often used in combination with alcohol. Rohypnol ("roofies," "rope," "forget pill"), GHB (gamma hydroxybutyrate, or "liquid X," "Grievous Bodily Harm," "easy lay," "Mickey Finn"), and ketamine ("K," "Special K," "cat valium") have all been used to facilitate rape. Rohypnol and GHB are difficult-to-detect drugs that depress the central nervous system. Ketamine can cause dreamlike states, hallucinations, delirium, amnesia, and impaired motor function. These drugs are often introduced to unsuspecting women through alcoholic drinks to render them unconscious and vulnerable to rape. This problem is so serious that the U.S. Congress passed the Drug-Induced Rape Prevention and Pun-

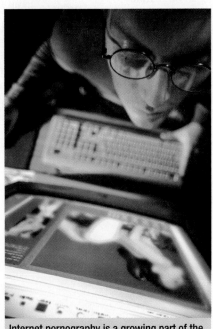

Internet pornography is a growing part of the multibillion-dollar pornographic industry.

ishment Act of 1996 to increase federal penalties for using drugs to facilitate sexual assault. The dangers of these drugs are discussed in more detail in Chapter 13.

# The Sex Industry

Throughout history, sex has been a prominent theme in art, literature, and the media. But when do depictions of the human body and human sexual behaviors cross the line from art to pornography, from story to exploitation, from sales tool to public perversion? These are difficult distinctions to make, and they challenge us at every level. Two particularly problematic aspects of the sex industry are pornography and prostitution.

**Pornography** refers to any visual or literary depictions of sexual activity intended to be sexually arousing. An Internet tracking firm recently reported that pornographic websites make up 12 percent (4.2 million) of total websites and that over 40 percent of Internet users in the United States visit adult sites each month.[21] The pornography industry—which includes the Internet, video sales and rentals, cable, pay-per-view, in-room viewing, phone sex, exotic dance clubs, computer games, and magazines—generates revenues of $13.33 billion annually in the United States, $2.8 billion of which is from online sources.[22] Clearly, pornography is a booming industry supported by millions of consumers. Why, then, is it so controversial? The fear many people have is that viewing pornographic materials leads to negative attitudes toward women, sexual aggression, and sexual violence. Current evidence suggests that pornography does not lead to sexual violence or predatory behavior in normal, healthy adults, but in those individuals who have preexisting negative attitudes toward women, this may be a legitimate concern.[23]

**pornography** Visual or literary depictions of sexual activity intended to be sexually arousing.
**prostitution** The practice of engaging in sexual acts for money.

**Prostitution,** the practice of engaging in sexual acts for money, is a widespread industry in the United States and around the world. Estimating the revenue generated by the prostitution industry in the United States is difficult, as most activity is illegal. Several countries have legalized prostitution, but in the United States it is legal only in selected counties in the state of Nevada. Illegal sex workers often struggle with substance abuse, sexual violence, and STIs. Countries that have legalized prostitution have made progress in regulating the industry and reducing these risks. In many parts of the world, the term *sex worker* or *commercial sex worker* is used to redefine commercial sex, not as the social or psychological characteristic of a class of women, but as an income-generating activity or form of employment for women and men.

# Responsible and Satisfying Sexual Behavior

Our sexuality is a fascinating, complex, contradictory, and sometimes frustrating aspect of our lives. Healthy sexuality doesn't happen by chance. It is a product of assimilating information and skills, of exploring values and beliefs, and of making responsible and informed choices. Healthy and responsible sexuality includes the following.

● **Good communication as the foundation.** Open and honest communication with your partner is the basis for establishing respect, trust, and intimacy. Do you communicate with your partner in caring and respectful ways? Can you share your thoughts and emotions freely with your partner? Do you talk about being sexually active and what that means? Can you share your sexual history with your partner? Do you discuss contraception and disease prevention? Are you able to communicate what you like and don't like? All of these are components of the open communication that accompanies healthy responsible sexuality.

● **Acknowledging that you are a sexual person.** People who can see and accept themselves as sexual beings are more likely to make informed decisions and take responsible actions. If you see yourself as a potentially sexual person, you will plan ahead for contraception and disease prevention. If you are comfortable being a sexually active person, you will not need or want your sexual experiences clouded by alcohol or other drug use. If you choose not to be sexually active, you do so consciously, as a personal decision based on your convictions. Even if you are not sexually active, it is important to acknowledge that sex is a natural aspect of everyone's life and to recognize that you are in charge of your own decisions about your sexuality.

● **Understanding sexual structures and their functions.** If you understand how your body works, sexual pleasure and response will not be mysterious events. You will be able to pleasure yourself as well as communicate to your partner

how best to please you. You will understand how pregnancy and STIs can be prevented. You will be able to recognize sexual dysfunction and take responsible actions to address the problem.

● **Accepting and embracing your gender identity and your sexual orientation.** "Being comfortable in your own skin" is an old saying that is particularly relevant when it comes to sexuality. It is difficult to feel sexually satisfied if you are conflicted about your gender identity or sexual orientation. You should explore and address questions and feelings you may have about either your gender identity or your sexual orientation. Having good communication skills, acknowledging that you are a sexual person, and understanding your sexual structures and their functions will allow you to complete this task.

See the **Skills for Behavior Change** box for tips on taking steps toward healthy sexuality.

## Skills for Behavior Change

### Taking Steps toward Healthy Sexuality

Healthy and responsible sexuality means having information and skills, exploring values and beliefs, and making responsible and informed choices. The following tips can help you:

✳ Give some thought to your own sexuality. Do you choose to be sexually active now, or are you more comfortable waiting?

✳ Get to know sexual structures and their functions in order to make communicating easier, and sex better.

✳ If you have a partner now, sit down and talk about your sexual relationship. Are you both comfortable and satisfied with all aspects of the relationship? Discuss what you like and don't like.

✳ Explore and address any questions and feelings you may have about either your gender identity or your sexual orientation.

# Assess Yourself

## What Are Your Sexual Attitudes and Preferences?

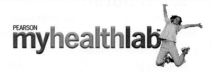

Fill out this assessment online at www.pearsonhighered.com/myhealthlab or www.pearsonhighered.com/donatelle.

### 1 What Are Your Attitudes about Sexual Differences?

Sexuality and sexual differences can be uncomfortable or difficult topics for many people. To complete this assessment, think about your attitudes regarding sexual differences and indicate how comfortable you would be in the following situations.

Completely Comfortable ① ② ③ ④ ⑤ Not at All Comfortable

1. Your close same-sex friend reveals to you his preference for same-sex partners. ① ② ③ ④ ⑤
2. Your roommate tells you that she likes sexual encounters that involve three or more partners at one time. ① ② ③ ④ ⑤
3. Your sister tells you that she would like to have a sex-change operation. ① ② ③ ④ ⑤
4. Your 85-year-old grandfather reveals that he is sexually active with his 85-year-old female partner. ① ② ③ ④ ⑤
5. A male friend reveals that, although he is primarily heterosexual, he occasionally has sex with other men. ① ② ③ ④ ⑤
6. Your lab partner, who looks and acts like a man, reveals that he is transgendered. ① ② ③ ④ ⑤
7. Your blind date tells you that he occasionally likes to engage in sadomasochistic sexual play. ① ② ③ ④ ⑤
8. Two women from your health class invite you to attend their commitment ceremony. ① ② ③ ④ ⑤
9. Your best friend reveals that she has made a personal commitment not to engage in sexual activity until marriage. ① ② ③ ④ ⑤
10. The person with whom you are romantically involved asks you to tell him your sexual fantasies. ① ② ③ ④ ⑤
11. Your divorced mother reveals that she is dating a man who is your age. ① ② ③ ④ ⑤
12. Your partner says he would like to try anal sex. ① ② ③ ④ ⑤
13. Your roommate believes it is important to be a virgin until marriage but engages in oral sex with her partner. ① ② ③ ④ ⑤
14. Two of your classmates invite you over for "porn" night. ① ② ③ ④ ⑤
15. Your best friend confides in you that he couldn't get an erection the last time he wanted to have intercourse. ① ② ③ ④ ⑤
16. You walk in on your partner as he is trying on one of your dresses and heels. ① ② ③ ④ ⑤
17. You go out dancing with friends at a gay bar and run into two women from your residence hall. ① ② ③ ④ ⑤
18. Your sister and her husband share with you that their first child was born with intersex. ① ② ③ ④ ⑤
19. A same-sex acquaintance hits on you at a party. ① ② ③ ④ ⑤
20. Your housemate asks how often you masturbate and if you own a vibrator. ① ② ③ ④ ⑤

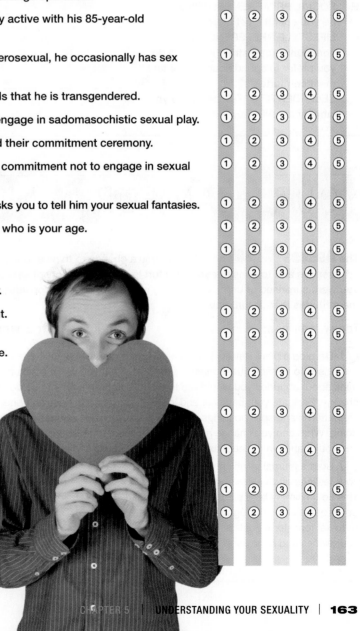

# 2 What Are Your Personal Preferences Relating to Your Sexuality?

Sexual orientation and sexual preferences encompass issues of attraction, behavior, fantasies, emotional closeness, socializing, lifestyle, and self-identification. To complete this worksheet, use the scales provided below and choose a number for each of the three aspects of your life: your past, your present, and your ideal. Remember that there are no right or wrong answers.

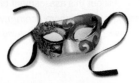

| | Past (Your Entire Life up to 1 Year Ago) | Present (Past 12 Months) | Ideal (If You Could Order Your Life Any Way You Wanted) |
|---|---|---|---|
| **A. SEXUAL ATTRACTION:** To whom are you sexually attracted? | _____ | _____ | _____ |
| **B. SEXUAL BEHAVIOR:** With whom do you have sex? | _____ | _____ | _____ |
| **C. SEXUAL FANTASIES:** Whom do you fantasize about? | _____ | _____ | _____ |
| **D. EMOTIONAL PREFERENCE:** Whom do you feel more drawn to or close to emotionally? | _____ | _____ | _____ |
| **E. SOCIAL PREFERENCE:** With whom do you spend most of your social life? | _____ | _____ | _____ |
| **F. LIFESTYLE PREFERENCE:** In which community (gay, straight, mixed) do you prefer to spend your time or feel most comfortable? | _____ | _____ | _____ |
| **G. SELF-IDENTIFICATION:** How do you label or identify yourself? | _____ | _____ | _____ |

**Scale for A–E**

0 = other sex only
1 = other sex mostly
2 = other sex somewhat more
3 = both sexes equally
4 = same sex somewhat more
5 = same sex mostly
6 = same sex only

**Scale for F and G**

0 = heterosexual only
1 = heterosexual mostly
2 = heterosexual somewhat more
3 = equally heterosexual and homosexual
4 = homosexual somewhat more
5 = homosexual mostly
6 = homosexual only

**Source:** *The Bisexual Option* by Fritz Klein. Copyright 1993 by HAWORTH PRESS/ TAYLOR & FRANCIS - BOOKS. Reproduced with permission of HAWORTH PRESS/ TAYLOR & FRANCIS - BOOKS in the format Textbook via Copyright Clearance Center.

# YOUR PLAN FOR CHANGE

The **Assess Yourself** activity gave you a chance to think about your own sexual preferences and to consider your comfort level with a variety of sexual situations. If you were surprised or unhappy with any of your responses, consider ways to change the attitudes that disturb you.

### Today, you can:

○ Develop a plan. Review your responses to the first questionnaire and think about attitudes you would like to change. Evaluate your behavior and identify patterns and specific things you are doing. What can you change now? What can you change in the near future?

○ Start a journal in which you explore your feelings and beliefs about sexuality. This could simply be a place for you to jot down questions or thoughts as they arise or to set long-term goals and examine your values and behaviors.

### Within the next 2 weeks, you can:

○ If you are in a sexual relationship, establish a time to sit down with your partner and have an honest and open discussion about sex. Before the discussion, think about what you would like to discuss and how you will bring it up. Are there sexual issues between you that need to be addressed? Are both you and your partner satisfied with the nature of your sexual relationship?

○ Take steps to be more responsible about your sexuality. If you have had unprotected sex in the recent past, make an appointment to be tested for STIs. If you have found yourself without contraception, stop by a drugstore and purchase several packages of condoms. If you feel your sexual decision making is sometimes impaired by drugs or alcohol, set goals to limit and control your use of these substances.

### By the end of the semester, you can:

○ Develop a greater understanding of and tolerance for people with different sexual values and lifestyles. Learn about different viewpoints by doing library research, attending group meetings on campus, or becoming better friends with sexually diverse people.

○ Expand your own sense of gender identity. Consider taking a class or workshop in an activity or subject area that you traditionally associate with the opposite gender. Volunteer with a group that focuses on issues relating to the opposite gender.

# Summary

* The major structures of the female sexual anatomy include the mons pubis, labia minora and majora, clitoris, vagina, uterus, cervix, fallopian tubes, and ovaries. The major structures of the male sexual anatomy are the penis, scrotum, testes, epididymides, vasa deferentia, ejaculatory ducts, urethra, and the accessory glands (seminal vesicles, prostate gland, and Cowper's glands).

* Physiologically, both males and females experience four stages of sexual response: excitement/arousal, plateau, orgasm, and resolution.

* *Sexual identity* is determined by the interaction of genetic, physiological, and environmental factors. Biological sex, gender identity, gender roles, and sexual orientation are all blended into our sexual identity.

* *Sexual orientation* refers to a person's enduring emotional, romantic, sexual, or affectionate attraction to other persons. Gay, lesbian, and bisexual persons are repeatedly the targets of sexual prejudice. *Sexual prejudice* refers to negative attitudes and hostile actions directed at a social group and its members.

* People can express themselves sexually in a variety of ways, including celibacy, autoerotic behaviors, kissing and erotic touch, manual stimulation, oral–genital stimulation, vaginal intercourse, and anal intercourse. Variant sexual behaviors are those that most people do not engage in. Some variant sexual behaviors are potentially harmful to others and are therefore illegal in at least some states.

* Sexual dysfunctions can be classified into disorders of sexual desire, sexual arousal, orgasm, sexual performance, and sexual pain. Drug use can also lead to sexual dysfunction.

* Sex is a multibillion-dollar industry in the United States and throughout the world. Pornography and prostitution are two aspects of the sex industry that have varying degrees of legality in different countries and in selected counties in the state of Nevada.

* Responsible and satisfying sexuality involves good communication, recognition of yourself as a sexual being, understanding sexual structures and functions, and acceptance of your gender identity and sexual orientation.

# Pop Quiz

1. Your personal inner sense of maleness or femaleness is known as your
   a. sexual identity.
   b. sexual orientation.
   c. gender identity.
   d. gender.

2. Intimacy is what type of romantic feeling?
   a. Romantic love
   b. Sensual feelings
   c. Empty commitment love
   d. Mutual feelings of emotional closeness

3. The most sensitive or erotic spot in the female genital region is the
   a. mons pubis.
   b. vagina.
   c. clitoris.
   d. labia.

4. When a woman is ovulating,
   a. she has released an egg cell.
   b. she is experiencing menstrual bleeding.
   c. an egg has been fertilized and she is pregnant.
   d. None of the above

5. Which of the following is *not* true about a woman's menstrual cycle?
   a. All women will experience premenstrual syndrome (PMS).
   b. The estrogen levels drop during ovulation.

   c. The hypothalamus monitors the hormone levels in the blood.
   d. The endometrium becomes engorged with blood and causes bleeding if the ovum is not fertilized.

6. A condition in which a woman experiences pain when menstruating is known as
   a. premenstrual syndrome.
   b. dysmenorrhea.
   c. premenstrual dysphoric disorder.
   d. amenorrhea.

7. What is the role of testosterone in the male reproductive system?
   a. It is used to produce sperm for reproduction.
   b. It is the hormone that stimulates development of secondary male sex characteristics.
   c. It allows the penis to harden during sexual arousal.
   d. It secretes the seminal fluid preceding ejaculation.

8. The preejaculate fluid that sometimes results before a man ejaculates comes from which gland in the male reproductive system?
   a. Prostate gland
   b. Cowper's glands
   c. Vas deferens
   d. Testicles

9. Individuals who are sexually attracted to both sexes are identified as
   a. heterosexual.
   b. bisexual.
   c. homosexual.
   d. intersex.

10. Fellatio is the oral stimulation of the
    a. male genitals.
    b. female genitals.
    c. anal region.
    d. mouth and tongue.

*Answers to these questions can be found on page A-1.*

# Think about It!

1. How have gender roles changed over your lifetime? Do you view the changes as positive for both men and women?
2. Have you ever discussed what it was like going through puberty (development of secondary sex characteristics) with your friends? Did you understand what was going on and why?
3. What criteria do you use to determine "normal" sexual behavior? What criteria should we use to determine healthful sexual practice?
4. If scientists are able to establish the combination of factors that interact to produce homosexual, heterosexual, or bisexual orientation, will that put an end to antigay prejudice? Why or why not?
5. How can we remove the stigma that surrounds sexual dysfunction so that individuals feel more comfortable seeking help? Are men and women affected differently by sexual dysfunction?
6. Have you ever watched pornography? What prompted your viewing? How did you feel about the experience?

# Accessing Your Health on the Internet

The following websites explore further topics and issues related to personal health. For links to the websites below, visit the Companion Website for *Access to Health,* 12th Edition, at www.pearsonhighered.com/donatelle.

1. *American Association of Sex Educators, Counselors, and Therapists (AASECT).* AASECT is a professional organization that provides standards of practice for treatment of sexual issues and disorders. www.aasect.org

2. *SmarterSex.org.* This site, created by the peer education group BACCHUS network, presents student-friendly information on sexual health targeted at 18- to 24-year-olds. www.smartersex.org

3. *Go Ask Alice.* Columbia University Health Services provides this interactive question-and-answer resource. "Alice" is available to answer questions about any health-related issues, including relationships, nutrition and diet, exercise, drugs, sex, alcohol, and stress. www.goaskalice.columbia.edu

4. *Sexuality Information and Education Council of the United States (SIECUS).* SIECUS provides information, guidelines, and materials for advancement of healthy and proper sex education. www.siecus.org

5. *Advocates for Youth.* Here, you can find current news, policy updates, research, and other resources about the sexual health of and choices particular to high school and college-aged students. www.advocatesforyouth.org

# References

1. S. E. Anderson, G. E. Dallal, and A. Must, "Relative Weight and Race Influence Average Age at Menarche: Results from Two Nationally Representative Surveys of U.S. Girls Studied 25 Years Apart," *Pediatrics* 111, no. 4 (2003): 844–50; H. Baer, G. Colditz, W. Willet, and J. Dorgan, "Adiposity and Sex Hormones in Girls," *Cancer Epidemiology Biomarkers Preview* 16, no. 9 (2007): 1880–08; L. Shi, S. Wudy, A. Buyken, M. Hartmann, and T. Remer, "Body Fat and Animal Protein Intakes Are Associated with Adrenal Androgen Secretion in Children," *American Journal of Clinical Nutrition* 90, no. 5 (2009): 1321–28; K. K. Ong et al., "Infancy Weight Gain Predicts Childhood Body Fat and Age at Menarche in Girls," *Journal of Clinical Endocrinology & Metabolism* no. 94 (2009): 1527–32.
2. Mayo Clinic Staff, "Menstrual Cramps," 2007, www.mayoclinic.com/Health/Menstrual-Cramps/Ds00506.
3. National Institutes of Health, *Facts about Menopausal Hormone Therapy* (NIH Publication no. 05-5200: 2005), Available at www.nhlbi.nih.gov/health/women/pht_facts.htm.
4. N. Siegfried et al., "HIV and Male Circumcision—A Systematic Review with the Assessment of Quality of Studies," *The Lancet—Infectious Diseases* 5, no. 3 (2005): 165–73; A. Bertran et al., "Randomized, Controlled Intervention Trial of Male Circumcision for Reduction of HIV Transmission Risk: The ANRS 1265 Trial," *PLoS Medicine* 2, no. 11 (2005): 1112–22; B. G. Williams et al., "The Potential Impact of Male Circumcision on HIV in Sub-Saharan Africa," *PLoS Medicine* 3, no. 7 (2006): e262; B. P. Homeier, "Circumcision," Paper presented at KidsHealth for Parents, Nemours Foundation, January 2005, Available at http://kidshealth.org/parent/system/surgical/circumcision.html; Mayo Clinic Staff, "Circumcision (Male): Why It's Done," February 2010, www.mayoclinic.com/health/circumcision/MY01023/DSECTION=why-its-done.
5. Mayo Clinic Staff, "Male Menopause: Myth or Reality?" June 25, 2009, www.mayoclinic.com/health/male-menopause/MC00058.
6. Ibid.
7. Consortium on the Management of Disorders of Sexual Development, *Handbook for Parents* (Rohnert Park, CA: Intersex Society of North America, 2006), Available at http://dsdguidelines.org.
8. Federal Bureau of Investigation, "Hate Crime Statistics, 2008," May 2010, www.fbi.gov/about-us/cjis/ucr/hate-crime/2008.
9. G. F. Kelly, "Sexual Individuality and Sexual Values," in *Sexuality Today: The Human Perspective,* 9th ed. (New York: McGraw-Hill, 2008).
10. Ibid.
11. J. A. Higgins, J. Trussell, N. B. Moore, and J. K. Davidson, "Young Adult Sexual Health: Current and Prior Sexual Behaviours among Non-Hispanic White U.S. College Students," *Sexual Health* 7, no. 1 (2010): 35–43.
12. American College Health Association, *American College Health Association—National College Health Assessment II (ACHA-NCHA II) Reference Group Data Report Fall 2009* (Baltimore: American College Health Association, 2010), Available at www.acha-ncha.org/reports_ACHA-NCHAII.html.
13. Ibid.
14. Ibid.
15. G. F. Kelly, "Sexual Individuality and Sexual Values," 2008.
16. Medline Plus, "Sexual Problems Overview: Medline Plus," Updated May 2010, www.nlm.nih.gov/medlineplus/ency/article/001951.htm.

17. Mayo Clinic Staff, "Erectile Dysfunction," January 2010, www.mayoclinic.com/health/erectile-dysfunction/DS00162.
18. National Kidney and Urological Diseases Information Clearinghouse, "Erectile Dysfunction," 2009, http://kidney.niddk.nih.gov/kudiseases/pubs/impotence/index.htm.
19. Medline Plus, "Sexual Problems Overview: Medline Plus," Updated May 2010.
20. K. M. Smith and F. Romanelli, "Recreational Use and Misuse of Phosphodiesterase 5 Inhibitors," *Journal of the American Pharmacists Association* 45, no. 1 (2005): 63–75; R. Kloner, "Erectile Dysfunction and Hypertension," *International Journal of Impotence Research* 19, no. 3 (2007): 296–302.
21. J. Ropelato, "Internet Pornography Statistics," TopTenREVIEWS, Inc., Accessed June 2010, www.internet-filter-review.toptenreviews.com/internet-pornography-statistics.html.
22. Ibid.
23. B. Paul, "Predicting Internet Pornography Use and Arousal: The Role of Individual Difference Variables," *Journal of Sex Research* 46, no. 4 (2009): 344–57; D. Kingston, N. Malamuth, P. Fedoroff, and W. Marchall, "The Importance of Individual Differences in Pornography Use: Theoretical Perspectives and Implications for Treating Sexual Offenders," *Journal of Sex Research* 46 no. 2/3 (2009): 216–32; B. A. Wilson et al., "Predicting Responses to Sexually Aggressive Stories: The Role of Consent, Interest in Sexual Aggression, and Overall Sexual Interest," *Journal of Sex Research* 39, no. 4 (2002): 275–83; M. T. Whitty and W. A. Fisher, "The Sexy Side of the Internet: An Examination of Sexual Activities and Materials in Cyberspace," In *Psychological Aspects of Cyberspace: Theory, Research, Applications,* ed. A. Barak (Cambridge, UK: Cambridge University Press, 2008), 185–208; A. McKee, "The Relationship between Attitudes towards Women, Consumption of Pornography, and Other Demographic Variables in a Survey of 1,023 Consumers of Pornography," *International Journal of Sexual Health* 19 (2007): 31–45.

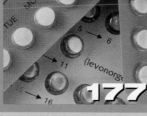

**177**

Does the birth control pill cause any side effects?

**183**

What is emergency contraception?

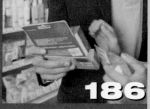

**186**

How do I choose a method of birth control?

# Considering Your Reproductive Choices

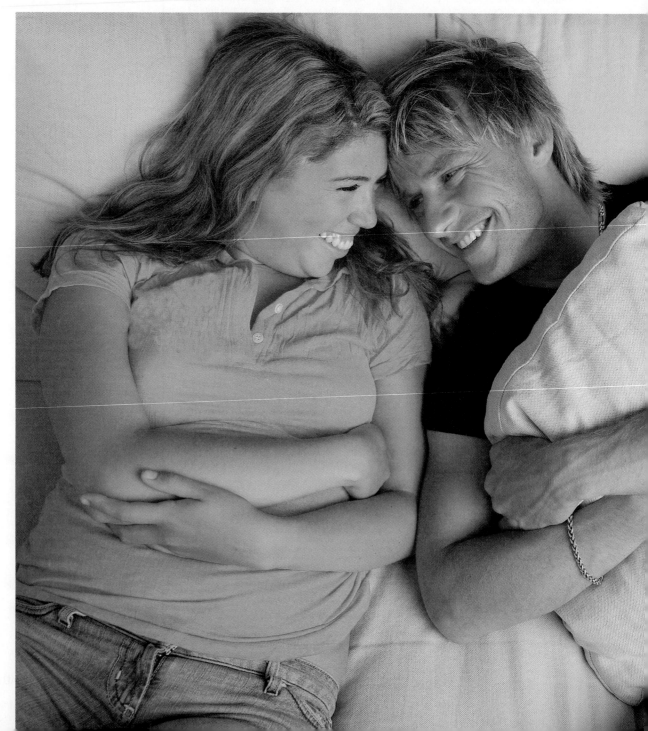

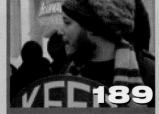

189

Where do Americans stand today on the issue of abortion?

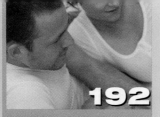

192

How can I prepare to be a parent?

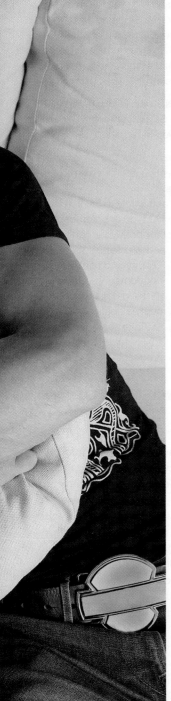

## Objectives

✴ Compare the different types of contraceptive methods and their effectiveness in preventing pregnancy and sexually transmitted infections.

✴ Summarize the legal decisions surrounding abortion and the various types of abortion procedures.

✴ Discuss key issues to consider when planning a pregnancy.

✴ Explain the importance of prenatal care and the physical and emotional aspects of pregnancy.

✴ Describe the basic stages of childbirth and the methods and complications that can arise during labor and delivery.

✴ Review primary causes of and possible solutions to infertility.

Today, we not only understand the intimate details of reproduction, but also possess technologies that can control or enhance our **fertility.** Along with information and technological advances comes choice, which goes hand in hand with responsibility. Choosing whether and when to have children is one of our greatest responsibilities. A woman and her partner have much to consider before planning or risking a pregnancy. Children transform people's lives. They require a lifelong personal commitment of love and nurturing. Before having children, ask yourself: Are you physically, emotionally, and financially prepared to care for another human being right now?

One measure of maturity is the ability to discuss reproduction and birth control with your sexual partner before engaging in sexual activity. Men often assume that their partners are taking care of birth control. (See the **Gender & Health** box on page 170 for more on this topic.) Women often feel that broaching the topic implies that they are promiscuous. Both may feel that bringing up the subject interferes with romance and spontaneity.

Too often, no one brings up the topic, and unprotected sex is the result. In fact, in a recent survey, only 52 percent of college students (55% of college women and 48% of college men) reported having used a method of contraception the last time they had sexual intercourse.[1] The sad result is too many unwanted pregnancies and sexually transmitted infections. If you're thinking about becoming sexually active, or you already are, but have not used birth control, make time to see a doctor or go to your health clinic to discuss getting contraceptives. Discussing the topic with your health care provider or your sexual partner will be easier and less embarrassing if you understand human reproduction and contraception and honestly consider your attitudes toward these matters. This chapter gives you some background to get you started on practicing safer sex.

**fertility** A person's ability to reproduce.
**contraception (birth control)** Methods of preventing conception.
**conception** The fertilization of an ovum by a sperm.

# Basic Principles of Birth Control

The term **birth control** (also called **contraception**) refers to methods of preventing conception. **Conception** occurs when a sperm fertilizes an egg. This usually takes place in a woman's fallopian tube. The following conditions are necessary for conception:

**1. A viable egg.** A sexually mature woman will release one egg (sometimes more) from one of her two ovaries once every 28 days, on average. Eggs remain viable for 24 to 36 hours after their release from the ovary into the fallopian tubes.

**2. A viable sperm.** Each ejaculation contains between 200 and 500 million sperm cells. Once sperm reach the fallopian

# Increasing Men's Involvement in Reproductive and Sexual Health

The sexual health needs of young men have been largely overlooked in the field of reproductive health. Much of the focus of prevention of teen pregnancy, sexually transmitted infections (STIs), and HIV/AIDS has been directed primarily at women. On our college campuses the emphasis of the sexual health messages we send out to the community or the discussions we have in the student health centers too often have focused mainly on women. We often miss the opportunity to emphasize the importance of shared responsibility for sexual health. There are several reasons for this: Men seek health care less often, so the opportunity for conversations regarding sexual health issues occurs less frequently, and we often incorrectly assume that men are not interested in sexual health issues. However, the development of healthy sexual relationships and reproductive health necessitates that both men and women have access to information. So, how can we involve more men in responsible sexual decision making?

To achieve the goal of having more males more aware of sexual health issues and involved in sexual health decisions, programs and environments need to be created that allow men to make healthy and well-informed decisions about their sexual health and sexual behavior. How can this be done?

✱ Create male-friendly clinics. Hire male health workers who can be advocates and role models for healthy behaviors. Have clinical programs that have a visible male focus. Train staff in male reproductive sexual health issues.
✱ Educate males about gender roles and how those roles can create

barriers to clear communication about sex and sexual expectations and get in the way of the development of healthy relationships.
✱ Provide male involvement programs that include educational programs, workshops, or one-on-one educational sessions. These workshops or sessions need to provide skill-based education to empower men to learn the correct way to put on a condom, and to practice communication skills for negotiation of safer sex. Most important, the workshops should be a safe space for males to ask questions about relationships and to express their feelings about their experiences. Incentives such as food, movie passes, or gift cards can help get men to a program or workshop.
✱ Train male peers to be health workers. They are often received better than a clinician.
✱ Develop marketing materials directed at men that present men as proactive about their sexual health.

But, men have to take their own responsibility for getting educated about sex, too, right? So, what can men do to become better involved in reproductive health?

✱ Initiate discussions with your partner about contraception and/or your sexual health histories.
✱ Take an active role in helping decide what type of contraception is best for both your partner and yourself.
✱ Buy and use condoms.
✱ Help pay for contraceptive costs.
✱ Take shared responsibility for an unintended pregnancy.

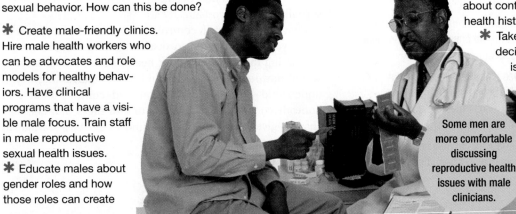

Some men are more comfortable discussing reproductive health issues with male clinicians.

tubes they survive an average of 48 to 72 hours—and can survive up to a week.

**3. Access to the egg by the sperm.** To reach the egg, sperm must travel up the vagina, through the cervical opening into the uterus, and from there to the fallopian tubes.

**perfect-use failure rate** The number of pregnancies (per 100 users) that are likely to occur in the first year of use of a particular birth control method if the method is used consistently and correctly.

Birth control methods prevent conception by interfering with one of these three conditions. Different methods offer varying degrees of control over when and whether

pregnancy occurs. Society has searched for a simple, infallible, and risk-free way to prevent pregnancy since people first associated sexual activity with pregnancy. We have not yet found one.

To evaluate the effectiveness of a particular contraceptive method, you must be familiar with two concepts: perfect-use failure rate and typical-use failure rate. **Perfect-use failure rate** refers to the number of pregnancies that are likely to occur in the first year of use (per 100 users of the method) if the method is used absolutely perfectly—that is, without any error. The **typical-use failure rate** refers to the number of pregnancies that are likely to occur in the first year of use

| TABLE 6.1 | Top Reported Means of Contraception Sexually Active College Students or Their Partner Used the Last Time They Had Intercourse | | |
|---|---|---|---|
| Method | Male | Female | Total |
| *Any form of hormonal contraceptive (pills, injection, patch, ring, implant) excluding IUD* | 70.2% | 68.5% | 69.1% |
| Male condom | 69.2% | 58.2% | 61.8% |
| Birth control pills (monthly or extended cycle) | 58.8% | 58.8% | 58.7% |
| *Male condom plus another method* | 49.3% | 43.0% | 45.0% |
| Withdrawal | 24.8% | 26.7% | 26.1% |
| *Any two or more methods (excluding male condoms)* | 26.0% | 25.7% | 25.7% |
| Fertility awareness (calendar, mucus, basal body temperature) | 5.2% | 6.0% | 5.7% |
| Spermicide (foam, jelly, cream) | 7.3% | 4.5% | 5.4% |
| Intrauterine device (IUD) | 3.9% | 5.3% | 4.9% |
| Vaginal ring | 4.3% | 4.7% | 4.6% |

*Note:* Survey respondents could select more than one method. Italicized rows are aggregates of the data.

**Source:** Data are from American College Health Association, *American College Health Association—National College Health Assessment II (ACHA-NCHA II): Reference Group Data Report Fall 2009* (Baltimore: ACHA, 2010).

with typical use—that is, with the normal number of errors, memory lapses, and incorrect or incomplete use. The typical-use information is much more practical in helping people make informed decisions about contraceptive methods.

Present methods of contraception fall into several categories. **Barrier methods** block the egg and sperm from joining. **Hormonal methods** introduce synthetic hormones into the woman's system that prevent ovulation, thicken cervical mucus, or prevent a fertilized egg from implanting. Surgical methods can prevent pregnancy permanently. Other methods may involve temporary or permanent abstinence or planning intercourse in accordance with fertility patterns. Table 6.1 lists the most popular forms of contraception among sexually active college students today.

Some contraceptive methods can also protect, to some degree, against **sexually transmitted infections (STIs),** which you'll learn more about in Chapter 14. This is an important factor to

consider in choosing a contraceptive. Table 6.2 on page 172 summarizes the effectiveness, STI protection, frequency of use, and costs of various methods.

# Barrier Methods

Barrier methods work on the simple principle of preventing sperm from ever reaching the egg by use of a physical or chemical barrier during intercourse. Some barrier methods prevent semen from having any contact with the woman's body, and others prevent sperm from going past the cervix. In addition, many barrier methods contain or are used in combination with a substance that kills sperm.

## The Male Condom

The **male condom** is a thin sheath designed to cover the erect penis and catch semen before it enters the vagina. Most male condoms are made of latex, although condoms made of polyurethane or lambskin also are available. Condoms come in a wide variety of styles. All may be purchased in pharmacies, supermarkets, public

**typical-use failure rate** The number of pregnancies (per 100 users) that are likely to occur in the first year of use of a particular birth control method if the method's use is not consistent or always correct.

**barrier methods** Contraceptive methods that block the meeting of egg and sperm by means of a physical barrier (such as condom, diaphragm, or cervical cap), a chemical barrier (such as spermicide), or both.

**hormonal methods** Contraceptive methods that introduce synthetic hormones into the woman's system to prevent ovulation, thicken cervical mucus, or prevent a fertilized egg from implanting.

**sexually transmitted infections (STIs)** Infectious diseases caused by pathogens transmitted through some form of intimate, usually sexual, contact.

**male condom** A single-use sheath of thin latex or other material designed to fit over an erect penis and to catch semen upon ejaculation.

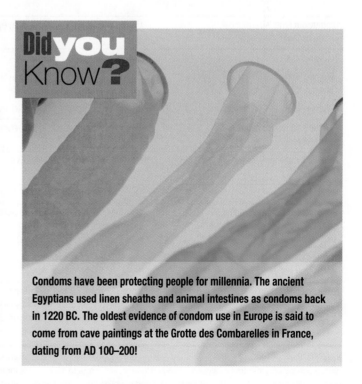

**Did you Know?**

Condoms have been protecting people for millennia. The ancient Egyptians used linen sheaths and animal intestines as condoms back in 1220 BC. The oldest evidence of condom use in Europe is said to come from cave paintings at the Grotte des Combarelles in France, dating from AD 100–200!

TABLE

6.2

**Contraceptive Effectiveness, STI Protection, Frequency of Use, and Cost**

| Method | Failure Rate | | STI Protection | Frequency of Use | Cost |
|---|---|---|---|---|---|
| | Typical Use | Perfect Use | | | |
| Continuous abstinence | 0 | 0 | Yes | N/A | None |
| Implanon | 0.05 | 0.05 | No | Inserted every 3 years | $400–$600/exam, device, and insertion; $75–$250 for removal |
| Male sterilization | 0.15 | 0.1 | No | Done once | $350–$1,000/interview, counseling, examination, operation, and follow-up sperm count |
| Female sterilization | 0.5 | 0.5 | No | Done once | $1,500–$6,000/interview, counseling, examination, operation, and follow-up |
| IUD (intrauterine device) | | | | | |
| ParaGard (copper T) | 0.8 | 0.6 | No | Inserted every 10 years | $175–$500/exam, insertion, and follow-up visit |
| Mirena (LNG-IUS) | 0.2 | 0.2 | No | Inserted every 5 years | $175–$500/exam, insertion, and follow-up visit |
| Depo-Provera | 3 | 0.3 | No | Injected every 12 weeks | $30–$75/3-month injection; $35–$175 for initial exam; $20–$40 for further visits to clinician for shots |
| Oral contraceptives (combined pill and progestin-only pill) | 8 | 0.3 | No | Take daily | $15–$35 monthly pill pack at drugstores, often less at clinics; $35–$175 for initial exam |
| Ortho Evra patch | 8 | 0.3 | No | Applied weekly | $30–$40/month at drugstores; often less at clinics, $35–$175 for initial exam |
| NuvaRing | 8 | 0.3 | No | Inserted every 4 weeks | $30–$35/month at drugstores, often less at clinics; $35–$175 for initial exam |
| Cervical cap (FemCap) (with spermicidal cream or jelly) | | | | | |
| Women who have never given birth | 14 | 4 | Some | Used every time | $15–$75 for cap; $50–$200 for initial exam; $8–$17/supplies of spermicide jelly or cream |
| Women who have given birth | 32 | No data | Some | Used every time | |
| Male condom (without spermicides) | 15 | 2 | Some | Used every time | $0.50 and up/condom—some family planning centers give them away or charge very little; available in drugstores, family planning clinics, some supermarkets, and vending machines |
| Diaphragm (with spermicidal cream or jelly) | 16 | 6 | Some | Used every time | $15–$75 for diaphragm; $50–$200 for initial exam; $8–$17/supplies of spermicide jelly or cream |
| Today sponge | | | | | |
| Women who have never given birth | 16 | 9 | No | Used every time | $7.50–$9/package of three sponges; available at family planning centers, drugstores, online, and in some supermarkets |
| Women who have given birth | 32 | 20 | No | Used every time | |
| Female condom (without spermicides) | 21 | 5 | Some | Used every time | $2.50/condom; available at family planning centers, drugstores, and in some supermarkets |
| Fertility awareness–based methods | 25 | 12 | No | Followed every month | $10–$12 for temperature kits; charts and classes often free in health centers and churches |
| Withdrawal | 27 | 4 | No | Used every time | None |
| Spermicides (foams, creams, gels, vaginal suppositories, and vaginal film) | 29 | 18 | No | Used every time | $8–$17/applicator kits of foam and gel ($4–$8 refills); film and suppositories are priced similarly; available at family planning clinics, drugstores, and some supermarkets |
| No contraceptive | 85 | 85 | No | N/A | None |
| Emergency contraceptive pill | Treatment initiated within 72 hours after unprotected intercourse reduces the risk of pregnancy by 75%–89% (with no protection against STIs). Costs depend on what services are needed: $10–$45/Plan B, available over the counter to women 18 and older; $20–$50/one pack of combination pills; $50–$70/two packs of progestin-only pills; $35–$150/visit with health care provider; $10–$20/pregnancy test. | | | | |

**Note:** "Failure Rate" refers to the number of unintended pregnancies per 100 women during the first year of use. "Typical Use" refers to failure rates for men and women whose use is not consistent or always correct. "Perfect Use" refers to failure rates for those whose use is consistent and always correct.
Some family planning clinics charge for services and supplies on a sliding scale according to income.

**Source:** Adapted from R. A. Hatcher et al., *Contraceptive Technology*, 19th rev. ed. Copyright © 2007 Contraceptive Technology Communications, Inc.

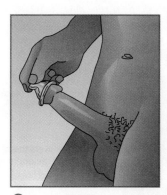
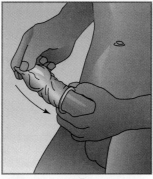
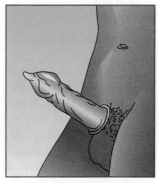
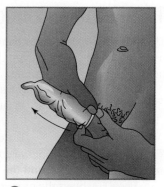

**1** Pinch the air out of the top half-inch of the condom to allow room for semen.

**2** Holding the tip of the condom with one hand, use the other hand to unroll it onto the penis.

**3** Unroll the condom all the way to the base of the penis, smoothing out any air bubbles.

**4** After ejaculation, hold the condom around the base until the penis is totally withdrawn to avoid spilling any semen.

FIGURE 6.1 **How to Use a Male Condom**

bathrooms, and many health clinics. A new condom must be used for each act of vaginal, oral, or anal intercourse.

A condom must be rolled onto the penis before the penis touches the vagina, and it must be held in place when removing the penis from the vagina after ejaculation (see **Figure 6.1**). Condoms come with or without **spermicide** and with or without lubrication. Spermicide can cause

# 80–90%

**That's the reduction in risk of STI transmission provided by latex condoms, according to several research studies.**

irritation for some users, and there is no evidence that using it with condoms reduces the risk of pregnancy. If desired, users can lubricate their own condoms with contraceptive foams, creams, and jellies or other water-based lubricants. Never use products such as baby oil, cold cream, petroleum jelly, vaginal yeast infection medications, or body lotion with a condom. These products contain mineral oil and will cause the latex to disintegrate.

Condoms are less effective and more likely to break during intercourse if they are old or improperly stored. To maintain effectiveness, store them in a cool place (not in a wallet or hip pocket), and inspect them for small tears before use. Discard all condoms that have passed their expiration date.

**"Why Should I Care?"**

Even if you use another method for contraception, it's a good idea to use a condom as well for protection against STIs. You don't want to get an STI—not only can they be unpleasant right now, but some of them can stay with you for life and cause lasting harm to your health and your fertility. Not to mention wreaking havoc on your love life!

**Advantages** When used consistently and correctly, condoms can be up to 98 percent effective. The condom is the only temporary means of birth control available for men, and latex and polyurethane condoms are the only barriers that effectively prevent the spread of HIV (the virus that causes AIDS) and some STIs. ("Skin" condoms, made from lamb intestines, are not effective against STIs.) Many people choose condoms because they are inexpensive and readily available without a prescription, and their use is limited to times of sexual activity, with no negative health effects. Some men find condoms help them stay erect longer or help prevent premature ejaculation.

**spermicide** Substance designed to kill sperm.

**Disadvantages** The easy availability of condoms is accompanied by considerable potential for user error; as a result, the typical use effectiveness of condoms in preventing pregnancy is around 85 percent. Improper use of a condom can lead to breakage, leakage, or slipping, potentially exposing the users to STI transmission or an unintended pregnancy. Even when used perfectly, a condom doesn't protect against transmission of STIs that may have external areas of infection (e.g., herpes). For some people, a condom ruins the spontaneity of sex because stopping to put it on may break the mood. Others report that the condom decreases sensation. These inconveniences and perceptions contribute to improper use or avoidance of condoms altogether. Partners who apply a condom as part of foreplay are generally more successful with this form of birth control. As a new condom is required for each act of intercourse, some users find it difficult to be sure to have a condom available when needed.

## The Female Condom

The **female condom** (brand name, Reality Condom) is a single-use, soft, loose-fitting polyurethane sheath meant for internal vaginal use. It is designed as one unit with two flexible rings. One ring lies inside the sheath and serves as an insertion mechanism and internal anchor. The other ring remains outside the vagina once the device is inserted and protects the labia and the base of the penis from infection. **Figure 6.2** shows the proper use of the female condom.

**female condom** A single-use polyurethane sheath for internal use during vaginal or anal intercourse to catch semen on ejaculation.

**Advantages** Used consistently and correctly, female condoms can be up to 95 percent effective. They also can prevent the spread of HIV and other STIs, including those that can be transmitted by external genital contact. The female condom can be inserted up to 8 hours in advance, so its use doesn't have to interrupt lovemaking. Some women choose to use the female condom because it gives them more personal control over pregnancy prevention and STI protection, or because they cannot rely on their partner to use a male condom. Because the polyurethane is thin and pliable, there is less loss of sensation with the female condom than there is with the latex male condom. The female condom is relatively inexpensive, readily available without a prescription, and causes no negative health effects.

**Disadvantages** As with the male condom, there is potential for user error with the female condom, including possible breaking, slipping, or leaking, all of which could lead to STI transmission or an unintended pregnancy. Because of the potential problems, the typical use effectiveness of the female condom is 79 percent. Some people dislike using the female condom because they feel it is disruptive, noisy, odd looking, or difficult to use. Some women have reported external or vaginal irritation from using the female condom. A new condom is required for each act of intercourse, so users may not always have one available when needed. The female condom can be used effectively for anal sex, but it is difficult to use in this manner and can be painful. There is also the risk of rectal bleeding, which increases the risk of contracting HIV. Therefore, it's better to use the male condom with plenty of lubricant for anal sex.

## Jellies, Creams, Foams, Suppositories, and Film

Like condoms, some other barrier methods—jellies, creams, foams, suppositories, and film—do not require a prescription. They are referred to as spermicides—substances designed to kill sperm. The active ingredient in most of them is nonoxynol-9 (N-9).

Jellies and creams are packaged in tubes, and foams are available in aerosol cans. All have applicators designed for insertion into the vagina. They must be inserted far enough

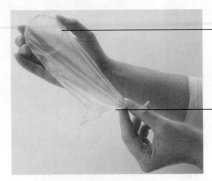

Inner ring is used for insertion and to help hold the sheath in place during intercourse.

Outer ring covers the area around the opening of the vagina.

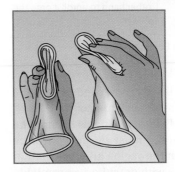

1 Grasp the flexible inner ring at the closed end of the condom, and squeeze it between your thumb and second or middle finger so it becomes long and narrow.

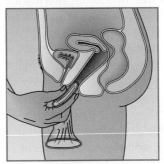

2 Choose a comfortable position for insertion: squatting, with one leg raised, or sitting or lying down. While squeezing the ring, insert the closed end of the condom into your vagina.

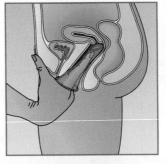

3 Placing your index finger inside of the condom, gently push the inner ring up as far as it will go. Be sure the sheath is not twisted. The outer ring should remain outside of the vagina.

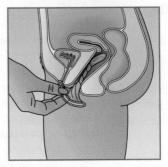

4 During intercourse, be sure that the penis is not entering on the side, between the sheath and the vaginal wall. When removing the condom, twist the outer ring so that no semen leaks out.

**FIGURE 6.2 How to Use a Female Condom**

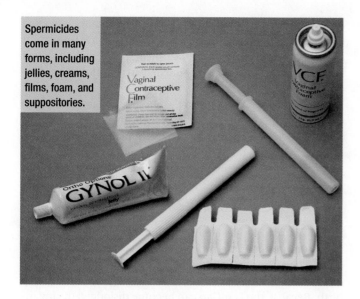

Spermicides come in many forms, including jellies, creams, films, foam, and suppositories.

Like condoms, spermicides are inexpensive, do not require a prescription or pelvic examination, and are readily available over the counter. They are simple to use and their use is limited to the time of sexual activity.

**Disadvantages** Spermicides can be messy and must be reapplied for each act of intercourse. Some people experience irritation or allergic reactions to spermicides, and recent studies indicate that spermicides containing N-9 are not effective in preventing transmission of STIs such as gonorrhea, chlamydia, and HIV. In fact, frequent use of N-9 spermicides has been shown to cause irritation and breaks in the mucous layer or skin of the genital tract, creating a point of entry for viruses and bacteria that cause disease.[2] Spermicides containing N-9 have also been associated with increased risk of urinary tract infection.

## The Diaphragm with Spermicidal Jelly or Cream

Invented in the mid-nineteenth century, the **diaphragm** was the first widely used birth control method for women. The device is a soft, shallow cup made of thin latex rubber. Its flexible, rubber-coated ring is designed to fit snugly behind the pubic bone in front of the cervix and over the back of the cervix on the other side so it blocks access to the uterus. Diaphragms must be used with spermicidal cream or jelly, which is applied to the inside of the diaphragm before it is inserted, up to 6 hours before intercourse. The diaphragm holds the spermicide in place, creating a physical and chemical barrier against sperm (Figure 6.3). Diaphragms are manufactured in different sizes and must be fitted to the woman by a trained practitioner, who should make sure the user knows how to insert her diaphragm correctly before leaving the practitioner's office.

> **diaphragm** A latex, cup-shaped device designed to cover the cervix and block access to the uterus; should always be used with spermicide.

to cover the cervix, thus providing both a chemical barrier that kills sperm and a physical barrier that stops sperm from continuing toward an egg.

Suppositories are waxy capsules that are inserted deep into the vagina, where they melt. They must be inserted 10 to 20 minutes before intercourse to have time to melt, but no longer than 1 hour prior to intercourse, or they lose their effectiveness. Additional contraceptive chemicals must be applied for each subsequent act of intercourse.

Vaginal contraceptive film is another method of spermicide delivery. A thin film infused with spermicidal gel is inserted into the vagina so that it covers the cervix. The film dissolves into a spermicidal gel that is effective for up to 3 hours. As with other spermicides, a new film must be inserted for each act of intercourse.

**Advantages** Spermicides are most effective when used in conjunction with another barrier method (condom, diaphragm, etc.); used alone they offer only 71 percent (typical use) to 82 percent (perfect use) effectiveness at preventing pregnancy.

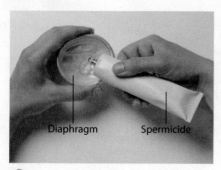

❶ Place spermicidal jelly or cream inside the diaphragm and all around the rim.

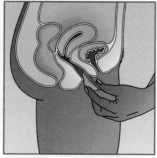

❷ Fold the diaphragm in half and insert dome-side down (spermicide-side up) into the vagina, pushing it along the back wall as far as it will go.

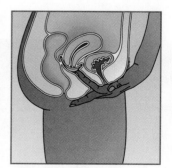

❸ Position the diaphragm with the cervix completely covered and the front rim tucked up against your pubic bone; you should be able to feel your cervix through the rubber dome.

FIGURE 6.3 **The Proper Use and Placement of a Diaphragm**

**Advantages** If used consistently and correctly, diaphragms can be 94 percent effective in preventing pregnancy. When used with spermicidal jelly or cream, the diaphragm also offers significant protection against gonorrhea and possibly chlamydia and human papillomavirus (HPV). After the initial prescription and fitting, the only ongoing expense involved with diaphragm use is spermicide. Because the diaphragm can be inserted up to 6 hours in advance and used for multiple acts of intercourse, some users may find it less disruptive than other barrier methods.

**cervical cap** A small cup made of latex or silicone that is designed to fit snugly over the entire cervix.

**toxic shock syndrome (TSS)** A potentially life-threatening disease that occurs when specific bacterial toxins multiply and spread to the bloodstream, most commonly through improper use of tampons, diaphragms, or cervical caps.

**Today sponge** A contraceptive device, made of polyurethane foam and containing nonoxynol-9, that fits over the cervix to create a barrier against sperm.

**Disadvantages** Although the diaphragm can be left in place for multiple acts of intercourse, additional spermicide must be applied before each time, and the diaphragm must then stay in place for 6 to 8 hours after intercourse to allow the chemical to kill any sperm remaining in the vagina. Some women find inserting the device can be awkward, especially if the woman is rushed. When inserted incorrectly, diaphragms are much less effective. It is also possible for a diaphragm to slip out of place, be difficult to remove, or require refitting by a physician (e.g., following a pregnancy or a significant weight gain or loss).

## The Cervical Cap with Spermicidal Jelly or Cream

One of the oldest methods used to prevent pregnancy, early **cervical caps** were made from beeswax, silver, or copper. The currently available FemCap is a clear silicone cup that fits snugly over the entire cervix. It comes in three sizes and must be fitted by a practitioner. The FemCap is designed for use with spermicidal jelly or cream. It is held in place by suction created during application and works by blocking sperm from the uterus.

**Advantages** Cervical caps can be reasonably effective (86%) with typical use. They also may offer some protection against transmission of gonorrhea, HPV, and possibly chlamydia. They are relatively inexpensive, as the only ongoing cost is for the spermicide.

The FemCap can be inserted up to 6 hours prior to intercourse, making it potentially less disruptive than other barrier methods. The device must be left in place for 6 to 8 hours afterward, but after that time period, if removed and cleaned, it can be reinserted immediately. Because the FemCap is made of silicon rubber, not latex, it is a suitable alternative for people who are allergic to latex.

**Disadvantages** The FemCap is somewhat more difficult to insert than a diaphragm because of its smaller size. Like a diaphragm, it requires an initial fitting and may require subsequent refitting if a woman's cervix size changes, as after giving birth. Because the FemCap can become dislodged during intercourse, placement must be checked frequently. The device cannot be used during the menstrual period or for longer than 48 hours because of the risk of **toxic shock syndrome (TSS).** Some women report unpleasant vaginal odors after use.

## The Sponge

The **Today Sponge** is made of polyurethane foam and contains nonoxynol-9. Prior to insertion, the sponge must be moistened with water to activate the spermicide. It is then folded and inserted deep into the vagina, where it fits over the cervix and creates a barrier against sperm.

**Advantages** The sponge is fairly effective (91% perfect use; 84% typical use) when used consistently and correctly. A main advantage of the sponge is convenience, because it does not

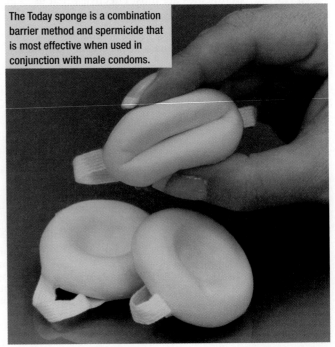

The Today sponge is a combination barrier method and spermicide that is most effective when used in conjunction with male condoms.

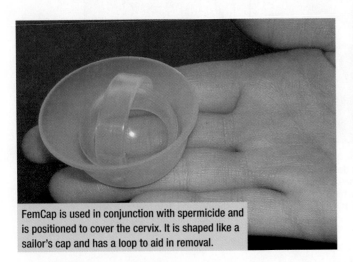

FemCap is used in conjunction with spermicide and is positioned to cover the cervix. It is shaped like a sailor's cap and has a loop to aid in removal.

require a trip to the doctor for fitting. Protection begins immediately on insertion and lasts for up to 24 hours. There is no need to reapply spermicide or insert a new sponge for any subsequent acts of intercourse within the same 24-hour period; it must be left in place for at least 6 hours after the last intercourse. Like the diaphragm and cervical cap, the sponge offers limited protection from some STIs.

**Disadvantages** The sponge is less effective for women who have previously given birth (80% perfect use; 68% typical use). Allergic reactions, such as irritation of the vagina, are more common with the sponge than with other barrier methods. Should the vaginal lining become irritated, the risk of yeast infections and other STIs may increase. Some cases of TSS have been reported in women using the sponge; the same precautions should be taken as with the diaphragm and cervical cap. In addition, some women find the sponge difficult or messy to remove.

# Hormonal Methods

The term *hormonal contraception* refers to birth control that contains synthetic estrogen and/or progestin. These ingredients are similar to the hormones estrogen and progesterone, which a woman's ovaries produce naturally for the process of ovulation and the menstrual cycle. In recent years, hormonal contraception has become available in a variety of forms (transdermal, injection, and oral). All forms require a prescription from a health care provider.

Hormonal contraception alters a woman's biochemistry, preventing ovulation (release of the egg) from taking place and producing changes that make it more difficult for the sperm to reach the egg if ovulation does occur. Some hormonal contraceptives contain both estrogen and progestin (synthetic progesterone), and several products contain just progestin. Synthetic estrogen works to prevent the ovaries from releasing an egg. If no egg is released, there is nothing to be fertilized by sperm and pregnancy cannot occur. Progestin works to thicken the cervical mucus, which hinders the movement of the sperm, inhibits the egg's ability to travel through the fallopian tubes, and suppresses the sperm's ability to unite with the egg. Progestin also alters the uterine lining, which renders the egg unlikely to implant in the uterine wall.

## Oral Contraceptives

**Oral contraceptive** pills were first marketed in the United States in 1960. Their convenience quickly made them the most widely used reversible method of fertility control. Most modern pills are up to 99 percent effective at preventing pregnancy with perfect use. Today, oral contraceptives are the most commonly used birth control method among college women.[3]

Most oral contraceptives work through the combined effects of synthetic estrogen and progestin (*combination*

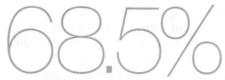

**68.5%** of sexually active female college students use **some form of hormonal contraception (pills, shot, patch, ring, or implant).**

*pills*). Combination pills are taken in a cycle. At the end of each 3-week cycle, the user discontinues the drug or takes placebo pills for 1 week. The resultant drop in hormones causes the uterine lining to disintegrate, and the user will have a menstrual period, usually within 1 to 3 days. Menstrual flow is generally lighter than it is for women who don't use the pill, because the hormones in the pill prevent thick endometrial buildup.

Several new types of pills have extended cycles, such as the 91-day Seasonale and Seasonique. A woman using this regimen takes active pills for 12 weeks, followed by 1 week of placebos. Under this cycle, women can expect to have a menstrual period every 3 months. Data indicate that women do have an increased occurrence of spotting or bleeding in the first few cycles.[4] Lybrel, another extended-cycle pill, is taken continuously for 1 year, thus eliminating menstruation completely.

**oral contraceptives** Pills containing synthetic hormones that prevent ovulation by regulating hormones.

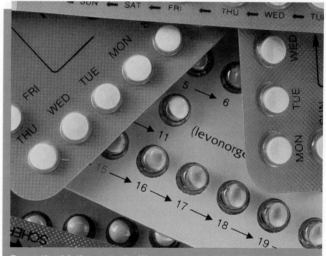

**Does the birth control pill cause any side effects?**

There are many different brands and regimens of oral contraceptives available to women today, some of which are associated with various health benefits such as reducing acne or symptoms of PMS (premenstrual syndrome). Some women experience minor side effects from pill use—the most common being headaches, breast tenderness, nausea, and breakthrough bleeding—but these usually clear up within 2 to 3 months. If you experience any side effects from pill use, talk to your health care provider about them, as she may be able to recommend another brand of pill or method of birth control that will work better for you.

**Advantages** Combination pills are highly effective at preventing pregnancy: 99.7 percent with perfect use and 92 percent with typical use. It is easier to achieve perfect use with pills than it is with barrier contraceptives, as there is less room for user error. Aside from its effectiveness, much of the pill's popularity is due to its convenience and discreetness. Users like the fact that it does not interrupt or interfere with lovemaking, which can lead to enhanced sexual enjoyment.

In addition to preventing pregnancy, the pill may lessen menstrual difficulties, such as cramps and premenstrual syndrome (PMS). Oral contraceptives also lower the risk of several health conditions, including endometrial and ovarian cancers, noncancerous breast disease, osteoporosis, ovarian cysts, pelvic inflammatory disease (PID), and iron-deficiency anemia.[5] There are many different brands of combination pills on the market, some of which contain progestins that offer additional benefits, such as reducing acne or minimizing fluid retention. Less-expensive generic versions are also available for many brands. With the extended-cycle pills, the major additional benefit is the reduction in or absence of menstruation and any cramps or PMS symptoms associated with it. Users of these pills also like that they don't need to remember when to stop or start a cycle of pills, or when to use placebos.

**Disadvantages** The estrogen in combination pills is associated with the risk of several serious health problems, including blood clots (which can lead to strokes or heart attacks) and an increased risk of high blood pressure. The risk is low for most healthy women under the age of 35 who do not smoke; it increases with age and especially with cigarette smoking. See **Figure 6.4** for early warning signs of complications associated with oral contraceptives.

Different brands of pills can cause varying minor side effects. Some of the most common are spotting between periods (particularly with extended cycle regimens), breast tenderness, and nausea and vomiting. With most pills, these side effects clear up within a few months. Other, less common potential side effects include a change in sexual desire, acne, weight gain, and hair loss or growth. Because there are so many brands available, most women who wish to use the pill are able to find one that works for them without causing unpleasant side effects.

Apart from the risk factors and potential side effects associated with the pill, its greatest disadvantage is that it must be taken every day. If a woman misses one pill, she should use an alternative form of contraception for the remainder of that cycle. A backup method of birth control is also necessary during the first week of use. After a woman discontinues the pill, return of fertility may be delayed, but the pill is not known to cause infertility. Another drawback is that the pill does not protect against STIs. Cost may also be a problem for some women (see the **Consumer Health** box at right), whereas some teenagers report that the requirement to have a complete gynecological examination in order to get a prescription for the pill is a huge obstacle.

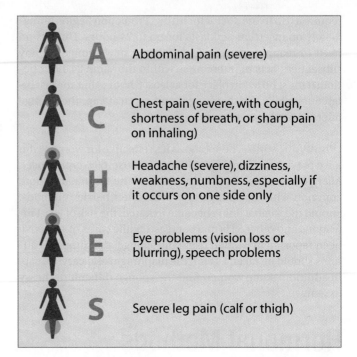

FIGURE $6.4$ **Early Warning Signs of Medical Complications for Users of the Birth Control Pill**

**Source:** Adapted from R. A. Hatcher et al., *Contraceptive Technology*, 19th ed. Copyright © 2007 Contraceptive Technology Communications, Inc.

## Progestin-Only Pills

Progestin-only pills (or minipills) contain small doses of progestin and no estrogen. These pills are taken continuously (there are no placebo pills included in each pack). Because these pills do not contain estrogen, women taking them may ovulate, but the progestin prevents pregnancy by thickening cervical mucus and by interfering with implantation of a fertilized egg.

**Advantages** Progestin-only pills are a good choice for women who are at high risk for estrogen-related side effects or who cannot take estrogen-containing pills because of diabetes, high blood pressure, or other cardiovascular conditions. They also can be used safely by women who are older than age 35 and by women who are currently breast-feeding. The effectiveness rate of these pills is 96 percent with perfect use, which is slightly lower than that of estrogen-containing pills. Progestin-only pills share some of the health benefits associated with combination pills, and they carry no estrogen-related cardiovascular risks. Also, some of the typical side effects of combination pills, including nausea and breast tenderness, usually do not occur with progestin-only pills. With progestin-only pills, women's menstrual periods generally become lighter or stop altogether.

**Disadvantages** Because of the lower dose of hormones in progestin-only pills, it is especially important that they be taken at the same time each day. If a woman takes a pill 3 or

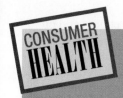
# THE FIGHT FOR AFFORDABLE BIRTH CONTROL ON COLLEGE CAMPUSES

Today's college students pay considerably more for contraceptives than those of even 5 years ago. For almost 20 years, college health centers could buy prescription drugs, including contraceptives, at deep discounts. Known as "nominal pricing," this arrangement allowed pharmaceutical companies to sell their products to certain charitable groups, including university health centers and some family planning centers, at very low (nominal) prices, without having to offer the same discounts to states' Medicaid programs. University health centers then passed along the savings to students.

All was well until accusations arose that some drug companies were abusing the exemption. In 2005, as part of its Deficit Reduction Act of 2005, U.S. Congress narrowed the definition of those who could qualify and, in the process, precluded legitimate charitable sales to university health centers and family planning centers that are not part of the Title X program. Family planning centers supported by Title X were not directly affected by this change and were still able to receive nominal prices. As stockpiles of discounted drugs ran out, payments shot up: Students saw the price of oral contraceptives rise from $5 to $10 per month to $30 to $50, and some campus pharmacies have stopped stocking contraceptives altogether, forcing students to go to outside pharmacies and pay out of pocket or with private insurance.

In 2007, Planned Parenthood Federation of America began a nationwide grassroots campaign to restore the exemption for university health centers and family planning centers. These efforts paid off in early 2009 when Congress passed legislation to make birth control affordable again. The provision, included in the 2009 Omnibus Appropriations Act, restores the exemption and eliminates one major disincentive to offering steep discounts to university health centers. But other disincentives for manufacturers remain, and whether this change will lead them to lower prices on college campuses remains to be seen.

**Source:** The Fight for Affordable Birth Control on College Campuses, adapted from H. D. Boonstra et al., "The Challenge in Helping Young Adults Better Manage Their Reproductive Lives," *Guttmacher Policy Review,* 2009, 12(2):16. Used with permission.

---

more hours later than usual, she will need to use a backup method of contraception for the next 48 hours. The most common side effect of progestin-only pills is irregular menstrual bleeding or spotting. Less common side effects include mood changes, changes in sex drive, and headaches. As with all oral contraceptives, progestin-only pills do not protect against STI transmission.

## Contraceptive Skin Patch

**Ortho Evra** is a square transdermal adhesive patch. It is as thin as a plastic strip bandage, is worn for 1 week, and is replaced on the same day of the week for 3 consecutive weeks; the fourth week is patch free. Ortho Evra works by delivering continuous levels of estrogen and progestin through the skin and into the bloodstream. The patch can be worn on one of four areas of the body: buttocks, abdomen, upper torso (front and back, excluding the breasts), or upper outer arm.

**Advantages** Ortho Evra is 99.7 percent effective with perfect use. As with other hormonal methods, there is less room for user error than there is with barrier methods. Women who choose to use the patch often do so because they find it easier to remember than taking a daily pill, and they like the fact that they need to change the patch only once a week. Ortho Evra probably offers similar potential health benefits as combination pills (reduction in risk of certain cancers and diseases, lessening of PMS symptoms, etc.). Like other hormonal methods, the patch regulates a woman's menstrual cycle.

**Disadvantages** Using the patch requires an initial exam and prescription, weekly patch changes, and the ongoing monthly expense of patch purchase. There is currently no generic version. A backup method is required during the first week of use. Similar to other hormonal methods of birth control, the patch offers no protection against HIV or other STIs. Some women experience minor side effects such as those associated with combination pills. The estrogen in the patch is associated with cardiovascular risks, particularly in women who smoke and women who are over the age of 35. In 2005, amidst evidence that the patch may increase a woman's risk for life-threatening blood clots, the U.S. Food and Drug Administration (FDA) mandated an additional warning label explaining that patch use exposes women to about 60 percent more total estrogen than if they were taking a typical combination pill. In April 2010, the FDA released another warning for users, indicating more conclusive evidence of an increased risk of blood clots among regular users.[6]

**Ortho Evra** A patch that releases hormones similar to those in oral contraceptives; each patch is worn for 1 week.

Ortho Evra is an adhesive patch that delivers estrogen and progestin through the skin for 3 weeks.

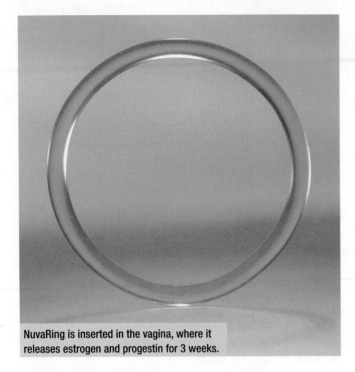

NuvaRing is inserted in the vagina, where it releases estrogen and progestin for 3 weeks.

## Vaginal Contraceptive Ring

**NuvaRing** is a soft, flexible plastic hormonal contraceptive ring about 2 inches in diameter. The user inserts the ring into her vagina, leaves it in place for 3 weeks, and removes it for 1 week for her menstrual period. Once the ring is inserted, it releases a steady flow of estrogen and progestin.

**NuvaRing** A soft, flexible ring inserted into the vagina that releases hormones, preventing pregnancy.
**Depo-Provera** An injectable method of birth control that lasts for 3 months.

**Advantages** When used properly, the ring is 99.7 percent effective. Advantages of NuvaRing include less likelihood of user error, protection against pregnancy for 1 month, no pill to take daily or patch to change weekly, no need to be fitted by a clinician, no requirement to use spermicide, and rapid return of fertility when use is stopped. It also exposes the user to a lower dosage of estrogen than do the patch and some combination pills, so it may have fewer estrogen-related side effects. It probably offers some of the same potential health benefits as combination pills, and, like other hormonal contraceptives, it regulates a woman's menstrual cycle.

**Disadvantages** NuvaRing requires an initial exam and prescription, monthly ring changes, and the ongoing monthly expense of purchasing the ring (there is currently no generic version). A backup method must be used during the first week, and the ring provides no protection against STI transmission. Like combina-

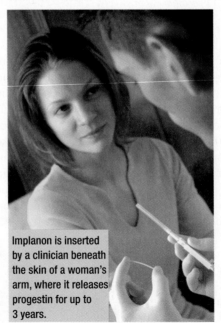

Implanon is inserted by a clinician beneath the skin of a woman's arm, where it releases progestin for up to 3 years.

tion pills, the ring poses possible minor side effects, and potentially more serious health risks for some women. Possible side effects unique to the ring include increased vaginal discharge and vaginal irritation or infection. Oil-based vaginal medicines to treat yeast infections cannot be used when the ring is in place; and a diaphragm or cervical cap cannot be used as a backup method for contraception.

## Contraceptive Injections

**Depo-Provera** is a long-acting progestin that is injected intramuscularly every 3 months by a health care provider. Researchers believe that the drug prevents ovulation.

**Advantages** Depo-Provera takes effect within 24 hours of the first shot so there is usually no need to use a backup method. There is little room for user error with the shot (as it is administered by a clinician every 3 months): with perfect use the shot is 99.7 percent effective, and with typical use it is 97 percent effective. Some women feel Depo-Provera encourages sexual spontaneity, because they do not have to remember to take a pill or insert a device. With continued use of this method, a woman's menstrual periods become lighter and may eventually stop altogether. There are no estrogen-related health risks associated with Depo-Provera, and it offers the same potential health benefits as progestin-only pills. Unlike estrogen-containing hormonal methods, Depo-Provera can be used by women who are breast-feeding.

**Disadvantages** Using Depo-Provera requires an initial exam and prescription, as well as follow-up visits every 3 months to have the shot administered. It offers no protection against transmission of STIs. The main disadvantage of Depo-Provera use is irregular bleeding, which can be troublesome at first, but within a year, most women are amenorrheic (have no menstrual periods). Weight gain (an average of 5 pounds in the first year) is common. Depo-Provera comes with a warning that prolonged use is linked with loss of bone density. Other possible side effects include dizziness, nervousness, and headache. Unlike other methods of contraception, this method cannot be stopped immediately if problems arise, and the drug and its side effects may linger for up to 6 months after the last shot. Also, after the final injection, it may take women who wish to get pregnant up to a year to conceive.

## Contraceptive Implants

A single-rod implantable contraceptive, Implanon, is a small (about the size of a matchstick) soft plastic capsule that is inserted just beneath the skin on the inner side of a woman's upper underarm by a health care provider. Implanon continually releases a low, steady dose of progestin for up to 3 years, suppressing ovulation during that time.

**Advantages** After insertion, Implanon is generally not visible, making it a discreet method of birth control. The main advantages of Implanon are that it is highly effective (99.95%), it is not subject to user error, and it needs to be replaced only once every 3 years. It has similar benefits as other progestin-only forms of contraception, including the lightening or cessation of menstrual periods, the lack of estrogen-related side effects, and safety for use by breast-feeding women. Fertility usually returns quickly after removal of the implant.

**Disadvantages** Insertion and removal of Implanon must be performed by a clinician. There is a higher initial cost for this method, and it may not be covered by all health plans. Potential minor side effects include irritation, allergic reaction, swelling, or scarring around the area of insertion, and there is also a possibility of infection or complications with removal. As with other progestin-only contraceptives, users can experience irregular bleeding. Implanon offers no protection against transmission of STIs, and it may require a backup method during the first week of use.

# Intrauterine Contraceptives

The **intrauterine device (IUD)** is a small plastic, flexible device, with a nylon string attached, that is placed in the uterus through the cervix and left there for 5 to 10 years at a time. The exact mechanism by which it works is not clearly understood, but researchers believe IUDs affect the way sperm and egg move, thereby preventing fertilization and/or affecting the lining of the uterus to prevent a fertilized ovum from implanting. The IUD was once extremely popular in the United States; however, most brands were removed from the market because of serious complications such as pelvic inflammatory disease and infertility. Worldwide, the IUD is again very popular, but has not experienced the same resurgence of popularity among U.S. women.

## ParaGard and Mirena IUDs

Two IUDs are currently available in the United States. *ParaGard* is a T-shaped plastic device with copper wrapped around the shaft. It does not contain any hormones and can be left in place for 10 years before replacement. A newer IUD, *Mirena*, is effective for 5 years and releases small amounts of progestin. A physician must

Mirena IUD is a flexible plastic device inserted by a clinician into a woman's uterus, where it releases progestin for up to 5 years.

fit and insert an IUD. One or two strings extend from the IUD into the vagina so the user can check to make sure that her IUD is in place. The device is removed by a practitioner when desired.

**Advantages** The IUD is a safe, discreet, and highly effective method of birth control (99.4%). It is effective immediately and needs to be replaced only every 10 years (ParaGard) or every 5 years (Mirena). ParaGard has the benefit of containing no hormones at all, and so having none of the potential negative health impacts of hormonal contraceptives (this also makes it an especially environmentally friendly form of birth control—see the **Be Healthy, Be Green** box on page 182). Mirena, on the other hand, probably offers some of the same potential health benefits as other progestin-only methods. Both IUDs can be used by breast-feeding women. With Mirena, periods become lighter or stop altogether. The IUDs are fully reversible; after removal, there is usually no delay in return of fertility. Both of these methods offer sexual spontaneity, as there is no need to keep supplies on hand or to interrupt lovemaking. The devices begin working immediately and there is a low incidence of side effects. The IUD can be removed at any time by a clinician.

> **intrauterine device (IUD)** A device, often T-shaped, that is implanted in the uterus to prevent pregnancy.
> **emergency contraceptive pills (ECPs)** Drugs taken within 3 days after unprotected intercourse to prevent fertilization or implantation.

**Disadvantages** Disadvantages of IUDs include possible discomfort, cost of insertion, and potential complications. Also, the IUD does not protect against STIs. In some women, the device can cause heavy menstrual flow and severe cramps for the first few months. With Mirena, menstrual periods tend to become shorter and lighter over time. Other side effects include acne, headaches, nausea, breast tenderness, mood changes, uterine cramps, and backache, which seems to occur most often in women who have never been pregnant. Women using IUDs have a higher risk of benign ovarian cysts. The devices are not usually recommended for use by women who have never had children because of an increased incidence of side effects and risk of infection with possible resultant infertility.

# Emergency Contraception

Emergency contraception is the use of a contraceptive to prevent pregnancy after unprotected intercourse, a sexual assault, or the failure of another birth control method. Combination estrogen-progestin pills and progestin-only pills are two common types of **emergency contraceptive pills (ECPs).**

# BE HEALTHY, BE GREEN

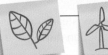

## What's the Most Environmentally Friendly Form of Contraceptive?

There must be a "green" form of contraceptive, right? This seems like a simple question, until you factor in what actually makes a form of birth control environmentally friendly. For it's not just about how much trash, including wrappers and dispensers, a given contraceptive generates, it's also about how effective that birth control is at preventing pregnancy, and thus the birth of another resource-using human being. You also have to think about whether the contraceptive is going to protect you against sexually transmitted infections (STIs), because, for the sake of Earth's health, you don't want to contract and spread communicable diseases.

You might think that because they are reusable, barrier forms of birth control such as the diaphragm would be the most "green." With a typical-use failure rate of 16 percent, though, the chances of pregnancy are great relative to other methods. And diaphragms don't provide protection against all STIs.

OK, then how about condoms? Male condoms are 85 percent effective against pregnancy with typical use. That's a better rate, but condoms aren't reusable. However, they take up only a tiny amount of space in the landfill, and latex condoms are said to be biodegradable with time. When you weigh the minuscule amounts of landfill they take up against the enormous amount of emissions a new human would create, the condom looks pretty good. In addition, they protect well against STIs. Just be sure not to flush condoms down the toilet. They might clog up your plumbing, and flushing also increases the chances that your condom may end up littering a beach or polluting the ocean.

What about hormonal methods such as birth control pills, injections, patches, rings, implants, and some intrauterine devices (IUDs)? Do they affect the environment? There's been quite a lot of research and debate about whether the progestins and estrogen in birth control—known in environmental circles as "endocrine disruptors"—can be damaging to the environment and to the health of others. Like many medications, these hormones can end up in our waterways—primarily through excretion (women pass some of the hormones in their urine), but also through improper disposal (i.e., flushing unused medication down a toilet). Once the hormones are in the waterways, they may cause harm to wildlife. For example, scientists in Washington State and Ontario, Canada, among other places, have discovered that fish in the waterways are displaying abnormalities—most notably, male fish are showing female characteristics. These abnormalities have been linked again and again to the hormone estrogen leaking into the water through sewage treatment systems.

Given these concerns, hormonal methods may not seem very environmentally friendly. Still, hormonal methods of birth control can be very effective in preventing pregnancy (92% with typical use)—and curtailing unintended pregnancies and overpopulation is the biggest environmental benefit of any birth control method. And women excrete natural estrogens in their urine, too, meaning that eliminating hormonal contraceptives wouldn't stop all estrogens from ending up in our

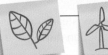

The copper-bearing IUD, ParaGard, is one of the most environmentally friendly birth control options.

waterways—the only way to do that would be installing better sewage treatment systems. So, if you feel that the ease of use and reliability of hormonal methods make them the best birth control option for you at this time in your life, it's probably best to go ahead and use them. Remember, though, hormonal methods do not protect against STIs.

Probably the best reversible method of birth control, from an environmental standpoint, is the copper IUD. It's made from a plentiful resource, it lasts 10 years, and it's 99 percent effective with typical use. However, it may not be a good option for everyone; in women who have not given birth, there is a greater chance of them naturally expelling the IUD, which obviously makes it ineffective. The IUD also offers no protection against STIs.

From an environmental point of view, sterilization is a great option: no waste, except whatever waste there is from the one-time surgical procedure, and no new humans to create an environmental impact. But, if your reproductive years are ahead of you, the chances are that's not an attractive option right now, as it's permanent. And no, it doesn't protect you against STIs!

What's the bottom line? Given that overpopulation is one of the greatest environmental problems facing the world today, simply using contraceptives at all is an environmentally sound choice when you are not ready to have a child. So use whichever method is best for you and your health, but use SOMETHING!

**Sources:** M. Kuster, M. López de Alda, and D. Barceló, "Estrogens and Progestogens in Wastewater, Sludge, Sediments, and Soil," in *Water Pollution: Emerging Organic Pollution in Waste Waters and Sludge,* vol. 2 (Heidelberg: Springer Berlin, 2005),1–24; A. Filby et al., "Health Impacts of Estrogens in the Environment, Considering Complex Mixture Effects," *Environmental Health Perspectives* 115, no. 12 (2007): 1704–10; K. Kidd et al., "Collapse of a Fish Population after Exposure to a Synthetic Estrogen," *Proceedings of the National Academy of Sciences* 104, no. 21 (2007): 8897–901.

Pills used for emergency contraception are sometimes referred to as "morning-after pills." They are not the same as the "abortion pill," although the two are often confused. Emergency contraception contains the same type of hormones as regular birth control pills and is used after unprotected intercourse but before a woman misses her period. A woman taking ECPs does so to prevent pregnancy; the method will not work if she is already pregnant, nor will it harm an existing pregnancy. In contrast, Mifeprex or mifepristone (formerly known as RU-486), the *early abortion pill,* is used to terminate a pregnancy that is already established—it is taken after a woman is sure she is pregnant, having already taken a pregnancy test with a positive result. It and other methods of abortion are discussed in more detail later in the chapter.

The ECPs prevent pregnancy the same way as other hormonal contraceptives: They delay or inhibit ovulation, inhibit fertilization, or block implantation of a fertilized egg, depending on the phase of the woman's menstrual cycle. Although ECPs use the same hormones as birth control pills, not all brands of birth control pills can be used for emergency contraception. When taken within 24 hours, ECPs reduce the risk of pregnancy by up to 95 percent; when taken 2 to 5 days later, ECPs reduce the risk of pregnancy by 75 to 89 percent.[7]

In August 2006, the FDA approved the over-the-counter sale of Plan B, one brand of emergency contraceptive pills, in the United States to women aged 18 and older. The age limit has since been lowered to 17; for women under 17, a prescription is still required. Nine states have enacted laws that permit a pharmacist to provide emergency contraception to customers under 17 without a prescription under certain conditions; seven states have laws allowing pharmacists to distribute it to minors if they are working in collaboration with a physician under state-approved protocols.[8]

Plan B is a progestin-only pill whose first dose should be taken as soon as possible (but not later than 120 hours, or 5 days) after unprotected intercourse. A second pill follows 12 hours after the first pill. Next Choice is a generic equivalent of Plan B now available for sale over the counter. Overall, Plan B and Next Choice reduce pregnancy risk by about as much as other ECPs that require a prescription. Although Plan B is still available at some pharmacies and health centers, it is being phased out and replaced by Plan B One-Step, which contains only 1 pill.

Widespread availability of emergency contraception has the potential to significantly affect the rates of unintended pregnancies and abortions, particularly among teenagers. In 2006, the rate of teen pregnancy in the United States began to increase for the first time in decades, reaching a rate of over 42 per 1,000 before declining again in 2008.[9] Researchers estimate that widespread use of ECPs could prevent 1.7 million unintended pregnancies and 800,000 abortions each year in the United States.[10] Although ECPs are no substitute for taking proper precautions before having sex (such as using latex condoms with a spermicide), their potential for reducing the rate of unintended pregnancy and ultimately abortion is very strong. According to recent surveys, 67 percent of all college health centers provide emergency contraception and 13.4 percent of sexually active college students reported using (or reported their partner had used) it within the past school year.[11]

# Behavioral Methods

Some methods of contraception rely on one or both partners altering their sexual behavior. In general, these methods require more self-control, diligence, and commitment, making them more prone to user error than hormonal and barrier methods.

## Withdrawal

**Withdrawal,** also called *coitus interruptus,* involves removing the penis from the vagina just prior to ejaculation. In the 2009 American Health College Association's National College Heath Assessment (ACHA-NCHA), approximately 26 percent of respondents reported that withdrawal was their method of birth control the last time they had sexual intercourse.[12] This statistic is startlingly high, considering the very high risk of pregnancy or contracting an STI associated with this method of birth control.

**withdrawal** A method of contraception that involves withdrawing the penis from the vagina before ejaculation; also called *coitus interruptus.*

### Advantages and Disadvantages Although withdrawal can be practiced when there is absolutely no other contraceptive available, it is highly unreliable, even with "perfect" use, because there can be up to half a million sperm in the drop of fluid at the tip of the penis *before* ejaculation. Timing withdrawal is also difficult, and males concentrating on accurate timing may not be able to relax and enjoy intercourse. Withdrawal offers no protection against the transmission of STIs and requires a high degree of self-control, experience, and trust.

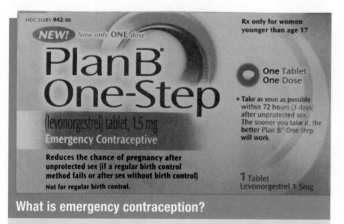

NDC 51285-942-88
Rx only for women younger than age 17
NEW! Now only ONE dose
**Plan B One-Step**
(levonorgestrel) tablet, 1.5 mg
Emergency Contraceptive
Reduces the chance of pregnancy after unprotected sex (if a regular birth control method fails or after sex without birth control)
Not for regular birth control.
One Tablet One Dose
• Take as soon as possible within 72 hours (3 days) after unprotected sex. The sooner you take it, the better Plan B° One-Step will work.
1 Tablet
Levonorgestrel 1.5mg

**What is emergency contraception?**

Emergency contraception is the use of a contraceptive—usually hormone-containing pills—after an act of unprotected intercourse. Plan B One-Step and Next Choice are the two brands of emergency contraceptive currently available without a prescription to American consumers aged 17 or older. When taken within 120 hours of unprotected intercourse, they reduce the risk of pregnancy by 75 to 89%.

# Abstinence and "Outercourse"

Strictly defined, *abstinence* means "deliberately avoiding intercourse." This definition would allow one to engage in such forms of sexual intimacy as massage, kissing, and solitary masturbation. However, many people today have broadened the definition of abstinence to include all forms of sexual contact, even those that do not culminate in sexual intercourse. Couples who go a step further than massage and kissing and engage in activities such as oral–genital sex and mutual masturbation are sometimes said to be engaging in "outercourse."

**Advantages and Disadvantages** Abstinence is the only method of avoiding pregnancy that is 100 percent effective. It is also the only method that is 100 percent effective against transmitting disease. Like abstinence, outercourse can be 100 percent effective for birth control as long as the male does not ejaculate near the vaginal opening. Unlike abstinence, however, outercourse is not 100 percent effective against STIs. Oral–genital contact can transmit disease, although the practice can be made safer by using a condom on the penis or a latex barrier, such as a dental dam, on the vaginal opening. Both abstinence and outercourse may be difficult for couples to sustain over long periods of time.

# Fertility Awareness Methods

**Fertility awareness methods (FAMs)** of birth control rely on altering sexual behavior during certain times of the month (Figure 6.5). These techniques require observing female fertile periods and abstaining from sexual intercourse (or any penis–vagina contact) during these times.

**fertility awareness methods (FAMs)** Several types of birth control that require alteration of sexual behavior rather than chemical or physical intervention in the reproductive process.

Fertility awareness methods rely on knowledge of basic physiology. A released ovum can survive for up to 48 hours after ovulation. Sperm can live for as long as 5 days in the vagina. Natural methods of birth control teach women to recognize their fertile times. Some of the more common forms include the following:

● **Cervical mucus method.** The cervical mucus method requires women to examine the consistency and color of their normal vaginal secretions. Prior to ovulation, vaginal mucus becomes gelatinous and stretchy, and normal vaginal secretions may increase. To prevent pregnancy, partners must avoid sexual activity involving penis–vagina contact while this mucus is present and for several days afterward.

● **Body temperature method.** The body temperature method relies on the fact that the woman's basal body temperature rises between 0.4 and 0.8 degree after ovulation has occurred. For this method to be effective, the woman must chart her temperature for several months to learn to recognize her body's temperature fluctuations. To prevent pregnancy, partners must abstain from penis–vagina contact before the temperature rise until several days after the temperature rise is observed.

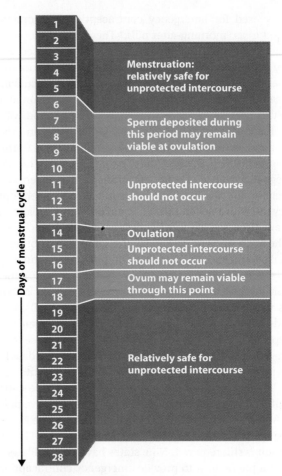

FIGURE 6.5 **The Fertility Cycle**
Fertility awareness methods (FAMs) can combine the use of a calendar, the cervical mucus method, and body temperature measurements to identify the fertile period. It is important to remember that most women do not have a consistent 28-day cycle.

● **Calendar method.** The calendar method requires the woman to record the exact number of days in her menstrual cycle. Because few women menstruate with complete regularity, this method involves keeping a record of the menstrual cycle for 12 months, during which time some other method of birth control must be used. This method assumes that ovulation occurs during the midpoint of the cycle. To prevent pregnancy, the couple must abstain from penis–vagina contact during the fertile time.

**Advantages and Disadvantages** Fertility awareness methods are the only forms of birth control that comply with certain religious teachings, including those of the Roman Catholic Church. They don't require a medical visit or prescription, and there are no negative health effects. Women who are untrained in these techniques run a high risk of unintended pregnancy; anyone interested in using them is advised to take a class. Classes are often offered for free by health centers and churches, and there is only minimal expense for supplies. The effectiveness of fertility awareness methods depends on diligence, commitment, and self-discipline; they are only 75 percent effective with typical use. These methods offer no STI protection, and they may not work for women with irregular menstrual cycles.

# Surgical Methods

In the United States, **sterilization** has become the second leading method of contraception for women of all ages and the leading method of contraception among married women.[13] Because sterilization is permanent, anyone considering it should think through possibilities such as divorce and remarriage or a future improvement in financial status that might make a pregnancy realistic or desirable.

## Female Sterilization

One method of sterilization for women is **tubal ligation,** a surgical procedure in which the fallopian tubes are sealed shut to block sperms' access to released eggs (see Figure 6.6). The operation is usually done laparoscopically in a hospital on an outpatient basis. The procedure usually takes less than an hour, and the patient is generally allowed to return home within a short time.

A tubal ligation does not affect ovarian and uterine function. The woman's menstrual cycle continues, and released eggs simply disintegrate and are absorbed by the lymphatic system. As soon as her incision heals, the woman may resume sexual intercourse with no fear of pregnancy.

A newer sterilization procedure, Essure, involves the placement of small microcoils into the fallopian tubes via the vagina. The entire procedure takes about 35 minutes and can be performed in a physician's office. Once in place, the microcoils expand to the shape of the fallopian tubes. The coils promote the growth of scar tissue around the device and lead to the fallopian tubes becoming blocked. Like traditional forms of tubal ligation, Essure is permanent. It is recommended for women who cannot have a tubal ligation because of chronic health conditions such as obesity or heart disease.

Adiana is another new, minimally invasive method of blocking a woman's fallopian tubes. A small flexible instrument is used to place a soft insert about the size of a grain of rice into each fallopian tube. The body's tissue begins to grow on and around the insert and eventually blocks the fallopian tubes. The insertion can be performed in a clinician's office in about 15 minutes.

A **hysterectomy,** or removal of the uterus, is a method of sterilization requiring major surgery. It is usually done only when a woman's uterus is diseased or damaged.

**sterilization** Permanent fertility control achieved through surgical procedures.
**tubal ligation** Sterilization of the woman that involves the cutting and tying off or cauterizing of the fallopian tubes.
**hysterectomy** Surgical removal of the uterus.
**vasectomy** Sterilization of the man that involves the cutting and tying off of both vasa deferentia.

**Advantages** The main advantage to female sterilization is that it is highly effective and permanent. After the one-time expense and operation or procedure, there is no other cost or ongoing action required. Sterilization has no negative effect on a woman's sex drive. A potential advantage of the Essure and Adiana methods is that they do not require an incision.

**Disadvantages** As with any surgery, there are risks involved with a tubal ligation. Although rare, possible complications include infection, pulmonary embolism, hemorrhage, anesthesia complications, and ectopic pregnancy. Essure and Adiana do not require an incision, so the immediate risks are lower; however, because these are relatively new techniques, the long-term risks are unknown. Sterilization offers no protection against STI transmission, and is initially expensive. The procedure is permanent and should be used only if both partners are certain they do not want more children.

## Male Sterilization

Sterilization in men is less complicated than it is in women. A **vasectomy** is frequently done on an outpatient basis, using a local anesthetic (see Figure 6.7). This procedure involves making a small incision in the side of the scrotum to expose a vas deferens, cutting the vas deferens and either tying off or cauterizing the ends, then repeating this on the other side.

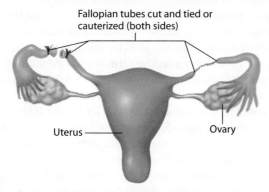

Fallopian tubes cut and tied or cauterized (both sides)

Uterus

Ovary

**FIGURE** 6.6 **Female Sterilization: Tubal Ligation**
In a tubal ligation, both fallopian tubes are cut and tied or sealed shut. This surgery is usually performed laparoscopically.

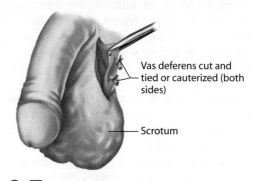

Vas deferens cut and tied or cauterized (both sides)

Scrotum

**FIGURE** 6.7 **Male Sterilization: Vasectomy**
In a vasectomy, the surgeon makes an incision in the scrotum, then locates and cuts the vasa deferentia, either sealing or tying both sides shut.

Many men are reluctant to consider sterilization because they fear the operation will affect their sexual performance. However, a vasectomy in no way affects sexual response. Because sperm constitute only a small percentage of the semen, the amount of ejaculate is not changed significantly. The testes continue to produce sperm, but the sperm can no longer enter the ejaculatory duct. Any sperm that are manufactured disintegrate and are absorbed into the lymphatic system.

**Advantages** A vasectomy is a highly effective and permanent means of preventing pregnancy: After 1 year, the pregnancy rate in women whose partners have had vasectomies is 0.15 percent.[14] A vasectomy is a fairly simple outpatient procedure requiring minimal recovery time, and after the one-time expense and operation, there is no other cost or ongoing action required. A vasectomy has no negative effect on a man's sex drive or sexual performance.

**Disadvantages** In addition to its initial expense, male sterilization offers no protection against STI transmission. Also, a vasectomy is not immediately effective in preventing pregnancy. Because sperm are stored in other areas of the reproductive system besides the vasa deferentia, couples must use alternative methods of birth control for at least 1 month after the vasectomy. The man must check with his physician (who will do a semen analysis) to determine when unprotected intercourse can take place. As with any surgery, there are some risks involved with a vasectomy. In a small percentage of cases, serious complications occur, such as formation of a blood clot in the scrotum, infection, or inflammatory reactions. Very infrequently the vas deferens may create a new path, negating the procedure.

# Choosing a Method of Contraception

With all the options available, how does a person or a couple decide what method of contraception is best? Take some time to research the various methods, ask questions of your health care provider, and be honest with yourself about your own preferences. Questions to ask yourself are included below. Also, see the **Student Health Today** box on page 188 for tips on talking about contraception with your partner.

● **How comfortable would I be using a particular method?** If you aren't at ease with a method, you may not use it consistently, and it probably will not be a reliable choice for you. Think about whether the method may cause discomfort for you or your partner, and consider your own comfort level with touching your body. For women, some methods, such as the diaphragm, sponge, or NuvaRing, require inserting an apparatus into the vagina and taking it out. For men, using a condom requires rolling it onto the penis.

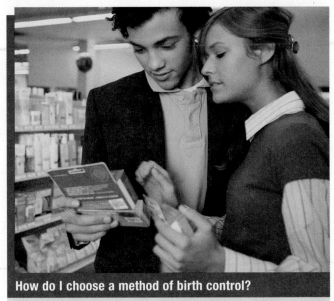

**How do I choose a method of birth control?**

There are many different methods of birth control on the market: barrier methods, hormonal methods, surgical methods, and other options. When you choose a method, you'll need to consider several factors, including cost, comfort level, convenience, and health risks. All of these factors together will influence your ability to consistently and correctly use the contraceptive and prevent unwanted pregnancy.

● **Will this method be convenient for me and my partner?** Some methods require more effort than do others. Be honest with yourself about how likely you are to use the method consistently. Are you willing to interrupt lovemaking, to abstain from sex during certain times of the month, or to take a pill every day? You may feel condoms are easy and convenient to use, or you may prefer something that requires little ongoing thought, such as Depo-Provera or an IUD.

● **Am I at risk for the transmission of STIs?** If you have multiple sex partners or are uncertain about the sexual history or disease status of your current sex partner, then you are at risk for transmission of STIs and HIV. Latex and polyurethane condoms (both male and female) are the *only* birth control method that protects against STIs and HIV (although some other barrier methods offer limited protection). They reduce your risk of STIs as well as HIV. Condoms alone are not a highly effective birth control method; to avoid both STI infection and pregnancy, combine a condom with a more effective birth control method.

● **Do I want to have a biological child in the future?** If you are unsure about your plans for future childbearing, you should use a temporary birth control method, rather than a permanent one such as sterilization. Keep in mind that you may regret choosing a permanent method if you are young, if you have few or no children, if you are choosing this method because your partner wants you to, or if you believe this option will fix relationship problems. If you know you want to have children in the future, consider how soon that will be, as some methods, such as Depo-Provera, will cause a delay in return to fertility.

- **How would an unplanned pregnancy affect my life?** If an unplanned pregnancy would be a potentially devastating event for you, or would have a serious impact on your plans for the future, then you should choose a highly effective birth control method, for example, the pill, patch, ring, implant, or IUD. If, however, you are in a stable relationship, have a reliable source of income, are planning to have children in the future, and would embrace a pregnancy should it occur now, then you may be comfortable with a less reliable method such as the diaphragm, cervical cap, or spermicides.
- **What are my religious and moral values?** Fertility awareness methods are a good option if you are morally or spiritually opposed to using certain other birth control methods. When both partners are motivated to use these methods, they can be successful at preventing unintended pregnancy. If you are considering this option, sign up for a class to get specific training using the method effectively.
- **How much will the birth control method cost?** Some contraceptive methods involve an initial outlay of money and few continuing costs (e.g., sterilization, IUD), whereas others are fairly inexpensive but must be purchased repeatedly (e.g., condoms, spermicides, monthly pill prescriptions). You should consider whether a method will be cost effective for you in the long run. Remember that any prescription methods require routine checkups, which may involve some cost to you.
- **Do I have any health factors that could limit my choice?** Hormonal birth control methods can pose potential health risks to women with certain preexisting conditions, such as high blood pressure, a history of stroke or blood clots, liver disease, migraines, or diabetes. You should discuss this issue with your health care provider when considering birth control methods. In addition, women who smoke or are over the age of 35 are at risk from complications of combination hormonal contraceptives. Breast-feeding women can use progestin-only methods, but should avoid methods containing estrogen. Men and women with latex allergies may need to use polyurethane or plastic barrier methods.
- **Are there any additional benefits I'd like to get from my contraceptive?** Hormonal birth control methods can have desirable secondary effects, such as the reduction of acne and the lessening of premenstrual symptoms. Certain pills are marketed as having specific effects, so it is possible to choose one that is known to clear skin or reduce mood changes caused by menstruation. Hormonal birth control methods are also associated with reduced risks of certain cancers. Extended-cycle pills and some progestin-only methods cause menstrual periods to be less frequent or to stop altogether, which some women find desirable. Condoms carry the added health benefit of protecting against STIs.

## what do you think?

Who do you think is responsible for deciding which method of contraception should be used in a sexual relationship? ● What are some examples of good opportunities for you and your partner to discuss contraceptives? ● What do you think are the biggest barriers in our society to the use of condoms?

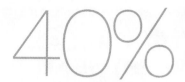 **of pregnancies that occur each year are unintended.**

# Abortion

Women obtain abortions for a variety of reasons. The vast majority of abortions occur because of unintended pregnancies.[15] As we know, even the best birth control methods can fail. In addition, some pregnancies are terminated because they are a consequence of rape or incest. Other reasons commonly cited are not being ready financially or emotionally to care for a child at that time.[16] When an unwanted pregnancy does occur, a woman must decide whether to terminate it, carry it to term and keep the baby, or carry it to term and give the baby up for adoption. This is a personal decision that each woman must make, based on her personal beliefs, values, and resources, and after carefully considering all alternatives.

In 1973, the landmark U.S. Supreme Court decision in *Roe v. Wade* stated that the "right to privacy . . . founded on the Fourteenth Amendment's concept of personal liberty . . . is broad enough to encompass a woman's decision whether or not to terminate her pregnancy."[17] The decision maintained that during the first trimester of pregnancy, a woman and her practitioner have the right to terminate the pregnancy through **abortion** without legal restrictions. It allowed individual states to set conditions for second-trimester abortions. Third-trimester abortions were ruled illegal unless the mother's life or health was in danger. Prior to the legalization of first- and second-trimester abortions, women wishing to terminate a pregnancy had to travel to a country where the procedure was legal, consult an illegal abortionist, or perform their own abortions. These procedures sometimes led to death from hemorrhage or infection, or infertility from internal scarring.

**abortion** The termination of a pregnancy by expulsion or removal of an embryo or fetus from the uterus.

## The Debate over Abortion

Abortion is a highly charged and politically thorny issue in American society. Pro-choice individuals feel that it is a woman's right to make decisions about her own body and health, including the decision to continue or terminate a pregnancy. On the other side of the issue, pro-life individuals believe that the embryo or fetus is a human being with rights that must be protected. The political debate continues as pro-life groups lobby for laws prohibiting the use of public funds for abortion and abortion counseling at the same time that pro-choice groups lobby for laws that make abortions more widely available. At times, violence has arisen as a result of this controversy, in the form of attacks on clinics or on individual physicians who perform abortions.

In recent years, new legislation has given states the right to impose certain restrictions on abortions. The procedure

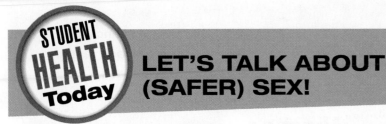
# LET'S TALK ABOUT (SAFER) SEX!

Communication is key to a healthy relationship, and it is especially so between those who are sexually intimate. It can be challenging to talk to your partner about using protection during sexual activity, but don't let embarrassment put your health at risk. The person that you're thinking about having sex with may or may not initially agree about using a condom or dental dam, so it's helpful to be prepared to discuss your concerns ahead of time. Research shows that individuals who set aside the time to have a conversation about safer sex are more likely to use condoms or dental dams during sexual activity. Remember: Communicating about sex is all about getting the most from your sex life, and getting it safely.

## WHY COMMUNICATING ABOUT SEX IS ESSENTIAL

Open sexual health communication is a sign of care and respect for your own body and your partner's. It empowers both of you to be assertive about your individual needs, likes, limits, and desires in the sexual relationship. Open communication also creates a safe environment to ask about your partner's sexual history, sexually transmitted infection (STI) testing, and sexual expectations.

You may feel awkward or uncomfortable discussing sex, and you may believe that talking beforehand ruins the naturalness or spontaneity of sex. Some people are concerned that their partner will misinterpret the conversation and feel accused of infidelity, distrust, promiscuity, or lack of love in the relationship. Try to address these concerns in an honest and open manner. And remember: Sexual communication is about protecting *both* of your bodies and ensuring that you are clear about your needs and concerns.

If you are afraid that talking about sex beforehand is going to make your partner think you don't trust him or her, take some time to examine the strength of your relationship. Trust is about being open and honest. If you're afraid to talk with your partner, the chances are you actually don't trust your partner and you might be better off with a partner you do trust.

## FINDING THE TIME AND PLACE FOR SEXUAL COMMUNICATION

Before you talk with your partner, it's a good idea to talk with your health care provider about your options for practicing safer sex.

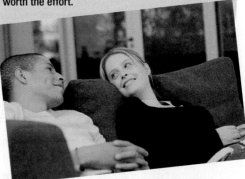

Don't let embarrassment put your health at risk! Talking about safer sex may be tough, but it is worth the effort.

Remember, you need to think about getting pregnant *and* avoiding STIs.

With your partner, try to find a time and place where you are both comfortable, free of distractions, and you have time to have a full conversation. It's generally better to have this conversation outside of the bedroom, so that you're not pressured by the heat of the moment to do things you don't want to do.

## FINDING THE WORDS FOR CONDOM/DENTAL DAM NEGOTIATION

In the table below are some examples of how you can address the potential excuses from your partner when you talk about using a condom or dental dam.

| Excuse | Answer |
|---|---|
| *Don't you trust me?* | *It's not an issue of trust; people can have sexually transmitted infections and not know it.* |
| *It doesn't feel as good with a condom/dental dam.* | *I'll feel more relaxed; if I'm more relaxed, I can make it feel better for you. We can also use lubricant to increase sensation for both of us.* |
| *I don't have a condom with me.* | *I do.* |
| *It's up to you.* | *It's your health. It should be your decision, too.* |
| *I'm on the pill; you don't need a condom.* | *I'd like to use one anyway. It will help to protect us from infections that we may not know we have.* |
| *Putting it on interrupts everything.* | *Not if I help put it on.* |
| *I guess you don't really love me.* | *I do, but I'm not willing to risk our futures to prove it.* |
| *I will pull out in time.* | *Pre-ejaculate can still cause pregnancy and spread STIs.* |
| *I'm allergic to latex.* | *No problem, Student Health Services has a wide assortment of nonlatex condoms and dental dams available FREE of charge.* |
| *But I love you.* | *Then you'll help us protect ourselves.* |
| *Just this once.* | *Once is all it takes.* |

*(continued)*

Although there is no perfect response for every situation, these may provide you the tools necessary for effective sexual health negotiation.

**TIPS TO BOOST YOUR CONFIDENCE IN NEGOTIATING SAFER SEX**

✳ It can be helpful to have condoms and/or dental dams around, so when things start to really heat up you will be ready.

✳ Talk to your partner about using protection before getting intimate. This will help both of you be more comfortable and prepared to use a condom or dental dam when the time comes.

✳ Practice makes perfect. The best way to learn how to use condoms correctly and guarantee their effectiveness is to practice putting them on yourself or your partner. A staggering 98 percent of all "condom malfunctions" (breaks, leaks, tears, slips) are due to user error. The two most essential keys to using a condom are *consistently* and *correctly*.

✳ If you are concerned about the interruption of using either condoms or dental dams, try to incorporate them into your foreplay. By helping your partner put on protection together, you both will stay aroused and in the moment.

**Sources:** M. K. Casey, L. Timmermann, M. Allen, S. Krahn, and K. L. Turkiewicz, "Response and Self-Efficacy in Condom Use: A Meta-Analysis of This Important Element of AIDS Education and Prevention," *Southern Communication Journal* 74, no. 1 (2009): 57–78; A. G. Lam, A. Mak, P. D. Lindsay, and S. T. Russell, "What Really Works? An Exploratory Study of Condom Negotiation Strategies," *AIDS Education and Prevention* 16, no. 2 (2004): 160–71.

cannot be performed in publicly funded clinics in some states, and other states have laws requiring parental notification before a teenager can obtain an abortion. In 2009, 14 states and the District of Columbia enacted 21 pro-choice measures, and another 14 states enacted 29 anti-choice measures. However, 17 states and the District of Columbia currently use public funds for women in poverty who seek an abortion.[18]

On the federal level, the U.S. Congress has banned access to abortion for virtually all women who receive health care through the federal government. Since the Federal Abortion Ban was signed in 2003, it has been challenged by the American Civil Liberties Union (ACLU), the National Abortion Federation, Planned Parenthood, and the Center for Reproductive Rights in federal courts across the country on the grounds that it is unconstitutional. The two main reasons for these claims are that the broad language could ban abortion as early as the twelfth week in pregnancy and that it does not include exceptions to protect women's health.[19] The U.S. Supreme Court struck down an identical law as unconstitutional in 2000, and the ban was found unconstitutional by six federal courts before the Supreme Court ruled in 2007 that the ban was constitutional and could be enforced.[20] This decision represented a monumental departure from prior cases, and with it the Court effectively eliminated one of *Roe v. Wade*'s core protections: that a woman's health must always be paramount. For a discussion of how contraception and abortion are perceived in different countries, see the **Health in a Diverse World** box on page 191.

## Emotional Aspects of Abortion

The best scientific evidence published indicates that among adult women who have an unplanned pregnancy, the risk of mental health problems is no greater if they have an abortion than if they deliver a baby. Although a variety of feelings such as regret, guilt, sadness, relief, and happiness are normal, no evidence has shown that an abortion causes long-term negative mental health outcomes.[21] Researchers found that the best predictor of a woman's emotional well-being following an abortion was her emotional well-being prior to the procedure.[22] The factors that place a woman at higher risk for negative psychological responses following an abortion include the following: perception of stigma, need for secrecy, low levels of social support for the abortion decision, prior history of mental health issues, low self-esteem, and avoidance and denial coping strategies.[23] The majority of women who have an abortion are able to view abortion as one of life's events. Certainly the presence of a support network and the assistance of mental health professionals are helpful to any woman who is struggling with the emotional aspects of her abortion decision.

## Methods of Abortion

The choice of abortion procedure is determined by how many weeks the woman has been pregnant. Length of pregnancy is calculated from the first day of her last menstrual period.

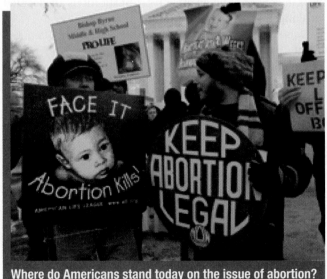

**Where do Americans stand today on the issue of abortion?**

Abortion continues to be a controversial and emotional issue in the United States. In recent polls, roughly 20% of the population have favored unrestricted access, 20% have favored a complete ban, and 60% have fallen somewhere between these two extremes.

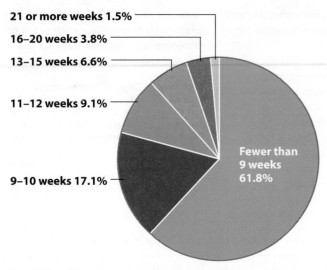

- 21 or more weeks 1.5%
- 16–20 weeks 3.8%
- 13–15 weeks 6.6%
- 11–12 weeks 9.1%
- 9–10 weeks 17.1%

Fewer than 9 weeks 61.8%

**FIGURE 6.8 When Women Have Abortions (in weeks from the last menstrual period)**

**Source:** Guttmacher Institute, *Facts on Induced Abortion in the United States, In Brief,* New York: Guttmacher Institute, 2010, www.guttmacher.org/pubs/fb_induced_abortion.pdf, Accessed May 6, 2010.

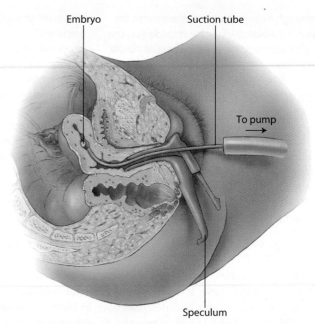

Embryo    Suction tube

To pump

Speculum

**FIGURE 6.9 Suction Curettage Abortion**
This procedure, in which a long tube with gentle suction is used to remove fetal tissue from the uterine walls, can be performed up to the twelfth week of pregnancy.

**Surgical Abortions** If performed during the first trimester of pregnancy, abortion presents a relatively low health risk to the mother. About 88 percent of abortions occur during the first 12 weeks of pregnancy (see **Figure 6.8**).[24] The most commonly used method of first-trimester abortion is **suction curettage** (Figure 6.9). Approximately 87 percent of abortions in the United States are done using this procedure, which is usually performed under a local anesthetic. The cervix is dilated with instruments or by placing laminaria, a sterile seaweed product, in the cervical canal. The laminaria is left in place for a few hours or overnight and slowly dilates the cervix. After it is removed, a long tube is inserted into the uterus through the cervix, and gentle suction removes fetal tissue from the uterine walls.

Pregnancies that progress into the second trimester (after week 12) can be terminated through **dilation and evacuation (D&E).** For this procedure, the cervix is dilated for 1 to 2 days, and a combination of instruments and vacuum aspiration is used to empty the uterus. Second-trimester abortions may be done under general anesthetic. The D&E can be performed on an outpatient basis (usually in the physician's office), with or without pain medication. Generally, however, the woman is given a mild tranquilizer to help her relax. This procedure may cause moderate to severe uterine cramping and blood loss. After a D&E, a return visit to the clinician is an important follow-up.

**suction curettage** An abortion technique that uses gentle suction to remove fetal tissue from the uterus.

**dilation and evacuation (D&E)** An abortion technique that uses a combination of instruments and vacuum aspiration; fetal tissue is both sucked and scraped out of the uterus.

**induction abortion** An abortion technique in which chemicals are injected into the uterus through the uterine wall; labor begins, and the woman delivers a dead fetus.

**hysterotomy** The surgical removal of the fetus from the uterus.

**intact dilation and extraction (D&X)** A late-term abortion procedure in which the body of the fetus is extracted up to the head and then the contents of the cranium are aspirated.

Two other methods used in second-trimester abortions, although less common than D&E, are prostaglandin and saline **induction abortions.** Prostaglandin hormones or saline solution are injected into the uterus, which kills the fetus and initiates labor contractions. After 24 to 48 hours, the fetus and placenta are expelled from the uterus. A **hysterotomy,** or surgical removal of the fetus from the uterus, may be used during emergencies, when the mother's life is in danger, or when other types of abortions are deemed too dangerous.

One surgical method that abortion opponents target is **intact dilation and extraction (D&X),** sometimes referred to by the nonmedical term *partial-birth abortion.* The dilation and extraction procedure is used after 21 weeks of gestation. This procedure is rarely performed but is considered when other abortion methods could injure the mother and when there are severe fetal abnormalities. Two days before the procedure, laminaria is inserted vaginally to dilate the cervix. The water should break on the third day, and the woman should return to the clinic. The fetus is rotated to a breech (feet first) position, and forceps are used to pull the legs, shoulders, and arms through the birth canal. The head is collapsed to allow it to pass through the cervix. Then the fetus is completely removed.

The risks associated with surgical abortion include infection, incomplete abortion (when parts of the placenta remain in the uterus), missed abortion, excessive bleeding, and cervical and uterine trauma. Follow-up and attention to danger signs decrease the chances of long-term problems.

The mortality rate for women undergoing first-trimester abortions in the United States averages 1 death per every

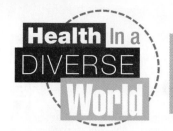
## CONTRACEPTIVE USE AND THE INCIDENCE OF ABORTION WORLDWIDE

Approximately 208 million pregnancies occur throughout the world every year, more than a third of which are unintended. Worldwide, about one-fifth of all pregnancies end in induced abortion, although reports have indicated a decline in the overall number of abortions in recent decades. This decline has been greater in developed nations than it has in developing ones. In developed nations, where almost all abortions are safe and legal, the incidence of the procedure dropped from 39 per 1,000 women aged 15 to 44 in 1995 to 26 per 1,000 women aged 15 to 44 in 2003. In developing nations, the rate declined from 34 to 29 in the same period of time. The world's population is largely concentrated in developing nations, and consequently most abortions occur in those countries—35 million annually— often in places where abortion is illegal and access to contraception is limited.

The primary cause of abortion is unplanned pregnancy. Whether abortion is legal or not has little to do with its overall incidence. The abortion rate in Africa, where abortion is illegal in most countries, is the same as the rate in Europe, where abortion is generally legal. Abortions performed illegally are usually

unsafe; 70,000 women die of complications from unsafe abortions each year, nearly all in developing nations where abortion is illegal. Worldwide, 48 percent of all abortions are unsafe; however, only 8 percent of abortions in developed nations are unsafe, compared to 55 percent in developing nations.

When abortion is legalized in a country, it also becomes safer. For example, after expanding the legalization of abortion in 1996, South Africa experienced a 52 percent reduction in the incidence of infection resulting from abortion. The general global trend is to remove legal restrictions on abortion: Since 1995, 17 countries have liberalized their abortion laws, compared to only 3 countries that have tightened them.

Access to voluntary family planning services, including contraception, is essential in helping to reduce the number of unintended pregnancies and, consequently, the incidence of abortion. When modern contraceptives are unavailable, women often turn to abortion to end unwanted pregnancy. Countries where contraceptive use is most prevalent usually have lower abortion rates.

The lowest abortion rates are in western Europe, where abortion is legal and

contraceptives are widely accepted and available at low cost. In eastern Europe and the former Soviet Union, abortion rates were high throughout the cold war, when it was free and was the only reliable method of fertility control available to most women. Modern contraceptives manufactured in the West were not available to these women until the fall of the Soviet Union. Since that time, contraceptives have become prevalent in eastern Europe and the former Soviet bloc countries, such that the abortion rate dropped 50 percent between 1995 and 2003. However, because of economic pressure to keep families small, the ratio of abortions to live births in eastern Europe is still the highest in the world: 105 abortions for every 100 live births.

**Sources:** Guttmacher Institute and WHO, "Issues in Brief: Facts on Induced Abortion Worldwide," 2009, www.guttmacher.org/pubs/fb_IAW.html; S. Cohen, "Facts and Consequences: Legality, Incidence and Safety of Abortion Worldwide," *Guttmacher Policy Review* 12, no. 4 (2009); S. Cohen, "New Data on Abortion Incidence, Safety Illuminate Key Aspects of Worldwide Abortion Rate," *Guttmacher Policy Review* 10, no. 4 (2007); G. Sedgh et al., "Legal Abortions Worldwide: Incidence and Recent Trends," *International Family Planning Perspectives* 33, no. 3 (2007).

---

1,000,000 procedures at 8 or fewer weeks. The risk of death increases with the length of pregnancy. At 16 to 20 weeks, the mortality rate is 1 per 29,000; at 21 weeks or more, it increases to 1 per 11,000.[25] This higher rate later in the pregnancy is due to the increased risk of uterine perforation, bleeding, infection, and incomplete abortion; these things can happen because the uterine wall becomes thinner as the pregnancy progresses.

**Medical Abortions** Unlike surgical abortions, a **medical abortion** is performed without entering the uterus. Mifepristone, formerly known as RU-486 and currently sold in the United States under the brand name Mifeprex, is a steroid hormone that induces abortion by blocking the action of progesterone, the hormone produced by the ovaries and placenta that maintains the lining of the uterus. As a result, the

uterine lining and the embryo are expelled from the uterus, terminating the pregnancy.

Mifepristone's nickname, "the abortion pill," may imply an easy process. However, this treatment actually involves more steps than a suction curettage abortion, which takes approximately 15 minutes followed by a physical recovery of about 1 day. With mifepristone, a first visit to the clinic involves a physical exam and a dose of three tablets, which may cause minor side effects such as nausea, headaches, weakness, and fatigue. The patient returns 2 days later for a dose of prostaglandins (misoprostol; brand name Cytotec), which causes uterine contractions that expel the fertilized egg. The patient is required to stay under observation at the clinic for 4 hours and to make a follow-up visit 12 days later.[26]

**medical abortion** The termination of a pregnancy during its first 9 weeks using hormonal medications that cause the embryo to be expelled from the uterus.

Ninety-two percent of women who use mifepristone during the first 9 weeks of pregnancy will experience a complete abortion.[27] The side effects are similar to those reported during heavy menstruation and include cramping, minor pain, and nausea. Approximately 1 in 1,000 women requires a blood transfusion because of severe bleeding. The procedure does not require hospitalization; women may be treated on an outpatient basis.

# Planning a Pregnancy

The many methods available to control fertility give you choices that did not exist when your parents—and even you—were born. If you are in the process of deciding whether or not to have children, take the time to evaluate your emotions, finances, and physical health.

## Emotional Health

First and foremost, consider why you want to have a child. To fulfill an inner need to carry on the family? Because it's expected? Other reasons? Then, consider the responsibilities involved with becoming a parent. Are you ready to make all the sacrifices necessary to bear and raise a child? Can you care for this new human being in a loving and nurturing manner?

**preconception care** Medical care received prior to becoming pregnant that helps a woman assess and address potential maternal health issues.

If you feel that you are ready to be a parent, the next step is preparation. You can prepare for this change in your life in several ways: Read about parenthood, take classes, talk to parents of children of all ages, spend time with friends' children, and join a support group. If you choose to adopt, you will find many support groups available to you as well.

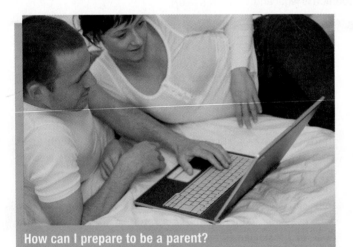

**How can I prepare to be a parent?**

Preparing to become a parent requires thoughtful evaluation of one's emotional, physical, social, and financial well-being. Both prospective mothers and prospective fathers should be willing to implement healthy change where needed to ready themselves for bringing a child into the world.

## Preparing for Pregnancy

Before becoming pregnant, parents-to-be should take stock of, and possibly improve, their own health to help ensure the health of their child. Among the most important factors to consider are the following:

### FOR WOMEN:
* If you smoke, drink alcohol, or use drugs, stop.
* Reduce or eliminate your caffeine intake.
* Maintain a healthy weight; lose or gain weight if necessary.
* Avoid X rays and environmental chemicals, such as lawn and garden herbicides and pesticides.
* Take prenatal vitamins, which are especially important in providing adequate folic acid.

### FOR MEN:
* If you smoke, quit.
* Drink alcohol only in moderation, and avoid drug use.
* Get checked for sexually transmitted infections and seek treatment if you have one.
* Avoid exposure to toxic chemicals in your work or home environment.
* Maintain a healthy weight; lose or gain weight if necessary.

## Maternal Health

Before becoming pregnant, a woman should have a thorough medical examination. **Preconception care** should include an assessment of potential complications that could occur during pregnancy. Medical problems such as diabetes and high blood pressure should be discussed, as well as any genetic disorders that run in the family. Additional suggestions for preparing for a healthy pregnancy can be found in the **Skills for Behavior Change** box above.

## Paternal Health

It is common wisdom that mothers-to-be should steer clear of toxic chemicals that can cause birth defects, should eat a healthy diet, and should stop smoking and drinking alcohol. Now, similar precautions are recommended for fathers-to-be. New research suggests that a man's exposure to chemicals influences not only his ability to father a child, but also the future health of his child.

Fathers-to-be have been overlooked in past preconception and prenatal studies for several reasons. Researchers assumed that the genetic damage leading to birth defects and other health problems occurred while a child was in the mother's womb or were caused by random errors of nature. After all, they reasoned, that's where embryonic and fetal development takes place. Conventional medical wisdom also held that defective-looking sperm (those with misshapen heads, crooked tails, or retarded swimming ability) were incapable of fertilizing an egg. However, scientists have recently discovered that how sperm look has little to do with how they act. Misshapen sperm can penetrate an egg, and they do not necessarily carry defective genetic goods. More-over, sperm that look healthy and swim well can be the true genetic culprits. DNA fluorescent markers have identified normal-looking, yet genetically flawed, sperm that carry too many or too few chromosomes. Fathers contribute the extra chromosome 21 in about 3 percent of children with Down syndrome, which causes mental retardation, and the extra X chromosome in 50 percent of boys with Klinefelter's syndrome, which causes abnormal sexual development.[28] Prader-Willi syndrome, a disorder characterized by retarda-tion and obesity, occurs because certain paternal genes that should be expressed are not.[29]

Although some birth defects are caused by random errors of nature, it now appears that some disorders can be traced to sperm damaged by chemicals. Sperm are naturally vulner-able to toxic assault and genetic damage. Many drugs and ingested chemicals can readily invade the testes from the bloodstream; others ambush sperm after they leave the testes and pass through the epididymides, where they mature and are stored. By one route or another, half of 100 chemicals studied so far (including by-products of cigarette smoke) apparently harm sperm.[30]

## Financial Evaluation

Finances are another important consideration. Are you pre-pared to go out to dinner less often, forgo a new pair of shoes, or drive an older car? These are important questions to ask yourself when considering the financial aspects of being a parent. Can you afford to give your child the life you would like him or her to enjoy?

First, check your medical insurance: Does it provide preg-nancy benefits? If not, you can expect to pay, on average, $14,000 for a normal delivery and up to $25,000 for a cesarean section birth. These costs don't include prenatal medical care, and complications can also increase the cost substantially. Both partners should investigate their employ-ers' policies concerning parental leave, including length of leave available and conditions for returning to work.

The U.S. Department of Agriculture estimates that it can cost between $11,610 and $13,480 annually for a middle-class married couple to raise a child (housing costs and food are the two largest expenditures).[31] These costs tend to increase with the age of the child. It is also more expensive to raise a child in the urban Northeast than in the South and rural areas. These figures do not include college, which can now run over $40,000 per year at a private institution, with room and board. Also consider the cost and availability of quality child care. How much family assistance can you realistically expect with a new baby, and is nonfamily child care available? How much does full-time child care cost? Prices vary by region and type of care. According to the National Association of Child Care Resource and Referral Agencies (NACCRRA), day care costs for an infant in the United States range from $4,560 to $15,895 a year.[32]

## Contingency Planning

A final consideration is how to provide for the child should something happen to you and your partner. If both of you were to die while the child is young, do you have relatives or close friends who would raise the child? If you have more than one child, would they have to be split up or could they be kept together? Although unpleasant to think about, this sort of contingency planning is crucial. Children who lose their parents are heartbroken and confused. A prearranged plan of action will smooth their transition into new families.

# Pregnancy

Pregnancy is an important event in a woman's life. The actions taken before, as well as behaviors engaged in during, pregnancy can significantly affect the health of both infant and mother.

## Preconception Care

Every woman should be thinking about her health whether or not she is planning a pregnancy. The birth of a healthy baby depends in part on the mother's preconception health. Preconception care focuses on the conditions and risk fac-tors that could affect a woman if she becomes pregnant, as well as the factors that can affect a fetus or infant. These include factors such as taking prescription drugs or drinking alcohol. The key to promoting preconception health is to combine the best medical care, healthy behaviors, strong support, and safe environments at home and at work.[33] Dur-ing a preconception care visit, a clinician talks with the woman about any conditions she might have, such as dia-betes or high blood presssure, and finds out whether the woman has had any problems with prior pregnancies. The clinician will check to make sure the woman's immuniza-tions are up to date, and will encourage her to eliminate alcohol consumption and tobacco use, and to follow a healthy diet.

Why is preconception care so important? Prenatal care, which usually begins at week 11 or 12 of a pregnancy, comes too late to prevent a number of serious maternal and child health problems in the United States. The fetus is most susceptible to developing certain problems in the first 4 to 10 weeks after conception, before prenatal care is normally initiated. Because many women are not aware that they are pregnant until after this critical period of time, they are unable to reduce the risks to their own and to their baby's health unless intervention begins before conception.[34]

# The Process of Pregnancy

The process of pregnancy begins the moment a sperm fertilizes an ovum in the fallopian tubes (Figure 6.10). From there, the single fertilized cell, now called a *zygote*, multiplies and becomes a sphere-shaped cluster of cells called a *blastocyst* that travels toward the uterus, a journey that may take 3 to 4 days. Upon arrival, the embryo burrows into the thick, spongy endometrium (implantation) and is nourished from this carefully prepared lining.

**human chorionic gonadotropin (HCG)** Hormone detectable in blood or urine samples of a mother within the first few weeks of pregnancy.

**Pregnancy Testing** A woman may suspect she is pregnant before she takes a pregnancy test. A pregnancy test scheduled in a medical office or birth control clinic will confirm the pregnancy. Women who wish to know immediately can purchase home pregnancy test kits, sold over the counter in drugstores. A positive test is based on the secretion of **human chorionic gonadotropin (HCG),** which is found in the woman's urine. Home test kits contain a small sample of red blood cells coated with HCG antibodies to which the user adds a small amount of urine (HCG is also detectable in blood). If the concentration of HCG is great enough, it will clump together with the HCG antibodies, indicating that the user is pregnant.

Home pregnancy tests can be used as early as 2 weeks after conception and are about 85 to 95 percent reliable. Instructions must be followed carefully. If the test is done too early in the pregnancy, it may show a false negative. Other causes of false negatives are unclean test tubes, ingestion of certain drugs, and vaginal or urinary tract infections. Accuracy also depends on the quality of the test itself and the user's ability to perform it and interpret the results. Blood tests administered and analyzed by a medical laboratory are more accurate.

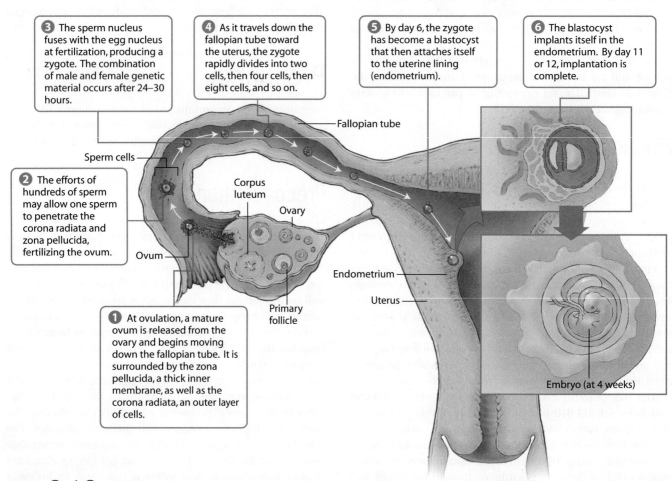

**3** The sperm nucleus fuses with the egg nucleus at fertilization, producing a zygote. The combination of male and female genetic material occurs after 24–30 hours.

**4** As it travels down the fallopian tube toward the uterus, the zygote rapidly divides into two cells, then four cells, then eight cells, and so on.

**5** By day 6, the zygote has become a blastocyst that then attaches itself to the uterine lining (endometrium).

**6** The blastocyst implants itself in the endometrium. By day 11 or 12, implantation is complete.

**2** The efforts of hundreds of sperm may allow one sperm to penetrate the corona radiata and zona pellucida, fertilizing the ovum.

**1** At ovulation, a mature ovum is released from the ovary and begins moving down the fallopian tube. It is surrounded by the zona pellucida, a thick inner membrane, as well as the corona radiata, an outer layer of cells.

Fallopian tube
Sperm cells
Corpus luteum
Ovary
Ovum
Primary follicle
Endometrium
Uterus
Embryo (at 4 weeks)

FIGURE 6.10 **Fertilization**
Fertilization usually occurs in the upper third of the fallopian tube, and implantation in the uterus takes place about 6 days later.

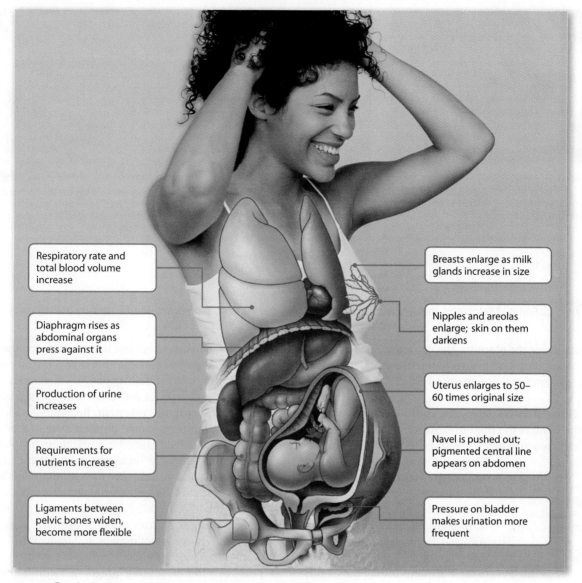

Respiratory rate and total blood volume increase

Diaphragm rises as abdominal organs press against it

Production of urine increases

Requirements for nutrients increase

Ligaments between pelvic bones widen, become more flexible

Breasts enlarge as milk glands increase in size

Nipples and areolas enlarge; skin on them darkens

Uterus enlarges to 50–60 times original size

Navel is pushed out; pigmented central line appears on abdomen

Pressure on bladder makes urination more frequent

FIGURE 6.11 **Changes in a Woman's Body during Pregnancy**

**Early Signs of Pregnancy** A woman's body undergoes substantial changes during the course of a pregnancy (Figure 6.11). The first sign of pregnancy is usually a missed menstrual period (although some women "spot" in early pregnancy, which may be mistaken for a period). Other signs include breast tenderness, emotional upset, extreme fatigue, sleeplessness, and nausea and vomiting (especially in the morning).

Pregnancy typically lasts 40 weeks and is divided into three phases, or **trimesters,** of approximately 3 months each. The due date is calculated from the expectant mother's last menstrual period.

**The First Trimester** During the first trimester, few noticeable changes occur in the mother's body. She may urinate more frequently and experience morning sickness, swollen breasts, or undue fatigue. These symptoms may not be frequent or severe, so she may not even realize she is pregnant unless she takes a pregnancy test.

During the first 2 months after conception, the **embryo** differentiates and develops its various organ systems, beginning with the nervous and circulatory systems. At the start of the third month, the embryo is called a **fetus,** indicating that all organ systems are in place. For the rest of the pregnancy, growth and refinement occur in each major body system so that they can function independently, yet in coordination with all the others, at birth. The photos in **Figure 6.12** on page 196 illustrate physical changes during fetal development.

**The Second Trimester** At the beginning of the second trimester, physical changes in the mother become more visible. Her breasts swell, and her waistline thickens. During this time, the fetus makes greater demands on the mother's

**trimester** A 3-month segment of pregnancy; used to describe specific developmental changes that occur in the embryo or fetus.
**embryo** The fertilized egg from conception until the end of 2 months' development.
**fetus** The word for a developing baby from the third month of pregnancy until birth.

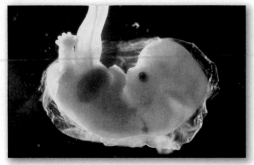

**a** A human embryo during the first trimester. The embryonic period lasts from the third to the eighth week of development. By the end of the embryonic period, all organs have formed.

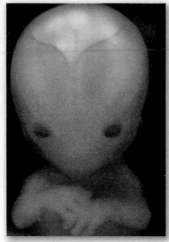

**b** A human fetus during the second trimester. Growth during the fetal period is very rapid.

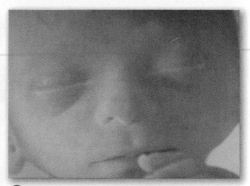

**c** A human fetus during the third trimester. By the end of the fetal period, the growth rate of the head has slowed relative to the growth rate of the rest of the body.

FIGURE 6.12 **Series of Fetoscopic Photographs Showing Development in the First, Second, and Third Trimesters of Pregnancy**

body. In particular, the **placenta,** the network of blood vessels that carries nutrients and oxygen to the fetus and fetal waste products to the mother, becomes well established.

**The Third Trimester** From the end of the sixth month through the ninth is the third trimester. This is the period of greatest fetal growth, when the fetus gains most of its weight. During this time, the fetus must get large amounts of calcium, iron, and nitrogen from food the mother eats. Approximately 85 percent of the calcium and iron the mother digests goes into the fetal bloodstream.

> **placenta** The network of blood vessels connected to the umbilical cord that carries nutrients, oxygen, and wastes between the developing infant and the mother.

Although the fetus may live if it is born during the seventh month, it needs the layer of fat it acquires during the eighth month and time for the organs (especially the respiratory and digestive organs) to develop fully. Infants born prematurely usually require intensive medical care.

**Emotional Changes** Of course, the process of pregnancy involves much more than the changes in a woman's body and the developing fetus. Many important emotional changes occur from the time a woman learns she is pregnant through the "fourth trimester" (the first 6 weeks of an infant's life outside the uterus). Throughout pregnancy, women may experience fear of complications, anxiety about becoming a parent, and wonder and excitement over the developing baby.

## Prenatal Care

A successful pregnancy depends on a mother who takes good care of herself and her fetus. Good nutrition and exercise; avoiding drugs, alcohol, and other harmful substances; and regular medical checkups from the beginning of pregnancy are essential. Early detection of fetal abnormalities, identifi-

cation of high-risk mothers and infants, and a complication-free pregnancy are the major purposes of prenatal care.

A woman should carefully choose a practitioner who will attend her pregnancy and delivery. If possible, she should do this before she becomes pregnant. Recommendations from friends and from one's family physician are a good starting point. Also she should consider a practitioner's philosophy about pain management during labor, experience handling complications, and willingness to accommodate her personal beliefs on these issues. Several different types of practitioners are qualified to care for a woman through pregnancy, birth, and the postpartum period, including obstetrician-gynecologists, family practitioners, and midwives (Table 6.3).

Ideally, a woman should begin medical checkups as soon as possible after becoming pregnant (within the first 3 months). This early care reduces infant mortality and low birth weight. On the first visit, the practitioner should obtain a complete medical history of the mother and her family and note any hereditary conditions that could put a woman or her fetus at risk. Regular checkups to measure weight gain and blood pressure and to monitor the fetus's size and position should continue throughout the pregnancy. The American College of Obstetricians and Gynecologists recommends seven or eight prenatal visits for women with low-risk pregnancies. Unfortunately, prenatal care is not available to everyone. Native American and African American women have the lowest rates of prenatal care in the United States.[35]

**Nutrition and Exercise** Pregnant women need additional protein, calories, vitamins, and minerals, so specific dietary needs and guidance should be discussed with the practitioner. Special attention should be paid to getting enough folic acid (found in dark leafy greens), iron (dried fruits, meats, legumes, liver, egg yolks), calcium (nonfat or low-fat dairy products and some canned fish), and fluids.

## Choosing a Prenatal Care Practitioner

| Practitioner/Description | Advantages | Disadvantages |
|---|---|---|
| **Obstetrician/Gynecologist:** an MD who specializes in obstetrics (care of a woman and child during pregnancy, birth, and the postpartum period) and gynecology (care of the reproductive system of women). | Trained to handle all types of pregnancy- and delivery-related emergencies. | Generally can perform deliveries only in a hospital setting. Cannot serve as the baby's physician after birth. |
| **Family Practitioner:** an MD or nurse practitioner who provides comprehensive care for people of all ages. | No need to change physicians; can refer to a specialist if necessary, can serve as the baby's physician after birth. | Some provide pregnancy care only to low-risk pregnancies; rarely perform home births. |
| **Midwife:** an experienced practitioner who can assist with pregnancies and deliveries. Midwives can oversee delivery of babies in nonhospital birthing sites, such as home deliveries or birthing centers. Most strive to help women have a natural childbirth experience. | | |
| *Certified Nurse Midwife:* An RN with specialized training in pregnancy and delivery; most work in private practice or in conjunction with physicians. | Certified nurse midwives have formal training and accreditation. They may work with physicians and have access to traditional medical facilities. | Cannot provide any medication; need to refer to clinician when the pregnancy is deemed high risk. |
| *Lay Midwives:* An uncertified or unlicensed midwife who was educated through informal routes such as self-study or apprenticeship rather than through a formal program. | Midwives tend to view pregnancy and childbirth as a family event. They may offer more personal attention than an MD would. Home birth can lower costs. | Cannot administer any medication; would need to refer to a clinician. May not have extensive training in handling an emergency. Women should carefully evaluate the credentials of a prospective lay midwife. |

Vitamin supplements can correct some deficiencies, but there is no substitute for a well-balanced diet. Babies born to poorly nourished mothers run high risks of substandard mental and physical development. Folic acid, when consumed before and during early pregnancy, reduces the risk of spina bifida, a congenital birth defect resulting from failure of the spinal column to close. Manufacturers of breads, pastas, rice, and other grain products are now required to add folic acid to their foods to reduce neural tube defects in newborns.

Weight gain during pregnancy helps nourish a growing baby. For a woman of normal weight before pregnancy, the recommended gain during pregnancy is 25 to 35 pounds. For obese or overweight women, weight gain of 15 to 25 pounds is recommended. Underweight women can gain 28 to 40 pounds, and women carrying twins should gain about 35 to 45 pounds. Gaining too much or too little weight can lead to complications. With higher weight gains, women may develop gestational diabetes, hypertension, or increased risk of delivery complications. Gaining too little increases the chance of a low–birth weight baby.

Of the total number of pounds gained during pregnancy, about 6 to 8 are the baby. The baby's birth weight is important, because low birth weight can mean health problems during labor and the baby's first few months. Pregnancy is not the time for a woman to think about losing weight—doing so may endanger the fetus.

As in all other stages of life, exercise is an important factor in overall maternal health during pregnancy. Regular exercise is recommended for pregnant women; however, they should consult their practitioner before starting any exercise program. Exercise can help control weight, make labor easier, and help with a faster recovery due to increased strength and endurance. Physical activity includes regular, moderate physical activity such as brisk walking and/or swimming. For the most part, women can usually maintain their pre-pregnancy level of activity. While pregnant, you should avoid doing any activity that involves lying on your back or that puts you at risk of falling or having an abdominal injury, such as horseback riding, soccer, or basketball.

**Drugs and Alcohol** A woman should avoid all types of drugs during pregnancy. Even common over-the-counter medications such as aspirin and some beverages such as coffee and tea can damage a developing fetus. During the first 3 months of pregnancy, the

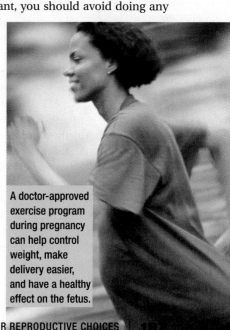

A doctor-approved exercise program during pregnancy can help control weight, make delivery easier, and have a healthy effect on the fetus.

fetus is especially subject to the **teratogenic** (birth defect–causing) effects of drugs, environmental chemicals, X rays, or diseases. The fetus can also develop an addiction to or tolerance for drugs that the mother is using.

Maternal consumption of alcohol is detrimental to a growing fetus. Symptoms of **fetal alcohol syndrome (FAS)** include mental retardation, slowed nerve reflexes, and small head size. The exact amount of alcohol that causes FAS is not known; therefore, researchers recommend total abstinence during pregnancy.

### Smoking

Tobacco use, and smoking in particular, harms every phase of reproduction. Women who smoke have more difficulty becoming pregnant and have a higher risk of being infertile. Women who smoke during pregnancy have a greater chance of complications, premature births, low–birth weight infants, stillbirth, and infant mortality.[36] Smoking restricts the blood supply to the developing fetus and thus limits oxygen and nutrition delivery and waste removal. Tobacco use appears to be a significant factor in the development of cleft lip and palate.

Studies also show that secondhand smoke is detrimental. The exposed fetus is likely to experience low birth weight, increased susceptibility to childhood diseases, and sudden infant death syndrome.[37] Tobacco smoke clearly has an influence throughout the pregnancy cycle and should be avoided by any woman who is or wishes to become pregnant.

### Other Teratogens

A pregnant woman should avoid exposure to X rays, toxic chemicals, heavy metals, pesticides, gases, and other hazardous compounds. She should not clean cat-litter boxes, because cat feces can contain organisms that cause **toxoplasmosis**. If a pregnant woman contracts this disease, her baby may be stillborn or suffer mental retardation or other birth defects.

If she has never had rubella (German measles), a woman should be immunized for it prior to becoming pregnant. A rubella infection can kill the fetus or cause blindness or hearing disorders in the infant. Sexually transmitted infections such as genital herpes or HIV are also risk factors. A woman should inform her physician of any infectious condition so proper precautions and treatment can be taken. The physician may want to deliver the baby by cesarean section, especially if a woman has active lesions. Contact with an active herpes infection during birth can be fatal to the baby.

**teratogenic** Causing birth defects; may refer to drugs, environmental chemicals, X rays, or diseases.
**fetal alcohol syndrome (FAS)** A collection of symptoms, including mental retardation, that can appear in infants of women who drink alcohol during pregnancy.
**toxoplasmosis** A disease caused by an organism found in cat feces that, when contracted by a pregnant woman, may result in stillbirth or an infant with mental retardation or birth defects.
**Down syndrome** A genetic disorder characterized by mental retardation and a variety of physical abnormalities.
**ultrasonography (ultrasound)** A common prenatal test that uses high-frequency sound waves to create a visual image of the fetus.
**chorionic villus sampling (CVS)** A prenatal test that involves snipping tissue from the fetal sac to be analyzed for genetic defects.

Several recent studies have shown that caffeine can significantly increase the risk of miscarriage and stillbirth.[38] Based on these and other studies, women who are pregnant are advised to cut back on their caffeine consumption. Pregnant women who need to drink caffeine-containing beverages should try to limit it to one cup per day, but preferably women should avoid caffeine during pregnancy.

### Maternal Age

The average age at which a woman has her first child has been creeping up, and today, a woman who becomes pregnant after age 35 has plenty of company. Although births to women in their twenties are declining, the rate of first births to women between the ages of 30 and 39 are the highest reported in four decades, and births to women over 39 have increased by more than 70 percent since 1990.[39] Many doctors note that older mothers tend to be more conscientious about following medical advice during pregnancy and are more psychologically mature and ready to include an infant in their family than are some younger women.

Statistically, the chances of having a baby with birth defects do rise after the age of 35. Researchers believe that there is a decline in both the quality and viability of eggs after this age. The incidence of **Down syndrome** increases with the mother's age.[40] Another concern is that a woman's fertility begins to decline as she ages. Fewer than 10 percent of women in their early twenties have issues with infertility, compared to nearly 30 percent in their early forties.

### Prenatal Testing and Screening

Modern technology enables medical practitioners to detect health defects in a fetus as early as the fourteenth to eighteenth weeks of pregnancy. One common test is **ultrasonography** or **ultrasound,** which uses high-frequency sound waves to create a *sonogram,* or visual image, of the fetus in the uterus. The sonogram is used to determine the fetus's size and position. Knowing the baby's position helps health care providers perform other tests and deliver the infant. Sonograms can also detect birth defects in the central nervous and digestive systems.

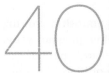 genetic abnormalities can be identified through amniocentesis, the most common being Down syndrome.

**Chorionic villus sampling (CVS)** involves snipping tissue from the developing fetal sac. Chorionic villus sampling can be used at 10 to 12 weeks of pregnancy. This is an attractive option for couples who are at high risk for having a baby with Down syndrome or a debilitating hereditary disease.

The **triple marker screen (TMS)** is a maternal blood test that is optimally conducted between the sixteenth and eighteenth weeks of pregnancy. The TMS is a screening test, not a diagnostic tool; it can detect susceptibility for a birth defect or genetic abnormality but is not meant to confirm a diagnosis of any condition.

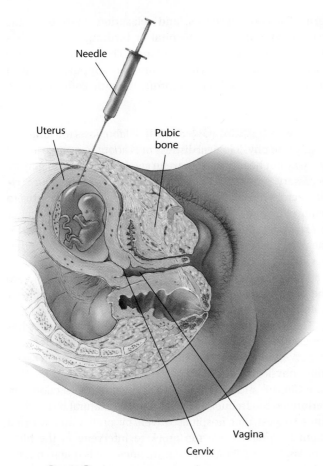

Needle

Uterus

Pubic bone

Vagina

Cervix

FIGURE 6.13 **Amniocentesis**
The process of amniocentesis, in which a long needle is used to withdraw a small amount of amniotic fluid for genetic analysis, can detect certain congenital problems as well as the fetus's sex.

**Amniocentesis** is a common testing procedure that is strongly recommended for women over age 35. This test involves inserting a long needle through the mother's abdominal and uterine walls into the **amniotic sac,** the protective pouch surrounding the fetus. The needle draws out 3 to 4 teaspoons of fluid, which is analyzed for genetic information about the baby (Figure 6.13). Amniocentesis can be performed between weeks 14 and 18.

If any of these tests reveals a serious birth defect, parents are advised to undergo genetic counseling. In the case of a chromosomal abnormality such as Down syndrome, the parents are usually offered the option of a therapeutic abortion. Some parents choose this option; others research the disability and decide to go ahead with the pregnancy.

## what do you think?
Would you want to know if you or your partner were carrying a child with a genetic birth defect or other abnormality? ● Would you consider having your own genes tested before starting a family? ● What would you do if both you and your partner were carriers of a genetic disorder that could be passed to your children?

# Childbirth

Prospective parents need to make several key decisions long before the baby is born. These include where to have the baby, whether to use drugs during labor and delivery, which childbirth method to choose, and whether to breast-feed or bottle-feed. Answering these questions in advance will ensure a smoother passage into parenthood.

## Labor and Delivery

During the few weeks preceding delivery, the baby normally shifts to a head-down position, and the cervix begins to dilate (widen). The junction of the pubic bones loosens to permit expansion of the pelvic girdle during birth. The exact mechanisms that initiate labor are unknown. A change in the hormones in the fetus and mother cause strong uterine contractions to occur, signaling the beginning of labor. Another common early signal is the breaking of the amniotic sac, which causes a rush of fluid from the vagina (commonly referred to as "water breaking").

The birth process has three stages, described in Figure 6.14 on page 200, which can last from several hours to more than a day. In some cases, the attending practitioner may perform an *episiotomy,* a straight incision in the mother's perineum (the area between the vulva and the anus), toward the end of the second stage to prevent the baby's head from tearing vaginal tissues and to speed the baby's exit from the vagina. Upon exit, the baby takes its first breath, which is generally accompanied by a loud wail. After delivery, the attending practitioner assesses the baby's overall condition, cleans the baby's mucus-filled breathing passages, and ties and severs the umbilical cord. The mother's uterus continues to contract in the third stage of labor until the placenta is expelled.

**triple marker screen (TMS)** A maternal blood test that can be used to help identify fetuses with certain birth defects and genetic abnormalities.
**amniocentesis** A medical test in which a small amount of fluid is drawn from the amniotic sac to test for Down syndrome and other genetic diseases.
**amniotic sac** The protective pouch surrounding the fetus.

**Managing Labor** Painkilling medications given to the mother during labor can cause sluggish responses in the newborn and other complications. For this reason, many women choose drug-free labor and delivery—but it is important to keep a flexible attitude about pain

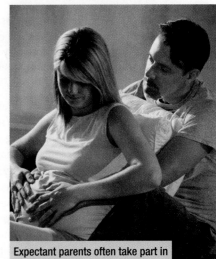

Expectant parents often take part in childbirth classes to learn what to expect during labor and delivery and to practice techniques for breathing and relaxation during labor.

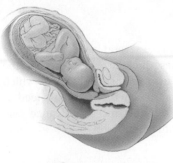

**①** **Stage I: Dilation of the cervix** Contractions in the abdomen and lower back push the baby downward, putting pressure on the cervix and dilating it. The first stage of labor may last from a couple of hours to more than a day for a first birth, but it is usually much shorter during subsequent births.

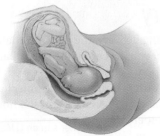

**②** **End of Stage I: Transition** The cervix becomes fully dilated, and the baby's head begins to move into the vagina (birth canal). Contractions usually come quickly during transition, which generally lasts 30 minutes or less.

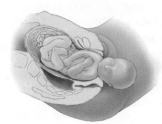

**③** **Stage II: Expulsion** Once the cervix has become fully dilated, contractions become rhythmic, strong, and more intense as the uterus pushes the baby headfirst through the birth canal. The expulsion stage lasts 1 to 4 hours and concludes when the infant is finally pushed out of the mother's body.

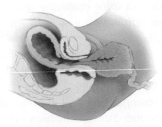

**④** **Stage III: Delivery of the placenta** In the third stage, the placenta detaches from the uterus and is expelled through the birth canal. This stage is usually completed within 30 minutes after delivery.

FIGURE 6.14 **The Birth Process**
The entire process of labor and delivery usually takes from 2 to 36 hours. Labor is generally longer for a woman's first delivery and shorter for subsequent births.

relief, because each labor is different. Use of painkilling medication during a delivery is not a sign of weakness. One person is not a "success" for delivering without medication and another a "failure" for using medical measures. Remember, pain is to be expected. In fact, many experts say that the pain of labor is the most difficult in the human experience. There is no one right answer for managing that pain.

The Lamaze method is the most popular technique of childbirth preparation in the United States. It discourages the use of drugs; prelabor classes teach the mother to control her pain through special breathing pat-

**cesarean section (C-section)** A surgical birthing procedure in which a baby is removed through an incision made in the mother's abdominal and uterine walls.

**preeclampsia** A complication in pregnancy characterized by high blood pressure, protein in the urine, and edema.

terns, focusing exercises, and relaxation. Lamaze births usually take place in a hospital or birthing center with a physician or midwife in attendance. The partner (or labor coach) assists by giving emotional support, physical comfort, and coaching for proper breath control during contractions.

**Cesarean Section (C-Section)** If labor lasts too long or if a baby is in physiological distress or is about to exit the uterus any way but headfirst, a **cesarean section (C-section)** may be necessary. This surgical procedure involves making an incision across the mother's abdomen and through the uterus to remove the baby. A C-section may also be performed if labor is extremely difficult, maternal blood pressure falls rapidly, the placenta separates from the uterus too soon, the mother has diabetes, or other problems occur. A C-section can be traumatic for the mother if she is not prepared for it. Risks are the same as for any major abdominal surgery, and recovery from birth takes considerably longer after a C-section.

The rate of delivery by C-section in the United States has increased from 5 percent in the mid-1960s to 32 percent in 2007.[41] Although this procedure is necessary in certain cases, some physicians and critics, including the Centers for Disease Control and Prevention (CDC), feel that C-sections are performed too frequently in this country. Natural birth advocates suggest that hospitals driven by profits and worried about malpractice are too quick to intervene in the birth process. Some doctors say that the increase is due to maternal demand: busy mothers who want to schedule their deliveries. It has also been reported that late preterm delivery (34 to 36 weeks) increased from 7.3 to 8.9 percent between 1990 and 2004 in the United States.[42] It is not clear how much of that is because of maternal choice.

# Complications of Pregnancy and Childbirth

Pregnancy carries the risk for potential complications and problems that can interfere with the proper development of the fetus or threaten the health of the mother and child. Some complications may result from a preexisting health condition of the mother, such as diabetes or an STI, whereas others can develop during pregnancy and may result from physiological problems, genetic abnormalities, or exposure to teratogens.

**Preeclampsia and Eclampsia** **Preeclampsia** is a condition that is characterized by high blood pressure, protein in the urine, and edema (fluid retention), which usually causes swelling of the hands and face. Symptoms may include sudden weight gain, headache, nausea or vomiting, changes in vision, racing pulse, mental confusion, and stomach or right shoulder pain. If preeclampsia is not treated, it can cause strokes and seizures, a condition called *eclampsia*. Potential problems can include liver and kidney damage, internal bleeding, stroke, poor fetal growth, and fetal and maternal death.

Preeclampsia tends to occur in the late second or third trimester. The cause is unknown; however, the incidence of preeclampsia is higher in first-time mothers; women over 40 or under 18 years of age; women carrying multiple fetuses; and women with a history of chronic hypertension, diabetes, kidney disorder, or previous history of preeclampsia. Family history of preeclampsia is also a risk factor, whether the history is on the man's or woman's side. Treatment for preeclampsia ranges from bed rest and monitoring for mild cases to hospitalization and close monitoring for more severe cases.

**Miscarriage** Unfortunately not every pregnancy ends in delivery. In fact, in the United States, between 15 to 20 percent of pregnancies end in **miscarriage** (also referred to as *spontaneous abortion*).[43] Most miscarriages occur during the first trimester.

Reasons for miscarriage vary. In some cases, the fertilized egg has failed to divide correctly. In others, genetic abnormalities, maternal illness, or infections are responsible. Maternal hormonal imbalance may also cause a miscarriage, as may a weak cervix, toxic chemicals in the environment, or physical trauma to the mother. In most cases, the cause is not known.

**Rh Factor** A blood incompatibility between mother and fetus can cause **Rh factor** problems, sometimes resulting in miscarriage. Rh is a blood protein, and problems occur when the mother is Rh-negative and the fetus is Rh-positive. During a first birth, some of the baby's blood passes into the mother's bloodstream. An Rh-negative mother may manufacture antibodies to destroy the Rh-positive blood introduced into her bloodstream at the time of birth. Her first baby will be unaffected, but subsequent babies with positive Rh factor will be at risk for a severe anemia called *hemolytic disease*, because the mother's Rh antibodies will attack the fetus's red blood cells.

Prevention is preferable to treatment. Women with Rh-negative blood should be injected with a medication called RhoGAM within 72 hours after any birth, miscarriage, or abortion. The injection prevents the mother from developing Rh antibodies.

**Ectopic Pregnancy** The implantation of a fertilized egg outside the uterus, usually in the fallopian tube or occasionally in the pelvic cavity, is called an **ectopic pregnancy.** Because these structures are not capable of expanding and nourishing a developing fetus, the pregnancy must be terminated surgically, or a miscarriage will occur. Ectopic pregnancy is generally accompanied by pain in the lower abdomen or aching in the shoulders as the blood flows up toward the diaphragm. If bleeding is significant, blood pressure drops, and the woman can go into shock. If an ectopic pregnancy progresses undiagnosed and untreated, the fallopian tube will rupture, which puts the woman at great risk of hemorrhage, peritonitis (infection in the abdomen), and even death. Ectopic pregnancy occurs at a rate of 19.7 cases per

1,000 pregnancies in North America and is a leading cause of maternal mortality in the first trimester.[44]

We do know that ectopic pregnancy is a potential side effect of pelvic inflammatory disease, which has become increasingly common in recent years. The scarring or blockage of the fallopian tubes that is characteristic of this disease prevents the fertilized egg from passing to the uterus.

**Stillbirth** One of the most traumatic events a couple can face is a **stillbirth.** Stillbirth is the death of a fetus *after* the twentieth week of pregnancy but before delivery. A stillborn baby is born dead, often for no apparent reason. Each year in the United States, there is about 1 stillbirth in every 160 births.[45] Birth defects, placental problems, poor fetal growth, infections, and umbilical cord accidents are all factors that may contribute to the baby's death.

**miscarriage** Loss of the fetus before it is viable; also called *spontaneous abortion*.

**Rh factor** A blood protein related to the production of antibodies; if an Rh-negative mother is pregnant with an Rh-positive fetus, the mother may manufacture antibodies that can kill the fetus, causing miscarriage.

**ectopic pregnancy** Implantation of a fertilized egg outside the uterus, usually in a fallopian tube; a medical emergency that can end in death from hemorrhage or peritonitis.

**stillbirth** The birth of a dead baby.

**postpartum depression** Energy depletion, anxiety, mood swings, and depression that women may feel during the postpartum period.

## The Postpartum Period

The postpartum period typically lasts 4 to 6 weeks after delivery. During this period, many women experience fluctuating emotions. For many new mothers, the physical stress of labor, dehydration and blood loss, and other stresses challenge their stamina. Many new mothers experience what is called the "baby blues," characterized by periods of sadness, anxiety, headache, sleep disturbances, and irritability. For most women, these symptoms disappear after a short while. About 10 percent of new mothers experience **postpartum depression,** a more disabling syndrome characterized by mood swings, lack of energy, crying, guilt, and depression. It can happen any time within the first year after childbirth. Mothers who experience postpartum depression should seek professional treatment. Counseling and sometimes medication are two of the most common types of treatment.[46]

**Breast-Feeding** Although the new mother's milk will not begin to flow for 2 or more days after delivery, her breasts secrete a yellow fluid called *colostrum*. Because colostrum contains vital antibodies to help fight infection, the newborn should be allowed to suckle.

The American Academy of Pediatrics strongly recommends that infants be breast-fed for at least 6 months and ideally for 12 months. Scientific findings indicate there are many advantages to breast-feeding. Breast-fed babies have fewer illnesses and a much lower hospitalization rate, because breast milk contains maternal antibodies and immunological cells that stimulate the infant's immune system. When breast-fed babies do get sick, they recover more quickly. They are also less likely to be obese than babies fed on formulas, and they have fewer allergies. They may even be more intelligent: A new study finds

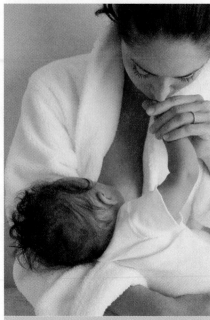
In addition to its numerous health benefits, breast-feeding enhances the development of intimate bonds between mother and child.

that the longer a baby was breast-fed, the higher the IQ will be in adulthood. Researchers theorize that breast milk contains substances that enhance brain development.[47] There is also a potential environmental advantage to breast-feeding. Compounds found in baby bottles, including bisphenol-A, are under intense scrutiny following research suggesting they can lead to health problems.[48]

This does not mean that breast milk is the only way to nourish a baby. Some women are unable or unwilling to breast-feed; women with certain medical conditions or receiving certain medications are advised not to breast-feed. Prepared formulas can provide nourishment that allows a baby to grow and thrive. When deciding whether to breast- or bottle-feed, mothers must consider their own desires and preferences, too. Both feeding methods can supply the physical and emotional closeness so essential to the parent–child relationship.

**Infant Mortality** After birth, infant death can be caused by birth defects, low birth weight, injuries, or unknown causes. In the United States, the unexpected death of a child under 1 year of age, for no apparent reason, is called **sudden infant death syndrome (SIDS).** Sudden infant death syndrome is the leading cause of death for children aged 1 month to 1 year and is responsible for about 2,500 deaths a year.[49] It is not a specific disease; rather, it is ruled a cause of death after all other possibilities are ruled out. A SIDS death is sudden and silent; death occurs quickly, often during sleep, with no signs of suffering.

The exact cause of SIDS is unknown, but researchers have discovered trends in SIDS deaths that may help them understand this mysterious fatal problem. For instance:[50]

- SIDS is the leading cause of death in babies after 1 month of age, and most SIDS deaths occur in babies less than 6 months old.
- Babies placed to sleep on their backs are less likely to die from SIDS than those placed on their stomachs to sleep.
- Babies are more likely to die from SIDS when they are placed on or covered by soft bedding.

**sudden infant death syndrome (SIDS)** The sudden death of an infant under 1 year of age for no apparent reason.
**infertility** Inability to conceive after a year or more of trying.

- African American babies are twice as likely to die from SIDS as are white babies.
- American Indian babies are nearly three times more likely to die of SIDS than white babies.

The American Academy of Pediatrics is the sponsor of the Back to Sleep educational campaign that provides parents the following advice when putting a baby down to sleep: Lay infants down on their backs; place them on a firm sleep surface; keep soft objects, toys and bedding out of the sleep area; don't allow smoking around the baby; and give the baby a clean, dry pacifier.

# Infertility

For the couple desperately wishing to conceive, the road to parenthood may be frustrating. An estimated 1 in 6 American couples experiences **infertility,** usually defined as the inability to conceive after trying for a year or more. In the United States, it affects about 10 to 20 percent of the reproductive-age population. Although the focus is often on women, in about 20 percent of cases, infertility is due to a cause involving only the male partner, and in about 30 to 40 percent of cases, infertility is due to causes involving both partners.[51] Because of the likelihood of this, it is important for both partners to be evaluated.

## 10%
of infertility cases have no known cause.

Reasons for the high level of infertility in the United States today include the trend toward delaying childbirth (as a woman gets older, she is less likely to conceive), endometriosis, the rising incidence of pelvic inflammatory disease, and low sperm count. Environmental contaminants known as *endocrine disrupters,* such as some pesticides and emissions from burning plastics, appear to affect fertility in both men and women. Stress and anxiety, both in general and about fertility, can also interfere with getting pregnant. The linked diseases of obesity and diabetes that are currently affecting our country also have reproductive implications.

## Causes in Women

Most cases of infertility in women result from problems with ovulation. The most common cause for female infertility is polycystic ovary syndrome (PCOS). A woman's ovaries have follicles, which are tiny, fluid-filled sacs that hold the eggs. When an egg is mature, the follicle breaks open to release the egg so it can travel to the uterus for fertilization. In women with PCOS, immature follicles bunch together to form large cysts or lumps. The eggs mature within the bunched follicles, but the follicles don't break open to release them. As a result, women with PCOS often don't have menstrual periods, or they have periods infrequently. Because the eggs are not released, most women with PCOS have trouble getting pregnant. Researchers estimate that 5 to 10 percent of women of childbearing age—as many as 5 million women in the United States—have PCOS.[52]

In some women the ovaries stop functioning before natural menopause, a condition called *premature ovarian failure*. Other causes of infertility include **endometriosis.** With this very painful disorder, parts of the endometrial lining of the uterus implant outside the uterus and block the fallopian tubes. The disorder can be treated surgically or with hormonal therapy.

**Pelvic inflammatory disease (PID)** is a serious infection that scars the fallopian tubes and blocks sperm migration. (See Chapter 14 for more on PID.) Infection-causing bacteria (chlamydia or gonorrhea) can silently invade the fallopian tubes, causing normal tissue to turn into scar tissue. This scar tissue blocks or interrupts the normal movement of eggs into the uterus. If the fallopian tubes are totally blocked by scar tissue, sperm cannot fertilize an egg, and the woman becomes infertile. Infertility also can occur if the fallopian tubes are partially blocked or even slightly damaged. About 1 in 10 women with PID becomes infertile, and if a woman has multiple episodes of PID, her chances of becoming infertile increase.[53]

## Causes in Men

Among men, the single largest fertility problem is **low sperm count.**[54] Although only one viable sperm is needed for fertilization, research has shown that all the other sperm in the ejaculate aid in the fertilization process. There are normally 60 to 80 million sperm per milliliter of semen. When the count drops below 20 million, fertility declines.

Low sperm count may be attributable to environmental factors (such as exposure of the scrotum to intense heat or cold, radiation, or altitude) or even to wearing excessively tight underwear or outerwear. However, other factors, such as the mumps virus, can damage the cells that make sperm. Varicose veins above one or both testicles can also render men infertile.

## Infertility Treatments

Medical treatment can identify the cause of infertility in about 90 percent of cases. The chances of becoming pregnant after the cause has been determined range from 30 to 70 percent, depending on the reason for infertility.[55] The countless tests and the invasion of privacy that characterize some couples' efforts to conceive can put stress on an otherwise strong, healthy relationship. A good physician or fertility team will take the time to ascertain the couple's level of motivation.

Workups to determine the cause of infertility can be expensive, and the costs are not usually covered by insurance companies. Fertility workups for men include a sperm count, a test for sperm motility, and an analysis of any disease processes present. Women are thoroughly examined by an obstetrician-gynecologist to determine the composition of cervical mucus and evidence of tubal scarring or endometriosis.

**Fertility Drugs** Fertility drugs stimulate ovulation in women who are not ovulating. Sixty to eighty percent of women who use these drugs will begin to ovulate; of those who ovulate, about half will conceive.[56] Fertility drugs can have many side effects, including headaches, irritability, restlessness, depression, fatigue, edema (fluid retention), abnormal uterine bleeding, breast tenderness, vasomotor flushes (hot flashes), and visual difficulties. Women using fertility drugs are also at increased risk of developing multiple ovarian cysts (fluid-filled growths) and liver damage. The drugs sometimes trigger the release of more than one egg. Thus a woman treated with one of these drugs has a 1 in 10 chance of having multiple births. Most such births are twins, but triplets and even quadruplets are not uncommon.

**Alternative Insemination** Another treatment option is **alternative insemination** (also known as *artificial insemination*) of a woman with her partner's sperm. The couple may also choose insemination by an anonymous donor through a sperm bank. The sperm are medically screened, classified according to the donor's physical characteristics (for example, blond hair, blue eyes), and then frozen for future use.

**Assisted Reproductive Technology (ART)** Assisted reproductive technology (ART) describes several different medical procedures that help a woman become pregnant. The most common type of ART is **in vitro fertilization (IVF)**; during IVF, eggs and sperm are mixed in a laboratory dish to fertilize, and some of the fertilized eggs (zygotes) are then transferred to the woman's uterus.

Other types of assisted reproductive technologies include

- **Intracytoplasmic sperm injection (ICSI),** which involves the injection of a single sperm into an egg. The fertilized egg is then placed in the woman's uterus or fallopian tube. Used with IVF, ICSI is often a successful treatment for men with impaired sperm.
- **Gamete intrafallopian transfer (GIFT),** which involves collecting eggs from the ovaries, then placing them into

**endometriosis** A disorder in which uterine lining tissue establishes itself outside the uterus; the leading cause of infertility in women in the United States.

**pelvic inflammatory disease (PID)** An infection that scars the fallopian tubes and consequently blocks sperm migration, causing infertility.

**low sperm count** A sperm count below 20 million sperm per milliliter of semen; the leading cause of infertility in men.

**alternative insemination** Fertilization accomplished by depositing a partner's or a donor's semen into a woman's vagina via a thin tube; almost always done in a doctor's office.

**in vitro fertilization (IVF)** Fertilization of an egg in a nutrient medium and subsequent transfer back to the mother's body.

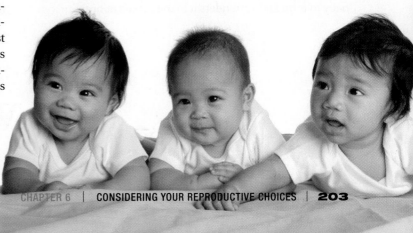

a thin flexible tube with the sperm. This is then injected into the woman's fallopian tubes, where fertilization takes place.

- **Zygote intrafallopian transfer (ZIFT),** which combines IVF and GIFT. Eggs and sperm are mixed outside of the body. The fertilized eggs (zygotes) are then returned to the fallopian tubes, through which they travel to the uterus.

**Other Treatments for Infertility** In *nonsurgical embryo transfer,* a donor egg is fertilized by the man's sperm and implanted in the woman's uterus. In *embryo transfer,* an ovum from a donor is artificially inseminated by the man's sperm, allowed to stay in the donor's body for a time, and then transplanted into the woman's body. Infertile couples have another alternative—embryo adoption programs. Fertility treatments such as IVF often produce excess fertilized eggs that a couple may choose to donate for other infertile couples to adopt.

The ethical and moral questions surrounding experimental infertility treatments are staggering. Before moving forward with any of these treatments, individuals must ask themselves a few important questions: Has infertility been absolutely confirmed? Are reputable infertility counseling services accessible? Have they explored all possible alternatives and considered potential risks? Have all parties examined their attitudes, values, and beliefs about conceiving a child in this manner? Finally, they need to consider what and how they will tell the child about their method of conception.

## what do you think?

If you or your partner had infertility problems, how much time and money would you be willing to invest in treatment? ● Do you think that single women should have equal access to alternative methods of insemination? ● What about lesbian couples—should they have equal access to alternative methods of insemination? ● Do you think single women, single men, gay couples, and lesbian couples should have equal opportunities to adopt? ● How do you think society views these types of adoptions?

## Surrogate Motherhood

The good news is that many infertile couples are able to conceive after treatment. The rest decide to live without children, to adopt, or to attempt surrogate motherhood. In the latter option, the couple hires a woman to be alternatively inseminated by the male partner. The surrogate then carries the baby to term and surrenders it to the couple at birth.

Couples considering surrogate motherhood are advised to consult a lawyer regarding contracts. Most of these legal documents stipulate that the surrogate mother must undergo amniocentesis and that if the fetus is defective, she must consent to an abortion. In that case, or if the surrogate miscarries, she is reimbursed for her time and expenses. The prospective parents must also agree to take the baby if it is carried to term, even if it is unhealthy or has physical abnormalities.

## Adoption

Adoption serves several important purposes in American society. It provides a way for individuals and couples who may not be able or have decided not to have children to form a legal parental relationship with a nonbiological child. As such, it benefits children whose birth parents are unable or unwilling to raise them and provides adults who are unable to conceive or carry a pregnancy to term a means to bring children into their families. It is estimated that approximately 2 percent of the adult population has adopted children.[57]

What are the characteristics of people who adopt? According to the most recent national survey, 2.3 percent of men have adopted children compared to 1.1 percent of women.[58] In addition, higher percentages of people over the age of 30 have adopted, compared to people aged 18 to 29. Adoption is also more common among people who are currently or formerly married, who have given birth or fathered a child, and who have ever used infertility services. In general, adoptive mothers are older than non-adoptive mothers. Eighty-one percent of adoptive mothers are in the 35- to 44-year-old age range compared with 52 percent of non-adoptive mothers.[59]

There are two types of adoption: *confidential* and *open.* In confidential adoption, the birth parents and the adoptive parents never know each other. Adoptive parents are given only basic information about the birth parents, such as medical background, that they need in order to care for the child. In open adoption, birth parents and adoptive parents know some things about each other. There are different levels of openness. Both parties must agree to this plan, and it is not available in every state.

Increasingly, couples are choosing to adopt children from other countries. In 2009, U.S. families adopted nearly 13,000 foreign-born children.[60] The cost of intercountry adoption varies from approximately $10,000 to more than $30,000, including agency fees, dossier and immigration processing fees, and court costs.[61] However, it may be a good alternative for many couples, especially those who want to adopt an infant rather than an older child.

## Are You Comfortable with Your Contraception?

PEARSON
**myhealthlab**

Fill out this assessment online at www.pearsonhighered.com/myhealthlab or www.pearsonhighered.com/donatelle.

These questions will help you assess whether your current method of contraception or one you may consider using in the future will be effective for you. Answering yes to any of these questions predicts potential problems. If you have more than a few yes responses, consider talking to a health care provider, counselor, partner, or friend to decide whether to use this method or how to use it so that it will really be effective.

Method of contraception you use now or are considering:

_____

1. Have I or my partner ever become pregnant while using this method? Ⓨ Ⓝ

2. Am I afraid of using this method? Ⓨ Ⓝ

3. Would I really rather not use this method? Ⓨ Ⓝ

4. Will I have trouble remembering to use this method? Ⓨ Ⓝ

5. Will I have trouble using this method correctly? Ⓨ Ⓝ

6. Does this method make menstrual periods longer or more painful for me or my partner? Ⓨ Ⓝ

7. Does this method cost more than I can afford? Ⓨ Ⓝ

8. Could this method cause serious complications? Ⓨ Ⓝ

9. Am I, or is my partner, opposed to this method because of any religious or moral beliefs? Ⓨ Ⓝ

10. Will using this method embarrass me or my partner? Ⓨ Ⓝ

11. Will I enjoy intercourse less because of this method? Ⓨ Ⓝ

12. Am I at risk of being exposed to HIV or other sexually transmitted infections if I use this method? Ⓨ Ⓝ

Total number of yes answers: _____

**Source:** Adapted from R. A. Hatcher et al., *Contraceptive Technology,* 19th ed. Copyright © 2007 Contraceptive Technology Communications, Inc.

## YOUR PLAN FOR CHANGE

The **Assess yourself** activity gave you the chance to assess your comfort and confidence with a contraceptive method you are using now or may use in the future. Depending on the results, you may consider changing your birth control method.

**Today, you can:**

◯ Visit your local drugstore and study the forms of contraception that are available without a prescription. Think about which of them you would consider using and why.

◯ If you are not currently using any contraception or are not in a sexual relationship but might become sexually active, purchase a package of condoms (or pick up a few free samples from your campus health center) to keep on hand just in case.

**Within the next 2 weeks, you can:**

◯ Make an appointment for a checkup with your health care provider. Be sure to ask him or her any questions you have about contraception.

◯ Sit down with your partner and discuss contraception. Decide who will be responsible and which form will work best for you.

**By the end of the semester, you can:**

◯ Periodically reevaluate whether your new or continued contraception is still effective for you. Review your experiences, and take note of any consistent problems you may have encountered.

◯ Always keep a backup form of contraception on hand. Check this supply periodically and throw out and replace any supplies that have expired.

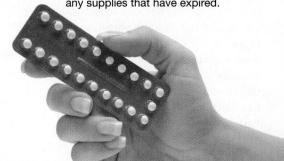

## Summary

* Latex or polyurethane male condoms and female condoms, when used correctly for oral sex or intercourse, provide the most effective protection in preventing sexually transmitted infections (STIs). Other contraceptive methods include spermicides, the diaphragm, the cervical cap, the Today sponge, oral contraceptives, Ortho Evra, NuvaRing, Depo-Provera, Implanon, and intrauterine devices. Emergency contraception may be used within 72 hours of unprotected intercourse or the failure of another contraceptive method. Fertility awareness methods rely on altering sexual practices to avoid pregnancy, as do abstinence, outercourse, and withdrawal. Whereas all these methods of contraception are reversible, sterilization is permanent.
* Abortion is legal in the United States through the second trimester. Abortion methods include suction curettage, dilation and evacuation (D&E), intact dilation and extraction (D&X), hysterotomy, induction abortion, and medical abortions.
* Parenting is a demanding job that requires careful planning. Prospective parents must consider emotional health, maternal and paternal health, financial plans, and contingency planning.
* Full-term pregnancy covers three trimesters. Prenatal care includes a complete physical exam within the first trimester, follow-up checkups throughout the pregnancy, healthy nutrition and exercise, and avoidance of all substances that could have teratogenic effects on the fetus. Prenatal tests, including ultrasonography, chorionic villus sampling, triple marker screening, and amniocentesis, can be used to detect birth defects during pregnancy.
* Childbirth occurs in three stages. Partners should jointly choose a labor method early in the pregnancy to be better prepared when labor occurs. Possible complications of pregnancy and childbirth include preeclampsia and eclampsia, miscarriage, Rh factor problems, ectopic pregnancy, and stillbirth.
* Infertility in women may be caused by pelvic inflammatory disease (PID) or endometriosis. In men, it may be caused by low sperm count. Treatments may include fertility drugs, alternative insemination, in vitro fertilization (IVF), assisted reproductive technology (ART), nonsurgical embryo transfer, embryo transfer, and embryo adoption programs. Surrogate motherhood and adoption are also options.

## Pop Quiz

1. What type of lubricant could you safely use with a latex condom?
   a. Mineral oil
   b. Water-based lubricant
   c. Body lotion
   d. Petroleum jelly

2. Which of the following is a barrier contraceptive?
   a. Seasonale
   b. FemCap
   c. Ortho Evra
   d. Contraceptive patch

3. What is the most commonly used method of first-trimester abortion?
   a. Suction curettage
   b. Dilation and evacuation (D&E)
   c. Medical abortion
   d. Induction abortion

4. What is meant by the *failure rate* of contraceptive use?
   a. The number of times a woman fails to get pregnant when she wanted to
   b. The number of times a woman gets pregnant when she did not want to
   c. The number of pregnancies that occurs for women using a particular method of birth control
   d. The reliability of alternative methods of birth control that do not use condoms

5. Toxic chemicals, pesticides, X rays, and other hazardous compounds that cause birth defects are referred to as
   a. carcinogens.
   b. teratogens.
   c. mutants.
   d. environmental assaults.

6. In an ectopic pregnancy, the fertilized egg implants itself in the woman's
   a. fallopian tube.
   b. uterus.
   c. vagina.
   d. ovaries.

7. What is the recommended pregnancy weight gain for a woman who is at a healthy weight before pregnancy?
   a. 15 to 20 pounds
   b. 20 to 30 pounds
   c. 25 to 35 pounds
   d. 30 to 45 pounds

8. What prenatal test involves snipping tissue from the developing fetal sac?
   a. Fetoscopy
   b. Ultrasound
   c. Amniocentesis
   d. Chorionic villus sampling

9. Why is it recommended not to use condoms made of lambskin?
   a. They are less elastic than latex condoms.
   b. They cannot be stored for as long as latex condoms.
   c. They do not protect against the transmission of STIs.
   d. They are likely to cause allergic reactions.

10. The number of American couples who experience infertility is
    a. 1 in 6.
    b. 1 in 24.
    c. 1 in 60.
    d. 1 in 100.

*Answers to these questions can be found on page A-1.*

# Think about It!

1. List the most effective contraceptive methods. What are their drawbacks? What medical conditions would keep a person from using each one? What are the characteristics of the methods you think would be most effective for you? Why do you consider them most effective for you?

2. What are the various methods of abortion? What are the two opposing viewpoints concerning abortion? What is *Roe v. Wade,* and what impact has it had on the abortion debate in the United States?

3. What are the most important considerations in deciding whether the time is right to become a parent? If you choose to have children, what factors will you consider regarding the number of children to have?

4. Discuss the growth of the fetus through the three trimesters. What medical checkups or tests should be done during each trimester?

5. Discuss the emotional aspects of pregnancy. What types of emotional reactions are common in each trimester and in the postpartum period (the "fourth trimester")?

6. If you and your partner are unable to have children, what alternative methods of conception would you consider? Would you consider adoption?

# Accessing Your Health on the Internet

The following websites explore further topics and issues related to personal health. For links to these websites below, visit the Companion Website for *Access to Health,* 12th Edition, at www.pearsonhighered.com/donatelle.

1. *Guttmacher Institute.* This is a nonprofit organization focused on sexual and reproductive health research, policy analysis, and public education. www.guttmacher.org

2. *Association of Reproductive Health Professionals.* This organization was originally founded by Alan Guttmacher as the educational arm of Planned Parenthood. Now an independent organization, it provides education for health care professionals and the general public. The Patient Resources portion of the website includes information on various methods of birth control and an interactive tool to help you choose a method that will work for you. www.arhp.org

3. *The American Pregnancy Association.* This is a national organization offering a wealth of resources to promote reproductive and pregnancy wellness. The website includes educational materials and information on the latest research. www.americanpregnancy.org

4. *Choosing Wisely birth control selection tool.* This interactive tool provided by the Society of Obstetricians and Gynaecologists of Canada helps you evaluate what type of birth control would best suit your needs. The questionnaire is quick and easy to use, and provides thorough information about the available contraceptive methods. www.sexualityandu.ca/trialdp/index.aspx

5. *Planned Parenthood.* This site offers a range of up-to-date information on sexual health issues, such as birth control, the decision of when and whether to have a child, sexually transmitted infections, and safer sex. www.plannedparenthood.org

6. *Sexuality Information and Education Council of the United States.* Information, guidelines, and materials for the advancement of sexuality education are all found here. The site advocates the right of individuals to make responsible sexual choices. www.siecus.org

7. *International Council on Infertility Information Dissemination.* This site includes current research and information on infertility. www.inciid.org

# References

1. American College Health Association, *American College Health Association—National College Health Assessment II: Reference Group Data Report Fall 2009* (Baltimore: American College Health Association, 2010). Available at www.acha-ncha.org/reports_ACHA-NCHAII.html.

2. R. A. Hatcher et al., *Contraceptive Technology,* 19th rev. ed. (New York: Ardent Media, 2007), 299.

3. American College Health Association, *American College Health Association—National College Health Assessment II,* 2010.

4. Drug Information Online, Drugs.Com, "Seasonale," www.drugs.com/seasonale.html, Accessed May, 2010.

5. R. A. Hatcher et al., *Contraceptive Technology,* 2007; R. Burkman et al., "Safety Concerns and Health Benefits Associated with Oral Contraception," *American Journal of Obstetrics and Gynecology* 190, no. 4 Suppl S (2004): S5–S22.

6. U.S. Food and Drug Administration, "Safety Labeling Changes Approved By FDA Center for Drug Evaluation and Research (CDER)—April 2010: Ortho Evra (Norelgestromin/Ethinyl Estradiol) Transdermal System," Updated May 2010, www.fda.gov/Safety/MedWatch/SafetyInformation/ucm211821.htm.

7. Office of Population Research & Association of Reproductive Health Professionals, Emergency Contraception Website "Answers to Frequently Asked Questions about Effectiveness," Updated March 2010, http://ec.princeton.edu/questions/eceffect.html.

8. Guttmacher Institute, *State Policies in Brief: As of October 1, 2010: Emergency Contraception.* Guttmacher Institute, October 2010, Available at www.guttmacher.org/statecenter/spibs.

9. J. Allen, "U.S. Teen Pregnancy Rate Up after 10-Year Decline," Reuters, January 2010, www.reuters.com/article/idUSN2519492420100126?loomia_ow=t0:s0:a49:g43:rl; B. Hamilton, J. Martin, and S. Ventura, "Births: Preliminary Data for 2008," *National Vital Statistics Reports* 58, no. 16 (Hyattsville, MD: National Center for Health Statistics, 2010): DHHS Publication no. (PHS) 2010-1120.

10. H. Boonstra, "Emergency Contraception: The Need to Increase Public Awareness," *Guttmacher Rep Public Policy* 5 (2002): 3–6.

11. R. Brening, A. Dalve-Endres, and K. Patrick, "Emergency Contraception Pills(ECPs): Current Trends in United States College Health Centers," *Contraception* 67, no. 6 (2003): 449–56; American College Health Association, *American College Health Association—National College Health Assessment II*, 2010.

12. American College Health Association, *American College Health Association—National College Health Assessment II*, 2010.

13. D. Bensyl et al., "Contraceptive Use—United States and Territories, Behavioral Risk Factor Surveillance System, 2002," *Morbidity and Mortality Weekly Report* 54 (SS6; November 18, 2005): 1–72.

14. R. A. Hatcher et al., *Contraceptive Technology*, 2007.

15. American Psychological Association, Task Force on Mental Health and Abortion, *Report of the Task Force on Mental Health and Abortion* (Washington, DC: American Psychological Association, 2008), Available at www.apa.org/pi/women/programs/abortion.

16. Ibid.

17. Boston Women's Health Collective, *Our Bodies, Ourselves: A New Edition for a New Era* (New York: Simon & Schuster, 2005).

18. NARAL Pro-Choice America Foundation, *Who Decides? The Status of Women's Reproductive Rights in the United States* (Washington, DC: NARAL Pro-Choice America Foundation, 2010), Available at www.prochoiceamerica.org/media/publications/who-decides; Guttmacher Institute, *State Policies in Brief: As of November 1, 2010: State Funding of Abortion under Medicaid*, Guttmacher Institute, November 2010, Available at www.guttmacher.org/statecenter/spibs.

19. NARAL Pro Choice America, "The Bush Administration's Federal Abortion Ban," January 2010, Available at www.naral.org/media/publications.

20. Guttmacher Institute, "Supreme Court Upholds Federal Abortion Ban, Opens Door for Further Restrictions by States," *Guttmacher Policy Review* 10, no. 2 (2007): 19.

21. American Psychological Association, Task Force on Mental Health and Abortion, *Report of the Task Force on Mental Health and Abortion*, 2008.

22. Ibid.

23. Ibid.

24. Guttmacher Institute, *Facts on Induced Abortion in the United States, In Brief*, May 2010, www.guttmacher.org/pubs/fb_induced_abortion.html.

25. Ibid.

26. Planned Parenthood, "The Difference between Emergency Contraception Pills and Medication Abortion," December 2006, www.plannedparenthood.org/resources/research-papers/difference-between-emergency-contraception-medication-abortion-6138.htm.

27. Ibid.

28. Mayo Clinic Staff, "Down Syndrome: Causes," MayoClinic.com, April 2009, www.mayoclinic.com/health/down-syndrome/ds00182/dsection=causes; National Human Genome Research Institute, "Learning about Klinefelter Syndrome," Reviewed June 2010, www.genome.gov/19519068.

29. Mayo Clinic Staff, "Prader-Willi Syndrome: Causes," MayoClinic.com, April 2009, www.mayoclinic.com/health/prader-willi-syndrome/DS00922/DSECTION=causes.

30. Donald Wigle et. al., "Epidemiologic Evidence of Relationships between Reproductive and Child Health Outcomes and Environmental Chemical Contaminants," *Journal of Toxicology* 11, no. 5-6 (2008): 373–517.

31. M. Lino, *Expenditures on Children by Families, 2009* (Alexandria, VA: U.S. Department of Agriculture, Center for Nutrition Policy and Promotion, 2010), Available at www.cnpp.usda.gov/ExpendituresonChildrenbyFamilies.htm.

32. National Association of Child Care Resource and Referral Agencies. *Parents and the High Price of Childcare, 2009 Update* (2009), Available at www.naccrra.org/publications/naccrra-publications.

33. Centers for Disease Control and Prevention, "Preconception Care Questions and Answers," April 2006, www.cdc.gov/ncbddd/preconception/QandA.htm.

34. Ibid.

35. National Center for Health Statistics, *Health, United States, 2009: With Special Feature on Medical Technology* (Hyattsville, MD: U.S. Government Printing Office, 2010), Available at www.cdc.gov/nchs/hus.htm.

36. National Center for Chronic Disease Prevention and Health Promotion, "Tobacco Use and Pregnancy," Modified May 2009, www.cdc.gov/reproductivehealth/TobaccoUsePregnancy/index.htm.

37. M. Kharrazi et al., "Environmental Tobacco Smoke and Pregnancy Outcome," *Epidemiology* 15, no. 6 (November 2006): 660–70.

38. D. Greenwood et al., "Caffeine Intake during Pregnancy, Late Miscarriage, and Stillbirth," *European Journal of Epidemiology* 25, no. 4 (2010): 275–80; B. Zhang et al., "Risk Factors for Unexplained Recurrent Spontaneous Abortion in a Population from Southern China," *International Journal of Gynaecology and Obstetrics* 108, no. 2 (2010): 135–38; A. Pollack, L. Buck, R. Sundarem, and K. Lum, "Caffeine Consumption and Miscarriage: A Prospective Cohort Study," *Fertility and Sterility* 93, no. 1 (2010): 304–06.

39. U.S. Department of Health and Human Services, Health Resources and Services Administration, Maternal and Child Health Bureau, *Child Health USA 2008–2009* (Rockville, MD: U.S. Department of Health and Human Services, 2009), Available at http://mchb.hrsa.gov/chusa08.

40. National Institute of Child Health and Human Development, "Down Syndrome," Updated March 2010, www.nichd.nih.gov/health/topics/down_syndrome.cfm.

41. F. Menacker and B. Hamilton, "Recent Trends in Cesarean Delivery in the United States," NCHS Data Brief no. 35 (Hyattsville, MD: National Center for Health Statistics, 2010), DHHS Publication no. (PHS) 2010–1209, Available at www.cdc.gov/nchs/data/databriefs/db35.htm.

42. Ibid.

43. E. Puscheck, "Early Pregnancy Loss," eMedicine from WebMD, Updated February 2010, http://emedicine.medscape.com/article/266317-overview.

44. J. Tenore, "Ectopic Pregnancy," *American Family Physician* 60 (2000): 1080–88.

45. March of Dimes, "Loss and Grief: Stillbirth," February 2010, www.marchofdimes.com/Baby/loss_stillbirth.html.

46. U.S. Department of Health and Human Services, Office on Women's Health, "Frequently Asked Questions: Depression During and After Pregnancy," Updated March 2009, www.womenshealth.gov/faq/depression-pregnancy.cfm.

47. American Pregnancy Association, "What's in Breast Milk?" Updated August 2006, www.americanpregnancy.org/firstyearoflife/whatsinbreastmilk.html.

48. A. Gardner, "Report Shows Dangerous Chemical Can Leach from Baby Bottles," *U.S. News & World Report*, February 7, 2008.

49. National Institute on Child and Human Development, "Research on Sudden Infant Death Syndrome," Updated October 2009,

www.nichd.nih.gov/womenshealth/
research/pregbirth/sids.cfm.

50. Ibid.

51. Mayo Clinic Staff, MayoClinic.com, "Infertility: Causes," June 2009, www.mayoclinic
.com/health/infertility/DS00310/
DSECTION=causes.

52. U.S. Department of Health and Human
Services, Office on Women's Health, "Frequently Asked Questions: Polycystic Ovary
Syndrome (PCOS)," Updated March 2010,
www.womenshealth.gov/faq/polycystic
-ovary-syndrome.cfm.

53. Centers for Disease Control and Prevention (CDC), "Pelvic Inflammatory Disease

CDC Fact Sheet," Modified April 2008,
www.cdc.gov/std/PID/STDFact-PID.htm.

54. Centers for Disease Control and Prevention (CDC), "Assisted Reproductive Technology," Reviewed November 2009, www
.cdc.gov/ART.

55. Ibid.

56. WebMD Medical Reference, "Fertility
Drugs," Reviewed February 2010, www
.webmd.com/infertility-and-reproduction/
guide/fertility-drugs.

57. J. Jones, "Who Adopts? Characteristics of
Women and Men Who Have Adopted Children," NCHS Data Brief no. 12 (Hyattsville,
MD: National Center for Health Statistics,

2009) DHHS Publication No. (PHS)
2009–1209, Available at www.cdc.gov/
nchs/data/databriefs/db12.htm.

58. Ibid.

59. Ibid.

60. Intercountry Adoption, Office of Children's
Issues, U.S. Department of State, "Total
Adoptions to the United States," Accessed
May 2010, http://adoption.state.gov/
news/total_chart.html.

61. Intercountry Adoption, Office of Children's
Issues, U.S. Department of State, "How to
Adopt" Accessed May 2010, http://
adoption.state.gov/about/how.html.

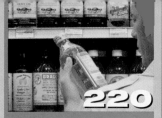
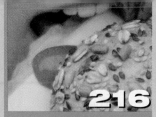
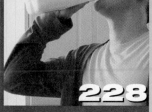
7

# Eating for a Healthier You

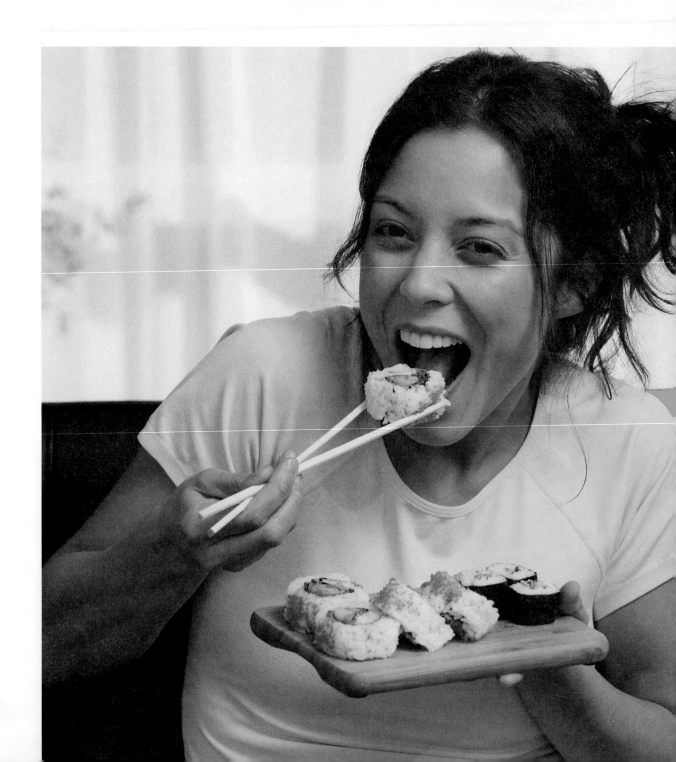

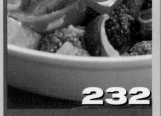
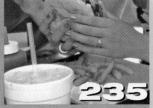

**232** Are vegetarian diets healthy?

**235** How can I eat well when I'm in a hurry?

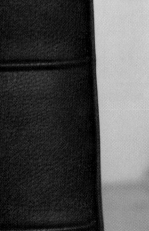

## Objectives

✳ Understand the factors that influence decisions about nutrition.

✳ List the six classes of nutrients, and explain the primary functions of each and their roles in maintaining long-term health.

✳ Discuss how to eat healthfully, including what is a healthful diet, how to use the MyPyramid Plan, information about supplement use, and reading food labels.

✳ Discuss the unique challenges that college students face when trying to eat healthy foods and the actions they can take to eat healthfully.

✳ Explain food safety concerns facing Americans and people in other regions of the world.

Advice about food can come at us from all directions: from newspaper headlines, popular magazines, cooking shows, and friends and neighbors. It seems everyone is eager to offer "expert" advice, but this advice can often be contradictory. For example, Dr. Atkins' recommendations for a diet high in protein and fat but low in carbohydrates contradict the advice of experts such as Dr. Dean Ornish and the American Heart Association—experts who advocate for low-fat diets. Knowing what to eat, how much to eat, and how to choose from a media-driven array of food and nutrition advice can be mind-boggling. For some, this can cause a phenomenon known as *eating anxiety* and lead to a lifetime of cycling on and off diets.[1] Why does something that can be so good, ultimately end up being a problem for so many of us? What influences our eating habits and how can we learn to eat more healthfully?

The answers to these questions aren't as simple as they may seem. When was the last time you ate because you felt true hunger pangs? True **hunger** occurs when there is a lack of basic foods. When we are hungry, our brains initiate a physiological response that prompts us to seek food for the energy and **nutrients** that our bodies require to maintain proper functioning. Most people in the United States don't know true hunger—most of us eat because of our **appetite**, a learned psychological desire to consume food. Hunger and appetite are not the only forces involved in our physiological drive to eat. Other factors include cultural and social meanings attached to food, convenience and advertising, habit or custom, emotional eating, perceived nutritional value, social interaction, and financial means.

**Nutrition** is the science that investigates the relationship between physiological function and the essential elements of the foods we eat. With an understanding of nutrition, you will be able to distinguish fact from fiction about trends in nutrition. Your health depends largely on what you eat, how much you eat, and the amount of exercise that you get throughout your life. The next few chapters focus on fundamental principles of nutrition, weight management, and exercise.

**hunger** The physiological impulse to seek food, prompted by the lack or shortage of basic foods needed to provide the energy and nutrients that support health.

**nutrients** The constituents of food that sustain humans physiologically: proteins, carbohydrates, fats, vitamins, minerals, and water.

**appetite** The desire to eat; normally accompanies hunger but is more psychological than physiological.

**nutrition** The science that investigates the relationship between physiological function and the essential elements of foods eaten.

### "Why Should I Care?"

The nutritional choices you make during college can have both immediate and lasting effects on your health. Thousands of studies associate what we eat with chronic diseases such as diabetes, heart disease, hypertension, stroke, and many types of cancer.

# Essential Nutrients for Health

Food provides the chemicals we need for activity and body maintenance. Our bodies cannot synthesize certain *essential nutrients* (or cannot synthesize them in adequate amounts)—we must obtain them from the foods we eat. Before the body can use foods, the digestive system must break down the larger food particles into smaller, more usable forms. The sequence of functions by which the body breaks down foods and either absorbs or excretes them is known as the **digestive process** (Figure 7.1).

**digestive process** The process by which the body breaks down foods and either absorbs or excretes them.

**calorie** A unit of measure that indicates the amount of energy obtained from a particular food.

**dehydration** Abnormal depletion of body fluids; a result of lack of water.

## Calories

A *kilocalorie* is a unit of measure used to quantify the amount of energy in food that the body can use. A **calorie** is also a unit of measure—technically, 1 kilocalorie is equal to 1,000 calories. Most nutrition labels use the word *calories* to refer to kilocalories. As such, we will use the word *calorie* throughout this chapter as we indicate energy levels of foods. *Energy* is defined as the capacity to do work. We derive energy from the energy-containing nutrients in the foods we eat. These energy-containing nutrients—protein, carbohydrate, and fat—provide calories. Vitamins, minerals, and water do not. Table 7.1 shows the caloric needs for various individuals.

## Water: A Crucial Nutrient

Humans can survive much longer without food than without water. The average person can go for weeks without certain vitamins and minerals before experiencing serious deficiency symptoms. However, **dehydration,** or abnormal depletion of body fluids, can cause serious problems within a matter of

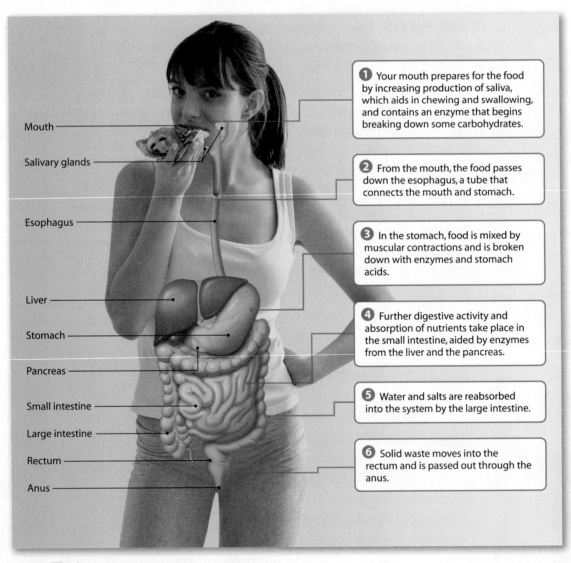

Mouth
Salivary glands
Esophagus
Liver
Stomach
Pancreas
Small intestine
Large intestine
Rectum
Anus

1 Your mouth prepares for the food by increasing production of saliva, which aids in chewing and swallowing, and contains an enzyme that begins breaking down some carbohydrates.

2 From the mouth, the food passes down the esophagus, a tube that connects the mouth and stomach.

3 In the stomach, food is mixed by muscular contractions and is broken down with enzymes and stomach acids.

4 Further digestive activity and absorption of nutrients take place in the small intestine, aided by enzymes from the liver and the pancreas.

5 Water and salts are reabsorbed into the system by the large intestine.

6 Solid waste moves into the rectum and is passed out through the anus.

FIGURE 7.1 **The Digestive Process**
The entire digestive process takes approximately 24 hours.

| TABLE 7.1 Estimated Daily Calorie Needs | | | |
|---|---|---|---|
| | Calorie Range | | |
| | Sedentary[a] | | Active[b] |
| **Children** | | | |
| 2–3 years old | 1,000 | → | 1,400 |
| **Females** | | | |
| 4–8 years old | 1,200 | → | 1,800 |
| 9–13 | 1,600 | → | 2,200 |
| 14–18 | 1,800 | → | 2,400 |
| 19–30 | 2,000 | → | 2,400 |
| 31–50 | 1,800 | → | 2,200 |
| 51+ | 1,600 | → | 2,200 |
| **Males** | | | |
| 4–8 years old | 1,400 | → | 2,000 |
| 9–13 | 1,800 | → | 2,600 |
| 14–18 | 2,200 | → | 3,200 |
| 19–30 | 2,400 | → | 3,000 |
| 31–50 | 2,200 | → | 3,000 |
| 51+ | 2,000 | → | 2,800 |

[a] A lifestyle that includes only the light physical activity associated with typical day-to-day life.

[b] A lifestyle that includes physical activity equivalent to walking more than 3 miles per day at 3 to 4 miles per hour, in addition to the light physical activity associated with typical day-to-day life.

**Source:** Center for Nutrition Policy and Promotion, April 2005, www.MyPyramid.gov.

hours, and death after a few days. Too much water can also pose a serious risk to your health. This condition is known as *hyponatremia,* and is characterized by low sodium levels.

The human body consists of 50 to 60 percent water by weight. The water in our system bathes cells, aids in fluid and electrolyte balance, maintains pH balance, and transports molecules and cells throughout the body. Water is the major component of our blood, which carries oxygen and nutrients to the tissues, removes metabolic wastes, and is responsible for maintaining cells in working order.

Individual needs for water vary drastically according to dietary factors, age, size, overall health, environmental temperature and humidity levels, and exercise. For the most part, scientists now refute the conventional wisdom that you need to drink eight glasses of water per day.[2] The latest Dietary Reference Intakes on water suggest that most people can meet their hydration needs simply by eating a healthy diet and drinking in response to thirst. The general recommendations for women are approximately 11 cups of total water from all beverages and foods each day and for men an average of 16 cups.[3]

We usually get the fluids we need each day through the food we eat and the water and other beverages we consume.

About 20 percent of our daily water needs are met through the food we eat. In fact, fruits and vegetables are 80 to 95 percent water, meats are more than 50 percent water, and even dry bread and cheese are about 35 percent water! Contrary to popular opinion, caffeinated drinks, including coffee, tea, and soda, also count toward total fluid intake for those who regularly consume them. Caffeinated beverages have not been found to dehydrate people whose bodies are used to caffeine.

Of course, there are situations in which a person needs to take in additional fluids in order to stay properly hydrated. It is important to drink extra fluids when you have a fever or an illness in which there is vomiting or diarrhea. Anyone with kidney function problems or who tends to develop kidney stones may need more water, as may people with diabetes or cystic fibrosis. The elderly and very young also may have increased water needs. When the weather heats up, or when you exercise, work, or engage in other activities in which you sweat profusely, extra water is needed to keep your body's core temperature within a normal range. If you are an athlete and wonder about water consumption, visit the American College of Sports Medicine's website (www.acsm.org) to view its guidelines on exercise and fluid replacement.[4] The focus on drinking water to meet hydration needs has contributed to the bottled water boom currently taking place in the United States. See the **Be Healthy, Be Green** box on page 214 for an exploration of the environmental problems associated with bottled water and for some more ecofriendly ways to stay hydrated.

# Proteins

Next to water, **proteins** are the most abundant substances in the human body. Proteins are major components of nearly every cell and have been called the "body builders" because of their role in developing and repairing bone, muscle, skin, and blood cells. They are the key elements of antibodies that protect us from disease, of enzymes that

**78.1** grams of protein is what the average American consumes daily—much more than the recommended amount.

control chemical activities in the body, and of hormones that regulate body functions. Proteins help transport iron, oxygen, and nutrients to all body cells and supply another source of energy to cells when fats and carbohydrates are not available. Adequate amounts of protein in the diet are vital to many body functions and ultimately to survival.

Your body breaks down proteins into smaller nitrogen-containing molecules known as **amino acids,** the building blocks of protein. Nine of the 20 different amino acids are termed

**proteins** The essential constituents of nearly all body cells; necessary for the development and repair of bone, muscle, skin, and blood; the key elements of antibodies, enzymes, and hormones.

**amino acids** The nitrogen-containing building blocks of protein.

## Bottled Water Boom: Who Pays the Price?

Globally, factories are churning out bottled water at unprecedented rates. Conservative estimates are that bottled water is now our second most popular drink, right behind soda, with over $100 billion in sales each year. In 1976, annual per person consumption of bottled water was just 1.6 gallons. By 2009, annual per person consumption had grown to 27.6 gallons. The United States is the world leader in bottled water consumption with approximately 8,500 million gallons produced in 2009, followed by Mexico with 6,900 gallons and China with 5,700 gallons.

We may imagine that bottled water comes from medicinal mountain streams or aquifers that ensure purity, but the fact is that most of the water sold in bottles comes from municipal water supplies, sometimes with extra minerals being added, or with an extra step in purification. If it was just your money going down the drain and you could afford it, it wouldn't be so worrisome. However, the environmental consequences of bottled water are significant. Consider the following:

✳ Around the world, factories are using more than 18 million barrels of oil and up to 130 billion gallons of fresh water to quench our bottled water thirst. When you include the resource cost of transporting bottled water, it is estimated that the total amount of energy required to create and transport every bottle is the equivalent of filling the bottle one-quarter full of oil.
✳ In general, systems such as reverse osmosis purifiers use about 2 liters of fresh water running through a system to realize 1 liter of bottled water.
✳ In 2006, more than 900,000 tons of plastic were used to package 8 billion gallons of bottled water.

✳ There is a growing concern about negative health risks from certain chemicals found in plastic bottles that can leach into the water, particularly *bisphenol-A (BPA)*. Research has suggested links between BPA and negative estrogen-related effects, including breast enlargement in young boys, some forms of cancer, early onset of puberty, and increased risk for type 2 diabetes.
✳ Tap water in the United States is among the safest in the world, largely because community water supplies are subject to strict and constant monitoring required by the Safe Drinking Act, whereas bottled water is considered a "food" and requires much less frequent monitoring for safety and quality by the U.S. Food and Drug Administration or individual state oversight.
✳ Nationwide, less than 15 percent of discarded bottles are recycled.
✳ Companies taking part in the bottled water boom are buying water supplies throughout the world for financial gain, leaving entire populations vulnerable to water shortages.

You can help to curb the personal and global environmental threats caused by bottled water use:

✳ Don't buy bottled water unless it's absolutely necessary. Instead, purchase a stainless steel or glass container and use it again and again. Look for a container with a wide mouth so that you can wash and dry it regularly.
✳ When you have parties, use covered pitchers of ice water and recyclable paper cups, rather than serving bottles or using plastic cups.
✳ Buy an inexpensive water filter to help remove the taste of chlorine from tap water. Refrigerate your water jug as a means of improving taste and clarity.
✳ Recycle any plastic bottles you use or come across. Many states offer 5 cent deposits on beverage bottles and cans as an incentive to increase recycling efforts.
✳ Become involved in initiatives to ensure quality tap water in your community. Ask questions about the filters being used, the chemicals and minerals that are removed, and the chemicals and minerals that remain.
✳ Encourage your campus to install water dispensers rather than providing bottled water in vending machines. You can find out more about reducing bottled water use on your campus in the "Beyond the Bottle at Brown Campaign Guide," prepared by Brown University, available at www.beyondthebottle.org.

Purchasing a stainless steel bottle that you can reuse is a better choice than buying plastic bottles every day.

**Sources:** Sierra Club, "Bottled Water: Learning the Facts and Taking Action," 2008, www.sierraclub.org/committees/cac/water/bottled_water/bottled_water.pdf; Oregon State University, "Bottled Water Boom Has Environmental Drawbacks," Media Release, 2007, http://oregonstate.edu/dept/ncs/newsarch/2007/May07/bottledwater.html; J. Rodwan Jr., "Bottled Water Statistic 2009: Challenging Circumstances Persist: U.S. and International Developments and Statistics," *Bottled Water Reporter* 50, no. 3 (2010): 10–16, Available at www.bottledwater.org/content/455/bottled-water-reporter.

---

**essential amino acids,** which means the body must obtain them from the diet; the other 11 can be produced by the body. Dietary protein that supplies all the essential amino acids is called **complete (high-quality) protein.** Typically, protein from animal products is complete. For proteins to be complete, they also must be present in digestible form and in amounts proportional to body requirements. When we consume foods that are deficient in some of the essential amino acids, the total amount of protein that can be synthesized from the other amino acids is decreased.

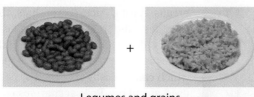

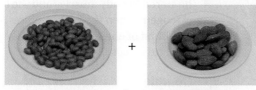

Legumes and grains

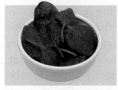

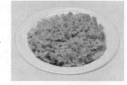

Legumes and nuts and seeds

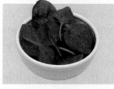

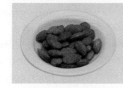

Green leafy vegetables and grains

Green leafy vegetables and nuts and seeds

FIGURE 7.2 **Complementary Proteins**
Eaten in the right combination, plant-based foods can provide complementary proteins and all essential amino acids.

What about plant sources of protein? Proteins from plant sources are often **incomplete proteins** in that they may lack one or two of the essential amino acids. However, it is easy for the non–meat eater to combine plant foods effectively and eat complementary sources of plant protein **(Figure 7.2)**. Plant sources of protein fall into three general categories: *legumes* (beans, peas, peanuts, and soy products), *grains* (e.g., wheat, corn, rice, and oats), and *nuts and seeds*. Certain vegetables, such as leafy green vegetables and broccoli, also contribute valuable plant proteins. Mixing two or more foods from each of these categories during the same meal will provide all the essential amino acids necessary to ensure adequate protein absorption.

Although protein deficiency poses a threat to the global population (see the **Health in a Diverse World** box on page 217), few Americans suffer from protein deficiencies. In fact, the average American consumes more than 78 grams of protein daily, and much of this comes from high-fat animal flesh and dairy products.[5] The recommended daily protein intake for adults is only 0.8 gram (g) per kilogram (kg) of body weight. To calculate your protein needs: Divide your body weight (in pounds) by 2.2 to get your weight in kilograms, then multiply by 0.8. The result is your recommended protein intake per day. The typical recommendation is that in a 2,000-calorie diet, 10 to 35 percent of calories should come from lean protein, for a total average of 50 to 175 grams per day (a 6-ounce steak contains 53 grams of protein—more than the daily needs of an average-sized woman!).

A person might need to eat extra protein if she is pregnant, fighting off a serious infection, recovering from surgery or blood loss, or recovering from burns. In these instances, proteins that are lost to cellular repair and development need to be replaced. There is considerable controversy over whether someone in high-level physical training needs additional protein to build and repair muscle fibers or whether normal daily requirements should suffice. In addition, a sedentary person or one who gets little exercise may find it easier to stay in energy balance if more of his calories come from protein and fewer come from carbohydrates. Why? Because proteins make a person feel full and satisfied for a longer period of time.

**essential amino acids** Nine of the basic nitrogen-containing building blocks of protein, which must be obtained from foods to ensure health.
**complete (high-quality) proteins** Proteins that contain all nine of the essential amino acids.
**incomplete proteins** Proteins that lack one or more of the essential amino acids.
**carbohydrates** Basic nutrients that supply the body with glucose, the energy form most commonly used to sustain normal activity.
**simple carbohydrates** A major type of carbohydrate, which provides short-term energy; also called *simple sugars*.
**complex carbohydrates** A major type of carbohydrate, which provides sustained energy.
**monosaccharides** Simple sugars that contain only one molecule of sugar.

# Carbohydrates

**Carbohydrates** supply us with the energy needed to sustain normal daily activity. The human body metabolizes carbohydrates more quickly and efficiently than it does proteins for a quick source of energy for the body. Carbohydrates are easily converted to glucose, the fuel for the body's cells. Carbohydrates also play an important role in the functioning of internal organs, the nervous system, and muscles. They are the best fuel for endurance athletics because they provide both an immediate and a time-released energy source; they are digested easily and then consistently metabolized in the bloodstream. There are two major types of carbohydrates: **simple carbohydrates** or *simple sugars,* which are found naturally in fruits and many vegetables, and **complex carbohydrates,** which are found in grains, cereals, and vegetables.

1/3 of the calories Americans consume come from junk foods with no nutritional value such as sweets, soft drinks, and alcoholic beverages.

**Simple Carbohydrates** A typical American diet contains large amounts of simple carbohydrates. The most common form is *glucose.* Eventually, the human body converts all types of simple sugars to glucose to provide energy to cells. Another simple sugar is *fructose* (commonly called *fruit sugar*), which is found in fruits and berries. Glucose and fructose are **monosaccharides.**

**Disaccharides** are combinations of two monosaccharides. Perhaps the best-known example is *sucrose* (granulated table sugar). *Lactose* (milk sugar), found in milk and milk products, and *maltose* (malt sugar) are other examples of common disaccharides. Disaccharides must be broken down into monosaccharides before the body can use them.

Americans typically consume far too many refined carbohydrates (i.e., carbohydrates containing only sugars and starches, discussed below), which have few health benefits and are a major factor in our growing epidemic of overweight and obesity. Many of the simple sugars in these foods come from *added sugars,* sweeteners that are put in during processing to flavor foods, make sodas taste good, and ease our craving for sweets. A classic example is the amount of added sugar in one can of soda: more than 10 teaspoons per can! All that refined sugar can cause tooth decay and put on pounds.

Sugar is found in high amounts in a wide range of food products. Such diverse items as ketchup, barbecue sauce, and flavored coffee creamers derive 30 to 65 percent of their calories from sugar. Knowing what foods contain these sugars, considering the amounts you consume each day that are hidden in foods, and then trying to reduce these levels can be a great way to reduce excess weight. Read food labels carefully before purchasing. If *sugar* or one of its aliases (including *high fructose corn syrup* and *cornstarch*) appears near the top of the ingredients list, then that product contains a lot of sugar and is probably not your best nutritional bet. Also, most labels list the amount of sugar as a percentage of total calories.

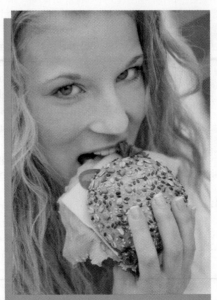

**Why are whole grains better than refined grains?**

Whole-grain foods contain fiber, a crucial form of carbohydrate that protects against some gastrointestinal disorders and reduces risk for certain cancers. Fiber is also associated with lowered blood cholesterol levels; studies have shown that eating 2.5 servings of whole grains per day can reduce cardiovascular disease risk by as much as 21%. But are people getting the message? One nutrition survey showed that only 8% of U.S. adults consume three or more servings of whole grains each day, and 42% ate no whole grains at all on a given day.

### Complex Carbohydrates: Starches and Glycogen

Complex carbohydrates, or **polysaccharides,** are formed by long chains of monosaccharides. Like disaccharides, they must be broken down into simple sugars before the body can use them. *Starches, glycogen,* and *fiber* are the main types of complex carbohydrates.

**Starches** make up the majority of the complex carbohydrate group and come from flours, breads, pasta, rice, corn, oats, barley, potatoes, and related foods. The body breaks down these complex carbohydrates into the monosaccharide glucose, which can be easily absorbed by cells and used as energy. Polysaccharides can also be stored in body muscles and the liver as **glycogen.** When the body requires a sudden burst of energy, it breaks down glycogen into glucose.

### Complex Carbohydrates: Fiber

**Fiber,** sometimes referred to as "bulk" or "roughage," is the indigestible portion of plant foods that helps move foods through the digestive system, delays absorption of cholesterol and other nutrients, and softens stools by absorbing water. Dietary fiber is found only in plant foods, such as fruits, vegetables, nuts, and grains. The Food and Nutrition Board of the Institute of Medicine makes three fiber distinctions: dietary fiber, functional fiber, and total fiber.[6] *Dietary fiber* comprises the nondigestible parts of plants—the leaves, stems, and seeds. *Functional fiber* consists of nondigestible forms of carbohydrates that may come from plants or may be manufactured in the laboratory and have known health benefits. *Total fiber* is the sum of dietary fiber and functional fiber in a person's diet.

A more user-friendly classification of fiber types is either *soluble* or *insoluble.* Soluble fibers, such as pectins, gums, and mucilages, dissolve in water, form gel-like substances, and can be digested easily by bacteria in the colon. Major food sources of soluble fiber include citrus fruits, berries, oat bran, dried beans (e.g., kidney, garbanzo, pinto, and navy beans), and some vegetables. Insoluble fibers, such as lignins and cellulose, are those that typically do not dissolve in water and that cannot be fermented by bacteria in the colon. They are found in most fruits and vegetables, and in **whole grains,** such as brown rice, wheat, bran, and whole-grain breads and cereals (see **Figure 7.3**). Find out more about the benefits of fiber in the **Student Health Today** box on page 219.

Despite growing evidence supporting the benefits of whole grains and high-fiber diets, intake among the general public remains low. Most experts believe that Americans should double their current consumption of dietary fiber—to 20 to 35 grams per day for most people and perhaps to 40 to 50 grams for others. What's the best way to increase your intake of dietary fiber? Eat fewer refined or processed carbohydrates in favor of more whole grains, fruits, vegetables, legumes, nuts, and seeds. As with most nutritional advice, however, too much of a good thing can pose problems. Sudden increases in

**disaccharides** Combinations of two monosaccharides.
**polysaccharides** Complex carbohydrates formed by the combination of long chains of monosaccharides.
**starch** Polysaccharide that is the storage form of glucose in plants.
**glycogen** The polysaccharide form in which glucose is stored in the liver and, to a lesser extent, in muscles.
**fiber** The indigestible portion of plant foods that helps move food through the digestive system and softens stools by absorbing water.
**whole grains** Grains that are milled in their complete form, and so include the bran, germ, and endosperm, with only the husk removed.

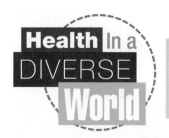

## Global Nutrition: Threats to World Populations

Although it's widely accepted that in general good nutrition means stronger immune systems, better productivity, fewer illnesses, and better health, millions of people in the developed and developing world suffer from food scarcity, food insecurity, and malnutrition. Just how much of an impact does poor nutrition have on the health of global populations? Consider the following:

※ Poor nutrition contributes to 1 out of 2 deaths (53%) associated with infectious diseases among children under age 5 in developing countries.
※ One out of 4 preschool children suffers from undernutrition in the global population.
※ One in 3 people in developing countries is affected by vitamin and mineral deficiencies and therefore are at greater risk for infection, birth defects, and impaired physical and intellectual development.
※ In the United States, nearly 15 percent of the population suffers from

*food insecurity,* meaning that they are unable to provide sufficient food for themselves or their families.

Ironically, at the same time that food insecurity and insufficient food levels plague the world, the global population is also seeing a dramatic increase in other forms of malnutrition. These are characterized by obesity and the long-term implications of unbalanced dietary and lifestyle practices that result in chronic diseases such as cardiovascular disease, cancer, and diabetes. Although we often think that obesity is a problem of excess and affluence, this isn't always the case. In fact, obesity flourishes in populations where acute hunger also persists.

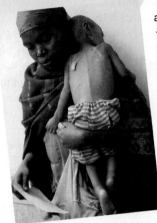

Drought, high food prices, and political unrest all contribute to the severe malnutrition experienced by millions of people worldwide.

※ Two out of 3 overweight and obese people now live in developing countries, the vast majority in emerging markets and transition economies.
※ Under- and overnutrition problems and diet-related chronic diseases (including obesity-related diseases) account for more than half of the world's diseases and hundreds of millions of dollars in public expenditure to combat them.

**Sources:** World Health Organization, "Nutrition: Challenges," Accessed April 2010, www.who.int/nutrition/challenges/en/index.html; M. Nord, M. Andrews, and S. Carlson, *Household Food Security in the United States, 2008,* Economic Research Report no. 83, U.S. Department of Agriculture, Economic Research Service, November 2009, www.ers.usda.gov/Publications/ERR83.

---

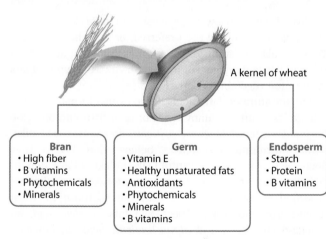

A kernel of wheat

**Bran**
• High fiber
• B vitamins
• Phytochemicals
• Minerals

**Germ**
• Vitamin E
• Healthy unsaturated fats
• Antioxidants
• Phytochemicals
• Minerals
• B vitamins

**Endosperm**
• Starch
• Protein
• B vitamins

FIGURE 7.3 **Anatomy of a Whole Grain**
Whole grains are more nutritious than refined grains, because they contain the bran, germ, and endosperm of the seed—sources of fiber, vitamins, minerals, and beneficial phytochemicals (chemical compounds that occur naturally in plants).
Source: Adapted from Blake, Joan Salge; Munoz, Kathy D.; Volpe, Stella, *Nutrition: From Science to You,* 1st, © 2010. Printed and Electronically reproduced by permission of Pearson Education, Inc., Upper Saddle River, New Jersey.

dietary fiber may cause flatulence (intestinal gas), cramping, or bloating. Consume plenty of water or other (sugar-free!) liquids to reduce such side effects.

## Fats

**Fats** are perhaps the most misunderstood of the body's required nutrients. Fats are the most energy-dense source of calories in our diet. Fats play a vital role in maintaining healthy skin and hair, insulating body organs against shock, maintaining body temperature, and promoting healthy cell function. Fats make foods taste better and carry the fat-soluble vitamins A, D, E, and K to the cells. They also provide a concentrated form of energy in the absence of sufficient amounts of carbohydrates and make you feel full after eating. If fats perform all these functions, why are we constantly urged to cut back on them? Because some fats are less healthy than others and because excessive consumption of fats can lead to weight gain.

**fats** Basic nutrients composed of carbon and hydrogen atoms; needed for the proper functioning of cells, insulation of body organs against shock, maintenance of body temperature, and healthy skin and hair.

**Triglycerides,** which make up about 95 percent of total body fat, are the most common form of fat circulating in the blood. When we consume too many calories from any source, the liver converts the excess into triglycerides, which are stored throughout our bodies. The remaining 5 percent of body fat is composed of substances such as **cholesterol.** The ratio of total cholesterol to a group of compounds called **high-density lipoproteins (HDLs)** is important to determining risk for heart disease. Lipoproteins facilitate the transport of cholesterol in the blood. High-density lipoproteins are capable of transporting more cholesterol than are **low-density lipoproteins (LDLs).** Whereas LDLs transport cholesterol to the body's cells, HDLs transport circulating cholesterol to the liver for metabolism and elimination from the body. People with a high percentage of HDLs appear to be at lower risk for developing cholesterol-clogged arteries. See Chapter 15 for more on the role cholesterol plays in cardiovascular health.

### "Why Should I Care?"

Cholesterol can accumulate on the inner walls of arteries and narrow the channels through which blood flows. This buildup, called plaque, is a major cause of *atherosclerosis,* a component of cardiovascular disease.

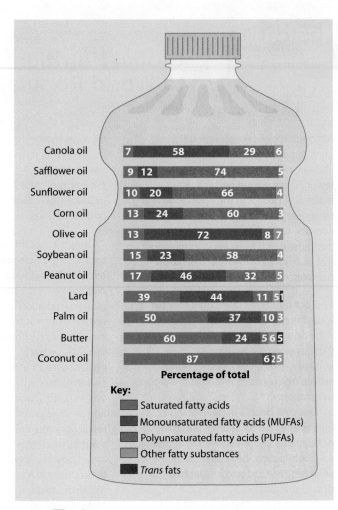

FIGURE 7.4 **Percentages of Saturated, Polyunsaturated, Monounsaturated, and *Trans* Fats in Common Vegetable Oils**

**Types of Dietary Fats** Fat molecules include *fatty acid* chains of carbon and hydrogen atoms. Fatty acid chains that cannot hold any more hydrogen in their chemical structure are called **saturated fats.** They generally come from animal sources, such as meat, dairy, and poultry products, and are solid at room temperature. **Unsaturated fats** have room for additional hydrogen atoms in their chemical structure, and are liquid at room temperature. They come from plants and include most vegetable oils.

The terms *monounsaturated fatty acids* (*MUFAs*) and *polyunsaturated fatty acids* (*PUFAs*) refer to the relative number of hydrogen atoms that are missing in a fatty acid chain. Peanut and olive oils are high in monounsaturated fats. Corn, sunflower, and safflower oils are high in polyunsaturated fats.

There is currently a great deal of controversy about which type of unsaturated fat is most beneficial. Monounsaturated fatty acids, such

as olive oil, seem to lower LDL levels and increase HDL levels and thus are currently the preferred, or least harmful, fats. They are also resistant to oxidation, a process that leads to cell and tissue damage. For a breakdown of the types of fats in common vegetable oils, see **Figure 7.4.**

Polyunsaturated fatty acids come in two forms: *omega-3 fatty acids* (found in many types of fatty fish) and *omega-6 fatty acids* (found in corn, soybean, and cottonseed oils). Some nutritional researchers believe that PUFAs may decrease levels of both harmful LDL cholesterol and beneficial HDL cholesterol. However, there are two PUFAs that are classified as *essential fatty acids*—that is, those we must receive from our diets. These two fats, *linoleic acid,* an omega-6 fatty acid, and *alpha-linolenic acid,* an omega-3 fatty acid, are needed to make hormone-like compounds that control immune function, pain perception, and inflammation, to name a few key benefits.[7]

It is believed that early humans ate a diet of approximately equal portions of omega-6 to omega-3. Today, Americans consume a ratio of approximately 10:1 omega-6 fats to omega-3 fats, and most experts agree that we need a more balanced approach.[8] Recently, an American Heart Associa-

**triglycerides** The most common form of fat in the body; excess calories consumed are converted into triglycerides and stored as body fat.

**cholesterol** A form of fat circulating in the blood that can accumulate on the inner walls of arteries, causing a narrowing of the channel through which blood flows.

**high-density lipoproteins (HDLs)** Compounds that facilitate the transport of cholesterol in the blood to the liver for metabolism and elimination from the body.

**low-density lipoproteins (LDLs)** Compounds that facilitate the transport of cholesterol in the blood to the body's cells.

**saturated fats** Fats that are unable to hold any more hydrogen in their chemical structure; derived mostly from animal sources; solid at room temperature.

**unsaturated fats** Fats that do have room for more hydrogen in their chemical structure; derived mostly from plants; liquid at room temperature.

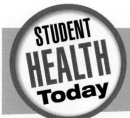

# WHY FIBER IS YOUR FRIEND

Getting enough fiber may seem like something only your grandparents need to be concerned about, but getting the recommended amount of fiber in your diet now can help you feel your best right now, and avoid disease in the future. Research supports many benefits of fiber:

* **Protection against colon and rectal cancer.** One of the leading causes of cancer deaths in the United States, colorectal cancer is much rarer in countries whose populations eat diets high in fiber and low in animal fat. Several studies have contributed to the theory that fiber-rich diets, particularly those including insoluble fiber, prevent the development of precancerous growths.

* **Protection against constipation.** Insoluble fiber acts like a sponge. When consumed with adequate fluids, it absorbs moisture and produces softer, bulkier stools that are easily passed.

* **Protection against diverticulosis.** Diverticulosis is a condition in which tiny bulges or pouches form on the large intestinal wall. These bulges can become irritated and cause chronic pain if under strain from constipation. Insoluble fiber helps to reduce constipation and discomfort.

* **Protection against heart disease.** Many studies have indicated that soluble fiber helps reduce blood cholesterol, primarily by lowering low-density lipoprotein (LDL: "bad") cholesterol.

* **Protection against type 2 diabetes.** Some studies suggest that soluble fiber improves control of blood sugar and can reduce the need for insulin or medication in people with type 2 diabetes.

* **Protection against obesity.** Because most high-fiber foods are high in carbohydrates and low in fat, they help control caloric intake. Many take longer to chew, which slows you down at the table, and fiber stays in the digestive tract longer than other nutrients, making you feel full sooner. So fiber can help you succeed in your weight-loss efforts.

Below are some ways for you to incorporate more fiber into your daily diet:

* Whenever possible, select whole-grain breads, especially those that are low in fat and sugars. Choose breads with 3 or more grams of fiber per serving. Read labels—just because bread is brown doesn't mean it is better for you. Make sure what you buy and consume actually are whole-grain products.

* Eat whole, unpeeled fruits and vegetables rather than drinking their juices. The fiber in the whole fruit tends to slow blood sugar increases and helps you feel full longer.

* Substitute whole-grain pastas, bagels, and pizza crust for the refined, white flour versions.

* Add wheat crumbs or grains to meat loaf and burgers to increase fiber intake.

* Toast grains to bring out their nutty flavor and make foods more appealing.

* Sprinkle ground flaxseed on cereals, yogurt, and salads, or add to casseroles, burgers, and baked goods. Flaxseed has a mild flavor and is also high in beneficial fatty acids.

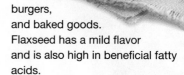

Cereal can be a good source of whole grains and fiber.

**Sources:** K. Maki et al., "Whole-Grain Ready-to-Eat Oat Cereal, as Part of a Dietary Program for Weight Loss, Reduces Low-Density Lipoprotein Cholesterol in Adults with Overweight and Obesity More than a Dietary Program Including Low-Fiber Control Foods," *Journal of the American Dietetic Association* 110, no. 2 (2010): 205–14; National Cholesterol Education Program Expert Panel, *Detection, Evaluation, and Treatment of High Cholesterol in Adults (Adult Treatment Panel III). Final Report*, U.S. Department of Health and Human Services, National Heart, Lung, and Blood Institute, NIH Publication no. 02-5215, 2002, Available at www.nhlbi.nih.gov/guidelines/cholesterol; E. J. Brunner et al., "Dietary Patterns and 15 Year Risks of Major Coronary Events, Diabetes and Mortality," *American Journal of Clinical Nutrition* 87, no. 5 (2008): 1414–21; A. E. Millen et al., "Fruit and Vegetable Intake and Prevalence of Colorectal Adenoma in Cancer Screening Trial," *American Journal of Clinical Nutrition* 86, no. 6 (2007): 1754–64; P. Newby et al., "Intake of Whole Grains, Refined Grains and Cereal Fiber Measured with 7-d Diet Records and Associations with Risk Factors for Chronic Disease," *American Journal of Clinical Nutrition* 86, no. 6 (2007): 1745–53.

tion advisory panel stated concern over people reducing omega-6 when instead the focus should be on limiting saturated fat in the diet.[9] Generally, about 20 to 35 percent of calories should come from fat, with 5 to 10 percent coming from omega-6 fatty acids.

**Avoiding *Trans* Fatty Acids** For decades, Americans shunned butter, certain cuts of red meat, and other foods because of the saturated fats found in them. What they didn't know is that foods low in saturated fat, such as margarine, could be just as harmful. As early as the 1990s Dutch researchers reported that a form of fat known as *trans* fats increased LDL cholesterol levels while decreasing HDL cholesterol levels.[10] In a more recent study, researchers concluded that just a 2 percent caloric intake of *trans* fats was associated with a 23 percent increased risk for heart disease and a 47 percent increased chance of sudden cardiac death.[11]

What are ***trans* fats (*trans* fatty acids)**? *Trans* fats are fatty acids that are produced by adding hydrogen molecules to liquid oil to make the oil into a solid. Unlike regular fats and oils, these "partially hydrogenated" fats stay solid or semisolid at room temperature. They change

***trans* fats (*trans* fatty acids)**
Fatty acids that are produced when polyunsaturated oils are hydrogenated to make them more solid.

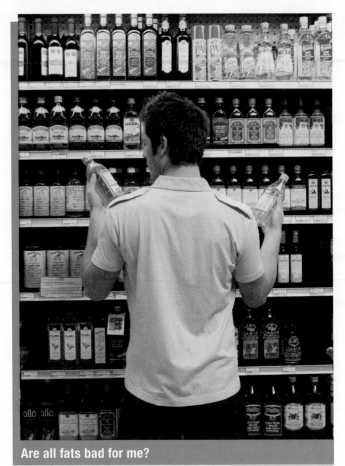

**Are all fats bad for me?**

All fats are not the same, and your body needs some fat to function healthily. Try to reduce saturated fats, those that come in meat, dairy, and poultry products; avoid *trans* fats, those that can come in stick margarine, commercially baked goods, and deep-fried foods; and replace these with monounsaturated fats, such as those in peanut and olive oils.

into irregular shapes at the molecular level, priming them to clog up arteries. *Trans* fats have been used in margarines, many commercial baked goods, and restaurant deep-fried foods.

# 228,000

deaths related to coronary heart disease could be averted each year by reducing Americans' consumption of *trans* fats, according to some estimates.

In 2006, the U.S. Food and Drug Administration (FDA) began to require *trans* fat labeling on all foods. In July 2008, California took bold steps by becoming the first state to ban *trans* fats from restaurant food. In January 2010, the California ban took effect, meaning that all oils, margarines, and shortenings used for frying must contain less than 0.5 percent *trans* fat per serving.[12] Bans have also been implemented in several cities, including New York City and Philadelphia, as well as parts of Maryland. Today, *trans* fats are being removed from most foods, and, if they *are* present,

they must be clearly indicated. If you see the words *partially hydrogenated oils, fractionated oils, shortening, lard,* or *hydrogenation* on a food label, then *trans* fats are present.

**New Fat Advice: Is More Fat Ever Better?** Although most of this section has promoted the long-term recommendation to reduce saturated fat; avoid *trans* fatty acids; and eat more monounsaturated fats, omega-3 fatty acids, and omega-6 fatty acids, some researchers worry that we have gone too far in our anti-fat frenzy. In fact, some studies have shown that when comparing low-fat diets to other diets, there are few improvements in weight loss and blood fat measures.[13]

The bottom line for fat intake is that moderation is the key. Remember that no more than 7 to 10 percent of your total calories should come from saturated fat and that no more than 35 percent should come from all forms of fat. In general, switching to beneficial fats without increasing total fat intake is a good idea. Enjoying a healthy intake of dietary fat doesn't have to be difficult or confusing. Follow these guidelines to add more healthy fats to your diet:

● Eat fatty fish (bluefish, herring, mackerel, salmon, sardines, or tuna) at least twice weekly. The **Be Healthy, Be Green** box at right provides tips for making sustainable seafood choices to fulfill your need for omega-3 fatty acids.
● Substitute soy and canola oils for corn, safflower, and sunflower oils. Keep using olive oil, too.
● Add healthy doses of green leafy vegetables, walnuts, walnut oil, and ground flaxseed to your diet.

Follow these guidelines to help reduce your overall intake of less healthy fats:

● Read the Nutrition Facts Panel on foods to find out how much fat is in your food. Remember that no more than 10 percent of your total calories should come from saturated fat, and no more than 30 percent should come from all forms of fat.
● Use olive oil for baking and sautéing.
● Chill soups and stews and scrape off any fat that hardens on top, and then reheat to serve.
● Fill up on fruits and vegetables.
● Hold the creams and sauces.
● Avoid margarine products with *trans* fatty acids. Whenever possible, opt for other condiments on your bread, such as fresh vegetable spreads, sugar-free jams, fat-free cheese, and other healthy toppings.
● Choose lean meats, fish, or skinless poultry. Broil or bake whenever possible. Drain off fat after cooking.
● Choose fewer cold cuts, bacon, sausages, hot dogs, and organ meats.

# BE HEALTHY, BE GREEN

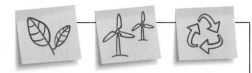

## Toward Sustainable Seafood

The U.S. Department of Agriculture recommends consuming fish two or three times per week to reduce saturated fat and cholesterol levels, and to increase omega-3 fatty acid levels. However, there are many environmental concerns surrounding the seafood industry today that call into question the sustainability and safety of such consumption. More than 70 percent of the world's natural fishing grounds have been overfished, and whole stretches of the oceans are, in fact, dead zones, where fish and shellfish can no longer live. The 2010 oil spill in the Gulf of Mexico is likely to exacerbate seafood shortages and contamination of precious fishing grounds for years to come.

In an effort to counteract the loss of wild fish populations, increasing numbers of fish are being farmed, which poses additional health risks and environmental concerns. Some farmed fish are laden with antibiotics, while highly concentrated levels of parasites and bacteria from fish farm runoff may enter the ocean and river fish populations through adjacent waterways. There are other reasons to think carefully about your farmed fish alternatives. Farmed salmon, for example, are often fed wild fish, resulting in a net loss of fish from the sea.

At the same time that fish populations are threatened, high levels of chemicals, parasites, bacteria, and toxins are also being found in many of the fish available on the market. Mercury, a waste product of many industries, binds to proteins and stays in an animal's body, accumulating as it moves up the food chain; in humans, mercury can cause damage to the nervous system and kidneys, and cause birth defects and developmental problems in fetuses and children. Polychlorinated biphenyls (PCBs), chemicals that can build up in the fatty tissue of fish, are another cause of major concern.

*So what is a savvy fish consumer to do?* Knowing where your fish are caught and the methods by which they are caught is important. Several major environmental groups have developed guides to inform consumers of safe and sustainable seafood choices. The guide shown here provides general national guidelines for seafood available for purchase in the United States. This guide is also available as a free iPhone application, or can be accessed on other mobile devices at http://mobile.seafoodwatch.org. Another great resource is the FishPhone service offered by the Blue Ocean Institute. Simply send a text message to 30644 with the word FISH and the type of fish you want to know about, and it will send you information about whether it is safe to eat. Remember: Your consumer choices make a difference. Purchasing seafood from environmentally responsible sources will support fisheries and fish farms that are healthier for you and the environment.

| **BEST CHOICES** | **GOOD ALTERNATIVES** | **AVOID** | **Support Ocean-Friendly Seafood** |
|---|---|---|---|
| Arctic Char (farmed)<br>Barramundi (US farmed)<br>Catfish (US farmed)<br>Clams (farmed)<br>Cobia (US farmed)<br>Cod: Pacific (Alaska longline)*<br>Crab: Dungeness, Stone<br>Halibut: Pacific⁺<br>Lobster: Spiny (US)<br>Mussels (farmed)<br>Oysters (farmed)<br>Sablefish/Black Cod (Alaska⁺ or British Columbia)<br>Salmon (Alaska wild)⁺<br>Scallops: Bay (farmed)<br>Shrimp, Pink (Oregon)*<br>Striped Bass (farmed or wild*)<br>Tilapia (US farmed)<br>Trout: Rainbow (farmed)<br>Tuna: Albacore (troll/pole, US⁺ or British Columbia)<br>Tuna: Skipjack (troll/pole) | Caviar, Sturgeon (US farmed)<br>Clams (wild)<br>Cod: Pacific (US trawled)<br>Crab: Blue*, King (US), Snow<br>Flounders, Soles (Pacific)<br>Herring: Atlantic<br>Lobster: American/Maine<br>Mahi Mahi/Dolphinfish (US)<br>Oysters (wild)*<br>Pollock (Alaska wild)⁺<br>Salmon (Washington wild)*<br>Sablefish/Black Cod (California, Oregon, or Washington)<br>Scallops: Sea (wild)<br>Shrimp (US, Canada)<br>Squid<br>Swai, Basa (farmed)<br>Swordfish (US)*<br>Tilapia (Central America, farmed)<br>Tuna: Bigeye, Yellowfin (troll/pole)<br>Tuna: Canned Skipjack and Albacore* | Caviar, Sturgeon* (imported wild)<br>Chilean Seabass/Toothfish*<br>Cobia (imported farmed)<br>Cod: Atlantic, imported Pacific<br>Flounders, Halibut, Soles (Atlantic)<br>Groupers*<br>Lobster: Spiny (Caribbean)<br>Mahi Mahi/Dolphinfish (imported)<br>Marlin: Blue*, Striped*<br>Monkfish<br>Orange Roughy*<br>Salmon (farmed, including Atlantic)*<br>Sharks*, Skates<br>Shrimp (imported)<br>Snapper: Red<br>Swordfish (imported)*<br>Tilapia (Asia farmed)<br>Tuna: Albacore, Bigeye, Yellowfin (longline)*<br>Tuna: Bluefin*, Tongol, Canned (except Albacore and Skipjack)<br>Yellowtail (imported, farmed) | **Best Choices** are abundant, well-managed and caught or farmed in environmentally friendly ways.<br><br>**Good Alternatives** are an option, but there are concerns with how they're caught or farmed — or with the health of their habitat due to other human impacts.<br><br>**Avoid** for now as these items are caught or farmed in ways that harm other marine life or the environment.<br><br>**Key**<br>✳ Limit consumption due to concerns about mercury or other contaminants. Visit www.edf.org/seafoodhealth<br>✦ Some or all of this fishery is certified as sustainable to the Marine Stewardship Council standard. Visit www.msc.org<br><br>Seafood may appear in more than one column |

**Sustainable Seafood Guide**

**Source:** Monterey Bay Aquarium Seafood Watch, *National Sustainable Seafood Guide, January 2010.* Copyright © 2010, Monterey Bay Aquarium. www.montereybayaquarium.org/cr/cr_seafoodwatch/download.aspx. Used with permission.

TABLE

7.2 | A Guide to Water-Soluble Vitamins

| Vitamin Name and Recommended Intake | Reliable Food Sources | Primary Functions | Toxicity/Deficiency Symptoms |
|---|---|---|---|
| Thiamin (vitamin B$_1$)<br><br>RDA: Men = 1.2 mg/day<br><br>Women = 1.1 mg/day | Pork, fortified cereals, enriched rice and pasta, peas, tuna, legumes | Required as enzyme cofactor for carbohydrate and amino acid metabolism | *Toxicity:* none known<br><br>*Deficiency:* beriberi, fatigue, apathy, decreased memory, confusion, irritability, muscle weakness |
| Riboflavin (vitamin B$_2$)<br><br>RDA: Men = 1.3 mg/day<br><br>Women = 1.1 mg/day | Beef liver, shrimp, milk and dairy foods, fortified cereals, enriched breads and grains | Required as enzyme cofactor for carbohydrate and fat metabolism | *Toxicity:* none known<br><br>*Deficiency:* ariboflavinosis, swollen mouth and throat, seborrheic dermatitis, anemia |
| Niacin, nicotinamide, nicotinic acid<br><br>RDA: Men = 16 mg/day<br><br>Women = 14 mg/day<br><br>UL = 35 mg/day | Beef liver, most cuts of meat/fish/poultry, fortified cereals, enriched breads and grains, canned tomato products | Required for carbohydrate and fat metabolism; plays role in DNA replication and repair and cell differentiation | *Toxicity:* flushing, liver damage, glucose intolerance, blurred vision differentiation<br><br>*Deficiency:* pellagra; vomiting, constipation, or diarrhea; apathy |
| Vitamin B$_6$ (pyridoxine, pyridoxal, pyridoxamine)<br><br>RDA: Men and women 19–50 = 1.3 mg/day<br><br>Men > 50 = 1.7 mg/day<br><br>Women > 50 = 1.5 mg/day<br><br>UL = 100 mg/day | Chickpeas (garbanzo beans), most cuts of meat/fish/poultry, fortified cereals, white potatoes | Required as enzyme cofactor for carbohydrate and amino acid metabolism; assists synthesis of blood cells | *Toxicity:* nerve damage, skin lesions<br><br>*Deficiency:* anemia; seborrheic dermatitis; depression, confusion, and convulsions |
| Folate (folic acid)<br><br>RDA: Men = 400 μg/day<br><br>Women = 400 μg/day<br><br>UL = 1,000 μg/day | Fortified cereals, enriched breads and grains, spinach, legumes (lentils, chickpeas, pinto beans), greens (spinach, romaine lettuce), liver | Required as enzyme cofactor for amino acid metabolism; required for DNA synthesis; involved in metabolism of homocysteine | *Toxicity:* masks symptoms of vitamin B$_{12}$ deficiency, specifically signs of nerve damage<br><br>*Deficiency:* macrocytic anemia; neural tube defects in a developing fetus; elevated homocysteine levels |
| Vitamin B$_{12}$ (cobalamin)<br><br>RDA: Men = 2.4 μg/day<br><br>Women = 2.4 μg/day | Shellfish, all cuts of meat/fish/poultry, milk and dairy foods, fortified cereals | Assists with formation of blood; required for healthy nervous system function; involved as enzyme cofactor in metabolism of homocysteine | *Toxicity:* none known<br><br>*Deficiency:* pernicious anemia; tingling and numbness of extremities; nerve damage; memory loss, disorientation, and dementia |
| Pantothenic acid<br><br>AI: Men = 5 mg/day<br><br>Women = 5 mg/day | Meat/fish/poultry, shiitake mushrooms, fortified cereals, egg yolks | Assists with fat metabolism | *Toxicity:* none known<br><br>*Deficiency:* rare |
| Biotin<br><br>RDA: Men = 30 μg/day<br><br>Women = 30 μg/day | Nuts, egg yolks | Involved as enzyme cofactor in carbohydrate, fat, and protein metabolism | *Toxicity:* none known<br><br>*Deficiency:* rare |
| Vitamin C (ascorbic acid)<br><br>RDA: Men = 90 mg/day<br><br>Women = 75 mg/day<br><br>Smokers = 35 mg more per day than RDA<br><br>UL = 2,000 mg | Sweet peppers, citrus fruits and juices, broccoli, strawberries, kiwi | Antioxidant in extracellular fluid and lungs; regenerates oxidized vitamin E; assists with collagen synthesis; enhances immune function; assists in synthesis of hormones, neurotransmitters, and DNA; enhances iron absorption | *Toxicity:* nausea and diarrhea, nosebleeds, increased oxidative damage, increased formation of kidney stones in people with kidney disease<br><br>*Deficiency:* scurvy, bone pain and fractures, depression, and anemia |

*Note:* RDA = Recommended Daily Allowance; AI = Adequate Intakes; UL = Tolerable Upper Level Intakes. Values are for all adults aged 19 and older, except as noted. Values increase among women who are pregnant or lactating.

**Source:** Thompson, Janice; Manore, Melinda, *Nutrition: An Applied Approach,* 2d, © 2009. Printed and Electronically reproduced by permission of Pearson Education, Inc., Upper Saddle River, New Jersey.

TABLE
7.3 | **A Guide to Fat-Soluble Vitamins**

| Vitamin Name and Recommended Intake | Reliable Food Sources | Primary Functions | Toxicity/Deficiency Symptoms |
|---|---|---|---|
| Vitamin A (retinol, retinal, retinoic acid)<br><br>RDA: Men = 900 µg<br><br>Women = 700 µg<br><br>UL = 3,000 µg/day | Preformed retinol: beef and chicken liver, egg yolks, milk<br>Carotenoid precursors: spinach, carrots, mango, apricots, cantaloupe, pumpkin, yams | Required for ability of eyes to adjust to changes in light; protects color vision; assists cell differentiation; required for sperm production in men and fertilization in women; contributes to healthy bone and healthy immune system | *Toxicity:* fatigue; bone and joint pain; spontaneous abortion and birth defects of fetuses in pregnant women; nausea and diarrhea; liver damage; nervous system damage; blurred vision; hair loss; skin disorders<br>*Deficiency:* night blindness, xerophthalmia; impaired growth, immunity, and reproductive function |
| Vitamin D (cholecalciferol)<br><br>AI (assumes that person does not get adequate sun exposure):<br>Adult 19–50 = 5 µg/day<br>Adult 50–70 = 10 µg/day<br>Adult > 70 = 15 µg/day<br>UL = 50 µg/day | Canned salmon and mackerel, milk, fortified cereals | Regulates blood calcium levels; maintains bone health; assists cell differentiation | *Toxicity:* hypercalcemia<br>*Deficiency:* rickets in children; osteomalacia and/or osteoporosis in adults |
| Vitamin E (tocopherol)<br><br>RDA: Men = 15 mg/day<br><br>Women = 15 mg/day<br><br>UL = 1,000 mg/day | Sunflower seeds, almonds, vegetable oils, fortified cereals | As a powerful antioxidant, protects cell membranes, polyunsaturated fatty acids, and vitamin A from oxidation; protects white blood cells; enhances immune function; improves absorption of vitamin A | *Toxicity:* rare<br>*Deficiency:* hemolytic anemia; impairment of nerve, muscle, and immune function |
| Vitamin K (phylloquinone, menaquinone, menadione)<br><br>AI: Men = 120 µg/day<br><br>Women = 90 µg/day | Kale, spinach, turnip greens, brussels sprouts | Serves as a coenzyme during production of specific proteins that assist in blood coagulation and bone metabolism | *Toxicity:* none known<br>*Deficiency:* impaired blood clotting; possible effect on bone health |

*Note:* RDA = Recommended Daily Allowance; AI = Adequate Intakes; UL = Tolerable Upper Level Intakes. Values are for all adults aged 19 and older, except as noted. Values increase among women who are pregnant or lactating.

**Source:** Adapted from Thompson, Janice; Manore, Melinda, *Nutrition: An Applied Approach,* 2nd, © 2009. Printed and Electronically reproduced by permission of Pearson Education, Inc., Upper Saddle River, New Jersey.

- Select nonfat and low-fat dairy products.
- When cooking, use substitutes for butter, margarine, oils, sour cream, mayonnaise, and full-fat salad dressings. Chicken or beef broth, fresh herbs, wine, vinegar, and low-calorie dressings provide flavor with less fat.

# Vitamins

**Vitamins** are potent and essential organic compounds that promote growth and help maintain life and health. Every minute of every day, vitamins help maintain nerves and skin, produce blood cells, build bones and teeth, heal wounds, and convert food energy to body energy—and they do all this without adding any calories to your diet.

Vitamins can be classified as either *fat soluble,* which means they are absorbed through the intestinal tract with the help of fats, or *water soluble,* which means they are dissolved easily in water. Vitamins A, D, E, and K are fat soluble; B-complex vitamins and vitamin C are water soluble. Fat-soluble vitamins tend to be stored in the body, and toxic accumulations in the liver may cause cirrhosis-like symptoms. Water-soluble vitamins generally are excreted and cause few toxicity problems. See Tables 7.2 and 7.3 at left and above for more information on the functions and potential dangers of specific vitamins.

**vitamins** Essential organic compounds that promote growth and reproduction and help maintain life and health.

**functional foods** Foods believed to have specific health benefits and/or to prevent disease.

**Antioxidants** The old adage "you are what you eat" is indeed a motto to live by. Beneficial foods are termed **functional foods** based on the ancient belief that eating the right foods

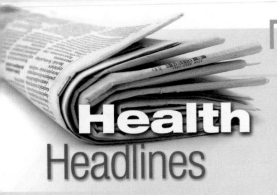

# Health Headlines

## FUNCTIONAL FOODS AND HEALTH CLAIMS

In the 1980s, health authorities in Japan recognized that if health costs were to be controlled, an improved quality of life must accompany longer life spans. It was at this time that the concept of functional foods was born. *Functional foods* are foods that may provide a health benefit beyond basic nutrition. Functional foods include a wide variety of foods that are believed to improve overall health, reduce disease, or minimize health concerns. For example, probiotics—live microorganisms found in, or added to, fermented foods that optimize the bacterial environment in our intestines—are currently receiving much attention as natural healers. Commonly, they are found in fermented milk products such as yogurt, and you will see them labeled as *Lactobacillus* or *Bifidobacterium* in a product's list of ingredients. Probiotics do not typically pose harm to healthy humans. However, if you have a compromised immune system you should consult with your doctor before using probiotics.

Other examples of functional foods include polyunsaturated fatty acids (PUFAs) and omega-3 fatty acids, found in walnuts and flax, which may contribute to heart health, and whole grains, found in whole-grain cereals, breads, and pastas, which may reduce risk of cardiovascular disease and some types of cancer, and may contribute to maintenance of healthy blood glucose levels.

In recent surveys, a significant number of Americans have indicated that they believe that some foods have benefits that extend beyond basic nutrition. When asked to identify the top functional foods, consumers listed fruits, vegetables, fish and fish oils, dairy (such as yogurt), fiber, teas, nuts, whole grains, oats, and vitamins and supplements. You may have noted that functional foods don't necessarily come in fancy packages. For example, fruits, vegetables, and fish are all considered functional foods.

If you want to incorporate more functional foods in your diet, there are a few things you should know about labeling. In the United States, the Food and Drug Administration (FDA) does not provide a specific definition or regulation for functional foods. Because of this, functional food categorization is determined by how the manufacturer chooses to market the products. The FDA allows for five types of health-related claims on food and dietary supplements:

✱ **Nutrient content claims** that indicate a specific nutrient is present at a certain level. For example, a product might say "High in fiber" or "Low in fat" or "This product contains 100 calories per serving." Nutrient content claims can use the following words: *More, Less, Fewer, Good Source Of, Free, Light, Lean, Extra Lean, High, Low, Reduced.*

✱ **Structure and function claims** that describe the effect that a dietary component has on the body. An example of a structure/function claim is "Calcium builds strong bones."

✱ **Dietary guidance claims** describe health benefits or health effects of a broad category of foods rather than a specific nutrient. An example is "Diets rich in fruits and vegetables may reduce the risks of some types of cancer."

✱ **Qualified health claims** convey a relationship between diet and the risk for disease. These must be approved by the FDA and supported by scientific research. You will

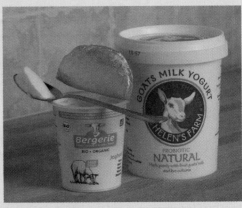

Many brands of yogurt and kefir (a fermented milk drink) are labeled with the message "live probiotic cultures."

find qualified health claims about cancer risk, cardiovascular disease, cognitive function, diabetes, and hypertension, for example, "Diets low in *sodium* may reduce the risk of high blood pressure, a disease associated with many factors." *High blood pressure* is another term for *hypertension*.

✱ **Health claims** confirm a relationship between components in the diet and the risk of disease or health. These must be approved by the FDA and supported by evidence. There are a number of health claims that are approved. For example, a whole-grain bread package may state, "In a low-fat diet, whole-grain foods like this bread may reduce the risk of heart disease."

Consider the foods that you buy currently. Do you use claims to assist your buying decisions? Health claims may assist you in selecting functional foods that meet your nutritional needs.

**Sources:** European Food Information Council (EUFIC), "Functional Foods," 2006, www.eufic.org/ article/en/page/BARCHIVE/expid/basics-functional -foods; International Food Information Council, "Background on Functional Foods Backgrounder," September 2009, www.foodinsight.org/Resources/ Detail.aspx?topic=Background_on_Functional _Foods; U.S. Food and Drug Administration, "Food Labeling Guide," Updated May 2009, www.fda.gov/ Food/GuidanceComplianceRegulatoryInformation/ GuidanceDocuments/FoodLabelingNutrition/ FoodLabelingGuide.

may not only prevent disease, but also cure some diseases (see the **Health Headlines** box above). Some of the most popular functional foods today are items containing **antioxidants** or other *phytochemicals* (from the Greek word meaning "plant"). Among the more commonly cited nutrients touted as providing a protective antioxidant effect are vitamin C, vitamin E, and beta-carotene, a precursor to vitamin A. These substances appear to protect people from the ravages of oxidative stress, a complex process in which *free radicals* (molecules with unpaired electrons that are produced in excess when the body is overly stressed) either damage or kill healthy cells, cell proteins, or genetic material in the cells. Free radical formation is a natural process that cannot be avoided, but antioxidants can combat it by producing enzymes that scavenge free radicals, slowing their formation, or by actually repairing oxidative stress damage.

Blueberries are a great source of antioxidants.

To date, many claims about the benefits of antioxidants in reducing the risk of heart disease, improving vision, and slowing the aging process have not been fully investigated, and conclusive statements about their true benefits are difficult to find. Large, longitudinal epidemiological studies support the hypothesis that antioxidants in foods, mostly fruits and vegetables, help protect against cognitive decline and risk of Parkinson's disease.[14] Other studies indicate that these vitamins, particularly when taken as supplements, have no effect on atherosclerosis.[15] Some studies indicate that when people's diets include foods rich in vitamin C, they seem to develop fewer cancers, but other studies detect no effect from dietary vitamin C.[16] Recent studies indicate that high-dose vitamin C given intravenously, rather than orally, may be effective in treating cancer and protecting from diseases affecting the central nervous system.[17]

Possible effects of vitamin E intake are even more controversial. Researchers have long theorized that because many cancers result from DNA damage, and because vitamin E appears to protect against DNA damage, vitamin E would also reduce cancer risk. Surprisingly, the great majority of studies have demonstrated no effect or, in some cases, a negative effect.[18] However, it can be difficult to compare studies on vitamin E because several different forms of vitamin E exist.

**Carotenoids** are part of the red, orange, and yellow pigments found in fruits and vegetables. They are fat soluble, transported in the blood by lipoproteins, and stored in the fatty tissues of the body. Beta-carotene, the most researched carotenoid, is a precursor of vitamin A. This means that vitamin A can be produced in the body from beta-carotene; like vitamin A, beta-carotene has antioxidant properties.

Although there are over 600 carotenoids in nature, two that have received a great deal of attention are *lycopene* (found in tomatoes, papaya, pink grapefruit, and guava) and *lutein* (found in green leafy vegetables such as spinach, broccoli, kale, and brussels sprouts). The National Cancer Institute and the American Cancer Society have endorsed lycopene as a possible factor in reducing the risk of cancer. A landmark study assessing the effects of tomato-based foods reported that men who ate ten or more servings of lycopene-rich foods per week had a 45 percent lower risk of prostate cancer.[19] However, subsequent research has questioned the benefits of lycopene, and some professional groups are modifying their endorsements of tomato-based products.[20] Lutein is most often touted as a means of

protecting the eyes, particularly from age-related macular degeneration (ARMD), a leading cause of blindness for people aged 65 and older.

**Folate** Folate is a form of vitamin B that is needed for DNA production in body cells. It is particularly important during fetal development; folate deficiencies during pregnancy can result in spina bifida, a birth defect in which a baby's spine and spinal cord are not fully developed. In 1998, the FDA began requiring that all bread, cereal, rice, and pasta products sold in the United States be fortified with folic acid, the synthetic form of folate. This practice, which boosts folate intake by an average of 100 micrograms daily, is intended to decrease the number of infants born with spina bifida and other neural tube defects.

Folate was widely studied in the late 1990s for its potential to decrease blood levels of *homocysteine* (an amino acid that has been linked to vascular diseases) and to protect against cardiovascular disease (CVD).[21] More recent research has raised questions about the benefits of the B vitamins in reducing the risks of CVD or stroke, leading researchers to question these earlier results.[22]

**antioxidants** Substances believed to protect against oxidative stress and resultant tissue damage at the cellular level.
**carotenoids** Fat-soluble plant pigments with antioxidant properties.
**minerals** Inorganic, indestructible elements that aid physiological processes.
**macrominerals** Minerals that the body needs in fairly large amounts.
**trace minerals** Minerals that the body needs in only very small amounts.

## Minerals

**Minerals** are the inorganic, indestructible elements that aid physiological processes within the body. Without minerals, vitamins could not be absorbed. Minerals are readily excreted and, with a few exceptions, are usually not toxic. **Macrominerals** are the minerals that the body needs in fairly large amounts: sodium, calcium, phosphorus, magnesium, potassium, sulfur, and chloride. **Trace minerals** include iron, zinc, manganese, copper, and iodine. Only very small amounts of trace minerals are needed, and serious problems may result if excesses or deficiencies occur (see Tables 7.4 and 7.5 on pages 226 and 227).

**Sodium** Sodium is necessary for the regulation of blood and body fluids, transmission of nerve impulses, heart activity, and certain metabolic functions. It enhances flavors, balances the bitterness of certain foods, acts as a preservative, and tenderizes meats, so it's often present in high quantities in many of the foods we eat. A common misconception is that salt and sodium are the same thing. However, table salt accounts for only 15 percent of sodium intake. The majority of sodium in our diet comes from highly processed foods

Even if you never use table salt, you still may be getting excess sodium in your diet.

TABLE
7.4 | **A Guide to Major Minerals**

| Mineral Name and Recommended Intake | Reliable Food Sources | Primary Functions | Toxicity/Deficiency Symptoms |
|---|---|---|---|
| Sodium<br><br>AI: Adults = 1.5 g/day (1,500 mg/day) | Table salt, pickles, most canned soups, snack foods, cured luncheon meats, canned tomato products | Fluid balance; acid–base balance; transmission of nerve impulses; muscle contraction | *Toxicity:* water retention, high blood pressure, loss of calcium<br><br>*Deficiency:* muscle cramps, dizziness, fatigue, nausea, vomiting, mental confusion |
| Potassium<br><br>AI: Adults = 4.7 g/day (4,700 mg/day) | Most fresh fruits and vegetables: potato, banana, tomato juice, orange juice, melon | Fluid balance; transmission of nerve impulses; muscle contraction | *Toxicity:* muscle weakness, vomiting, irregular heartbeat<br><br>*Deficiency:* muscle weakness, paralysis, mental confusion, irregular heartbeat |
| Phosphorus<br><br>RDA: Adults = 700 mg/day | Milk/cheese/ yogurt, soy milk and tofu, legumes (lentils, black beans), nuts (almonds, peanuts), poultry | Fluid balance; bone formation; component of ATP, which provides energy for our bodies | *Toxicity:* muscle spasms, convulsions, low blood calcium<br><br>*Deficiency:* muscle weakness, muscle damage, bone pain, dizziness |
| Chloride<br><br>AI: Adults = 2.3 g/day (2,300 mg/day) | Table salt | Fluid balance; transmission of nerve impulses; component of stomach acid (HCL); antibacterial | *Toxicity:* none known<br><br>*Deficiency:* dangerous blood acid–base imbalances, irregular heartbeat |
| Calcium<br><br>AI: Adults 19–50 = 1,000 mg/day<br><br>Adults > 50 = 1,200 mg/day<br><br>UL = 2,500 mg | Milk/yogurt/cheese (best absorbed form of calcium), sardines, collard greens and spinach, calcium-fortified juices | Primary component of bone; acid–base balance; transmission of nerve impulses; muscle contraction | *Toxicity:* mineral imbalances, shock, kidney failure, fatigue, mental confusion<br><br>*Deficiency:* osteoporosis, convulsions, heart failure |
| Magnesium<br><br>RDA: Men 19–30 = 400 mg/day<br><br>Men > 30 = 420 mg/day<br><br>Women 19–30 = 310 mg/day<br><br>Women > 30 = 320 mg/day<br><br>UL = 350 mg/day | Greens (spinach, kale, collards), whole grains, seeds, nuts, legumes (navy and black beans) | Component of bone; muscle contraction; assists more than 300 enzyme systems | *Toxicity:* none known<br><br>*Deficiency:* low blood calcium; muscle spasms or seizures; nausea; weakness; increased risk of chronic diseases such as heart disease, hypertension, osteoporosis, and type 2 diabetes |
| Sulfur<br><br>No DRI | Protein-rich foods | Component of certain B vitamins and amino acids; acid–base balance; detoxification in liver | *Toxicity:* none known<br><br>*Deficiency:* none known |

*Note:* RDA = Recommended Daily Allowance; AI = Adequate Intakes; UL = Tolerable Upper Level Intake. Values are for all adults aged 19 and older, except as noted.

**Source:** Thompson, Janice; Manore, Melinda, *Nutrition: An Applied Approach,* 2nd, © 2009. Printed and Electronically reproduced by permission of Pearson Education, Inc., Upper Saddle River, New Jersey.

that are infused with sodium to enhance flavor and preservation. Pickles, fast foods, salty snack foods, processed cheeses, canned soups and frozen dinners, many breads and bakery products, and smoked meats and sausages often contain several hundred milligrams of sodium per serving.

Many health professionals believe there is evidence that Americans need to reduce sodium.[23] The Institute of Medicine, the American Heart Association, the FDA, and the U.S. Department of Agriculture (USDA) are among the professional and governmental organizations that recommend that healthy people consume fewer than 2,300 milligrams of sodium each day. What does that really mean? For most of us, less than 1 teaspoon of table salt per day is all we need! The latest National Health and Nutrition Examination Survey (NHANES) estimated that the average American over 2 years of age consumes 3,436 milligrams per day.[24]

Why is high sodium intake a concern? Many experts believe that there is a link between excessive sodium intake

| Mineral Name and Recommended Intake | Reliable Food Sources | Primary Functions | Toxicity/Deficiency Symptoms |
|---|---|---|---|
| Selenium<br><br>RDA: Adults = 55 µg/day<br><br>UL = 400 µg/day | Nuts, shellfish, meat/fish/poultry, whole grains | Required for carbohydrate and fat metabolism | *Toxicity:* brittle hair and nails, skin rashes, nausea and vomiting, weakness, liver disease<br><br>*Deficiency:* specific forms of heart disease and arthritis, impaired immune function, muscle pain and wasting, depression, hostility |
| Fluoride<br><br>AI: Men = 4 mg/day<br><br>Women = 3 mg/day<br><br>UL = 2.2 mg/day for children 4–8 years; children > 8 years = 10 mg/day | Fluoridated water and other beverages made with this water | Development and maintenance of healthy teeth and bones | *Toxicity:* fluorosis of teeth and bones<br><br>*Deficiency:* dental caries, low bone density |
| Iodine<br><br>RDA: Adults = 150 µg/day<br><br>UL = 1,100 µg/day | Iodized salt and foods processed with iodized salt | Synthesis of thyroid hormones; temperature regulation; reproduction and growth | *Toxicity:* goiter<br><br>*Deficiency:* goiter, hypothyroidism, cretinism in infant of mother who is iodine deficient |
| Chromium<br><br>AI: Men 19–50 = 35 µg/day<br><br>Men > 50 = 30 µg/day<br><br>Women 19–50 = 25 µg/day<br><br>Women > 50 = 20 µg/day | Grains, meat/fish/poultry, some fruits and vegetables | Glucose transport; metabolism of DNA and RNA; immune function and growth | *Toxicity:* none known<br><br>*Deficiency:* elevated blood glucose and blood lipids, damage to brain and nervous system |
| Manganese<br><br>AI: Men = 2.3 mg/day<br><br>Women = 1.8 mg/day<br><br>UL = 11 mg/day for adults | Whole grains, nuts, legumes, some fruits and vegetables | Assists many enzyme systems; synthesis of protein found in bone and cartilage | *Toxicity:* impairment of neuromuscular system<br><br>*Deficiency:* impaired growth and reproductive function, reduced bone density, impaired glucose and lipid metabolism, skin rash |
| Iron<br><br>RDA: Men = 8 mg/day<br><br>Women 19–50 = 18 mg/day<br><br>Women > 50 = 8 mg/day | Meat/fish/poultry (best absorbed form of iron), fortified cereals, legumes, spinach | Component of hemoglobin in blood cells; component of myoglobin in muscle cells; assists many enzyme systems | *Toxicity:* nausea, vomiting, and diarrhea; dizziness, confusion; rapid heartbeat; organ damage; death<br><br>*Deficiency:* iron-deficiency microcytic anemia, hypochromic anemia |
| Zinc<br><br>RDA: Men 11 mg/day<br><br>Women = 8 mg/day<br><br>UL = 40 mg/day | Meat/fish/poultry (best absorbed form of zinc), fortified cereals, legumes | Assists more than 100 enzyme systems; immune system function; growth and sexual maturation; gene regulation | *Toxicity:* nausea, vomiting, and diarrhea; headaches; depressed immune function; reduced absorption of copper<br><br>*Deficiency:* growth retardation, delayed sexual maturation, eye and skin lesions, hair loss, increased incidence of illness and infection |
| Copper<br><br>RDA: Adults = 900 µg/day<br><br>UL = 10 mg/day | Shellfish, organ meats, nuts, legumes | Assists many enzyme systems; iron transport | *Toxicity:* nausea, vomiting, and diarrhea; liver damage<br><br>*Deficiency:* anemia, reduced levels of white blood cells, osteoporosis in infants and growing children |

*Note:* RDA = Recommended Daily Allowance; AI = Adequate Intakes; UL = Tolerable Upper Intake Level. Values are for all adults aged 19 and older, except as noted.

**Source:** Adapted from Thompson, Janice; Manore, Melinda, *Nutrition: An Applied Approach,* 2nd, © 2009. Printed and Electronically reproduced by permission of Pearson Education, Inc., Upper Saddle River, New Jersey.

## Shake Your Salt Habit

Take simple steps today to reduce your overall sodium intake:

* When buying packaged foods, choose low-sodium or salt-free products.
* At the movies, order popcorn without salt.
* Use kosher salt—it has 25 percent less sodium than regular table salt.
* Avoid adding salt to foods during cooking or at the table; instead, try using fresh or prepackaged herbs and spices to season foods.

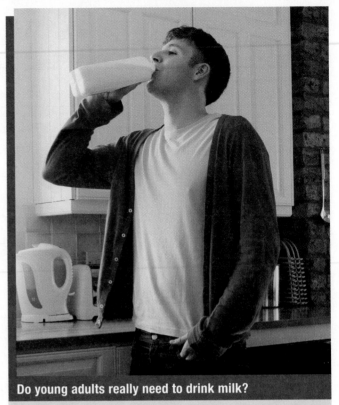

**Do young adults really need to drink milk?**

Consumption of calcium, one of the many nutrients in milk, is important for people of all ages. To build healthy bones and teeth, and to prevent bone loss later in life, you need to get enough calcium while you are young; women, in particular, should be sure to obtain adequate amounts. If you are one of those who do not drink milk, be sure you are getting enough calcium—at least 1,200 milligrams per day—through other sources.

and hypertension (high blood pressure). Although this theory is controversial, researchers recommend that hypertensive Americans cut back on sodium to reduce their risk for cardiovascular disorders, including stroke, debilitating bone fractures, and other health problems.[25] See the **Skills for Behavior Change** box above for tips on how to reduce your sodium intake.

**Calcium** Calcium plays a vital role in building strong bones and teeth, muscle contraction, blood clotting, nerve impulse transmission, regulating heartbeat, and fluid balance within cells. The issue of calcium consumption has gained national attention with the rising incidence of osteoporosis among older adults. Most Americans do not consume the recommended 1,000 to 1,200 milligrams of calcium per day.[26]

Milk is one of the richest sources of dietary calcium. Calcium-fortified orange juice and soy milk are good alternatives if you do not drink dairy milk. Many green leafy vegetables are good sources of calcium, but some contain oxalic acid, which makes their calcium harder to absorb. Spinach, chard, and beet greens are not particularly good sources of calcium, whereas broccoli, cauliflower, and many peas and beans offer good supplies.

It is generally best to take calcium throughout the day, consuming it with foods containing protein, vitamin D, and vitamin C for optimal absorption. Many dairy products are fortified with vitamin D, which is known to improve calcium absorption. We also know that sunlight increases the manufacture of vitamin D in the body and is therefore like an extra calcium source.

**anemia** Condition that results from the body's inability to produce hemoglobin.

Do you consume carbonated soft drinks? Be aware that the added phosphoric acid (phosphate) in these drinks can cause you to excrete extra calcium, which may result in calcium loss from your bones. One study of 2,500 men and women found that in women who consumed at least three cans of cola per week, even diet cola, bone density of the hip was 4 to 5 percent lower than in women who drank fewer than one cola per month. Colas did not seem to have the same effect on men.[27]

**Iron** Worldwide, iron deficiency is the most common nutrient deficiency, affecting more than 2 billion people, nearly 30 percent of the world's population. In the United States iron deficiency is less prevalent, but it is still the most common micronutrient deficiency.[28] How much iron do we need? Women aged 19 to 50 need about 18 milligrams per day, and men aged 19 to 50 need about 8 milligrams.

Iron deficiency frequently leads to *iron-deficiency anemia*. **Anemia** results from the body's inability to produce hemoglobin (the oxygen-carrying component of the blood). When iron-deficiency anemia occurs, body cells receive less oxygen, and carbon dioxide wastes are removed less efficiently. As a result, the iron-deficient person feels tired. Iron deficiency in the diet is not the only cause of anemia; anemia can also result from blood loss, cancer, ulcers, and other conditions.

Iron overload or iron toxicity due to ingesting too many iron-containing supplements is the leading cause of accidental poisoning in small children in the United States. Symptoms of toxicity include nausea, vomiting, diarrhea, rapid heartbeat, weak pulse, dizziness, shock, and confusion.

Excess iron intake has also been associated with other problems: A recent study of over 45,000 men indicated that those who consumed excess heme iron—the kind found in meat, seafood, and poultry—had a 20 percent higher risk of gallstones than those who consumed low-iron foods or got their iron from supplements.[29]

# How Can I Eat More Healthfully?

Now that you have some idea of your nutritional needs, let's discuss what a healthy diet looks like, how you can begin to meet your needs, and how you can meet the challenge of getting the foods you need on campus. This section gives you some practical advice for meeting your goals, and some tips for dealing with issues specific to eating in college.

## What Is a Healthful Diet?

Generally speaking, a healthful diet provides the combination of energy and nutrients needed to sustain proper functioning. A healthful diet should be

● **Adequate.** It provides enough of the energy, nutrients, and fiber to maintain health and essential body functions. Everyone's nutritional needs differ. For example, a small woman with a sedentary lifestyle may need only 1,700 calories of energy daily to support her body's functions, whereas a competitive bicyclist may need several thousand calories of energy to be fit for a race.

● **Moderate.** It often isn't what you eat that causes nutrition imbalance or weight gain—it's the amount you consume. Moderate caloric consumption, portion control, and awareness of the total amount of nutrients in the foods you eat are key aspects of dietary health.

● **Balanced.** Your diet should contain the proper combination of foods from different groups. Following the recommendations for the MyPyramid Plan described below should help you achieve balance.

● **Varied.** Eat many different foods each day. Variety keeps you interested and makes it less likely that your diet will contain nutrient deficiencies.

● **Nutrient dense.** *Nutrient density* refers to the proportion of vitamins, minerals, and other nutrients compared to the number of calories. The foods you eat should have the biggest nutritional bang for the calories consumed.

Trends indicate that Americans today overall eat more food than ever before. From 1970 to 2008, average calorie consumption increased from 2,157 to 2,673 calories per day

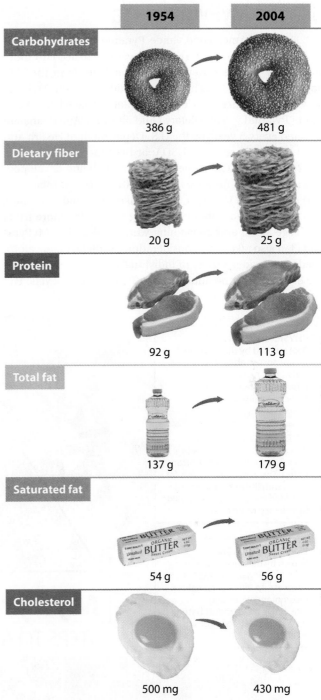

| | 1954 | 2004 |
|---|---|---|
| Carbohydrates | 386 g | 481 g |
| Dietary fiber | 20 g | 25 g |
| Protein | 92 g | 113 g |
| Total fat | 137 g | 179 g |
| Saturated fat | 54 g | 56 g |
| Cholesterol | 500 mg | 430 mg |

FIGURE 7.5 **Trends in Per Capita Nutrient Consumption**
Since 1954, Americans' daily caloric intake has increased by about 25%, as has daily consumption of carbohydrates, fiber, and protein. Daily total fat intake has increased by 30%.
**Source:** Data are from USDA Economic Research Service, Nutrient Availability, Updated February 2010, www.ers.usda.gov/Data/FoodConsumption/NutrientAvailIndex.htm.

(see **Figure 7.5**).[30] In general, it isn't the actual amounts of food, but the number of calories in the foods we choose to eat that has increased. When these trends are combined with our increasingly sedentary lifestyle, it is not surprising that we have seen a dramatic rise in obesity.

# Use the MyPyramid Plan

In 2005, the former Food Guide Pyramid created and promoted by the USDA underwent an overhaul to account more completely for the variety of nutritional needs in the U.S. population (Figure 7.6). This new pyramid, called the MyPyramid Plan (because it is customizable), replaced the Food Guide Pyramid.[31] The Dietary Guidelines for Americans are updated every 5 years by the U.S. Department of Health and Human Services and the USDA; at the time of this writing, the 2010 Dietary Guidelines are currently being developed, and are intended for release in late 2010.[32] The former pyramid emphasized variety in daily intake, but it did not reflect what we now know about restricting fats, eating more fruits and vegetables, and consuming whole grains. The MyPyramid Plan also takes into consideration the dietary and caloric needs for a wider variety of individuals, such as people over age 65, children, and adults with different activity levels. The MyPyramid Plan promotes personalizing dietary and exercise recommendations based on individual needs.

**Understand Serving Sizes** The MyPyramid Plan presents personalized dietary recommendations in terms of numbers of servings of particular nutrients. But how much is one serving? Is it different from a portion? Although these two terms are often used interchangeably, they actually mean very different things. A *serving* is the recommended amount you should consume, whereas a *portion* is the amount you choose to eat at any one time. Most of us select portions that are much bigger than recommended servings. In a survey conducted by the American Institute for Cancer Research, respondents were asked to estimate the standard servings defined by the old USDA Food Guide Pyramid for eight different foods. Only 1 percent of those surveyed correctly answered all serving size questions, and nearly 65 percent answered five or more of them incorrectly.[33] See

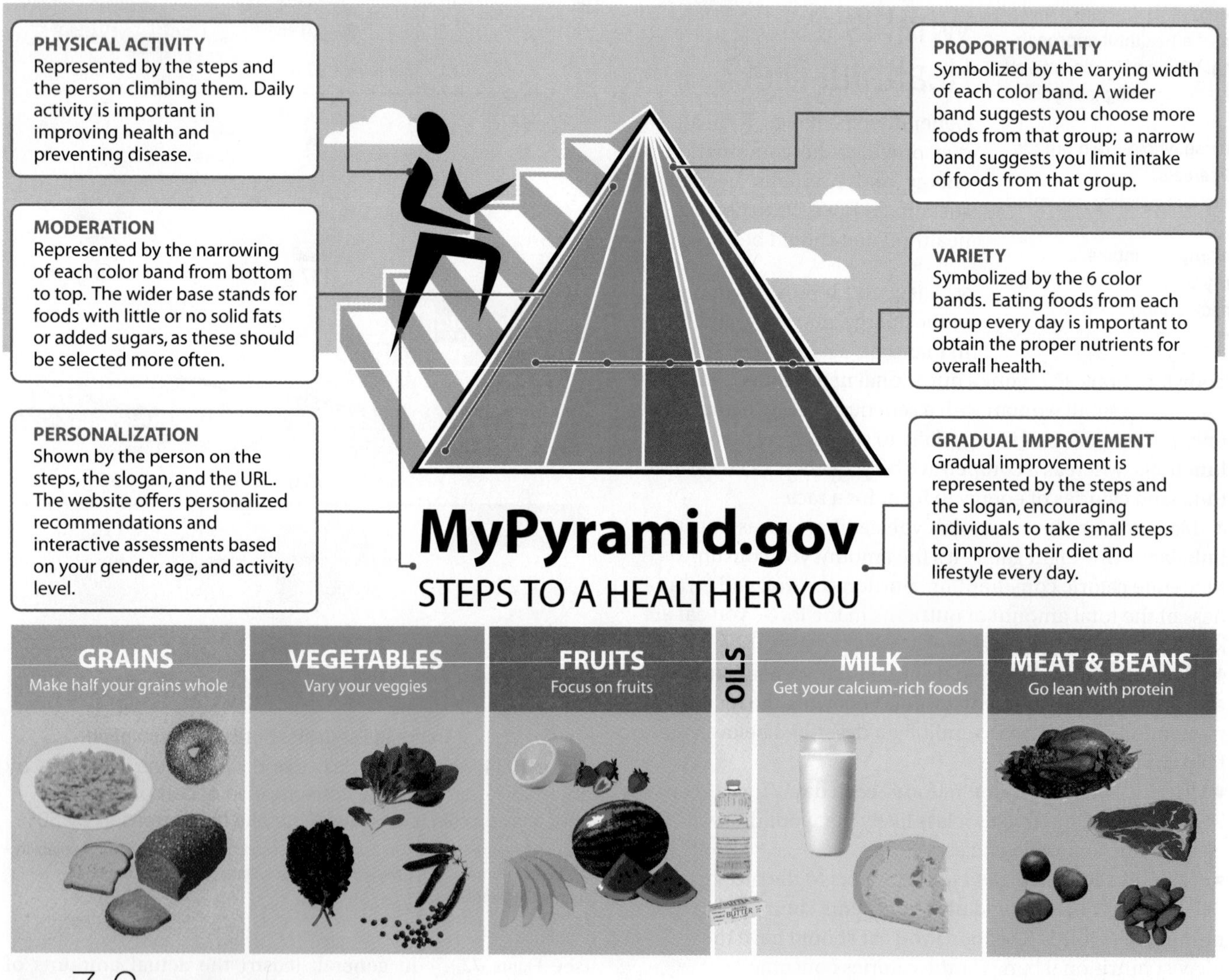

**PHYSICAL ACTIVITY**
Represented by the steps and the person climbing them. Daily activity is important in improving health and preventing disease.

**MODERATION**
Represented by the narrowing of each color band from bottom to top. The wider base stands for foods with little or no solid fats or added sugars, as these should be selected more often.

**PERSONALIZATION**
Shown by the person on the steps, the slogan, and the URL. The website offers personalized recommendations and interactive assessments based on your gender, age, and activity level.

**PROPORTIONALITY**
Symbolized by the varying width of each color band. A wider band suggests you choose more foods from that group; a narrow band suggests you limit intake of foods from that group.

**VARIETY**
Symbolized by the 6 color bands. Eating foods from each group every day is important to obtain the proper nutrients for overall health.

**GRADUAL IMPROVEMENT**
Gradual improvement is represented by the steps and the slogan, encouraging individuals to take small steps to improve their diet and lifestyle every day.

**MyPyramid.gov**
STEPS TO A HEALTHIER YOU

**GRAINS** Make half your grains whole

**VEGETABLES** Vary your veggies

**FRUITS** Focus on fruits

**OILS**

**MILK** Get your calcium-rich foods

**MEAT & BEANS** Go lean with protein

FIGURE 7.6 **MyPyramid Plan**
The USDA MyPyramid Plan takes a new approach to dietary and exercise recommendations. Each colored section of the pyramid represents a food group, with the needs of specific individuals in mind.
**Source:** U.S. Department of Agriculture, 2005, www.MyPyramid.gov.

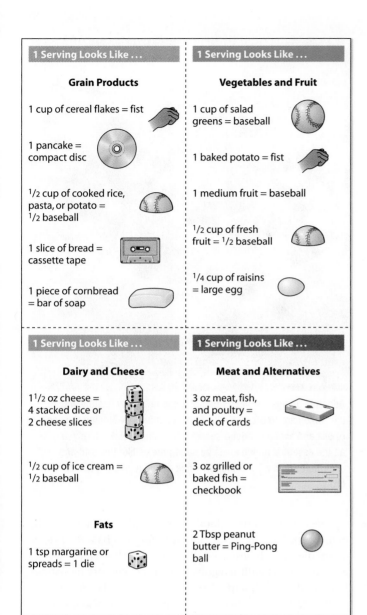

| 1 Serving Looks Like ... | |
|---|---|
| **Grain Products** | |
| 1 cup of cereal flakes = fist | |
| 1 pancake = compact disc | |
| 1/2 cup of cooked rice, pasta, or potato = 1/2 baseball | |
| 1 slice of bread = cassette tape | |
| 1 piece of cornbread = bar of soap | |

| 1 Serving Looks Like ... | |
|---|---|
| **Vegetables and Fruit** | |
| 1 cup of salad greens = baseball | |
| 1 baked potato = fist | |
| 1 medium fruit = baseball | |
| 1/2 cup of fresh fruit = 1/2 baseball | |
| 1/4 cup of raisins = large egg | |

| 1 Serving Looks Like ... | |
|---|---|
| **Dairy and Cheese** | |
| 1 1/2 oz cheese = 4 stacked dice or 2 cheese slices | |
| 1/2 cup of ice cream = 1/2 baseball | |
| **Fats** | |
| 1 tsp margarine or spreads = 1 die | |

| 1 Serving Looks Like ... | |
|---|---|
| **Meat and Alternatives** | |
| 3 oz meat, fish, and poultry = deck of cards | |
| 3 oz grilled or baked fish = checkbook | |
| 2 Tbsp peanut butter = Ping-Pong ball | |

**FIGURE 7.7 Serving Size Card**

One of the challenges of following a healthy diet is judging how big a portion size should be and how many servings you are really eating. The comparisons on this card can help you recall what a standard food serving looks like. For easy reference, photocopy or cut out this card, fold on the dotted lines, and keep it in your wallet. You can even laminate it for long-term use.

**Source:** National Heart, Lung and Blood Institute, "Serving Size Card," Accessed April 2010, http://hp2010.nhlbihin.net/portion/servingcard7.pdf.

Figure 7.7 for a handy pocket guide with tips on recognizing serving sizes.

Unfortunately, we don't always get a clear picture from food producers and advertisers about what a serving really is. Consider a bottle of soda: The food label may list one serving size as 8 fluid ounces and 100 calories. However, note the size of the entire bottle; if the bottle holds 20 ounces, drinking the whole thing serves up 250 calories.

Be sure to eat at least the lowest number of servings from the major food groups; you need them for the nutrients they provide. If you eat a large portion, count it as more than one serving. Figure 7.8 lists the suggested daily amount of food from each group for a variety of calorie intake levels.

**Eat Nutrient-Dense Foods** Although eating the proper number of servings from MyPyramid is important, it is also important to recognize that there are large caloric, fat, and energy differences among foods within a given food group. For example, fish and hot dogs provide vastly different nutrient levels per ounce. Fish provides less fat and more nutritional value per serving. It is important to eat foods that have a high nutritional value for their caloric content. Avoid "empty calories," that is, high-calorie foods that have little nutritional value.

**Discretionary Calories** Every day you must consume a certain number of nutrient-dense foods to maintain health. Because these foods tend to be lower in calories, your total caloric intake may be less than your total daily energy needs. Hence,

| | 1,200 | 1,400 | 1,600 | 1,800 | 2,000 | 2,200 | 2,400 | 2,600 | 2,800 | 3,000 |
|---|---|---|---|---|---|---|---|---|---|---|
| Fruits | 1 cup | 1.5 cups | 1.5 cups | 1.5 cups | 2 cups | 2 cups | 2 cups | 2 cups | 2.5 cups | 2.5 cups |
| Vegetables | 1.5 cups | 1.5 cups | 2 cups | 2.5 cups | 2.5 cups | 3 cups | 3 cups | 3.5 cups | 3.5 cups | 4 cups |
| Grains | 4 oz-eq. | 5 oz-eq. | 5 oz-eq. | 6 oz-eq. | 6 oz-eq. | 7 oz-eq. | 8 oz-eq. | 9 oz-eq. | 10 oz-eq. | 10 oz-eq. |
| Meat and beans | 3 oz-eq. | 4 oz-eq. | 5 oz-eq. | 5 oz-eq. | 5.5 oz-eq. | 6 oz-eq. | 6.5 oz-eq. | 6.5 oz-eq. | 7 oz-eq. | 7 oz-eq. |
| Milk | 2 cups | 2 cups | 3 cups | 3 cups | 3 cups | 3 cups | 3 cups | 3 cups | 3 cups | 3 cups |
| Oils | 4 tsp | 4 tsp | 5 tsp | 5 tsp | 6 tsp | 6 tsp | 7 tsp | 8 tsp | 8 tsp | 10 tsp |
| Discretionary calories | 171 | 171 | 132 | 195 | 267 | 290 | 362 | 410 | 426 | 512 |

**FIGURE 7.8 Nutritional Needs for Different Groups**

Once you've determined your daily calorie requirements (see Table 7.1 on page 213), use this chart to see how many servings of each food group you need per day to maintain good health.

**Source:** U.S. Department of Agriculture, 2005, www.MyPyramid.gov.

you may find yourself with a few *discretionary calories* to spend. Most of us have a very small discretionary calorie allowance at the end of the day. For example, suppose you need 2,000 calories to meet your daily energy requirement, and you've eaten wisely all day, choosing whole-grain, low-fat, and low-sugar foods that collectively provided 1,800 calories. This means you can spend the remaining 200 calories on what might be considered dietary indulgences. This might include an extra helping at dinner, a soda, a small serving of ice cream, or a higher fat cheese or meat than you would normally consume.

**Physical Activity** Strive to be physically active for at least 30 minutes daily, preferably with moderate to vigorous activity levels on most days. Physical activity does not mean you have to go to the gym, jog 3 miles a day, or hire a personal trainer. Any activity that gets your heart pumping (e.g., gardening, playing basketball, heavy yard work, and dancing) is a good way to get moving. For more on physical fitness, see Chapter 9.

## Vegetarianism: A Healthy Diet?

According to a 2009 poll conducted by the Vegetarian Resource Group, more than 3 percent of U.S. adults, approximately 6 to 8 million people, are vegetarians.[34] Other surveys have shown that nearly 23 million Americans are "vegetarian inclined," or "flexitarians," meaning that they are omnivores who are trying to eat more vegetarian meals and reducing meat consumption in favor of other "faceless" forms of protein.[35] The word **vegetarian** means different things to different people. See Table 7.6 for a complete listing of vegetarian types, and the things they eat.

**vegetarian** A person who follows a diet that excludes some or all animal products.

Why are so many moving toward meat and dairy reduction or elimination in their diets? Common reasons for pursuing a vegetarian lifestyle include concern for animal welfare, improving health, environmental concerns, natural

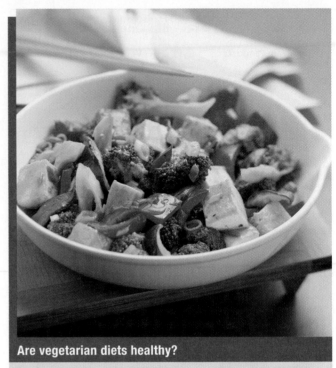

**Are vegetarian diets healthy?**

Adopting a vegan or vegetarian diet can be a very healthy way to eat. Take care to prepare your food healthfully by limiting the use of oils and avoiding added sugars and sodium. Make sure you get all the essential amino acids by eating meals like this tofu and vegetable stir-fry. To further enhance it, add a whole grain, such as brown rice.

approaches to wellness, food safety, weight loss, and weight maintenance. Generally, people who follow a balanced vegetarian diet weigh less and have better cholesterol levels, fewer problems with irregular bowel movements (constipation and diarrhea), and a lower risk of heart disease than do nonvegetarians. The benefits of vegetarianism also include a

TABLE
7.6 | **Types of Vegetarians**

| Type of Vegetarian | Does Eat | Doesn't Eat |
|---|---|---|
| Vegan | Vegetables, grains, fruits, nuts, seeds, and legumes | Meat, poultry, seafood, dairy products, eggs, any other animal-based products |
| Lacto-vegetarian | Vegetables, grains, fruits, nuts, seeds, legumes, and dairy products | Meat, poultry, seafood, and eggs |
| Ovo-vegetarian | Vegetables, grains, fruits, nuts, seeds, legumes, and eggs | Meat, poultry, seafood, and dairy products |
| Lacto-ovo-vegetarian | Vegetables, grains, fruits, nuts, seeds, legumes, dairy products, and eggs | Meat, poultry, and seafood |
| Pesco-vegetarian | Vegetables, grains, fruits, nuts, seeds, legumes, dairy products, eggs, and seafood | Meat and poultry |
| Semi-vegetarian (or "non–red meat eater") | Vegetables, grains, fruits, nuts, seeds, legumes, dairy products, eggs, seafood, and poultry (occasional) | Meat |

reduced risk of some cancers, particularly colon cancer, and a reduced risk of kidney disease.[36]

With proper information and food choices, vegetarianism provides a superb alternative to a high-fat, high-calorie, meat-based cuisine. Although in the past vegetarians often suffered from vitamin deficiencies, most vegetarians today are adept at combining the right types of foods and eating a variety of different foods to ensure proper nutrient intake. Vegan diets may be deficient in vitamins $B_2$ (riboflavin), $B_{12}$, and D. Vegans are also at risk for deficiencies of calcium, iron, zinc, and other minerals but can obtain these nutrients from supplements. Strict vegans have to pay much more attention to what they eat than the average person does, but by eating complementary combinations of plant products, they can receive adequate amounts of essential amino acids. In fact, whereas vegans typically get 50 to 60 grams of protein per day, lacto-ovo-vegetarians normally consume between 70 and 90 grams per day, well beyond the recommended amounts. Eating a full variety of grains, legumes, fruits, vegetables, and seeds each day will keep even the strictest vegetarian in excellent health. Pregnant women, older adults, sick people, and children who are vegans need to take special care to ensure that their diets are adequate. In all cases, seek advice from a health care professional if you have questions.

## what do you think?

Why are so many people becoming vegetarians? ● How easy is it to be a vegetarian on your campus? ● What concerns about vegetarianism would you be likely to have, if any?

## Read Food Labels

Historically, various government and scientific organizations developed dietary guidelines to reduce the public's risk of diseases from nutrient deficiency. Known as the **Recommended Dietary Allowances (RDAs)**, these guidelines have provided Americans and Canadians with recommended intake levels that meet the nutritional needs of about 97 percent of healthy individuals. In 1997, the U.S. Food and Nutrition Board expanded upon the RDAs by creating new *Dietary Reference Intakes (DRIs)*, a list of 26 nutrients essential to maintaining health. The DRIs identify and recommend maximum safe intake levels for healthy people and establish the amount of a nutrient needed to prevent deficiencies or to reduce the risk of chronic disease. The DRIs are considered the umbrella guidelines under which the following categories fall:

● *U.S. Recommended Dietary Allowances (USRDAs):* The reference standard for intake levels necessary to meet the nutritional needs of 97 to 98 percent of healthy individuals
● *Adequate Intake (AI):* The recommended average daily nutrient intake level by healthy people when there is not enough research to determine the full RDA

## 52%
**of U.S. adults take multivitamins, at an annual cost of over $23 billion.**

● *Tolerable Upper Intake Level (UL):* The highest amount of a nutrient that an individual can consume daily without the risk of adverse health effects

To help consumers determine the nutritional values of foods, the FDA and the USDA developed the *Reference Daily Intakes (RDIs)* and the *Daily Reference Values (DRVs)*. The RDIs are the recommended daily amounts of vitamins and minerals, also known as *macronutrients,* and the DRVs are the recommended amounts of macronutrients such as total fat, saturated fat, cholesterol, total carbohydrates, dietary fiber, sodium, potassium, and protein.

Confused by all of these values? Don't despair—many people are confused by all the numbers and percentages that make up food labels. Just remember this: Together, the RDIs and DRVs make up the **Daily Values (DVs).** These are the percentages that you will find listed as "% Daily Value" on food and supplement labels. In addition to the percentage of nutrients found in a serving of food, labels also include information on the serving size, calories, calories from fat per serving, and percentage of *trans* fats in a food. **Figure 7.9** on page 234 walks you through a typical food label.

**Recommended Dietary Allowances (RDAs)** The average daily intakes of energy and nutrients considered adequate to meet the needs of most healthy people in the United States under usual conditions. **Daily Values (DVs)** Percentages listed as "% DV" on food and supplement labels; made up of the RDIs and DRVs together. **dietary supplements** Vitamins and minerals taken by mouth that are intended to supplement existing diets.

## Supplements: Research on the Daily Dose

**Dietary supplements** are products—usually vitamins and minerals—taken by mouth and intended to supplement existing diets. Ingredients range from vitamins, minerals, and herbs to enzymes, amino acids, fatty acids, and organ tissues. They can come in tablet, capsule, liquid, powder, and other forms. Because of dietary supplements' potential for influencing health, their sales have skyrocketed in the past decades.

It is important to note that all dietary supplements are not regulated like other food and drug products. The FDA does not evaluate the safety and efficacy of supplements prior to their marketing; it can take action to remove a supplement from the market only after it has been proved harmful. Currently, the United States has no formal guidelines for supplement sale and safety, and supplement manufacturers are responsible for self-monitoring their activities.

But, do you really need to buy any of the myriad dietary supplements that are available? For years, health experts had touted the benefits of

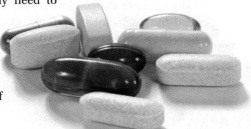

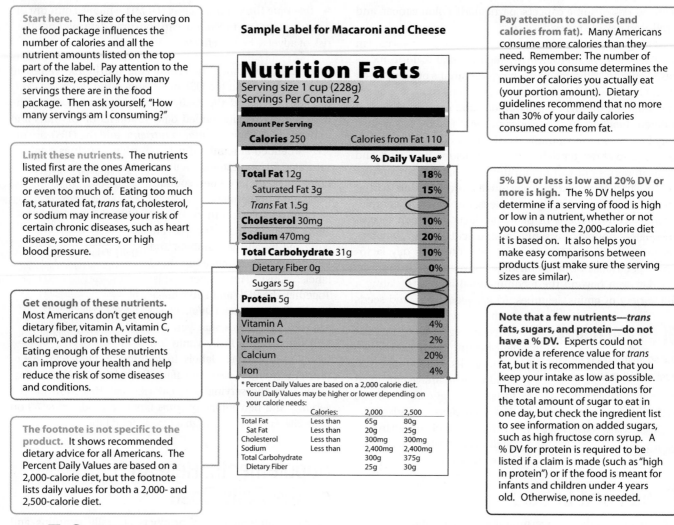

**FIGURE 7.9 Reading a Food Label**

**Source:** Center for Food Safety and Applied Nutrition, "A Key to Choosing Healthful Foods: Using the Nutrition Facts on the Food Label," Updated May 2009, www.fda.gov/Food/ResourcesForYou/Consumers/ucm079449.htm.

eating a balanced diet over popping a vitamin or mineral supplement, so it came as a surprise when a 2001 article in the *Journal of the American Medical Association* (*JAMA*) recommended that "a vitamin/mineral supplement a day just might be important in keeping the doctor away, particularly for some groups of people."[37] The article indicated that older adults, vegans, alcohol-dependent individuals, and patients with malabsorption problems may be at particular risk for deficiency of several vitamins. Although the article acknowledged a possible risk of overdosing on fat-soluble vitamins, it noted that preliminary research has linked inadequate amounts of vitamins $B_6$, $B_{12}$, D, and E and lycopene to chronic diseases, including coronary heart disease, cancer, and osteoporosis.

The scientific debate doesn't stop there. In a 2006 report issued by the National Institutes of Health, a 13-member panel of experts concluded that "the present evidence is insufficient to recommend either for or against the use of multivitamins and minerals by the American public to prevent chronic diseases."[38] More recently, Canadian researchers argued that some supplements should be considered over-the-counter medications. The research team recommends that vitamins A, E, D, folic acid, and niacin should be categorized as over-the-counter medications and that vitamin A be removed from multivitamins.[39]

## Eating Well in College

College students often face a challenge when trying to eat healthy foods. Some students live in dorms and do not have their own cooking or refrigeration facilities. Others live in crowded apartments where everyone forages in the refrigerator for everyone else's food. Still others eat at university food services where food choices may be overwhelming. Nearly all have financial and time constraints that make buying, preparing, and eating healthy food a difficult task. What's a student to do?

Many college students may find it hard to fit a well-balanced meal into the day, but eating breakfast and lunch are important if you are to keep energy levels up and get the most out of your classes. If your campus is like many others,

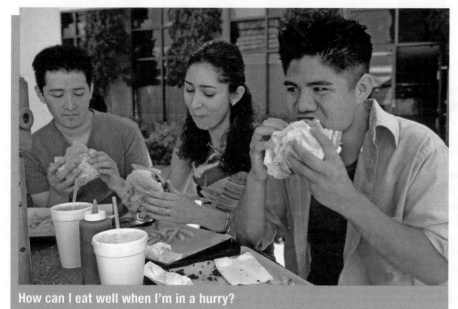

**How can I eat well when I'm in a hurry?**

Meals like this one may be convenient, but they are high in fat, calories, sodium, and refined carbohydrates. Even when you are short on time and money, it is possible—and worthwhile—to make healthier choices. If you are ordering fast food, opt for foods prepared by baking, roasting, or steaming; ask for the leanest meat option; and request that sauces, dressings, and gravies be served on the side.

- At least once per week, substitute a vegetable-based meat substitute into your fast-food choices. Most places now offer Gardenburgers, Boca burgers, and similar products, which provide excellent sources of protein and often have considerably less fat and fewer calories.

In the dining hall, try these ideas:

- Choose lean meats, grilled chicken, fish, or vegetable dishes. Avoid fried chicken, fatty cuts of red meat, or meat dishes smothered in creamy or oily sauce.
- Hit the salad bar and load up on leafy greens, beans, tuna, or tofu. Choose items such as avocado or nuts for a little "good" fat, and go easy on the dressing.
- Get creative: Choose items such as a baked potato with salsa, or add grilled chicken to your salad. Top toast with veggies, hummus, or grilled chicken or tuna.
- When choosing items from a made-to-order food station, ask the preparer to hold the butter or oil, mayonnaise, sour cream, or cheese- or cream-based sauces.
- Avoid going back for seconds and consuming large portions.
- If there is something you'd like but don't see in your dining hall, or if you are vegetarian and feel like your food choices are limited, speak to your food services manager and provide suggestions.
- Pass on high-calorie, low-nutrient foods such as sugary cereals, ice cream, and other sweet treats. Choose fruit or low-fat yogurt to satisfy your sweet tooth.

Maintaining a nutritious diet within the confines of student life can be challenging. However, if you take the time to plan healthy meals, you will find that you are eating better, enjoying it more, and actually saving money. The **Skills for Behavior Change** box on page 236 boils down healthy eating into some simple tips to follow, whereas the **Consumer Health** box on page 237 offers suggestions for ways to continue your healthy eating when dining out.

you've probably noticed a distinct move toward fast-food restaurants in your student unions. However, eating a complete breakfast that includes complex carbohydrates, protein, and healthy, unsaturated fat (such as a banana, peanut butter and whole-grain bread sandwich, or a dry fruit and nut mix without added sugar or salt) is key. If you are short on time you can bring these items to class to ensure your meals fit into your day. Generally speaking, you can eat more healthfully and for less money if you bring food from home or your campus dining hall. If you must eat fast food, follow the tips below to get more nutritional bang for your buck:

- Ask for nutritional analyses of items. Most fast-food chains now have them.
- Order salads, but be careful about what you add to them. Taco salads and Cobb salads are often high in fat, calories, and sodium. Ask for dressing on the side, and use it sparingly. Try the vinaigrette or low-fat dressings. Stay away from eggs and other high-fat add-ons, such as bacon bits, croutons, and crispy noodles.
- If you must have fries, check to see what type of oil is used to cook them. Avoid lard-based or other saturated-fat products and *trans* fats. Some fast-food restaurants offer baked "fries," which may be lower in fat.
- Avoid giant sizes, and refrain from ordering extra sauce, bacon, cheese, dressings, and other extras that add additional calories, sodium, carbohydrates, and fat.
- Limit beverages and foods that are high in added sugars. Common forms of added sugars include sucrose, glucose, fructose, maltose, dextrose, corn syrups, concentrated fruit juices, and honey.

## Is Organic for You?

Concerns about food safety, genetically modified foods, and the health impacts of chemicals used in the growth and production of food have led many people to turn to foods that are **organic**—foods and beverages developed, grown, or raised without the use of synthetic pesticides, chemicals, or hormones. As of 2002, any food sold in the United States as organic has to meet criteria set by the USDA under the National Organic Rule and can carry a USDA seal verifying products as "certified organic." Under this rule, a product that is certified may carry one of the following terms: "100 percent Organic" (100% compliance

**organic** Grown without use of pesticides, chemicals, or hormones.

## Healthy Eating Simplified

Messages from nutrition experts, marketing campaigns, and media blitzes may leave you scratching your head about how to eat healthfully. When it all starts to feel too complicated to be worthwhile, here are some simple tips to follow for health-conscious eating:

✳ You don't need foods from fancy packages to improve your health. Fruits, vegetables, and whole grains should make up the bulk of your diet. Shop the perimeter of the store and shop the bulk foods aisle.
✳ Let the plate method guide you. Your plate should be half vegetables, a quarter lean protein, and a quarter whole grains/bread. A serving of fruit should be dessert.
✳ Avoid or limit processed foods/packaged foods. This will assist you in limiting added sodium, sugar, and fat. If you can't make sense of the ingredients, don't eat it.
✳ Eat natural "snacks" such as dried fruit, nuts, fresh fruits, string cheese, yogurt without added sugar, hard-boiled eggs, and vegetables.
✳ Be mindful of your eating. Eat until you are satisfied but not overfull.
✳ Bring healthful foods with you when you head out the door. Whether to class, on a road trip, or going to work, you *can* control the foods that are available. Don't put yourself in a position to buy from a vending machine or convenience store.

**Source:** M. Pollan, *Food Rules: An Eater's Manual* (New York: Penguin Books, 2010).

In 2007, several reports by consumer groups questioned the nutrient value of organic foods. Some sources say that smaller organic farmers may have trouble getting their produce to market in the proper climate-controlled vehicles. As such, their foods might lose valuable nutrients while sitting in warm trucks or at a roadside stand compared to the refrigerated section of a local supermarket; or, as important, increased bacterial growth may occur.

Today, the word **locavore** has been coined to describe people who eat only food grown or produced locally, usually within close proximity to their homes. Farmers' markets or home-grown foods or those grown by independent farmers are thought to be fresher and to require far fewer resources to get them to market and keep them fresh for longer periods of time. Locavores believe that locally grown organic food is preferable to foods produced by large corporations or supermarket-based organic foods, as they make a smaller impact on the environment. Although there are many reasons organic farming is better for the environment, the fact that pesticides, herbicides, and other products are not used is perhaps the greatest benefit. The **Be Healthy, Be Green** box on page 238 discusses some of the issues surrounding food politics and agriculture in the United States.

# Food Safety: A Growing Concern

Eating unhealthy food is one thing. Eating food that has been contaminated with a pathogen, toxin, or other harmful substance is quite another. As outbreaks of salmonella in chicken and vegetables or *Escherichia coli* (*E. coli,* a potentially lethal bacterial pathogen) in spinach or beef periodically make the news, the food industry has come under fire. To convince us that their products are safe, some manufacturers have come up with "new and improved" ways of protecting our foods. What are the dangers of contaminated foods, and how well do food manufacturers' new strategies work? Let's find out.

## Foodborne Illnesses

Are you concerned that the chicken you are buying doesn't look pleasingly pink or that your "fresh" fish smells a little *too* fishy? You may have good reason to be worried. In increasing numbers, Americans are becoming sick from what they eat, and many of these illnesses are life threatening. Based on several studies conducted over the past 10 years, scientists estimate that foodborne pathogens sicken over 76 million people and cause some 400,000 hospitalizations and 5,000 deaths in the United States annually.[41] These numbers have remained fairly constant since 2004, despite increased attention to prevention in the United States.[42] Because most of us don't go to the doctor every time we feel ill, we may not make a connection between what we eat and later symptoms.

with organic criteria), "Organic" (must contain at least 95% organic materials), "Made with Organic Ingredients" (must contain at least 70% organic ingredients), or "Some Organic Ingredients" (contains less than 70% organic ingredients—usually listed individually). To be labeled with any of the above terms, the foods must be produced without hormones, antibiotics, herbicides, insecticides, chemical fertilizers, genetic modification, or germ-killing radiation. However, reliable monitoring systems to ensure credibility are still under development.

**locavore** A person who primarily eats food grown or produced locally.

Is buying organic really better for you? It is almost impossible to assess the health impact of organic versus nonorganic foods. Nevertheless, the market for organics has been increasing by more than 20 percent per year—five times faster than food sales in general. Where only a small subset of the population once bought organic, nearly all U.S. consumers now occasionally reach for something labeled organic. In 2010, annual organic food sales were estimated to be $25 billion.[40]

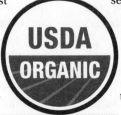

USDA label for certified organic foods.

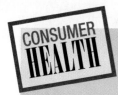

# What's Healthy on the Menu?

No matter what type of cuisine you enjoy, there will always be healthier and less healthy options on the menu. To help you order wisely, here are lighter options and high-fat pitfalls. "Best" choices contain fewer than 30 grams of fat, a generous meal's worth for an active, medium-sized woman. "Worst" choices have up to 100 grams of fat. Most college campuses offer an array of cuisines. This guide will help you make healthier choices.

## Italian
**Best** Pasta with red or white clam sauce
Spaghetti with marinara or tomato-and-meat sauce
**Worst** Eggplant parmigiana
Fettuccine Alfredo
Fried calamari
Lasagna
**Tips** Stick with plain bread instead of garlic bread made with butter or oil. Ask for the waiter's help in avoiding cream- or egg-based sauces. Try vegetarian pizza, and don't ask for extra cheese.

## Mexican
**Best** Bean burrito (no cheese)
Chicken fajitas
**Worst** Beef chimichanga
Quesadilla
Chile relleno
Refried beans
**Tips** Choose soft tortillas (not fried) with fresh salsa, not guacamole. Special-order grilled shrimp, fish, or chicken. Ask for beans made without lard or fat, and have cheeses and sour cream provided on the side or left out altogether.

## Chinese
**Best** Hot-and-sour soup
Stir-fried vegetables
Shrimp with garlic sauce
Szechuan shrimp
Wonton soup
**Worst** Crispy chicken
Kung pao chicken
Moo shu pork
Sweet-and-sour pork
**Tips** Share a stir-fry; help yourself to steamed rice. Ask for vegetables steamed or stir-fried with less oil. Order moo shu vegetables instead of pork. Avoid fried rice, breaded dishes, egg rolls and spring rolls, and items loaded with nuts. Avoid high-sodium sauces.

## Japanese
**Best** Steamed rice and vegetables
Tofu as a substitute for meat
Broiled or steamed chicken and fish
**Worst** Fried rice dishes
Miso (very high in sodium)
Tempura
**Tips** Avoid soy sauces. Use caution in eating sashimi (raw fish) and sushi dishes to avoid possible bacteria or parasites.

## Thai
**Best** Clear broth soups
Stir-fried chicken and vegetables
Grilled meats
**Worst** Coconut milk
Peanut sauces
Deep-fried dishes
**Tips** Avoid coconut-based curries. Ask for steamed, not fried, rice.

## Korean
**Best** Soups, like hot fish soup ("mehoontang") or stews ("chigae") or chigae also known as soft tofu soup
Kimchee-fermented cabbage
**Worst** Pork bulgogi
Barbeque
**Tips** Avoid high sugar and sodium BBQ and opt for dishes with lots of vegetables.

## Peruvian
**Best** Grilled fish
Steamed fish
Seafood
**Worst** Dishes with heavy milk
Deep-fried items
**Tips** Select boiled or steamed dishes, limit cheese and milk.

## Ethiopian
**Best** Vegetable stews
Lentils
Potatoes
**Worst** Ketfo (raw or rare beef)
Deep-fried foods
**Tips** Choose vegetables and lentils, fish, and leaner meats such as chicken and goat.

## Moroccan
**Best** Eggplant and tomato salads
Couscous
Fish and broth soups
**Worst** Pastilla or meat pie
Beef dishes
Pastry
**Tips** Look for tagines of slow-cooked lean meats and vegetables and avoid pastry and fried foods.

## Indian
**Best** Gobi aloo
Vegetables
Lentils
Roti
**Worst** Samosas (stuffed and fried vegetable turnover)
Butter chicken
Coconut oil
Ghee (clarified butter)
**Tips** Limit foods cooked in heavy coconut oil or ghee. Enjoy fish and modest amounts of white rice. Avoid dishes that are deep fried.

## American Breakfast
**Best** Hot or cold cereal with 2 percent milk
Pancakes or French toast with syrup
Scrambled eggs with hash browns and plain toast
**Worst** Belgian waffle with sausage
Sausage and eggs with biscuits and gravy
Ham-and-cheese omelet with hash browns and toast
**Tips** Ask for whole-grain cereal or shredded wheat with 2 percent milk or whole wheat toast without butter or margarine. Order omelets without cheese, and order fried eggs without bacon or sausage.

## Sandwiches
**Best** Ham and Swiss cheese
Roast beef
Turkey
**Worst** Tuna salad
Reuben
Submarine
**Tips** Ask for mustard; hold the mayonnaise and high-fat cheese. See if turkey-ham is available.

## Seafood
**Best** Broiled bass, halibut, or snapper
Grilled scallops
Steamed crab or lobster
**Worst** Fried seafood platter
Blackened catfish
**Tips** Order fish broiled, baked, grilled, or steamed—not pan fried or sautéed. Ask for lemon instead of tartar sauce. Avoid creamy and buttery sauces.

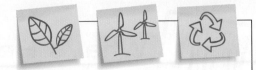

## Eating for a Healthy Environment

Food politics affect us all yet often they are not part of our consciousness. In recent years journalist Michael Pollan has brought the food politics conversation to the mainstream with his books, *The Omnivore's Dilemma*, *In Defense of Food*, and, most recently, *Food Rules*. Pollan's work has prompted the public and politicians alike to engage in discussion of our food and farm policies.

Much of the food politics debate focuses on controversies over which foods are best for you, for the environment, and for other living species. For example, a commonly cited estimate is that it takes up to 16 pounds of grain and soybeans to produce a pound of beef and that far too much water, land, and food-based resources are used in doing so. Proponents of this concept argue that it would be better to eat the grains and soybeans, rather than eating the cow fed on them. Critics of this estimate argue that these numbers are incorrect and that it's probably closer to 2.6 pounds of grain/soybean to 1 pound of beef; they feel that, nutritionally, lean beef is an efficient, environmentally friendly resource. Proponents of grass-fed beef argue for raising cattle and producing beef in a more humane and ecologically sound manner. Others argue that all food production takes a toll on the environment and that even crops raised for vegan diets can have a significant effect on wild animals, water supplies, soil nutrients, insects, and other aspects of a locale's ecology.

One of the most significant forces shaping the nature of food production in the United States, and its environmental and human impacts, is the Farm Bill, properly known as the Food, Conservation, and Energy Act, which is renewed every 5 years by Congress (most recent renewal in 2008). This is the primary agricultural and food policy tool of the federal government, and it is highly controversial among many groups. Essentially, the Farm Bill determines which crops the federal government will subsidize and at what levels. Critics argue that it benefits corporate farming and factory farms that have huge negative environmental impacts and disadvantages for the small, local, organic farmer. The Farm Bill also has the potential for having a major impact on food availability, pricing, and distribution in various geographical locations, including international trade venues.

The Farm Bill is composed of 15 titles that focus on governing most of the federally regulated agriculture programs. One of the Farm Bill's 15 titles includes income support for commodities such as wheat, feed grains, rice, and oilseeds. There are also titles relating to livestock, forestry, conservation, and rural development. Fruits and vegetables are considered specialty crops and receive little financial support except through the nutrition title of the bill.

How might the Farm Bill and other agricultural legislation affect you personally? Why might such a bill hinder the national movement toward buying organic foods, reducing pesticide and herbicide use, and buying local products? What food choices can you make to minimize your impact on the environment? There is no easy answer, but here are a few actions to consider to enhance your health and that of other species and the environment:

✳ Challenge yourself to a 100-mile diet. This means eating food that is shipped no farther than a 100-mile radius from where you live. Imagine the trip your food has been on even before it reaches your home. If your food is transported to your local store, there is always an environmental cost involved, for example, the fuel that is needed to transport that food. Compared to locally grown foods, the transportation of foods that make up an average meal uses up to 17 times more petroleum products and increases carbon dioxide emissions by the same amount. Shopping at local vendors such as a farmer's market or vegetable stand is a great way to start eating locally. By buying local food, you not only reduce the amount of fuel used to transport the food, but you also support local growers at the same time.

✳ Know where your meat comes from. Avoid large meat-producing superfarms where animals live in unhealthy conditions, where the potential for water and air pollution is great, or where animal abuse is present. Buy locally, from small farmers. Find out which ones have the best conditions for producing healthy animals and which ones follow humane slaughtering practices.

✳ Remember that food-producing groups have good reason to write biased reports on the benefits of their products. Get your information from solid research organizations, university groups, and government groups that are less likely to have strong lobbying interests influencing their positions on food production and consumption.

✳ If you feel frustrated by the cost of "healthy foods," particularly organic fruits and vegetables, remember that the Food, Conservation, and Energy Act is a reauthorization bill, that is, a bill that is reexamined and renewed roughly every 5 years by the federal government. Watch for the next renewal in 2012 and get involved in shaping our food landscape by becoming informed on the provisions of the bill, contacting your congressperson, and joining or organizing community education campaigns. Until then, vote for healthy foods with your food dollars.

TABLE
7.7

## Common Foodborne Illnesses

| Bacteria or Other Pathogen | Cases per Year | Description |
|---|---|---|
| *Salmonella* | 7,444 | Commonly found in the intestines of birds and in the intestines of reptiles and mammals, it can spread to humans through foods of animal origin. Infection by *Salmonella* usually consists of fever, diarrhea, and abdominal cramps. Salmonellosis can be life threatening if the bacteria invade the bloodstream, as is more likely in people with poor underlying health or weakened immune systems. |
| *Campylobacter* | 5,825 | Most raw poultry has *Campylobacter* in it, and this infection most frequently results from eating undercooked chicken or food that has been contaminated with juices from raw chicken. Infection causes fever, diarrhea, and abdominal cramps. |
| *Shigella* | 3,029 | A bacterium that is commonly found in human stool, its most likely route of infection is improper hand washing. Most people who are infected develop diarrhea, fever, and stomach cramps starting a day or two after they have been exposed to the bacteria. The diarrhea is often bloody. Shigellosis usually resolves in 5 to 7 days. |
| *Cryptosporidium* | 1,036 | A microscopic parasite that lives in the small intestine of humans and animals, "Crypto" is one of the most common causes of waterborne disease in the world. It is transmitted via the fecal-oral route. |
| *E. coli* O157:H7 | 718 | *E. coli* O157:H7 lives in the intestines of cattle and other livestock and can contaminate food and water that come in contact with animal feces. In humans, infection by *E. coli* O157:H7 causes severe and bloody diarrhea and painful abdominal cramps. In 3% to 5% of cases, complications including anemia, bleeding, and kidney failure can occur several weeks after the initial onset of symptoms. |
| *Listeria* | 135 | A bacterium that is found in soil and in water, *Listeria* can contaminate raw foods, such as vegetables and meat products, as well as food that has been processed. Healthy adults and children rarely become seriously ill, but the infection can be dangerous for people with weakened immune systems, older adults, pregnant women, and newborns. Symptoms include fever, muscle aches, and sometimes nausea or diarrhea. More serious symptoms can occur if the infection spreads to the nervous system. |

**Source:** Data are from Centers for Disease Control and Prevention "Preliminary FoodNet Data on the Incidence of Infection with Pathogens Transmitted Commonly Through Food—10 States, 2008," *Morbidity and Mortality Weekly Report* 58, no. 13 (April 10, 2009): 333–37.

Most foodborne infections and illnesses are caused by several common types of bacteria and viruses.[43] Table 7.7 lists some of the most common. Foodborne illnesses can also be caused by a toxin in food that was originally produced by a bacterium or other microbe in the food. These toxins can produce illness even if the microbes that produced them are no longer there. For example, botulism is caused by a deadly toxin produced by the bacterium *Clostridium botulinum.* This bacterium is widespread in soil, water, plants, and intestinal tracts, but it can grow only in environments with limited or no oxygen. Potential food sources include improperly canned food and vacuum-packed or tightly wrapped foods. Though rare, this illness is fatal if untreated, as the powerful neurotoxin causes paralysis and can lead to the cessation of breathing.

Signs of foodborne illnesses vary tremendously and usually include one or several symptoms: diarrhea, nausea, cramping, and vomiting. Depending on the amount and virulence of the pathogen, symptoms may appear as early as 30 minutes after eating contaminated food or as long as several days or weeks later. Most of the time, symptoms occur 5 to 8 hours after eating and last only a day or two. For certain populations, such as the very young; older adults; or people with severe illnesses such as cancer, diabetes, kidney disease, or AIDS, foodborne diseases can be fatal.

Several factors may contribute to the increase in foodborne illnesses. The movement away from a traditional meat-and-potato American diet to "heart-healthy" eating—increasing consumption of fruits, vegetables, and grains—has spurred demand for fresh foods that are not in season most of the year. This means that we must import fresh fruits and vegetables, thus putting ourselves at risk for ingesting exotic pathogens or even pesticides that have been banned in the United States for safety reasons. Depending on the season, up to 70 percent of the fruits and vegetables consumed in the United States come from Mexico. Although we are told when we travel to developing countries to "boil it, peel it, or don't eat it," we bring these foods into our kitchens at home and eat them, often without even washing them. Food can become contaminated by being

Many people worldwide enjoy sashimi and sushi. Use caution when eating, however, as raw fish can be a breeding ground for dangerous microbes.

watered with tainted water, fertilized with animal manure, picked by people who have not washed their hands properly after using the toilet, or by not being subjected to the same rigorous pesticide regulations as American-raised produce. To

give you an idea of the implications, studies have shown that *E. coli* can survive in cow manure for up to 70 days and can multiply in foods grown with manure unless heat or additives such as salt or preservatives are used to kill the microbes.[44] There are no regulations that prohibit farmers from using animal manure to fertilize crops. In addition, *E. coli* actually increases in summer months as cows await slaughter in crowded, overheated pens. This increases the chances of meat coming to market already contaminated.

**food irradiation** Treating foods with gamma radiation from radioactive cobalt, cesium, or other sources of X rays to kill microorganisms.

Other key factors associated with the increasing spread of foodborne diseases include the inadvertent introduction of pathogens into new geographic regions and insufficient education about food safety. Globalization of the food supply, climate change, and global warming are also factors that may influence increasing spread.

## Avoiding Risks in the Home

Part of the responsibility for preventing foodborne illness lies with consumers—more than 30 percent of all such illnesses result from unsafe handling of food at home. Fortunately, consumers can take several steps to reduce the likelihood of contaminating their food (see **Figure 7.10**). Among the most basic precautions are to wash your hands and to wash all produce before eating it. Also, avoid cross-contamination in

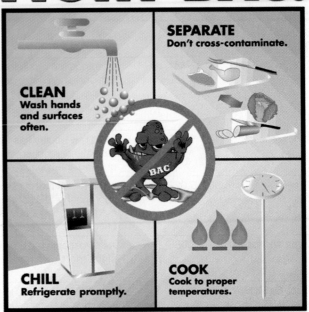

# FIGHT BAC!

CLEAN
Wash hands and surfaces often.

SEPARATE
Don't cross-contaminate.

CHILL
Refrigerate promptly.

COOK
Cook to proper temperatures.

## Keep Food Safe From Bacteria™

FIGURE 7.10 **The USDA's Fight BAC!**
This logo reminds consumers how to prevent foodborne illness.

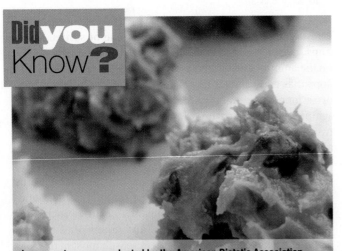

**Did you Know?**

In a recent survey conducted by the American Dietetic Association, college students indicated a high degree of confidence in their ability to handle food safely, yet, in the same survey 53% of students admitted to eating raw homemade cookie dough (which contains uncooked eggs, a potential source of salmonella), 33% said they ate fried eggs with soft or runny yolks, and 7% said they ate pink hamburger.

**Source:** Data are from C. Byrd-Bredbenner et al., "Risky Eating Behaviors of Young Adults—Implications for Food Safety Education," *Journal of the American Dietetic Association* 108, no. 3 (2008): 549–52.

the kitchen by using separate cutting boards and utensils for meats and produce. Temperature control is also important—refrigerators must be set at 40 degrees or less. Be sure to cook meats to the recommended temperature to kill contaminants before eating. Hot foods must be kept hot and cold foods kept cold in order to avoid unchecked bacterial growth. Eat leftovers within 3 days, and if you're unsure how long something has been sitting in the fridge, don't take chances. When in doubt, throw it out. See the **Skills for Behavior Change** box at right for more tips about reducing risk of foodborne illness when shopping for and preparing food.

## Food Irradiation

**Food irradiation** is a process that involves treating foods with invisible waves of energy that damage microorganisms. These energy waves are actually low doses of radiation, or ionizing energy, which breaks chemical bonds in the DNA of harmful bacteria, destroying the pathogens and keeping them from replicating. Essentially, the rays pass through the food without leaving any radioactive residue.[45]

Irradiation lengthens food products' shelf life and prevents the spread of deadly microorganisms, particularly in high-risk foods such as ground beef and pork. Thus, the minimal costs of irradiation should result in lower overall costs to

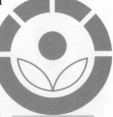

U.S. FDA label for irradiated foods.

## Reduce Your Risk for Foodborne Illness

* When shopping for fish, buy from markets that get their supplies from state-approved sources; check for cleanliness at the salad bar and at the meat and fish counters.

* Keep most cuts of meat, fish, and poultry in the refrigerator no more than 1 or 2 days. Check the shelf life of all products before buying. Use the sniff test—if fish smells really fishy, don't eat it.

* Use a meat thermometer to ensure that meats are completely cooked. Beef and lamb steaks and roasts should be cooked to at least 145°F; ground meat, pork chops, ribs, and egg dishes to 160°F; ground poultry and hot dogs to 165°F; chicken and turkey breasts to 170°F; and chicken and turkey legs, thighs, and whole birds to 180°F. Fish is done when the thickest part becomes opaque and the fish flakes easily when poked with a fork.

* Never leave cooked food standing on the stove or table for more than 2 hours.

* Never thaw frozen foods at room temperature. Put them in the refrigerator for a day to thaw or thaw in cold water, changing the water every 30 minutes.

* Wash your hands and countertop with soap and water when preparing food, particularly after handling meat, fish, or poultry.

* When freezing chicken or other raw foods, make sure juices can't spill over into ice cubes or into other areas of the refrigerator.

---

consumers and reduce the need for toxic chemicals now used to preserve foods and prevent contamination from external pathogens. Use of food irradiation is limited because of consumer concerns about safety, and because irradiation facilities are expensive to build. Still, food irradiation is now common in over 40 countries. Foods that have been irradiated are marked with the "radura" logo.

## Food Additives

Additives are substances added to food to reduce the risk of foodborne illness, prevent spoilage, and enhance the look and taste of foods. Additives can also enhance nutrient value, especially to benefit the general public. Examples include the fortification of milk with vitamin D and of grain products with folate. Although the FDA regulates additives according to effectiveness, safety, and ability to detect them in foods, consumers should take the time to determine what the additives are and whether there are alternatives. As a general rule, the fewer chemicals, colorants, and preservatives there are, the better the food is. Examples of common additives include the following:

- **Antimicrobial agents.** Substances such as salt, sugar, nitrates, and others that tend to make foods less hospitable for microbes.
- **Antioxidants.** Substances that reduce the loss of color and flavor due to exposure to oxygen. Vitamins C and E are among the antioxidants believed to reduce the risk of cancer and cardiovascular disease. The additives butylated hydroxyanisole (BHA) and butylated hydroxytoluene (BHT) are also antioxidants.
- **Artificial colors, nutrient additives, and flavor enhancers** such as MSG (monosodium glutamate).
- **Sulfites.** Used to preserve vegetable color; some people have severe allergic reactions to them.

## Food Allergy or Food Intolerance?

About 33 percent of people today *think* they have an allergy or avoid a certain food because they think they are allergic to it; however, only 4 to 8 percent of children and 2 percent of adults have a true food allergy. Still, there may be reason to be concerned. From 1997 through 2007 the prevalence of reported food allergies rose 18 percent.[46]

A **food allergy,** or hypersensitivity, is an abnormal response to a food that is triggered by the immune system. Symptoms of an allergic reaction vary in severity and may include a tingling sensation in the mouth; swelling of the lips, tongue, and throat; difficulty breathing; hives; vomiting; abdominal cramps; diarrhea; drop in blood pressure; loss of consciousness; and death. Approximately 200 deaths per year occur from the anaphylaxis (the acute systemic immune and inflammatory response) that occurs with allergic reactions. These symptoms may appear within seconds to hours after eating the foods to which one is allergic.[47]

In 2004, Congress passed the Food Allergen Labeling and Consumer Protection Act (FALCPA), which requires food manufacturers to label foods clearly to indicate the presence of (or possible contamination by) any of the 8 major food allergens: milk, eggs, peanuts, wheat, soy, tree nuts (walnuts, pecans, etc.), fish, and shellfish. Although over 160 foods have been identified as allergy triggers, these 8 foods account for 90 percent of all food allergies in the United States.[48]

**Celiac disease** is an inherited autoimmune disorder that affects digestive activity in the small intestine. Affecting over 3 million Americans, most of whom are undiagnosed, it is a growing problem particularly for

**food allergy** Overreaction by the body to normally harmless proteins, which are perceived as allergens. In response, the body produces antibodies, triggering allergic symptoms.

**celiac disease** An inherited autoimmune disorder affecting the digestive process of the small intestine and triggered by the consumption of gluten.

Peanuts are among the 8 most common food allergens: 0.6% of the general population are allergic to them, with slightly higher rates in children.

those under the age of 20.[49] When a person with celiac disease consumes gluten, a protein found in wheat, rye, and barley, the person's immune system attacks the small intestine and stops nutrient absorption. Pain, cramping, and other symptoms often follow in the short term. Untreated, celiac disease can lead to other health problems, such as osteoporosis, nutritional deficiencies, and cancer. Once a person is diagnosed with celiac disease, the best treatment is to avoid breads, pastas, and other foods containing gluten.

In contrast to allergies, **food intolerance** can cause you to have symptoms of gastric upset, but the upset is not the result of an immune system response. Probably the best example of a food intolerance is *lactose intolerance*, a problem that affects about 1 in every 10 adults. Lactase is an enzyme in the lining of the gut that degrades lactose, which is in dairy products. If you don't have enough lactase, you cannot digest lactose, and it remains in the gut to be used by bacteria. Gas is formed, and you experience bloating, abdominal pain, and sometimes diarrhea. Food intolerance also occurs in response to some food additives, such as the flavor enhancer MSG, certain dyes, sulfites, gluten, and other substances. In some cases, the food intolerance may have psychological triggers.

**food intolerance** Adverse effects resulting when people who lack the digestive chemicals needed to break down certain substances eat those substances.

**genetically modified (GM) foods** Foods derived from organisms whose DNA has been altered using genetic engineering techniques.

If you suspect that you have an actual allergic reaction to food, see an allergist to be tested to determine the source of the problem. Because there are several diseases that share symptoms with food allergies (ulcers and cancers of the gastrointestinal tract can cause vomiting, bloating, diarrhea, nausea, and pain), you should have persistent symptoms checked out as soon as possible. If particular foods seem to bother you consistently, look for alternatives or modify your diet. In true allergic instances, you may not be able to consume even the smallest amount of a substance safely.

## Genetically Modified Food Crops

Genetic modification involves the insertion or deletion of genes into the DNA of an organism. In the case of **genetically modified (GM) foods,** usually this genetic cutting and pasting is done to enhance production, for example, by making disease- or insect-resistant plants, improving yield, or controlling weeds. In addition, GM foods are sometimes created to improve the color and appearance of foods or to enhance specific nutrients. For example, in places where rice is a staple, GM technology has been used to create varieties with vitamin A and iron. In underdeveloped countries where vitamin A deficiency and iron-deficiency anemia are leading causes of morbidity and mortality, the addition of these nutrients can reduce disease. Another use under development is the production and delivery of vaccines through GM foods.

The first genetically modified food crop was a tomato called the FlavrSavr, which was developed to ripen without

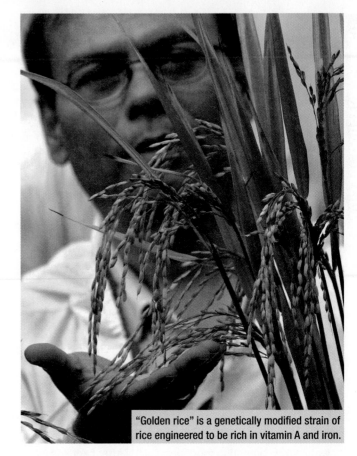

"Golden rice" is a genetically modified strain of rice engineered to be rich in vitamin A and iron.

getting soft, thereby increasing its shipping capacity and shelf life. Since the first crop was grown in 1996, U.S. farmers have widely accepted GM crops.[50] Soybeans and cotton are the most common GM crops, followed by corn. On our supermarket shelves, about 75 percent of the soy and about 40 percent of the corn used in processed foods are genetically modified. It seems consumers are generally accepting of GM foods. However, in a recent report in *New Scientist,* three strains of maize (corn) showed signs of causing liver and kidney toxicity.[51] These claims are refuted by producers but it does leave others questioning the safety of these foods.

The use of GM organisms and food has sparked much controversy among diverse groups. Some see the use of genetic engineering as too much meddling; others are concerned about seeds being controlled by large corporations; and organic farmers may be concerned about genetically modified seeds drifting into their fields. In addition, it has been suggested that GM foods may lead to an increase in allergens and antibiotic resistance.[52] According to the World Health Organization, no effects on human health have been shown from consumption of GM foods in countries that have approved their use.[53] However, a number of organizations would like to see greater regulation of GM foods and a number of lawsuits are pending. The debate surrounding GM foods is not likely to end soon; see the **Points of View** box at right for more on this debate.

# Genetically Modified Foods:
## BOON OR BANE?

If the population continues to expand and if plant diseases continue unchecked, soils are depleted, and our supply of traditional food sources is depleted by overconsumption and slow renewal, we may face severe food shortages in coming decades. Some scientists and food producers believe that genetically modified (GM) food crops could help solve problems of matching food supply to demand, but many other researchers and health advocates are opposed to the further development and widespread use of genetically modified foods, which they feel carry health risks and could have a negative impact on the ecosystem. Below are some of the main points for and against the development of GM organisms for food.

### Arguments for the Development of GM Foods

○ People have been manipulating food crops—primarily through selective breeding—since the beginning of agriculture. Genetic modification is fundamentally the same thing, just more precise.

○ Genetically modified seeds and products are tested for safety, and there has never been a substantiated claim for a human illness resulting from consumption of a GM food.

○ By modifying the DNA in foods that cause allergies, we may be able to prevent many foodborne allergies.

○ Genetically modified crops can have a positive impact on the environment. Current agricultural practices are very environmentally damaging, whereas insect- and weed-resistant GM crops will allow farmers to use far fewer chemical insecticides and herbicides.

○ Genetically modified crops have the potential to reduce world hunger: They can be created to grow more quickly than conventional crops, increasing productivity and allowing for faster cycling of crops, which means more food yield. In addition, nutrient-enhanced crops can address malnutrition, and crops engineered to resist spoiling or damage can allow for transportation to areas affected by drought or natural disaster.

○ Genetically modified crops are under development to produce and deliver vaccines. This is vitally important to protecting the health of people in developing nations and preventing epidemics.

### Arguments against the Development of GM Foods

○ Genetic modification is fundamentally different from and more problematic than selective breeding because it transfers genes between species in ways that could never happen naturally.

○ There haven't been enough independent studies of GM products to confirm that they are safe for consumption. Also, there are potential health risks if GM products approved for animal feed or other uses are mistakenly or inadvertently used in the production of food for human consumption.

○ The use of GM crops cannot be completely controlled, so they have the potential to damage the environment. Inadvertent cross-pollination could lead to the creation of "super weeds"; insect-resistant crops could harm insect species that are not pests; and insect- and disease-resistant crops could prompt the evolution of even more virulent species, which would then require more aggressive control measures, such as the increased use of chemical sprays.

○ There is the potential for genetic engineering to introduce allergens into otherwise nonallergenic foods.

○ Because corporations create and patent GM seeds, they will control the market, meaning that poor farmers in the developing world would become reliant on these corporations. This circumstance would be more likely to increase world hunger than to alleviate it.

○ Creating and patenting new life forms is unethical. The introduction of foreign genes into a plant—particularly genes taken from an animal—is offensive to many religious and cultural groups and upsets the balance of nature.

### Where Do You Stand?

○ Do you think GM foods are more helpful or harmful?

○ What are your greatest concerns over GM foods? What do you think are their greatest benefits?

○ In what ways could the creators of GM foods address the concerns of those opposed to them?

○ What sort of regulation do you think the government should have with regard to the creation, cultivation, and sale of GM foods?

○ Currently, there are no GM livestock; however, many livestock are fed GM feed or feed that includes additives and vaccines produced by GM microorganisms. Do you feel any differently about directly consuming GM crops versus eating the flesh, milk, or eggs of an animal that has been fed on GM crops?

○ If scientists were to develop GM livestock, would that alter your stance on any of these questions?

# Assess Yourself

## How Healthy Are Your Eating Habits?

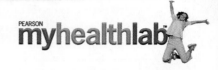

**1** Keep Track of Your Food Intake

Keep a food diary for 5 days, writing down everything you eat or drink. Be sure to include the approximate amount or portion size. Add up the number of servings from each of the major food groups on each day and enter them into the chart below.

Fill out this assessment online at www.pearsonhighered.com/myhealthlab or www.pearsonhighered.com/donatelle.

### Number of Servings of:

| | Day 1 | Day 2 | Day 3 | Day 4 | Day 5 | Average |
|---|---|---|---|---|---|---|
| **Fruits** | | | | | | |
| **Vegetables** | | | | | | |
| **Grains** | | | | | | |
| **Protein Foods** | | | | | | |
| **Dairy** | | | | | | |
| **Fats and Oils** | | | | | | |
| **Sweets** | | | | | | |

### 2A Does your diet have proportionality?

| | Yes | No |
|---|---|---|
| **1.** Are grains the main food choice at all your meals? | ○ | ○ |
| **2.** Do you often forget to eat vegetables? | ○ | ○ |
| **3.** Do you typically eat fewer than three pieces of fruit daily? | ○ | ○ |
| **4.** Do you often have fewer than 3 cups of milk daily? | ○ | ○ |
| **5.** Is the portion of meat, chicken, or fish the largest item on your dinner plate? | ○ | ○ |

### Scoring 2A

If you answered yes to three or more of these questions, your diet probably lacks proportionality. Review the recommendations in this chapter, particularly the MyPyramid guidelines, to learn how to balance your diet.

## 2 Evaluate Your Food Intake

Now compare your consumption patterns to the MyPyramid recommendations. Look at Table 7.1 (page 213) and Figure 7.8 (page 231) or visit www.mypyramid.gov/mypyramid/index.aspx to evaluate your daily caloric needs and the recommended consumption rates for the different food groups. How does your diet match up?

| | Less than the recommended amount | About equal to the recommended amount | More than the recommended amount |
|---|---|---|---|
| **1.** How does your daily fruit consumption compare to the recommendation for your age and activity level? | ○ | ○ | ○ |
| **2.** How does your daily vegetable consumption compare to the recommendation for your age and activity level? | ○ | ○ | ○ |
| **3.** How does your daily grain consumption compare to the recommendation for your age and activity level? | ○ | ○ | ○ |
| **4.** How does your daily protein food consumption compare to the recommendation for your age and activity level? | ○ | ○ | ○ |
| **5.** How does your daily fats and oils consumption compare to the recommendation for your age and activity level? | ○ | ○ | ○ |
| **6.** How does your daily consumption of discretionary calories (sweets) compare to the recommendation for your age and activity level? | ○ | ○ | ○ |

### Scoring

If you found that your food intake is consistent with the MyPyramid recommendations, congratulations! If, on the other hand, you are falling short in a major food group or are overdoing it in certain categories, consider taking steps to adopt healthier eating habits. There are some additional assessments at left and on the next page to help you figure out where your diet is lacking.

## 2B Are you getting enough fat-soluble vitamins in your diet?

Yes  No

1. Do you eat at least 1 cup of deep yellow or orange vegetables, such as carrots and sweet potatoes, or dark green vegetables, such as spinach, every day? ○ ○

2. Do you consume at least two glasses (8 ounces each) of milk daily? ○ ○

3. Do you eat a tablespoon of vegetable oil, such as corn or olive oil, daily? (Tip: Salad dressings, unless they are fat free, count!) ○ ○

4. Do you eat at least 1 cup of leafy green vegetables in your salad and/or put lettuce in your sandwich every day? ○ ○

### Scoring 2B

If you answered yes to all four questions, you are on your way to acing your fat-soluble vitamin needs! If you answered no to any of the questions, your diet needs some fine-tuning. Deep orange and dark green vegetables are excellent sources of vitamin A, and milk is an excellent choice for vitamin D. Vegetable oils provide vitamin E, and if you put them on top of your vitamin K–rich leafy green salad, you'll hit the vitamin jackpot.

## 2C Are you getting enough water-soluble vitamins in your diet?

Yes  No

1. Do you consume at least 1/2 cup of rice or pasta daily? ○ ○

2. Do you eat at least 1 cup of a ready-to-eat cereal or hot cereal every day? ○ ○

3. Do you have at least one slice of bread, a bagel, or a muffin daily? ○ ○

4. Do you enjoy a citrus fruit or fruit juice, such as an orange, a grapefruit, or orange juice every day? ○ ○

5. Do you have at least 1 cup of vegetables throughout your day? ○ ○

### Scoring 2C

If you answered yes to all of these questions, you are a vitamin B and C superstar! If you answered no to any of the questions, your diet could use some refinement. Rice, pasta, cereals, bread, and bread products are all excellent sources of B vitamins. Citrus fruits are a ringer for vitamin C. In fact, all vegetables can contribute to meeting your vitamin C needs daily.

**Source:** Adapted from J. Blake, *Nutrition and You* (San Francisco: Benjamin Cummings, 2008).

# YOUR PLAN FOR CHANGE

The **Assess yourself** activity gave you the chance to evaluate your current nutritional habits. Now that you have considered these results, you can decide whether you need to make changes in your daily eating for long-term health.

### Today, you can:

○ Start keeping a more detailed food log. Take note of the nutritional information of the various foods you eat and write down particulars about the number of calories, grams of fat, grams of sugar, milligrams of sodium, and so on of each food. Try to find specific weak spots: Are you consuming too many calories or too much salt or sugar? Do you eat too little calcium or iron?

○ Take a field trip to the grocery store. Forgo your fast-food dinner and instead spend some time in the produce section of the supermarket. Purchase your favorite fruits and vegetables, and try something new to expand your tastes.

### Within the next 2 weeks, you can:

○ Plan at least three meals that you can make at home or in your dorm room, and purchase the ingredients you'll need ahead of time. Something as simple as a chicken sandwich on whole-grain bread will be more nutritious, and probably cheaper, than heading out for a fast-food meal.

○ Start reading labels. Be aware of the amount of calories, sodium, sugars, and fats in prepared foods; aim to buy and consume those that are lower in all of these and are higher in calcium and fiber.

### By the end of the semester, you can:

○ Get in the habit of eating a healthy breakfast every morning. Combine whole grains, proteins, and fruit in your breakfast—for example, eat a bowl of cereal with milk and bananas or a cup of yogurt combined with granola and berries. Eating a healthy breakfast will jump-start your metabolism, prevent drops in blood glucose levels, and keep your brain and body performing at their best through those morning classes.

○ Commit to one or two healthful changes to your eating patterns for the rest of the semester. You might resolve to eat five servings of fruits and vegetables every day, to switch to low-fat or nonfat dairy products, to stop drinking soft drinks, or to use only olive oil in your cooking. Use your food diary to help you spot places where you can make healthier choices on a daily basis.

## Summary

✱ Recognizing that we eat for more reasons than just survival is the first step toward improving our nutritional habits.

✱ The essential nutrients include water, proteins, carbohydrates, fats, vitamins, and minerals. Water makes up 50 to 60 percent of our body weight and is necessary for nearly all life processes. Proteins are major components of our cells and are key elements of antibodies, enzymes, and hormones. Carbohydrates are our primary sources of energy. Fats play important roles in maintaining body temperature and cushioning and protecting organs. Vitamins are organic compounds, and minerals are inorganic compounds. We need both in relatively small amounts to maintain healthy body function.

✱ A healthy diet is adequate, moderate, balanced, varied, and nutrient dense. MyPyramid provides guidelines for healthy eating. These recommendations, developed by the USDA, place emphasis on personalization, proportionality, moderation, variety, physical activity, and gradual improvement. Vegetarianism can provide a healthy alternative for people wishing to eat less or no meat.

✱ Food labels provide information on the serving size, number of calories in a food, as well as the amounts of various nutrients and the percentage of recommended daily values those amounts represent.

✱ College students face unique challenges in eating healthfully. Learning to make better choices at fast-food restaurants, to eat healthfully on a budget, and to eat nutritionally in the dorm are all possible when you use the information in this chapter.

✱ Organic foods are grown and produced without the use of synthetic pesticides, chemicals, or hormones. The USDA offers certification of organics. These foods have become increasingly available and popular, as people take a greater interest in eating healthfully and sustainably.

✱ Foodborne illnesses, food irradiation, food additives, food allergies, food intolerances, GM foods, and other food safety and health concerns are becoming increasingly important to health-wise consumers. Recognizing potential risks and taking steps to prevent problems are part of a sound nutritional plan.

## Pop Quiz

1. Triglycerides make up about ___ percent of total body fat.
   a. 5
   b. 35
   c. 55
   d. 95

2. Which of the following foods would be considered a healthy, *nutrient-dense* food?
   a. nonfat milk
   b. cheddar cheese
   c. soft drink
   d. potato chips

3. What is the most crucial nutrient for life?
   a. water
   b. fiber
   c. minerals
   d. starch

4. Which of the following nutrients moves food through the digestive tract?
   a. water
   b. fiber
   c. minerals
   d. starch

5. Which of the following nutrients are required for the repair and growth of body tissue?
   a. carbohydrates
   b. proteins
   c. vitamins
   d. fats

6. What substance plays a vital role in maintaining healthy skin and hair, insulating body organs against shock, maintaining body temperature, and promoting healthy cell function?
   a. fats
   b. fibers
   c. proteins
   d. carbohydrates

7. Which vitamin maintains bone health?
   a. $B_{12}$
   b. D
   c. $B_6$
   d. Niacin

8. What is the most common nutrient deficiency worldwide?
   a. fat deficiency
   b. iron deficiency
   c. fiber deficiency
   d. calcium deficiency

9. Carrie eats dairy products, and eggs, but she does not eat fish or red meat. Carrie is considered a(n)
   a. vegan.
   b. lacto-ovo-vegetarian.
   c. ovo-vegetarian.
   d. pesco-vegetarian.

10. Which of the following fats is a healthier fat to include in the diet?
    a. *trans* fat
    b. saturated fat
    c. unsaturated fat
    d. hydrogenated fat

*Answers to these questions can be found on page A-1.*

## Think about It!

1. Which factors influence a person's dietary patterns and behaviors? What factors have been the greatest influences on your eating behaviors?

2. What are the six major food groups in MyPyramid? From which groups do you eat too few servings? What

can you do to increase or decrease your intake of selected food groups?

3. What are the major types of nutrients that you need to obtain from the foods you eat? What happens if you fail to get enough of some of them? Are there significant differences between men and women in particular areas of nutrition?

4. Distinguish between the different types of vegetarianism. Which types are most likely to lead to nutrient deficiencies? What can be done to ensure that even the most strict vegetarian receives enough of the major nutrients?

5. What are the major problems that many college students face when trying to eat the right foods? List five actions that you and your classmates could take immediately to improve your eating.

6. What are the major risks for foodborne illnesses, and what can you do to protect yourself?

7. How do food intolerances differ from true food allergies?

# Accessing Your Health on the Internet

The following websites explore further topics and issues related to personal health. For links to these websites, visit the Companion Website for *Access to Health,* 12th Edition, at www.pearsonhighered.com/donatelle.

1. *American Dietetic Association (ADA).* The ADA provides information on a full range of dietary topics, including sports nutrition, healthful cooking, and nutritional eating; the site also links to scientific publications and information on scholarships and public meetings. www.eatright.org

2. *U.S. Food and Drug Administration (FDA).* The FDA provides information for consumers and professionals in the areas of food safety, supplements, and medical devices. There are links to other sources of information about nutrition and food. www.fda.gov

3. *Food and Nutrition Information Center.* This site offers a wide variety of information related to food and nutrition. http://fnic.nal.usda.gov

4. *National Institutes of Health: Office of Dietary Supplements.* This is the site of the International Bibliographic Database of Information on Dietary Supplements (IBDIDS), updated quarterly. http://dietary-supplements.info.nih.gov

5. *U.S. Department of Agriculture (USDA).* The USDA offers a full discussion of the USDA's *Dietary Guidelines for Americans.* www.usda.gov

6. *Linus Pauling Institute.* This is a key U.S. research center for studies on macro- and micronutrients, and it is a leader in antioxidant research. http://lpi.oregonstate.edu

# References

1. F. Bruni, "Eating Anxiety: Is Anyone to Blame?" *The Atlantic,* September 8, 2009, Available at www.theatlantic.com/food/archive/2009/09/eating-anxiety-is-anyone-to-blame/24615.

2. D. Negoianu and S. Goldfarb, "Just Add Water," *Journal of the American Society of Nephrology* 19, no. 6 (2008): 1041–43; E. Jéquier and F. Constant, "Water as an Essential Nutrient: The Physiological Basis of Hydration," *European Journal of Clinical Nutrition* 64, no. 2 (2010): 115–23.

3. Institute of Medicine of the National Academies, Food and Nutrition Board, *Dietary Reference Intakes for Water, Potassium, Sodium, Chloride, and Sulfate* (Washington, DC: The National Academies Press, 2004), Available at http://iom.edu/Reports/2004/Dietary-Reference-Intakes-Water-Potassium-Sodium-Chloride-and-Sulfate.aspx.

4. ACSM, "Exercise and Fluid Replacement," *Medicine and Science in Sports and Exercise* 39, no. 2 (2007): 377–90.

5. U.S. Department of Agriculture, Agricultural Research Service, Beltsville Human Nutrition Research Center, Food Surveys Research Group (Beltsville, MD) and U.S. Department of Health and Human Services, Centers for Disease Control and Prevention, National Center for Health Statistics (Hyattsville, MD), *What We Eat in America, NHANES 2007–2008 Data: Table 1. Nutrient Intakes from Food: Mean Amounts Consumed per Individual by Gender and Age, in the United States,* 2007–2008, Revised August 2010, Available at www.ars.usda.gov/Services/docs.htm?docid=18349.

6. Institute of Medicine of the National Academies, "Dietary, Functional, and Total Fiber," in *Dietary Reference Intakes for Energy, Carbohydrate, Fiber, Fat, Fatty Acids, Cholesterol, Protein, and Amino Acids* (Washington, DC: The National Academies Press, 2005), 339–421, Available at www.nap.edu/openbook.php?isbn=0309085373.

7. N. D. Riediger, R. A. Othman, M. Suh, and M. H. Moghadasian, "A Systemic Review of the Roles of n-3 Fatty Acids in Health and Disease," *Journal of the American Dietetic Association* 109 (2009): 668–79; B. McKevith, "Review: Nutritional Aspects of Oilseeds," *Nutrition Bulletin* 30, no. 1 (2005): 13–14.

8. P. M. Kris-Etherton, W. S. Harris, and L. J. Appel, "Fish Consumption, Fish Oil, Omega-3 Fatty Acids, and Cardiovascular Disease," *Circulation* 106, no. 21 (2002): 2747–57.

9. W. Harris et al., "Omega-6 Fatty Acids and Risk for Cardiovascular Disease," *Circulation* 119 (2009): 902–907.

10. P. McKeigue, "*Trans* Fatty Acids and Coronary Heart Disease: Weighing the Evidence against Hardened Fat," *Lancet* 345, no. 8945 (1995): 269–70; W. C. Willwett et al., "Intake of *Trans* Fatty Acids and Risk of Coronary Heart Disease among Women," *Lancet* 341, no. 8845 (1993): 581–85.

11. W. Willett and D. Mozaffarian, "*Trans* Fats in Cardiac and Diabetes Risk: An Overview," *Current Cardiovascular Risk Reports* 1, no. 1 (2007): 16–23; S. E. Chiuve et al., "Intake of Total *Trans,* *Trans*-18:1, and *Trans*-18:2 Fatty Acids and Risk of Sudden Cardiac Death in Women," *American Heart Journal* 158, no. 5 (2009): 761–67; D. Mozaffarian et al., "*Trans* Fatty Acids and Cardiovascular Disease," *New England Journal of Medicine* 354 (2006): 1601–13.

12. C. Scott-Thomas, "Californian Trans Fat Ban Takes Effect," FoodNavigator-USA.com, January 4, 2010, www.foodnavigator-usa.com/Legislation/Californian-trans-fat-ban-takes-effect.

13. F. Sacks et al., "Comparison of Weight-Loss Diets with Different Compositions of Fat, Protein, and Carbohydrates," *New England Journal of Medicine* 360, no. 9 (2009): 859–73; M. Hession et al., "Systematic Review of Randomized Controlled Trials of Low-carbohydrate vs. Low-fat/Low-calorie Diets in the Management of Obesity and its Comorbidities," *Obesity Reviews* 10, no. 1 (2008): 36–50.

14. G. Bjelakovic et al., "Mortality in Randomized Trials of Antioxidant Supplements for

Primary and Secondary Prevention: Systematic Review and Meta-Analysis," *Journal of the American Medical Association* 297, no. 8 (2007): 842–57; J. H. Kang and F. Grodstein, "Plasma Carotenoids and Tocopherols and Cognitive Function: A Prospective Study," *Neurobiological Aging* 29, no. 9 (2008): 1394–1403.

15. J. May, "Ascorbic Acid Transporters in Health and Disease," Paper presented at the Linus Pauling Diet and Optimum Health Annual Conference (Portland, OR: May 2007).

16. D. Albanes, "Vitamin Supplements and Cancer Prevention: Where Do Randomized Controlled Trials Stand?" *Journal of the National Cancer Institute* 101, no. 1 (2009): 2–4; J. Lin et al., "Vitamins C and E and Beta Carotene Supplementation and Cancer Risk: A Randomized Controlled Trial," *Journal of the National Cancer Institute* 101, no. 1 (2009): 14–23.

17. M. Levine, "Pharmacologic Ascorbate Concentrations Selectively Kill Cancer Cells: Ascorbic Acid as a Pro-Drug for Ascorbate Radical and/or $H_2O_2$ Delivery to Tissues," Paper presented at the Linus Pauling Diet and Optimum Health Annual Conference (Portland, OR: May 2007); J. May, "Ascorbic Acid Transporters in Health and Disease," 2007.

18. C. M. Hasler et al., "Position Statement of the American Dietetic Association: Functional Foods," *Journal of the American Dietetic Association* 104, no. 5 (2004): 814–18; Linus Pauling Institute, Oregon State University, "Micronutrient Information Center: Vitamin E," Updated January 2009, http://lpi.oregonstate.edu/infocenter/vitamins/vitaminE.

19. J. Chan and E. Giovannucci, "Vegetables, Fruits, Associated Micronutrients and Risk of Prostate Cancer," *Epidemiology Review* 23, no. 1 (2001): 82–86.

20. E. Giovannucci, "Tomato Products, Lycopene, and Prostate Cancer: A Review of the Epidemiological Literature," *Journal of Nutrition* 135, no. 8 (2005): 2030S–2031S.

21. A. Chait et al., "Increased Dietary Micronutrients Decrease Serum Homocysteine Concentrations in Patients at High Risk of Cardiovascular Disease," *American Journal of Clinical Nutrition* 70, no. 5 (1999): 881–87.

22. A. D. Dangour et al., "Plasma Homocysteine, but Not Folate or Vitamin B-12, Predicts Mortality in Older People in the United Kingdom," *Journal of Nutrition* 138, no. 6 (2008): 1121–28; J. Manson et al., "A Randomized Trial of Folic Acid and B-Vitamins in the Secondary Prevention of Cardiovascular Events in Women: Results from the Women's Antioxidant and Folic Acid Cardiovascular Study (WAFACS),"

*Circulation* 114, no. 22 (2006): 2424; J. Manson et al., "A Randomized Factorial Trial of Vitamins C, E, and Beta-Carotene in the Secondary Prevention of Cardiovascular Events in Women: Results from the Women's Antioxidant Cardiovascular Study (WACS)," *Circulation* 114, no. 22 (2006): 2424.

23. L. J. Appel and C. A. Anderson, "Compelling Evidence for Public Health Action to Reduce Salt Intake," *New England Journal of Medicine* 362, no. 7 (2010): 650–52.

24. C. Ayala et al., "Application of Lower Sodium Intake Recommendations to Adults—United States, 1999–2006," *Morbidity and Mortality Weekly (MMWR)* 58, no. 11 (2009): 281–83.

25. H. Cohen et al., "Sodium Intake and Mortality in the NHANES II Follow-Up Study," *American Journal of Medicine* 119, no. 275 (2006): e7–e14; J. Feng et al., "Salt Intake and Cardiovascular Mortality," *American Journal of Medicine* 120, no. 1 (2007): e5–e7; H. Harpannen and E. Mervaala, "Sodium Intake and Hypertension," *Progress in Cardiovascular Diseases* 49, no. 2 (2006): 59–75.

26. J. Ma, R. Johns, and R. Stafford, "Americans Are Not Meeting Current Calcium Recommendations," *American Journal of Clinical Nutrition* 85 (2007): 1361–66.

27. K. Tucker et al., "Colas, but Not Other Carbonated Beverages, Are Associated with Low Bone Mineral Density in Older Women: The Framingham Osteoporosis Study," *American Journal of Clinical Nutrition* 84 (2006): 936–42.

28. World Health Organization, "Miconutrient Deficiencies: Iron Deficiency Anemia," www.who.int/nutrition/topics/ida/en/index.html, Accessed April 2010.

29. C. Tsai et al., "Heme and Non-Heme Iron Consumption and Risk of Gallstone Disease in Men," *American Journal of Clinical Nutrition* 85 (2007): 518–22.

30. U.S. Department of Agriculture, Economic Research Service, "U.S. Per Capita Loss-Adjusted Food Availability: Total Calories," Updated April 2010, www.ers.usda.gov/Data/FoodConsumption/app/reports/displayCommodities.aspx?reportName=Total+Calories&id=36#startForm.

31. U.S. Department of Health and Human Services and U.S. Department of Agriculture, *Dietary Guidelines for Americans,* 2005 (Washington, DC: Government Printing Office, 2005).

32. U.S. Department of Agriculture, Center for Nutrition Policy and Promotion, "Development of the 2010 *Dietary Guidelines,*" Modified July 2010, www.cnpp.usda.gov/DietaryGuidelines.htm.

33. B. Black, "Health Library: Just How Much Food Is on That Plate? Understanding Portion Control," Last reviewed February

2009, EBSCO Publishing, www.ebscohost.com/healthLibrary.

34. "How Many Vegetarians Are There?" Vegetarian Resource Group, Press Release, May, 15, 2009, www.vrg.org/press/2009poll.htm.

35. "Vegetarian Times Study Shows 7.3 Million Americans Are Vegetarians," *Vegetarian Times,* Press Release, April 15, 2008, www.vegetariantimes.com/features/667.

36. American Dietetic Association, "Position of the American Dietetic Association: Vegetarian Diets," *Journal of the American Dietetic Association* 109, no. 7 (2009): 1266–82.

37. K. M. Fairfield and R. H. Fletcher, "Vitamins for Chronic Disease Prevention in Adults: Scientific Review," *Journal of the American Medical Association* 287, no. 23 (2001): 3116–26.

38. "NIH State-of-the-Science Conference Statement on Multivitamin/Mineral Supplements and Chronic Disease Prevention," *Annals of Internal Medicine* 145, no. 5 (2006): 364–71.

39. A. L. Rogovik, S. Vohra, and R. D. Goldman, "Safety Considerations and Potential Interactions of Vitamins: Should Vitamins Be Considered Drugs?" *Annals of Pharmacotherapy* 44, no. 2 (2010): 311–24.

40. U.S. Department of Agriculture, Economic Research Services, "Organic Agriculture: Organic Market Overview," 2009, www.ers.usda.gov/briefing/organic/demand.htm.

41. National Center for Infectious Diseases, Division of Bacterial and Mycotic Diseases, "Food-Borne Illnesses," 2005, www.cdc.gov/ncidod/dbmd/diseaseinfo/foodborneinfections_g.htm.

42. Centers for Disease Control and Prevention, "Preliminary FoodNet Data on the Incidence of Infection with Pathogens Transmitted Commonly through Food—10 States, 2008," *Morbidity and Mortality Weekly Report* 58, no. 13 (April 10, 2009): 333–37.

43. National Center for Infectious Diseases, Division of Bacterial and Mycotic Diseases, "Food-Borne Illnesses," 2005.

44. National Center for Infectious Diseases, Division of Bacterial and Mycotic Diseases, "E. Coli," Modified March 2010, www.cdc.gov/ecoli; Centers for Disease Control and Prevention, "Preliminary FoodNet Data on the Incidence of Infection with Pathogens Transmitted Commonly through Food—10 States, 2008," 2009.

45. Iowa State University, "Food Irradiation: What Is It?" *Iowa State University Extension Newsletter,* Revised August 2006, www.extension.iastate.edu/foodsafety/irradiation.

46. A. M. Branum and S. L. Lukacs, "Food Allergy among U.S. Children: Trends in Prevalence and Hospitalizations," *National*

*Center for Health Statistics Data Brief,* no 10. (Hyattsville, MD: 2008).

47. Food Allergy and Anaphylaxis Network, "Food Allergy Facts and Statistics," 2008 Available at www.foodallergy.org/section/helpful-information.

48. Food Allergy and Anaphylaxis Network, "Advocacy: FALCPA FAQ," 2010, www.foodallergy.org/page/falcpa-faq.

49. University of Chicago Celiac Disease Center, *Celiac Disease Facts and Figures* (Chicago, University of Chicago Celiac Disease Center: 2010), Available at www.celiacdisease.net/factsheets.

50. U.S. Department of Agriculture, Economic Research Service, "Adoption of Genetically Engineered Crops in the U.S.," Updated July 2009, www.ers.usda.gov/Data/BiotechCrops.

51. A. Coghlan, "Engineered Maize Toxicity Claims Roundly Rebuffed," *New Scientist* 2744 (January 22, 2010).

52. A. Bakshi, "Potential Adverse Health Effects of Genetically Modified Crops," *Journal of Toxicology and Environmental Health Part B: Critical Reviews* 6, no. 3 (2003): 211–25.

53. World Health Organization, "20 Questions on Genetically Modified Foods," Accessed April 2010, www.who.int/foodsafety/publications/biotech/20questions/en.

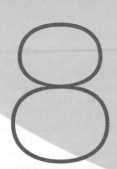

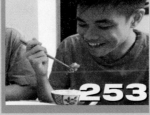
**253**
Do my genes have any effect on my weight?

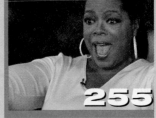
**255**
Why don't most diets succeed?

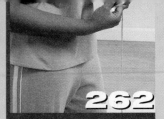
**262**
How can I tell if I am overweight or overfat?

# Reaching and Maintaining a Healthy Weight

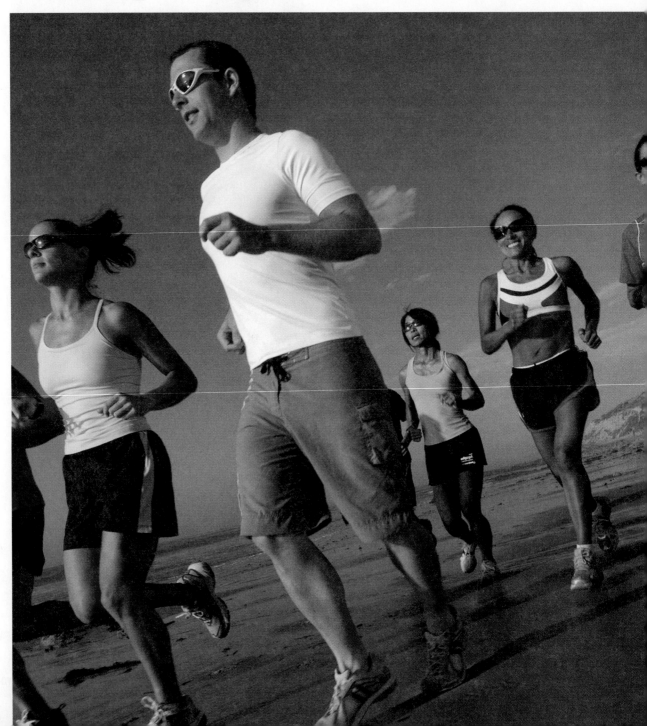

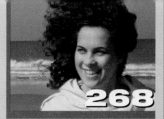

How important is exercise to weight management?

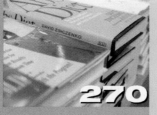

Is there a best way to lose weight?

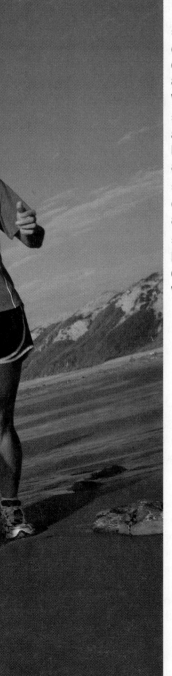

## Objectives

✳ Define *overweight* and *obesity,* describe the current epidemic of overweight/obesity in the United States, and understand risk factors associated with these weight problems.

✳ Describe factors that place people at risk for problems with obesity. Distinguish between factors that can and cannot be controlled.

✳ Discuss reliable options for determining percentage of body fat and a healthy weight for yourself.

✳ Discuss the roles of exercise, diet, lifestyle modification, fad diets, and other strategies of weight control, and which methods are most effective.

*The surge in obesity in this country is nothing short of a public health crisis that is threatening our children, our families, and our futures. In fact, the health consequences are so severe that medical experts have warned that our children could be on track to live shorter lives than their parents.*

—*First Lady Michelle Obama, Introduction of New Plan to Combat Overweight and Obesity, Press Conference, Alexandria, Virginia, January 28, 2010*

The United States currently has the dubious distinction of being among the fattest nations on Earth. Young and old, rich and poor, rural and urban, educated and uneducated Americans share one thing in common—they are fatter than virtually all previous generations. The word **obesogenic,** meaning "characterized by environments that promote increased food intake, nonhealthful foods and physical inactivity" has increasingly become an apt descriptor of our society. The U.S. maps in **Figure 8.1** on page 252 illustrate the increasing levels of obesity that have occurred in the past two decades. Indeed, the prevalence of obesity has tripled among children and doubled among adults in recent decades.[1] Research indicates that the rate of increase in obesity began to slow between 1999 and 2008 for many populations.[2] However, although the rate of increase has slowed, current rates are still extremely high, with more than 68 percent of U.S. adults overall (72.3% of men and 64.1% of women) considered to be *overweight* (having a body mass index [BMI] of 25.0–29.9) or *obese* (having a BMI of 30.0 or higher).[3]

This translates into over 72 million adults—32.2 percent of men and 35.5 percent of women—who are classified as obese. This has staggering implications for increased risks from heart disease, diabetes, and other health complications associated with obesity.[4] Research suggests that the prospect is even more bleak for certain populations within the United States. A recent study of American preschool children showed obesity rates of nearly 19 percent among children under age 4.[5] The rates are even more troubling when broken down by ethnicity: In the under-4 age group, nearly 32 percent of Native Americans/Native Alaskans, 22 percent of Hispanics, and nearly 21 percent of non-Hispanic blacks were found to be obese. Rates among non-Hispanic whites and Asian Americans were 16 percent and 13 percent, respectively. Other research points to higher obesity risks among adults of different ethnicities—most notably African American women, who have been found to have rates of overweight/obesity as high as 80 percent.[6] Similar racial disparities exist for both children and adolescents.[7]

Obesity is the second-to-top preventable cause of death in the United States, after smoking. Obesity and inactivity increase the risks from three of our leading killers: heart disease, cancer, and cerebrovascular ailments, including strokes.[8] In addition, some experts predict that the number of Americans diagnosed with diabetes, another major

> **obesogenic** Characterized by environments that promote increased food intake, nonhealthful foods, and physical inactivity; refers to conditions that lead people to become excessively fat.

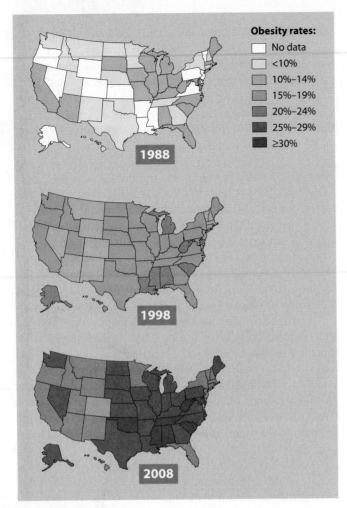

**Obesity rates:**
- No data
- <10%
- 10%–14%
- 15%–19%
- 20%–24%
- 25%–29%
- ≥30%

1988

1998

2008

FIGURE 8.1 **Obesity Trends among U.S. Adults, 1988, 1998, and 2008**
These maps indicate the percentage of population in each state that is considered obese, based on a body mass index of 30 or higher, or about 30 pounds overweight for a person 5 feet 4 inches tall.
**Source:** Centers for Disease Control and Prevention, "U.S. Obesity Trends: 1985–2008," 2009, www.cdc.gov/obesity/data/trends.html#State.

obesity-associated problem, will increase by 165 percent, from 15 million in 2005 to well over 30 million in 2030.[9] Other health risks associated with obesity include gallstones, sleep apnea, osteoarthritis, and several cancers. Figure 8.2 summarizes these and other potential health consequences of obesity.

Short- and long-term health consequences of obesity are not our only concern: The estimated annual cost of obesity in the United States exceeds $147 billion in medical expenses and lost productivity.[10] Overall, obese individuals average $1,500 more per year in medical costs, about 41 percent more than an average weight individual.[11] Of course, it is impossible to place a dollar value on a life lost prematurely due to diabetes, stroke, or heart attack or to assess the cost of the social isolation of and discrimination against overweight individuals. Of growing importance is the recognition that

obese individuals suffer significant disability during their lives, in terms of both mobility and activities of daily living.[12]

The United States is not alone. During the past 20 years, the world's population has grown progressively heavier. Globally, there are more than 1 billion overweight adults, at least 300 million of them obese.[13] Since 1980, rates have risen threefold or more in some areas of North America, the United Kingdom, eastern Europe, the Middle East, the Pacific Islands, Australasia, and China. Many developing regions of the world are demonstrating even faster rising rates of obesity.[14] The **Health in a Diverse World** box on page 254 looks at strategies to combat obesity around the globe, a problem sometimes referred to as *globesity*. This chapter will help you understand why we have such a weight problem in the United States and globally today and will provide you with simple strategies to help you manage your own weight. It will also help you understand contributors to obesity in various populations; what *underweight, normal weight, overweight,* and *obesity* really mean; and why managing your weight is essential to overall health and well-being.

# Factors Contributing to Overweight and Obesity

In a landmark 2005 report focused on our nation's health, the U.S. Surgeon General stated it quite plainly: "Overweight and obesity result from an energy imbalance. This means eating too many calories and not getting enough exercise."[15] However, since this report, many have criticized such a simplistic view of a multifaceted problem. If all it took was the willpower to eat less and exercise more, Americans would merely reevaluate their diets; cut calories; and exercise, exercise, exercise. Unfortunately, it's not that easy.

What factors predispose us to excess weight? Although diet and exercise are clearly two of the major contributors, other factors, including genetics and physiology, are also important. In addition, the environment you live in, eat in, exercise in, and play and work in has a significant influence on what you eat, how much you eat, and when you eat.[16]

## Genetic and Physiological Factors

Are some people born to be fat? Several factors appear to influence why one person becomes obese and another remains thin; genes, hormones, and other aspects of a person's physiology seem to interact with many of these factors.

**Body Type and Genes** Many scientists have explored the role of heredity in determining human body shape. In spite of decades of research, the exact role of genes in one's predisposition toward obesity remains in question. Children whose parents are obese also tend to be overweight. In fact, a family history of obesity has long been thought to increase one's chances of becoming obese based on countless observational studies. Early researchers found that adopted individuals

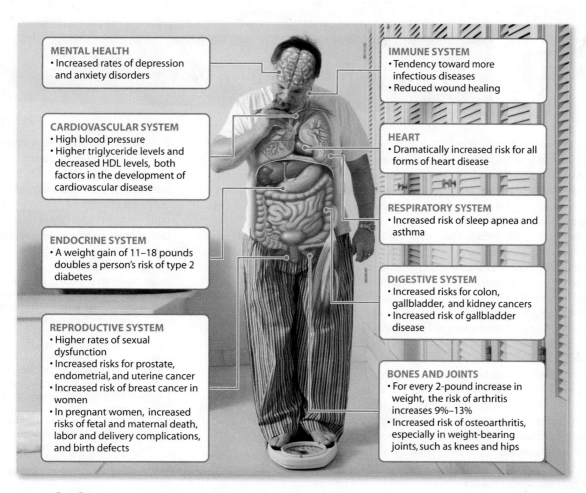

**MENTAL HEALTH**
• Increased rates of depression and anxiety disorders

**IMMUNE SYSTEM**
• Tendency toward more infectious diseases
• Reduced wound healing

**CARDIOVASCULAR SYSTEM**
• High blood pressure
• Higher triglyceride levels and decreased HDL levels, both factors in the development of cardiovascular disease

**HEART**
• Dramatically increased risk for all forms of heart disease

**ENDOCRINE SYSTEM**
• A weight gain of 11–18 pounds doubles a person's risk of type 2 diabetes

**RESPIRATORY SYSTEM**
• Increased risk of sleep apnea and asthma

**DIGESTIVE SYSTEM**
• Increased risks for colon, gallbladder, and kidney cancers
• Increased risk of gallbladder disease

**REPRODUCTIVE SYSTEM**
• Higher rates of sexual dysfunction
• Increased risks for prostate, endometrial, and uterine cancer
• Increased risk of breast cancer in women
• In pregnant women, increased risks of fetal and maternal death, labor and delivery complications, and birth defects

**BONES AND JOINTS**
• For every 2-pound increase in weight, the risk of arthritis increases 9%–13%
• Increased risk of osteoarthritis, especially in weight-bearing joints, such as knees and hips

**FIGURE 8.2 Potential Negative Health Effects of Overweight and Obesity**

tend to be similar in weight to their biological parents and that identical twins are twice as likely to weigh the same as are fraternal twins, even if they are raised separately.[17] Newer meta-analyses of twin studies indicate that although genetics seems to play a role in body composition, the environment plays a substantial role in one's obesity-prone future.[18]

Although the exact mechanism remains unknown, researchers continue to explore whether genes are important in setting metabolic rates, influencing how the body balances calories and energy, or causing us to crave certain foods.[19] Some researchers are now focusing on areas of the brain that may contribute to the desire to eat and satiety, as well as the role of hormones, genetic factors, and the environment.[20] In the past decades, more and more research has pointed to the fact that there are individual differences in the predisposition to

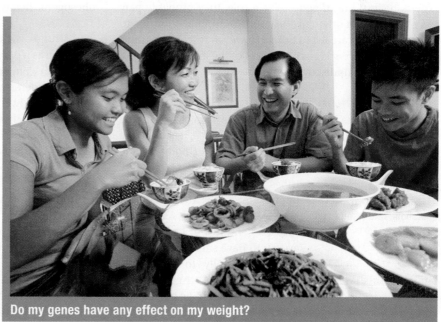

**Do my genes have any effect on my weight?**

Many factors help determine weight and body type, including heredity and genetic makeup, environment, and learned eating patterns, which are often connected to family habits.

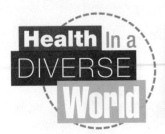

# Combating Globesity

The United States is not alone in being a "fat" country. During the past decade, epidemic rates of obesity and diabetes have emerged as global health problems. Today, more than 1.6 billion adults worldwide are overweight, and 400 million of them are obese. Add to that the 155 million children worldwide—20 million under age 5—who are overweight or obese and the vastness of the problem is clear. The World Health Organization (WHO) projects that by 2015 approximately 2.3 billion adults will be overweight and more than 700 million will be obese.

As the problems of obesity and overweight capture international attention, countries around the world are beginning to establish their own sets of policies and procedures to combat obesity. Consider these examples:

❋ In Great Britain, residents of some cities are being recruited to wear accelerometers that track movement and calories burned. Daily exercise is rewarded with coupons and even days off from work.
❋ In Germany, the equivalent of nearly $50 million is being spent on healthier school lunches and sports programs, as well as new, tougher nutritional standards.
❋ New Zealand has rules barring people who weigh too much from immigrating to the country, because such individuals would pose a potential burden to the health care system.
❋ In Japan, health officials check the waistlines of citizens over age 40, and those who are considered too fat undergo diet counseling. Failure to slim down can lead to fines.

What do you think? How do you feel about policies such as those listed above? Should governments try to regulate weight? How is the regulation of overweight and obesity similar to or different from that of other health-related behaviors such as smoking or drinking alcohol?

**Sources:** World Health Organization, *The World Health Report 2006: Working Together for Health* (Geneva: World Health Organization, 2006); P. Hossain, K. Bisher, and M. El Nahas, "Obesity and Diabetes in the Developing World—A Growing Challenge," *New England Journal of Medicine* 356, no. 3 (2007): 312–15; J. Levi et al., *F as in FAT: How Obesity Policies Are Failing in America 2009* (Washington, DC: Robert Wood Johnson Foundation and Trust for America's Health, 2009); P. Rowland, "Today: Too Fat for Surgery Tomorrow: Where Do We Draw the Line?" RedOrbit, 2006, www.redorbit.com/news/health/381336/today_too_fat_for_surgery_tomorrow_where_do_we_draw/index.html.

---

weight gain and that genetic variation, along with environmental influences, may increase risks of obesity. However, despite some positive indicators, a growing number of experts believe that if genes play a role, they probably play less of a role than originally believed. Those that continue to receive attention are listed below. However, researchers indicate that there are still many aspects of the genetic architecture that remain undiscovered.[21]

### Thrifty Gene Theory

One potential genetic basis for obesity that continues to gain traction comes from observational studies of certain Indian and African tribes. Labeled the "thrifty gene" theory, researchers note higher body fat and obesity levels in some of these tribes today than in the general population.[22] It is theorized that because their ancestors struggled through centuries of famine, they appear to have survived by adapting metabolically to periods of famine with slowed metabolism. Over time, ancestors may have passed on a genetic, hormonal, or metabolic predisposition toward fat storage that makes losing fat more difficult. If this thrifty gene hypothesis is true, certain people may be genetically programmed to burn fewer calories. Nevertheless, there is growing consensus that only 2 to 5 percent of child-

**basal metabolic rate (BMR)** The rate of energy expenditure by a body at complete rest in a neutral environment.
**resting metabolic rate (RMR)** The energy expenditure of the body under BMR conditions plus other daily sedentary activities.

hood obesity cases are caused by a defect that impairs function in a gene and that the common forms of childhood obesity seem to result from a predisposition that primarily favors obesogenic behaviors in an obesogenic environment.[23]

### Metabolic Rates

Although the number of calories you consume as a part of your daily energy supply is important in the weight-gain equation, several aspects of your metabolism also help determine whether you gain, maintain, or lose weight. Frankly, some of us seem to hang on to the calories we take in longer than others due to a variety of factors related to our metabolism. Each of us has an innate energy-burning capacity that hums along even when we are in the deepest levels of sleep. This **basal metabolic rate (BMR)** is the minimum rate at which the body uses energy when at complete rest in a neutrally temperate environment, activities such as digestion are not occurring, and the body is simply working to maintain basic vital functions. Technically, to measure BMR, a person would be awake, but all major stimuli, including stressors to the sympathetic nervous system, would be at rest. Usually, the best time to measure BMR is after 8 hours of sleep and after a 12-hour fast. A BMR for the average, healthy adult is usually between 1,200 and 1,800 calories per day.

A more commonly used, less restrictive, and more practical way of assessing your energy expenditure levels is the **resting metabolic rate (RMR).** Slightly higher than the BMR, the RMR includes the BMR plus any additional energy expended through daily sedentary activities such as food digestion, sitting, studying, or standing. The **exercise metabolic rate (EMR)** accounts for the remaining percentage of all daily calorie expenditures. It refers to the energy expenditure that occurs during physical activity. For most of us, these calories come from light daily activities, such as walking, climbing stairs, and mowing the lawn.

Your BMR (and RMR) can fluctuate considerably, with several factors influencing whether it slows down or speeds up. In general, the younger you are, the higher your BMR will be, partly because cells undergo rapid subdivision during periods of growth, an activity that consumes a good deal of energy. The BMR is highest during infancy, puberty, and pregnancy, when bodily changes are most rapid. After age 30, a person's BMR slows down by about 1 to 2 percent a year. Therefore, people over age 30 commonly find that they must work harder to burn off an extra helping of ice cream than they did in their teens. A slower BMR, coupled with less activity, shifting priorities (family and career become more important than fitness), and loss in muscle mass, contribute to the weight-gain of many middle-aged people.

Theories abound concerning the mechanisms that regulate metabolism and food intake. Some sources indicate that

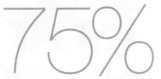

**75%** of dieters regain lost weight within 2 years of a major diet.

the hypothalamus (the part of the brain that regulates appetite) closely monitors levels of certain nutrients in the blood. When these levels fall, the brain signals us to eat. According to one theory, the monitoring system in obese people does not work properly, and the cues to eat are more frequent and intense than they are in people of normal weight.

Another theory is that thin people send more effective messages to the hypothalamus. This concept, called **adaptive thermogenesis,** states that thin people can consume large amounts of food without gaining weight because the appetite center of their brains speeds up metabolic activity to compensate for the increased consumption.

On the other side of the BMR equation is the **set point theory,** which suggests that our bodies fight to maintain our weight around a narrow range or at a set point. If we go on a drastic starvation diet or fast, our bodies slow down our BMR to conserve energy. Set point theory suggests that our own bodies may sabotage our weight loss efforts by holding on to calories as a form of protection. The good news is that set points can be changed; however, these changes may take time to be permanent. Healthy diet, steady weight loss, and exercise appear to be the best methods of sustaining weight loss.

**Yo-yo diets,** in which people repeatedly gain weight and then starve themselves to lose it all quickly, are doomed to fail. When dieters resume eating after their weight loss, their BMR is set lower, making it almost certain that they will regain the pounds they just lost. After repeated cycles of dieting and regaining weight, these people find it increasingly hard to lose weight and increasingly easy to regain it, so they become heavier and heavier.

**exercise metabolic rate (EMR)** The energy expenditure that occurs during exercise.

**adaptive thermogenesis** Theoretical mechanism by which the brain regulates metabolic activity according to caloric intake.

**set point theory** Theory that a form of internal thermostat controls our weight and fights to maintain this weight around a narrowly set range.

**yo-yo diets** Cycles in which people diet and regain weight.

**satiety** The feeling of fullness or satisfaction at the end of a meal.

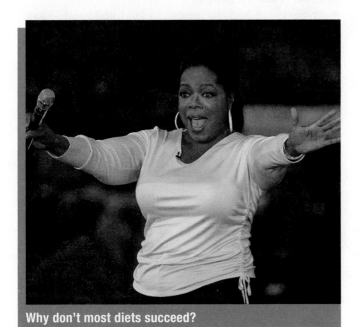

**Why don't most diets succeed?**

Just about any calorie-cutting diet can produce weight loss in the short term, often through water-weight loss. However, without improved nutrition and sustained exercise and activity, lost weight will return and the overall dieting process will have failed. Talk show host and media personality Oprah Winfrey has been candid about her struggles with this pattern of weight cycling, or yo-yo dieting. Such a pattern disrupts the body's metabolism and makes future weight loss more difficult and permanent changes even harder to maintain.

**Hormonal Influences: Ghrelin and Leptin** Obese people may be more likely than thin people to satisfy their appetite and eat for reasons other than nutrition.[24] Over the years, many people have attributed obesity to problems with their thyroid gland and resultant hormone imbalances that impeded their ability to burn calories. Today, most authorities agree that less than 2 percent of the obese population have a thyroid problem and can trace their weight problems to a metabolic or hormone imbalance.[25] However, researchers are increasingly convinced that hormones may have an impact on a person's ability to lose weight, control appetite, and sense fullness. In some instances, the problem with overconsumption may be related more to **satiety** than it is to appetite or hunger. People generally feel satiated, or full, when they have satisfied their nutritional needs and their stomach signals "no more."

One hormone that researchers suspect may influence satiety and play a role in our ability to keep weight off is *ghrelin,* sometimes referred to as "the hunger hormone," which is produced in the stomach. Researchers at the University of Washington studied a small group of obese people who had lost weight over a 6-month period.[26] They noted that ghrelin levels rose before every meal and fell drastically shortly afterward, suggesting that the hormone plays a role in appetite stimulation. Since that early research, ghrelin has been shown to be an important growth hormone that plays a key role in the regulation of appetite and food intake control, gastrointestinal motility, gastric acid secretion, endocrine and exocrine pancreatic secretions, glucose and lipid metabolism, and cardiovascular and immunologic processes.[27]

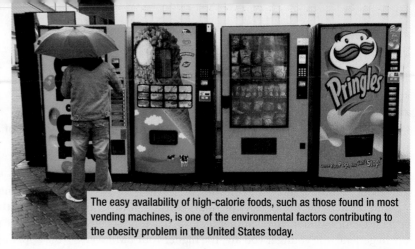

The easy availability of high-calorie foods, such as those found in most vending machines, is one of the environmental factors contributing to the obesity problem in the United States today.

Another hormone gaining increased attention and research is *leptin,* which has long been recognized as an appetite regulator in mammals. Leptin is produced by fat cells; its levels in the blood increase as fat tissue increases. Scientists believe leptin serves as a form of satiety signal, telling the brain when you are full.[28] When levels of leptin in the blood rise, appetite levels drop. Although obese people have adequate amounts of leptin and leptin receptors, the receptors do not seem to work properly. The exact reasons leptin levels seem to be high in obese individuals but appetite level is not suppressed remains a mystery. It may be simply that environmental cues are stronger than our hunger pangs. After all, how often do we eat due to time of day, the smells of food, or other cues, when we are not hungry at all?

**Fat Cells and Predisposition to Fatness** Some obese people may have excessive numbers of fat cells. An average-weight adult has approximately 25 to 35 billion fat cells, a moderately obese adult 60 to 100 billion, and an extremely obese adult as many as 200 billion.[29] This type of obesity, **hyperplasia,** usually appears in early childhood and perhaps, due to the mother's dietary habits, even prior to birth. The most critical periods for the development of hyperplasia seem to be the last 2 to 3 months of fetal development, the first year of life, and between the ages of 9 and 13. Central to this theory is the belief that the number of fat cells in a body does not increase appreciably during adulthood. However, the ability of each of these cells to swell (**hypertrophy**) and shrink does carry over into adulthood. People who add large numbers of fat cells to their bodies in childhood may be able to lose weight by decreasing the size of each cell in adulthood, but the total number of cells will remain the same. With the next calorie binge, the cells swell and sabotage weight-loss efforts. Weight gain may be tied to both the number of fat cells in the body and the capacity of individual cells to enlarge (see **Figure 8.3**).

**hyperplasia** A condition characterized by an excessive number of fat cells.
**hypertrophy** The act of swelling or increasing in size, as with cells.

# Environmental Factors

With all our twenty-first-century conveniences, environmental factors have come to play a large role in weight maintenance. Automobiles, remote controls, desk jobs, and long sessions on the Internet all cause us to sit more and move less, and this lack of physical activity causes a decrease in energy expenditure. Time our grandparents spent going for a walk after dinner we now spend watching our favorite television shows. Our culture also urges us to eat more. There is a long list of environmental factors believed to trigger our "eat" responses:[30]

- We are bombarded with advertising designed to increase energy intake—ads for high-calorie foods at a low price and marketing of super-sized portions (see the **Consumer Health** box at right).
- Prepackaged, high-fat meals; fast food; and sugar-laden soft drinks are all increasingly widespread. High-calorie drinks such as coffee lattes and energy drinks add to daily caloric intake.

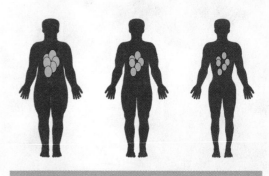

| | Before body weight reduction | Initial weight reduction | Second weight reduction |
|---|---|---|---|
| Body weight | 328 lb | 227 lb | 165 lb |
| Fat cell size | 0.9 µg/cell | 0.6 µg/cell | 0.2 µg/cell |
| Fat cell number | 75 billion | 75 billion | 75 billion |

FIGURE 8.3 **One Person at Various Stages of Weight Loss** Note that, according to the hyperplasia theory, the number of fat cells remains constant, but their size decreases when weight is lost.

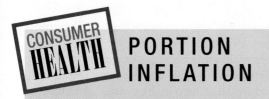
When you go out to your local restaurant, do you think your dinner looks the same as one your grandmother might have ordered 50 years ago? Would you be surprised to learn that today's serving portions are significantly larger than those of past decades? From burgers and fries to meat-and-potato or pasta meals, today's popular restaurant foods dwarf their earlier counterparts. For example, a 25-ounce prime-rib dinner served at one local steak chain contains nearly 3,000 calories and 150 grams of fat! That's half as many calories and more than three times the fat that most adults need in a whole day, and it's just the meat part of the meal.

What accounts for increased portion sizes? Restaurant owners might say that they are only giving customers what they want.

This may be true, but it's also true that bigger portions justify higher prices, which increase an owner's bottom line.

Many researchers believe that the main reason Americans are gaining weight is that people no longer recognize a normal serving size. The National Heart, Lung, and Blood Institute has developed a pair of "Portion Distortion" quizzes that show how today's portions compare with those of 20 years ago. Test yourself online at http://hp2010.nhlbihin .net/portion to see whether you can guess the differences between today's meals and those previously considered normal.

To make sure you're not overeating when you dine out, follow these strategies:

✳ Order the smallest size available. Focus on taste, not quantity. Get used to eating less and enjoy what you eat.
✳ Take your time, and let your fullness indicator have a chance to kick in while there is still time to quit.
✳ Dip your food in dressings, gravies, and sauces on the side rather than pouring these extra calories over the top.
✳ Order an appetizer as your main meal.
✳ Split your main entrée with a friend, and order a side salad for each of you. Alternatively, eat only half your dinner and take the rest home for another day.

✳ Avoid buffets and all-you-can-eat establishments.
✳ Skip dessert or split one among several people.

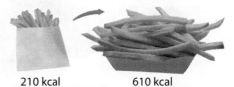

**Today's bloated portions.**

**Source:** Data are from National Heart, Lung, and Blood Institute, "Portion Distortion," Accessed August 2009, http://hp2010.nhlbihin.net/portion.

• The number of working women has grown, leading to greater consumption of restaurant meals, fast foods, and convenience foods. As society eats out more, higher-calorie, high-fat foods become the norm, and increased weight is the result.
• Bottle-feeding infants may increase energy intake relative to breast-feeding.
• Misleading food labels confuse consumers about portion and serving sizes.
• The opportunities and locations for eating have increased. Fast-food restaurants, cafes, vending machines, and quick-stop markets are everywhere, offering easy access to high-calorie foods and beverages. Meals, mini-meals, and snacks have become common diversions for many of us.
• Larger dishes, cups, and serving utensils mask serving sizes and lead to increased calorie and fat intake.

## what do you think?

In addition to those listed, can you think of other factors in your particular environment that might contribute to obesity? ● What actions could you take to reduce your risk for each of these factors?

**Early Sabotage: A Youthful Start on Obesity** Children have always loved junk food, from sugary sweets and beverages to fat-laden chips and salty French fries. However, today's youth tend to eat larger portions and, from their earliest years, exercise less than any previous generation.[31] Video games, television, cell phones, and the Internet often keep them exercising their fingers more than any other part of their bodies, and children are subject to the same environmental, social, and cultural factors that influence obesity in their elders.

In addition, youth are at risk because of factors that are only beginning to be understood. Epidemiological studies suggest that maternal undernutrition, obesity, and diabetes during gestation and lactation are strong predictors of obesity in children.[32] Research also shows that race and ethnicity seem to be intricately interwoven with environmental factors in increasing risks to young people by as much as three times in selected populations, most notably among Native Americans/Alaska Natives, Hispanics, and African Americans.[33]

Obese kids not only suffer from the potential physical problems of obesity, they also often face weight-related

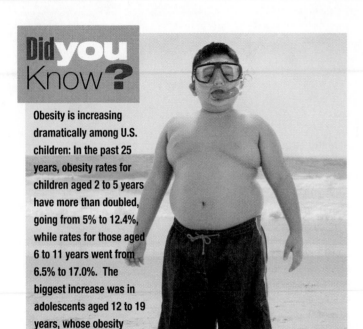
affluent people to exercise.[36] New research suggests that the more educated you are, the lower your body mass index and overall obesity profile are likely to be. In a study of comparative international data, highly educated men and, in particular, highly educated women in the United States have a lower average BMI than their less-educated counterparts. Likewise, higher educational levels are directly related to less overweight and obesity among European men, and even more so, among women. Educational inequalities in overweight and obesity were largest among Mediterranean women.[37]

## Lifestyle Factors

Athough heredity, metabolism, and environment all have an impact on weight management, the increasingly high rate of overweight and obesity in the past decades is largely due to the way we live our lives. In general, Americans are eating more and moving less than ever before, and becoming over-fat as a result. Weight management can be much harder when it feels like a chore (the **Skills for Behavior Change** box below offers some ideas for making exercising and healthy eating more fun).

Of all the factors affecting obesity, perhaps the most critical is the relationship between activity level and calorie intake. Obesity rates are rising, but aren't more people exercising than ever before? Although the many advertisements

stigma and hateful comments about their size from their peers (see the **Health Headlines** box at right).[34] As a result, overweight and obese children may suffer lasting blows to their self-esteem, feelings of social acceptance, and emotional health, affecting personal identity and fostering mistrust and fear of others.

## Psychosocial and Economic Factors

The relationship of weight problems to deeply rooted emotional insecurities, needs, and wants remains uncertain. Food often is used as a reward for good behavior in childhood. As adults face unemployment, broken relationships, financial uncertainty, fears about health, and other problems, the bright spot in the day is often "what's on the table for dinner" or "we're going to that restaurant tonight." Again, the research underlying this theory is controversial. What is certain is that eating tends to be a focal point of people's lives; it has become a social ritual associated with companionship, celebration, and enjoyment. For many people, the psychosocial aspect of the eating experience is a major obstacle to successful weight control.

Socioeconomic factors can provide obstacles or aids to weight control, as well. When economic times are tough, people tend to eat more inexpensive, high-calorie processed foods.[35] Unsafe neighborhoods and poor infrastructure (lack of recreational areas, for example) make it difficult for less-

**Skills for Behavior Change**

### Finding the Fun in Healthy Eating and Exercise

Managing your weight—eating right and exercising—may not be that exciting an idea to you. However, with a little creativity, you can make it a fun, positive part of your life that you look forward to. Here are some tips for doing that:

✳ **Cook and eat with friends.** You can share the responsibility for making the meal while you spend time with people you like.
✳ **Experiment with new foods**—variety is the spice of life!
✳ **Invite an international student over for dinner and cook together.**
✳ **Vary your exercise routine**—either change the exercise itself or change your location. Even small changes can breathe life into an old routine.
✳ **Try something new:** Join a team for the social aspects in addition to exercise, or decide to run a long foot race for the challenge, or learn how to skateboard for fun.

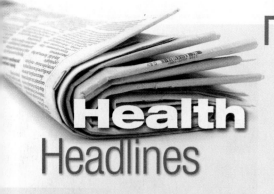

# OBESITY STIGMA GROWS ALONG WITH OUR WAISTLINES

As the obesity epidemic in the United States has gained media attention in recent years, there is also a growing trend to bring up obesity as a cause of other ills of our society. For example, high rates of obesity are considered a major contributor to rising health care costs for everyone, and, according to a summary of recent transportation research by Jacobson and King, "obese people contribute more than their thinner compatriots to food scarcity and global warming, given that they eat more and require more transportation energy (over 1 billion extra gallons/year to carry their extra weight) to move themselves around." When such reports are picked up by the national media, the findings get simplified and the headlines become more sensationalist and accusatory. The tacit message is that fat people cause problems for the rest of us.

Although there may be truth behind the claims and value in their ability to increase public health awareness, in the end, shaming people who are overweight or obese, making fun of them, or discriminating against them in work and social life isn't going to motivate them to be thin. In fact, embarrassment and shame may be the very things that keep some overweight and obese people out of the gym, or drive them to eat excessively to numb their feelings. A recent study of college students showed that having more experience with weight stigma and vicious or subtle attacks on their weight actually makes people less likely to exercise.

*Weight stigma* or *bias* refers to negative weight-related attitudes toward an overweight or obese individual. It can be subtle or overt with examples ranging from negative stereotyping, social rejection

and prejudice, to physical aggression. According to the experts, weight bias exists because of pervasive societal beliefs that shame will motivate people to diet and lose weight. Our culture also sanctions the overt expression of weight bias by placing value on thinness and perpetuating societal messages that obesity is the mark of a defective person, blaming the victim rather than addressing environmental conditions that lead to obesity.

An extension of weight bias in our society is *weight discrimination,* or the unequal, unfair treatment of people because of weight. Weight discrimination might mean being qualified for a job but not being hired because of your weight, or receiving unequal treatment in health care, being denied scholarships or awards due to appearance, or not being allowed to get a loan or rent a particular car or home. Documented weight discrimination is on the rise in the United States, with a 66 percent increase noted between 1995 and 2006, affecting up to 12 percent of the population.

Weight bias and discrimination can have a major impact on a person's mental, social, intellectual, economic, and physical health. Common consequences include:

✳ Depression, anxiety, low self-esteem, poor body image, and suicidal acts and thoughts
✳ Social rejection, poor quality of relationships, and lower socioeconomic status
✳ Binge eating and unhealthy weight-control practices, or coping with stigma by eating more, refusing to diet, and avoiding physical activity
✳ Avoidance of friends and family members due to embarrassment or problems finding suitable clothing
✳ Fewer promotions, lower salaries, more frequent firings or suspensions, and difficulty finding jobs
✳ Difficulty being accepted into academic programs and worse academic outcomes
✳ Lack of adequate health care due to doctors spending less time with and doing fewer interventions on overweight patients, and doctor reluctance to perform preventive health screenings
✳ Reluctance to visit the doctor and get necessary preventive health care services

Currently, the United States has no federal laws that protect overweight or obese individuals from discrimination and,

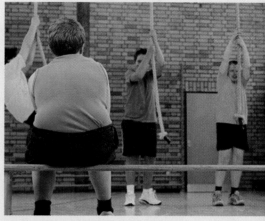

Stigmatization against people who are obese can contribute to depression and low self-esteem.

as of this writing, only one state, Michigan, has state laws that prohibit discrimination against overweight and obese individuals. There are many people who argue that making weight discrimination illegal would lead to countless irresolvable court cases. Others argue that weight discrimination laws are just as necessary as disability protection and anti-hate laws, and would have an equally positive impact on society.

What do you think? Should there be laws against obesity stigma and discrimination? Do you think treating obese people differently—by requiring them to pay higher health care premiums or purchase a second airline seat, or excluding them from certain jobs and social settings—is ever justified? Besides enacting laws, what do you think can be done to address weight stigma and discrimination in our society?

**Sources:** S. Jacobson and D. King, "Measuring the Potential for Automobile Fuel Savings in the U.S.: The Impact of Obesity," *Transportation Research Part D: Transport and the Environment* 14, no. 1 (2009): 6–13; R. Puhl and C. Heuer, "Obesity Stigma: Important Considerations for Public Health," *American Journal of Public Health* 100, no. 6 (2010): 1019–28; L. Vartanian and J. Shaprow, "Effects of Weight Stigma on Exercise Motivation and Behavior: A Preliminary Investigation among College-Aged Females," *Journal of Health Psychology* 13, no. 1 (2008): 131–38; R. Puhl, Obesity Action Coalition, "Weight Discrimination: A Socially Acceptable Injustice," 2010, www.obesityaction.org/magazine/oacnews12/obesityanddiscrimination.php; R. Puhl and C. Heuer, "The Stigma of Obesity: A Review and Update," *Obesity* 17, no. 5 (2009): 941–64; T. Andreyeva, R. Puhl, and K. Brownell, "Changes in Perceived Weight Discrimination among Americans, 1995–1996 through 2004–2006," *Obesity* 16, no. 5 (2008): 1129–34; Rudd Center for Food Policy and Obesity, Yale University, *Rudd Report: Weight Bias: A Social Justice Issue: Policy Brief* (New Haven, CT: Rudd Center for Food Policy and Obesity, 2009), Available at www.yaleruddcenter.org/briefs.aspx.

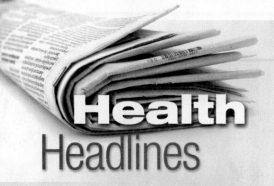

# Health Headlines

## IS SITTING MAKING YOU FAT?

While reading this chapter, watching TV, eating meals, driving or riding to and from campus, sitting in the classroom, working at our computers, visiting with friends—it always seems as though we're looking for the best chair or most comfortable spot to sit . . . sit . . . and sit some more. But why not? As long as you exercise regularly there shouldn't be any harm in sitting the rest of the time, right? Not so fast, say the experts.

Rather than focusing only on how much formal exercise we get in each day, health and fitness experts have begun to focus on the flip side of how much time we spend sitting. How many of us do our exercise routines and then "veg" or go into "slo-mo" mode for much of the rest of day? It's that time spent sitting in classes, watching TV, eating meals, studying, surfing the Internet, playing computer games, or chatting on Facebook that ultimately sabotages our best efforts at weight control. The bottom line is, if the body isn't moving, it's not burning very many calories.

The term *sitting behavior* has surfaced as an apt way for experts to explain the negative effects of our seeming preoccu-

pation with the chairs of our lives. New research indicates that there is a dose-response association between sitting time and mortality from all causes and from cardiovascular disease, independent of leisure-time activity—that is, the more time you spend sitting, the worse your health is likely to be, regardless of whether you exercise or not. Because muscle activity burns energy, passive sitting is one of the worst things you can do if you are trying to burn calories. If you stood up while reading this chapter, the large and small muscle groups in your legs would be constantly moving, trying to hold your balance and keep you from falling over onto the floor. That simple action would burn more calories. If you also got up to get a glass of water at a fountain farther down the hall, clenched your fists, flexed your muscles, twisted your torso or swung your arms, or ran up or downstairs to go to the bathroom, you'd burn even more calories for each small muscle group that is awakened from its little nap while you were sitting.

Recent research suggests that we should make an effort to balance light-intensity activities and sedentary behaviors throughout our days. What if instead of spending all of our effort on getting in 30 minutes of exercise each day, we focused more on the little things we can do to burn calories 24/7? What if workplaces were designed to get people up and moving and using larger muscle groups at various intervals throughout the day? How about standing to use your computer rather than sitting, or riding a stationary bike at a comfortable speed while watching TV or reading your textbooks? What if you rocked in a chair

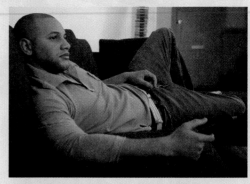

Americans today spend 15 or more hours each day sitting—and many of us have the weight problems to prove it!

while watching TV, or didn't let yourself sit down anywhere other than in classes for the first 5 or 6 hours of the day? Try it! These little extra bouts of movement may make a big difference in daily calories burned, weight management, and overall health.

**Sources:** D. Dunstan et al., "Television Viewing Time and Mortality: The Australian Diabetes, Obesity and Lifestyle Study (AusDiab)," *Circulation* 121 (2010): 384–91; G. Duntun et al., "Joint Associations of Physical Activity and Sedentary Behaviors with Body Mass Index: Results from a Time Use Survey of U.S. Adults," *International Journal of Obesity* 33 (2010): 1427–36; N. Owen, A. Bauman, and W. Brown, "Too Much Sitting: A Novel and Important Predictor of Chronic Disease Risk?" *British Journal of Sports Medicine* 43, no. 2 (2009): 81–83; S. A. Anderssen et al., "Changes in Physical Activity Behavior and the Development of Body Mass Index during the Last 30 Years in Norway," *Scandinavian Journal of Medicine and Science in Sports* 18, no. 3 (2008): 309–17; P. Katzmarzyk, P. T. Church, C. L. Craig, and C. Bouchard, "Sitting Time and Mortality from All Causes, Cardiovascular Diseases, and Cancer," *Medicine and Science in Sports and Exercise* 41, no. 5 (2009): 998–1005; 2655–67.

for sports equipment and the popularity of athletes may give the impression that Americans love a good workout, the facts are not so clear. One big problem in determining activity levels is that data are largely based on self-report and people also overestimate their daily exercise level and intensity. Complicating this is a hodgepodge of terminology for determining activity levels. It is difficult to determine which measures of fitness were actually used and how indicative of overall health these may ultimately be. Data from the National Health Interview Survey show that 4 in 10 adults in the United States *never* engage in any exercise, sports, or physically active hobbies in their leisure time.[38] Based on the most recent data, using leisure-time activity as a measure, only 35 percent of adults aged 18 and over reported regular activity.[39] See the **Health Headlines** box above for an exploration of the idea of "sitting behavior" and its impact on health.

Do you know people who seemingly can eat whatever they want without gaining weight? With few exceptions, if you were to follow them around for a typical day and monitor the level and intensity of their activity, you would discover the reason. Even if their schedule does not include jogging or intense exercise, it probably includes a high level of activity. Walking up a flight of stairs rather than taking the elevator, speeding up the pace while mowing the lawn, getting up to change the TV channel rather than using the remote, and doing housework all burn extra calories.

# Assessing Body Weight and Body Composition

What weight is healthiest for you? Everyone has his or her own ideal weight, based on individual variables such as body structure, height, and fat distribution. Traditionally, experts used measurement techniques such as height–weight charts to determine whether an individual fell into the ideal weight, overweight, or obese category. However, these charts can be misleading because they don't take body composition—that is, a person's ratio of fat to lean muscle—or fat distribution into account. In fact, weight can be a deceptive indicator. Many extremely muscular athletes would be considered overweight based on traditional height–weight charts, whereas many young women might think their weight is normal based on charts, only to be shocked to discover that 35 to 40 percent of their weight is body fat! More accurate measures of evaluating healthy weight and disease risk focus on a person's percentage of body fat, and how that fat is distributed in his or her body.

Many people worry about becoming fat, but some fat is essential for healthy body functioning. Fat regulates body temperature, cushions and insulates organs and tissues, and is the

body's main source of stored energy. Body fat is composed of two types: essential fat and storage fat. *Essential fat* is that fat necessary for maintenance of life and reproductive functions. *Storage fat,* the nonessential fat that many of us try to shed, makes up the remainder of our fat reserves.

## Overweight and Obesity

In general, **overweight** is increased body weight due to excess fat that exceeds healthy recommendations, whereas **obesity** refers to body weight that greatly exceeds health recommendations. Traditionally, *overweight* was defined as being 1 to 19 percent above one's ideal weight, based on a standard height–weight chart, and *obesity* was defined as being 20 percent or more above one's ideal weight. **Morbidly obese** people are 100 percent or more above their ideal weight. Experts now usually define *overweight* and *obesity* in terms of BMI, a measure discussed below, or percentage of body fat, as determined by some of the methods we'll discuss shortly. Although opinion varies somewhat, most experts agree that men's bodies should contain between 8 and 20 percent total body fat, and women should be within the range of 20 to 30 percent. At various ages and stages of life, these ranges also vary, but generally, men who exceed 22 percent body fat and women who exceed 35 percent are considered overweight (see Table 8.1).

## Underweight

There are percentages of body fat below which a person is considered **underweight,** and health is compromised. In men, this lower limit is approximately 3 to 7 percent of total body weight and in women it is approximately 8 to 15 percent. Extremely low body fat can cause a host of problems including hair loss, visual disturbances, skin problems, a tendency

**overweight** Having a body weight more than 10 percent above healthy recommended levels; in an adult, having a BMI of 25 to 29.
**obesity** A body weight more than 20 percent above healthy recommended levels; in an adult, a BMI of 30 or more.
**morbidly obese** Having a body weight 100 percent or more above healthy recommended levels; in an adult, having a BMI of 40 or more.
**underweight** Having a body weight more than 10 percent below healthy recommended levels; in an adult, having a BMI below 18.5.

**TABLE 8.1** | **Body Fat Percentage Recommendations for Men and Women***

|  | Recommended | Overweight | Obese |
|---|---|---|---|
| **Men** | ≤34 years old: 8%–22% | ≤34 years old: 23%–25% | ≤34 years old: 25% |
|  | >35 years old: 10%–25% | >35 years old: 26%–28% | >35 years old: 28% |
| **Women** | ≤34 years old: 20%–35% | ≤34 years old: 36%–38% | ≤34 years old: 38% |
|  | 35–55 years old: 23%–38% | >35 years old: 39%–40% | >35 years old: 40% |
|  | >55 years old: 25%–38% |  |  |

*Assumes nonathletes. For athletes, recommended body fat is 5 to 15 percent for men and 12 to 22 percent for women. Please note that there are no agreed-upon national standards for recommended body fat percentage.

**Source:** American College of Sports Medicine, *ACSM's Resource Manual for Guidelines for Exercise Testing and Prescription,* 5th ed. (Baltimore: Lippincott Williams & Wilkins, 2006). Copyright © 2006 ACSM. Reprinted by permission of Wolters/Kluwer http://lww.com.

to fracture bones easily, digestive system disturbances, heart irregularities, gastrointestinal problems, difficulties in maintaining body temperature, and amenorrhea (in women). Problems with being underweight and having a percentage of body fat that is too low are on the increase today, particularly as our culture's obsession with appearance continues. See Focus On: Enhancing Your Body Image beginning on page 280 for an in-depth discussion of eating disorders and body image issues.

## Body Mass Index (BMI)

Although people have a general sense that BMI is an indicator of how "fat" a person is, most do not really know what it is assessing. **Body mass index (BMI)** is a description of body weight relative to height, numbers that are highly correlated with your total body fat. Body mass index is not gender specific, and it does not directly measure percentage of body fat, but it provides a more accurate measure of overweight and obesity than weight alone.[40] Find your BMI in inches and pounds in Figure 8.4, or calculate your BMI now by dividing your weight in kilograms by height in meters squared. The mathematical formula is

$$BMI = weight (kg)/height \ squared \ (m^2)$$

A BMI calculator is also available at the National Heart, Lung, and Blood Institute's website at http://nhlbisupport.com/bmi/bmicalc.htm.

Desirable BMI levels may vary with age and by sex; however, most BMI tables for adults do not account for such variables. *Healthy weights* are defined as those with BMIs of 18.5 to 25, the range of lowest statistical health risk.[41] A BMI of 25 to 29.9 indicates overweight and potentially significant health risks. A BMI of 30 or above is classified as obese, whereas a BMI of 40 or higher is morbidly obese.[42] Nearly 3 percent of obese men and almost 7 percent of obese women are morbidly obese.[43]

Although useful, BMI levels don't account for the fact that muscle weighs more than fat and a well-muscled person could weigh enough to be classified as obese according to his or her BMI, nor are bone mass and water weight considered in BMI calculations. For people who are under 5 feet tall, are highly muscled, or are older and have little muscle mass, BMI levels can be inaccurate. More precise methods of determining body fat, described below, should be used for these individuals.

**body mass index (BMI)** A number calculated from a person's weight and height that is used to assess risk for possible present or future health problems.

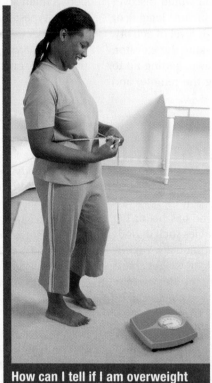

**How can I tell if I am overweight or overfat?**

Observing the way you look and how your clothes fit can give you a general idea of whether you weigh more or less than in the past. But for evaluating your weight and body fat levels in terms of potential health risks, it's best to use more scientific measures, such as BMI, waist circumference, waist-to-hip ratio, or a technician-administered body composition test.

# 34%

of American adults have a BMI of 30 or higher, and are therefore classified as obese.

**Youth and BMI** Although the labels *obese* and *morbidly obese* have been used for years for adults, there is growing concern about the long-term consequences of pinning these potentially stigmatizing labels on children.[44] BMI ranges above a normal weight for children and teens are often labeled differently, as "at risk of overweight" and "overweight," to avoid the sense of shame such words may cause. In addition, BMI ranges for children and teens are defined so that they take into account normal differences in body fat between boys and girls and the differences in body fat that occur at various ages. After BMI is calculated, the BMI number is plotted on the Centers for Disease Control and Prevention (CDC) BMI-for-age growth charts (for either girls or boys) to obtain a percentile ranking. Percentiles are the most commonly used indicator to assess the size and growth patterns of individual children in the United States. The percentile indicates the relative position of the child's BMI number among children of the same sex and age.[45]

# Waist Circumference and Ratio Measurements

Knowing where your fat is carried may be more important than knowing how much you carry. Men and postmenopausal women tend to store fat in the upper regions of the body, particularly in the abdominal area. Premenopausal women usually store fat in the lower regions of their bodies, particularly the hips, buttocks, and thighs. Waist circumference measurement is increasingly recognized as a useful tool in assessing abdominal fat, which is considered more threatening to health than fat in other regions of the body. In particular, as waist circumference increases, there is a greater risk for diabetes, cardiovascular disease, and stroke. A waistline greater than 40 inches (102 centimeters) in men and 35 inches (88 centimeters) in women may be particularly indicative of

| BMI | 19 | 20 | 21 | 22 | 23 | 24 | 25 | 26 | 27 | 28 | 29 | 30 | 31 | 32 | 33 | 34 | 35 | 36 | 37 | 38 | 39 | 40 | 41 | 42 |
|---|---|---|---|---|---|---|---|---|---|---|---|---|---|---|---|---|---|---|---|---|---|---|---|---|
| **Height** | | | | | | | **Weight in pounds** | | | | | | | | | | | | | | | | | |
| 4'10" | 91 | 96 | 100 | 105 | 110 | 115 | 119 | 124 | 129 | 134 | 138 | 143 | 148 | 153 | 158 | 162 | 167 | 172 | 177 | 181 | 186 | 191 | 196 | 201 |
| 4'11" | 94 | 99 | 104 | 109 | 114 | 119 | 124 | 128 | 133 | 138 | 143 | 148 | 153 | 158 | 163 | 168 | 173 | 178 | 183 | 188 | 193 | 198 | 203 | 208 |
| 5' | 97 | 102 | 107 | 112 | 118 | 123 | 128 | 133 | 138 | 143 | 148 | 153 | 158 | 163 | 168 | 174 | 179 | 184 | 189 | 194 | 199 | 204 | 209 | 215 |
| 5'1" | 100 | 106 | 111 | 116 | 122 | 127 | 132 | 137 | 143 | 148 | 153 | 158 | 164 | 169 | 174 | 180 | 185 | 190 | 195 | 201 | 206 | 211 | 217 | 222 |
| 5'2" | 104 | 109 | 115 | 120 | 126 | 131 | 136 | 142 | 147 | 153 | 158 | 164 | 169 | 175 | 180 | 186 | 191 | 196 | 202 | 207 | 213 | 218 | 224 | 229 |
| 5'3" | 107 | 113 | 118 | 124 | 130 | 135 | 141 | 146 | 152 | 158 | 163 | 169 | 175 | 180 | 186 | 191 | 197 | 203 | 208 | 214 | 220 | 225 | 231 | 237 |
| 5'4" | 110 | 116 | 122 | 128 | 134 | 140 | 145 | 151 | 157 | 163 | 169 | 175 | 180 | 186 | 192 | 197 | 204 | 209 | 215 | 221 | 227 | 232 | 238 | 244 |
| 5'5" | 114 | 120 | 126 | 132 | 138 | 144 | 150 | 156 | 162 | 168 | 174 | 180 | 186 | 192 | 198 | 204 | 210 | 216 | 222 | 228 | 234 | 240 | 246 | 252 |
| 5'6" | 118 | 124 | 130 | 136 | 142 | 148 | 155 | 161 | 167 | 173 | 179 | 186 | 192 | 198 | 204 | 210 | 216 | 223 | 229 | 235 | 241 | 247 | 253 | 260 |
| 5'7" | 121 | 127 | 134 | 140 | 146 | 153 | 159 | 166 | 172 | 178 | 185 | 191 | 198 | 204 | 211 | 217 | 223 | 230 | 236 | 242 | 249 | 255 | 261 | 268 |
| 5'8" | 125 | 131 | 138 | 144 | 151 | 158 | 164 | 171 | 177 | 184 | 190 | 197 | 204 | 210 | 216 | 223 | 230 | 236 | 243 | 249 | 256 | 262 | 269 | 276 |
| 5'9" | 128 | 135 | 142 | 149 | 155 | 162 | 169 | 176 | 182 | 189 | 196 | 203 | 210 | 216 | 223 | 230 | 236 | 243 | 250 | 257 | 263 | 270 | 277 | 284 |
| 5'10" | 132 | 139 | 146 | 153 | 160 | 167 | 174 | 181 | 188 | 195 | 202 | 209 | 216 | 222 | 229 | 236 | 243 | 250 | 257 | 264 | 271 | 278 | 285 | 292 |
| 5'11" | 136 | 143 | 150 | 157 | 165 | 172 | 179 | 186 | 193 | 200 | 208 | 215 | 222 | 229 | 236 | 243 | 250 | 257 | 265 | 272 | 279 | 286 | 293 | 301 |
| 6' | 140 | 147 | 154 | 162 | 169 | 177 | 184 | 191 | 199 | 206 | 213 | 221 | 228 | 235 | 242 | 250 | 258 | 265 | 272 | 279 | 287 | 294 | 302 | 309 |
| 6'1" | 144 | 151 | 159 | 166 | 174 | 182 | 189 | 197 | 204 | 212 | 219 | 227 | 235 | 242 | 250 | 257 | 265 | 275 | 280 | 288 | 295 | 302 | 310 | 318 |
| 6'2" | 148 | 155 | 163 | 171 | 179 | 186 | 194 | 202 | 210 | 218 | 225 | 233 | 241 | 249 | 256 | 264 | 272 | 280 | 287 | 295 | 303 | 311 | 319 | 326 |
| 6'3" | 152 | 160 | 168 | 176 | 184 | 193 | 200 | 208 | 216 | 224 | 232 | 240 | 248 | 256 | 264 | 272 | 279 | 287 | 295 | 303 | 311 | 319 | 327 | 335 |
| 6'4" | 156 | 164 | 172 | 180 | 189 | 197 | 205 | 213 | 221 | 230 | 238 | 246 | 254 | 263 | 271 | 279 | 287 | 295 | 304 | 312 | 320 | 328 | 336 | 344 |

|  Healthy weight<br>BMI 18.5–24.9  |  Overweight<br>BMI 25–29.9  |  Obese<br>BMI 30–39.9  |  Morbidly obese<br>BMI ≥40  |
|---|---|---|---|

FIGURE 8.4 **Body Mass Index (BMI)**

Locate your height, read across to find your weight, then read up to determine your BMI. Any weight less than those listed for a given height would yield a BMI of less than 18.5, classified as underweight.

**Source:** National Institutes of Health/National Heart, Lung, and Blood Institute (NHLBI). *Evidence Report of Clinical Guidelines on the Identification, Evaluation, and Treatment of Overweight and Obesity in Adults*, 1998, www.nhlbi.nih.gov/guidelines/obesity/ob_gdlns.htm.

greater health risk.[46] If a person is less than 5 feet tall or has a BMI of 35 or above, waist circumference standards used for the general population might not apply.

The **waist-to-hip ratio** measures regional fat distribution. A waist-to-hip ratio greater than 1 in men and 0.8 in women indicates increased health risks.[47] Although used extensively in the past, waist-to-hip ratios are used less often today with BMI and waist circumference being the preferred measures of health risk for many.

# Measures of Body Fat

There are numerous ways besides BMI calculations and waist measurements to assess whether your body fat levels are too high. One low-tech way is simply to look in the mirror or consider how your clothes fit now compared with how they fit the last season you wore them. For

**waist-to-hip ratio** Waist circumference divided by hip circumference; a high ratio indicates increased health risks due to unhealthy fat distribution.

**Underwater (hydrostatic) weighing:**
Measures the amount of water a person displaces when completely submerged. Fat tissue is less dense than muscle or bone, so body fat can be computed within a 2%–3% margin of error by comparing weight underwater and out of water.

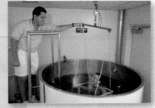

**Skinfolds:**
Involves "pinching" a person's fold of skin (with its underlying layer of fat) at various locations of the body. The fold is measured using a specially designed caliper. When performed by a skilled technician, it can estimate body fat with an error of 3%–4%.

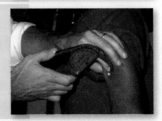

**Bioelectrical impedance analysis (BIA):**
Involves sending a very low level of electrical current through a person's body. As lean body mass is made up of mostly water, the rate at which the electricity is conducted gives an indication of a person's lean body mass and body fat. Under the best circumstances, BIA can estimate body fat with an error of 3%–4%.

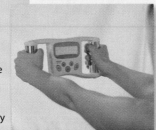

**Dual-energy X-ray absorptiometry (DXA):**
The technology is based on using very-low-level X ray to differentiate between bone tissue, soft (or lean) tissue, and fat (or adipose) tissue. The margin of error for predicting body fat is 2%–4%.

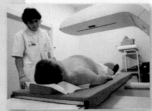

**Bod Pod:**
Uses air displacement to measure body composition. This machine is a large, egg-shaped chamber made from fiberglass. The person being measured sits in the machine wearing a swimsuit. The door is closed and the machine measures how much air is displaced. That value is used to calculate body fat, with a 2%–3% margin of error.

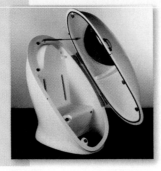

FIGURE 8.5 **Overview of Various Body Composition Assessment Methods**

**Source:** Adapted from J. Thompson and M. Manore, *Nutrition: An Applied Approach*, 2nd, © 2009. Printed and Electronically reproduced by permission of Pearson Education, Inc., Upper Saddle River, New Jersey.

those who wish to take a more precise measurement of their percentage of body fat, more accurate techniques are available, several of which are described and depicted in Figure 8.5. These methods usually involve the help of a skilled professional and typically must be done in a lab or clinical setting. Before undergoing any procedure, make sure you understand the expense, potential for accuracy, risks, and training of the tester. Also, consider why you are seeking this assessment and what you plan to do with the results.

# Managing Your Weight

At some point in our lives, almost all of us will decide to lose weight or modify our diet. Many will have mixed success. Failure is often related to thinking about losing weight in terms of short-term "dieting" rather than carefully analyzing individual risks for obesity and adjusting long-term eating behaviors (such as developing the habit of healthy snacking; see the Skills for Behavior Change box below). Low-calorie diets produce only temporary losses and may actually lead to disordered binge eating or related problems.[48] Repeated bouts of restrictive dieting may be physiologically harmful; moreover, the sense of failure we experience each time we don't meet our goal can exact far-reaching psychological costs. Drugs and intensive counseling can contribute to positive weight

## Tips for Sensible Snacking

✷ **Keep healthy munchies around.** Buy 100 percent whole wheat breads, and if you need something to spice that up, use low-fat or soy cheese, low-fat cream cheese, peanut butter, hummus, or other healthy favorites. Some baked crackers or chips are low in fat and calories and high in fiber. Look for these on your grocery shelves.

✷ **Keep "crunchies" on hand.** Apples, pears, green pepper sticks, popcorn, carrots, and celery all are good choices. Wash the fruits and vegetables and cut them up to carry with you; eat them when a snack attack comes on.

✷ **Quench your thirst with hot drinks.** Hot tea, heated milk, plain or decaffeinated coffee, hot chocolate made with nonfat milk or water, or soup broths will help keep you satisfied.

✷ **Choose natural beverages.** Drink plain water, 100 percent juice in small quantities, or other low-sugar choices to satisfy your thirst. Avoid certain juices, energy drinks, and soft drinks that have added sugars, low fiber, and no protein. Usually, they are high in calories and low in longer-term satisfaction.

✷ **Eat nuts instead of candy.** Although nuts are relatively high in calories, they are also loaded with healthy fats and make a healthy snack when consumed in moderation.

✷ **If you must have a piece of chocolate, keep it small.** Note that dark chocolate is better than milk chocolate or white chocolate because of its antioxidant content.

✷ **Avoid high-calorie energy bars.** Eat these only if you are exercising hard and don't have an opportunity to eat a regular meal. If you buy energy bars, look for ones with a good mixture of fiber and protein and that are low in fat and calories.

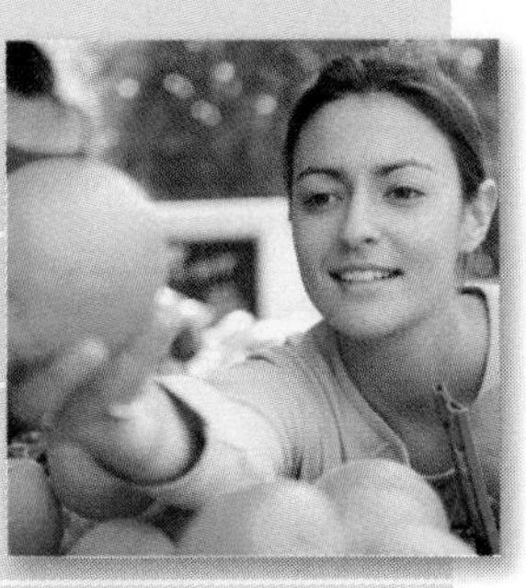

| If your trigger is ... | then → | try this strategy ... |
|---|---|---|
| A stressful situation | | Acknowledge and address feelings of anxiety or stress, and develop stress management techniques to practice daily. |
| Feeling angry or upset | | Analyze your emotions and look for a noneating activity to deal with them, such as taking a quick walk or calling a friend. |
| A certain time of day | | Change your eating schedule to avoid skipping or delaying meals and overeating later; make a plan of what you'll eat ahead of time to avoid impulse or emotional eating. |
| Pressure from friends and family | | Have a response ready to help you refuse food you do not want, or look for healthy alternatives you can eat instead when in social settings. |
| Being in an environment where food is available | | Avoid the environment that causes you to want to eat: Sit far away from the food at meetings, take a different route to class to avoid passing the vending machines, shop from a list and only when you aren't hungry, arrange nonfood outings with your friends. |
| Feeling bored and tired | | Identify the times when you feel low energy and fill them with activities other than eating, such as exercise breaks; cultivate a new interest or hobby that keeps your mind and hands busy. |
| The sight and smell of food | | Stop buying high-calorie foods that tempt you to snack, or store them in an inconvenient place, out of sight; avoid walking past or sitting or standing near the table of tempting treats at a meeting, party, or other gathering. |
| Eating mindlessly or inattentively | | Turn off all distractions, including phones, computers, television, and radio, and eat more slowly, savoring your food and putting your fork down between bites so you can become aware of when your hunger is satisfied. |
| Feeling deprived | | Allow yourself to eat "indulgences" in moderation, so you won't crave them; focus on balancing your calorie input to calorie output. |
| Eating out of habit | | Establish a new routine to circumvent the old, such as taking a new route to class so you don't feel compelled to stop at your favorite fast-food restaurant on the way. |
| Watching television | | Look for something else to occupy your hands and body while your mind is engaged with the screen: Ride an exercise bike, do stretching exercises, doodle on a pad of paper, or learn to knit. |

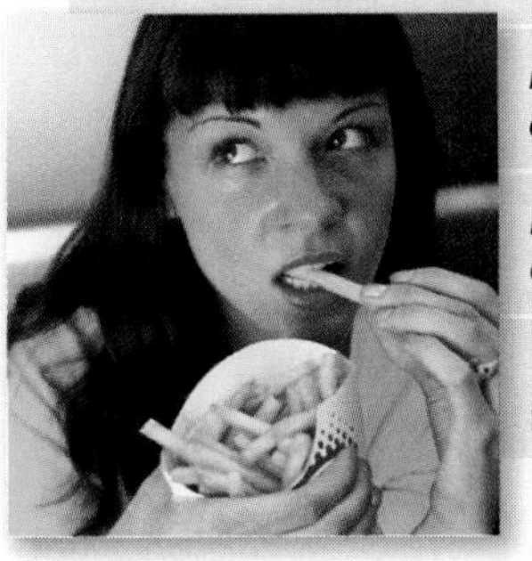

**FIGURE 8.6 Avoid Trigger-Happy Eating**
Learn what triggers your "eat" response—and what stops it—by keeping a daily log.

## Improving Your Eating Habits

Before you can change a behavior, such as unhealthy eating habits, you must first determine what causes (or "triggers") it. Many people find it helpful to keep a chart of their eating patterns: when they feel like eating, where they are when they decide to eat, the amount of time they spend eating, other activities they engage in during the meal (watching television or reading), whether they eat alone or with others, what and how much they consume, and how they felt before they took their first bite. If you keep a detailed daily log of eating triggers for at least a week, you will discover useful clues about what in your environment or your emotional makeup causes you to want food. Typically, these dietary triggers center on patterns and problems in everyday living rather than on real hunger pangs. Many people eat compulsively when stressed; however, for other people, the same circumstances diminish their appetite, causing them to lose weight. See Figure 8.6 for ways you can adjust your eating triggers and snack more healthfully in order to manage your weight.

Once you have evaluated your behaviors and determined your triggers, you can begin to devise a plan for improved eating. If you are unsure of where to start, seek assistance from reputable sources in selecting a dietary plan that is nutritious and easy to follow, such as the MyPyramid Plan discussed in Chapter 7. Registered dietitians, some physicians (not all doctors have a strong background in nutrition), health educators

loss, but even then, many people regain weight after treatment. Maintaining a healthful body takes constant attention and nurturing over the course of your lifetime.

TABLE
8.2
**Analyzing Popular Diet Books**

| Diet Book | Author Credentials | Claims | What You Eat | Science Validity | Cautions |
|---|---|---|---|---|---|
| *The Best Life Diet*, revised and updated | Bob Greene (Oprah Winfrey's personal fitness trainer) | • Prepares "festive foods" <br> • Watch weight go away <br> • Emphasis on lifestyle change | • Three phases <br> 1. Adopt healthy habits and increase activity; regular meals; no food before bed; ditch problem foods <br> 2. Weekly weigh-ins; get rid of emotional eating <br> 3. Rest of life | • Sensible multipronged approach <br> • Sticks to good science <br> • No quick weight loss | • None evident |
| *The Complete Beck Diet for Life: The Five-Stage Program for Permanent Weight Loss* | Judith S. Beck, PhD | • Teaches self-motivation <br> • Teaches how to handle hunger and cravings <br> • Teaches how to create time for dieting | • Five-stage program <br> • Meal plans <br> • 1,600–2,400 daily calories <br> • Recipes | • Sensible approach <br> • Well-balanced meals <br> • Flexible "bonus" calories <br> • Behavior based | • None evident |
| *The Flexitarian Diet: The Mostly Vegetarian Way to Lose Weight, Be Healthier, Prevent Disease, and Add Years to Your Life* | Dawn Jackson Blatner, RD, LDN | • Be healthier <br> • Prevent disease; add years to your life | • 5 × 5 Flex Plan <br> • Vegetarian <br> • Occasional meat, poultry, fish | • In the beginning, small amounts of meat allowed | • No direction on how to wean self off meat <br> • No step-by-step instruction on how to include meat in a mostly vegetarian diet |
| *You: On a Diet: The Owner's Manual for Waist Management* | Michael F. Roizen, MD and Mehmet C. Oz, MD | • Shaves inches off waistline: 2 inches in 2 weeks | • 14-Day Rebooting Plan <br> • Whole grains <br> • Nuts <br> • Lean meat <br> • Fish | • Simplified science <br> • Daily exercise <br> • Strength training <br> • Describes how emotions, hormones, and other variables affect eating behaviors | • 2 inches in 2 weeks are mostly water <br> • Inch mentality not as relevant as BMI and health |
| *Dr. Shapiro's Picture Perfect Weight Loss 30-Day Plan* | Howard Shapiro, DO | • Teaches "a way of eating" <br> • Focus on calorie density of certain foods | • Free choice of foods <br> • Comparisons of high-calorie choices and low-calorie options | • Sound approach | • None evident <br> • Calorie density isn't the only key criterion |
| *Your Big Fat Boyfriend: How to Stay Thin When Dating a Diet Disaster* | Jenna Bergen | • How to eat healthfully when dining at not-so-healthy places <br> • Healthy recipes | • Humorous solutions to unhealthy situations <br> • Simple formulas | • Lacking nutrition and scientific research | • Only for target audiences, i.e., young women with no medical conditions |
| *The All-New Atkins Advantage: The 12-Week Low-Carb Program to Lose Weight, Achieve Peak Fitness and Health, and Maximize Your Willpower to Reach Life Goals* | Stuart L. Trager, MD, with Colette Heimowitz, MSc | • Achieve peak fitness and health <br> • Maximize will power | • 12-week meal plan <br> • 20–80 grams of net carbohydrates <br> • Multivitamin supplement recommended | • Vague approach | • Unproven claims to control cravings <br> • Misleading regarding intake of saturated fats <br> • Eating fewer whole grains, fruits, and vegetables reduces natural vitamins and minerals <br> • Emphasis on carbohydrate cuts is questionable |

*Continued on next page*

| Diet Book | Author Credentials | Claims | What You Eat | Science Validity | Cautions |
|-----------|-------------------|--------|--------------|------------------|----------|
| *The Biggest Loser: The Weight Loss Program to Transform Your Body, Health, and Life—Adapted from NBC's Hit Show!* | Maggie Greenwood-Robinson, PhD, et al. | • Lower cholesterol<br>• Strengthen body | 4-3-2-1 Daily Pyramid:<br>• 4 servings of fruits and vegetables<br>• 3 servings of proteins<br>• 2 servings of whole grains<br>• 1 200 calories from "extra" category | • Sensible approach<br>• Gaining health through diet and exercise<br>• Explains how to choose healthy, low-fat foods | • Does not explain how to choose daily calorie intake range<br>• Fewer than 1,200 calories puts body in semistarvation mode<br>• Makes it difficult to obtain necessary vitamins and nutrients |
| *Skinny Bitch* | Rory Freedman and Kim Barnouin | • Makes you feel clean, healthy, energized, and pure | • Natural foods<br>• Vegan diet<br>• Fresh, organic, and raw vegetables<br>• Vegetable protein<br>• Limited fruits | • Challenges widely accepted and well-researched science<br>• Opposes current scientific evidence | • No recipes<br>• Verbally abusive language used |
| *The Mayo Clinic Diet: Eat Well, Enjoy Life, Lose Weight* | Mayo Foundation for Medical Education and Research | • Lifestyle approach<br>• Long-term success | • Reduce calories and fats<br>• Increase fruits and vegetables<br>• Lean protein | • Sound and sensible, based on ADA recommendations<br>• Lifestyle emphasis<br>• Creative strategies to remove barriers and ensure success | • Short on detail<br>• Large print |

**Source:** Adapted from American Dietetic Association's Diet and Lifestyle Book Reviews, Available at www.eatright.org/Media/content.aspx?id=6442452236#E-H.

and exercise physiologists with nutritional training, and other health professionals can provide reliable information. Beware of people who call themselves nutritionists. There is no such official designation. Avoid weight-loss programs that promise quick, "miracle" results or that are run by "trainees," often people with short courses on nutrition and exercise that are designed to sell products or services.

Before engaging in any weight-loss program, ask about the credentials of the adviser; assess the nutrient value of the prescribed diet; verify that dietary guidelines are consistent with reliable nutrition research; and analyze the suitability of the diet to your tastes, budget, and lifestyle. Any diet that requires radical behavior changes or sets up artificial dietary programs through prepackaged products that don't teach you how to eat healthfully is likely to fail. Supplements and fad diets that claim fast weight loss will invariably mean fast weight regain. The most successful plans allow you to make food choices in real-world settings and

do not ask you to sacrifice everything you enjoy. See Table 8.2 for an analysis of some of the popular diet books being marketed today. For information on other books, check out the regularly updated list of the diet book reviews on the American Dietetic Association website at www.eatright.org.

**"Why Should I Care?"**

It may be easy to grab a fast-food meal and go, but unless you are very physically active, your body will likely store that "supersized" meal as fat, which is anything but easy to lose. Remember—it takes only 3,500 unused calories to create a pound of body fat, so eating 500 extra calories a day—less than the average hamburger—can lead to a pound of weight gain in just a week's time.

## Understanding Calories and Energy Balance

A *calorie* is a unit of measure that indicates the amount of energy gained from food or expended through activity. Each time you consume 3,500 calories more than your body needs to maintain weight, you gain a pound of storage fat. Conversely, each time your body expends an extra 3,500 calories, you lose a pound of fat. If you consume 140 calories (the amount in one can of regular soda) more than you need every single day and make no other changes in diet or activity, you would gain 1 pound in 25 days (3,500 calories ÷ 140 calories/day = 25 days). Even when you think you

# 3,500

calories equal approximately
1 pound of body fat.

are watching fat intake by ordering your Starbucks vanilla latte with skim milk, you are still consuming a whopping 230 calories with every 16 ounces. Assuming you start having the same drink every day and do nothing else differently, you'll gain 1 pound every 15 days! Conversely, if you walk for 30 minutes each day at a pace of 15 minutes per mile (172 calories burned) in addition to your regular activities, you would lose 1 pound in 20 days (3,500 calories ÷ 172 calories/day = 20.3 days). This is an example of the concept of energy balance described in Figure 8.7. Of course, these are generic formulas. If you weigh more, you will burn more calories moving your body through the same exercise routine than someone who is thinner.

## Including Exercise

Increasing BMR, RMR, or EMR levels will help burn calories. Any increase in the intensity, frequency, and duration of daily exercise levels can have a significant impact on total calorie expenditure.

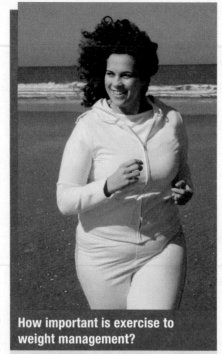

**How important is exercise to weight management?**

Participating in daily physical activity is key to managing your weight. Go for a jog on your own for some quiet time, or join a soccer game for social, fast-moving fun, but get out there and move!

Physical activity makes a greater contribution to metabolic rate when large muscle groups are used. The energy spent on physical activity is the energy used to move the body's muscles and the extra energy used to speed up heartbeat and respiration rate. The number of calories spent depends on three factors:

**1.** The number and proportion of muscles used
**2.** The amount of weight moved
**3.** The length of time the activity takes

An activity involving both the arms and legs burns more calories than one involving only the legs. An activity performed by a heavy person burns more calories than the same activity performed by a lighter person. And an activity performed for 40 minutes requires twice as much energy as the same activity performed for only 20 minutes. Thus, an obese person walking for 1 mile burns more calories than does a slim person walking the same distance. It also may take overweight people longer to walk the mile, which means that they are burning energy for a longer time and therefore expending more overall calories than the thin walkers.

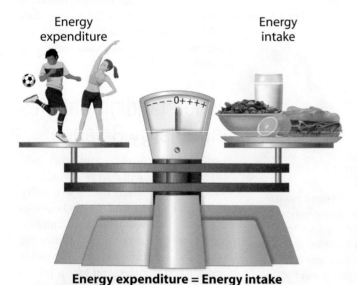

**Energy expenditure = Energy intake**

FIGURE 8.7 **The Concept of Energy Balance**
If you consume more calories than you burn, you will gain weight. If you burn more than you consume, you will lose weight. If both are equal, your weight will not change, according to this concept.

## Keeping Weight Control in Perspective

Weight loss is difficult for many people and may require supportive friends, relatives, and community resources, plus extraordinary efforts to prime the body for burning extra calories. People of the same age, sex, height, and weight can have differences of as much as 1,000 calories a day in RMR—this may explain why one person's gluttony is another's starvation. Other factors such as depression, stress, culture, and available foods can also affect a person's ability to lose weight. Being overweight does not mean people are weak willed or lazy.

To reach and maintain the weight at which you will be healthy and feel your best, you must develop a program of exercise and healthy eating behaviors that will work for you now and over the long term. Remember that you didn't gain your weight in 1 week, so you're not likely to lose it all in the week or two before spring break. It is unrealistic and potentially dangerous to punish your body by trying to lose weight in a short period of time. Instead, try to lose a healthy 1 to 2 pounds during the first week, and stay with this slow and easy regimen. Making permanent changes to your lifestyle by adding exercise and cutting back on calories to expend about 500 calories more than you consume each day will help you lose weight at a rate of 1 pound per week. See the Skills for Behavior Change box for strategies to make your weight management program succeed.

## Keys to Successful Weight Management

The key to successful weight management is finding a sustainable way to control what you eat and to make exercise a priority. First:

✳ Write down the things that you think are positive about your diet and exercise behaviors. Then write down the things that need changing. For each change you need to make, list three or four small things you could change right now.
✳ Ask yourself some key questions. Why do you want to make this change right now? What are your ultimate goals?
✳ What resources are available on your campus or in your community where you could go for help? Out of your friends and family members, who will help you?
✳ Keep a food and exercise log for 2 or 3 days. Note the good things you are doing, the things that need improvement, and the triggers you need to address.
✳ Talk with your health care provider about any medical conditions you have or medicines you take.

### MAKE A PLAN

✳ Set realistic short- and long-term goals.
✳ Establish a plan. What are the diet and exercise changes you can make this week? Once you do 1 week, plot a course for 2 weeks, and so on.
✳ Look for balance. Remember that it is calories taken in and burned over time that make the difference.

### CHANGE YOUR HABITS

✳ Be adventurous. Expand your usual meals and snacks to enjoy a wide variety of different options.
✳ Do not constantly deprive yourself or set unrealistic guidelines.
✳ Notice whether you are hungry before starting a meal. Eat slowly, noting when you start to feel full, and STOP before you are full.
✳ Eat breakfast. This will prevent you from being too hungry and overeating at lunch.
✳ Keep healthful snacks on hand for when you get hungry.

### INCORPORATE EXERCISE

✳ Be active and slowly increase your time, speed, distance, or resistance levels.
✳ Vary your physical activity. Find activities that you really love and try things you haven't tried before.
✳ Find an exercise partner to help you stay motivated.
✳ Make it a fun break. Go for a walk in a place that interests you. Tune in to your surroundings to take your mind off of your sweating and heavy breathing!

# Considering Drastic Weight-Loss Measures

When nothing seems to work, people often become frustrated and may take significant risks to lose weight. Dramatic weight loss may be recommended in cases of extreme health risk. However, even in such situations, drastic dietary, pharmacological, or surgical measures should be considered carefully and discussed with several knowledgeable health professionals.

**Very-Low-Calorie Diets** In severe cases of obesity that are not responsive to traditional dietary strategies, medically supervised, powdered formulas with daily values of 400 to 700 calories plus vitamin and mineral supplements may be given to patients. Such **very-low-calorie diets (VLCDs)** should never be undertaken without strict medical supervision. These severe diets do not teach healthy eating and persons who manage to lose weight on them may experience significant weight regain. More important, fasting, starvation diets, and other forms of VLCDs have been shown to cause significant health risks and can, in fact, be deadly. Problems associated with any form of severe caloric restriction include blood sugar imbalance, cold intolerance, constipation, decreased BMR, dehydration, diarrhea, emotional problems, fatigue, headaches, heart irregularities, kidney infections and failure, loss of lean body tissue, weakness, and the potential for coma and death.

One particularly dangerous potential complication of VLCDs or starvation diets is *ketoacidosis*. After a prolonged period of inadequate carbohydrate or food intake, the body will have depleted its immediate energy stores and will begin metabolizing fat stores through *ketogenesis* in order to supply the brain and nervous system with an alternative fuel known as *ketones*. Ketogenesis is one of the body's normal processes for metabolizing fat and may help provide energy to the brain during times of fasting, low carbohydrate intake, or vigorous exercise. However, ketones may also suppress appetite and cause dehydration at a time when a person should feel hungry and seek out food. The condition of having increased levels of ketones in the body is *ketosis*; if enough ketones accumulate in the blood, it may lead to *ketoacdiosis,* in which the blood becomes more acidic.[49] People with untreated type 1 diabetes and individuals with anorexia nervosa or bulimia nervosa are at risk of developing ketoacidotic symptoms as damage to body tissues begins.

**very-low-calorie diets (VLCDs)** Diets with a daily caloric value of 400 to 700 calories.

If fasting continues, the body will turn to its last resort—protein—for energy, breaking down muscle and organ tissue to stay alive. As this occurs, the body loses weight rapidly. At the same time, it also loses significant water stores. Eventually, the body begins to run out of liver tissue, heart muscle, and so on. Within about 10 days after the typical adult begins a complete fast, the body will have depleted its energy stores, and death may occur.

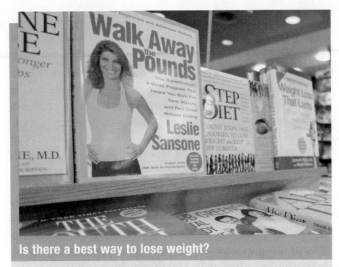

**Is there a best way to lose weight?**

There are hundreds of weight-loss plans currently being marketed commercially, but no one plan is a miracle fix. Ultimately, the best way to lose weight is by evaluating and modifying your own eating and exercising behaviors. Enlisting the aid of a registered dietitian or other reliable health professional can help you craft a healthy plan that will work for you.

**Drug Treatment** Individuals looking for help in losing weight often turn to thousands of commercially marketed weight-loss supplements, which are available on the Internet and at drug and health food stores. U.S. Food and Drug Administration (FDA) approval is not required for over-the-counter "diet aids" or supplements, and many manufacturers simply feed off people's desperation. Most of these supplements contain stimulants such as caffeine or diuretics, and their effectiveness in promoting weight loss has been largely untested and unproved by any scientific studies. In many cases, the only thing that users lose is money they might have put to better use. Virtually all persons who used diet pills in review studies regained their weight once they stopped taking them.[50]

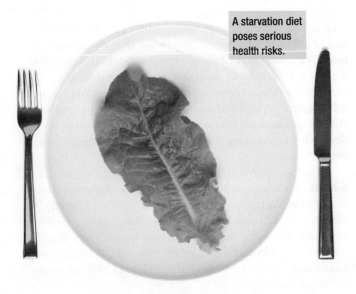

A starvation diet poses serious health risks.

In contrast, FDA-approved diet pills have historically been available only by prescription. These lines were blurred in 2007 when the FDA approved the first over-the-counter weight loss pill—a half-strength version of the prescription drug orlistat (brand name Xenical), marketed as Alli. This drug inhibits the action of lipase, an enzyme that helps the body to digest fats, causing about 30 percent of fats consumed to pass through the digestive system undigested, leading to reduced overall caloric intake. Known side effects of orlistat include gas with watery fecal discharge; oily stools and spotting; frequent, often unexpected, bowel movements; and possible deficiencies of fat-soluble vitamins. There have also been several FDA warnings issued about fake Alli products being sold at reduced prices online.

In general, diet pills have not been proved to be all that effective when used alone. When used as part of a long-term, comprehensive weight-loss program, these drugs can potentially help those who are severely obese lose up to 10 percent of their weight and maintain the loss. The challenge is to develop an effective drug that can be used over time without adverse effects or abuse, and no such drug currently exists. A classic example of supposedly safe drugs that were later found to have dangerous side effects are Pondimin and Redux, known as *fen-phen* (from their chemical names fenfluramine and phentermine), two of the most widely prescribed diet drugs in U.S. history.[51] When they were found to damage heart valves and contribute to pulmonary hypertension, a massive recall and lawsuit ensued.

Some currently available diet drugs and supplements that you should view with caution include the following:

- **Sibutramine (Meridia).** This prescription-only medication suppresses appetite by inhibiting the uptake of serotonin in the brain. It works best with a reduced-calorie diet and exercise, but side effects are not to be taken lightly. They include dry mouth, headache, constipation, insomnia, and high blood pressure. Although research has shown positive effects on blood glucose control, the FDA has issued warnings about use of Meridia for people who have hypertension or heart disease.[52]
- **Hoodia gordonii.** This cactus-like plant native to Africa is a purported appetite suppressant. No convincing evidence has been shown for or against it; to date, it is not FDA approved and has not been tested in clinical trials.[53] Supplements containing *Hoodia gordonii* have become popular in recent years, and there are many off-market brands produced, including some that contain more unproven ingredients such as bitter orange and other stimulants.
- **Herbal weight-loss aids.** In attempts to fight the battle of the bulge, many people turn to potentially unsafe herbal remedies. Products containing *Ephedra* can cause rapid heart rate, tremors, seizures, insomnia, headaches, and raised blood pressure, all without significant effects on long-term weight control. *St. John's wort* and other alternative medicines

reported to enhance serotonin, suppress appetite, and reduce the side effects of depression have not been shown to be effective in weight loss, either.

**Surgery** When all else fails, particularly for people who are severely overweight and have weight-related diseases such as diabetes or hypertension, a person may be a candidate for weight-loss surgery. Generally, these surgeries fall into one of two major categories: *restrictive surgeries,* such as gastric banding, that limit food intake, and *malabsorption surgeries* that decrease the absorption of food into the body, such as *gastric bypass* (Figure 8.8). Each type of surgery has its own benefits and risks. To select the best option, a physician will consider that operation's benefits and risks along with many other factors, including the patient's BMI, eating behaviors, obesity-related health conditions, and previous operations. Some health advocates have proposed that obesity be classified as a disability (see the **Points of View** box on page 272), which could potentially affect a physician's decision on recommending surgery.

In gastric banding and other restrictive surgeries, the surgeon uses an inflatable band to partition off part of the stomach. The band is wrapped around that part of the stomach and is pulled tight, like a belt, leaving only a small opening between the two parts of the stomach. The upper part of the stomach is smaller, so the person feels full more quickly, and food digestion slows so that the person also feels full longer. Although the bands are designed to stay in place, they can be removed surgically. They can also be inflated to different levels to adjust the amount of restriction.

In contrast to the restrictive surgeries, gastric bypass is designed to drastically decrease the amount of food a person can eat and absorb. Results are fast and dramatic, but there are many risks, including blood clots in the legs, a leak in a staple line in the stomach, pneumonia, infection, and death. Because the stomach pouch that remains after surgery is so

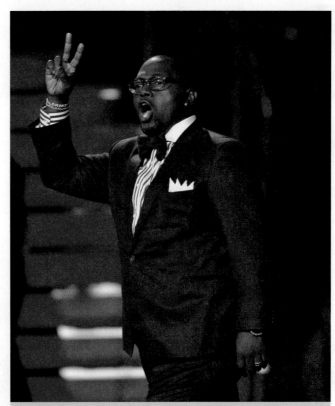

*American Idol* judge and record producer Randy Jackson underwent gastric bypass surgery in 2003 after being diagnosed with type 2 diabetes. He has since lost 110 pounds.

small (about the size of a lime), the person can drink only a few tablespoons of liquid and consume only a very small amount of food at a time. For this reason, possible side effects include nausea and vomiting (if the person consumes too much), vitamin and mineral deficiencies, and dehydration (if the patient cannot eat or drink enough).

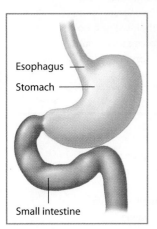

Esophagus

Stomach

Small intestine

**a** Normal anatomy

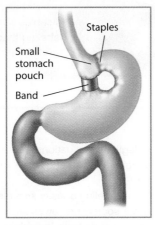

Small stomach pouch

Staples

Band

**b** Vertical banded gastroplasty

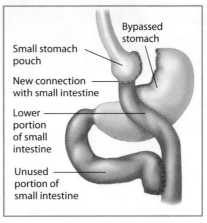

Small stomach pouch

Bypassed stomach

New connection with small intestine

Lower portion of small intestine

Unused portion of small intestine

**c** Gastric bypass

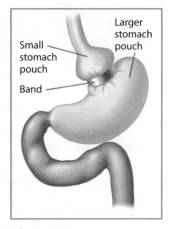

Small stomach pouch

Larger stomach pouch

Band

**d** Gastric banding

FIGURE 8.8 **Weight-Loss Surgery Alters the Normal Anatomy of the Stomach**

**Source:** Adapted from J. Thompson and M. Manore, *Nutrition: An Applied Approach,* 2nd, © 2009. Printed and Electronically reproduced by permission of Pearson Education, Inc., Upper Saddle River, New Jersey.

# Obesity:
## IS IT A DISABILITY?

There is no question that obesity can lead to health problems and difficulty performing activities of daily living. A person who is 150 to 200 pounds overweight can have difficulty walking, running, getting out of a chair, and doing simple daily tasks. But does that mean that obesity constitutes a disability? Obesity is generally not considered a disability under the federal Americans with Disabilities Act (ADA), which defines *disability* as "a physical or mental impairment that substantially limits one or more of the major life activities of [an] individual."

To be covered by the ADA, an obese person must have a body mass index (BMI) of over 40 or be at least 100 pounds overweight, as well as an underlying disorder that caused the obesity. These strict criteria means that the ADA currently receives few complaints relating to obesity. However, some people believe obesity should be considered a disability that legally entitles individuals to certain health benefits and other accommodations. Other people believe that labeling obesity as a disability would add to its stigma and create more problems than it would solve.

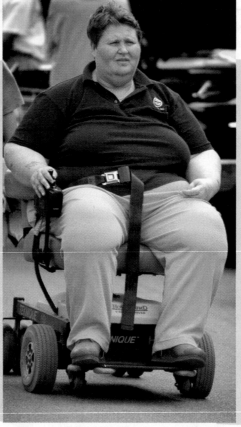

### Arguments Favoring Disability Status for Obese People

◯ Labeling obesity as a disability would provide obese individuals with better insurance coverage.

◯ A disability label would protect the rights of obese individuals against discrimination based on their weight.

◯ Obesity truly can involve physical disability: An obese person can have many related medical conditions including arthritis, increased blood pressure, diabetes, diabetic-related vascular diseases, and a weakened cardiovascular system. All of these conditions can lead to the need for walkers, wheelchairs, and other mobility devices, as well as special health accommodations at home or in the workplace.

### Arguments Opposing Disability Status for Obese People

◯ Doctors are worried that defining obesity as a disability would make them vulnerable to lawsuits from obese patients who don't want their doctors to discuss their weight. The threat of such lawsuits would prevent doctors from discussing obesity with their overweight patients and recommending specific actions.

◯ Rather than labeling obesity as a disability and adding to its stigma, issues of unfair insurance or job practices could be handled with antidiscrimination laws.

◯ Not all obese people are disabled by their weight, so labeling them as such would be discriminatory.

### Where Do You Stand?

◯ In your opinion, what positive results could come from classifying overweight or obese individuals as disabled?

◯ What negative consequences do you foresee from classifying overweight or obese people as disabled?

◯ How would you determine whether an individual is disabled because of his or her weight?

◯ Are there legitimate situations where a person who is overweight or obese should be labeled as disabled?

◯ Do you think labeling obesity as a disability would alter the way our society perceives and behaves toward overweight and obese individuals? If so, in what way?

Aftercare for gastric surgery patients often includes counseling to help them cope with the urge to eat after the ability to eat normal portions has been removed, as well as other adjustment problems. Keep in mind that it is always best to lose weight by eating a healthy diet and getting regular physical activity. Ironically, even after undergoing surgery, people must learn to eat healthy foods and exercise. Otherwise, they can continue to gain weight, even returning to their original weight.

Recent research has demonstrated exciting, unexpected results from gastric surgeries: Even prior to weight loss, patients have shown complete remission of type 2 diabetes in the majority of cases, with drastic reductions in blood glucose levels in others.[54] In one study, nearly 99 percent of the morbidly obese who had gastric bypass and had a previous history of type 2 diabetes were free of the disease after surgery, even before they began to lose weight. This finding has caused much excitement in the scientific community as researchers explore surgical options for prevention of diabetes in other populations.[55] For those at high risk from these diseases, these benefits may factor in to surgical decisions in the future.

Unlike restrictive and malabsorption surgeries, which facilitate overall weight loss, *liposuction* is a surgical procedure in which fat cells are removed from specific areas of the body. Generally, liposuction is considered cosmetic surgery rather than weight-loss surgery and is used for spot reducing and body contouring. Although this technique has garnered much attention, it too is not without risk: Infections, severe scarring, and even death have resulted. In many cases, people who have liposuction regain fat in those areas or require multiple surgeries to repair lumpy, irregular surfaces from which the fat was removed.

## Trying to Gain Weight

For some people, trying to gain weight is a challenge for a variety of metabolic, hereditary, psychological, and other reasons. If you are one of these individuals, the first priority is to determine why you cannot gain weight. Perhaps you're an athlete and you burn more calories than you manage to eat. Perhaps you're stressed out and skipping meals to increase study time. Among older adults, the senses of taste and smell may decline, which makes food taste different and therefore less pleasurable to eat. Visual problems and other disabilities may make meals more difficult to prepare, and dental problems may make eating more difficult. People who engage in extreme energy-burning sports and exercise routines may be at risk for caloric and nutritional deficiencies, which can lead not only to weight loss, but to immune system problems and organ dysfunction; weakness, which leads to falls and fractures; slower recovery from diseases; and a host of other problems as well. (See the **Skills for Behavior Change** box for several weight-gaining strategies.) People who are too thin need to take the same steps as those who are overweight or obese to find out what their healthy weight is and attain that weight.

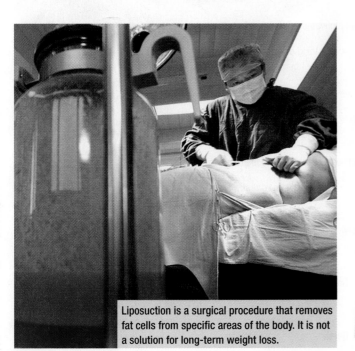

Liposuction is a surgical procedure that removes fat cells from specific areas of the body. It is not a solution for long-term weight loss.

**Skills for Behavior Change**

## Tips for Gaining Weight

* Eat at regularly scheduled times.
* Eat more frequently, spend more time eating, eat high-calorie foods first if you fill up fast, and always start with the main course.
* Take time to shop, to cook, and to eat slowly.
* Put extra spreads such as peanut butter, cream cheese, or cheese on your foods. Make your sandwiches with extra-thick slices of bread and add more filling. Take seconds whenever possible, and eat high-calorie, nutrient-dense snacks such as nuts, cheese, whole-grain tortilla chips, and guacamole during the day.
* Supplement your diet. Add high-calorie drinks that have a healthy balance of nutrients, such as whole milk.
* Try to eat with people you are comfortable with. Avoid people who you feel are analyzing what you eat or make you feel as if you should eat less.
* If you are sedentary, be aware that exercise can increase appetite. If you are exercising, or exercising to extremes, moderate your activities until you've gained some weight.
* Avoid diuretics, laxatives, and other medications that cause you to lose body fluids and nutrients.
* Relax. Many people who are underweight operate at high gear most of the time. Slow down, get more rest, and control stress.

# Assess yourself

## Are You Ready for Weight Loss?

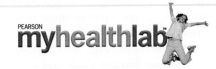

How well do your attitudes equip you for a weight-loss program? For each question, circle the answer that best describes your attitude. As you complete sections 2–5, tally your score and analyze it according to the scoring guide.

Fill out this assessment online at www.pearsonhighered.com/myhealthlab or www.pearsonhighered.com/donatelle.

## 1 Diet History

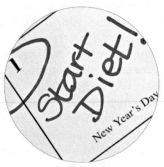

**A. How many times in the past year have you been on a diet?**

| 0 times | 1–3 times | 4–10 times | 11–20 times | More than 20 |

**B. What is the most weight you lost on any of these diets?**

| 0 lb | 1–5 lb | 6–10 lb | 11–20 lb | More than 20 lb |

**C. How long did you stay at the new lower weight?**

| Less than 1 mo | 2–3 mo | 4–6 mo | 6–12 mo | Over 1 yr |

**D. Put a check mark by each dieting method you have tried:**

____ Skipping breakfast     ____ Skipping lunch or dinner     ____ Taking over-the-counter appetite suppressants

____ Counting calories     ____ Cutting out most fats     ____ Cutting out most carbohydrates

____ Increasing regular exercise     ____ Taking weight-loss supplements     ____ Cutting out all snacks

____ Using meal replacements such as Slim Fast     ____ Taking prescription appetite suppressants     ____ Taking laxatives

____ Inducing vomiting     ____ Other _____

## 2 Readiness to Start a Weight-Loss Program

If you are thinking about starting a weight-loss program, answer questions A–F.

**A. How motivated are you to lose weight?**

| 1 | 2 | 3 | 4 | 5 |
| Not at all motivated | Slightly motivated | Somewhat motivated | Quite motivated | Extremely motivated |

**B. How certain are you that you will stay committed to a weight-loss program long enough to reach your goal?**

| 1 | 2 | 3 | 4 | 5 |
| Not at all certain | Slightly certain | Somewhat certain | Quite certain | Extremely certain |

**C. Taking into account other stresses in your life (school, work, and relationships), to what extent can you tolerate the effort required to stick to your diet plan?**

| 1 | 2 | 3 | 4 | 5 |
| Cannot tolerate | Can tolerate somewhat | Uncertain | Can tolerate well | Can tolerate easily |

**D. Assuming you should lose no more than 1 to 2 pounds per week, have you allotted a realistic amount of time for weight loss?**

| 1 | 2 | 3 | 4 | 5 |
| Very unrealistic | Somewhat unrealistic | Moderately realistic | Somewhat realistic | Very realistic |

**E. While dieting, do you fantasize about eating your favorite foods?**

| 1 | 2 | 3 | 4 | 5 |
| Always | Frequently | Occasionally | Rarely | Never |

**F. While dieting, do you feel deprived, angry, upset?**

| 1 | 2 | 3 | 4 | 5 |
| Always | Frequently | Occasionally | Rarely | Never |

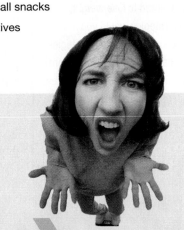

**Total your scores** from questions A–F and circle your score category.

**6 to 16:** This may not be a good time for you to start a diet. Inadequate motivation and commitment and unrealistic goals could block your progress. Think about what contributes to your unreadiness. What are some of the factors? Consider changing these factors before undertaking a diet.

**17 to 23:** You may be nearly ready to begin a program but should think about ways to boost your readiness.

**24 to 30:** The path is clear—you can decide how to lose weight in a safe, effective way.

# 3 Hunger, Appetite, and Eating

Think about your hunger and the cues that stimulate your appetite or eating, and then answer questions A–C.

A. When food comes up in conversation or in something you read, do you want to eat, even if you are not hungry?

| 1 | 2 | 3 | 4 | 5 |
|---|---|---|---|---|
| Never | Rarely | Occasionally | Frequently | Always |

B. How often do you eat for a reason other than physical hunger?

| 1 | 2 | 3 | 4 | 5 |
|---|---|---|---|---|
| Never | Rarely | Occasionally | Frequently | Always |

C. When your favorite foods are around the house, do you succumb to eating them between meals?

| 1 | 2 | 3 | 4 | 5 |
|---|---|---|---|---|
| Never | Rarely | Occasionally | Frequently | Always |

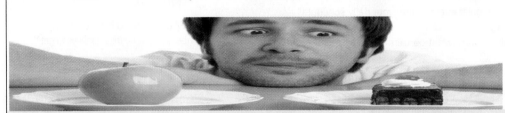

## Total your scores

from questions A–C and circle your score category.

**3 to 6:** You might occasionally eat more than you should, but it is due more to your own attitudes than to temptation and other environmental cues. Controlling your own attitudes toward hunger and eating may help you.

**7 to 9:** You may have a moderate tendency to eat just because food is available. Losing weight may be easier for you if you try to resist external cues and eat only when you are physically hungry.

**10 to 15:** Some or much of your eating may be in response to thinking about food or exposing yourself to temptations to eat. Think of ways to minimize your exposure to temptations so you eat only in response to physical hunger.

# 4 Controlling Overeating

How good are you at controlling overeating when you are on a diet? Answer questions A–C.

A. A friend talks you into going out to a restaurant for a midday meal instead of eating a brown-bag lunch. As a result, for the rest of the day, you:

| 1 | 2 | 3 | 4 | 5 |
|---|---|---|---|---|
| Would eat much less | Would eat somewhat less | Would make no difference | Would eat somewhat more | Would eat much more |

B. You "break" your diet by eating a fattening, "forbidden" food. As a result, for the rest of the day, you:

| 1 | 2 | 3 | 4 | 5 |
|---|---|---|---|---|
| Would eat much less | Would eat somewhat less | Would make no difference | Would eat somewhat more | Would eat much more |

C. You have been following your diet faithfully and decide to test yourself by taking a bite of something you consider a treat. As a result, for the rest of the day, you:

| 1 | 2 | 3 | 4 | 5 |
|---|---|---|---|---|
| Would eat much less | Would eat somewhat less | Would make no difference | Would eat somewhat more | Would eat much more |

## Total your scores

from questions A–C and circle your score category.

**3 to 7:** You recover rapidly from mistakes. However, if you frequently alternate between out-of-control eating and very strict dieting, you may have a serious eating problem and should get professional help.

**8 to 11:** You do not seem to let unplanned eating disrupt your program. This is a flexible, balanced approach.

**12 to 15:** You may be prone to overeating after an event breaks your control or throws you off track. Your reaction to these problem-causing events could use improvement.

# 5 Emotional Eating

Consider the effects of your emotions on your eating behaviors, and answer questions A–C.

A. Do you eat more than you would like to when you have negative feelings such as anxiety, depression, anger, or loneliness?

| 1 | 2 | 3 | 4 | 5 |
|---|---|---|---|---|
| Never | Rarely | Occasionally | Frequently | Always |

B. Do you have trouble controlling your eating when you have positive feelings (i.e., do you celebrate feeling good by eating)?

| 1 | 2 | 3 | 4 | 5 |
|---|---|---|---|---|
| Never | Rarely | Occasionally | Frequently | Always |

C. When you have unpleasant interactions with others in your life or after a difficult day at work, do you eat more than you'd like?

| 1 | 2 | 3 | 4 | 5 |
|---|---|---|---|---|
| Never | Rarely | Occasionally | Frequently | Always |

## Total your scores

from questions A–C and circle your score category.

**3 to 8:** You do not appear to let your emotions affect your eating.

**9 to 11:** You sometimes eat in response to emotional highs and lows. Monitor this behavior to learn when and why it occurs, and be prepared to find alternative activities to respond to your emotions.

**12 to 15:** Emotional ups and downs can stimulate your eating. Try to deal with the feelings that trigger the eating and find other ways to express them.

# 6 Exercise Patterns and Attitudes

Exercise is key for weight loss. Think about your attitudes toward it, and answer questions A–D.

**A. How often do you exercise?**

| 1 | 2 | 3 | 4 | 5 |
|---|---|---|---|---|
| Never | Rarely | Occasionally | Somewhat frequently | Frequently |

**B. How confident are you that you can exercise regularly?**

| 1 | 2 | 3 | 4 | 5 |
|---|---|---|---|---|
| Not at all confident | Slightly confident | Somewhat confident | Highly confident | Completely confident |

**C. When you think about exercise, do you develop a positive or negative picture in your mind?**

| 1 | 2 | 3 | 4 | 5 |
|---|---|---|---|---|
| Completely negative | Somewhat negative | Neutral | Somewhat positive | Completely positive |

**D. How certain are you that you can work regular exercise into your daily schedule?**

| 1 | 2 | 3 | 4 | 5 |
|---|---|---|---|---|
| Not at all certain | Slightly certain | Somewhat certain | Quite certain | Extremely certain |

## Total your scores

from questions A–D and circle your score category.

**4 to 10:** You're probably not exercising as regularly as you should. Determine whether it is your attitude about exercise or your lifestyle that is blocking your way, then change what you must and put on those walking shoes!

**11 to 16:** You need to feel more positive about exercise so you can do it more often. Think of ways to be more active that are fun and fit your lifestyle.

**17 to 20:** The path is clear for you to be active. Now think of ways to get motivated.

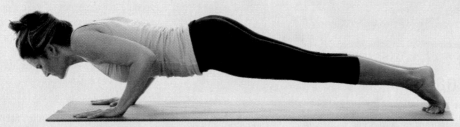

**Source:** Reprinted with permission from *Psychology Today Magazine*. (Copyright © 1989 Sussex Publishers, LLC).

# YOUR PLAN FOR CHANGE

The **Assess yourself** activity identifies six areas of importance in determining your readiness for weight loss. If you wish to lose weight to improve your health, understanding your attitudes about food and exercise will help you succeed in your plan.

## Today, you can:

◯ Set "SMART" goals for weight loss and give them a reality check: Are they **s**pecific, **m**easurable, **a**chievable, **r**elevant, and **t**ime-oriented? For example, rather than aiming to lose 15 pounds this month (which probably wouldn't be healthy or achievable), set a comfortable goal to lose 5 pounds. Realistic goals will encourage weight-loss success by boosting your confidence in your ability to make lifelong healthy changes.

◯ Begin keeping a food log and identifying the triggers that influence your eating habits. Think about what you can do to eliminate or reduce the influence of your two most common food triggers.

## Within the next 2 weeks, you can:

◯ Get in the habit of incorporating more fruits, vegetables, and whole grains in your diet and eating less fat. The next time you make dinner, look at the proportions on your plate. If vegetables and whole grains do not take up most of the space, substitute 1 cup of the meat, pasta, or cheese in your meal with 1 cup of legumes, salad greens, or a favorite vegetable. You'll reduce the number of calories while eating the same amount of food!

◯ Aim to incorporate more exercise into your daily routine. Visit your campus rec center or a local gym, and familiarize yourself with the equipment and facilities that are available. Try a new machine or sports activity, and experiment until you find a form of exercise you really enjoy.

## By the end of the semester, you can:

◯ Get in the habit of grocery shopping every week and buying healthy, nutritious foods while avoiding high-fat, high-sugar, or overly processed foods. As you make healthy foods more available and unhealthy foods less available, you'll find it easier to eat better.

◯ Chart your progress and reward yourself as you meet your goals. If your goal is to lose weight and you successfully take off 10 pounds, reward yourself with a new pair of jeans or other article of clothing (which will likely fit better than before!).

## Summary

* Overweight, obesity, and weight-related health problems have reached epidemic levels in the United States. *Globesity,* or global rates of obesity, is also on an epidemic rise, particularly among the developing regions of the world. Obesogenic behaviors in an obesogenic environment are key reasons for our weight-related problems.

* Societal costs from obesity include increased health care costs, lowered worker productivity, low self-esteem, increased depression, discrimination, and obesity-related stigma. Individual health risks from overweight and obesity include a variety of disabling and deadly chronic diseases and increased risks for certain infectious diseases.

* Many factors contribute to one's risk for obesity, including environmental factors, poverty, education level, genetics, developmental factors, endocrine influences, psychosocial factors, eating cues, metabolic changes, and lifestyle.

* Percentage of body fat is a reliable indicator for levels of overweight and obesity. There are many different methods of assessing body fat. Body mass index (BMI) is one of the most commonly accepted measures of weight based on height. *Overweight* is most commonly defined as a BMI of 25 to 29, and *obesity* as a BMI of 30 or greater. Waist circumference, or the amount of fat in the belly region, is believed to be related to the risk for several chronic diseases, particularly type 2 diabetes.

* Exercise, dieting, diet pills, surgery, and other strategies are used to maintain or lose weight. However, sensible eating behavior and aerobic exercise and exercise that builds muscle mass offer the best options for weight loss and maintenance.

## Pop Quiz

1. The proportion of your total weight made up of fat is called
   a. body composition.
   b. lean mass.
   c. percentage of body fat.
   d. BMI.

2. All of the following statements are true EXCEPT which?
   a. A slowing basal metabolic rate may contribute to weight gain after age 30.
   b. Hormones are increasingly implicated in hunger impulses and eating behavior.
   c. The more muscles you have, the fewer calories you will burn.
   d. Overweight and obesity among young adults can have serious health consequences even before you reach middle age.

3. All of the following statements about BMI are true EXCEPT which?
   a. BMI is based on height and weight measurements.
   b. BMI is accurate for everyone, including athletes with high amounts of muscle mass.
   c. Very low and very high BMI scores are associated with greater risk of mortality.
   d. BMI stands for "body mass index."

4. Which of the following BMI ratings is considered overweight?
   a. 20
   b. 25
   c. 30
   d. 35

5. Which of the following body circumferences is most strongly associated with risk of heart disease and diabetes?
   a. Hip circumference
   b. Chest circumference
   c. Waist circumference
   d. Thigh circumference

6. One pound of additional body fat is created through consuming how many extra calories?
   a. 1,500 calories
   b. 3,500 calories
   c. 5,000 calories
   d. 7,000 calories

7. To lose weight, you must establish a(n)
   a. negative caloric balance.
   b. isocaloric balance.
   c. positive caloric balance.
   d. set point.

8. The rate at which your body consumes food energy to sustain basic functions is your
   a. basal metabolic rate.
   b. resting metabolic rate.
   c. body mass index.
   d. set point.

9. Successful weight maintainers are most likely to do which of the following?
   a. Eat two large meals a day before 1 PM
   b. Skip meals
   c. Drink diet sodas
   d. Eat high-volume but low-calorie density foods

10. Successful, healthy weight loss is characterized by
    a. a lifelong pattern of healthful eating and exercise.
    b. cutting out all fats and carbohydrates and eating a lean, mean, high-protein diet.
    c. never eating foods that are considered bad for you and rigidly adhering to a plan.
    d. a pattern of repeatedly losing and regaining weight.

*Answers to these questions can be found on page A-1.*

## Think about It!

1. Discuss the pressures, if any, you feel to change your body's shape.

Do these pressures come from media, family, friends, and other external sources, or from concern for your personal health?

2. Are you satisfied with your body weight right now? Why or why not? Are other members of your family suffering from weight-related health problems? How much do you worry that you will have a similar problem in the next 10 years? 20 years?

3. Which measurement would you choose to assess your fat levels? Why?

4. List the risk factors for your being overweight or obese right now. Which seem most likely to determine whether you will be obese in middle age?

5. Why do you think that obesity rates are rising in both developed and less-developed regions of the world? What strategies can we take collectively and individually to reduce risks of obesity?

## Accessing Your Health on the Internet

The following websites explore further topics and issues related to personal health. For links to these websites, visit the Companion Website for *Access to Health*, 12th Edition, at www.pearsonhighered.com/donatelle.

1. *American Dietetic Association*. This site includes recommended dietary guidelines and other current information about weight control. www.eatright.org

2. *Duke University Diet and Fitness Center*. This site includes information about one of the best programs in the country focused on helping people live healthier, fuller lives through weight control and lifestyle change. www.dukedietcenter.org

3. *F as in Fat: How Obesity Policies Are Failing in America*. This report provides an excellent summary of the current status of obesity, obesity policies, and programs in the United

States, as well as suggestions for new strategies and policies to reduce risks. http://healthyamericans.org/reports/obesity2009

4. *Weight Control Information Network*. This is an excellent resource for diet and weight-control information. http://win.niddk.nih.gov/index.htm

5. *The Rudd Center for Foods Policy and Obesity*. This website provides excellent information on the latest in obesity research, public policy, and ways we can stop the obesity epidemic at the community level. www.yaleruddcenter.org

## References

1. U.S. Department of Health and Human Services, *The Surgeon General's Vision for a Healthy and Fit Nation* (Rockville, MD: U.S. Department of Health and Human Services, Office of the Surgeon General, 2010), Available at www.surgeongeneral.gov/library/obesityvision.

2. K. M. Flegal et al., "Prevalence and Trends in Obesity among U.S. Adults, 1999–2008," *Journal of the American Medical Association* 303, no. 3 (2010): 235–41.

3. Ibid.

4. S. Steward et al., "Forecasting the Effects of Obesity and Smoking on U.S. Life Expectancy," *New England Journal of Medicine* 361, no. 23 (2009): 2252–60.

5. S. Anderson and R. Whitaker, "Prevalence of Obesity among U.S. Preschool Children in Different Racial and Ethnic Groups," *Archives of Pediatrics and Adolescent Medicine* 163, no. 4 (2009): 344–48.

6. C. Ogden, "Disparities in Obesity Prevalence in the United States: Black Women at Risk," *American Journal of Clinical Nutrition* 89, no. 4 (2009): 1001–02.

7. C. Ogden et al., "Prevalence of High Body Mass Index in U.S. Children and Adolescents, 2007–2008," *JAMA: The Journal of the American Medical Association* 303, no. 3 (2010): 242–49.

8. K. M. Flegal and B. I. Graubard, "Estimates of Excess Deaths Associated with Body Mass Index and Other Anthropometric Variables," *American Journal of Clinical Nutrition* 89, no. 4 (2009): 1213–19; J. P. Reis et al., "Comparison of Overall Obesity and Body Fat Distribution in Predicting Risk of Mortality," *Obesity* 17, no. 6 (2009): 1232–39; J. P. Reis et al., "Overall Obesity and Abdominal Adiposity as Predictors of Mortality in U.S. White and Black Adults,"

*Annals of Epidemiology* 19, no. 2 (2009): 2134–42.

9. N. Pandey and V. Gupta, "Trends in Diabetes," *Lancet* 369, no. 14 (2007): 1256–57.

10. E. Finkelstein et al., "Annual Medical Spending Attributable to Obesity: Payer- and Service-Specific Estimates," *Health Affairs* 28, no. 5 (2009): w822–w831.

11. J. Bhattacharya and K. Bundorf, "The Incidence of the Healthcare Costs of Obesity," *Journal of Health Economics* 28, no. 3 (2009): 649–58.

12. K. Butcher and K. Park, "Obesity, Disability, and the Labor Force," *Economic Perspectives* 32, no. 1 (2008): 2–16; H. Chen and X. Guo, "Obesity and Functional Disability in Elderly Americans," *Journal of the American Geriatrics Society* 56, no. 4 (2008): 689–94; A. Peeters et al., "Adult Obesity and the Burden of Disability throughout Life," *Obesity Research* 12, no. 7 (2004): 1145–51.

13. World Health Organization, "Global Strategy on Diet, Physical Activity and Health: Obesity and Overweight," 2009, www.who.int/dietphysicalactivity/publications/facts/obesity/en.

14. Ibid.

15. U.S. Department of Health and Human Services, *Surgeon General's Call to Action to Prevent and Decrease Overweight and Obesity* (Washington, DC: USOHHS, 2005), Available at www.surgeongeneral.gov/topics/obesity/calltoaction/toc.htm.

16. J. Spence et al., "Relation between Local Food Environments and Obesity among Adults," *BMC Public Health* 9, no. 1 (2009): 192.

17. D. Cummings and M. Schwartz, "Genetics and Pathophysiology of Human Obesity," *Annual Review of Medicine* 54 (2003): 453–71.

18. K. Silventoinen et al., "The Genetic and Environmental Influences on Childhood Obesity: A Systematic Review of Twin and Adoption Studies," *International Journal of Obesity* 34, no. 1 (2010): 29–40.

19. S. Li et al., "Cumulative and Predictive Value of Common Obesity—Susceptibility Variants Identified by Genome-wide Association Studies," *American Journal of Clinical Nutrition* 91, no. 1 (2010): 184–90.

20. H. Chang, "Scientists Probe the Role of the Brain in Obesity," *Journal of the American Medical Association* 303, no. 1 (2010): 19–20.

21. C. Bouchard, "Defining the Genetic Architecture of the Predisposition to Obesity: A Challenging but Not Insurmountable Task," *American Journal of Clinical Nutrition* 91, no. 1 (2010): 5–6.

22. C. Bouchard, "Thrifty Gene Hypothesis: Maybe Everyone Is Right?" *International Journal of Obesity* 32, no. 4 (2008): 25–27; R. Stoger, "The Thrifty Epigenotype: An

Acquired and Heritable Predisposition for Obesity and Diabetes?" *Bioessays* 30, no. 2 (2008): 156–66.

23. C. Bouchard, "Defining the Genetic Architecture of the Predisposition to Obesity," 2010; S. Li et al., "Cumulative and Predictive Value of Common Obesity," 2010.

24. E. Schuer et al., "Activation in Brain Energy Regulation and Reward Centers by Food Cues Varies with Choice of Visual Stimulation," *International Journal of Obesity* 33, no. 6 (2009): 653–61.

25. T. Reinehr et al., "Thyroid Hormones and Their Relation to Weight Status," *Hormone Research* 70, no. 1 (2008): 51–57.

26. D. E. Cummings et al., "Plasma Ghrelin Levels after Diet-Induced Weight Loss or Gastric Bypass Surgery," *New England Journal of Medicine* 346, no. 21 (2002): 1623–30.

27. C. DeVriese et al., "Focus on the Short- and Long-Term Effects of Ghrelin on Energy Homeostasis," *Nutrition* 26, no. 6 (2010): 579–84; T. Castaneda et al., "Ghrelin in the Regulation of Body Weight and Metabolism," *Frontiers in Neuroendocrinology* 31, no. 1 (2010): 44–60.

28. V. Paracchini et al., "Genetics of Leptin and Obesity: A HuGE Review," *American Journal of Epidemiology* 162, no. 2 (2005): 101–14; Y. Friedlander et al., "Leptin, Insulin, and Obesity-Related Phenotypes: Genetic Influences on Levels and Longitudinal Changes," *Obesity* 17, no. 7 (2009): 1458–60.

29. L. K. Mahan and S. Escott-Stump, *Krause's Food, Nutrition, and Diet Therapy* (New York: W. B. Saunders, 2000).

30. J. Spence et al., "Relation between Local Food Environments and Obesity among Adults," 2009; T. Harder et al., "Duration of Breast Feeding and Risk of Overweight," *American Journal of Epidemiology* 162, no. 5 (2005): 397–403; M. Wang et al., "Changes in Neighbourhood Food Store Environment, Food Behaviour, and Body Mass Index, 1981–1990," *Public Health Nutrition* 11, no. 9 (2008): 963–70; R. Havermans et al., "Food Liking, Food Wanting, and Sensory Specific Satiety," *Appetite.* 52, no. 1 (2009): 222–25; J. Smith and T. Ditschun, "Controlling Satiety: How Environmental Factors Influence Food Intake," *Trends in Food Science and Technology* 20, nos. 6–7 (2009): 271–77.

31. M. Treuth et al., "A Longitudinal Study of Sedentary Behavior and Overweight in Adolescent Girls," *Obesity* 17, no. 5 (2009): 1003–08.

32. B. Levin, "Synergy of Nurture and Nature in the Development of Childhood Obesity," *International Journal of Obesity* 33, Suppl 1 (2009): S53–S56.

33. S. Anderson and R. Whitaker, "Prevalence of Obesity among U.S. Preschool Children in Different Racial and Ethnic Groups," 2009.

34. R. Puhl and C. Heuer, "Obesity Stigma: Important Considerations for Public Health," *American Journal of Public Health* 100, no. 6 (2010): 1019–28; W. Craig et al., "Understanding and Addressing Obesity and Victimization in Youth," *Obesity and Weight Management* 6, no. 1 (2010): 12–16.

35. M. Beydoun et al., "The Association of Fast Food, Fruit, and Vegetable Prices with Dietary Intakes among U.S. Adults: Is There Modification by Family Income?" *Social Science and Medicine* 66, no. 11 (2008): 2218–29; J. Tillotson, "Americans' Food Shopping in Today's Lousy Economy," *Nutrition Today* 44, no. 5 (2009): 218–21.

36. F. Li et al., "Built Environment, Adiposity, and Physical Activity in Adults Aged 50–75," *American Journal of Preventive Medicine* 35, no. 1 (2008): 38–46.

37. A. Roskam et al., "Comparative Appraisal of Educational Inequalities in Overweight and Obesity among Adults in 19 European Countries," *International Journal of Epidemiology* 39, no. 2 (2010): 392–404.

38. Centers for Disease Control and Prevention, "U.S. Physical Activity Statistics," Updated February 2010, www.cdc.gov/nccdphp/dnpa/physical/stats/index.htm; National Center for Health Statistics, "Prevalence of Sedentary Leisure Time Behavior among Adults in the United States," Updated February 2010, www.cdc.gov/nchs/data/hestat/sedentary/sedentary.htm.

39. C. Schoenborn and P. Adams, "Health Behaviors of Adults, United States: 2005–2007," National Center for Health Statistics, *Vital Health Statistics* 10, no. 245 (2010).

40. American Heart Association, "Body Composition Tests," 2010, www.americanheart.org/presenter.jhtml?identifier=4489.

41. Obesity Society, "What Is Obesity?" Accessed November 2009, www.obesity.org/information/what_is_obesity.asp.

42. Centers for Disease Control and Prevention, "Defining Overweight and Obesity," Updated June 2010, www.cdc.gov/obesity/defining.html.

43. K. Flegal et al., "Prevalence and Trends in Obesity among U.S. Adults, 1999–2008," 2010.

44. J. Hill and H. Wyatt, "Is It OK to Call Children Obese?" *Obesity Management* 2, no. 4 (2006): 131–32.

45. Centers for Disease Control and Prevention, "About BMI for Children and Teens," Updated January 2009, www.cdc.gov/healthyweight/assessing/bmi/childrens_BMI/about_childrens_BMI.html.

46. National Heart, Lung, and Blood Institute, "Classification of Overweight and Obesity by BMI, Waist Circumference and Associated Disease Risks," 2009, www.nhlbi.nih.gov/health/public/heart/obesity/lose_wt/bmi_dis.htm.

47. Rush University, "Waist to Hip Ratio Calculator," Accessed May 2010, www.rush.edu/itools/hip/hipcalc.html.

48. F. Fernandez-Aranda et al., "Individual and Family Eating Patterns during Childhood and Early Adolescence: An Analysis of Associated Eating Disorder Factors," *Appetite* 49, no. 2 (2007): 476–85.

49. J. Thompson and M. Manore, *Nutrition: An Applied Approach,* 2d ed. (San Francisco: Benjamin Cummings, 2009), 126.

50. D. Rucker et al., "Long-Term Pharmacotherapy for Obesity and Overweight: Updated Meta-Analysis," *British Medical Journal* 335, no. 7631 (2007): 1194–99.

51. U.S. Food and Drug Administration, "Fen-Phen Safety Update Information," Updated September 2009, www.fda.gov/Drugs/DrugSafety/PostmarketDrugSafetyInformationforPatientsandProviders/ucm072820.htm.

52. U.S. Food and Drug Administration, "Follow-Up to the November 2009 Early Communication about an Ongoing Safety Review of Sibutramine, Marketed as Meridia," January 2010, www.fda.gov/Drugs/DrugSafety/PostmarketDrugSafetyInformationforPatientsandProviders/DrugSafetyInformationforHeathcareProfessionals/ucm198206.htm.

53. ConsumerSearch, "Diet Pills: Reviews," 2008, www.consumersearch.com/diet-pills.

54. F. Rubino et al., "Metabolic Surgery to Treat Type 2 Diabetes: Clinical Outcomes and Mechanisms of Action," *Annual Review of Medicine* 61 (2010): 393–411; E. Karra et al., "Mechanisms Facilitating Weight Loss and Resolution of Type 2 Diabetes Following Bariatric Surgery," *Trends in Endocrinology and Metabolism* 21, no. 6 (2010): 227–344.

55. C. Mottin et al., "Behavior of Type 2 Diabetes Mellitus in Morbid Obese Patients Submitted to Gastric Bypass," *Obesity Surgery* 18, no. 2 (2008): 179–82.

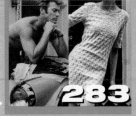
**283** Is the media's obsession with appearance a new phenomenon?

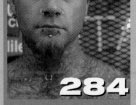
**284** Do people who keep changing their looks really hate their bodies?

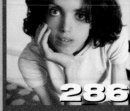
**286** Can eating disorders lead to a person's death?

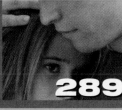
**289** How can I talk to a friend about an eating disorder?

# FOCUS ON

## Enhancing Your Body Image

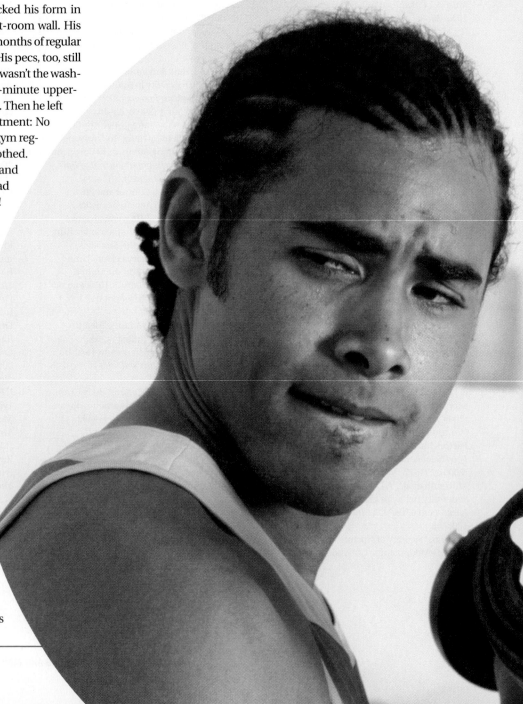

As he began his arm curls, Ali checked his form in the full-length mirror on the weight-room wall. His biceps were bulking up, but after 6 months of regular weight training, he expected more. His pecs, too, still lacked definition, and his abdomen wasn't the washboard he envisioned. So after a 45-minute upper-body workout, he added 200 sit-ups. Then he left the gym to shower back at his apartment: No way was he going to risk any of the gym regulars seeing his flabby torso unclothed. But by the time Ali got home and looked in the mirror, frustration had turned to anger. He was just too fat! To punish himself for his slow progress, instead of taking a shower, he put on his Nikes and went for a 4-mile run.

When you look in the mirror, do you like what you see? If you feel disappointed, frustrated, or even angry like Ali, you're not alone. A spate of recent studies is revealing that a majority of adults are dissatisfied with their bodies. For instance, a study of men in the United States, Austria, and France found that the ideal bodies they envisioned for themselves were an average of 28 pounds more muscular than their actual bodies. Most adult women—80 percent in one study—are also dissatisfied with their appearance, but for a different reason: Most want to lose weight.[1] Tragically, negative feelings about one's body can contribute to disordered eating, excessive exercise, and other behaviors that can threaten your health—and your life. Having a healthy body image is a key indicator of self-esteem, and can contribute to reduced stress, an increased sense of personal empowerment, and more joyful living.

# What Is Body Image?

This chapter focuses on body image because it's so fundamental to our sense of who we are. Consider the fact that mirrors made from polished stone have been found at archaeological sites dat-

> Dissatisfaction with one's appearance and shape is an all-too-common feeling in today's society that can foster unhealthy attitudes and thought patterns, as well as disordered eating and exercising behaviors.

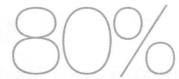

## 80%

**of adult American women report dissatisfaction with their appearance.**

ing from before 6000 BCE; humans have been viewing themselves for millennia.[2] But the term **body image** refers to more than just what you see when you look in a mirror. The National Eating Disorders Association (NEDA) identifies several additional components of body image:[3]

- How you see yourself in your mind
- What you believe about your own appearance (including your memories, assumptions, and generalizations)
- How you feel about your body, including your height, shape, and weight
- How you sense and control your body as you move

NEDA identifies a *negative body image* as either a distorted perception of your shape, or feelings of discomfort, shame, or anxiety about your body. You may be convinced that only other people are attractive, whereas your own body is a sign of personal failure. Does this attitude remind you of Ali? It should, because he clearly exhibits signs of a negative body image. In contrast, NEDA describes a *positive body image* as a true perception of your appearance: You see yourself as you really are. You understand that everyone is different, and you celebrate your uniqueness—including your "flaws," which you know have nothing to do with your value as a person.

Is your body image negative or positive—or is it somewhere in between? Researchers at the University of Arizona have developed a body image continuum that may help you decide (see **Figure 1**). Like a spectrum of light, a continuum represents a series of stages that aren't entirely distinct. Notice that the continuum identifies behaviors associated with particular states, from total dissociation with one's body to body acceptance and body ownership.

# Many Factors Influence Body Image

You're not born with a body image, but you do begin to develop one at an early age as you compare yourself against images you see in the world around you, and interpret the responses of family members and peers to your appearance. Let's look more closely at the factors that probably played a role in the development of your body image.

## The Media and Popular Culture

Today images of six-pack loaded actors such as Taylor Lautner send young women to the movies in hoards and snapshots of emaciated celebrities such as Lindsay Lohan and Paris Hilton dominate the tabloids and sell magazines. The images and celebrities in the media set the standard for what we find attractive, leading some people to go to dangerous extremes to have the biggest biceps or fit into size 2 jeans. Most of us think of this obsession with appearance as a recent phenomenon. The truth is, it has long been part of American culture. During the early twentieth century, while men idolized the hearty outdoorsman President Teddy Roosevelt, women pulled their corsets ever tighter to achieve unrealistically tiny waists. In the 1920s and 1930s, men emulated the burly cops and robbers in gangster films, while women dieted and bound their breasts to achieve the boyish "flapper" look. After World War II, both men and women strove for a healthy, wholesome appearance, but by the 1960s, tough-guys like Clint Eastwood and Marlon Brando were the male ideal, whereas rail-thin supermodel Twiggy embodied the nation's standard of female beauty.

Today, more than 66 percent of Americans are overweight or obese; thus, a significant disconnect exists between the media's idealized images of male and female bodies and the typical American body.[4] At the same time, the media—in the form of television, the Internet, movies, and print publications—is a

---

**body image** Most fundamentally, how you see yourself when you look in a mirror or picture yourself in your mind and how you feel about your body.

| Body hate/ dissociation | Distorted body image | Body preoccupied/ obsessed | Body acceptance | Body ownership |
|---|---|---|---|---|
| I often feel separated and distant from my body—as if it belongs to someone else. | I spend a significant amount of time exercising and dieting to change my body. | I spend a significant amount of time viewing my body in the mirror. | I base my body image equally on social norms and my own self-concept. | My body is beautiful to me. |
| I don't see anything positive or even neutral about my body shape and size. | My body shape and size keep me from dating or finding someone who will treat me the way I want to be treated. | I spend a significant amount of time comparing my body to others. | I pay attention to my body and my appearance because it is important to me, but it only occupies a small part of my day. | My feelings about my body are not influenced by society's concept of an ideal body shape. |
| I don't believe others when they tell me I look OK. | I have considered changing or have changed my body shape and size through surgical means so I can accept myself. | I have days when I feel fat. | I nourish my body so it has the strength and energy to achieve my physical goals. | I know that the significant others in my life will always find me attractive. |
| I hate the way I look in the mirror and often isolate myself from others. | | I am preoccupied with my body. | | |
| | | I accept society's ideal body shape and size as the best body shape and size. | | |

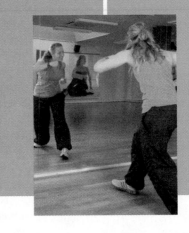

FIGURE 1 Body Image Continuum

This is part of a two-part continuum, the second part of which is shown in Figure 2. Individuals whose responses fall to the far left side of the continuum have a highly negative body image, whereas responses to the right indicate a positive body image.

**Source:** Adapted from Smiley/King/Avery, Campus Health Service. Original continuum, C. Schislak, *Preventive Medicine and Public Health.* Copyright © 1997 Arizona Board of Regents. Used with permission.

more powerful and pervasive presence than ever before. In fact, one study of more than 4,000 television commercials revealed that approximately one out of every four sends some sort of "attractiveness message."[5] Thus, Americans are bombarded daily with messages telling us that we just don't measure up.

**Family, Community, and Cultural Groups** The members of society with whom we most often interact—our family members, friends, and others—strongly influence the way we see ourselves. Parents are especially influential in body image development. For instance, it's common and natural for fathers of adolescent girls to experience feelings of discomfort related to their daughters' changing bodies. If they are

able to navigate these feelings successfully, and validate the acceptability of their daughters' appearance throughout puberty, it's likely that they'll help their daughters maintain a positive body image. In contrast, if they verbalize or indicate even subtle judgments about their daughters' changing bodies, girls may begin to question how members of the opposite sex view their bodies in general. In addition, mothers who model body acceptance or body ownership may be more likely to foster a similar positive body image in their daughters, whereas mothers who are frustrated with or ashamed of their bodies may have a greater chance of fostering these attitudes in their daughters.

Interactions with siblings and other relatives, peers, teachers, coworkers,

and other community members can also influence body image development. For instance, peer harassment (teasing and bullying) is widely acknowledged to contribute to a negative body image. Moreover, associations within one's cultural group appear to influence body image. For example, studies have found that European American females experience the highest rates of body dissatisfaction, and as a minority group becomes more acculturated into the mainstream, the body dissatisfaction levels of women in that group increase.[6]

Body image also reflects the larger culture in which you live. In parts of Africa, for example, obesity has been associated with abundance, erotic desirability, and fertility. Girls in Mauritania traditionally were force-fed to

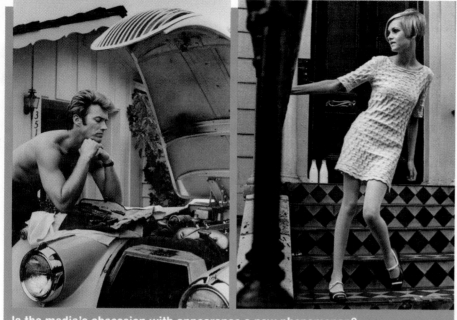

**Is the media's obsession with appearance a new phenomenon?**

Although the exact nature of the "in" look may change from generation to generation, unrealistic images of both male and female celebrities are nothing new. For example, in the 1960s, images of brawny film stars such as Clint Eastwood and ultrathin models such as Twiggy dominated the media.

increase their body size in order to signal a family's wealth, although the practice has become much less common in recent years.[7]

**Physiological and Psychological Factors** Recent neurological research has suggested that people who have been diagnosed with a body image disorder show differences in the brain's ability to regulate chemicals called *neurotransmitters*, which are linked to mood.[8] Poor regulation of neurotransmitters is also involved in depression and in anxiety disorders, including obsessive-compulsive disorder (see Chapter 2). One study linked distortions in body image to a malfunctioning in the brain's visual processing region that was revealed by MRI scanning.[9]

## How Can I Build a More Positive Body Image?

If you want to develop a more positive body image, your first step might be to bust some toxic myths and challenge some commonly held attitudes in con-

temporary society. Have you been accepting these four myths?[10] How would you answer the questions that accompany them?

**Myth 1:** How you look is more important than who you are. Do you think your weight is important in defining who you are? How much does your weight matter to your success? How much does it matter to you to have friends who are thin and attractive? How important do you think being thin is in trying to attract your ideal partner?

**Myth 2:** Anyone can be slender and attractive if they work at it. When you see someone who is extremely thin, what assumptions do you make about that person? When you see someone who is overweight or obese, what assumptions do you make? Have you ever berated

yourself for not having the "willpower" to change some aspect of your body?

**Myth 3:** Extreme dieting is an effective weight-loss strategy. Do you believe in trying fad diets or "quick-weight-loss" products? How far would you be willing to go to attain the "perfect" body?

**Myth 4:** Appearance is more important than health. How do you evaluate whether a person is healthy? Do you believe it's possible for overweight people to be healthy? Is your desire to change some aspect of your body motivated by health reasons or by concerns about appearance?

To learn ways to bust these toxic myths and attitudes, and to build a more positive body image, check out the **Skills for Behavior Change** box on page 284.

## Some People Develop Body Image Disorders

Although most Americans are dissatisfied with some aspect of their appearance, very few have a true body image disorder. However, several diagnosable body image disorders affect a small percentage of the population. Let's look at two of the most common.

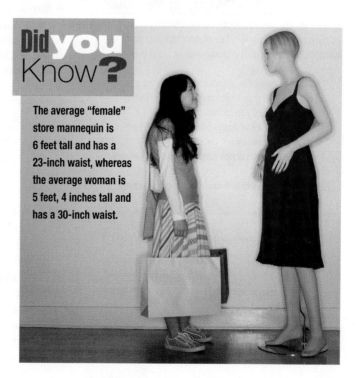

**Did you Know?**

The average "female" store mannequin is 6 feet tall and has a 23-inch waist, whereas the average woman is 5 feet, 4 inches tall and has a 30-inch waist.

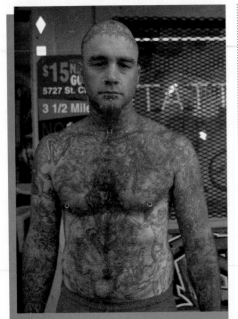

**Do people who keep changing their looks really hate their bodies?**

It's not always easy to spot people who are highly dissatisfied with their bodies, as they don't necessarily stick out in a crowd. For instance, people who cover their bodies with tattoos may have a strong sense of self-esteem. On the other hand, extreme tattooing can be an outward sign of a severe body image disturbance known as *body dysmorphic disorder*.

## What's 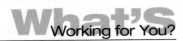 Working for You?

Maybe you're already focusing on building a positive body image. Below is a list of some behaviors that contribute to a positive body image. Which of these is true for you?

☐ I surround myself with people who are supportive of me and help to build me up, rather than being critical of me or others.

☐ I ignore media messages that put an emphasis on physical appearances.

☐ I wear clothes that are comfortable and make me feel good.

☐ I remind myself that beauty is not just outer appearance.

### Body Dysmorphic Disorder (BDD)

Approximately 1 percent of people in the United States suffer from **body dysmorphic disorder (BDD)**.[11] Persons with

**body dysmorphic disorder (BDD)** Psychological disorder characterized by an obsession with a minor or imagined flaw in appearance.

# Ten Steps to a Positive Body Image

One list cannot automatically tell you how to turn negative body thoughts into a positive body image, but it can help you think about new ways of looking more healthfully and happily at yourself and your body. The more you do that, the more likely you are to feel good about who you are and the body you naturally have.

✳ **Step 1.** Appreciate all that your body can do. Every day your body carries you closer to your dreams. Celebrate all of the amazing things your body does for you—running, dancing, breathing, laughing, dreaming.

✳ **Step 2.** Keep a list of things you like about yourself—things that aren't related to how much you weigh or how you look. Read your list often. Add to it as you become aware of more things to like about yourself.

✳ **Step 3.** Remind yourself that true beauty is not simply skin deep. When you feel good about yourself and who you are, you carry yourself with a sense of confidence, self-acceptance, and openness that makes you beautiful. Beauty is a state of mind, not a state of your body.

✳ **Step 4.** Look at yourself as a whole person. When you see yourself in a mirror or in your mind, choose not to focus on specific body parts. See yourself as you want others to see you—as a whole person.

✳ **Step 5.** Surround yourself with positive people. It is easier to feel good about yourself and your body when you are around others who are supportive and who recognize the importance of liking yourself just as you naturally are.

✳ **Step 6.** Shut down those voices in your head that tell you your body is not "right" or that you are a "bad" person. You can overpower those negative thoughts with positive ones.

✳ **Step 7.** Wear clothes that are comfortable and that make you feel good about your body. Work with your body, not against it.

✳ **Step 8.** Become a critical viewer of social and media messages. Pay attention to images, slogans, or attitudes that make you feel bad about yourself or your body. Protest these messages: Write a letter to the advertiser or talk back to the image or message.

✳ **Step 9.** Do something nice for yourself—something that lets your body know you appreciate it. Take a bubble bath, make time for a nap, or find a peaceful place outside to relax.

✳ **Step 10.** Use the time and energy that you might have spent worrying about food, calories, and your weight to do something to help others. Sometimes reaching out to other people can help you feel better about yourself and can make a positive change in our world.

**Source:** Reprinted with permission from the National Eating Disorders Association, www.NationalEatingDisorders.org.

BDD are obsessively concerned with their appearance, and have a distorted view of their own body shape, body size, weight, perceived lack of muscles, facial blemishes, size of body parts, and so on. Although the precise cause of the disorder isn't known, an anxiety disorder such as obsessive-compulsive disorder is often present as well. (Anxiety disorders are discussed in Chapter 2.)

Contributing factors may include genetic susceptibility, childhood teasing, physical or sexual abuse, low self-esteem, and rigid sociocultural expectations of beauty.[12]

People with BDD may try to fix their perceived flaws through abuse of steroids, excessive bodybuilding, repeated cosmetic surgeries, extreme tattooing, or other appearance-altering behaviors. It is estimated that 10 percent of people seeking dermatology or cosmetic treatments have BDD.[13] Not only do such actions fail to address the underlying problem, but they are actually considered diagnostic signs of BDD. In contrast, psychiatric treatment, including psychotherapy and/or antidepressant medications, is often successful.

**Social Physique Anxiety** An emerging problem, seen in both young men and women, is **social physique anxiety (SPA).** Consider this a concern about your appearance taken to the extreme: The desire to "look good" is so strong that it has a destructive and sometimes disabling effect on the person's ability to function effectively in relationships and interactions with others. People suffering from SPA may spend a disproportionate amount of time fixating on their bodies, working out, and performing tasks that are ego centered and self-directed, rather than focusing on interpersonal relationships and general tasks.[14] Experts speculate that this anxiety may contribute to disordered eating behaviors (discussed below).

# What Is Disordered Eating?

As we've seen, people with a negative body image can fixate on a wide range of physical "flaws," from thinning hair to flat feet. Still, the "flaw" that causes

**social physique anxiety (SPA)** A desire to look good that has a destructive effect on a person's ability to function well in social interactions and relationships.
**disordered eating** A pattern of atypical eating behaviors that is used to achieve or maintain a lower body weight.

distress to the majority of people with negative body image is overweight.

Some people channel their anxiety about their weight into self-defeating thoughts and harmful behaviors. Check out the eating issues continuum in **Figure 2**: The far left identifies a pattern of thoughts and behaviors associated with **disordered eating.** These behaviors can include chronic dieting, abuse of diet pills and laxatives, self-induced vomiting, and many others.

| Eating disordered | Disruptive eating patterns | Food preoccupied/obsessed | Concerned well | Food is not an issue |
|---|---|---|---|---|
| I regularly stuff myself and then exercise, vomit, or use diet pills or laxatives to get rid of the food or calories.<br><br>My friends and family tell me I am too thin.<br><br>I am terrified of eating fatty foods.<br><br>When I let myself eat, I have a hard time controlling the amount of food I eat.<br><br>I am afraid to eat in front of others. | I have tried diet pills, laxatives, vomiting, or extra time exercising in order to lose or maintain my weight.<br><br>I have fasted or avoided eating for long periods of time in order to lose or maintain my weight.<br><br>I feel strong when I can restrict how much I eat.<br><br>Eating more than I wanted to makes me feel out of control. | I think about food a lot.<br><br>I feel I don't eat well most of the time.<br><br>It's hard for me to enjoy eating with others.<br><br>I feel ashamed when I eat more than others or more than what I feel I should be eating.<br><br>I am afraid of getting fat.<br><br>I wish I could change how much I want to eat and what I am hungry for. | I pay attention to what I eat in order to maintain a healthy body.<br><br>I may weigh more than what I like, but I enjoy eating and balance my pleasure with eating with my concern for a healthy body.<br><br>I am moderate and flexible in goals for eating well.<br><br>I try to follow the USDA's Dietary Guidelines for healthy eating. | I am not concerned about what others think regarding what and how much I eat.<br><br>When I am upset or depressed, I eat whatever I am hungry for without any guilt or shame.<br><br>Food is an important part of my life but only occupies a small part of my time. |

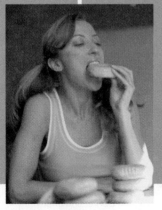 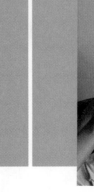 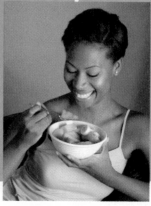

FIGURE 2 **Eating Issues Continuum**
This second part of the continuum shown in Figure 1 suggests that the progression from normal eating to eating disorders occurs on a continuum.

**Source:** Adapted from Smiley/King/Avery, Campus Health Service. Original continuum, C. Schislak, *Preventive Medicine and Public Health.* Copyright © 1997 Arizona Board of Regents. Used with permission.

# Some People Develop Eating Disorders

Only some people who exhibit disordered eating patterns progress to a clinical **eating disorder.** The diagnosis of an eating disorder can be applied only by a physician to a patient who exhibits severe disturbances in thoughts, behavior, and body functioning—disturbances that can prove fatal. These diagnostic criteria are defined by the American Psychiatric Association (APA), which in 2010 revised its categories of eating disorders to include binge-eating disorder. The APA-defined eating disorders are *anorexia nervosa, bulimia nervosa, binge-eating disorder,* and a cluster of less distinct conditions collectively referred to as *eating disorders not otherwise specified* (*EDNOS*).

In the United States, as many as 24 million people of all ages meet the established criteria for an eating disorder.[15] Although anorexia nervosa and bulimia nervosa affect people primarily in their teens and twenties, increasing numbers of children as young as 6 have been diagnosed, as have women as old as 76. In 2009, 3.2 percent of college students reported that they were dealing with either anorexia or bulimia.[16] Disordered eating and eating disorders are also common among athletes, affecting up to 62 percent of college athletes in sports such as gymnastics, wrestling, swimming, and figure skating.[17]

Eating disorders are on the rise among men, who currently represent up to 25 percent of anorexia and bulimia patients and almost 40 percent of binge eaters (a category within EDNOS).[18] Many men suffering from eating disorders fail to seek treatment, because these illnesses are traditionally thought of as being a woman's problem, and treatment centers are often geared toward women.

What factors put individuals at risk? Eating disorders are very complex, and despite scientific research to try to understand them, their biological, behavioral, and social underpinnings remain elusive. Many people with these disorders feel disenfranchised in other aspects of their lives, and try to gain a sense of control through food. Many are clinically depressed, suffer from obsessive-compulsive disorder, or have other psychiatric problems. In addition, studies have shown that individuals with low self-esteem, negative body image, and a high tendency for perfectionism are at risk.[19] Figure 3 shows how individual and social factors can interact to increase the risk of an eating disorder.

## Anorexia Nervosa

**Anorexia nervosa** is a persistent, chronic eating disorder characterized by deliberate food restriction and severe, life-threatening weight loss. It involves self-starvation motivated by an intense fear of gaining weight along with an extremely distorted body image. Initially, most people with anorexia nervosa lose weight by reducing total food intake, particularly of high-calorie foods. Eventually, they progress to restricting their intake of almost all foods. The little they do eat, they may purge through vomiting or using laxatives. Although they lose weight, people with anorexia nervosa never seem to feel thin enough and constantly identify body parts that are "too fat."

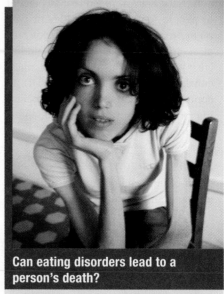

**Can eating disorders lead to a person's death?**

People with anorexia nervosa put themselves at risk for starving to death. In addition, they may die from sudden cardiac arrest caused by electrolyte imbalances; this is also a risk for people with bulimia nervosa. About 20% to 25% of people with a serious eating disorder die from it.

It is estimated that between 0.5 and 3.7 percent of females suffer from anorexia nervosa in their lifetime.[20] The revised APA criteria for anorexia nervosa are as follows:[21]

- Refusal to maintain body weight at or above a minimally normal weight for age and height

---

**eating disorder** A psychiatric disorder characterized by severe disturbances in body image and eating behaviors.

**anorexia nervosa** Eating disorder characterized by excessive preoccupation with food, self-starvation, or extreme exercising to achieve weight loss.

---

**Sociocultural factors**
- Family and personal relationships
- History of being teased
- History of abuse
- Cultural norms
- Media influences
- Economic status

**Psychological factors**
- Low self-esteem
- Feelings of inadequacy or lack of control
- Unhealthy body image
- Perfectionism
- Lack of coping skills

**Biological factors**
- Inherited personality traits
- Genes that affect hunger, satiety, and body weight
- Depression or anxiety
- Brain chemistry

FIGURE 3 **Factors That Contribute to Eating Disorders**

- Intense fear of gaining weight or becoming fat, even though considered underweight by all medical criteria
- Disturbance in the way in which one's body weight or shape is experienced, undue influence of body weight or shape on self-evaluation, or denial of the seriousness of the current low body weight

Physical symptoms and negative health consequences associated with anorexia nervosa are illustrated in **Figure 4**. Because it involves starvation and can lead to heart attacks and seizures, anorexia nervosa has the highest death rate (20%) of any psychological illness.

The causes of anorexia nervosa are complex and variable. Many people with anorexia have other coexisting psychiatric problems, including low self-esteem, depression, an anxiety disorder such as obsessive-compulsive disorder, and substance abuse. Some people have a history of being physically or sexually abused, and others have troubled interpersonal relationships with family members. Cultural norms that value people on the basis of their appearance and glorify thinness are of course a factor, as is weight-based teasing and weight bias.[22] Physical factors are thought to include an imbalance of neurotransmitters and genetic susceptibility.[23]

**Bulimia Nervosa** Individuals with **bulimia nervosa** often binge on huge amounts of food and then engage in some kind of purging, or "compensatory behavior," such as vomiting, taking laxatives, or exercising excessively, to lose the calories they have just consumed. People with bulimia are obsessed with their bodies, weight gain, and appearance, but unlike those with anorexia, their problem is often "hidden" from the public eye because their

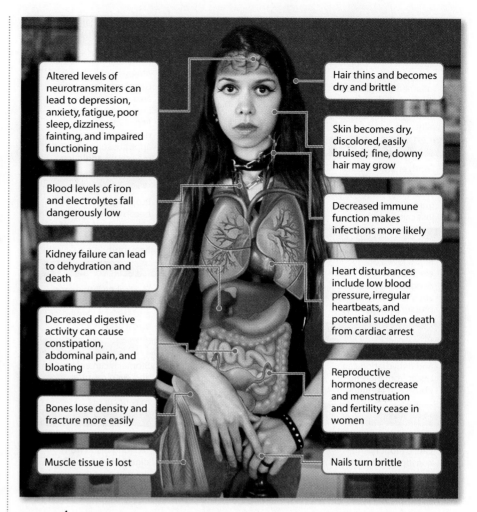

Altered levels of neurotransmitters can lead to depression, anxiety, fatigue, poor sleep, dizziness, fainting, and impaired functioning

Blood levels of iron and electrolytes fall dangerously low

Kidney failure can lead to dehydration and death

Decreased digestive activity can cause constipation, abdominal pain, and bloating

Bones lose density and fracture more easily

Muscle tissue is lost

Hair thins and becomes dry and brittle

Skin becomes dry, discolored, easily bruised; fine, downy hair may grow

Decreased immune function makes infections more likely

Heart disturbances include low blood pressure, irregular heartbeats, and potential sudden death from cardiac arrest

Reproductive hormones decrease and menstruation and fertility cease in women

Nails turn brittle

FIGURE 4 **What Anorexia Nervosa Can Do to the Body**

weight may fall within a normal range or they may be overweight.

Up to 3 percent of adolescents and young women are bulimic; rates among men are about 10 percent of the rate among women.[24] The revised APA diagnostic criteria for bulimia nervosa are as follows:[25]

- Recurrent episodes of binge eating (defined as eating, in a discrete period of time, an amount of food that is larger than most people would eat during a similar period of time and under simi-

lar circumstances, and experiencing a sense of lack of control over eating during the episode)
- Recurrent inappropriate compensatory behavior to prevent weight gain, such as self-induced vomiting; misuse of laxatives, diuretics, or other medications; fasting; or excessive exercise
- Binge eating and inappropriate compensatory behavior occurs on average at least once a week for 3 months
- Body shape and weight unduly influence self-evaluation
- The disturbance does not occur exclusively during episodes of anorexia nervosa

**bulimia nervosa** Eating disorder characterized by binge eating followed by inappropriate measures, such as vomiting, to prevent weight gain.

1 million **American males are estimated to struggle with some form of eating disorder.**

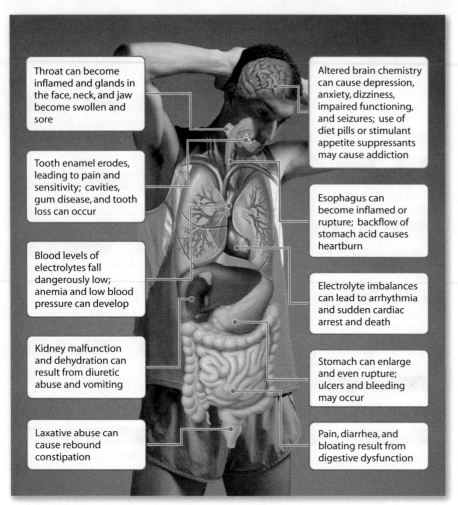

- Throat can become inflamed and glands in the face, neck, and jaw become swollen and sore

- Tooth enamel erodes, leading to pain and sensitivity; cavities, gum disease, and tooth loss can occur

- Blood levels of electrolytes fall dangerously low; anemia and low blood pressure can develop

- Kidney malfunction and dehydration can result from diuretic abuse and vomiting

- Laxative abuse can cause rebound constipation

- Altered brain chemistry can cause depression, anxiety, dizziness, impaired functioning, and seizures; use of diet pills or stimulant appetite suppressants may cause addiction

- Esophagus can become inflamed or rupture; backflow of stomach acid causes heartburn

- Electrolyte imbalances can lead to arrhythmia and sudden cardiac arrest and death

- Stomach can enlarge and even rupture; ulcers and bleeding may occur

- Pain, diarrhea, and bloating result from digestive dysfunction

FIGURE 5 **What Bulimia Nervosa Can Do to the Body**

Physical symptoms and negative health consequences associated with bulimia nervosa are shown in **Figure 5**. One of the more common symptoms of bulimia is tooth erosion, which results from the excessive vomiting associated with this disorder. Bulimics who vomit are also at risk for electrolyte imbalances and dehydration, both of which can contribute to a heart attack and sudden death.

A combination of genetic and environmental factors is thought to cause bulimia nervosa.[26] A family history of obesity, an underlying anxiety disorder, and an imbalance in neurotransmitters are all possible contributing factors. In support of the role of neurotransmitters,

**binge-eating disorder** A type of eating disorder characterized by binge eating once a week or more, but not typically followed by a compensatory behavior.

a recent study showed that brain circuitry involved in regulating impulsive behavior seems to be less active in women with bulimia than in normal women.[27] However, it is impossible at this point to determine whether such differences exist before bulimia develops or arise as a consequence of the disorder.

**Binge-Eating Disorder** Individuals with **binge-eating disorder** gorge like their bulimic counterparts but do not take excessive measures to lose the weight that they gain. Thus, they are often clinically obese. As in bulimia, binge-eating episodes are typically characterized by eating large amounts of food rapidly, even when not feeling hungry, and feeling guilty or depressed after overeating.[28]

A national survey on eating disorders conducted by Harvard-affiliated McLean Hospital reported that binge-eating disorder is more prevalent than either anorexia nervosa or bulimia nervosa. The survey showed that 3.5 percent of women and 2 percent of men experience binge-eating disorder at some point in their lives.[29] The revised APA criteria for binge-eating disorder are as follows:[30]

- Recurrent episodes of binge eating (defined as eating, in a discrete period of time, an amount of food that is larger than most people would eat during a similar period of time and under similar circumstances, and experiencing a sense of lack of control over eating during the episode)
- The binge-eating episodes are associated with three (or more) of the following: (1) eating much more rapidly than normal; (2) eating until feeling uncomfortably full; (3) eating large amounts of food when not feeling physically hungry; (4) eating alone

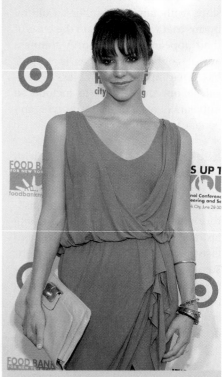

Katharine McPhee, the well-known singer, actress, and former *American Idol* contestant, has publicly discussed her past battles with bulimia and her successful recovery from the eating disorder. She continues to share her story to help other young women.

because of embarrassment over how much one is eating; (5) feeling disgusted with oneself, depressed, or very guilty after overeating
• Marked distress regarding binge eating is present
• The binge eating occurs, on average, at least once a week for 3 months
• The binge eating is not associated with the recurrent use of inappropriate compensatory behavior (i.e., purging) and does not occur exclusively during the course of bulimia nervosa or anorexia nervosa

**Some Eating Disorders Are Not Easily Classified** The APA recognizes that some patterns of disordered eating qualify as a legitimate psychiatric illness but don't fit into the strict diagnostic criteria for either anorexia, bulimia, or binge-eating disorder. These are the **eating disorders not otherwise specified (EDNOS).** This group of disorders can include night eating syndrome and recurrent purging in the absence of binge eating.

**Treatment for Eating Disorders**
Because eating disorders are caused by a combination of many factors, spanning many years of development, there are no quick or simple solutions. The bad news is that without treatment, approximately 20 percent of people with a serious eating disorder will die from it; with treatment, long-term full recovery rates range from 44 to 76 percent for anorexia nervosa and from 50 to 70 percent for bulimia nervosa.[31]

Treatment often focuses first on reducing the threat to life; once the patient is stabilized, long-term therapy focuses on the psychological, social, environmental, and physiological factors that have led to the problem. Therapy allows the patient to work on adopting new eating behaviors, building self-confidence, and finding other ways to deal with life's problems. Support groups can help the family and the individual learn to foster positive actions and interactions. Treatment of an underlying anxiety disorder or depression may also be a focus.

**what do you think?**
Is the national attention to the obesity epidemic likely to worsen the problems with eating disorders? Why or why not? ● What do you think can be done to increase awareness of eating disorders in the United States? ● Can you think of ways that eating disorders can effectively be prevented?

## How Can You Help Someone with Disordered Eating?

Although every situation is different, there are several things you can do if you suspect someone you know is struggling with disordered eating:[32]

• **Learn** as much as you can about disordered eating through books, articles, brochures, and trustworthy websites.

• **Know the differences** between facts and myths about weight, nutrition, and exercise. Being armed with this information can help you reason against any inaccurate ideas that your friend may be using as excuses to maintain a disordered eating pattern.

• **Be honest.** Talk openly and honestly about your concerns with your friend who is struggling with eating problems. Avoiding it or ignoring it is not the solution.

• **Be caring, but be firm.** Caring about your friend does not mean allowing him or her to manipulate you. Your friend must be responsible for his or her actions and the consequences of those actions. Avoid making rules or promises that you cannot or will not uphold, such as, "I promise not to tell

**eating disorders not otherwise specified (EDNOS)** Eating disorders that are a true psychiatric illness but do not fit the strict diagnostic criteria for anorexia nervosa, bulimia nervosa, or binge-eating disorder.

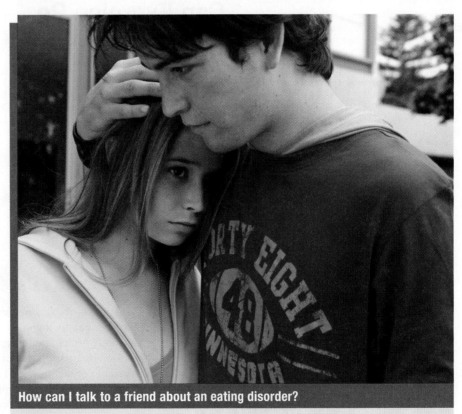

**How can I talk to a friend about an eating disorder?**

When talking to a friend about an eating disorder or disordered eating patterns, avoid casting blame, preaching, or offering unsolicited advice. Instead, be a good listener, let the person know that you care, and offer your support.

anyone," or, "If you do this one more time, I'll never talk to you again."

● **Compliment** your friend's personality, successes, or accomplishments.

● **Be a good role model** in regard to healthy eating, exercise, and self-acceptance.

● **Tell someone.** It may seem difficult to know when, if at all, to tell someone else about your concerns. Your friend needs as much support as possible, the sooner the better. Don't wait until the situation is so severe that your friend's life is in danger. Addressing disordered eating patterns in their beginning stages offers your friend the best chance for working through these issues and becoming healthy again.

## Can Eating Disorders Be Prevented?

As you've learned, eating disorders arise from a variety of physical, emo-

---

**compulsive exercise** Disorder characterized by a compulsion to engage in excessive amounts of exercise, and feelings of guilt and anxiety if the level of exercise is perceived as inadequate.

**muscle dysmorphia** Body image disorder in which men believe that their body is insufficiently lean or muscular.

---

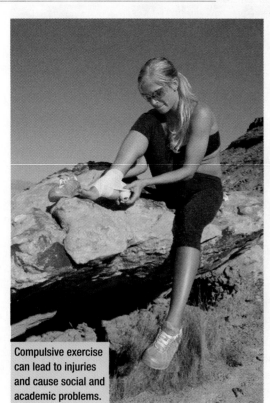

Compulsive exercise can lead to injuries and cause social and academic problems.

tional, social, and familial issues, all of which need to be addressed for effective prevention and treatment. Effective prevention must not only warn the public about the signs, symptoms, and dangers of eating disorders, but must also address the following:[33]

● Our cultural obsession with slenderness as a physical, psychological, and moral issue

● The roles of men and women in our society

● The development of people's self-esteem and self-respect in a variety of areas (school, work, community service, hobbies) that transcend physical appearance

Eating-disorders prevention programs are offered on many college campuses, and typically involve professionals with expertise in the field of eating disorders. Ideally, these provide opportunities for students to meet confidentially with mental health care providers.

## Can Exercise Be Unhealthy?

Although exercise is generally beneficial to health, in excess it can be a problem. In addition to being a common compensatory behavior used by people with anorexia or bulimia, exercise can become a compulsion, or contribute to either of two more complex disorders: muscle dysmorphia and the female athlete triad.

**"Why Should I Care?"**

Although exercising is generally beneficial to your health, doing it compulsively can lead to broken bones, joint injuries, and even depression—all of which can put you out of commission for the other things you enjoy. Remember that moderation is essential and taking rest days is important to your health.

## Some People Develop Exercise Disorders

A recent study of almost 600 college students revealed that 18 percent met the criteria for **compulsive exercise.**[34] Also called *anorexia athletica*, compulsive exercise is characterized not by a *desire* to exercise but a *compulsion* to do so. That is, the person struggles with guilt and anxiety if he or she doesn't work out. Compulsive exercisers, like people with eating disorders, often define their self-worth externally. They overexercise in order to feel more in control of their lives. Disordered eating or a true eating disorder is often part of the picture.

Compulsive exercise can contribute to a variety of other problems, including injuries to joints and broken bones. It can also put significant stress on the heart, especially if combined with disordered eating. Psychologically, people who engage in compulsive exercise are often plagued by anxiety and/or depression. Their social life and academic success can suffer as they fixate more and more on exercise.

**Muscle Dysmorphia** **Muscle dysmorphia** appears to be a relatively new form of body image disturbance and exercise disorder among men in which a man believes that his body is insufficiently lean or muscular.[35] Men with muscle dysmorphia believe that they look "puny," when in reality they look normal or may even be unusually muscular. As a result of their adherence to a meticulous diet, their time-consuming workout schedule, and their shame over their perceived appearance flaws, they may neglect important social or occupational activities. Other behaviors characteristic of muscle dysmorphia include comparing oneself unfavorably to others, checking one's appearance in the mirror, and camouflaging

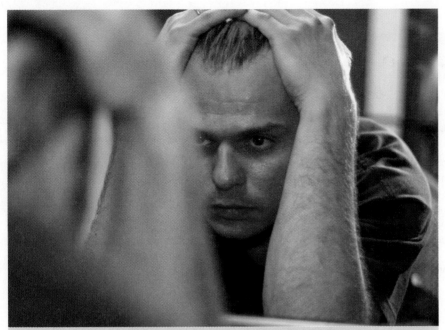
Men with muscle dysmorphia may have unusually muscular bodies but suffer from very low self-esteem.

one's appearance. Men with muscle dysmorphia also have higher rates of substance abuse and suicide than other men.[36]

**The Female Athlete Triad** Female athletes in competitive sports often strive for perfection. In an effort to be the best, they may do more damage than good, and put themselves at risk for developing a syndrome called the **female athlete triad.** *Triad* means "three," and the three interrelated problems are as follows (Figure 6):[37]

● Low energy intake, typically prompted by disordered eating behaviors
● Menstrual dysfunction such as amenorrhea
● Poor bone density

How does the female athlete triad develop, and what makes it so dangerous? First, a chronic pattern of low energy intake and intensive exercise alters normal body functions. For example, when an athlete restricts her eating, she can deplete her body stores of nutrients essential to health. At the same time, her body will begin to burn its stores of fat tissue for energy. Adequate body fat is essential to maintaining healthy levels of the female reproductive hormone *estrogen*; when an athlete isn't getting enough food, estrogen levels decline. This can manifest as amenorrhea: The body is using all calories to keep the athlete alive, and nonessential body functions such as menstruation cease. In addition, fat-soluble vitamins, calcium, and estrogen are all essential for dense, healthy bones, so their depletion weakens the athlete's bones, leaving her at high risk for fracture.

Not all athletes are equally prone to the female athlete triad: It is particularly prevalent in women who participate in highly competitive individual sports or activities that emphasize leanness and require the wearing of body-contouring clothing. Gymnasts, figure skaters, cross-country runners, and ballet dancers are among those at highest risk for the female athlete triad.

Warning signs of the female athlete triad include dry skin; light-headedness/fainting; lanugo (fine, downy hair covering the body); multiple injuries; and changes in endurance, strength, or speed. In addition, behaviors associated with the disorder include preoccupation with food and weight, compulsive exercising, use of weight-loss products or laxatives, trips to the bathroom during or immediately after eating, a decreased ability to concentrate, self-criticism, anxiety, and depression. Treatment can be challenging, and requires a multidisciplinary approach involving the athlete's coach and trainer, a sports medicine team, psychologist, and other professionals, as well as family members and friends.

**female athlete triad** A syndrome of three interrelated health problems seen in some female athletes: disordered eating, amenorrhea, and poor bone density.

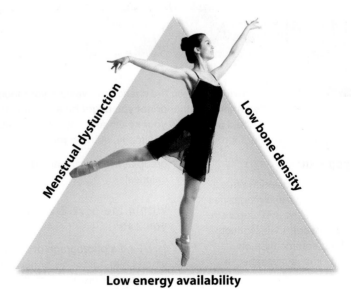

FIGURE 6 **The Female Athlete Triad**
The female athlete triad is a cluster of three interrelated health problems.

## Are Your Efforts to Be Thin Sensible— Or Spinning Out of Control?

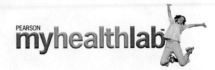

PEARSON
## myhealthlab™

Fill out this assessment online at www.pearsonhighered.com/myhealthlab or www.pearsonhighered.com/donatelle.

On one hand, just because you weigh yourself, count calories, or work out every day, don't jump to the conclusion that you have any of the health concerns discussed in this chapter. On the other hand, efforts to lose a few pounds can spiral out of control. To find out whether your efforts to be thin are harmful to you, take the following quiz from the National Eating Disorders Association (NEDA).

1. I constantly calculate numbers of fat grams and calories. **T F**

2. I weigh myself often and find myself obsessed with the number on the scale. **T F**

3. I exercise to burn calories and not for health or enjoyment. **T F**

4. I sometimes feel out of control while eating. **T F**

5. I often go on extreme diets. **T F**

6. I engage in rituals to get me through mealtimes and/or secretively binge. **T F**

7. Weight loss, dieting, and controlling my food intake have become my major concerns. **T F**

8. I feel ashamed, disgusted, or guilty after eating. **T F**

9. I constantly worry about the weight, shape, and/or size of my body. **T F**

10. I feel my identity and value are based on how I look or how much I weigh. **T F**

If any of these statements is true for you, you could be dealing with disordered eating. If so, talk about it! Tell a friend, parent, teacher, coach, youth group leader, doctor, counselor, or nutritionist what you're going through. Check out the NEDA's Sharing with EEEase handout at www.nationaleatingdisorders.org/nedaDir/files/documents/handouts/ShEEEase.pdf for help planning what to say the first time you talk to someone about your eating and exercise habits.

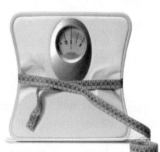

**Source:** Reprinted with permission from the National Eating Disorders Association, www.NationalEatingDisorders.org.

---

# YOUR PLAN FOR CHANGE

The **Assess yourself** activity gave you the chance to evaluate your feelings about your body, and to determine whether or not you might be engaging in eating or exercise behaviors that could undermine your health and happiness. Below are some steps you can take to improve your body image, starting today.

### Today, you can:

○ Talk back to the media. Write letters to advertisers and magazines that depict unhealthy and unrealistic body types. Boycott their products or start a blog commenting on harmful body image messages in the media.

○ Visit www.mypyramid.gov and print out your personalized food plan. Just for today, eat the recommended number of servings from every food group at every meal, and don't count calories!

### Within the next 2 weeks, you can:

○ Find a photograph of a person you admire *not* for his or her appearance, but for his or her contribution to humanity. Paste it up next to your mirror to remind yourself that true beauty comes from within and benefits others.

○ Start a diary. Each day, record one thing you are grateful for that has nothing to do with your appearance. At the end of each day, record one small thing you did to make someone's world a little brighter.

### By the end of the semester, you can:

○ Establish a group of friends who support you for who you are, not what you look like, and who get the same support from you. Form a group on a favorite social-networking site, and keep in touch, especially when you start to feel troubled by self-defeating thoughts or have the urge to engage in unhealthy eating or exercise behaviors.

○ Borrow from the library or purchase one of the many books on body image now available, and read it!

# References

1. H. G. Pope Jr. et al., "Body Image Perception among Men in Three Countries," *American Journal of Psychiatry* 157 (2000): 1297–1301; National Eating Disorders Association, "Statistics: Eating Disorders and Their Precursors," 2005, www.nationaleatingdisorders.org/information-resources/general-information.php#facts-statistics.

2. J. M. Enoch, "History of Mirrors Dating Back 8,000 Years," *Optometry and Vision Science* 83, no. 10 (2006): 775–81.

3. National Eating Disorders Association, "Body Image," 2005, Available at www.nationaleatingdisorders.org/information-resources/general-information.php#body-image-issues.

4. Centers for Disease Control and Prevention, "U.S. Obesity Trends 1985 to 2008," Updated November 2009, www.cdc.gov/obesity/data/trends.html.

5. National Eating Disorders Association, "The Media, Body Image, and Eating Disorders," 2005, www.nationaleatingdisorders.org/information-resources/general-information.php#body-image-issues.

6. S. Grogan, *Body Image: Understanding Body Dissatisfaction in Men, Women, and Children*, 2nd ed. (New York: Psychology Press, 2008), 159–61.

7. Associated Press, "Mauritania Struggles with Love of Fat Women," 2007, www.msnbc.msn.com/id/18141550.

8. Mayo Clinic Staff, "Body Dysmorphic Disorder," 2008, www.mayoclinic.com/health/body-dysmorphic-disorder/DS00559.

9. J. D. Feusner et al., "Visual Information Processing of Faces in Body Dysmorphic Disorder," *Archives of General Psychiatry* 64, no. 12 (2007): 1417–25.

10. K. Kater, "Building Healthy Body Esteem," *Healthy Body Image: Teaching Kids to Eat and Love Their Bodies Too* (Seattle: National Eating Disorders Association, 2005), Available at www.bodyimagehealth.org.

11. Mayo Clinic Staff, "Body Dysmorphic Disorder," 2008.

12. Mayo Clinic Staff, "Body Dysmorphic Disorder," 2008; KidsHealth, "Body Dysmorphic Disorder," 2007, http://kidshealth.org/parent/emotions/feelings/bdd.html.

13. Mayo Clinic Staff, "Body Dysmorphic Disorder," 2008.

14. G. Flett and P. Hewitt, "The Perils of Perfectionism in Sports and Exercise," *Current Directions in Psychological Science* 14, no. 1 (2005): 14–22; P. Crocker et al., "Examining Current Ideal Discrepancy Scores and Exercise Motivations as Predictors of Social Physique Anxiety in Exercising Females," *Journal of Sport Behavior* 28 (2005): 63–72.

15. Disordered Eating, UK, "Eating Disorders Statistics (U.S.)," 2010, www.disordered-eating.co.uk/eating-disorders-statistics/eating-disorders-statistics-us.html; National Eating Disorder Association, "Statistics: Eating Disorders and Their Precursors," 2005, www.nationaleatingdisorders.org/information-resources/general-information.php#facts-statistics.

16. American College Health Association, *National College Health Assessment Assessment II: Reference Group Executive Summary Fall 2009* (Linthicum, MD: American College Health Association, 2010), Available at www.acha-ncha.org/reports_ACHA-NCHAII.html.

17. K. Beals and A. Hill, "The Prevalence of Disordered Eating, Menstrual Dysfunction, and Low Bone Mineral Density among U.S. Collegiate Athletes," *International Journal of Sport Nutrition and Exercise Metabolism* 16, no. 3 (2006): 1–23; L. Ronco, "The Female Athlete Triad: When Women Push Their Limits in High-Performance Sports," *American Fitness* 25, no. 2 (2007): 22–24.

18. E. Bernstein, "Men, Boys Lack Options to Treat Eating Disorders," *Wall Street Journal* (April 17, 2007): D1–D2.

19. S. Forsberg and J. Lock, "The Relationship between Perfectionism, Eating Disorders and Athletes: A Review," *Minerva Pediatrica* 58, no. 6 (2006): 525–34.

20. K. Beals and A. Hill, "The Prevalence of Disordered Eating," 2006.

21. American Psychiatric Association, "DSM-5 Development: Proposed Revision: 307.1 Anorexia Nervosa," Updated October 2010, www.dsm5.org/ProposedRevisions/Pages/proposedrevision.aspx?rid=24.

22. A. L. Ahern et al., "Internalization of the Ultra-Thin Ideal: Positive Implicit Associations with Underweight Fashion Models Are Associated with Drive for Thinness in Young Women," *Eating Disorders* 16, no. 4 (2008): 294–307; M. Eisenberg and D. Neumark-Sztainer, "Peer Harassment and Disordered Eating," *International Journal of Adolescent Medicine and Health* 20, no. 2 (2008): 155–64.

23. National Eating Disorders Association, "Factors That May Contribute to Eating Disorders," 2004, www.nationaleatingdisorders.org/information-resources/general-information.php#causes-eating-disorders.

24. National Alliance on Mental Illness, "Bulimia Nervosa," 2010, www.nami.org/template.cfm?Section=by_illness&template=/ContentManagement/ContentDisplay.cfm&ContentID=65839.

25. American Psychiatric Association, "DSM-5 Development: Proposed Revision: 307.51 Bulimia Nervosa," Updated October 2010, www.dsm5.org/ProposedRevisions/Pages/proposedrevision.aspx?rid=25.

26. National Alliance on Mental Illness, "Bulimia Nervosa," 2010.

27. R. Marsh et al, "Deficient Activity in the Neural Systems That Mediate Self-Regulatory Control in Bulimia Nervosa," *Archives of General Psychiatry* 66, no. 1 (2009): 51–63.

28. J. Manwaring et al., "Risk Factors and Patterns of Onset in Binge Eating Disorder," *International Journal of Eating Disorders* 39, no. 2 (2005): 101–07.

29. J. Hudson et al., "The Prevalence and Correlates of Eating Disorders in the National Comorbidity Survey Replication," *Biological Psychiatry* 61, no. 3 (2007): 348–58.

30. American Psychiatric Association, "DSM-5 Development: Proposed Revision: Binge Eating Disorder," Updated October 2010, www.dsm5.org/ProposedRevisions/Pages/proposedrevision.aspx?rid=372.

31. K. N. Franco, Cleveland Clinic Center for Continuing Education, "Eating Disorders," www.clevelandclinicmeded.com/medicalpubs/diseasemanagement/psychiatry-psychology/eating-disorders, Accessed July 2010; Mirasol Eating Disorder Recovery Centers, "Eating Disorder Statistics," www.mirasol.net/eating-disorders/information/eating-disorder-statistics.php, Accessed July 2010.

32. National Eating Disorders Association, "How to Help a Friend with Eating and Body Image Issues," 2005, www.nationaleatingdisorders.org/information-resources/family-and-friends.php.

33. National Eating Disorders Association, "Eating Disorders Can Be Prevented!" 2005, www.nationaleatingdisorders.org/information-resources/general-information.php.

34. J. Guidi et al., "The Prevalence of Compulsive Eating and Exercise among College Students: An Exploratory Study," *Psychiatry Research* 165, nos. 1–2 (2009): 154–62.

35. C. G. Pope et al., "Clinical Features of Muscle Dysmorphia among Males with Body Dysmorphic Disorder," *Body Image* 2, no. 4 (2005): 395–400.

36. Ibid.

37. A. Nattiv et al., "American College of Sports Medicine Position Stand: The Female Athlete Triad," *Medicine and Science in Sports and Exercise* 39, no. 10 (2007): 1867–82.

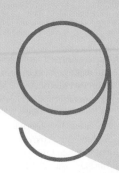

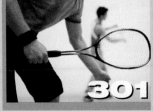

**301**

Can physical activity really reduce stress?

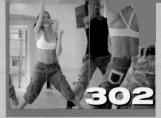

**302**

How can I motivate myself to be more physically active?

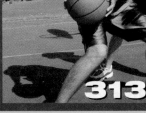

**313**

Why is core strength training important?

# Improving Your Physical Fitness

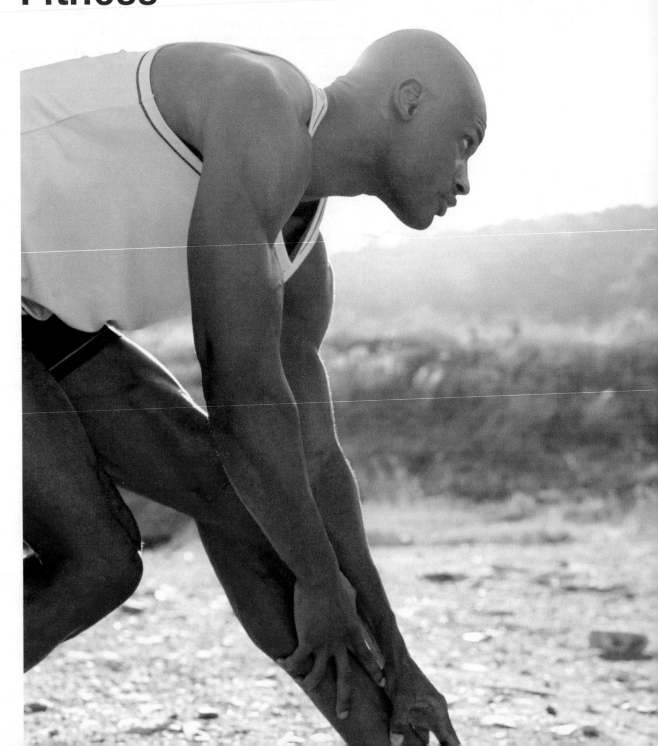

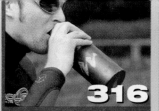

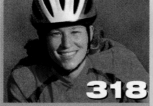

How much do I need to drink before, during, and after physical activity?

What can I do to avoid injury when I am physically active?

## Objectives

✳ Describe physical activity for health, for fitness, and for performance.

✳ Identify the motivating factors for getting physically fit, including benefits, fitness goals, and obstacles to overcome.

✳ Design a program that works for you, incorporating the key components of a personal fitness program.

✳ Understand and be able to use the FITT principle and to apply it to the different components of physical fitness.

✳ Summarize ways to prevent and treat common injuries related to physical activity.

Most Americans are aware of the wide range of physical, social, and mental health benefits of physical activity and that they should be more physically active. The physiological changes in the body that result from regular physical activity reduce the likelihood of coronary artery disease, high blood pressure, type 2 diabetes, obesity, and other chronic diseases. Further, engaging in physical activity regularly helps to control stress, increases self-esteem, and contributes to that "feel-good" feeling. It is no surprise that physical activity is often viewed as a panacea for health and disease prevention![1]

Despite the fact that they know the importance of physical activity for their health and wellness, most people are not sufficiently active for optimal health benefits. Recent statistics indicate that 25.4 percent of American adults do not engage in any leisure-time physical activity, or activity done during one's "down" time.[2] The growing percentage of Americans who live physically inactive lives (that is, perform no physical activity of low, moderate, or high intensity or engage in less than 10 minutes total per week of moderate or vigorous intensity lifestyle activities) has been linked to the current high incidences of obesity, type 2 diabetes, and other chronic and mental health diseases.[3]

In general, college students are more physically active than older adults are, but a recent survey indicated that 60 percent of college women and 50 percent of college men do not meet recommended guidelines for engaging in moderate or vigorous physical activities.[4] In another study, only 47 percent of men and 28 percent of women between the ages of 18 and 24 said they performed any strengthening activities or calisthenics in their leisure time.[5]

College is a great time to develop positive physical activity attitudes and behaviors that can increase the quality and quantity of your life. Now is the time to get moving. It may not be easy to change a sedentary lifestyle, but is definitely worth every effort made. This chapter will provide you with knowledge and strategies to help you get moving.

## what do you think?

Why do you think most college students aren't more physically active? ● Why do you think women are less likely than men to obtain sufficient levels of physical activity? ● Do you think your college or university years are a good time to become more physically active? Why or why not?

**27%** of American adults aged 18 and over report doing strength-training activities in their leisure time. Among all age groups except those aged 65 to 74 years, men are more likely than women to engage in leisure-time strengthening activities.

# Physical Activity for Health, Fitness, and Performance

**Physical activity** refers to all body movements produced by skeletal muscles resulting in substantial increases in energy expenditure.[6] Walking, swimming, strength training, dancing, and doing yoga are examples of physical activity. Physical activities can vary by intensity. For example, walking to class typically requires little effort, while walking to class uphill is more intense and harder to do. There are three general categories of physical activity defined by the purpose for which they are done: physical activity for health, physical activity for physical fitness, and physical activity for performance.

**Exercise** refers to a particular kind of physical activity. Although all exercise is physical activity, not all physical activity would be considered exercise. For example, walking from your car to class is physical activity, whereas going for a brisk 30-minute walk is considered exercise. *Exercise* is defined as planned, structured, and repetitive bodily movement done to improve or maintain one or more components of physical fitness, such as cardiorespiratory endurance, muscular strength or endurance, or flexibility.[7]

**physical activity** Refers to all body movements produced by skeletal muscles resulting in substantial increases in energy expenditure.

**exercise** Planned, structured, and repetitive bodily movement done to improve or maintain one or more components of physical fitness.

**physical fitness** Refers to a set of attributes that allow you to perform moderate- to vigorous-intensity physical activities on a regular basis without getting too tired and with energy left over to handle physical or mental emergencies.

**cardiorespiratory fitness** The ability of the heart, lungs, and blood vessels to supply oxygen to skeletal muscles during sustained physical activity.

**aerobic exercise** Any type of exercise that increases heart rate.

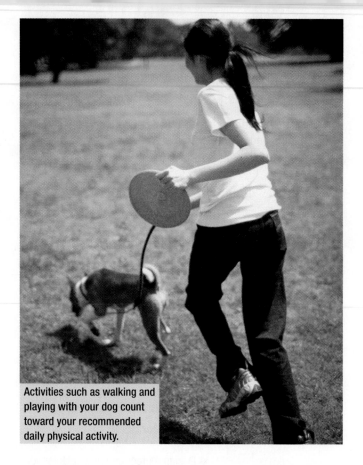

Activities such as walking and playing with your dog count toward your recommended daily physical activity.

## Physical Activity for Health

From a major review of research on physical activity and health, researchers concluded that "there is irrefutable evidence of the effectiveness of regular physical activity in the primary and secondary prevention of several chronic diseases (e.g., cardiovascular disease, diabetes, cancer, hypertension, obesity, depression, and osteoporosis, and premature death)."[8] Adding more physical activity to your day, like walking or cycling to school, can benefit your health. In fact, if all Americans followed the 2008 Physical Activity Guidelines (see Table 9.1) it is estimated that about one-third of deaths related to coronary heart disease; one-quarter of deaths related to stroke and osteoporosis; one-fifth of deaths related to colon cancer, high blood pressure, and type 2 diabetes; and one-seventh of deaths related to breast cancer could be prevented.[9]

## Physical Activity for Physical Fitness

**Physical fitness** refers to a set of attributes that is either health or performance related. The health-related attributes—cardiorespiratory fitness, muscular strength and endurance, flexibility, and body composition—allow you to perform moderate- to vigorous-intensity physical activities on a regular basis without getting too tired and with energy left over to handle physical or mental emergencies. Figure 9.1 identifies the major health-related components of physical fitness.

**Cardiorespiratory Fitness** **Cardiorespiratory fitness** refers to the ability of the heart, lungs, and blood vessels to function efficiently. The primary category of physical activity known to improve cardiorespiratory fitness is **aerobic exercise.** The word *aerobic* means "with oxygen" and describes any type of

It is important for all people, including those with disabilities, to develop optimal levels of physical fitness to participate in physical activities they enjoy—including competitive sports.

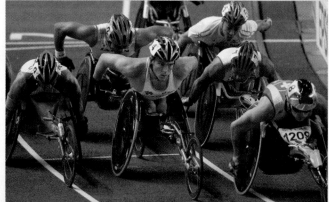

TABLE

9.1

## 2008 Physical Activity Guidelines for Americans

|  | Key Guidelines for Health* | For Additional Fitness or Weight Loss Benefits* | PLUS |
|---|---|---|---|
| Adults | 150 min/week moderate-intensity<br>**OR**<br>75 min/week of vigorous-intensity<br>**OR**<br>Equivalent combination of moderate- and vigorous-intensity (i.e., 100 min moderate-intensity + 25 min vigorous-intensity) | 300 min/week moderate-intensity<br>**OR**<br>150 min/week of vigorous-intensity<br>**OR**<br>Equivalent combination of moderate- and vigorous-intensity (i.e., 200 min moderate-intensity + 50 min vigorous-intensity)<br>**OR**<br>More than the previously described amounts | Muscle strengthening activities for ALL the major muscle groups at least 2 days/week |
| Older Adults | If unable to follow above guidelines, then as much physical activity as their condition allows | If unable to follow above guidelines, then as much physical activity as their condition allows | In addition to muscle strengthening activities, exercise to improve balance |
| Children and Youth | 60 min or more of moderate- or vigorous-intensity physical activity at least 3 days/week | At least 60 min of moderate- or vigorous-intensity physical activity on every day of the week | Include muscle strengthening activities at least 3 days/week<br>Include bone-strengthening activities at least 3 days per week |

*Accumulate this physical activity in sessions of 10 minutes or more at one time.

**Source:** Office of Disease Prevention and Health Promotion, U.S. Department of Health and Human Services, *2008 Physical Activity Guidelines for Americans: Be Active, Healthy, and Happy!* ODPHP Publication no. U0036 (Washington, DC: U.S. Department of Health and Human Services, 2008), Available at www.health.gov/paguidelines.

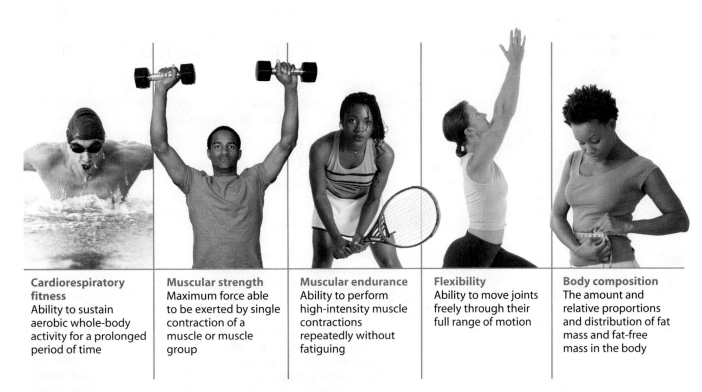

**Cardiorespiratory fitness**
Ability to sustain aerobic whole-body activity for a prolonged period of time

**Muscular strength**
Maximum force able to be exerted by single contraction of a muscle or muscle group

**Muscular endurance**
Ability to perform high-intensity muscle contractions repeatedly without fatiguing

**Flexibility**
Ability to move joints freely through their full range of motion

**Body composition**
The amount and relative proportions and distribution of fat mass and fat-free mass in the body

FIGURE 9.1 **Components of Physical Fitness**

**aerobic capacity (or power)**
The functional status of the cardiorespiratory system; refers specifically to the volume of oxygen the muscles consume during exercise.
**muscular strength** The amount of force that a muscle is capable of exerting in one contraction.
**muscular endurance** A muscle's ability to exert force repeatedly without fatiguing or the ability to sustain a muscular contraction for a length of time.
**flexibility** The range of motion, or the amount of movement possible, at a particular joint or series of joints.
**body composition** Describes the relative proportions of fat and lean (muscle, bone, water, organs) tissues in the body.

exercise that increases your heart rate. Aerobic activities such as swimming, cycling, and jogging are among the best exercises for improving or maintaining cardiorespiratory fitness.

The fitness of one's cardiorespiratory system is assessed by measuring **aerobic capacity (or power),** the volume of oxygen the muscles consume during exercise. Maximal aerobic power (commonly written as $VO_{2max}$) is defined as the maximal volume of oxygen that the muscles consume during exercise. The most common measure of maximal aerobic capacity is a walk- or run-test on a treadmill. For greatest accuracy, this is done in a lab, and requires special equipment and technicians to measure the precise amount of oxygen entering and exiting the body during the exercise session. Submaximal tests can be used in the classroom or field to get a more general sense of one's cardiorespiratory fitness; one such test, the 1.5-mile run-test, is described in the **Assess Yourself** box on page 324.

**Muscular Strength** Muscular strength refers to the amount of force a muscle or group of muscles is capable of exerting in one contraction. The most common way to assess the strength of a particular muscle group is to measure the maximum amount of weight you can move one time (and no more) or your one repetition maximum (1 RM).

**Muscular Endurance** Muscular endurance is the ability of a muscle or group of muscles to exert force repeatedly without fatigue or the ability to sustain a muscular contraction. The more repetitions you can perform successfully (e.g., push-ups) or the longer you can hold a certain position (e.g., flexed arm hang), the greater your muscular endurance. General muscular endurance is most often measured from the number of curl-ups or push-ups an individual can do; these tests are both described in the Assess Yourself box on pages 321 and 322.

**Flexibility** Flexibility refers to the range of motion, or the amount of movement possible, at a particular joint or series of joints: the greater the range of motion, the greater the flexibility. Various tests measure the flexibility of the body's joints, including range of motion tests for specific joints. One of the most common measures of general flexibility is the sit-and-reach test, described in the Assess Yourself box on page 323.

**Body Composition** Body composition is the fifth and final component of a comprehensive fitness program. Body composition describes the relative proportions and distribution of fat and lean (muscle, bone, water, organs) tissues in the body. For more details on body composition, including its measurement, see Chapter 8.

## Physical Activity for Performance

People who participate in athletics undertake specific exercises to increase speed, power, agility, coordination, and the other performance-related attributes of physical fitness. Although many recreational exercisers use interval training to improve their speed, power, and cardiorespiratory fitness, performance training is safest for those individuals who already have a high physical fitness level.

# Getting Motivated and Committing to Your Physical Fitness

The first step in starting a physical fitness program is identifying your goals for that program. Then you should consider the things that might get in the way of your achievement of those goals. Once you have contemplated these factors, you are ready to create your individual exercise program to meet your physical fitness goals. Before we start, and to help you get motivated, let's take a look at the many physical and psychological benefits of physical activity.

## What Are the Health Benefits of Regular Physical Activity?

Regular participation in physical activity improves more than 50 different physiological, metabolic, and psychological aspects of human life. Figure 9.2 summarizes some of these major health-related benefits.

**"Why Should I Care?"**

Being physically active reduces your risk for many chronic diseases. Maybe that doesn't seem like an immediate concern, but remember, there are also a lot more immediate benefits to staying physically fit—regular activity can help improve your physical appearance and your sense of self-esteem, protect you from infectious disease, reduce your stress levels, and even improve your sleep and your ability to concentrate. All that, and it's fun, too—so drop the excuses and get out and play!

**Reduced Risk of Cardiovascular Diseases** Aerobic exercise is good for the heart and lungs and reduces the risk for heart-related diseases. It improves blood flow and eases the performance of everyday tasks. Regular exercise makes the cardiovascular and respiratory systems more efficient by strengthening the heart muscle, enabling more blood to be pumped with each stroke, and increasing the

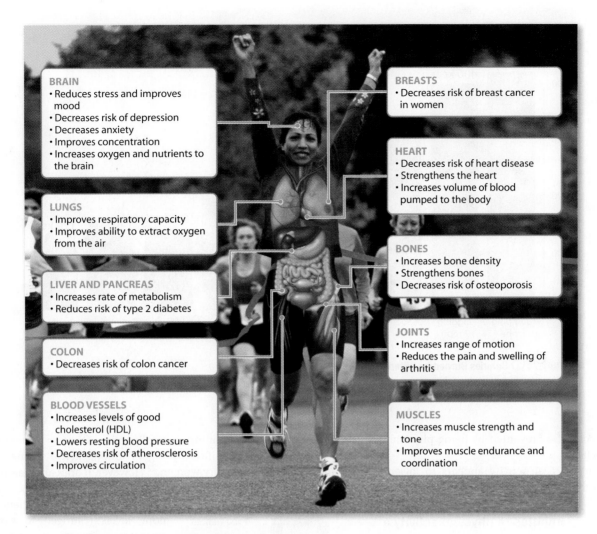

FIGURE 9.2 **Some Health Benefits of Regular Exercise**

**BRAIN**
- Reduces stress and improves mood
- Decreases risk of depression
- Decreases anxiety
- Improves concentration
- Increases oxygen and nutrients to the brain

**LUNGS**
- Improves respiratory capacity
- Improves ability to extract oxygen from the air

**LIVER AND PANCREAS**
- Increases rate of metabolism
- Reduces risk of type 2 diabetes

**COLON**
- Decreases risk of colon cancer

**BLOOD VESSELS**
- Increases levels of good cholesterol (HDL)
- Lowers resting blood pressure
- Decreases risk of atherosclerosis
- Improves circulation

**BREASTS**
- Decreases risk of breast cancer in women

**HEART**
- Decreases risk of heart disease
- Strengthens the heart
- Increases volume of blood pumped to the body

**BONES**
- Increases bone density
- Strengthens bones
- Decreases risk of osteoporosis

**JOINTS**
- Increases range of motion
- Reduces the pain and swelling of arthritis

**MUSCLES**
- Increases muscle strength and tone
- Improves muscle endurance and coordination

number of *capillaries* (small blood vessels that allow gas exchange between blood and surrounding tissues) in trained skeletal muscles, which supply more blood to working muscles. Exercise also improves the respiratory system by increasing the amount of oxygen that is inhaled and distributed to body tissues.[10]

Regular physical activity can reduce hypertension, or chronic high blood pressure, a form of cardiovascular disease and a significant risk factor for coronary heart disease and stroke (see Chapter 15).[11] Regular aerobic exercise also reduces low-density lipoproteins (LDLs, or "bad" cholesterol), total cholesterol, and triglycerides (a blood fat), thus reducing plaque buildup in the arteries while increasing high-density lipoproteins (HDLs, or "good" cholesterol), which are associated with lower risk for coronary artery disease.[12]

**Reduced Risk of Metabolic Syndrome and Type 2 Diabetes** Being regularly physically active reduces the risk of metabolic syndrome, a combination of heart disease and diabetes risk factors that produces a synergistic increase in risk.[13] Specifically, metabolic syndrome includes high blood pressure, abdominal obesity, low levels of HDLs, high levels of triglycerides, and impaired glucose tolerance.[14] Regular participation in moderate-intensity physical activities reduces risk for each factor individually and collectively.[15]

Research indicates that a healthy dietary intake combined with sufficient physical activity could prevent many of the current cases of type 2 diabetes.[16] In a major national clinical trial, researchers found that exercising 150 minutes per week while eating fewer calories and less fat could prevent or delay the onset of type 2 diabetes.[17] For more on diabetes prevention and management, see Focus On: Minimizing Your Risk for Diabetes beginning on page 514.

**Reduced Cancer Risk** After decades of research, most cancer epidemiologists believe that the majority of cancers are preventable and can be avoided by healthier lifestyle and environmental choices.[18] In fact, a report recently released by the World Cancer Research Fund in conjunction with the American Institute for Cancer Research, stated that two-thirds of all cancers could be prevented based on lifestyle changes.[19] Specific to a physically active lifestyle, one-third of

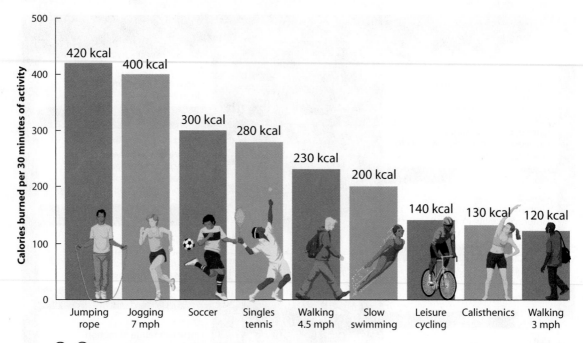

FIGURE 9.3 **Calories Burned by Different Activities**
The harder you exercise, the more energy you expend. Estimated calories burned for various moderate and vigorous activities are listed for a 30-minute bout of activity.

cancers could be prevented by being physically active and eating well.

Regular physical activity appears to lower the risk for some specific types of cancer, particularly breast cancer.

**30** minutes of physical activity a day—all at one time or in three 10-minute sessions—provides health benefits.

Research on exercise and breast cancer risk has found that the earlier in life a woman starts to exercise, the lower her breast cancer risk.[20] Further, regular exercise is also associated with lower risk for colon and rectal cancers.[21] One must keep in mind that just as there may be multiple causes of cancer, there are also many possible factors involved in its prevention.

**Improved Bone Mass and Reduced Risk of Osteoporosis** A common affliction for older people is *osteoporosis,* a disease characterized by low bone mass and deterioration of bone tissue, which increases fracture risk. Regular weight-bearing and strength-building physical activities are recommended to maintain bone health and prevent osteoporotic fractures. Although men and women are both negatively affected by osteoporosis, it is more common in women. Women (and men) have much

to gain by remaining physically active as they age—bone mass levels are significantly higher among active women than among sedentary women.[22] However, it appears that the full bone-related benefits of physical activity can only be achieved with sufficient hormone levels (estrogen in women; testosterone in men) and adequate calcium, vitamin D, and total caloric intakes.[23]

If you want to lose weight, you need to move more and move often!

**Improved Weight Management**
For many people, the desire to lose weight is the main reason for their physical activity. On the most basic level, physical activity requires your body to generate energy through calorie expenditure; if calories expended exceeds calories consumed over a span of time, the net result will be weight loss. Some activities are more intense or vigorous than others, and result in more calories used; Figure 9.3 shows the caloric cost of various activities when done for 30 minutes.

In addition to the calories expended during activity, physical activity has a direct positive effect on metabolic rate, keeping it elevated for several hours following vigorous physical activities (see also Chapter 8). This increase in metabolic rate can reduce body fat and increase lean muscle mass. Further, regular physical activity may lead to body composition changes that favor weight management. Specifically, lean body mass is often increased as a result of regular exercise. Given that lean body mass is more metabolically active than fat tissue, there is an overall increase in metabolic rate and enhanced calorie burning. In addition to helping you lose weight, increased physical activity also improves your chances of maintaining the weight loss.[24]

**Improved Immunity** Research shows that regular moderate-intensity physical activity reduces individual susceptibility to disease.[25] Just how physical activity alters immunity is not well understood. We do know that moderate-intensity physical activity temporarily increases the number of white blood cells (WBCs), which are responsible for fighting infection.[26] Often the relationship of physical activity to immunity, or more specifically to disease susceptibility, is described as a J-shaped curve. In other words, susceptibility to disease decreases with moderate activity, but then increases as you move to more extreme levels of physical activity or exercise or if you continue to exercise without adequate recovery time.[27] Athletes engaging in marathon-type events or very intense physical training programs have been shown to be at greater risk for upper respiratory tract infections (cold and flu).[28]

**Improved Mental Health** Most people who engage in regular physical activity are likely to notice the psychological benefits, such as feeling better about oneself and an overall sense of well-being. Although these mental health benefits are difficult to quantify, they are frequently mentioned as reasons for continuing to be physically active.

Regular physical activity tones and develops muscles, and can reduce or maintain body fat, thus improving a person's physical appearance. This improvement often results in increased self-esteem. Thus, physical activity contributes to mental health in more than one way. Learning new skills, developing increased ability and capacity in recreational activities, and sticking with a physical activity plan also improve self-esteem.

**Improved Stress Management** Regular vigorous exercise has been shown to "burn off" the chemical by-products of the stress response and increase endorphins, giving your mood a natural boost. Elimination of these stress hormones reduces the stress response by accelerating the neurological system's return to a balanced state.[29] For this reason, regular physical activity of moderate to vigorous intensity should be an integral component of your stress management plan.

**Longer Life Span** Experts have long debated the relationship between physical activity and longevity. In one study of over 5,000 middle-aged and older Americans, researchers found that those who engaged in moderate to high levels of activity lived 1.3 to 3.7 years longer than those who did less.[30] Furthermore, individuals who were physically active at a more intense level outlived sedentary subjects by 3.5 to 3.7 years.

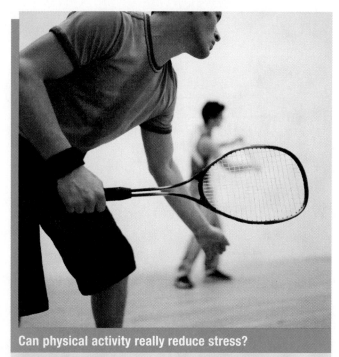

**Can physical activity really reduce stress?**

You bet it can! Physical activity actually stimulates the stress response, but a physically fit body adapts efficiently to the *eustress* of exercise, and as a result is better able to tolerate and effectively manage *distress* of all kinds. In fact a more physically fit body has a lower stress response and more effectively clears the chemical by-products associated with the stress response.

## Identifying Your Physical Fitness Goals

There are many reasons for wanting to be more physically active and become more physically fit, including the many health benefits listed above. By taking some time to reflect on your personal circumstances, goals, and desires regarding physical fitness, you will probably find it easier to come up with a plan you can stick to. Are you interested in becoming more physically active to be better at sports? To feel better about your body? To manage your stress? Or is it to improve your health and reduce your risk of chronic diseases? Perhaps your most vital goal will be to commit to your physical fitness for the long haul—to establish a realistic schedule of diverse physical activities that you can maintain and enjoy throughout your life.

## Overcoming Common Obstacles to Physical Activity

There are many excuses people give to explain why they do not exercise, ranging from personal ("I do not have time") to environmental ("I do not have a safe place to be active"). Some people may be reluctant to exercise if they are overweight, are embarrassed to work out with their more "fit" friends, or feel they lack the knowledge and skills required.

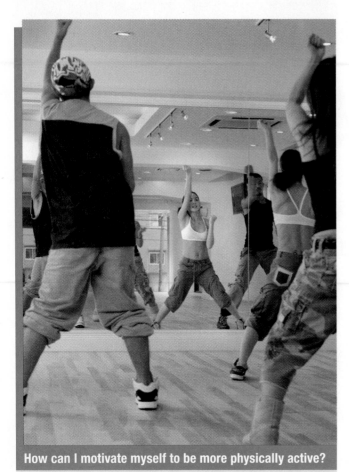

**How can I motivate myself to be more physically active?**

One great way to motivate yourself is to sign up for an exercise class. Find something that interests you—dance, yoga, aerobics, martial arts, acrobatics—and get yourself involved. The structure, schedule, social interaction, and challenge of learning a new skill can be terrific motivators that make exercising and being physically active exciting and fun.

What keeps you from being more physically active? Is it time? Do you lack a support group? Is the fitness center location inconvenient, or do you lack money for a membership or equipment? Perhaps you are ready to begin but do not know how to start. Think about your obstacles and write them down. Once you honestly evaluate why you are not as physically active as you want to be, review Table 9.2 for suggestions on overcoming your hurdles.

There was a time when women had to overcome the additional obstacle of society's frowning on their exercising and participating in recreational sports. Hard to imagine, right? See the **Gender & Health** box at right for more on this topic.

# Incorporating Fitness into Your Life

When designing your program, there are several factors to consider in order to boost your chances of achieving your physical fitness goals. First, choose activities that are appropriate for

TABLE

9.2 | **Overcoming Obstacles to Physical Activity**

| Obstacle | Possible Solution |
|---|---|
| Lack of time | • Look at your schedule. Where can you find 30-min time slots? Perhaps you need to focus on shorter times (10 min or more) throughout the day. |
| | • Multitask. Read while riding an exercise bike or listen to lecture tapes while walking. |
| | • Be physically active during your lunch and study breaks as well as between classes. Skip rope or throw a Frisbee with a friend. |
| | • Select activities that require less time, such as brisk walking or jogging. |
| | • Ride your bike to class, or park (or get off the bus) farther from your destination. |
| Social influence | • Invite family and friends to be active with you. |
| | • Join a class to meet new people. |
| | • Explain the importance of exercise and your commitment to physical activity to people who may not support your efforts. |
| | • Find a role model to support your efforts. |
| | • Plan for physically active dates—go dancing or bowling. |
| Lack of motivation, willpower, or energy | • Schedule your workout time just as you would any other important commitment. |
| | • Enlist the help of an exercise partner to make you accountable for working out. |
| | • Give yourself an incentive. |
| | • Schedule your workouts when you feel most energetic. |
| | • Remind yourself that exercise gives you more energy. |
| | • Get things ready for your workout; for example, if you choose to walk in the morning, set out your walking clothes the night before. Or pack your gym bag before going to bed. |
| Lack of resources | • Select an activity that requires minimal equipment, such as walking, jogging, jumping rope, or calisthenics. |
| | • Identify inexpensive resources on campus or in the community. |
| | • Use active forms of transportation. |
| | • Take advantage of no-cost opportunities, such as playing catch in the park/green space on campus. |

**Source:** Adapted from National Center for Chronic Disease Prevention and Health Promotion, "How Can I Overcome Barriers to Physical Activity?" Updated May 2010, www.cdc.gov/physicalactivity/everyone/getactive/barriers.html.

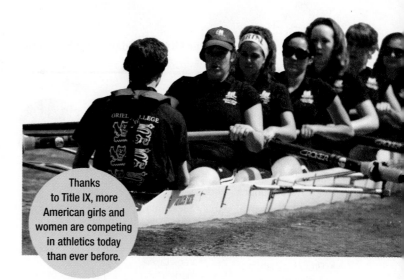

## Gender&Health

# Title IX in Athletics

Physical activity is good for everyone's health, but research shows that boys and men are more physically active than girls and women, beginning in elementary school and throughout adult life. A national survey found that 73 percent of high school–aged boys report regular physical activity, compared with 60 percent of girls. Also, almost 50 percent of girls reported *not* playing on a sports team, compared with only 38 percent of boys. Gender differences in participation are also reported in college-aged men and women. According to the American College Health Association (ACHA) National College Health Assessment, fewer women than men report participating in regular exercise 3 or more days per week.

Why such differences? In the past, women were not encouraged to be physically active because it was thought that physical exertion would cause damage to their bodies, especially their reproductive organs. Women were also thought to be physiologically incapable of feats such as weight lifting or endurance running. Even though it is now well known and accepted that physical activity is necessary for the optimal growth and development of girls (and boys) and optimal health and wellness of woman (and men) of all ages, girls and women still do not participate at the same rate as boys and men.

Supporting women's efforts to get into sports, a piece of legislation, Title IX, was put in place in the early 1970s to guarantee equal access for women and men to federally funded education programs. In addition to requiring that girls and women have equal opportunities for and access to academic and extracurricular programs, Title IX requires that they have equal opportunity to participate in athletic programs. In a progress report on Title IX, the U.S. Department of Education stated that in the first 25 years since Title IX was enacted, there was a fourfold increase in the participation of women in intercollegiate sports.

Thanks to Title IX, more American girls and women are competing in athletics today than ever before.

✳ In 1995, women made up 37 percent of athletes in college, compared to 15 percent in 1972.
✳ In 1996, girls constituted 39 percent of high school athletes, compared to 7.5 percent in 1971.
✳ U.S. women won 19 Olympic medals in the 1996 Summer Olympic Games—more than in any previous year's Olympics.

Clearly, when given a chance, women will participate and achieve in sports. With Title IX, women are guaranteed a chance to do so.

**Sources:** Centers for Disease Control and Prevention, "Behavioral Risk Factor Surveillance System Prevalence Data," *Physical Activity,* 2007, http://apps.nccd.cdc.gov/BRFSS; American College Health Association, *American College Health Association—National College Health Assessment II (ACHA-NCHA II) Reference Group Executive Summary Fall 2009* (Linthicum, MD: American College Health Association, 2009); N. Schuler, "Once Upon a Time before Title IX," Women's Sports Foundation, 2010, www.womenssportsfoundation.org/Content/Articles/Issues/History/O/Once-Upon-A-Time-Before-Title-IX.aspx; U.S. Department of Education, Office for Civil Rights, *Title IX: 25 Years of Progress* (Washington, DC: U.S. Department of Education, 1997), Available at http://www2.ed.gov/pubs/TitleIX/index.html.

---

you, that you genuinely like doing, and that are convenient. For example, choose jogging because you like to run and there are beautiful trails nearby versus swimming when you do not really like the water and the pool is difficult to get to. Likewise, choose activities that are suitable for your current fitness level. If you are overweight or obese and have not exercised in months, do not sign up for the advanced aerobics classes. Start slow, plan fun activities, and progress to more challenging physical activities as your physical fitness improves. You may choose to simply walk more in an attempt to achieve the recommended goal of 10,000 steps per day; keep track with a pedometer (or step counter; see Table 9.3 on page 304 for more on this handy gadget and other fitness equipment you may consider purchasing or using at a health club). Try to make exercise a part of your routine by incorporating it into something you already have to do—such as getting to class or work. See the **Be Healthy, Be Green** box on page 305 for more on this topic.

# Fitness Program Components

A well-designed program should improve or maintain cardiorespiratory fitness, muscular strength and endurance, flexibility, and body composition. But what should you do when you go to exercise? A comprehensive workout would include a warm-up, cardiorespiratory and/or resistance training, and then a cool-down to finish the session. Each of these is described in more detail below.

## Warm-Up

The primary purpose of the warm-up is to prepare the body physically and mentally for the cardiorespiratory and/or resistance training that is to follow. Generally, a warm-up

TABLE
9.3    **Some Popular Fitness Gadgets and Equipment**

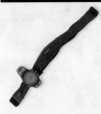
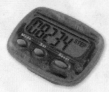
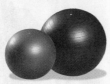
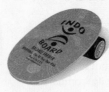
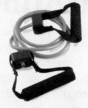

### Heart Rate Monitor

A chest strap with a watch device that measures heart rate during training.

- Provides instant and continuous feedback about the intensity of your workout.
- Strap must fit well; can be cumbersome (most women tuck the strap under the bottom strap of their sport bra).

Cost: $50–$200

### Pedometer

A battery-operated device, usually worn on your belt, that measures the number of steps taken. Some models also monitor calories, distance, and speed.

- Great motivation and feedback regarding the recommended 10,000 steps per day.
- Must be calibrated for your height, weight, and stride length.

Cost: $25–$50

### Stability Ball

Ball made of burst-resistant vinyl that can be used for strengthening core muscles, or to improve flexibility.

- Balls must be inflated correctly to be most effective.

Cost: $25–$50

### Balance Board

A board with a rounded bottom that can be used to improve balance, core muscle strength, and flexibility.

- Great for improving agility, coordination, reaction skills, and ankle strength.
- Can be difficult initially for new users. Caution new users with weak ankles, as there is risk of straining ligaments and tendons with excessive use.

Cost: $40–$80

### Resistance Band

Rubber or elastic material, sometimes with handles that can be used to build muscular strength and endurance. Also can be used in yoga or Pilates to provide assistance in flexibility training.

- Improves muscular strength and endurance, balance, coordination, and, flexibility.
- Lightweight, durable, and portable.

Cost: $5–$15

### Medicine Ball

A heavy ball, about 14" in diameter used in rehabilitation and strength training.

Weight varies from 2 to 25 lb. Some made with handles.

- Can be used effectively in plyometric training to increase explosive power.
- Also used to develop core body strength.
- If used incorrectly, there is potential for lower back injuries.

Cost: $10–$150

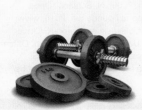
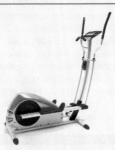
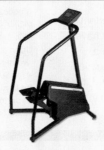
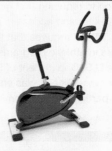
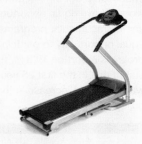

### Free Weights

Rubber, plastic, or metal dumbbells or barbells, often with adjustable weight; can be used with a weight bench.

- Traditional method for building muscular strength and endurance.
- A full set allows you to increase resistance as you train, allowing for greater improvements in muscular strength.
- Potential for injury if form is incorrect; must concentrate on body alignment and ensuring sufficient core body strength.

Cost: $10–$300

### Elliptical Trainer

A stationary exercise machine that simulates walking or running without impact on the bones and joints. Some machines include arm movements.

- Nonimpact; less wear and tear on the joints and risk of shin splints.
- Readout and programs vary.

Cost: $300–$4,000

### Stair Climber

A stationary exercise machine that provides a low-impact lower-body workout via stair climbing.

- Nonimpact; less wear and tear on the joints and risk of shin splints.
- Various programs are available.

Cost: $200–$3,000

### Stationary Bike

A lower-body exercise machine designed to simulate bike riding.

- Generally easy to use; does not require balance.
- Comes with varied resistance programs.
- Recumbent styles offer less strain on back and knees and are useful for individuals struggling with back pain.

Cost: $200–$2,000

### Treadmill

Exercise machine for walking or running on a moving platform while remaining in one place.

- Generally easy to use; comes with an emergency shutoff.
- Different models have varied readouts and programmability.
- Lower impact on joints than running on most pavements.

Cost: $500–$4,000

# BE HEALTHY, BE GREEN

## Transport Yourself!

Before we became a car culture, much of our transportation was human powered. Bicycling and walking historically were important means of transportation and recreation in the United States. These modes not only helped keep people in good physical shape, but they also had little or no impact on the environment. Even in the first few decades after the automobile started to be popularized, people continued to get around under their own power. Since World War II, however, the development of automobile-oriented communities has led to a steady decline of bicycling and walking. Currently, only about 10 percent of trips are made by foot or bike.

The more we use our cars to get around, the more congested our roads, the more polluted our air, and the more sedentary our lives become. That is why many people are now embracing a movement toward more active transportation. *Active transportation* means getting out of your car and using your own power to get from place to place—whether walking, riding a bike, skateboarding, or roller skating. The following are just a few of the many reasons to make active transportation a bigger part of your life:

✱ **You will be adding more exercise into your daily routine.** People who walk, bike, or use other active forms of transportation to complete errands are physically active.

✱ **Walking or biking can save you money.** With rising gas prices and parking fees, in addition to increasing car mainte-

nance and insurance costs, fewer automobile trips could add up to considerable savings. During the course of a year, regular bicycle commuters who ride 5 miles to work can save about $500 on fuel and more than $1,000 on other expenses related to driving.

✱ **Walking or biking may save you time!** Cycling is usually the fastest mode of travel door to door for distances up to 5 or 6 miles in city centers. Walking is simpler and faster for distances of about a mile.

✱ **You will enjoy being outdoors.** Research is emerging on the physical and mental health benefits of nature and being outdoors. So much of what we do is inside, with recirculated air and artificial lighting, that our bodies are deficient in fresh air and sunlight.

✱ **You will be making a significant contribution to the reduction of air pollution.** Driving less means fewer pollutants being emitted into the air. Leaving your car at home just two days a week will reduce greenhouse gas emissions by an average of 1,600 pounds per year.

✱ **You will help reduce traffic.** The average traveler now wastes the equivalent of a full work week stuck in traffic every year. Having more active commuters means fewer cars on the roads and less traffic congestion.

✱ **You will contribute to global health.** Annually, personal transportation

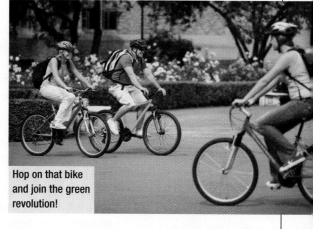

Hop on that bike and join the green revolution!

accounts for the consumption of approximately 136 billion gallons of gasoline, or the production of 1.2 billion tons of carbon dioxide. Reducing vehicle trips will help reduce overall greenhouse gas emissions and reduce the need to source more fossil fuel.

**Sources:** T. Gotschi and K. Mills, *Active Transportation for America: The Case for Increased Federal Investment in Bicycling and Walking* (Washington, DC: Rails to Trails Conservancy, 2008), Available at www.railstotrails.org/ourwork/advocacy/activetransportation/makingthecase; D. Shinkle and A. Teigens, *Encouraging Bicycling and Walking: The State Legislative Role* (Washington, DC: National Conference of State Legislatures, 2008), Available at www.americantrails.org/resources/trans/Encourage-Bicycling-Walking-State-Legislative-Role.html; U.S. Environmental Protection Agency, "Climate Change: What You Can Do—On the Road," Updated May 2010, www.epa.gov/climatechange/wycd/road.html.

---

involves large body movements, followed by light stretching of the muscle groups to be used. A warm-up usually lasts 5 to 15 minutes, but is shorter when you are geared up and ready to go and longer when you are struggling with your motivation to get moving. The important thing is to listen to your body and to take the time needed to prepare it for more intense activity. The warm-up provides a transition from rest to physical activity by slowly increasing heart rate, blood pressure, breathing rate, and body temperature. These gradual changes improve joint lubrication, as well as increase

muscles' and tendons' elasticity and flexibility, facilitating performance during the next stage of the workout.

## Cardiorespiratory and/or Resistance Training

Immediately following your warm-up, move into the next stage of your workout. This stage may involve cardiorespiratory training or resistance training or a little of both. If you are in a fitness center setting, you may choose to use one or more of the aerobic training devices for the recommended time frame. Before or after cardiorespiratory training, you may choose to follow your prescribed program for strength and endurance training. Regardless of what you choose, the bulk of the workout occurs in this section and can last 20 to 30 minutes or more.

## Cool-Down

Just as you ease into a workout with a warm-up, you should slowly transition from activity to rest. A cool-down is an essential component of a fitness program involving another 5 to 15 minutes of activity. Generally it starts with 5 to 10 minutes of moderate- to low-intensity activity followed by 5 to 10 minutes of stretching exercises. Because of the body's increased temperature, the cool-down is an excellent time to stretch to improve flexibility. The purpose of the cool-down is to gradually reduce your heart rate, blood pressure, and body temperature to pre-exercising levels. In addition, the cool-down reduces the risk of blood pooling in the extremities and facilitates quicker recovery between exercise sessions.

**FITT** Acronym for Frequency, Intensity, Time, and Type; the terms that describe the essential components of a program or plan to improve a parameter of physical fitness.
**frequency** As part of the FITT prescription, refers to how many days per week a person should exercise to improve a parameter of physical fitness.
**intensity** As part of the FITT prescription, refers to how hard or how much effort is needed when a person exercises to improve a parameter of physical fitness.

# Creating Your Own Fitness Program: The FITT Principle

Now that you've set appropriate and realistic goals and are motivated to improve your physical fitness, the next step is to learn about the fitness recommendations and principles involved so that you can begin devising your own workout plan. What is the best approach to take? What do you have to do? Where should you start? Assuming your intention is to improve your health-related physical fitness (although the principles can also be applied to performance-related physical fitness), the **FITT (Frequency, Intensity, Time, and Type)** principle should be used to define your exercise program. Each part of the FITT principle (Figure 9.4) is explained here:

● Exercise **frequency** refers to the number of times per week you need to engage in particular exercises to achieve the desired level of physical fitness in a particular component.

● **Intensity** refers to how hard your workout must be to achieve the desired level of physical fitness.

| | Cardiorespiratory endurance | Muscular strength and endurance | Flexibility |
|---|---|---|---|
| **F**requency | 3–5 days per week | 2–4 days per week | Minimally 2–3 days per week; optimally daily |
| **I**ntensity | 70%–90% of maximum heart rate | Strength: >60% of 1RM<br>Endurance: <60% of 1RM | To the point of tension |
| **T**ime | 20–30+ minutes | Strength: 2–6 reps, 1–3 sets<br>Endurance: 10–15 reps, 2–6 sets | 10–30 seconds per stretch, 2–3 repetitions |
| **T**ype | Any rhythmic, continuous, vigorous activity | Resistance training (with body weight and/or external resistance) | Stretching, dance, yoga, gymnastics |

FIGURE 9.4 **The FITT Principle Applied to Cardiorespiratory Fitness, Muscular Strength and Endurance, and Flexibility**

- How much **time,** or the *duration,* refers to how many minutes or repetitions of an exercise are required at a specified intensity during any one session to attain the desired level of physical fitness for each component.
- **Type** refers to what kind of exercises should be performed to improve the various components of physical fitness.

## The FITT Principle for Cardiorespiratory Fitness

The most effective aerobic exercises for building cardiorespiratory fitness are total body activities involving the large muscle groups of your body. The FITT prescription for cardiorespiratory fitness includes 3 to 5 days per week of vigorous, rhythmic, continuous activity, at 70 to 90 percent of maximal heart rate, for 20 to 30 minutes.[31]

**Frequency** To improve your cardiorespiratory fitness, you must vigorously exercise at least three times a week. If you are a newcomer to exercise, you can still make improvements by doing less intense exercise but doing it more days a week, following the recommendations from the Centers for Disease Control and Prevention (CDC) and the American College of Sports Medicine (ACSM) for moderate physical activity 5 days a week (refer to Table 9.1 on page 297).

**Intensity** The most common methods used to determine the intensity of cardiorespiratory endurance exercises are target heart rate, rating of perceived exertion, and the talk test. The exercise intensity required to improve cardiorespiratory endurance is a heart rate between 70 and 90 percent of your maximum heart rate. To calculate this **target heart rate,** subtract your age from 220 (males) or 226 (females). This results in your maximum heart rate. Your target heart rate would be 70 to 90 percent of your maximum heart rate. For example, if you are a 20-year-old male, your estimated maximum heart rate is 200 (220 − 20 = 200). Your target heart rate would be somewhere between 140 (200 × 0.70 = 140) and 180 (200 × 0.90 = 180) beats per minute. Figure 9.5 shows a range of target heart rates.

Take your pulse during your workout to determine how close you are to your target heart rate. Lightly place your index and middle fingers (not your thumb) over one of the major arteries in your neck, or on the artery on the inside of your wrist (Figure 9.6). Start counting your pulse immediately after you stop exercising, as your heart rate decreases rapidly. Using a watch or a clock, take your pulse for 6 seconds (the first pulse is "0") and multiply this number by 10 (add a zero to your count) to get the number of beats per minute.

Another way of determining the intensity of cardiorespiratory exercise intensity is to use Borg's rating of perceived exertion (RPE) scale. Perceived exertion refers to how hard you feel you are working, which you might base on your heart rate, breathing rate, sweating, and level of fatigue. This scale uses a rating from 6 (no exertion at all) to 20 (maximal exertion). An RPE of 12 to 16 is generally recommended for training the cardiorespiratory system.

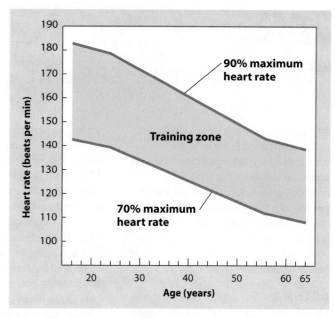

FIGURE $9.5$ **Target Heart Rate Ranges**
These ranges are based on calculating the maximum heart rate as 220 − age and the training zone as 70% to 90% of maximum heart rate. Individuals with low fitness levels should start below or at the low end of these ranges.

The easiest, but least scientific, method of measuring cardiorespiratory exercise intensity is the "talk test." A heart rate of 70 percent of maximum is also called the "conversational" level of exercise, because you are able to talk with a partner while exercising.[32] If you are breathing so hard that talking is difficult, the intensity of your exercise is too high. Conversely, if you are able to sing or laugh heartily while exercising, the intensity of your exercise is insufficient for maintaining and/or improving cardiorespiratory fitness.

**time** As part of the FITT prescription, refers to how long a person needs to exercise each time to improve a parameter of physical fitness.
**type** As part of the FITT prescription, refers to what kind of exercises a person needs to do to improve a parameter of physical fitness.
**target heart rate** The heart rate range of aerobic exercise that leads to improved cardiorespiratory fitness (i.e., 70% to 90% of maximal heart rate).

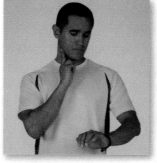 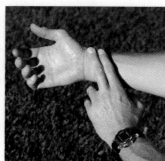

ⓐ Carotid pulse        ⓑ Radial pulse

FIGURE $9.6$ **Taking a Pulse**
Palpation of the carotid (neck) or radial (wrist) artery is a simple way of determining heart rate.

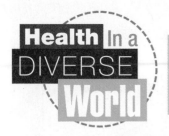
# PHYSICAL ACTIVITY AND EXERCISE FOR SPECIAL POPULATIONS

All individuals benefit from a physically active lifestyle, regardless of the physical and/or mental challenges they face. For some, modifications to the FITT prescription may be suggested. For people with the special considerations mentioned below, as for all individuals, it is recommended that you consult with your physician before beginning an exercise program.

## ASTHMA

Regular physical activity provides the following benefits for individuals with asthma:

**1.** Strengthens the respiratory muscles, making it easier to breathe
**2.** Improves immune system functioning
**3.** Helps in weight maintenance (preventing weight gain is important as obesity increases the difficulty of exercising with asthma)

If you have asthma, talk to your physician before you begin your exercise plan. Prior to engaging in exercise, ensure that your asthma is under control. If not, exercise could be dangerous. Ask about adjusting your medications (your doctor may recommend you use your inhaler 15 minutes prior to exercise, for example). When exercising, keep your inhaler nearby—in your pocket, for example. Warm up and cool down properly; it is particularly important that you allow your lungs and breathing rate to adjust slowly. Protect yourself from your asthma triggers when exercising. Finally, if you have symptoms while exercising, stop and use your inhaler; if an asthma attack persists, call 9-1-1.

## OBESITY

Limitations such as heat intolerance, shortness of breath during physical activity, lack of flexibility, frequent musculoskeletal injuries, and difficulty with balance in weight-bearing activities need to be addressed. Programs for individuals who are obese should emphasize physical activities that can be sustained

for longer periods of time (30+ minutes) such as walking, swimming, or bicycling, with caution recommended for performing these activities in hot or humid environments. Although it is recommended to start slow (5 to 10 minutes of activity) and at a lower intensity (55% to 65% of maximal heart rate), the ultimate goal is to obtain at least 30 minutes per exercise session resulting in 150 to 250 minutes per week. Regardless of weight loss, evidence suggests that individuals who are obese improve their health with cardiorespiratory and resistance training activities.

## CORONARY HEART DISEASE

Although regular physical activity reduces risk of coronary heart disease, vigorous-intensity activity acutely increases risk of sudden cardiac death and myocardial infarction (heart attack). Physical activity in the form of cardiorespiratory exercises improves the functional capacity and reduces the clinical symptoms in individuals with coronary heart disease. However, given the variation in individuals with coronary heart disease, it is not possible to provide a generic exercise prescription. Thus, the recommendation is for individuals with coronary heart disease to consult their physicians.

## HYPERTENSION

Physical activity is an integral component for the prevention and treatment of hypertension. Using the FITT prescription, individuals who are hypertensive should engage in physical activity on most, if not all, days of the week, at a moderate intensity (12 to 13 on the Borg RPE scale), for 30 minutes or more.

## DIABETES

Physical activity benefits individuals with diabetes in a number of ways:

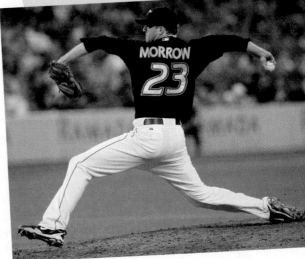

Athletes like Brandon Morrow, a Major League Baseball pitcher and a type 1 diabetic, are living proof that chronic conditions needn't prevent you from achieving your physical activity goals.

**1.** Controls blood glucose (for individuals with type 2) by improving transport into the cells
**2.** Controls body weight
**3.** Reduces risk for heart disease, critical for individuals with diabetes because they are at greater risk for heart disease

Before individuals with type 1 diabetes engage in physical activity, they must learn how to manage their resting blood glucose levels. The recommendations for their physical activity then are similar to those for individuals without diabetes; however, their physical activity should be daily so they can more easily manage their blood glucose. Further, individuals with type 1 diabetes should have an exercise partner, eat 1 to 3 hours prior to the activity; eat a snack composed of complex carbohydrates after the activity; avoid late-evening physical activities; and monitor their blood glucose before, during, and after the activity.

*(Continued on next page)*

The most important factor for individuals with type 2 diabetes is the time or length of their physical activity. Because a critical objective of the management of type 2 diabetes is reduction of body fat (obesity), the recommendations for time are longer—reaching 60 minutes per session. For sessions of this length, it is prudent to reduce the intensity of the activity to a target heart rate range of 40 to 60 percent of maximal heart rate.

### OLDER ADULTS

Engaging in a physically active lifestyle increases life expectancy by limiting the development and progression of chronic diseases and disabling conditions. As such, the general recommendation for older adults is to engage in regular physical activity. The recommendations made in the 2008 Physical Activity Guidelines for Americans can be followed. For individuals with disabling conditions such as arthritis, osteoarthritis, and other musculoskeletal problems, non–weight-bearing activities, such as cycling and swimming or other water exercises, are recommended.

**Sources:** J. E. Donnelly et al., "American College of Sports Medicine Position Stand: Appropriate Physical Activity Intervention Strategies for Weight Loss, and Prevention of Weight Regain for Adults," *Medicine and Science in Sports and Exercise* 41, no. 2 (2009): 459–71; L. S. Pescatello et al., "American College of Sports Medicine Position Stand: Exercise and Hyptertension," *Medicine and Science in Sports and Exercise* 36, no. 3 (2004): 533–53; B. A. Franklin et al., "American College of Sports Medicine and American Heart Association Joint Position Stand: Exercise and Acute Cardiovascular Events: Placing the Risks into Perspective, *Medicine and Science in Sports and Exercise* 39, no. 5 (2007): 886–97; W. J. Chodzko-Zajko et al., "American College of Sports Medicine Position Stand: Exercise and Physical Activity for Older Adults," *Medicine and Science in Sports and Exercise* 41, no. 7 (2009): 1510–30; The Canadian Lung Association, "Asthma: Exercise and Asthma," Updated April 2010, www.lung.ca/diseases -maladies/asthma-asthme/exercise-exercice/ index_e.php.

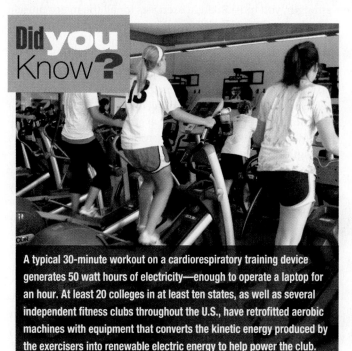

**Did you Know?**

A typical 30-minute workout on a cardiorespiratory training device generates 50 watt hours of electricity—enough to operate a laptop for an hour. At least 20 colleges in at least ten states, as well as several independent fitness clubs throughout the U.S., have retrofitted aerobic machines with equipment that converts the kinetic energy produced by the exercisers into renewable electric energy to help power the club.

**Time** For cardiorespiratory fitness benefits, the ACSM recommends that vigorous activities (70% to 90% of heart rate maximum) be performed for at least 20 minutes at a time, and moderate activities (50% to 70% of heart rate maximum) for at least 30 minutes.[33] See also the **Health in a Diverse World** box for more specific recommendations for individuals with chronic diseases or conditions that require alterations to the FITT prescription.

**Type** Any sort of rhythmic, continuous, and vigorous physical activity that can be done for 20 or more minutes will improve cardiorespiratory fitness. Examples include walking briskly, cycling, jogging, fitness classes, and swimming.

## The FITT Principle for Muscular Strength and Endurance

The FITT prescription for muscular strength and endurance includes 2 to 4 days per week of exercises that train the major muscle groups, using enough sets and repetitions and enough resistance to maintain or improve muscular strength and endurance.[34]

**Frequency** For frequency, performing eight to ten exercises that train the major muscle groups 2 to 4 days a week is recommended. It is believed that overloading the muscles, a normal part of resistance training described below, causes microscopic tears in muscle fibers, and the rebuilding process that increases the muscle's size and capacity takes about 24 to 48 hours. Thus, resistance-training exercise programs should include at least one day of rest between workouts before the same muscles are overloaded again. But don't wait too long between workouts—one of the important principles of strength training is the idea of *reversibility.* Reversibility means that if you stop exercising, then the body responds by deconditioning. Even after as little as 4 days without training, muscles begin to revert to their untrained state.[35] The saying "use it or lose it" applies!

**Intensity** To determine the intensity of exercise needed to improve muscular strength and endurance, you need to know the maximum amount of weight you can lift (or move) in one contraction. This value is called your **one repetition maximum (1 RM)** and can be individually determined or predicted from a 10 RM test. Once your 1 RM is determined, it is used as the basis for intensity recommendations for improving muscular strength and endurance. Muscular strength is improved when resistance loads are greater than 60 percent of your 1 RM,

**one repetition maximum (1 RM)** The amount of weight or resistance that can be lifted or moved only once.

whereas muscular endurance is improved using loads less than 60 percent of your 1 RM.

Everyone begins a resistance-training program at an initial level of strength. To become stronger, you must *overload* your muscles, that is, regularly create a degree of tension in your muscles that is greater than what you are accustomed to. Overloading them forces your muscles to adapt by getting larger, stronger, and capable of producing more tension. If you "underload" your muscles, you will not increase strength. If you create too great an overload, you may experience muscle injury, muscle fatigue, and potentially a loss in strength. Once your strength goal is reached, no further overload is necessary; your challenge at that point is to maintain your level of strength by engaging in a regular (once or twice per week) total-body resistance exercise program.

**Time** The time recommended for muscular strength and endurance exercises is measured not in minutes of exercise, but rather in repetitions and sets. The types of demands that you put on your body will result in the kind of adaptation that will follow.

- **Sets and repetitions.** To increase muscular strength, you need higher intensity and fewer repetitions and sets: Use a resistance of at least 60 percent of your 1RM, performing two to six repetitions per set, with one to three sets performed overall. If improving muscular endurance is your goal, use less resistance and more repetitions and sets. The recommendations for improving muscular endurance are to perform two to six sets of 10 to 15 repetitions using a resistance that is less than 60 percent of your 1RM.

- **Rest periods.** The amount of rest between exercises is key to an effective strength-training workout. Resting between exercises can reduce fatigue and help with performance and safety in subsequent sets. A rest period of 2 to 3 minutes is recommended for multiple-joint exercises that use large-muscle groups (e.g., squats with overhead presses) and a rest period of 1 to 2 minutes for single-joint exercises or for strength exercises using machines. It should be pointed out that this "rest period" refers specifically to the muscle group being exercised and it is possible to alternate muscle groups, thus taking advantage of your time available to train. For example, you can alternate a set of push-ups with curl-ups, as the muscle groups worked in one set can rest while you are working the other muscle groups.

**Type** To improve muscular strength or endurance, resistance training is most often recommended either using your

own body weight or devices that provide a fixed, variable, or accommodating load or resistance (see Table 9.4). Some cardiorespiratory training activities also enhance muscular endurance as thousands of repetitions are performed during a 20-minute (or longer) workout using relatively low resistance when jogging, or training on an exercise device such as a stationary bicycle, rowing machine, or stair-climbing machine.

When selecting the type of strength-training exercises to do, there are several important principles to bear in mind. The first of these is *specificity*. According to the specificity principle, the effects of resistance-exercise training are specific to the muscles exercised; only the muscle or muscle group that is overloaded responds to the demands placed upon it. For example, if you regularly do curls, the muscles involved—your biceps—will become larger and stronger, but the other muscles in your body do not change. This sort of training may put opposing muscle groups—in this case the triceps—at increased risk for injury. To improve total body strength, you must include exercises for all the major muscle groups. You must also ensure that your overload is sufficient to increase strength and not only endurance.

Another important concept to consider is *exercise selection*. Exercises that work a single joint (e.g., chest presses) are effective for building specific muscle strength, while multiple-joint exercises (e.g., a squat coupled with an overhead press) are more effective for increasing overall muscle strength. The ACSM recommends that both exercise types be included in a strength-training program, with an emphasis on multiple-joint exercises for maximizing muscle strength.[36]

Finally, for optimal training effects, it is important to pay attention to *exercise order*. When training all major muscle groups in a single workout, complete large-muscle group exercises before small-muscle group exercises, multiple-joint exercises before single-joint exercises, and high-intensity exercises before lower-intensity exercises.

> Resistance training to improve muscular strength and endurance can be done with free weights, machines, or even your own body weight.

## The FITT Principle for Flexibility

Although often overshadowed by cardiorespiratory and muscular strength and endurance training, flexibility is important. Improving your flexibility not only enhances the efficiency of your movements, it can enhance your sense of well-being, help you manage your stress effectively, and

TABLE
9.4 | **Methods of Providing Exercise Resistance**

| 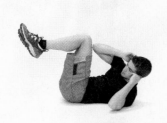 | 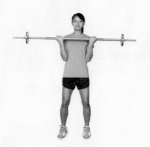 | 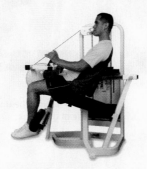 | 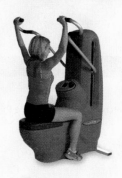 |
|---|---|---|---|
| **Body Weight Resistance (Calisthenics)** | **Fixed Resistance** | **Variable Resistance** | **Accommodating Resistance** |
| • Using your own body weight to develop muscular strength and endurance.<br>• Improves overall muscular fitness—and in particular core body strength and overall muscle tone. | • Provides a constant resistance throughout the full range of movement.<br>• Requires balance and coordination; promotes development of core body strength. | • Resistance is altered so that the muscle's effort is consistent throughout the full range of motion.<br>• Provides more controlled motion and isolates certain muscle groups. | • Sometimes called isokinetic machines; they maintain a constant speed throughout the range of motion.<br>• Requires a maximal effort as the machine controls the speed of exercise.<br>• Often used for rehabilitation after injury. |
| **Examples:** Push-ups, pull-ups, curl-ups, dips, leg raises, chair sits, etc. | **Examples:** Free weights such as barbells and dumbbells. | **Examples:** Specific machines in gyms, some home models available, such as Nautilus or Bowflex machines. | **Examples:** Specific machines in rehabilitation facilities and gyms. |

prevent or reduce pain in your joints as well. Further, inflexible muscles are susceptible to injury, and flexibility training is effective in reducing the incidence and severity of lower back problems and muscle or tendon injuries that can occur during sports and everyday physical activities.[37] Improved flexibility also means less tension and pressure on joints, resulting in less joint pain and joint deterioration.[38]

**Frequency** The FITT principle calls for a minimum of 2 to 3 days per week for flexibility training; even better is daily training.

**Intensity** Flexibility has the least formal method for identifying the intensity required for improvement. Specifically, the recommendations are that you perform or hold static (still) stretching positions at the "point of tension." This "point of tension" is individually determined. You should be able to feel tension or mild discomfort in the muscle(s) you are stretching, but the stretch should not hurt.[39]

**Time** The time recommended to improve flexibility is based upon time per stretch. Once you are in a static stretching position, you should hold at the "point of tension" for 10 to 30 seconds for each stretch and repeat two or three times in close succession.[40]

**Type** The most effective exercises for building flexibility fitness involve stretching of the major muscle groups of your body when the body is already warm, as it is after cardiorespiratory activities. The safest exercises for improving flexibility involve **static stretching.** Static stretching techniques slowly and gradually lengthen a muscle or group of muscles and their tendons. The primary strategy is to decrease the resistance to stretch (tension) within a tight muscle targeted for increased range of motion.[41] To do this, you repeatedly stretch the muscle and its two tendons of attachment to elongate them. With each repetition of a static stretch, your range of motion improves temporarily due to the slightly lessened sensitivity of tension receptors in the stretched muscles, and when done regularly, range of motion increases.[42] Figure 9.7 illustrates some basics stretching exercises to increase flexibility.

**static stretching** Stretching techniques that slowly and gradually lengthen a muscle or group of muscles and their tendons.

## What If I Have Been Inactive for a While?

If you have been physically inactive for the past few months or longer, the frequency, intensity, and time of your exercise sessions should begin at the lower end of the recommendations.

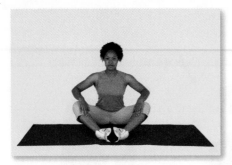

(a) Stretching the inside of the thighs

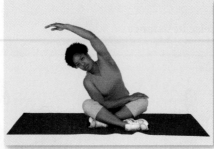

(b) Stretching the upper arm and the side of the trunk

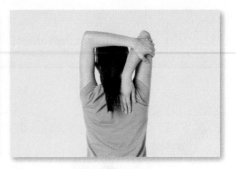

(c) Stretching the triceps

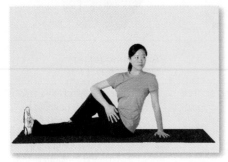

(d) Stretching the trunk and the hip

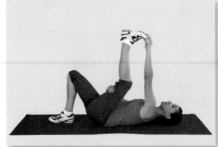

(e) Stretching the hip, back of the thigh, and the calf

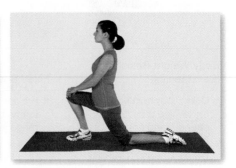

(f) Stretching the front of the thigh and the hip flexor

FIGURE 9.7 **Stretching Exercises to Improve Flexibility and Prevent Injury**
Use these stretches as part of your warm-up and cool-down. Hold each stretch for 10 to 30 seconds, and repeat two to three times for each limb.

This is known as *preconditioning,* and it can ease individuals into a workout regime with a minimum of soreness. For example, you might start your cardiorespiratory exercises with a target heart rate between 40 and 50 percent of maximum. You might focus your resistance-training program first on muscular endurance training or training with little or no resistance with an emphasis on developing proper technique and proper body alignment. And, you should start at the lower range of time.

## Developing a Progressive Plan Using the FITT Principle

As your physical fitness improves, you will need to adjust the frequency, intensity, time, and type of exercise that you do to continue to improve and/or to maintain the level of physical fitness attained. Generally it is recommended that you begin an exercise regimen by picking an exercise and gradually increasing frequency of workouts. For week 1, you may exercise on 3 days, moving to 4 days in week 3 or 4 and so on. Once you are working out 5 or more days per week and that seems comfortable, then you increase the length of each workout. It is recommended that you increase the time of exercise by 10 percent.[43] For example, for your cardiorespiratory training, if you are accustomed to walking for 20

minutes, then you would add 2 minutes to your walking time (20 min × 0.10 = 2 min) so that you walk for a total of 22 minutes. You continue adding 10 percent until you reach the recommended amount of 30 minutes. Once you have adjusted to these time changes and are working out 5 days per week, then it is recommended that you increase the intensity of your workout. Again it is recommended to increase the intensity gradually, using a 10 percent increase as your guideline. So, if you start with a target heart rate of 70 percent of your heart rate maximum (which, as previously shown, was 140 beats per minute for a 20-year-old male), then you would increase that by 1 to 2 beats per minute (140 beats/min × 0.10 = 1.4 beats per min).

For type of exercise, the focus is on variation, a fundamental principle in strength training that is also relevant to cardiorespiratory fitness and flexibility training. This principle identifies the need for changes in one or more parts of your workout, not only to produce a higher level of physical fitness (because different muscle groups are used) but also to keep you motivated and interested enough to continue training regularly.

In addition to progressively adjusting your workouts, it is important to reevaluate your overall physical fitness goals and action plan monthly to ensure that you are still motivated and that the plan is working for you. A mistake many people make when they decide to become more

## Plan It, Start It, Stick with It!

The most successful physical activity program is one that is realistic and appropriate for your skill level and needs.

✳ **Start slow.** If you have been physically inactive for a while or are a first-time exerciser, any type and amount of physical activity is a step in the right direction. Keep in mind that it is an achievement to get to the fitness center or to put your sneakers on for a walk! Make sure you start slowly—in fact, 5 minutes of walking or exercise may be plenty—letting your body adapt so that your new physical activity or exercise does not cause excess pain the next day (a real reaction to using muscles you have not used much or as intensely before). Do not be discouraged; you will be able to increase your activity each week and soon you will be on your way to meeting the physical activity recommendations and your personal physical fitness goals!

✳ **Make only one lifestyle change at a time.** It is not realistic to change everything at once. Further, success with one behavioral change will increase your belief in yourself and encourage you to make other positive changes.

✳ **Set reasonable expectations for yourself and your physical fitness program.** You will not become "fit" overnight. It takes several months to really feel the benefits of your physical activity. Be patient, there will be a day soon where you will think, "Wow, I feel and look great!"

✳ **Choose a specific time to exercise and stick with it.** Learning to establish priorities and keeping to a schedule are vital steps toward improved fitness. Try exercising at different times of the day to learn what schedule works best for you. Yet, be flexible, so if something comes up that you cannot work around, you will find time later that day or evening to do some physical activity. Be careful of an all-or-none attitude.

✳ **Keep a record of your progress.** Include the intensity, time, and type of physical activities and your emotions and personal achievements.

✳ **Take lapses in stride.** Sometimes life gets in the way. Learn how to start again and do not despair; your commitment to physical fitness has ebbs and flows like most everything else in life.

# Pulling It All Together: Activities That Develop Core Strength and Multiple Components of Fitness

Some forms of activity—including three styles of exercise that have become increasingly popular in the United States in recent years, yoga, tai chi, and Pilates—have the potential to improve several components of physical fitness. In addition to improving flexibility, these types of exercise increase muscular strength and endurance—particularly of the core—balance, coordination, and agility. They also focus on the mind–body connection through concentration on breathing and body position. Some people see these activities as strongly connected to the development of their spiritual health, particularly when time is spent relaxing, breathing deeply, and trying to clear the mind. For more on enhancing

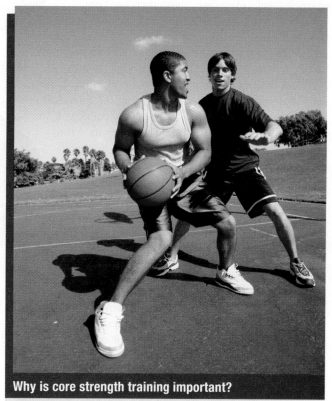

**Why is core strength training important?**

Your core muscles are essential for supporting your spine in everything you do—from standing to sitting, from dancing to playing basketball. Core muscles work together to effectively transmit forces between your upper and lower body, allowing you to twist, jump, lift, bend, and change directions. While weak core muscles can lead to back pain, strong core muscles can prevent back pain and lead to increased physical performance in all of your activities.

physically active (or to make any other behavior change) is putting so much effort into getting started that they allow their efforts to dwindle once in the action phase. Evaluate your progress, make changes if necessary, and continue to reevaluate regularly. The **Skills for Behavior Change** box offers more tips on starting and sticking with an exercise plan.

spiritual health through movement, see Focus on: Cultivating Your Spiritual Health beginning on page 60.

# Core Strength Training

Before we explore yoga, tai chi, and Pilates, let's consider core strength for a moment. The body's core muscles are the foundation for all movement.[44] These muscles include the deep back and abdominal muscles that attach to the spine and pelvis. The contraction of these muscles provides the basis of support for movements of the upper and lower body and powerful movements of the extremities. A weak core generally results in poor posture, low back pain, and muscle injuries. A strong core provides a more stable center of gravity and as a result more stable platform for movements, thus reducing the chance of injury.

You can develop core strength by doing various exercises including calisthenics, yoga, or Pilates. Holding yourself in a front or reverse plank ("up" and reverse of a push-up position) and holding or doing abdominal curl-ups are examples of exercises that increase core strength. Increasing core strength does not happen from one single exercise, but rather from a structured regime of postures and exercises.[45] Recently, the use of instability devices (stability ball, wobble boards, etc.) and exercises to train the core have become popular.[46] Although research suggests instability training is effective for improving core strength and reducing back pain, it should not replace traditional programs completely, but rather be used in conjunction with and become part of the FITT prescription.[47]

# Yoga

Yoga originated in India about 5,000 years ago. It blends the mental and physical aspects of exercise, a union of mind and body that participants often find relaxing and satisfying. If done regularly, yoga improves flexibility, vitality, posture, agility, balance, coordination, and muscular strength and endurance. Many people report an improved sense of general well-being, too.

The practice of yoga focuses attention on controlled breathing as well as physical exercise and incorporates a complex array of static stretching exercises expressed as postures (*asanas*). During a session, participants move to different asanas and hold them for 30 seconds or longer. Asanas, singly or in combination, can be changed and adpated for young and old or to accommodate physical limitations or disabilities. Asanas can also be combined to provide well-conditioned athletes with a challenging workout!

Some forms of yoga are more meditative in their practice (see Chapter 3), whereas other forms, such as Ashtanga and Bikram, are more athletic. *Ashtanga yoga*, also called "power yoga," is an energetic form of yoga that focuses on a series of poses done in a continuous, repeated flow, with controlled breathing. *Bikram yoga*, also known as *hot yoga*, is unique in that classes are held in rooms heated to 105°F. The theory behind this practice is that performing yoga in a "hot" environment allows the muscles to easily stretch to their point of tension with a greater potential for increasing flexibility.

# Tai Chi

Tai chi is an ancient Chinese form of exercise that combines stretching, balance, muscular endurance, coordination, and meditation. It increases range of motion and flexibility while reducing muscular tension. Based on Qigong, a Taoist philosophy dedicated to spiritual growth and good health, tai chi was developed about AD 1000 by monks who wanted to defend themselves against bandits and warlords. It involves a series of positions called *forms* that are performed continuously. Tai chi is often described as "meditation in motion" because it promotes serenity through gentle movements, connecting the mind and body.

Tai chi and other styles of exercise that strengthen core body muscles can also enhance flexibility and help lower stress levels.

# Pilates

Pilates was developed by Joseph Pilates in 1926 as an exercise style that combines stretching with movement against resistance, frequently aided by devices such as tension springs or heavy rubber bands. It teaches body awareness, good posture, and easy, graceful body movements. Further it improves flexibility, coordination, core strength, muscle tone, and economy of motion.

Pilates differs from yoga and tai chi in that it includes a component specifically designed to increase strength. The method consists of a sequence of carefully performed movements. Some are carried out on specially designed equipment, whereas others can be performed on mats. Each exercise stretches and strengthens the muscles involved and has a specific breathing pattern associated with it.

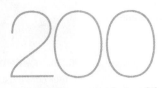

**200**

**yoga postures exist, with 50 practiced regularly.**

# Nutrition and Exercise

To make the most of your workouts, follow the recommendations from the MyPyramid Plan, and make sure that you eat sufficient carbohydrates, the body's main source of fuel (see Chapter 7 for more details). Your body stores carbohydrates as glycogen primarily in the muscles and liver and then uses this stored glycogen for energy when you are physically active. Fats are also an important source of energy, packing more than double the energy per gram compared to carbohydrates. Protein plays a role in muscle repair and growth, but is not normally a source of energy. Another important nutrient to consider is water or fluids.

When you eat is almost as important as what you eat. Eating a large meal before exercising can cause upset stomach, cramping, and diarrhea, because your muscles have to compete with your digestive system for energy. Eat larger meals at least 4 hours before you begin exercising. Smaller meals (snacks) can be eaten about an hour before activity. Not eating at all before a workout can cause low blood sugar levels that in turn cause weakness and slower reaction times. It is also important to refuel after your workout. Help your muscles recover and prepare for the next bout of activity by eating a snack or meal that contains plenty of carbohydrates and a little protein too. Today there is a burgeoning market for dietary supplements that claim to deliver the nutrients needed for muscle recovery, as well as some that include additional "performance-enhancing" ingredients; see Table 9.5 for a list of some of the most popular performance-enhancing drugs and supplements, their purported benefits, and associated risks.

In addition to eating well, staying hydrated is also crucial for active individuals to maintain a healthy, fully functional body. How much fluid do you need to stay well hydrated? Keep in mind that the goal of fluid replacement is to prevent excessive dehydration (greater than 2% loss of body weight).

## TABLE 9.5 Performance-Enhancing Dietary Supplements and Drugs—Their Uses and Effects

|  | Primary Uses | Side Effects |
| --- | --- | --- |
| **Creatine** <br> Naturally occurring compound that helps supply energy to muscle | • To improve postworkout recovery <br> • To increase muscle mass <br> • To increase strength <br> • To increase power | • Weight gain, nausea, muscle cramps. <br> • Large doses have a negative effect on the kidneys |
| **Ephedra and ephedrine** <br> Stimulant that constricts blood vessels and increases blood pressure and heart rate | • Weight loss <br> • Increased performance | • Nausea, vomiting <br> • Anxiety and mood changes <br> • Hyperactivity <br> • In rare cases, seizures, heart attack, stroke, psychotic episodes |
| **Anabolic steroids** <br> Synthetic versions of the hormone testosterone | • To improve strength, power, and speed <br> • To increase muscle mass | • In adolescents, stops bone growth; therefore reduced adult height <br> • Masculinization of females; feminization of males <br> • Mood swings <br> • Severe acne, particularly on the back <br> • Sexual dysfunction <br> • Aggressive behavior <br> • Potential heart and liver damage |
| **Steroid precursors** <br> Substances that the body converts into anabolic steroids, e.g., androstenedione (andro), dehydroepiandrosterone (DHEA) | • Converted in the body to anabolic steroids to increase muscle mass | • In addition to side effects noted with anabolic steroids: <br> • Body hair growth, increased risk of pancreatic cancer |
| **Human growth hormone** <br> Naturally occurring hormone secreted by the pituitary gland that is essential for body growth | • Anti-aging agent <br> • To improve performance <br> • To increase muscle mass | • Structural changes to the face <br> • Increased risk of high blood pressure <br> • Potential for congestive heart failure |

**Sources:** Mayo Clinic Staff, "Performance-Enhancing Drugs and Your Teen Athlete," MayoClinic.com, January 2009, www.mayoclinic.com/health/performance-enhancing-drugs/SM00045; Office of Diversion Control, Drug and Chemical Evaluation Section, "Drugs and Chemicals of Concern: Human Growth Hormone," August 2009, www.deadiversion.usdoj.gov/drugs_concern/hgh.htm; Office of Dietary Supplements, National Institutes of Health, "Ephedra and Ephedrine Alkaloids for Weight Loss and Athletic Performance," Updated July 2004, http://ods.od.nih.gov/factsheets/EphedraandEphedrine.

The ACSM and the National Athletic Trainers Association recommend consuming 5 to 7 mL per kg body weight (approximately 0.7 to 1.07 oz per 10 lb body weight) 4 hours prior to exercise.[48] Drinking fluids during exercise is also important, but it is difficult to provide guidelines for how much or when because intake should be based on time, intensity, and type of activity performed. A good way to monitor how much fluid you need to replace is to weigh yourself before and after your workout. The difference in weight is how much you should drink. So, for example, if you lost 2 pounds during a training session, you should drink 32 ounces of fluid.[49]

What are the best fluids to drink? For exercise sessions lasting less than 1 hour, plain water is sufficient for rehydration. If your exercise session exceeds 1 hour—and you sweat profusely—consider a sports drink containing electrolytes. The electrolytes in these products are minerals and ions such as sodium and potassium that are needed for proper functioning of your nervous and muscular systems. Replacing electrolytes is particularly important for endurance athletes engaging in long bouts of exercise or competition. In endurance events lasting more than 4 hours, an athlete's over-consumption of plain water can dilute the sodium concentration in the blood with potentially fatal results, an effect called **hyponatremia** or **water intoxication.** See the Student Health Today box at right for more on what to drink when you work out.

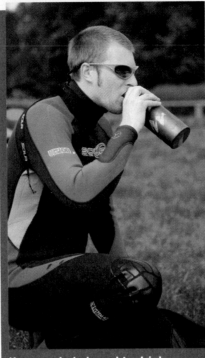

**How much do I need to drink before, during, and after physical activity?**

The American College of Sports Medicine and the National Athletic Trainers' Association recommend consuming 14 to 22 ounces of fluid several hours prior to exercise and about 6 to 12 ounces per 15 to 20 minutes during—assuming you are sweating.

# Fitness-Related Injuries

There are two basic types of fitness-related injuries: traumatic and overuse injuries. **Traumatic injuries** occur suddenly and violently, typically by accident. Typical traumatic injuries are broken bones, torn ligaments and muscles, contusions, and lacerations. Many traumatic injuries are unavoidable—for example, spraining your ankle by landing on another person's foot after jumping up for a rebound in basketball. Others are preventable through proper training, appropriate equipment and clothing, and common sense. If your traumatic injury causes a noticeable loss of function and immediate pain or

**hyponatremia** or **water intoxication** The overconsumption of water, which leads to a dilution of sodium concentration in the blood with potentially fatal results.

**traumatic injuries** Injuries that are accidental and occur suddenly and violently.

**overuse injuries** Injuries that result from the cumulative effects of day-after-day stresses placed on tendons, muscles, and joints.

pain that does not go away after 30 minutes, consult a physician.

Overtraining is the most frequent cause of injuries related to physical fitness training. Doing too much intense exercise, too much exercise without variation, or not allowing for sufficient rest and recovery time can increase the likelihood of **overuse injuries.** Overuse injuries occur because of the cumulative, day-after-day stresses placed on tendons, muscles, and joints.

## Common Overuse Injuries

Common sites of overuse injuries are the hip, knee, shoulder, and elbow joints. Three of the most common overuse injuries are plantar fasciitis, shin splints, and runner's knee.

**Plantar Fasciitis** *Plantar fasciitis* is an inflammation of the plantar fascia, a broad band of dense, inelastic tissue (fascia) that runs from the heel to the toe on the bottom of your foot. The main function of the plantar fascia is to protect the nerves, blood vessels, and muscles of the foot from injury. In repetitive weight-bearing physical activities such as walking and running, the plantar fascia may become inflamed. Common symptoms are pain and tenderness under the ball of the foot, at the heel, or at both locations.[50] The pain of plantar fasciitis is particularly noticeable during your first steps in the morning. If not treated properly, this injury may progress to the point that weight-bearing activities are too painful to endure.

**Shin Splints** *Shin splints* is a general term for any pain that occurs on the front part of the lower legs, and the term is used to describe more than 20 different medical conditions. The most common type of shin splints occurs along the inner side of the tibia and is usually a combination of muscle irritation and irritation of the tissues that attach the muscles to the bone. Specific pain on the tibia or on the fibula (the adjacent smaller bone) should be examined for a possible stress fracture.

Sedentary people who start a new weight-bearing physical activity program are at the greatest risk for shin splints, although even well-conditioned aerobic exercisers who rapidly increase their distance or pace may also be at risk.[51] Running and exercise classes are the most frequent cause of shin splints, but those who do a great deal of walking (such as postal carriers and restaurant workers) may also develop them.

**Runner's Knee** *Runner's knee* describes a series of problems involving the muscles, tendons, and ligaments of the

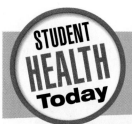

# SPORTS DRINKS OR CHOCOLATE MILK: WHICH TO USE AFTER A WORKOUT?

You know it is important to replenish fluids following a workout, but you may not be sure what the best choice is for you. Generally, water is the best fluid to choose before, during, and after a workout. However, there are situations in which you might need to choose something different.

The rationale for drinking fluids other than water ranges from preference to the physiological need to replenish lost nutrients. Most sports drinks are absorbed as effectively as water, and some are absorbed better than juice, another popular thirst-quencher. Some people are likely to consume more when their drink is flavored, a point that may be significant in ensuring proper hydration. Keep in mind, however, that the intent of sports drinks is to replenish electrolytes lost through perspiration, as well as to quickly replenish glycogen or energy stores. When perspiration is profuse (that is, 60 minutes or more of sweating), sports drinks may be necessary to replace lost electrolytes. However, if you have been physically active for a shorter duration or your exercise is not accompanied by heavy sweating, a sports drink is not needed and may add unnecessary calories to your diet. For a shorter, easier workout, water can probably meet your needs.

Recently, research has been given to milk and its potential to hydrate the body and replenish nutrients. Milk is a liquid that not only hydrates but also is a source of the electrolytes sodium and potassium, as well as carbohydrates and protein. Consuming carbohydrates after exercise will help replenish muscle and liver glycogen stores and stimulate muscle protein synthesis, while consuming protein immediately after exercise rather than several hours later results in greater muscle protein synthesis. The protein in milk, whey protein, is ideal because it contains all of the essential amino acids and is rapidly absorbed by the body. Although there are many commercial shakes and drinks available to provide the desired combination of carbohydrates and protein, low-fat chocolate milk is a cheaper alternative that will provide you with the nutrients your body needs to hydrate, repair, and recover after exercise.

For hydration, electrolytes, carbohydrates, and protein, low-fat chocolate milk may be the ideal post-workout drink.

**Sources:** J. R. Karp et al., "Chocolate Milk as Post-Exercise Recovery Aid," *International Journal of Sport Nutrition and Exercise Metabolism* 16, no. 1 (2006): 78–91; T. K. Morris and E. Stevenson, "Improved Endurance Capacity Following Chocolate Milk Consumption Compared with 2 Commercially Available Sport Drinks," *Applied Physiology, Nutrition, and Metabolism* 34, no. 1 (2009): 78–82; B. D. Roy, "Milk: The New Sports Drink? A Review," *Journal of the International Society of Sports Nutrition* 2, no. 5 (2008): 15.

---

knee. The most common cause is abnormal movements of the patella (or kneecap).[52] Women are more commonly affected because their wider pelvis results in a lateral pull on the patella by the muscles that act on the knee. In women (and some men), this causes irritation to the cartilage on the back of the patella as well as to the nearby tendons and ligaments. The main symptom is the pain experienced when downward pressure is applied to the kneecap after the knee is straightened fully. Additional symptoms include pain, swelling, redness, and tenderness around the patella, and a dull aching pain in the center of the knee.[53]

Applying ice to an injury such as a sprain can help relieve pain and reduce swelling, but never apply the ice directly to the skin, as that could lead to frostbite.

## Treatment of Fitness-Training Related Injuries

First-aid treatment for virtually all fitness-training related injuries involves **RICE: r**est, **i**ce, **c**ompression, and **e**levation. *Rest* is required to avoid further irritation of the injured body part. *Ice* is applied to relieve pain and constrict the blood vessels to reduce internal or external bleeding. To prevent frostbite, wrap the ice or cold pack in a layer of wet toweling or elastic bandage before applying to your skin. A new injury should be iced for approximately 20 minutes every hour for the first 24 to 72 hours. *Compression* of the injured body part can be accomplished with a 4- or 6-inch-wide

**RICE** Acronym for the standard first aid treatment for virtually all traumatic and overuse injuries: **r**est, **i**ce, **c**ompression, and **e**levation.

elastic bandage; this applies indirect pressure to damaged blood vessels to help stop bleeding. Be careful, though, that the compression wrap does not interfere with normal blood flow. Throbbing or pain indicates that the compression wrap should be loosened. *Elevation* of an injured extremity above the level of your heart also helps to control internal or external bleeding by making the blood flow upward to reach the injured area.

## Preventing Injuries

There are steps you can take to reduce your risk of overuse or traumatic injuries. Using common sense and identifying and using only the proper gear and equipment can help you avoid an injury. Varying your physical activties throughout the week, setting appropriate and realistic short- and long-term goals will also help. It is important to listen to your body when working out. Warning signs include muscle stiffness and soreness, bone and joint pains, and whole-body fatigue that simply does not go away.

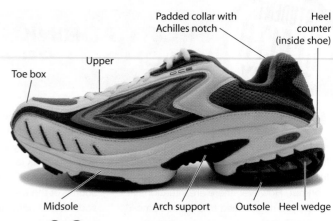

FIGURE $9.8$ **Anatomy of a Running Shoe**
A good running shoe should fit comfortably; allow room for your toes to move; have a firm, but flexible midsole; and have a firm grip on your heel to prevent slipping

**Appropriate Footwear** Proper footwear can decrease the likelihood of foot, knee, or back injuries. Biomechanics research has revealed that running is a collision sport—with each stride, the runner's foot collides with the ground with a force three to five times the runner's body weight.[54] The force not absorbed by the running shoe is transmitted upward into the foot, leg, thigh, and back. Our bodies can absorb forces such as these but may be injured by the cumulative effect of repetitive impacts (such as running 40 miles per week). Thus, the shoes' ability to absorb shock is critical—not just for those who run, but for anyone engaged in weight-bearing activities.

In addition to providing shock absorption, an athletic shoe should provide a good fit for maximal comfort and performance—see also Figure 9.8. To get the best fit, shop at a sports or fitness specialty store where there is a large selection to choose from and there are salespeople available who are trained in properly fitting athletic shoes. Try on shoes later in the day when your feet are largest, and check to make sure there is a little extra room in the toe and that the width is appropriate. Because different activities place different stresses on your feet and joints, you should choose shoes specifically designed for your sport or activity. Shoes of any type should be replaced once they lose their cushioning.

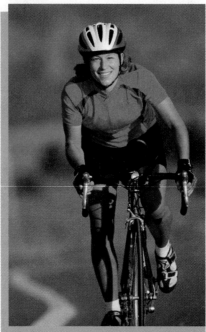

**What can I do to avoid injury when I am physically active?**

Reducing risk for exercise-related injuries requires common sense and some preventative measures. Wear protective gear, such as helmets, knee pads, elbow pads, eyewear, and supportive footwear, that is appropriate for your activity. Vary your activities to avoid overuse injuries. Dress for the weather, try to avoid exercising in extreme conditions, and always stay properly hydrated. Finally, respect your personal physical limitations, listen to your body, and respond effectively to it.

Continuing to use a shoe that is worn out will increase your risk of injury.

**Appropriate Protective Equipment** It is essential to use well-fitted, appropriate protective equipment for your physical activities. For some activities, that means choosing what is best for you and your body. For example, the use of the "right" racquet with the "right" tension helps prevent the general inflammatory condition known as "tennis elbow." Other activities require specialized protective equipment to reduce your chances of injuries. For example, eye injuries can occur in virtually all physical activities, although some are more risky than others. As many as 90 percent of the eye injuries resulting from racquetball and squash could be prevented by wearing appropriate eye protection—for example, goggles with polycarbonate lenses.[55]

Wearing a helmet while bicycle riding is an important safety precaution. An estimated 45 to 88 percent of head injuries among cyclists can be prevented by wearing a helmet. More than 60 percent of college students who rode a bike in the past 12 months also reported never wearing a helmet (40%) or wearing one only rarely.[56] The direct medical costs from cyclists' failure to wear helmets is an estimated $81 million a year.[57] Cyclists aren't the only ones who should be wearing helmets. People who skateboard, use kick-scooters, ski, in-line skate, play contact sports,

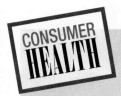

# SHOPPING FOR FITNESS: FACILITIES, EQUIPMENT, AND CLOTHING

Do you really need to belong to the best gym in town or have the latest equipment and fashionable clothing to meet your physical fitness goals? The short answer is no. You can achieve your personal physical fitness goals without becoming a member of a fitness or wellness center, without buying equipment, and without spending lots of money on the latest fitness fashions. All you need is a good pair of shoes, comfortable clothing to suit the environment you will be physically active in, your own body to use as resistance, and a safe place for activity. However, you may enjoy the outing or experience created by going to a fitness or wellness center or prefer to have some exercise equipment in your home and you may be in need of new exercise clothing. The following will help guide your selections.

## CHOOSING FACILITIES

✳ Visit several facilities before making a decision—and if possible during the time when you intend to use them (so you can see how busy or crowded they are at that time).
✳ Determine the hours of operation—are these convenient for you?
✳ Consider the exercise classes offered. What is the

schedule? Can you try one out?
✳ Consider the equipment. What do they have? Is it sufficient to cover your training needs (i.e., aerobic exercise machines, resistance-training equipment including both free weights and machines, mats, and other items to assist with stretching)?
✳ Consider the location. How convenient is it (i.e., on your way to or from work or school, close to your home)?
✳ Consider the personnel (including training in first aid and CPR), options for working with a personal trainer, and how friendly and approachable they are.
✳ Consider the financial implications. What membership benefits, student rates, or other discounts are available? Steer clear of clubs that pressure you for a long-term commitment and do not offer trial memberships or grace periods that allow you to get a refund.

## BUYING EQUIPMENT

✳ Ignore claims that an exercise device provides lasting "no sweat" results in a short time.
✳ Question claims that an exercise device can target or burn fat.
✳ Read the fine print. Advertised results may be based on more than just using a

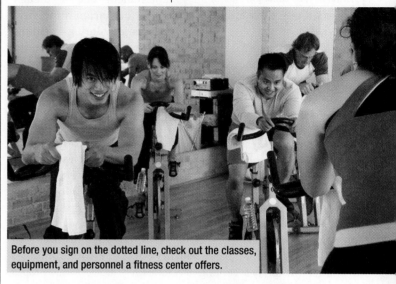

Before you sign on the dotted line, check out the classes, equipment, and personnel a fitness center offers.

machine; they may also involve caloric restriction.
✳ Be skeptical of testimonials and before-and-after pictures of satisfied customers.
✳ Calculate the cost including shipping and handling fees, sales tax, delivery and setup charges, or long-term commitments.
✳ Obtain details on warranties, guarantees, and return policies.
✳ Try the equipment at a gym if you can or borrow it from someone.
✳ Consider how this piece of equipment will fit in your home. Where will you store it? Will you be able to get to it easily?
✳ Check out consumer reports or online resources for the best product ratings and reviews.

## BUYING EXERCISE CLOTHING

✳ Choose your exercise clothing based on comfort, not looks.
✳ Consider the environment (temperature, humidity, ventilation) when making your selection.
✳ Dress in layers, ensuring that your skin can breathe in the cold (see also Exercising in the Cold, page 320).
✳ Dress to allow for optimal heat dissipation in hot and humid environments (see also Exercising in the Heat, below).
✳ Ensure your clothing is well fitted—neither too loose nor too tight to allow for freedom of movement.
✳ Choose clothing that helps you to feel good about yourself and the activity you are undertaking.

or snowboard should also wear helmets. Look for helmets that meet the standards established by the American National Standards Institute or the Snell Memorial Foundation. The **Consumer Health** box above offers suggestions on evaluating and choosing a fitness center, equipment, and fitness clothing.

**Exercising in the Heat** Exercising in hot or humid weather increases your risk of a heat-related injury. In these conditions, your body's rate of heat production can exceed its ability to cool. The three different heat stress illnesses, progressive in their level of severity, are heat cramps, heat exhaustion, and heatstroke.

**Heat cramps** (heat-related involuntary and forcible muscle contractions that cannot be relaxed), the least serious problem, can usually be prevented by adequate fluid replacement and a dietary intake that includes the electrolytes lost during sweating.

**Heat exhaustion** is actually a mild form of shock, in which the blood pools in the arms and legs away from the brain and major organs of the body. It is caused by excessive water loss because of intense or prolonged exercise or work in a hot and/or humid environment. Symptoms of heat exhaustion include nausea, headache, fatigue, dizziness and faintness, and, paradoxically, "goosebumps" and chills. When suffering from heat exhaustion, your skin will be cool and moist. **Heatstroke,** often called *sunstroke,* is a life-threatening emergency condition with a 20 to 70 percent death rate.[58] Heatstroke occurs during vigorous exercise when the body's heat production significantly exceeds its cooling capacities. Core body temperature can rise from normal (98.6°F) to 105°F to 110°F within minutes after the body's cooling mechanism shuts down. A rapid increase in core body temperature can cause brain damage, permanent disability, and death. Common signs of heatstroke are dry, hot, and usually red skin; very high body temperature; and rapid heart rate. If you experience any of the symptoms of heat illness mentioned here, stop exercising immediately, move to the shade or a cool spot to rest, and drink plenty of cool fluids.

You can prevent heat stress by following certain precautions. First, acclimatize yourself to hot or humid climates. The process of heat acclimatization, which increases your body's cooling efficiency, requires about 10 to 14 days of gradually increased physical activity in the hot environment. Second, reduce your risk of dehydration by replacing fluids before, during, and after exercise. Third, wear clothing appropriate for the activity and the environment—for example, light-colored nylon shorts and a mesh tank top. Finally, use common sense—for example, on a day when the temperature is 85°F and the humidity is around 80 percent, postpone your lunchtime run until the evening when it is cooler.

Heat stress illnesses may also occur in situations in which the danger is not so obvious. Serious or fatal heat stroke may result from prolonged immersion in a sauna, hot tub, or steam bath or from exercising in a plastic or rubber head-to-toe "sauna suit." Similarly, exercising or training in the heat with lots of heavy clothing

**heat cramps** Involuntary and forcible muscle contractions that occur during or following exercise in hot and/or humid weather.

**heat exhaustion** A heat stress illness caused by significant dehydration resulting from exercise in hot and/or humid conditions.

**heatstroke** A deadly heat stress illness resulting from dehydration and overexertion in hot and/or humid conditions.

**hypothermia** Potentially fatal condition caused by abnormally low body core temperature.

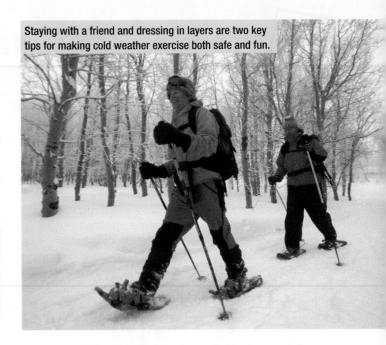

Staying with a friend and dressing in layers are two key tips for making cold weather exercise both safe and fun.

and equipment, such as a football uniform, including the helmet, puts an individual at risk.[59]

**Exercising in the Cold** When you exercise in cool weather, especially in windy conditions, your body's rate of heat loss is frequently greater than its rate of heat production. These conditions may lead to **hypothermia**—a potentially fatal condition resulting from abnormally low body core temperature. Temperatures need not be frigid for hypothermia to occur; it can also result from prolonged, vigorous exercise in 40°F to 50°F temperatures, particularly if there is rain, snow, or a strong wind.

As body core temperature drops from the normal 98.6°F to about 93.2°F, shivering begins. Shivering—the involuntary contraction of nearly every muscle in the body—increases body temperature by using the heat given off by muscle activity. You may also experience cold hands and feet, poor judgment, apathy, and amnesia. Shivering ceases in most hypothermia victims as body core temperatures drop to between 87°F and 90°F, a sign that the body has lost its ability to generate heat. Death usually occurs at body core temperatures between 75°F and 80°F.[60]

To prevent hypothermia, analyze weather conditions before engaging in your planned outdoor physical activity. Remember that wind and humidity are as significant as temperature. Have a friend join you for your cold-weather outdoor activities and wear layers of appropriate clothing to prevent excessive heat loss (polypropylene or woolen undergarments, a windproof outer garment, and a wool hat and gloves). Keep your head, hands, and feet warm. Finally, do not allow yourself to become dehydrated.[61] See also the ACSM Position Stand regarding the prevention of injuries during exercise in the cold.[62]

# How Physically Fit Are You?

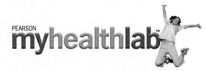

## 1 Evaluating Your Muscular Strength and Endurance (the Partial Curl-Up and Push-Up Tests)

The most commonly used tests for muscular strength and endurance are partial curl-ups and push-ups. Other less commonly used tests include the grip strength and vertical jump tests. Generally, the best measure of strength alone is 1 RM. However, this measurement is not recommended for individuals who have been sedentary for a long time or are new to resistance training.

## 1A CURL-UPS

**The partial curl-up measures the muscular strength and endurance of the abdominal musculature. In the partial curl-up, the trunk is raised no more than 30 to 40 degrees above the mat so that the shoulders are raised about 6 to 10 in. off the floor. A full sit-up is not used because of the stress placed on the lower back.**

Description/Procedure: Lie on a mat with your arms by your sides, palms flat on the mat, elbows straight, and fingers extended. Bend your knees at a 90-degree angle. Your instructor or partner will mark your starting finger position with a piece of masking tape aligned with the tip of each middle finger. He or she will also mark with tape your ending position, 10 cm or 3 in. away from the first piece of tape—one ending position tape for each hand.

Set a metronome to 50 beats per minute and curl up at this slow, controlled pace: one curl-up every two beats (25 curl-ups per min). Curl your head and upper back upward, lifting your shoulder blades off the mat (your trunk should make a 30-degree angle with the mat) and reaching your arms forward

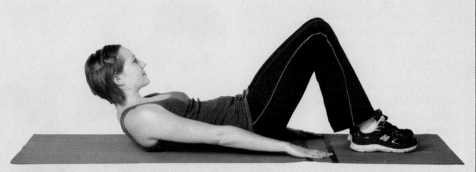

### Healthy Musculoskeletal Fitness: Norms and Health Benefit Zones: Curl-Ups

| Men | Excellent | Very Good | Good | Fair | Needs Improvement |
|---|---|---|---|---|---|
| Ages 20–29 | 25 | 21–24 | 16–20 | 11–15 | ≤10 |
| Ages 30–39 | 25 | 18–24 | 15–17 | 11–14 | ≤10 |
| Ages 40–49 | 25 | 18–24 | 13–17 | 6–12 | ≤5 |
| Ages 50–59 | 25 | 17–24 | 11–16 | 8–10 | ≤7 |
| Ages 60–69 | 25 | 16–24 | 11–15 | 6–10 | ≤5 |

| Women | Excellent | Very Good | Good | Fair | Needs Improvement |
|---|---|---|---|---|---|
| Ages 20–29 | 25 | 18–24 | 14–17 | 5–13 | ≤4 |
| Ages 30–39 | 25 | 19–24 | 10–18 | 6–9 | ≤5 |
| Ages 40–49 | 25 | 19–24 | 11–18 | 4–10 | ≤3 |
| Ages 50–59 | 25 | 19–24 | 10–18 | 6–9 | ≤5 |
| Ages 60–69 | 25 | 17–24 | 8–16 | 3–7 | ≤2 |

**Source:** Adapted from *Canadian Physical Activity, Fitness & Lifestyle Approach: CSEP-Health & Fitness Program's Appraisal and Counselling Strategy*, 3rd edition, © 2003. Reprinted with permission from the Canadian Society for Exercise Physiology.

along the mat to touch the ending tape. Then curl back down so that your upper back and shoulders touch the floor. During the entire curl-up, your fingers, feet, and buttocks should stay on the mat. Your partner will count the number of correct repetitions you complete. Perform as many curl-ups as you can in 1 minute without pausing, to a maximum of 25.

# 1B PUSH-UPS

Push-ups provide a measure of the muscular endurance of the upper body, including the shoulders, arms, and chest. There is no time limit for performing push-ups. The norms for men performing the test are based on a full push-up; the norms for women are based on a modified "knee push-up."

**Description/Procedure:** Start by positioning yourself on the ground in the standard "down" position (hands pointing forward and under the shoulder, back straight, head up, using the toes as the pivotal point) or in the modified "knee push-up" position (legs together, lower leg in contact with mat with ankles flexed, back straight, hands shoulder width apart, head up, using the knees as the pivotal point). Push yourself up by straightening your elbows and then lower your body back to the "down" position, until your chin touches the mat. Keep your back straight at all times and do not allow your stomach to contact the mat.

The maximal number of push-ups you can perform consecutively without rest is counted as your score. Stop the test when you are straining forcibly or are unable to maintain the appropriate technique within two repetitions.

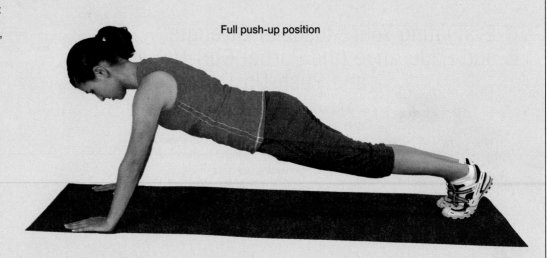

Full push-up position

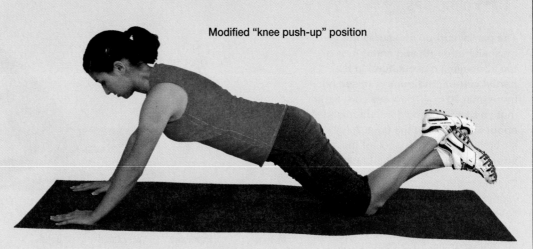

Modified "knee push-up" position

## Healthy Musculoskeletal Fitness: Norms and Health Benefit Zones: Push-Ups

| Men | Excellent | Very Good | Good | Fair | Needs Improvement |
|---|---|---|---|---|---|
| Ages 20–29 | ≥36 | 29–35 | 22–28 | 17–21 | ≤16 |
| Ages 30–39 | ≥30 | 22–29 | 17–21 | 12–16 | ≤11 |
| Ages 40–49 | ≥25 | 17–24 | 13–16 | 10–12 | ≤9 |
| Ages 50–59 | ≥21 | 13–20 | 10–12 | 7–9 | ≤6 |
| Ages 60–69 | ≥18 | 11–17 | 8–10 | 5–7 | ≤4 |
| **Women** | **Excellent** | **Very Good** | **Good** | **Fair** | **Needs Improvement** |
| Ages 20–29 | ≥30 | 21–29 | 15–20 | 10–14 | ≤9 |
| Ages 30–39 | ≥27 | 20–26 | 13–19 | 8–12 | ≤7 |
| Ages 40–49 | ≥24 | 15–23 | 11–14 | 5–10 | ≤4 |
| Ages 50–59 | ≥21 | 11–20 | 7–10 | 2–6 | ≤1 |
| Ages 60–69 | ≥17 | 12–16 | 5–11 | 2–4 | ≤1 |

**Source:** Adapted from *Canadian Physical Activity, Fitness & Lifestyle Approach: CSEP-Health & Fitness Program's Appraisal and Counselling Strategy,* 3rd edition, © 2003. Reprinted with permission from the Canadian Society for Exercise Physiology.

# 2 Evaluating Your Flexibility (the Sit-and-Reach Test)

The sit-and-reach test measures the general flexibility of your lower back, hips, and hamstring muscles. For this test you will need a sit-and-reach box (also known as a flexometer). You can make your own box by locating a solid box about 30 cm (12 in.) tall. Fix a meter stick on top of the box so that the 26-cm mark is at the front edge of the box (that is, 26 cm of the ruler will extend past the front edge).

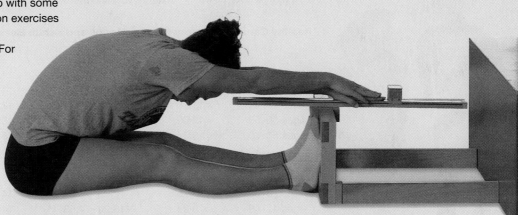

Description/Procedure: Warm up with some light activity and range-of-motion exercises and stretches for the joints and muscles that you will be using. For the test, start by sitting upright, straight-legged on a mat with your shoes removed and soles of the feet flat against the flexometer (sit-and-reach box) at the 26-cm mark. Inner edges of the soles are placed within 2 cm of the measuring scale.

Have a partner on hand to record your measurements. Stretch your arms out in front of you and, keeping the hands parallel to each other, slowly reach forward with both hands as far as possible, holding the position for approximately 2 seconds. Your fingertips should be in contact with the measuring portion (meter stick) of the sit-and-reach box. To facilitate a longer reach, exhale and drop your head between your arms while reaching forward. Keep your knees extended the whole time and breathe normally.

Your score is the most distant point (in centimeters) reached with the fingertips; have your partner make note of this number for you. Perform the test twice, record your best score, and compare it with the norms presented in the tables below.

**Healthy Musculoskeletal Fitness: Norms and Health Benefit Zones: Sit-and-Reach Test***

| Men | Excellent | Very Good | Good | Fair | Needs Improvement |
|---|---|---|---|---|---|
| Ages 20–29 | ≥40 cm | 34–39 cm | 30–33 cm | 25–29 cm | ≤24 cm |
| Ages 30–39 | ≥38 cm | 33–37 cm | 28–32 cm | 23–27 cm | ≤22 cm |
| Ages 40–49 | ≥35 cm | 29–34 cm | 24–28 cm | 18–23 cm | ≤17 cm |
| Ages 50–59 | ≥35 cm | 28–34 cm | 24–27 cm | 16–23 cm | ≤15 cm |
| Ages 60–69 | ≥33 cm | 25–32 cm | 20–24 cm | 15–19 cm | ≤14 cm |

| Women | Excellent | Very Good | Good | Fair | Needs Improvement |
|---|---|---|---|---|---|
| Ages 20–29 | ≥41 cm | 37–40 cm | 33–36 cm | 28–32 cm | ≤27 cm |
| Ages 30–39 | ≥41 cm | 36–40 cm | 32–35 cm | 27–31 cm | ≤26 cm |
| Ages 40–49 | ≥38 cm | 34–37 cm | 30–33 cm | 25–29 cm | ≤24 cm |
| Ages 50–59 | ≥39 cm | 33–38 cm | 30–32 cm | 25–29 cm | ≤24 cm |
| Ages 60–69 | ≥35 cm | 31–34 cm | 27–30 cm | 23–26 cm | ≤22 cm |

*Note: These norms are based on a sit-and-reach box in which the zero point is set at 26 cm. When using a box in which the zero point is set at 23 cm, subtract 3 cm from each value in this table.

Source: Adapted from *Canadian Physical Activity, Fitness & Lifestyle Approach: CSEP-Health & Fitness Program's Appraisal and Counselling Strategy,* 3rd edition, © 2003. Reprinted with permission from the Canadian Society for Exercise Physiology.

# 3 Evaluating Your Cardiorespiratory Fitness (the 1.5-Mile Run Test)

**The 1.5-mile run test assesses your cardiorespiratory fitness level.**

Description/Procedure: Use a track with a one-quarter-mile lap to perform this test. Using a stopwatch, determine how long it takes you to run 1.5 miles (6 laps using the inside lane). Do not eat a heavy meal for at least 2 to 3 hours prior to the test. Be sure to warm-up and stretch thoroughly prior to the test, and to cool-down

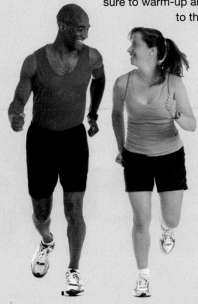

by walking slowly for about 5 minutes after you complete the run. It is best to pace yourself on this test; in other words, do not run your fastest when you start, but run a speed that you think you can continue for the entire test. If you become extremely fatigued during the test, slow your pace or walk— do not overstress yourself! If you feel faint or nauseated or experience any unusual pains in your upper body, stop and notify your instructor.

### Healthy Cardiorespiratory Fitness: Norms and Health Benefit Zones: 1.5-Mile Run Test

| Men | Excellent | Good | Fair | Poor |
|---|---|---|---|---|
| Ages 20–29 | <10:10 | 10:10–11:29 | 11:30–12:38 | >12:38 |
| Ages 30–39 | <10:47 | 10:47–11:54 | 11:55–12:58 | >12:58 |
| Ages 40–49 | <11:16 | 11:16–12:24 | 12:25–13:50 | >13:50 |
| Ages 50–59 | <12:09 | 12:09–13:35 | 13:36–15:06 | >15:06 |
| Ages 60–69 | <13:24 | 13:24–15:04 | 15:05–16:46 | >16:46 |
| **Women** | **Excellent** | **Good** | **Fair** | **Poor** |
| Ages 20–29 | <11:59 | 11:59–13:24 | 13:25–14:50 | >14:50 |
| Ages 30–39 | <12:25 | 12:25–14:08 | 14:09–15:43 | >15:43 |
| Ages 40–49 | <13:24 | 13:24–14:53 | 14:54–16:31 | >16:31 |
| Ages 50–59 | <14:35 | 14:35–16:35 | 16:36–18:18 | >18:18 |
| Ages 60–69 | <16:34 | 16:34–18:27 | 18:28–20:16 | >20:16 |

Source: Reprinted with permission from The Cooper Institute, Dallas, Texas from a book called "Physical Fitness Assessments and Norms for Adults and Law Enforcement." Available online at www.cooperinstitute.org.

# YOUR PLAN FOR CHANGE

The **Assessyourself** activity helped you determine your current level of physical fitness. Based on your results, you may decide that you should take steps to improve one or more components of your physical fitness.

### Today, you can:

◯ Visit your campus fitness facility and familiarize yourself with the equipment and resources. Find out what classes they offer, and take home a copy of the schedule.

◯ Walk between your classes; make an extra effort to take the long way to get from building to building. Use the stairs instead of the elevator or escalator.

◯ Take a stretch break. Spend 5 to 10 minutes in between homework projects or just before bed doing some whole-body stretches to release tension.

### Within the next 2 weeks, you can:

◯ Shop for comfortable workout clothes and appropriate athletic footwear.

◯ Look into group activities on your campus or in your community that you might enjoy.

◯ Ask a friend to join you in your workout once a week. Agree on a date and time in advance so you'll both be committed to following through.

◯ Plan for a physically active outing with a friend or date; perhaps you can go dancing or bowling, or shoot hoops. Use active transportation (i.e., walk or cycle) to get to a movie or go out for dinner.

### By the end of the semester, you can:

◯ Establish a regular routine of engaging in physical activity or exercise at least three times a week. Mark your exercise times on your calendar and keep a log to track your progress.

◯ Take your workouts to the next level. If you have been working out at home, try going to a gym or participating in an exercise class. If you are walking, perhaps try intermittent jogging or sign up for a fitness event such as a charity 5K.

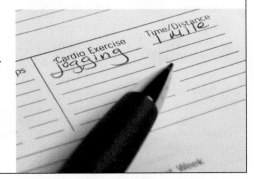

# Summary

* Benefits of regular physical activity include reduced risk of heart attack, some cancers, hypertension, and type 2 diabetes; and improved blood profile, bone mass, weight control, immunity to disease, mental health and stress management, and physical fitness. Regular physical activity can also increase life span.

* Planning to improve your physical fitness involves setting goals and designing a program to achieve these goals. A comprehensive workout repeated regularly will increase physical fitness and should include a warm-up with some light stretching activities, strength-development exercises, aerobic activities, and a cool-down period with a heavier emphasis on stretching exercises. The FITT principle can be used to develop a progressive program of physical fitness.

* For general health benefits, every adult should participate in moderate-intensity activities for 30 minutes at least 5 days a week. To improve cardiorespiratory fitness, you should engage in vigorous, continuous, and rhythmic activities 3 to 5 days per week at an exercise intensity of 70 to 90 percent of your maximum heart rate for 20 to 30 minutes.

* Three key principles for developing muscular strength and endurance are overload, specificity of training, and variation. Muscular strength is improved by engaging in resistance training exercises two to four times per week, using an intensity of greater than 60 percent of 1RM and completing one to three sets of two to six reps. Muscular endurance is improved by engaging in resistance training exercises two to four times per week, using an intensity of less than 60 percent of 1 RM and completing two to six sets of 10 to 15 reps.

* Flexibility is improved by engaging in two to three repetitions of static stretching exercises at least 2 to 3 days a week (and preferably daily) where each stretch is held for 10 to 30 seconds.

* Core strength training is important for maintaining full mobility and stability and for preventing back injury. The popular exercise forms of yoga, tai chi, and Pilates all develop core strength as well as flexibility, strength, and endurance.

* Fitness training-related injuries are generally caused by overuse or trauma; the most common are plantar fasciitis, shin splints, and runner's knee. Proper footwear and equipment can help prevent injuries. Exercise in the heat or cold requires special precautions.

# Pop Quiz

1. The maximum volume of oxygen consumed by the muscles during exercise defines
   a. target heart rate.
   b. muscular strength.
   c. aerobic capacity.
   d. muscular endurance.

2. What is physical fitness?
   a. The ability to respond to routine physical demands
   b. Having enough reserves after working out to cope with a sudden challenge
   c. Both aerobic and muscular strength
   d. All of the above

3. Type 2 diabetes can be prevented by
   a. reading about it.
   b. getting your blood sugar level tested.
   c. engaging in daily physical activity.
   d. It cannot be prevented.

4. Flexibility is the range of motion around
   a. specific bones.
   b. a joint or series of joints.
   c. the tendons.
   d. the muscles.

5. The "talk test" measures
   a. exercise intensity.
   b. exercise time.
   c. exercise frequency.
   d. exercise type.

6. An example of aerobic exercise is
   a. brisk walking.
   b. bench-pressing weights.
   c. stretching exercises.
   d. holding yoga poses.

7. Theresa wants to lower her ratio of fat to her total body weight. She wants to work on her
   a. flexibility.
   b. muscular endurance.
   c. muscular strength.
   d. body composition.

8. Miguel is a cross-country runner and is therefore able to sustain moderate-intensity, whole-body activity for extended periods of time. This ability relates to what component of physical fitness?
   a. Flexibility
   b. Body composition
   c. Cardiorespiratory fitness
   d. Muscular strength and endurance

9. Janice has been lifting 95 pounds while doing three sets of ten leg curls. To become stronger, she began lifting 105 pounds while doing leg curls. What principle of strength development does this represent?
   a. Reversibility
   b. Overload
   c. Flexibility
   d. Specificity of training

10. Overuse injuries can be prevented by
    a. monitoring the quantity and quality of your workouts.
    b. engaging in only one type of aerobic training.
    c. working out daily.
    d. working out with a friend.

*Answers to these questions can be found on page A-1.*

## Think about It!

1. How do you define *physical fitness*? What are the key components of a physical fitness program? What should you consider when planning and starting a physical fitness program?

2. What do you do to motivate yourself to engage in physical activity on a regular basis? What and who helps you to be physically active?

3. Describe the FITT prescription for cardiorespiratory fitness, muscular strength and endurance, and flexibility training.

4. Why is flexibility important in everyday activities? Why is it important in athletic performance?

5. Your roommate has decided to start running to improve his or her cardiorespiratory fitness. What advice would you give to make sure he or she gets off to a good start, does not get injured, and continues the program throughout the year?

6. Identify at least four physiological and psychological benefits of physical activity. How would you promote these benefits to non-exercisers?

## Accessing Your Health on the Internet

The following websites explore further topics and issues related to personal health. For links to the websites below, visit the Companion Website for *Access to Health*, 12th Edition, at www.pearsonhighered.com/donatelle.

1. *ACSM Online.* This site is the link to the American College of Sports Medicine and all its resources. www.acsm.org

2. *American Council on Exercise.* Information is found here on exercise and disease prevention. www.acefitness.org

3. *Centers for Disease Control and Prevention, National Center for Chronic Disease Prevention and Health Pro-* motion, *Division of Nutrition and Physical Activity.* This site is a great resource for current information on exercise and health. www.cdc.gov/nccdphp/dnpa

4. *National Strength and Conditioning Association.* This site is a resource for personal trainers and others interested in conditioning and fitness. www.nsca-lift.org

5. *The President's Council on Physical Fitness and Sports.* Look here for information on fitness programs. www.fitness.gov

## References

1. D. E. R. Warburton, C. Whitney Nicol, and S. S. D. Bredin, "Prescribing Exercise as Preventive Therapy," *Canadian Medical Association Journal,* 174, no. 7 (2006): 961–74. Erratum, 178, no. 6 (2008): 731–32.

2. Centers for Disease Control and Prevention, "Physical Activity Statistics," Updated February 2010, http://apps.nccd.cdc.gov/PASurveillance/StateSumResultV.asp; Centers for Disease Control and Prevention, "QuickStats: Percentage of Adults Aged ≥ 18 Years Who Engaged in Leisure Time Strengthening Activities, by Age Group and Sex— National Health Interview Survey, United States, 2008," *Morbidity and Mortality Weekly Report* 58, no. 34 (2009): 955.

3. Office of Disease Prevention and Health Promotion, U.S. Department of Health and Human Services, *2008 Physical Activity Guidelines for Americans: Be Active, Healthy, and Happy!* ODPHP Publication no. U0036 (Washington, DC: U.S. Department of Health and Human Services, 2008), Available at www.health.gov.paguidelines; Centers for Disease Control and Prevention, "Physical Activity Statistics: Definitions," Updated May 2007, www.cdc.gov/nccdphp/dnpa/physical/stats/definitions.htm; Centers for Disease Control and Prevention, "Physical Activity for Everyone: Physical Activity and Health," Updated May 2010, www.cdc.gov/nccdphp/dnpa/physical/everyone/health.

4. American College Health Association, *American College Health Association-National College Health Assessment II (ACHA-NCHA II) Reference Group Executive Summary Fall 2009* (Linthicum, MD: American College Health Association, 2009), Available at www.achancha.org/reports_ACHA-NCHAII.html.

5. Ibid.

6. W. L. Haskell et al., "Physical Activity and Public Health: Updated Recommendation for Adults from the American College of Sports Medicine and the American Heart Association," *Medicine and Science in Sports and Exercise* 39, no. 8 (2007): 1423–34; Office of Disease Prevention and Health Promotion, U.S. Department of Health and Human Services, *2008 Physical Activity Guidelines for Americans*, 2008.

7. W. L. Haskell et al., "Physical Activity and Public Health," 2007.

8. D. E. R. Warburton, C. Whitney Nicol, and S. S. D. Bredin, "Health Benefits of Physical Activity: The Evidence," *Canadian Medical Association Journal,* 174, no. 6 (2006): 801–09.

9. D. E. R. Warburton et al., "Evidence-Informed Physical Activity Guidelines for Canadian Adults," *Canadian Journal of Public Health* 98, Suppl. 2 (2007): S16–S68.

10. S. Plowman and D. Smith, *Exercise Physiology for Health, Fitness, and Performance.* 2d ed. reprint (Philadelphia: Lippincott Williams & Wilkins, 2008): 312–13.

11. W. L. Haskell et al., "Cardiovascular Benefits and Assessment of Physical Activity and Physical Fitness in Adults," *Medicine and Science in Sports and Exercise* 24, Suppl. 6 (1992): s201–S220.

12. American Heart Association, "About Cholesterol," Updated July 2010, www.heart.org/HEARTORG/Conditions/Cholesterol/AboutCholesterol/About-Cholesterol_UCM_001220_Article.jsp.

13. A. Mehta, "Management of Cardiovascular Risk Associated with Insulin Resistance, Diabetes, and the Metabolic Syndrome," *Postgraduate Medicine* 122, no. 3 (2010) 61–70.

14. Ibid.

15. U.S. Department of Health and Human Services, *2008 Physical Activity Guidelines for Americans: Be Active, Healthy, and Happy!*, 2008.

16. C. E. Tudor-Locke, R. C. Bell, and A. M. Meters, "Revisiting the Role of Physical Activity and Exercise in the Treatment of Type 2 Diabetes," *Canadian Journal of Applied Physiology* 25, no. 6 (2000): 466–92.

17. National Diabetes Information Clearinghouse, U.S. Department of Health and Human Services, *Diabetes Prevention Program (DPP),* NIH Publication no. 09–5099 (Bethesda, MD: National Diabetes Information Clearinghouse, 2008), Available at http://diabetes.niddk.nih.gov/dm/pubs/preventionprogram.

18. J. Peto, "Cancer Epidemiology in the Last Century and the Next Decade," *Nature* 411 (2001): 390–95.

19. World Cancer Research Fund/American Institute for Cancer Research, *Policy and Action for Cancer Prevention. Food, Nutrition, and Physical Activity: A Global*

*Perspective* (Washington, DC: American Institute for Cancer Research, 2009), www.dietandcancerreport.org/downloads/Policy_Report.pdf.

20. C. M. Friedenreich and A. E. Cust, "Physical Activity and Breast Cancer Risk: Impact of Timing, Type, and Dose of Activity and Population Subgroup Effects," *British Journal of Sports Medicine* 42, no. 8 (2008): 636–47.

21. World Cancer Research Fund/American Institute for Cancer Research, *Policy and Action for Cancer Prevention*, 2009; A. Shibata, K. Ishii, and K. Oka, "Psychological, Social, and Environmental Factors of Meeting Recommended Physical Activity Levels for Colon Cancer Prevention among Japanese Adults," *Journal of Science and Medicine in Sport* 12, no. 2 (2010): e155–e156; K. Y. Wolin, Y. Yan Y, G. A. Colditz, and I. M. Lee, "Physical Activity and Colon Cancer Prevention: A Meta-Analysis," *British Journal of Cancer* 100, no. 4 (2009): 611–16.

22. S. Tolomio et al., "Short-Term Adapted Physical Activity Program Improves Bone Quality in Osteopenic/Osteoporotic Postmenopausal Women," *Journal of Physical Activity and Health*, 5, no. 6 (2008): 844–53.

23. T. Post et al., "Bone Physiology, Disease and Treatment: Towards Disease System Analysis in Osteoporosis," *Clinical Pharmacokinetics*, 49, no. 2 (2010): 89–118.

24. J. G. Thomas and R. R. Wing, "Maintenance of Long-Term Weight Loss," *Medicine & Health Rhode Island* 92, no. 2 (2009): 56–57.

25. A. Koch, "Immune Response to Resistance Exercise," *American Journal of Lifestyle Medicine* 4, no. 3 (2010): 244–52.

26. MedLine Plus, National Institutes of Health, "Exercise and Immunity," Updated May 2010, www.nlm.nih.gov/medlineplus/ency/article/007165.htm.

27. Ibid.

28. M. Gleeson, "Immune Function in Sport and Exercise," *Journal of Applied Physiology* 103, no. 2 (2007): 693–99.

29. M. Cardinale et al., "Hormonal Responses to a Single Session of Wholebody Vibration Exercise in Older Individuals," *British Journal of Sports Medicine*, 44, no. 4 (2010): 284–88.

30. O. H. Franco et al., "Effects of Physical Activity on Life Expectancy with Cardiovascular Disease," *Archives of Internal Medicine* 165, no. 20 (2005): 2355–60.

31. W. L. Haskell et al., "Physical Activity and Public Health," 2007.

32. B. Stamford, "Tracking Your Heart Rate for Fitness," *The Physician and Sportsmedicine* 21, no. 3 (1993): 227–28.

33. W. L. Haskell et al., "Physical Activity and Public Health," 2007.

34. Ibid.

35. S. A. Herring et al., "The Team Physician and Conditioning of Athletes for Sports: A Consensus Statement," *Medicine and Science in Sports and Exercise* 33, 10 (2001): 1789–93.

36. N. A. Ratamess et al., "American College of Sports Medicine Position Stand: Progression Models in Resistance Training for Healthy Adults," *Medicine and Science in Sports and Exercise* 41, no. 3 (2009): 687–708.

37. L. Y. Lee, D. T. Lee, and J. Woo, "Tai Chi and Health-Related Quality of Life in Nursing Home Residents," *Journal of Nursing Scholarship* 41, no. 1 (2009): 35–43.

38. Arthritis Foundation, "Exercise and Arthritis: Introduction to Exercise," 2010, www.arthritis.org/conditions/exercise.

39. M. L. Pollack et al., "American College of Sports Medicine Position Stand: The Recommended Quantity and Quality of Exercise for Developing and Maintaining Cardiorespiratory and Muscular Fitness, and Flexibility in Healthy Adults," *Medicine & Science in Sports & Exercise* 30, no. 6 (1998): 975–91.

40. Ibid.

41. S. J. Hartley-O'Brien, "Six Mobilization Exercises for Active Range of Hip Flexion," *Research Quarterly for Exercise and Sport* 51, no. 4 (1980): 625–35.

42. K. Small, L. McNaughton, and M. Matthews, "A Systematic Review into the Efficacy of Static Stretching as Part of a Warm-Up for the Prevention of Exercise-Related Injury," *Research in Sports Medicine* 16, no. 3 (2008): 213–31.

43. M. L. Pollack et al., "American College of Sports Medicine Position Stand," 1998.

44. V. Baltzpoulos, "Isokinetic Dynamometry," in *Biomechanical Evaluation of Movement in Sport and Exercise: The British Association of Sport and Exercise Sciences Guidelines*, eds. C. Payton and R. Bartlett (New York: Routledge, 2008), 105.

45. J. R. Fowles, "What I Always Wanted to Know about Instability Training," *Applied Physiology, Nutrition, and Metabolism* 35, no. 1 (2010): 89–90: D. G. Behm, et al., "The Use of Instability to Train the Core Musculature," *Applied Physiology, Nutrition, and Metabolism*, 35, no. 1 (2010): 91–108.

46. J. R. Fowles, "What I Always Wanted to Know about Instability Training," 2010.

47. D. G. Behm et al., "Canadian Society for Exercise Physiology Position Stand: The Use of Instability to Train the Core in Athletic and Nonathletic Conditioning," *Applied Physiology, Nutrition, and Metabolism* 35, no. 1 (2010): 109–12.

48. M. N. Sawka, et al., "American College of Sports Medicine Position Stand: Exercise and Fluid Replacement," *Medicine and Science in Sports and Exercise* 39, no. 2 (2007): 377–90.

49. Ibid.

50. D. Ritchie, "Plantar Fasciitis: Treatment Pearls," American Academy of Podiatric Sports Medicine, Accessed July 2010, www.aapsm.org/plantar_fasciitis.html.

51. M. H. Moen et al., "Medial Tibial Stress Syndrome: A Critical Review," *Sports Medicine* 39, no. 7 (2009) 523–46.

52. D. M. Brody, "Running Injuries: Prevention and Management," *Clinical Symposia* 39, no. 3 (1987): 1–36.

53. M. A. Schiff, D. J. Caine, and R. O'Halloran, "Injury Prevention in Sport," *American Journal of Lifestyle Medicine* 4, no. 1 (2010): 42–64.

54. U. G. Kersting and G. P. Brüggemann, "Midsole Material-Related Force Control During Heel-Toe Running," *Research in Sports Medicine* 14, no. 1 (2006): 1–17.

55. American Academy of Ophthalmology, "Protective Eyewear," Updated February 2009, www.aao.org/eyesmart/injuries/eyewear.cfm.

56. American College Health Association, *American College Health Association-National College Health Assessment II*, 2009.

57. Bicycle Helmet Safety Institute, "Helmet-Related Statistics from Many Sources," Revised July 2010, www.helmets.org/stats.htm.

58. B. Q. Hafen and K. J. Karren, *Prehospital Emergency Care and Crisis Intervention*. 4th ed. (Englewood Cliffs, NJ: Prentice-Hall, 1992).

59. L. E. Armstrong et al., "The American Football Uniform: Uncompensable Heat Stress and Hyperthermic Exhaustion," *Journal of Athletic Training* 45, no. 2 (2010): 117–27.

60. R. Curtis, Princeton University Outdoor Action Program, "Hypothermia and Cold Weather Injuries, Outdoor Action Guide," National Ag Safety Database, Reviewed April 2002, www.nasdonline.org/document/1421/d001216/hypothermia-and-cold-weather-injuries-outdoor-action-guide.html.

61. American Council on Exercise, "Exercising in the Cold," 2010, www.acefitness.org/fitfacts/fitfacts_display.aspx?itemid=24.

62. J. W. Castellani et al., "American College of Sports Medicine Position Stand: Prevention of Cold Injuries during Exercise," *Medicine and Science in Sports and Exercise* 38, no. 11 (2006): 2012–29.

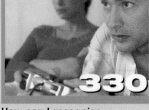
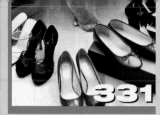
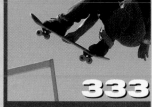
# 10

# Recognizing and Avoiding Addiction

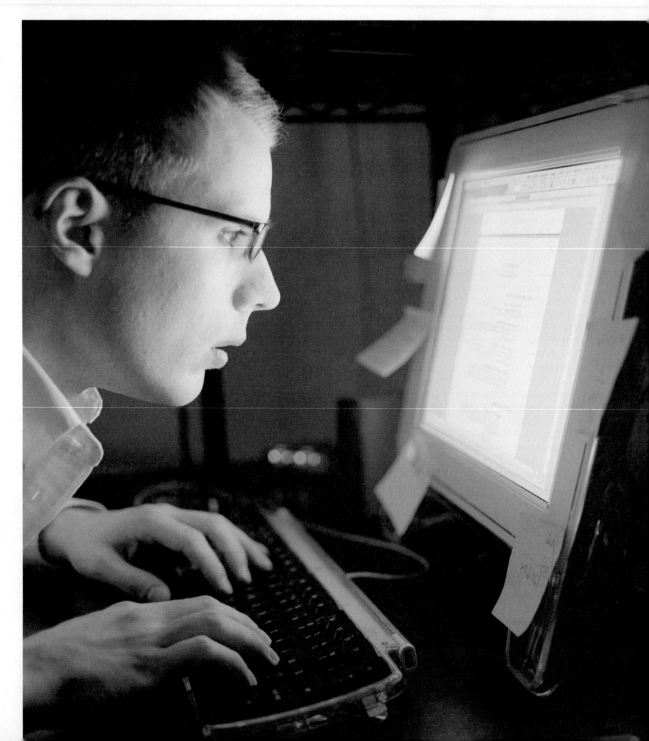

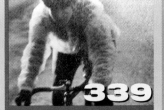
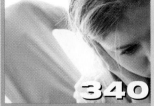

**339**

Is my roommate's constant exercising an addiction?

**340**

How can I approach someone who needs help and treatment?

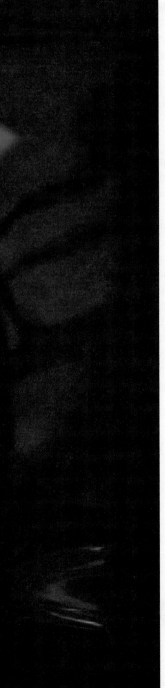

## Objectives

✳ Define and discuss *addiction.*

✳ Distinguish addictions from habits, and identify the signs of addiction.

✳ Discuss the addictive process, the physiology of addiction, the biopsychosocial model of addiction, as well as codependence.

✳ Describe types of addictions, including disordered gambling, compulsive buying, compulsive Internet or technology use, work addiction, compulsive exercise, and sexual addiction.

✳ Evaluate treatment and recovery options for addicts, including intervention, individual therapy, group therapy, family therapy, and 12-step programs.

These days, it's easy to find high-profile cases of compulsive and destructive behavior. Stories of celebrities and politicians struggling with addictions to alcohol, drugs, and sex are splashed in the headlines and profiled on TV news programs. But millions of "everyday" people throughout the world are waging their own battles with addiction as well. People with addictions can sometimes be unaware that they have a problem, because many potentially addictive activities may actually enhance the lives of those who engage in them moderately. In addition to alcohol and drugs, the most commonly recognized addictions include food, sex, relationships, shopping, work, exercise, gambling, and using the Internet.

## What Is Addiction?

**Addiction** is a persistent, compulsive dependence on a behavior or substance, including mood-altering behaviors or activities, despite ongoing negative consequences. Some researchers speak of two types of addictions: *substance addictions* (e.g., alcoholism, drug abuse, and smoking) and *process addictions* (e.g., gambling, spending, shopping, eating, and sexual activity). There is a growing recognition that many addicts, such as polydrug abusers, are addicted to more than one substance or process. Addictive behaviors initially provide a sense of pleasure or stability that is beyond the addict's power to achieve in other ways. Eventually, the addicted person needs to do the behavior in order to feel normal.

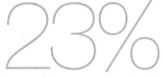

**23%** of college students meet the medical criteria for substance abuse or dependence.

**That's about triple the proportion in the general population.**

In this chapter, *addiction* is used interchangeably with *physiological addiction.* However, **physiological dependence,** the adaptive state that occurs with regular addictive behavior and results in withdrawal syndrome, is only one indicator of addiction. Psychological dynamics play an important role, which explains why behaviors not related to chemicals may also be additive. To be addictive, a behavior must have the potential to produce a positive mood change. Chemicals are responsible for the most profound addictions because they produce dramatic mood changes and cause cellular changes to which the body adapts so well that it eventually requires the chemical in order to function normally. Yet other behaviors, such as gambling, spending money,

**addiction** Persistent, compulsive dependence on a behavior or substance, including mood-altering behaviors or activities, despite ongoing negative consequences.
**physiological dependence** The adaptive state that occurs with regular addictive behavior and results in withdrawal syndrome.

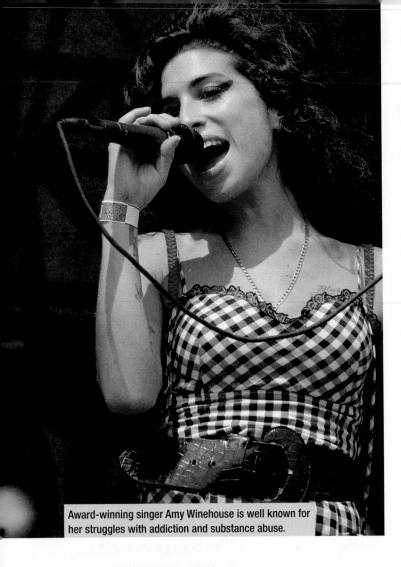

Award-winning singer Amy Winehouse is well known for her struggles with addiction and substance abuse.

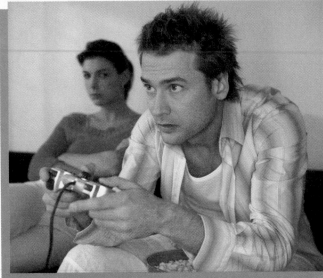

**How can I recognize addiction in a loved one or even myself?**

Addiction can be difficult to recognize or acknowledge. Symptoms to look for are an obsession or compulsion with a behavior or activity, a loss of control, and negative consequences as a result of the behavior. Another symptom, denial of a problem, may be easy to see in another person but difficult to recognize in yourself.

working, and sex, also create changes at the cellular level along with positive mood changes. A person with an intense, uncontrollable urge to continue engaging in a particular activity is said to have developed a psychological dependence. In fact, psychological and physiological dependence are so intertwined that it is not really possible to separate the two. Although the mechanism is not well understood, all forms of addiction probably reflect dysfunction of certain biochemical systems in the brain.[1]

Studies show that most animals share the same basic pleasure and reward circuits in the brain that turn on when they encounter addictive substances or engage in something pleasurable, such as eating or orgasm. We all engage in potentially addictive behaviors to some extent, because some are essential to our survival and are highly reinforcing, such as eating, drinking, and sex. At some point along the continuum, however, some individuals are not able to engage in these or other behaviors moderately—they become addicted.

Addiction has four common symptoms: (1) **compulsion,** which is characterized by **obsession,** or excessive preoccupation, with the behavior and an overwhelming need to perform it; (2) **loss of control,** or the inability to reliably predict whether any isolated occurrence of the behavior will be healthy or damaging; (3) **negative consequences,** such as physical damage, legal trouble, financial problems, academic failure, and family dissolution, which do not occur with healthy involvement in any behavior; and (4) **denial,** the inability to perceive that the behavior is self-destructive. These four components are present in all addictions, whether chemical or behavioral.

## Habit versus Addiction

How do we distinguish between a harmless habit and an addiction? Addiction certainly involves elements of **habit,** a repeated behavior in which the repetition may be unconscious. A habit can be annoying, but it can be broken without too much discomfort by simply becoming aware of its presence and choosing not to do it. Addiction also involves repetition of a behavior, but the repetition occurs by compulsion, and considerable discomfort is experienced if the behavior is not performed. Habits are behaviors that occur through choice and typically do not cause negative health

**compulsion** Preoccupation with a behavior and an overwhelming need to perform it.

**obsession** Excessive preoccupation with an addictive object or behavior.

**loss of control** Inability to reliably predict whether a particular instance of involvement with the addictive substance or behavior will be healthy or damaging.

**negative consequences** Severe problems associated with addiction, such as physical damage, legal trouble, financial problems, academic failure, or family dissolution.

**denial** Inability to perceive or accurately interpret the self-destructive effects of the addictive behavior.

**habit** A repeated behavior in which the repetition may be unconscious.

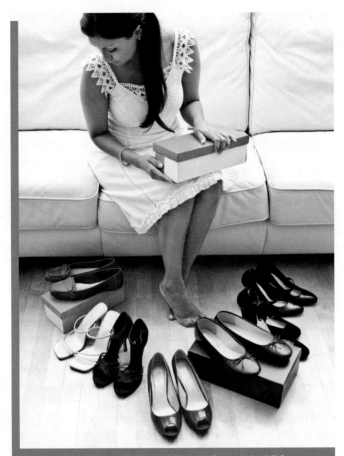

**What makes an addiction different from a habit?**

Once a person recognizes a habit and decides to change it, the habit can usually be broken. With an addiction, however, there is a sense of compulsion so strong that the addict is no longer in control of his or her behavior. For example, you may like to hit the stores when the latest fashions arrive, or spend time online hunting for bargains, but your shopping isn't considered an addiction unless you have lost control over where and when you shop—and how much—and you are experiencing negative impacts on the rest of your life as a result.

consequences. In contrast, no one decides to become addicted, even though people make choices that contribute to the development of an addiction.

To understand addiction, we must look beyond the amount and frequency of the behavior, because what happens when a person is involved in the behavior is far more meaningful. For example, someone who drinks only rarely and then engages in a night of heavy drinking may experience personality changes, blackouts (drug-induced amnesia), and other negative consequences (e.g., failing a test, missing an important appointment, getting into a fight) that would never have occurred otherwise. On the other hand, someone who has a few martinis every evening may never do anything out of character while under the influence of alcohol but may become irritable, manipulative, and aggressive without those regular drinks. For both of these people, alcohol appears to perform a function (mood control) that

they should be able to do without the aid of chemicals, which is a possible sign of addiction.

# Addiction Affects Family and Friends

The family and friends of an addicted person can suffer many negative consequences. Often they struggle with **codependence,** a self-defeating relationship pattern in which a person is "addicted to the addict." It is the primary outcome of dysfunctional relationships or families.

Codependence is defined by a pattern of behavior. Codependents find it hard to set healthy boundaries and often live in the chaotic, crisis-oriented mode that naturally occurs around addicts. They assume responsibility for meeting others' needs to the point that they subordinate or even cease being aware of their own needs. They may be unable to perceive their needs because they have repeatedly been taught that their needs are inappropriate or less important than someone else's. Although the word *codependent* is used less frequently today, treatment professionals still recognize the importance of helping addicts see how their behavior affects those around them and of working with family and friends to establish healthier relationships and boundaries.

Family and friends can play an important role in getting an addict to seek treatment. They are most helpful when they refuse to be enablers. **Enablers** are people who knowingly or unknowingly protect addicts from the natural consequences of their behavior. If they don't have to deal with the consequences, addicts cannot see the self-destructive nature of their behavior and will therefore continue it. Codependents are the primary enablers of their addicted loved ones, although anyone who has contact with an addict can be an enabler and thus contribute (perhaps powerfully) to continuation of the addictive behavior. Enablers are generally unaware that their behavior has this effect. In fact, enabling is rarely conscious and certainly not intentional.

**codependence** A self-defeating relationship pattern in which a person is "addicted to the addict."

**enablers** People who knowingly or unknowingly protect addicts from the natural consequences of their behavior.

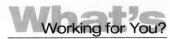
**what do you think?**

Why do you think friends and family members become enablers and codependents of people engaging in destructive behaviors? ● Have you ever confronted someone you were concerned about? If so, was the confrontation successful? ● What tips would you give someone who wants to confront a loved one about an addiction?

# How Addiction Develops

Addiction is a process that evolves over time. It begins when a person repeatedly seeks the illusion of relief to avoid unpleasant feelings or situations. This pattern is known as *nurturing through avoidance* and is a maladaptive way of taking care of emotional needs. As a person becomes increasingly dependent on the addictive behavior, there is a corresponding deterioration in relationships with family, friends, and coworkers; in performance at work or school; and in personal life. Eventually, addicts do not find the addictive behavior pleasurable but consider it preferable to the unhappy realities they are seeking to escape. Figure 10.1 illustrates the cycle of psychological addiction.

## The Physiology of Addiction

Virtually all intellectual, emotional, and behavioral functions occur as a result of biochemical interactions between nerve cells in the body. Biochemical messengers, called **neurotransmitters,** exert their influence at specific receptor sites on nerve cells. Drug use and chronic stress can alter these receptor sites and cause the production and breakdown of neurotransmitters. Some people's bodies naturally produce insufficient quantities of these neurotransmitters, which predisposes them to seeking out chemicals, such as alcohol, as substitutes or pursuing behaviors such as exercise that increase natural production. Thus, some may be "wired" to look for substances or experiences that increase pleasure or reduce discomfort, making them more susceptible to addiction.

**neurotransmitters** Biochemical messengers that bind to specific receptor sites on nerve cells.

**tolerance** Phenomenon in which progressively larger doses of a drug or more intense involvement in a behavior is needed to produce the desired effects.

**withdrawal** A series of temporary physical and biopsychosocial symptoms that occurs when an addict abruptly abstains from an addictive chemical or behavior.

### "Why Should I Care?"

Addictions of any kind limit your ability to make good decisions and maintain your focus, making it hard for you to meet your full potential as a student and as a member of the community. A seemingly harmless habit may actually be progressing into an addiction that prevents you from attending classes, meeting new people, or participating in other activities that you might find enjoyable.

Mood-altering substances and experiences produce **tolerance,** defined as a phenomenon in which progressively larger doses of a drug or more intense involvement in an experience are needed to obtain the desired effects. All of us develop some degree of tolerance to any mood-altering experience. But because addicts tend to seek intense mood-altering experiences, they eventually increase the amount and intensity to the point of causing negative side effects.

**Withdrawal** is another phenomenon associated with mood-altering experiences. The drug or activity replaces or causes an effect that the body should normally provide on its own. If the experience is repeated often enough, the body adjusts: It starts requiring the drug or experience to obtain the effect. Stopping the behavior will cause a withdrawal syndrome, because the body cannot naturally create the same effect as the drug. Mood-altering chemicals, for example, fill up the receptor sites for the body's natural "feel-good" neurotransmitters (endorphins) and nerve cells shut down production of these substances temporarily. When the drug use stops, those receptor sites sit empty, resulting in uncomfortable feelings that remain until the body resumes normal neurotransmitter production or the person consumes more of the drug.

Withdrawal symptoms of chemical dependencies are generally the opposite of the effects of the drugs. For example, a cocaine addict who feels a high while using the drug will experience a characteristic "crash" (depression and lethargy) when he stops taking it. Conversely, a heroin addict experiences drowsiness, slowed speech and reactions, and uninhibited behavior while using the drug. When withdrawing from heroin, the addict experiences anxiety, elevated heart rate, trembling, irritability, insomnia, and convulsions. Withdrawal symptoms for addictive behaviors are usually less dramatic. They typically involve

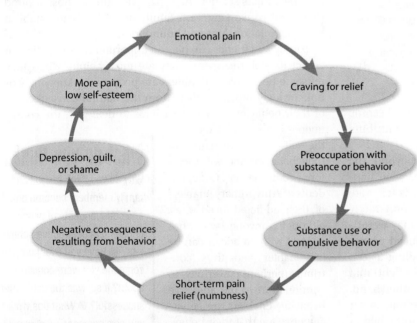

FIGURE 10.1 **Cycle of Psychological Addiction**

Source: From TURNER/SIZER/WHITNEY/WILKS. Life Choices, 2E. © 1992 Brooks/Cole, a part of Cengage Learning, Inc. Reproduced by permission. www.cengage.com/permissions.

psychological discomfort such as anxiety, depression, irritability, guilt, anger, and frustration, with an underlying preoccupation with or craving for the behavior. Withdrawal syndromes range from mild to severe. The most severe form is delirium tremens (DTs), which occurs in approximately 5 to 10 percent of dependent individuals withdrawing from alcohol.[2]

# The Biopsychosocial Model of Addiction

The most effective treatment today is being provided by those who rely on the **biopsychosocial model of addiction,** which proposes that addiction is caused by a variety of factors operating together. The biopsychosocial model was developed to explain the complex interaction between the biological, psychological, and social aspects of addiction. The complexity of addiction and consistent evidence of multiple contributing factors lead us to conclude that the problem is not the result of a single influence but rather of a variety of influences working together. Biological, psychological, and environmental factors all contribute to its development. Although one factor may play a larger role than another in a specific individual, it is rarely sufficient to explain an addiction. Figure 10.2 lists risk factors for addiction.

**Psychological Factors** A person's psychological makeup also factors into the potential for addiction. People with low self-esteem, a tendency toward risk-taking behavior, or poor

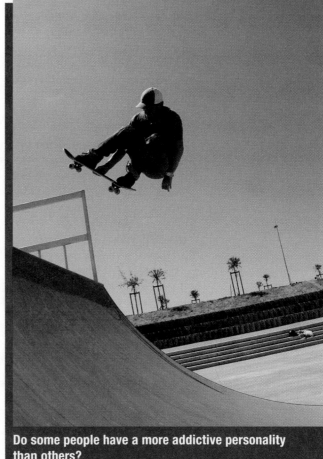

**Do some people have a more addictive personality than others?**

Psychological factors may make some people more prone to addiction than others. Having low self-esteem, poor coping skills, or a tendency toward risk-taking behavior may put you at higher risk of developing an addiction than someone without these traits.

coping skills are more likely to develop addictive patterns of behavior. Individuals who consistently look outside themselves for solutions and explanations for life events (who have an external locus of control) are more likely to experience addiction.

**Biological or Disease Influences** For many people, addiction is thought to be based in the brain and involves memory, motivation, and emotional state. The processes that control these aspects of brain function are thus logical subjects for genetic research into a biologically based risk for addiction, particularly to mood-altering substances. Studies show that drug addicts metabolize these substances differently than do nonaddicted people. Research suggests that genes affecting the activity of the neurotransmitters serotonin and GABA (gamma-aminobutyric acid) are likely involved in the risk

**Environmental factors**
• Ready access to the substance or experience
• Abusive or neglectful home environment
• Peer norms
• Membership in an oppressed or marginalized group
• Chronic or acute stressors

**Psychological factors**
• Low self-esteem
• External locus of control (looking outside oneself for solutions)
• Passivity
• Post-traumatic stress disorders (victims of abuse or other trauma)

**Biological factors**
• Unusual early response to the substance or experience
• Attention-deficit/hyperactivity disorder and other learning disabilities
• Biologically based mood disorders
• Addiction among biological family members

**FIGURE 10.2 Risk Factors for Addiction**

**biopsychosocial model of addiction** Theory of the relationship between an addict's biological (genetic) nature and psychological and environmental influences.

for alcoholism.[3] For example, a study found that college students with a particular variant of the serotonin transporter gene consumed more alcohol per occasion, drank expressly to become inebriated more often, and engaged more frequently in heavy drinking than students with another variant of the gene. The relationships between neurotransmitters and alcoholism are complex, however; not all studies have shown a connection between alcoholism risk and these genes.[4]

**social learning theory** Theory that people learn behaviors by watching role models—parents, caregivers, and significant others.

**process addictions** Behaviors such as disordered gambling, compulsive buying, compulsive Internet or technology use, work addiction, compulsive exercise, and sexual addiction that are known to be addictive because they are mood altering.

Studies also support a genetic influence on addiction. It has been known for centuries that alcoholism runs in families. Recent studies have confirmed that identical twins, who share the same genes, are about twice as likely as fraternal twins, who share an average of 50 percent of their genes, to resemble each other in terms of the presence of alcoholism. Studies also show that 50 to 60 percent of the risk for alcoholism is genetically determined for both men and women.[5]

**Environmental Influences** Cultural expectations and mores help determine whether people engage in certain behaviors. For example, although many native Italians use alcohol abundantly, there is a low incidence of alcoholism in this culture. Low rates of alcoholism typically exist in countries and cultures where children are gradually introduced to alcohol in diluted amounts, on special occasions, and within a strong family group. There is deep disapproval of intoxication, which is not viewed as socially acceptable, stylish, or funny.[6] Such cultural traditions and values are less widespread in the United States, where the incidence of alcohol addiction and alcohol-related problems is very high.

Societal attitudes and messages also influence addictive behavior. The media's emphasis on appearance and the ideal body plays a significant role in exercise addiction. Societal glorification of money and material achievement can lead to

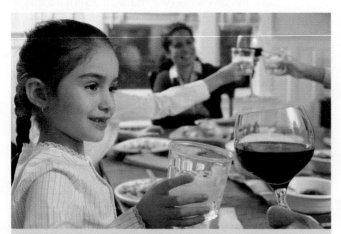

One predisposing factor for whether a person develops an addiction might be environmental influences such as the norms and cultural values he or she was taught during childhood.

work addiction, which is often admired. Societal changes, in turn, influence individual norms. People living in cities characterized by rapid social change or social disorganization often feel less connected to social, religious, and civic institutions. The resulting disenfranchisement leads to increased destructive behaviors, including addiction.[7]

**Social learning theory** proposes that people learn behaviors by watching role models—parents, caregivers, and significant others. The effects of modeling, imitation, and identification with behavior from early childhood on are well documented. Modeling is especially influential when it involves behavior that is mood altering. Many studies show that modeling by parents and by idolized celebrities exerts a profound influence on young people.[8]

On an individual level, major stressful life events, such as marriage, divorce, change in work status, and death of a loved one, may trigger addictive behaviors. Traumatic events in general often instigate addictive behaviors, as traumatized people seek to medicate their pain—pain they may not even be aware of because they've repressed it. One thing that makes addictive behaviors so powerfully attractive is that they reliably alleviate personal pain, at least for a short time. However, over the long-term, addictive behaviors actually cause more pain than they relieve.

Family members whose needs for love, security, and affirmation are not consistently met; who are refused permission to express their feelings, desires, or needs; and who frequently submerge their personalities to "keep the peace" are prone to addiction. Children whose parents are not consistently available to them (physically or emotionally); who are subjected to sexual abuse, physical abuse, neglect, or abandonment; or who receive inconsistent or disparaging messages about their self-worth may experience psychosocial or physical illness and addiction in adulthood.

# Addictive Behaviors

Thus far in this chapter, we have examined the fundamental concepts and processes of addiction and its associated problems. Clearly, tobacco, alcohol, and other drugs are addictive, and addictions to them create multiple problems for addicted individuals and for their families and society. Later chapters will discuss these specific substance-related addictions; here we will look at what are commonly called **process addictions**—behaviors known to be addictive because they are mood altering. Traditionally, the word *addiction* has been confined to use mainly with alcohol and other psychoactive substances. However, this is changing. New knowledge about the brain's reward system suggests that, as far as the brain is concerned, a reward is a reward, whether it is brought on by a chemical or a behavior.[9] When there is a reward, there is a risk that a vulnerable brain might get trapped in a compulsion. Examples of process addictions include disordered gambling, compulsive buying, compulsive Internet or technology use, work addiction, compulsive exercise, and sexual addiction.

# Disordered or Pathological Gambling

Gambling is a form of recreation and entertainment for millions of Americans. Most people who gamble do so casually and moderately to experience the excitement of anticipating a win. However, more than 2 million Americans suffer from pathological or **disordered gambling** and 6 million more are considered to be at risk for developing a gambling addiction.[10] The American Psychiatric Association (APA), which previously used the term *pathological gambling,* has proposed the term *disordered gambling* for this addiction and recognizes it as a mental disorder. As proposed for the APA's *Diagnostic and Statistical Manual of Mental Disorders,* 5th edition, (*DSM-V,* publishing in May 2013), the revised APA definition lists nine characteristic behaviors, including preoccupation with gambling, unsuccessful efforts to cut back or quit, using gambling to escape problems, and lying to family members to conceal the extent of involvement with gambling.

Gamblers and drug addicts describe many similar cravings and highs. A recent study supports what many experts believe to be true: that compulsive gambling is like drug addiction.[11] Compulsive gamblers in this study were found to have decreased blood flow to a key section of the brain's reward system. Much as it is for people who abuse drugs, it is thought that compulsive gamblers compensate for this deficiency in their brain's reward system by overdoing it and getting hooked.[12] Most compulsive gamblers state that they seek excitement even more than money. They place increasingly larger bets to obtain the desired level of excitement. Like drug addicts, compulsive gamblers live from fix to fix. Their subjective cravings can be as intense as those of drug abusers; they show tolerance in their need to increase the amount of their bets; and they experience highs rivaling that of a drug high. Up to half of compulsive gamblers show withdrawal symptoms similar to a mild form of drug withdrawal, including sleep disturbance, sweating, irritability, and craving.

**disordered gambling** Compulsive gambling that cannot be controlled.

Whereas casual gamblers can stop anytime they wish and are capable of seeing the necessity to do so, compulsive gamblers are unable to control the urge to gamble even in the face of devastating consequences: high debt; legal problems; and the loss of everything meaningful, including homes, families, jobs, health, and even their lives. See the **Skills for Behavior Change** box below for tips on keeping your own gambling in check.

## Did you Know?

The average tuition for a 4-year public university in 2009–2010 was $7,797. If you gamble and lose an average of $150 per week for a full year, you'll have spent your entire year's tuition!

**Source:** The College Board, *Trends in College Pricing, 2009* (New York: The College Board, 2010), Available at www.trends-collegeboard.com/college_pricing.

## Tips for Controlling Your Gambling

If gambling is taking over your life, it's probably best to give it up altogether. If you're not ready to give it up, here are some strategies to help you keep it in check.

### CONTROL YOUR CASH

Many gamblers find that they can't stop if they have cash in their pocket and an opportunity to bet. Many who stop gambling find limiting their access to cash is helpful. Here are some strategies:

* Don't keep large sums of cash.
* Carry only enough cash for the day's expenses.
* Have wages paid directly to a bank account.
* Pay bills by automatic transfer, check, or credit card.
* Tell family and friends what you're doing, and that they shouldn't lend you money.
* All cash flow must be "visible" on account printouts.
* Use automatic teller machines to provide limited amounts of cash per week.
* Avoid jobs that involve handling cash.

### FILL THE GAP

Problem gamblers may spend 10 to 20 hours or more a week gambling. They also spend a lot of time thinking and worrying about their gambling. When you give up gambling you need to fill the gap it leaves. There are lots of ways to do this:

* Set short- and long-term goals to work toward.
* Plan ahead, so you don't gamble because "there's nothing else to do."
* Spend more time studying.
* Spend more time with friends who do not gamble.
* Take a part-time job.
* Spend more time working out at the fitness or recreation center.
* Look at other things you can do to treat yourself (e.g., play games with friends, go to the movies).
* Start to do the things you may have stopped when you started to gamble too much.
* Learn how to relax. Try exercise, yoga, or meditation.

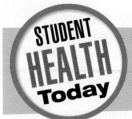
# GAMBLING AND COLLEGE STUDENTS

Although many people gamble occasionally without it ever becoming a problem, otherwise model students can find themselves caught up in the rush of making big bets and winning even bigger money. Consider John,* an ex–Lehigh University sophomore, the son of a Baptist minister, a former fraternity member, a former cellist in the university orchestra, and the former sophomore class president—the epitome of a responsible student active in the community and serving as a role model to the student body. When John was arrested for allegedly robbing the Wachovia Bank branch in Allentown, Pennsylvania, making off with $2,781, many wondered why such a good kid would be driven to such an act. According to the Associated Press, his lawyer stated that his client had run up about $5,000 in debt playing online poker. In a desperate move to feed his compulsive gambling addiction, John turned to bank robbery. He has since been sentenced to 22 months to 10 years in prison.

Compulsive gambling on college campuses has become a big concern for college administrators as gambling grows ever more popular among students. The National Collegiate Athletic Association (NCAA) estimates that each year during March Madness (the men's college basketball tournament), there are over 1.2 million active gambling pools, with over $2.5 billion gambled. More and more of these dollars come from the pockets of college students. There is growing evidence, in fact, that betting on college campuses is interfering with students' financial and academic futures. In a recent survey, approximately 60 percent of students reported they had gambled, almost 13 percent reported a significant loss of time, and 12 percent reported a significant loss of money. Consider the following:

❋ Almost 53 percent of college students have participated in most forms of gambling, including casino gambling, lottery tickets, racing, and sports betting in the past month.
❋ At least 78 percent of youths have placed a bet by the age of 18.
❋ An estimated 18 percent of men and 4 percent of women on college campuses could be classified as problem gamblers.
❋ The three most common reasons college students give for gambling are risk, excitement, and the chance to make money.

Although most college students who gamble are able to do so without developing a problem, warning signs of problem gambling include the following:

❋ Frequent talk about gambling; encouraging or challenging others to gamble
❋ Spending more time or money on gambling than can be afforded
❋ Borrowing money to gamble
❋ Selling sports-betting cards or organizing sports pools
❋ Possession of gambling paraphernalia such as lottery tickets or poker items
❋ Missing or being late for school, work, or family activities due to gambling
❋ Feeling sad, anxious, fearful, or angry about gambling losses

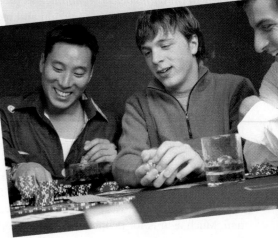

Call, fold, or raise? For increasing numbers of college students, gambling and the debts it can incur are becoming serious problems.

*Not his real name.

**Sources:** Task Force on College Gambling Policies, Division on Addictions at the Cambridge Health Alliance and the National Center for Responsible Gambling, *A Call to Action: Addressing College Gambling: Recommendations for Science-Based Policies and Programs* (Cambridge, MA: Cambridge Health Alliance and the National Center for Responsible Gambling, 2009), Available at www.ncrg.org/public_education/task-force-college-gambling-policies.cfm; W. DeJong et al., "Gambling: The New Addiction Crisis in Higher Education," *Alcohol, Tobacco, and Other Drugs Prevention File* 21, no. 1 (2006): 11–13; Massachusetts Council on Compulsive Gambling, *Students: Know the Limit* (Boston: Massachusetts Council on Compulsive Gambling, 2006), Available at www.masscompulsivegambling.org/paths/families.php; R. Schachter, "Targeting Student Gambling," *University Business* (January 2008): 35–38; J. Welte et al., "The Prevalence of Problem Gambling among U.S. Adolescents and Young Adults: Results from a National Survey," *Journal of Gambling Studies* 24, no. 2 (2008): 119–33.

**26%** of college men report gambling at least once a week, compared to 5.5% of college women.

Who is at risk for getting hooked on the rush of gambling? Men are more likely to have gambling problems than are women. Gambling prevalence is also higher among lower-income individuals, those who are divorced, African Americans, older adults, and individuals residing within 50 miles of a casino. Residents in southern states, where opportunities to gamble have increased significantly over the past 20 years, also have higher gambling rates.[13]

Gambling among college students appears to be on the rise across the nation. According to the latest results of the National Annenberg Risk Survey of Youth poll, conducted by the University of Pennsylvania's Annenburg Public Policy Center, weekly card playing increased from 12.7 percent in 2005 to 16.3 percent in 2006, reflecting the rise in card playing among college students.[14] What accounts for this trend? College students have easier access to gambling opportunities than ever before, with the advent of online gambling and a growing number of casinos, scratch tickets, lotteries, and sports betting networks. In particular, the largest boost has come from the increasing popularity of poker. Access to poker on the Internet and televised poker tournaments have revived the game, causing many young people to spend an unhealthy amount of time and money playing it. Some characteristics associated with gambling among college students include spending more time watching TV; using computers for nonacademic purposes; spending less time studying; earning lower grades; participating in intercollegiate athletics; and engaging in heavy, episodic drinking and using illicit drugs.[15] See the **Student Health Today** box at left for more on college students and gambling.

## Compulsive Buying Disorder

Compulsive buying has been estimated to affect up to 16 percent of the U.S. population.[16] In our society, people often use shopping as a way to make themselves feel better. However, for compulsive buyers, it does not make them feel any better but actually worse. Compulsive buying has many of the same characteristics as alcoholism, gambling, and other addictions. **Compulsive shoppers** are preoccupied with shopping and spending and exercise little control over their impulses to buy. Symptoms that signal that a person has crossed the line into compulsive buying include a preoccupation with shopping and spending, buying more than one of the same item, keeping items in the closet with the tags still attached, repeatedly buying much more than he or she needs or can afford, hiding purchases from relatives and loved ones, and experiencing feelings of euphoria and excitement when shopping.[17]

Compulsive buying disorders are reported to begin in a person's late teens and early twenties, coinciding with the age that people first establish credit and an independence from their parents. And because of easy buying capabilities via the Internet, it is likely that compulsive buyers can begin their adult life in substantial debt.

Compulsive buying can be seasonal, such as shopping during the winter months, to alleviate feelings of anxiety and depression. It can also occur when people feel depressed, lonely, or angry. Shopping and spending will not assure more love; increase self-esteem; or heal the hurts, regrets, stresses, and problems of daily living. It generally makes people feel worse because of the increased financial debt into which the person has sunk as a result of this addiction. Both compulsive gambling and buying can frequently lead to borrowing

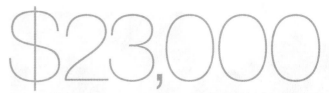

**$23,000** is the average amount of debt that a compulsive shopper owes.

to help support the addiction. People may borrow money repeatedly from family, friends, or institutions in spite of the problems doing so causes.

## Technology Addictions

As technology becomes an ever larger part of our daily lives, the risk of overexposure to it grows for people of all ages. Some people, in fact, become addicted to new technologies, such as smart phones, video games, personal digitial assistants (PDAs), networking sites, and the Internet in general. Have you ever opened your Web browser to check something quickly, and an hour later found yourself still blogging or checking your Facebook page? Do you have friends who seem more concerned with texting or surfing the Internet than with eating, going out, studying, or watching TV? These attitudes and behaviors are not unusual; many experts suggest that technology addiction is real and can present serious problems for those addicted. An estimated 5 to 10 percent of Internet users will likely experience **Internet addiction.** Younger people are also more likely to be addicted to the Internet than middle-aged users.[18] Approximately 11 percent of college students report that Internet use and computer games have interfered with their academic performance.[19]

**compulsive shoppers** People who are preoccupied with shopping and spending.

**Internet addiction** Compulsive use of the computer, PDA, cell phone, or other forms of technology to access the Internet for activities such as e-mail, games, shopping, or blogging.

What is normal Internet use? Because the Internet has been around a relatively short time, it is difficult to say. Studies suggest that some college students average 10 hours or so per week, and Web surfers can average 20 hours online without having

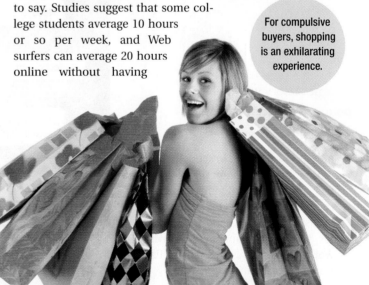

For compulsive buyers, shopping is an exhilarating experience.

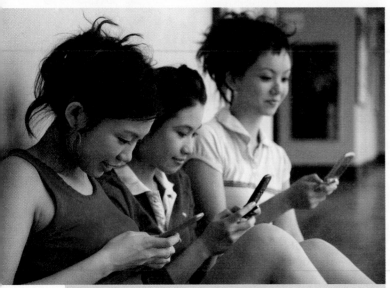
As the world goes wireless, many of us are becoming increasingly dependent on—and compulsive about—our technology.

major problems.[20] What you do online may be as important as how long you spend there. Some online activities, such as gaming and cybersex, seem to be more compelling and potentially addictive than others. As Internet use continues to increase, there are more applications and activities available than ever before. Some people find themselves texting constantly, while others update their status repeatedly on Facebook and other social networking sites. You may follow numerous Twitter feeds or engage in extended gaming sessions.

**work addiction** The compulsive use of work and the work persona to fulfill needs for intimacy, power, and success.

Internet addicts have multiple signs and symptoms, such as general disregard for one's health, sleep deprivation, depression, neglecting family and friends, lack of physical activity, euphoria when

# 5–10%
## of Internet users will likely experience Internet addiction.

online, lower grades in school, and poor job performance. Internet addicts may feel moody or uncomfortable when they are not online. Online addicts may be using their behavior to compensate for feelings of loneliness, marital or work problems, a poor social life, or financial problems.

# Work Addiction

In order to understand work addiction, we must understand the concept of healthy work. Healthy work provides a sense of identity; helps develop our strengths; and is a means of satisfaction, accomplishment, and mastery of problems. Healthy workers may work passionately for long hours. Although they have occasional projects that keep them away from family, friends, and personal interests for short periods of time, they generally maintain balance in their lives and full control of their schedules. Healthy work does not "consume" the worker.

Conversely, **work addiction** is the compulsive use of work and the work persona to fulfill needs of intimacy, power, and success. Work addicts usually set an intense work schedule, are unable to set boundaries regarding work, and feel driven to work even when they are away from work. Work addiction is more than being unable to relax when not doing something considered "productive."[21] The disorder is characterized by obsession, perfectionism, overachievement, anxiety, stress, anger, and burnout.[22] Work addicts may feel too busy to take care of their health needs, and there is some evidence work addiction may cause physical symptoms such as ulcers and chest pain or more chronic health conditions such as heart disease and asthmatic attacks. Figure 10.3 identifies other typical signs of work addiction.

Work addiction is found among all age, racial, and socioeconomic groups, but it typically develops in people in their forties and fifties. Male work addicts outnumber female work addicts, but this is changing as women gain more equality in the workforce. Most work addicts come from homes that were alcoholic, rigid, violent, or otherwise dysfunctional.

Work addiction can bring admiration from society at large, as addicts often excel in their professions. However, the

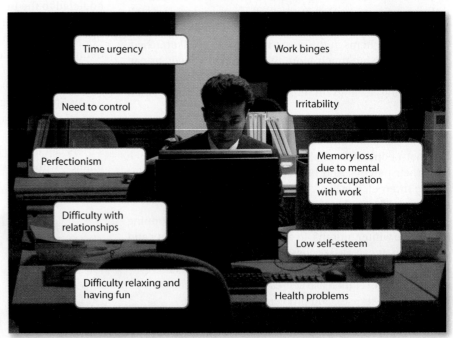

Time urgency

Work binges

Need to control

Irritability

Perfectionism

Memory loss due to mental preoccupation with work

Difficulty with relationships

Low self-esteem

Difficulty relaxing and having fun

Health problems

FIGURE 10.3 **Signs of Work Addiction**

negative effects on individuals and those around them are far reaching. Work addiction is a major source of marital discord and family breakup in addition to causing relationship problems with friends.[23]

## Exercise Addiction

It may seem odd that a personal health text that advocates exercise would also identify it as a potential addiction. Yet, as a powerful mood enhancer, exercise can be addictive. Firm statistics on the incidence of exercise addiction are not available, but one indication of its prevalence is that a large portion of Americans with the eating disorders anorexia nervosa and bulimia nervosa use exercise to purge instead of, or in addition to, self-induced vomiting.[24] **Exercise addicts** use exercise compulsively to try to meet needs—for nurturance, intimacy, self-esteem, and self-competency—that an object or activity cannot truly meet. Consequently, addictive or compulsive exercise results in negative consequences similar to those found in other addictions: alienation of family and friends, injuries from overdoing it, and a craving for more.

Traditionally, women have been perceived as being more at risk for exercise addiction. However, evidence is growing that more men are developing unhealthy exercise patterns. Media images promoting six-pack abs and lean, muscular bodies have influenced society's view of the masculine ideal. Meanwhile, more men are abusing steroids and overexercising to attain an ideal frame. *Muscle dysmorphia,* sometimes referred to as *bigarexia,* is a pathological preoccupation with being larger and more muscular.[25] Sufferers view themselves as small and weak even though they may be quite the opposite. Consequences of muscle dysmorphia include excessive weight lifting and exercising as well as steroid or supplement abuse. See Focus On: Enhancing Your Body Image beginning on page 280 for further discussion of these disorders and the body image issues associated with them.

## Sexual Addiction

Everyone needs love and intimacy, but the sexual practices of people addicted to sex involve neither. In **sexual addiction,** people confuse the intensity of physical arousal with intimacy.[26] They do not feel nurtured by the person with whom they have sex but by the activity itself. Likewise, they are incapable of nurturing another person because sex, not the person, is the object of their affection. In fact, people with sexual addictions do not necessarily seek partners to obtain

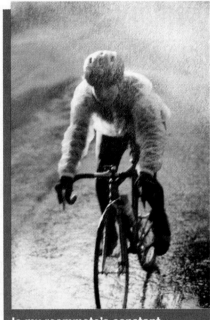

**Is my roommate's constant exercising an addiction?**

Obsession with a substance or behavior, even a generally positive activity such as exercise, can eventually develop into an addiction. If there are negative consequences from exercising, such as overuse injuries or withdrawal from friends and other activities, then addiction is a possibility.

sexual arousal; they may be satisfied by masturbation, whether alone or during phone sex or while reading or watching erotica. They may participate in a wide range of sexual activities, including affairs, sex with strangers, prostitution, voyeurism, exhibitionism, rape, incest, and pedophilia. People addicted to sex frequently experience crushing episodes of depression and anxiety, fueled by the fear of discovery. The toll that sexual addiction exacts is most clearly seen in loss of intimacy with loved ones, which frequently leads to family disintegration.

No group of people is more or less likely than another to become involved in sexual addictions. They affect men and women of all ages, including married and single people, and people of any sexual preference. Most people with sexual addictions share a similar background: a dysfunctional childhood family, often characterized by chemical dependency or other addictions. Many were physically and emotionally abused. People addicted to sex often have a history of sexual abuse. Sexual addiction has become a hot topic in recent months, as celebrities such as Tiger Woods and Jesse James have sought treatment for their problems through clinics specializing in these disorders.

## Multiple Addictions

Health professionals at addiction treatment centers often find that addicts depend on more than one chemical or behavior. Although addicts tend to have a favorite drug or behavior—one that is most effective at meeting their needs—as many as 60 percent of people in treatment have problems with more than one addiction. The figure may be as high as 75 percent for people addicted to chemicals. For example, alcohol addiction and eating disorders are commonly paired in women. Individuals trying to break a chemical dependency frequently resort to compulsive eating to keep themselves abstinent from drugs. Although multiple addictions certainly complicate recovery, they do not make it impossible. As with single addictions, recovery begins with the recognition that there is a problem.

**exercise addicts** People who exercise compulsively to try to meet needs of nurturance, intimacy, self-esteem, and self-competency.
**sexual addiction** Compulsive involvement in sexual activity.

## what do you think?

Do you think any behavior can be addictive? ● For example, can one be a chocolate addict, a study addict, or a shoe addict? Why or why not? ● What potential dangers lie in using the word *addiction* too loosely?

# Recovering from Addiction

Recovery from addiction is a lifelong process, starting with treatment of the addiction. Before treatment can begin, an individual must recognize the addiction. This can be difficult because of the power of denial—the inability to see the truth. Denial is the hallmark of addiction. It can be so powerful that intervention is sometimes necessary to break down the addict's defenses against recognizing the problem.

## Intervention

**Intervention** is a planned process of confrontation by people who are important to the addict, including spouses, parents, children, bosses, and friends. Its purpose is to break down the denial compassionately so that the person can see the addiction's destructive nature. Getting addicts to admit that they have a problem is not enough. They must come to perceive that the behavior is destructive and requires treatment.

> **intervention** A planned process of confronting an addict; carried out by close family, friends, and significant others.
>
> **abstinence** Refraining from a behavior.
>
> **detoxification** The early abstinence period during which an addict adjusts physically and cognitively to being free from the influences of the addiction.

Individual confrontation is difficult and often futile. However, an addict's defenses generally crumble when significant others collectively share their observations and concerns about the addict's behavior. Components of effective intervention include (1) emphasizing care and concern for the addicted person; (2) describing the behavior that is the cause for concern; (3) expressing how the behavior affects the addict, each person taking part in the intervention, and others; and (4) outlining specifically what you would like to see happen.

It is critical that those involved in the intervention clarify how they plan to end their enabling. For example, there have been instances where a wife has stated in public, or put notices in the local paper, that she will no longer cover bounced checks or be responsible for her gambling-addicted husband's antisocial behavior. Some spouses have even closed their joint bank accounts and opened personal accounts so they are not legally responsible for irresponsible acts. Whether these actions hold up under legal scrutiny may be dependent on state laws. Regardless of the type of intervention, all parties involved in the intervention should obtain advice about the legality of specific actions before jumping into a complicated situation. In addition, persons contemplating interventions must choose consequences they are ready to stick to if the addict refuses treatment. Significant others must also be ready to give support if the addict is willing to begin a recovery program.

Intervention is a serious step toward assisting someone who probably does not want help. It should therefore be well planned and rehearsed. Most addiction treatment centers have specialists on staff who can help plan an intervention. In addition, books on the subject are available for families and friends who are concerned about an addict. Once the problem has been recognized, recovery can begin.

## Treatment for Addiction

Treatment and recovery for any addiction generally begin with **abstinence**—refraining from the addictive behavior. Whereas complete abstinence is possible for people addicted to chemicals, it obviously is not feasible for people addicted to behaviors such as work and sex. For these addicts, abstinence means restoring balance to their lives through noncompulsive engagement in the behaviors, such as avoiding certain activities.

**Detoxification** refers to the early abstinence period during which an addict adjusts physically and cognitively to being free from the addiction's influence. It occurs in virtually every recovering addict, and, whereas it is uncomfortable for all addicts, it can be dangerous for some. This is primarily true for those addicted to chemicals, especially alcohol, heroin, and painkillers such as OxyContin. For these people, early abstinence may involve profound withdrawal

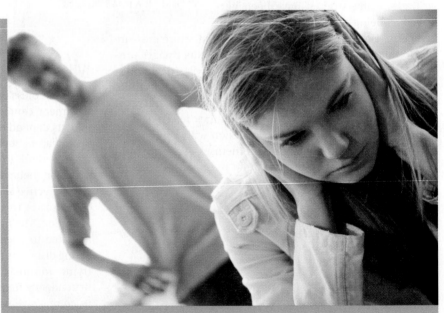

**How can I approach someone who needs help and treatment?**

Confronting a person about addiction is a difficult task, and one that usually requires intervention by a group of family members and friends. It is more effective for an addict to be faced with the facts from a group of the people most important to him or her than by one person. In a planned intervention, the goal is to break down the addict's denial compassionately and to get him or her to recognize the addiction's destructive nature. Most addiction treatment centers have specialists who can help plan an intervention.

symptoms that require medical supervision. Therefore, most inpatient treatment programs provide a pretreatment component of supervised detoxification to achieve abstinence safely before treatment begins.

Abstinence alone does little to change the psychological, biological, and environmental dynamics that underlie the addictive behavior. Without treatment, an addict is apt to relapse repeatedly or simply to change addictions. Treatment involves learning new ways of looking at oneself, others, and the world. It may require exploring a traumatic past so that psychological wounds can be healed. It also involves learning interdependence with significant others and new ways of taking care of oneself, physically and emotionally—and it involves developing communication skills and new ways of having fun.

**Finding a Quality Treatment Program** For a large number of addicts, recovery begins with a period of formal treatment. A good treatment program includes the following characteristics:

- Professional staff familiar with the specific addictive disorder for which help is being sought
- A flexible schedule of both inpatient and outpatient services
- Access to medical personnel who can assess the addict's health and treat all medical concerns as needed
- Medical supervision of addicts who are at high risk for a complicated detoxification
- Involvement of family members in the treatment process
- A coordinated team approach to treating addictive disorders (for example, medical personnel, counselors, psychotherapists, social workers, clergy, educators, dietitians, and fitness counselors)
- Both group and individual therapy options
- Peer-led support groups that encourage the addict to continue involvement after treatment ends
- Structured aftercare and relapse-prevention programs
- Accreditation by the Joint Commission (a national organization that accredits and certifies health care organizations and programs) and a license from the state in which it operates

Most programs apply a combination of family, individual, and group counseling, supplemented with attendance at a 12-step support group. Individuals may also wish to explore alternatives to 12-step groups. Organizations such as Rational Recovery and the Secular Organization for Sobriety provide support without the spiritual emphasis of 12-step groups such as Alcoholics Anonymous.

The National Institute on Alcohol Abuse and Alcoholism (NIAAA) completed Project MATCH (Matching Alcoholism Treatment to Client Heterogeneity), a large-scale study designed to determine if certain types of patients respond better to particular treatments.[27] The

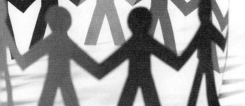

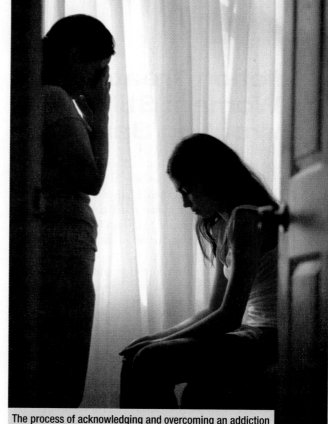

The process of acknowledging and overcoming an addiction is a long and difficult journey for everyone involved.

investigators studied three strategies: cognitive-behavior therapy, motivational psychology, and a facilitated 12-step program with sessions run by a therapist. Results showed that patients did equally well in each of the treatment approaches. This outcome was somewhat surprising, given that it has been common practice for treatment professionals to match patients to certain approaches. Researchers concluded that the focus, therefore, should simply be on selecting a competently run treatment program. Large-scale studies on other addictions have yet to occur. The **Gender & Health** box on page 342 describes factors that are important to address when treating female addicts.

# Relapse

**Relapse** is an isolated occurrence of or full return to addictive behavior. It is one of the defining characteristics of addiction. A person who does not relapse or have powerful urges to do so was probably not addicted in the first place. Addicts are set up to relapse long before they actually do so because of their tendency to meet change and other forms of stress in their lives with the same kind of denial they once used to justify their addictive behavior (for example, thinking, "I don't have a problem; I can handle this"). This sets off a series of events involving immediate or gradual abandonment of structured recovery plans. For example, the addict may quit attending support group

**relapse** The tendency to return to the addictive behavior after a period of abstinence.

# Addiction Treatment for Women: Still Confronting Barriers

The addiction treatment industry has traditionally been based on a model set up for males and has only recently begun to address the unique needs of women. Studies support the need for greater prevention efforts targeted specifically toward women at risk and gender-specific treatment for drug and alcohol dependence. Unfortunately, significant barriers remain for women seeking addiction treatment.

Although women entering treatment generally have fewer addiction-related legal problems (arrests for public intoxication or drug dealing, for example) than men, they face more psychological issues and family, financial, and medical problems. Research has shown that physical and sexual trauma followed by post-traumatic stress disorder are more common in drug-abusing women than men seeking treatment.

There are also practical barriers that women are faced with. Studies consistently indicate that the two primary barriers women face in successfully completing treatment are child care and transportation. One study found that women who were able to bring their children along with them to inpatient treatment were more likely to remain healthy 6 months after treatment. Additional barriers for women seeking addiction treatment include the following factors:

## INDIVIDUAL
* Lack of insurance or inadequate coverage
* Fear of losing child custody
* Low self-esteem and low sense of self-efficacy

## FAMILY
* Too many responsibilities
* Lack of family support for treatment
* Abuse in the family environment

## COMMUNITY
* Lack of support from employer
* Lack of gender-sensitive treatment options

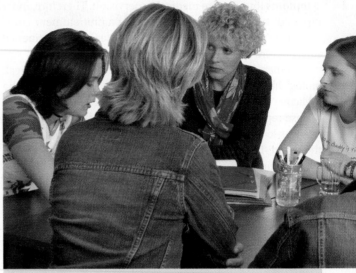

One important component of a woman-friendly treatment center is the existence of women-only counseling and therapy groups.

To address these barriers and provide effective assistance in overcoming addiction, a "women-friendly" treatment center should offer the following:

* Educational programs on self-worth, assertiveness, family issues, parenting, and anger management
* Women-only groups, especially for addressing issues of rape, incest, and abuse
* Networking with and support from other women in recovery
* Housing and day care

Clearly, many women have different treatment needs than men do. Finding a program that addresses these needs improves the likelihood of long-term success and recovery.

**Sources:** National Institute on Drug Abuse, National Institutes of Health, U.S. Department of Health and Human Services, *Principles of Drug Addiction Treatment: A Research Based Guide,* 2d ed., NIH Publication no. 09–4180 (Bethesda, MD: National Institute on Drug Abuse, 2009), Available at www .drugabuse.gov/PODAT/PODATIndex.html; W. Weschberg, S. Craddock, and R. Hubbard, "How Are Women Who Enter Substance Abuse Treatment Different than Men? A Gender Comparison from the Drug Abuse Treatment Outcome Study," *Drugs & Society* 13, no. 1 & 2 (1998): 97–115; C. A. Hernandez-Avila, B. J. Rounsaville, and H. R. Kranzler, "Opioid-, Cannabis-, and Alcohol-Dependent Women Show More Rapid Progression to Substance-Abuse Treatment," *Journal of Drug and Alcohol Dependence* 74, no. 3 (2004): 265–72.

---

meetings and slip into situations that previously triggered the addictive behavior.

Because those who facilitate treatment programs recognize this strong tendency to relapse, they routinely teach clients and significant others concepts of relapse prevention, including how to recognize the signs of imminent relapse and to develop a plan for responding to these signs. Without such a plan, recovering addicts are likely to relapse more frequently, more completely, and perhaps permanently.

Relapse should not be interpreted as failure to change or lack of desire to stay well. The appropriate response to relapse

is to remind addicts that they are addicted and to redirect them to the strategies that have previously worked for them. In addition to teaching skills, relapse prevention may involve aftercare planning such as connecting the recovering person with support groups, career counselors, or community services.

## what do you think?
Why do you think addicts resist seeking treatment, even when they may admit they have a problem? ● What factors need to be considered in helping addicted individuals prevent relapse?

## Are You Addicted?

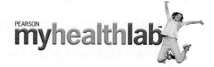

We may not always recognize addictive behaviors in ourselves or even our closest friends. This simple exercise will help you in two ways: (1) if you already know or strongly believe you are addicted to one of the behaviors below, this guide will assist you in identifying the areas in your life most affected by your compulsive behavior, and (2) if you're not sure whether you are addicted, this will help you determine the answer and assess the damage.

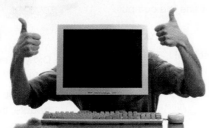

Fill out this assessment online at www.pearsonhighered.com/myhealthlab or www.pearsonhighered.com/donatelle.

### 1 Are You an Internet Addict?

Circle the answer that most closely describes your behavior.

| | Rarely | Occasionally | Frequently | Often | Always |
|---|---|---|---|---|---|
| 1. How often do you stay online longer than you intended? | 1 | 2 | 3 | 4 | 5 |
| 2. How often do you neglect household chores to spend more time online? | 1 | 2 | 3 | 4 | 5 |
| 3. How often do you prefer the excitement of the Internet to intimacy with your partner? | 1 | 2 | 3 | 4 | 5 |
| 4. How often do you form new relationships with people you meet online? | 1 | 2 | 3 | 4 | 5 |
| 5. How often do others in your life complain about the amount of time you spend online? | 1 | 2 | 3 | 4 | 5 |
| 6. How often do your grades or schoolwork suffer because of the amount of time you spend online? | 1 | 2 | 3 | 4 | 5 |
| 7. How often do you check your e-mail before something else that you need to do? | 1 | 2 | 3 | 4 | 5 |
| 8. How often does your job performance or productivity suffer because of the Internet? | 1 | 2 | 3 | 4 | 5 |
| 9. How often do you become defensive or secretive when someone asks you what you do online? | 1 | 2 | 3 | 4 | 5 |
| 10. How often do you block out disturbing thoughts about your life with soothing thoughts about the Internet? | 1 | 2 | 3 | 4 | 5 |
| 11. How often do you find yourself anticipating when you will go online again? | 1 | 2 | 3 | 4 | 5 |
| 12. How often do you fear that life without the Internet would be boring, empty, and joyless? | 1 | 2 | 3 | 4 | 5 |

| | Rarely | Occasionally | Frequently | Often | Always |
|---|---|---|---|---|---|
| 13. How often do you snap, yell, or act annoyed if someone bothers you while you are online? | 1 | 2 | 3 | 4 | 5 |
| 14. How often do you lose sleep to late-night log-ons? | 1 | 2 | 3 | 4 | 5 |
| 15. How often do you feel preoccupied with the Internet when offline or fantasize about being online? | 1 | 2 | 3 | 4 | 5 |
| 16. How often do you find yourself saying, "Just a few more minutes" when online? | 1 | 2 | 3 | 4 | 5 |
| 17. How often do you try to cut down the amount of time you spend online and fail? | 1 | 2 | 3 | 4 | 5 |
| 18. How often do you try hiding how long you've been online? | 1 | 2 | 3 | 4 | 5 |
| 19. How often do you choose to spend more time online rather than go out with others? | 1 | 2 | 3 | 4 | 5 |
| 20. How often do you feel depressed, moody, or nervous when you are offline? Do these feelings go away once you are back online? | 1 | 2 | 3 | 4 | 5 |

### Interpreting Your Scores for This Section

After you have answered all the questions, add the numbers you selected for each response to obtain a final score. The higher your score is, the greater your level of addiction is and the more problems your Internet usage causes.

**20–49 points:** You are an average Internet user. You may surf the Web a bit too long at times, but you have control over your usage.

**50–79 points:** You are experiencing occasional or frequent problems because of the Internet. You should consider the Internet's full impact on your life.

**80–100 points:** Your Internet usage is causing significant problems. You should evaluate the Internet's impact on your life and address the problems directly caused by it.

**Source:** Reprinted by permission of Dr. K. S. Young, director of the Center for Online and Internet Addiction, 2004, www.netaddiction.com.

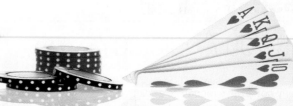

# 2 Are You a Compulsive Gambler?

Gamblers Anonymous offers the following questions to anyone who may have a gambling problem. These questions are provided to help an individual decide if he or she is a compulsive gambler and wants to stop gambling.

| | Yes | No |
|---|---|---|
| 1. Did you ever lose time from work or school due to gambling? | ○ | ○ |
| 2. Has gambling ever made your home life unhappy? | ○ | ○ |
| 3. Did gambling affect your reputation? | ○ | ○ |
| 4. Have you ever felt remorse after gambling? | ○ | ○ |
| 5. Did you ever gamble to get money with which to pay debts or otherwise solve financial difficulties? | ○ | ○ |
| 6. Did gambling cause a decrease in your ambition or efficiency? | ○ | ○ |
| 7. After losing did you feel you must return as soon as possible and win back your losses? | ○ | ○ |
| 8. After a win did you have a strong urge to return and win more? | ○ | ○ |
| 9. Did you often gamble until your last dollar was gone? | ○ | ○ |
| 10. Did you ever borrow to finance your gambling? | ○ | ○ |
| 11. Have you ever sold anything to finance gambling? | ○ | ○ |
| 12. Were you reluctant to use "gambling money" for normal expenditures? | ○ | ○ |
| 13. Did gambling make you careless of the welfare of yourself or your family? | ○ | ○ |

| | Yes | No |
|---|---|---|
| 14. Did you ever gamble longer than you had planned? | ○ | ○ |
| 15. Have you ever gambled to escape worry, trouble, boredom, or loneliness? | ○ | ○ |
| 16. Have you ever committed, or considered committing, an illegal act to finance gambling? | ○ | ○ |
| 17. Did gambling cause you to have difficulty in sleeping? | ○ | ○ |
| 18. Do arguments, disappointments, or frustrations create within you an urge to gamble? | ○ | ○ |
| 19. Did you ever have an urge to celebrate any good fortune by a few hours of gambling? | ○ | ○ |
| 20. Have you ever considered self-destruction or suicide as a result of your gambling? | ○ | ○ |

Most compulsive gamblers will answer yes to at least seven of these questions.

**Source:** Gamblers Anonymous, "Twenty Questions," www.gamblersanonymous .org/20questions.html. Used with permission.

# 3 Are You a Compulsive Buyer?

Answer true or false to each of the following questions:

| | True | False |
|---|---|---|
| 1. I often return items—at least one out of every four purchases. | ○ | ○ |
| 2. I've lied to my spouse, friends, or colleagues about the cost of things. | ○ | ○ |
| 3. I've had guilt, insomnia, fatigue, or a sense of hopelessness about my spending. | ○ | ○ |
| 4. I can correlate my overspending with overeating. | ○ | ○ |
| 5. My closet has four or more unworn items with the tags still hanging from them. | ○ | ○ |
| 6. I'm having trouble making ends meet. | ○ | ○ |

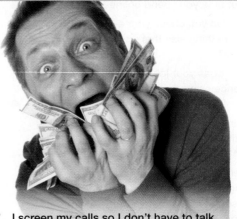

| | True | False |
|---|---|---|
| 7. I screen my calls so I don't have to talk to creditors. | ○ | ○ |
| 8. Shopping is my antidote to feeling bored, lonely, angry, or frustrated. | ○ | ○ |
| 9. When I shop, I can't return home empty-handed. | ○ | ○ |

| | True | False |
|---|---|---|
| 10. I've made false statements to creditors to get new lines of credit. | ○ | ○ |
| 11. My shopping habits have interfered with my work. | ○ | ○ |
| 12. My spending has caused problems in my marriage or my primary relationship. | ○ | ○ |
| 13. I feel uneasy if I've not shopped for several days. | ○ | ○ |
| 14. I spend over 30 percent of my income on nonmortgage debt. | ○ | ○ |
| 15. I have considered illegal or questionable means to raise money to support my shopping habits. | ○ | ○ |

| | True | False |
|---|---|---|
| 16. I've had issues with eating disorders or sexual, drug, or alcohol addictions. | ○ | ○ |
| 17. I repeatedly resolve not to spend, only to relapse and binge shop. | ○ | ○ |
| 18. I have to drive or wear status initials (e.g., BMW, DKNY, LV). | ○ | ○ |

## Interpreting Your Scores for This Section

Total your true responses and find your corresponding score below.

**1–3:** You have an indicator or two that trouble could be brewing around the corner, but you know your issues and are in a strong position to keep a check on things.

**4–6:** You're within shouting distance of having a problem. Make note of any marked changes in your shopping habits. Cognizance of your behavior is your most effective tool for keeping your spending in check.

**7–12:** You may be close to having a shopping addiction. Take a good look at the motivations driving your behavior. Know what money will buy for you, and get clear about what it won't. Consider seeking advice from a credit counselor or a therapist.

**13–18:** You likely have a shopping addiction, and it's time to get help. Check out www.debtorsanonymous.org. Relief is only a meeting away.

**Source:** S. Durling, "Am I a Compulsive Shopper?" Copyright © 2002, Available at www.sharondurling.com/Compulsive.htm.

# YOUR PLAN FOR CHANGE

The **Assessyourself** activity gave you a chance to evaluate signs of Internet, gambling, and shopping addictions. Depending on your results, you may need to take steps toward changing certain behaviors that could be detrimental to your health

### Today, you can:

○ Identify any problem areas in which you may have an addiction. Be honest with yourself about your behaviors and commit to addressing the issue. The first step in beating an addiction is admitting you have a problem.

○ Write a list of the things that contribute to the behavior you feel may be addictive. Include your reasons for engaging in the behavior and the things about it that are reinforcing. Why do you want to change it? Try to identify barriers that would make it hard to break away from the behavior or bring it under control. What would help you address these barriers?

### Within the next 2 weeks, you can:

○ Look into support groups in your area that could possibly help you, such as Gamblers Anonymous or Debtors Anonymous. Visit your student health center to find out about programs that may be available on campus.

○ Begin tracking your addictive behavior. Keep a log of dates, time spent engaging in the behavior, the way you are feeling, the amount of money spent (if pertinent), any other people involved, and anything else you think is relevant. Look for patterns in your log, such as particular times of day when you are most vulnerable to the addiction, a specific mood related to it, or certain people or places that trigger your compulsion.

### By the end of the semester, you can:

○ Take positive steps to address some of the patterns you noted in your log. Come up with a distraction to turn to when you begin feeling the addictive urge, and try to avoid settings or circumstances that trigger your addictive behavior.

○ Establish new limits for your addictive behavior and strive to enforce them for several days at a time. For example, this could mean setting a time limit on Internet use. Enlist a trusted friend to help you enforce these limits—for example, by making plans to play Frisbee after your allotted half hour of Internet surfing.

## Summary

* Addiction is the continued use of a substance or activity despite ongoing negative consequences. Addiction develops over time through a pattern known as *nurturing through avoidance*. Mood-altering substances and experiences produce biochemical reactions that make the body feel good; when they are absent, the person feels the effects of withdrawal. All addictions share four common symptoms: compulsion, loss of control, negative consequences, and denial.
* Habits are repeated behaviors, whereas addiction is behavior resulting from compulsion; without the behavior, the addict experiences withdrawal.
* Codependents are typically friends or family members who are "addicted to the addict." Enablers are people who knowingly or unknowingly protect addicts from the consequences of their behavior.
* The biopsychosocial model of addiction takes into account biological (genetic) factors as well as psychological and environmental influences in understanding the addiction process.
* Addictive behaviors include disordered gambling, compulsive buying, compulsive Internet or technology use, work addiction, compulsive exercise, and sexual addiction.
* Treatment begins with abstinence from the addictive behavior or substance, usually instituted through intervention by close family, friends, or other loved ones. Treatment programs may include individual, group, or family therapy, as well as 12-step programs.

## Pop Quiz

1. Which of the following is not a characteristic of addiction?
   a. Compulsion
   b. Loss of control
   c. Habit
   d. Withdrawal

2. Gina is addicted to the Internet. She is so preoccupied with surfing websites that she skips classes and misses important exams. What symptom of addiction does her preoccupation characterize?
   a. Denial
   b. Compulsion
   c. Loss of control
   d. Negative consequences

3. Which of the following is the definition of *denial*?
   a. The body's rejection of a drug or chemical
   b. The inability to perceive that a behavior is self-destructive
   c. The need to consume more drugs to get the same high
   d. A person's ability to handle a toxic amount of drugs in the body

4. Chemical dependency *relapse* refers to
   a. a person who is experiencing a blackout.
   b. a gap in one's drinking or drug-taking patterns.
   c. a full return to addictive behavior.
   d. the failure to change one's behavior.

5. People who excessively and compulsively exercise to meet needs of nurturance, intimacy, and self-esteem have a(n)
   a. money addiction.
   b. work addiction.
   c. buying addiction.
   d. exercise addiction.

6. When a person repeatedly seeks the illusion of relief to avoid unpleasant feelings, this pattern is known as
   a. neurotransmitter deficiency.
   b. nurturing through avoidance.
   c. a bad habit.
   d. compulsive behavior.

7. The current theory of addiction relies on the biopsychosocial model of addiction. This model proposes that most addictive conditions were influenced by
   a. biological or disease influences.
   b. genetic influences.
   c. environmental influences.
   d. All of the above

8. Chris is obsessed with his weight-lifting program and constantly checks to see if his six-pack abs and lean muscles are nicely sculpted. He suffers from
   a. anorexia.
   b. muscle dysmorphia.
   c. exercise addiction.
   d. tolerance.

9. The first step in treating an addiction is to
   a. organize an intervention.
   b. recognize the addiction.
   c. enter a rehabilitation facility.
   d. find a psychotherapist.

10. An individual who knowingly tries to protect an addict from natural consequences of his or her destructive behaviors is
    a. enabling.
    b. coddling.
    c. practicing intervention.
    d. controlling.

*Answers to these questions can be found on page A-1.*

## Think about It!

1. What factors distinguish a habit from an addiction? Is it possible for you to tell whether someone else is truly addicted?

2. Explain why the biopsychosocial model of addiction is a more effective model for treatment than a single-factor model.
3. Explain the potential genetic, environmental, and psychological risk factors for addiction.
4. Discuss how addiction affects family and friends. What role do family and friends play in helping the addict get help and maintain recovery?
5. What are some key components of an effective treatment program? Do the components vary for men and women? Why or why not?

# Accessing Your Health on the Internet

The following websites explore further topics and issues related to personal health. For links to the websites below, visit the Companion Website for *Access to Health*, 12th Edition, at www.pearsonhighered.com/donatelle.

1. *Center for Online and Internet Addiction.* This site provides information and assistance for those dealing with Internet addiction. www.netaddiction.com
2. *National Council on Problem Gambling.* This site provides information and help for people with gambling problems and their families, including a searchable directory for counselors. www.ncpgambling.org
3. *Keeping the Score (University of Missouri, Columbia).* This site provides pertinent information for college students regarding gambling. http://pip.students.missouri.edu/
4. *Society for the Advancement of Sexual Health.* This site provides information, resources, and a self-quiz relating to sexual addiction. www.sash.net

# References

1. R. Goldberg, *Drugs across the Spectrum*, 6th ed. (Belmont, CA: Brooks/Cole, 2009).
2. J. Kinney, *Loosening the Grip: A Handbook of Alcohol Information*, 9th ed. (Boston: McGraw-Hill, 2009), 175.
3. A. Agrawal et al., "Linkage Scan for Quantitative Traits Identifies New Regions of Interest for Substance Dependence in the Collaborative Study on the Genetics of Alcoholism (COGA) Sample," *Drug and Alcohol Dependence* 93, no. 1–2 (2008): 12–20.
4. A. I. Herman et al., "Serotonin Transporter Promoter Polymorphism and Differences in Alcohol Consumption Behavior in a College Student Population," *Alcohol and Alcoholism* 38, no. 5 (2003): 446–49.
5. A. Agrawal et al., "Linkage Scan for Quantitative Traits Identifies New Regions of Interest for Substance Dependence in the Collaborative Study on the Genetics of Alcoholism (COGA) Sample" 2008.
6. J. Kinney, *Loosening the Grip*, 2009, 106.
7. G. Hansen and P. Venturelli, *Drugs and Society*, 10th ed. (Sudbury, MA: Jones and Bartlett, 2009), 49.
8. Ibid, 4.
9. National Institute on Drug Abuse, National Institutes of Health, U.S. Department of Health and Human Services, *Drugs, Brains, and Behavior: The Science of Addiction*, NIH Publication no. 07-5605 (Bethesda, MD: National Institute on Drug Abuse, 2007), Available at www.nida.nih.gov/scienceofaddiction.
10. National Council on Problem Gambling, "FAQs—Problem Gamblers," www.ncpgambling.org/i4a/pages/index.cfm?pageid=3390, Accessed April 2010.
11. C. Holden, "Random Samples: Gambling as Addiction," *Science* 307, no. 5708 (2005): 349.
12. Ibid.
13. J. W. Welte et al., "Gambling Participation and Pathology in the United States: A Sociodemographic Analysis Using Classification Trees," *Addictive Behaviors* 29, no. 5 (2004): 983–89.
14. The Annenburg Public Policy Center, "Card Playing Trend in Young People Starts to Diverge," Press release, September 28, 2006, Available at www.annenbergpublicpolicycenter.org/PressReleases.aspx.
15. W. DeJong et al., "Gambling: The New Addiction Crisis in Higher Education," *Alcohol, Tobacco, and Other Drugs Prevention File* 21, no. 1 (2006): 11–13.
16. L. M. Koran et al., "Estimated Prevalence of Compulsive Buying Behavior in the United States," *American Journal of Psychiatry* 163, no. 10 (2006): 1806–12.
17. H. Tavares et al., "Compulsive Buying Disorder: A Review and Case Vignette." *Brazilian Journal of Psychiatry* 30, suppl. 1 (2008): S16–23; R. Engs, "How Can I Manage Compulsive Shopping and Spending Addiction (Shopoholism)?" Updated December 2006, www.indiana.edu/~engs/hints/shop.html.
18. C. Morrison and H .Gore, "The Relationship between Excessive Internet Use and Depression: A Questionnaire-Based Study of 1,319 Young People and Adults," *Psychopathology* 43, no. 2 (2010): 121–26. D. M. Wieland, "Computer Addiction: Implications for Nursing Psychotherapy Practice," *Perspectives in Psychiatric Care* 41, no. 4 (2005): 153–61.
19. American College Health Association, *American College Health Association—National College Health Assessment II: Reference Group Data Report Fall 2009* (Baltimore: American College Health Association, 2009), Available at www.acha-ncha.org/reports_ACHA-NCHAII.html.
20. A. C. Douglas, "Internet Addiction: Meta-Synthesis of Qualitative Research for the Decade 1996–2006," *Computers in Human Behavior* 24, no. 6 (2008): 3027–44.
21. C. Chamberlin and N. Zhang, "Workaholism, Health and Self-Acceptance," *Journal of Counseling and Development* 87, no. 2 (2009): 159–69.
22. Ibid.
23. Ibid.
24. B. Cook and H. A. Hausenblas, "The Role of Exercise Dependence for the Relationship between Exercise Behavior and Eating Pathology: Mediator or Moderator?," *Journal of Health Psychology* 13, no. 4 (2008): 495–502.
25. J. F. Morgan, *The Invisible Man: A Self-Help Guide for Men with Eating Disorders, Compulsive Exercise and Bigorexia* (New York: Routledge, 2008), 36.
26. C. Nakken, *The Addictive Personality: Understanding the Addictive Process and Compulsive Behavior* (Center City, MN: Hazelden, 1996).
27. S. Maisto, P. Clifford, and J. S. Tonigan, "Initial and Long-Term Alcohol Treatment Success: A 10-Year Study of the Project MATCH Albuquerque Sample," *Alcoholism: Clinical and Experimental Research* 26, no. 5 (2003).

# 11

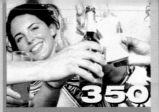

**350**

How much do college students really drink?

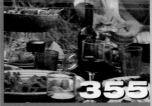

**355**

Why do some people feel the effects of alcohol more quickly than others?

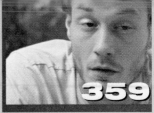

**359**

Is there any cure for a hangover?

# Drinking Alcohol Responsibly

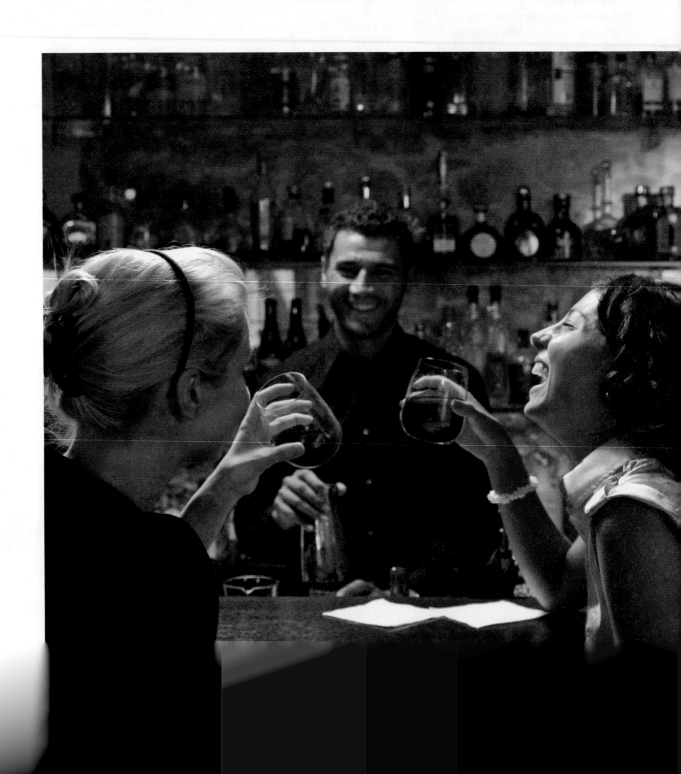

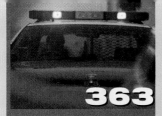

**363**

What are the legal consequences if you are caught drinking and driving?

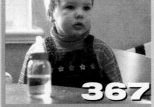

**367**

How does it affect you to grow up in a family with alcoholism?

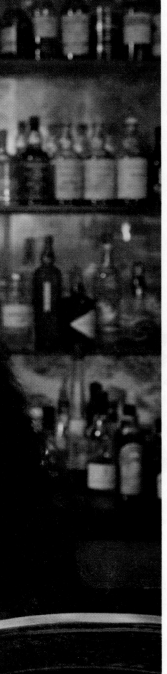

## Objectives

✳ Discuss the alcohol use patterns of college students and overall trends in consumption.

✳ Explain the physiological and behavioral effects of alcohol, including blood alcohol concentration, absorption, metabolism, and the immediate and long-term effects of excess alcohol consumption on your overall health.

✳ Learn practical strategies for drinking responsibly and coping effectively with campus and societal pressures to drink.

✳ Explain the symptoms and causes of alcoholism, its cost to society, and its effects on you, your friends, your family, and the community.

✳ Discuss the treatment of alcoholism, including the family's role, varied treatment methods, and whether alcoholics can be cured.

People all over the world and throughout history have used alcohol for everything from social gatherings to religious ceremonies. The consumption of alcoholic beverages is part of many traditions, and moderate use of alcohol can enhance celebrations or special times. College campuses are no exception. You can probably think of many instances of celebration on campus that involved alcohol.

Research even shows that very low levels of alcohol consumption, particularly red wine, may actually lower some health risks in older adults. Potential benefits include reduced risks of cardiovascular diseases and osteoporosis, though some critics of these studies argue that confounding factors, such as socioeconomic status, may account for the apparent benefits.[1] We need to remember, however, that although alcohol can sometimes play a positive role in some people's lives, it is first and foremost a chemical substance that affects physical and mental behavior. Alcohol is a drug, and if it is not used responsibly, it can become dangerous.

Alcohol is an important topic not just on campus, but in American society overall. Approximately half of all Americans consume alcoholic beverages regularly, while about 21 percent abstain from drinking alcohol altogether.[2] Among those who drink, consumption patterns vary. More men are regular drinkers and men typically drink more than women. White drinkers are more likely to drink daily or nearly daily than are nonwhites. As age increases, the number of people who consume alcohol regularly decreases.[3]

Alcohol consumption levels among Americans have declined steadily since the late 1970s. In 2007, the estimated annual per capita consumption was the equivalent of 2.31 gallons of pure alcohol per person.[4] (This is the same as drinking approximately 50 gallons of beer, 20 gallons of wine, or more than 4 gallons of distilled spirits.) This represents a substantial decrease from 2.64 gallons of pure alcohol per person in 1977. This downward trend has been tied to growing attention to weight, personal health, and physical activity. The alcohol industry has responded by introducing beers and wines with fewer calories and carbohydrates and with reduced alcohol content.

# 90%
**of the drinking population are infrequent, light, or moderate drinkers.**

In this chapter, we discuss the use of alcohol in the United States and on college campuses, and its effects on the body and on health. We also look at the hallmarks of responsible consumption, signs of alcohol dependency, and the health risks of irresponsible use. Finally, we discuss treatment and recovery from alcoholism.

# Alcohol Use on College Campuses

Alcohol is the most popular drug on college campuses, where over 70 percent of students report having consumed alcoholic beverages in the past 30 days (Figure 11.1).[5] In a new trend on college campuses, women's consumption of alcohol has come close to equaling men's.

Almost half of all college students engage in **heavy episodic (binge) drinking.** Over the years, there has been a lack of uniformity in defining the word *binge*. Recognizing this, in 2007, the National Advisory Council of the National Institute on Alcohol Abuse and Alcoholism (NIAAA) approved a new definition: "A binge is a pattern of drinking alcohol that brings blood alcohol concentration (BAC) to 0.08 gram-percent or above. For a typical adult, this pattern corresponds to consuming 5 or more drinks (male), or 4 or more drinks (female), in about 2 hours."[6] Therefore, students who might go out and drink only once a week are considered heavy episodic drinkers (binge drinkers) if they consume these amounts within 2 hours.

**heavy episodic (binge) drinking** A *binge* is a pattern of drinking alcohol that brings blood alcohol concentration (BAC) to 0.08 gram-percent or above; for a typical adult, this pattern corresponds to consuming five or more drinks (male) or four or more drinks (female) in about 2 hours.

Binge drinking is especially dangerous because it involves consuming a lot of alcohol in a very short period of time. This can quickly lead to extreme intoxication, unconsciousness, alcohol poisoning, and even death. Often, drinking competitions, celebrations or games, and hazing rituals encourage this type of drinking.

College is a critical time to become aware of and responsible for drinking. Many students are away from home, often for the first time, and are excited by their newfound independence. For some students, this independence and the rite of passage into the college culture are symbolized by alcohol use. For others, alcohol provides the answer to one of the most commonly heard statements on any college campus: "There is nothing to do." In addition, many students say they drink to have fun. "Having fun," which often means drinking simply to get drunk, may really be a way of coping with stress,

boredom, anxiety, or pressures created by academic and social demands.

A significant number of students experience negative consequences as a result of their alcohol consumption. According to the American College Health Association's National College Health Assessment, in the past 12 months approximately 50 percent of college students who drank experienced at least one negative consequence.[7] Thirty-one percent of students reported doing something they regretted after

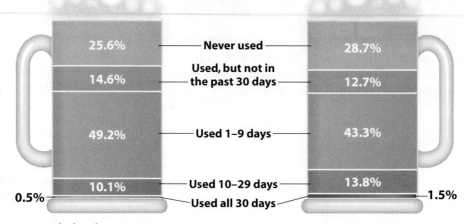

| Women | | Men |
|---|---|---|
| 25.6% | Never used | 28.7% |
| 14.6% | Used, but not in the past 30 days | 12.7% |
| 49.2% | Used 1–9 days | 43.3% |
| 10.1% | Used 10–29 days | 13.8% |
| 0.5% | Used all 30 days | 1.5% |

**FIGURE 11.1** College Students' Patterns of Alcohol Use in the Past 30 Days

**Source:** Data are from American College Health Association, *American College Health Association—National College Health Assessment II (ACHA-NCHA II) Reference Group Data Report Fall 2009* (Baltimore: American College Health Association, 2010).

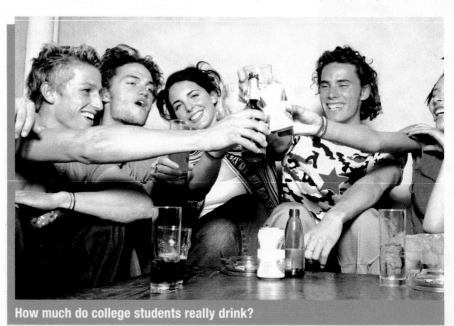

**How much do college students really drink?**

It may sometimes seem like your campus is crowded with heavy drinkers, but, in fact, most college students—about 61%—drink only occasionally, and 27% don't drink at all. However, college students have high rates of binge drinking; when they do drink, they tend to drink a lot. Irresponsible consumption of alcohol can easily result in disaster, so it is important for you to take control of when you drink, and how much.

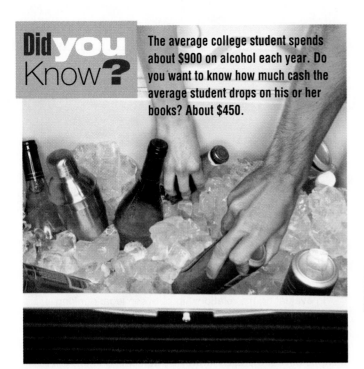

drinking; 27 percent forgot where they were or what they did; 15 percent physically injured themselves; and 15 percent had unprotected sex. In addition, 2 percent reported having had sex with someone without giving consent, and 0.5 percent reported having sex with someone without getting consent. Women were more likely to have someone use force or use the threat of force to have sex with them after they had been drinking.

On a more positive note, in the same survey, many college students reported always or usually practicing protective behaviors when consuming alcohol to reduce the risk of negative consequences as a result of their alcohol use. Seventy-seven percent of students reported eating before or during drinking, 84 percent reported staying with the same group of friends the entire time they drank, 82 percent reported using a designated driver, 66 percent kept track of how many drinks they consumed, and 41 percent determined in advance a set number of drinks they would not exceed.[8] It is important for students to recognize that if they consume alcohol, choices such as these can help reduce the risk of experiencing a negative consequence as a result of their drinking. The **Skills for Behavior Change** box provides additional strategies for drinking responsibly.

# High-Risk Drinking and College Students

There are, however, some students who don't drink responsibly. The stakes of doing so are high, because it poses a high risk for alcohol-related injuries and death. According to a recent study, 1,825 college students die each year because of alcohol-related unintentional injuries, including car accidents.[9] Unintentional injuries are the leading cause of death in the 18- to 24-year-old age group and alcohol is the leading contributing factor in those deaths. Consumption of alcohol is the number one cause of preventable death among undergraduate college students in the United States today.

Who are the students who drink heavily? Why are these students drinking so much, and what are their typical drinking behaviors? What impact does their drinking have, and what are college campuses doing to prevent this behavior? These are the questions we'll discuss in this section.

**Who Drinks?** It's likely that students who enter college will drink at some point, but there are groups of students who are more likely to drink more and more often. For example, students who believe that their parents approve of their drinking are more likely to drink and to report a drinking-related problem.[10] Students who drank heavily in high school are also at risk for heavy drinking in college.[11] Most students have tried alcohol in high school. By twelfth grade, 26 percent of high school students report engaging in binge drinking, and 55 percent report having been drunk, while another 12 percent report having had at least one full drink.[12]

**Why Do College Students Drink So Much?** Although everyone is at some risk for alcohol-related problems, college students seem to be particularly vulnerable. The college years bring more freedom, fewer restrictions, and many more

# POINTS OF VIEW

## The Drinking Age:
## IS THERE A RIGHT ONE?

In years prior to 1984, the drinking age varied from state to state. In some states, the drinking age was 18, some 19, and others 21. However, since 1984 when Congress passed the National Minimum Drinking Age Act, the drinking age in all states has been 21. In 2008, the Amethyst Initiative was founded by university and college presidents to call for the discussion of the current drinking age laws and whether the appropriate minimum legal drinking age should be younger than 21. Below are the major points from both sides of the issue.

### Arguments for Reducing the Legal Drinking Age

○ Alcohol education that mandates abstinence as the only legal option for those under age 21 has not resulted in significant constructive behavioral change among students.

○ Adults under 21 are deemed capable of voting, signing contracts, serving on juries, and enlisting in the military, but are told they are not mature enough to have a beer.

○ By choosing to use fake IDs, students make ethical compromises that erode respect for the law.

○ Binge drinking often occurs off campus to avoid detection of underage drinkers, which makes it more difficult when a drinker needs medical attention.

### Arguments for Keeping the Drinking Age 21

○ Higher drinking ages were associated with reduced consumption in 11 of 33 studies.

○ In evaluating the relationship between legal drinking ages and traffic crashes, 46 of 79 studies found higher drinking age was related to decreased traffic crashes.

○ Students are influenced to drink responsibly by their campus environment, so improving that environment will be more effective than changing the drinking age.

○ The public school system will be faced with an increased burden in dealing with those who are legal to drink and those who are not within the high school setting.

### Where Do You Stand?

○ What do you think the drinking age should be? What do you think the potential problems are that might be created by changing it and what issues might it solve?

○ Do you think that drinking ages should vary by state?

○ How do you think the laws should change for those who drink underage? Are laws effective deterrents?

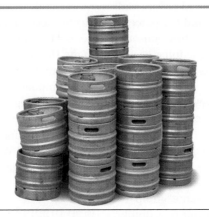

**Sources:** Amethyst Initiative, "Statement," 2008, www.amethystinitiative.org/statement; Washington State University, College Coalition for Substance Abuse Prevention, "Response to Amethyst Initiative," August 2008, http://ccsap .wsu.edu/default.asp?PageID=2718; K. Kiewra, "Binge Drinking: Harvard College Alcohol Study Calls for Changes at U.S. Colleges," Harvard School of Public Health, Accessed June 2010, www.hsph.harvard.edu/news/hphr/winter-2009/ winter09binge.html.

---

opportunities to party with friends. In addition to this new-found college freedom, there are several other factors that encourage students to drink in college:

● Many college and university students' customs (e.g., Greek rush or initiations), norms (e.g., reputation as party schools, tailgate parties at football games), and traditional celebrations (e.g., St. Patrick's Day, Mardi Gras) encourage alcohol use.

● Advertising and promotions from the alcoholic beverage industry target students.

● College students are particularly vulnerable to peer influence and have a strong need to be accepted by their peers.

● College women tend to care how much men want them to drink, and they tend to overestimate how much men prefer they consume. In a recent study, 26 percent of women stated that men would most likely want to be friends with a woman who drinks five or more drinks; 17 percent thought that men would be most attracted to that woman. Both estimates were almost double what men actually said.[13]

● Students believe that alcohol will make them feel better, less stressed, more sociable, and less self-conscious. The behaviors most commonly reported by students reflect these expectations: dancing, flirting, telling jokes, and laughing more frequently. The primary expectations of students going to bars and nightclubs are becoming intoxicated, socializing with friends, seeking romance or sex, and relieving problems or stress.[14]

● More than 80 percent of college students drink alcohol to celebrate their twenty-first birthday, and they consume an average of nearly 13 drinks, with estimated blood alcohol concentrations (BACs) of 19 percent and higher. See the **Points of View** box at left on the legal drinking age.

- Students drink as part of hazing rituals. The use of alcohol in hazing is most prevalent in Greek and varsity athletics organizations, with more than 50 percent of students involved in these activities reporting participation in a drinking game as a hazing activity.[15]

- The low price of alcohol, whether it is beer or liquor, is strongly related to higher rates of drinking and binging. In a recent study, students who paid the most money per gram of alcohol consumed the least amount of alcohol. The least intoxicated students paid $4.44 for 14 grams of alcohol (one 12-ounce beer, one 5-ounce glass of wine, or 1 ounce of liquor), whereas those students who were found to be the drunkest paid $1.81 for the same amount of alcohol. All-you-can-drink specials attract students who want to drink and get drunk.[16]

- Easy access to alcohol, often referred to as *density of alcohol outlets,* contributes to higher rates of binge drinking. Campus communities with a large number of bars and alcohol outlets have a higher rate of binge drinking than those with few bars and alcohol outlets in close vicinity to campus.[17]

**College Student Drinking Behavior** College students are more likely than their noncollegiate peers to drink recklessly and to engage in drinking games and other dangerous drinking practices. One such practice is **pre-gaming** (also called pre-loading or front-loading). Pre-gaming has become increasingly common on college campuses, and involves planned heavy drinking, usually in someone's home, apartment, or residence hall, prior to going out to a bar, nightclub, or sporting event. Sometimes it occurs prior to attending an event where alcohol is not available. In a recent study of pre-gaming, 55 percent of college men and 60 percent of college women drank before going to a bar or nightclub.[18] The goal of many pre-gamers is to get drunk. Some of the motivations for pre-gaming are to avoid paying for high-cost drinks, to socialize with friends, to reduce social anxiety, and to enhance male bonding. Pre-gamers have higher alcohol consumption during the evening and more negative consequences such as blackouts, hangover, passing out, and alcohol poisoning.

**What Is the Impact of Student Drinking?** Unfortunately, recent studies confirm what students have been experiencing for a long time—drinking and binge drinkers cause problems not only for themselves, but also for those around them. One study indicated that over 696,000 students between the ages of 18 and 24 were assaulted by another student who had been drinking.[19] There is significant evidence that campus rape is linked to binge drinking. Women from colleges with medium to high binge drinking rates are 1.5 times more at risk of being raped than those from schools with a low binge drinking rate. Although exact numbers are hard to find, estimates are that more than 97,000 students between the ages of 18 and 24 experience alcohol-related sexual assault or date rape each year in the United States.[20] The laws regarding sexual consent are clear: A person who is drunk or passed out cannot consent to sex. If you have sex with someone who is drunk or unconscious

(passed out), you are committing rape. Claiming you were also drunk when you had sex with someone who is intoxicated or unconscious will not absolve you of your legal and moral responsibility for this crime. For more on rape, see Chapter 19.

**pre-gaming** A strategy of drinking heavily at home before going out to an event or other location.

Other students report sleep and study disruptions, and vandalism of personal property. Approximately 25 percent of college students report negative academic consequences because of their drinking.[21] About 30 percent of students who drink and 68 percent of binge drinkers say they have missed a class because of alcohol use.[22] The more students drink the more likely they are to miss class, do poorly on tests and papers, have lower grade point averages (GPAs), and fall behind on their schoolwork. Some students may even drop out of school as a result of their drinking. **Figure 11.2** gives some examples of alcohol-related problems.

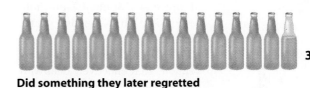

**31.4%**

**Did something they later regretted**

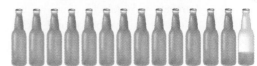

**26.8%**

**Forgot where they were or what they did**

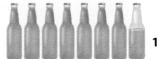

**15.2%**

**Had unprotected sex**

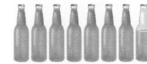

**15.1%**

**Physically injured self**

**3.7%**

**Got in trouble with the police**

**2.6%**

**Physically injured another person**

FIGURE 11.2 **Prevalence of Negative Consequences of Drinking among College Students, Past Year**

**Source:** Data are from American College Health Association, *American College Health Association—National College Health Assessment II (ACHA-NCHA II) Reference Group Data Report Fall 2009* (Baltimore: American College Health Association, 2010).

## Colleges' Efforts to Reduce Student Drinking

Some colleges are taking action to curb binge drinking and alcohol abuse by instituting strong policies against drinking. For example, university presidents have formed a leadership group to help control the problem of alcohol abuse. Many fraternities have elected to have "dry" houses. At the same time, schools are making more help available to students with drinking problems. Today, most campuses offer both individual and group counseling and are directing more attention toward preventing alcohol abuse. Student organizations such as BACCHUS (Boost Alcohol Consciousness Concerning the Health of University Students) promote responsible drinking and party hosting.

The NIAAA has studied interventions that effectively deal with the problem. Programs that have proven particularly effective include cognitive-behavioral skills training with *motivational interviewing,* a nonjudgmental approach to working with students to change behavior, and e-Interventions, which are electronically based alcohol education interventions using text messages.[23] Preventive podcasts and e-mails have become more common on campus.[24] Sending electronic twenty-first birthday cards about the negative consequences of excess drinking on that milestone birthday has actually shown to reduce the number of drinks taken and consequently resulted in lower BACs in women celebrating that day.[25]

Colleges and universities are also trying a *social norms* approach to reducing alcohol consumption, sending a consistent message to students about actual drinking behavior on campus. Many students perceive that their peers drink more than they actually do, which may cause them to feel pressured to drink more themselves. This misperception includes inaccurately estimating how much and how often students drink, and the actual consequences of students' drinking. In a national survey, for example, college students perceived that 60 percent of students used alcohol 10 to 30 days a month, but the actual use rate is 16 percent.[26] As a result of these social norms campaigns, heavy episodic alcohol consumption—binge drinking—has declined at campuses across the country.

**ethyl alcohol (ethanol)** An addictive drug produced by fermentation and found in many beverages.
**fermentation** The process whereby yeast organisms break down plant sugars to yield ethanol.
**distillation** The process whereby mash is subjected to high temperatures to release alcohol vapors, which are then condensed and mixed with water to make the final product.
**proof** A measure of the percentage of alcohol in a beverage.
**standard drink** The amount of any beverage that contains about 14 grams of pure alcohol (about 0.6 fluid ounce or 1.2 tablespoons).

# Alcohol in the Body

What do you need to know in order to reduce the likelihood of experiencing negative consequences as a result of your drinking? Learning about the metabolism and absorption of alcohol can help you understand how it affects each person differently and how it is possible to drink safely. It is also key in understanding how to avoid life-threatening circumstances such as alcohol poisoning. This information can be critical for your safety and that of your friends.

## The Chemistry and Potency of Alcohol

The intoxicating substance found in beer, wine, liquor, and liqueurs is **ethyl alcohol,** or **ethanol.** It is produced during a process called **fermentation,** in which yeast organisms break down plant sugars, yielding ethanol and carbon dioxide. Fermentation continues until the solution of plant sugars (called *mash*) reaches a concentration of 14 percent alcohol. For beers, ales, and wines, the process ends with fermentation. Manufacturers then add other ingredients that dilute the beverage's alcohol content. Hard liquor is produced through further processing called **distillation,** during which alcohol vapors are released from the mash at high temperatures. The vapors are then condensed and mixed with water to make the final product.

The **proof** of an alcoholic drink is a measure of the percentage of alcohol in the beverage and therefore the strength of the drink. Alcohol percentage by volume is half of the given proof. For example, 80 proof whiskey or scotch is 40 percent alcohol by volume. Lower-proof drinks will produce fewer alcohol effects than the same amount of higher-proof drinks will produce. Most wines are between 12 and 15 percent alcohol, and most beers are between 2 and 8 percent, depending on state laws and the type of beer.

When discussing alcohol consumption, researchers usually talk in terms of "standard drinks." As defined by the NIAAA, a **standard drink** is any drink that contains about 14 grams of pure alcohol (about 0.6 fluid ounce or 1.2 tablespoons; see Figure 11.3). The actual size of a standard drink depends on the proof: a 12-ounce can of beer and a 1.5-ounce shot of vodka are both considered one standard drink because they contain the same amount of alcohol—about 0.6 fluid ounce. If you are estimating your blood alcohol concentration using standard drinks as a measure (see the following sections), you need to keep in mind the size of your drinks as well as their proof. For example, you may have bought only one beer while you were at the ballpark last weekend, but if that beer came in a 22-ounce glass, then you actually consumed two standard drinks.

## Absorption and Metabolism

Unlike the molecules found in most foods and drugs, alcohol molecules are sufficiently small and fat soluble to be absorbed throughout the entire gastrointestinal system. A

| Standard drink equivalent (and % alcohol) | | Approximate number of standard drinks in: |
|---|---|---|
| 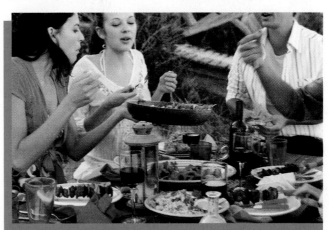 | Beer = 12 oz (~5% alcohol) | 12 oz = 1 <br> 16 oz = 1.3 <br> 22 oz = 2 <br> 40 oz = 3.3 |
| | Malt liquor = 8.5 oz (~7% alcohol) | 12 oz = 1.5 <br> 16 oz = 2 <br> 22 oz = 2.5 <br> 40 oz = 4.5 |
| | Table wine = 5 oz (~12% alcohol) | 750-mL (25-oz) bottle = 5 |
| | 80 proof spirits (gin, vodka, etc.) = 1.5 oz (~40% alcohol) | mixed drink = 1 or more* <br> pint (16 oz) = 11 <br> fifth (25 oz) = 17 <br> 1.75 L (59 oz) = 39 |

FIGURE 11.3 **What Is a Standard Drink?**

*Note: It can be difficult to estimate the number of standard drinks in a single mixed drink made with hard liquor. Depending on factors such as the type of spirits and the recipe, a mixed drink can contain from one to three or more standard drinks.

**Source:** Adapted from National Institute on Alcohol Abuse and Alcoholism, *Tips for Cutting Down on Drinking*, NIH Publication no. 07–3769 (Bethesda, MD: National Institutes of Health, 2007), http://pubs.niaaa.nih.gov/publications/Tips/tips.htm.

negligible amount of alcohol is absorbed through the mouth's lining. Approximately 20 percent of ingested alcohol diffuses through the stomach lining into the bloodstream, and nearly 80 percent passes through the lining of the upper third of the small intestine.

Several factors influence how quickly your body will absorb alcohol: the alcohol concentration in your drink, the amount of alcohol you consume, the amount of food in your stomach, your metabolism, weight, body mass index, and your mood. The higher the concentration of alcohol in your drink, the more rapidly it will be absorbed in your digestive tract. As a rule, wine and beer are absorbed more slowly than distilled beverages. "Fizzy" alcoholic beverages—such as champagne and carbonated wines—are absorbed more rapidly than those containing no sparkling additives. Carbonated beverages and drinks served with mixers cause the pyloric valve to relax, thereby emptying the stomach's contents more rapidly into the small intestine. Because the small intestine

absorbs the greatest amount of alcohol, carbonated beverages increase the rate of absorption. The **Health Headlines** box on page 356 discusses the effects of mixing energy drinks with alcohol.

The more alcohol you consume, the longer absorption takes. High concentrations of alcohol can irritate the digestive system, causing pylorospasm (spasm of the pyloric valve, the opening from the stomach into the small intestine). When the pyloric valve is closed, nothing can move from the stomach to the upper third of the small intestine, which slows absorption. If the irritation continues, it can cause vomiting. Alcohol also takes longer to absorb if there is food in your stomach, because the surface area exposed to alcohol is smaller, and because a full stomach retards the emptying of alcoholic beverages into the small intestine.

Mood is another factor, because emotions affect how long it takes for the stomach's contents to empty into the intestine. Powerful moods, such as stress and tension, are likely to cause the stomach to dump its contents into the small intestine faster. Alcohol is absorbed much more rapidly when people are tense than when they are relaxed.

Once it has been absorbed into the bloodstream, alcohol circulates throughout the body and is metabolized in the liver, where it is converted to *acetaldehyde* by the enzyme *alcohol dehydrogenase*. It is then rapidly oxidized to *acetate*, converted to carbon dioxide and water, and eventually excreted from the body. Acetaldehyde is a toxic chemical that can cause immediate symptoms, such as nausea and vomiting, as well as long-term effects such as liver damage. A very small portion of alcohol is excreted unchanged by the kidneys, lungs, and skin.

Alcohol contains 7 calories (kcal) per gram. This means that the average regular beer contains about 150 calories. Mixed drinks may contain more if they are combined with sugary

**Why do some people feel the effects of alcohol more quickly than others?**

Many factors influence how rapidly a person's body absorbs alcohol, and thus how quickly that person feels the effects of the alcohol. For example, eating while drinking slows down the absorption of alcohol into your bloodstream. Other relevant factors include gender, body weight, body composition, and mood.

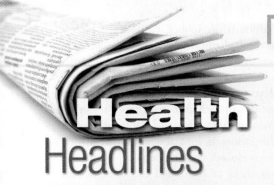

# Health Headlines

## ALCOHOL AND ENERGY DRINKS: A DANGEROUS MIX

Does this sound familiar to you? "Get It Up and Keep It Up" or "Party Like a Rockstar," or perhaps "Party Up"? Energy drinks are widely consumed on college campuses, with claims that Monster, Rockstar, Amp, Red Bull, and Full Throttle, among others, provide a burst of energy from caffeine and other plant-based stimulants and vitamins. Thirty-four percent of 18- to 24-year-olds are regular energy drink consumers. The drinks have been aggressively marketed on college campuses. For example, Red Bull gives away cases of the product to promote the drink.

The alcohol industry has used the popularity of energy drinks to promote its own products, introducing premixed alcohol and energy drink products such as Sparks, Rockstar 21, and Tilt. In addition, alcohol companies promote mixing energy drinks with alcohol products on their edgy websites. Captain Morgan, for example, promotes what it calls the "Ink Drop," which is a mix of rum and energy drink.

Over 28 percent of college students report mixing alcohol and energy drinks. White male students, athletes, fraternity or sorority or pledge members, and younger students are more likely to consume alcohol mixed energy drinks (AMEDs). Reasons students give for drinking AMEDs is to hide the flavor of the alcohol, and/or to drink more and not feel as drunk.

Because students often mix energy drinks with alcohol for the sake of masking the taste or effects of alcohol, these drinks can be particularly dangerous. Students who report consuming energy drinks tend to drink more than students who do not drink AMEDs (8.3 drinks vs. 6.1 drinks). Students also report not noticing the signs of intoxication (dizziness, fatigue, headache, and trouble walking) when they had consumed AMEDs. Students who reported drinking AMEDs

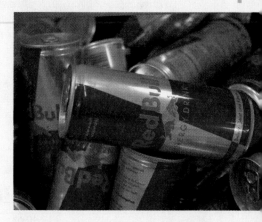

had an increased prevalence of several alcohol-related consequences of drinking. They were more likely to be taken advantage of sexually, and twice as likely to take advantage of someone sexually, ride with a drunk driver, be hurt or injured, or require medical treatment.

**Sources:** D. L. Thombs et al., "Event-level Analyses of Energy Drink Consumption and Alcohol Intoxication in Bar Patrons," *Addictive Behaviors* 35, no. 4 (2010): 325–30; M. C. O'Brien et al., "Caffeinated Cocktails: Energy Drink Consumption, High-Risk Drinking, and Alcohol-Related Consequences among College Students," *Society for Academic Emergency Medicine* 15 (2008): 1–8; Center for Science in the Public Interest, *Alcohol Policies Project Fact Sheet: Alcoholic Energy Drinks*, Updated September 2008, www.cspinet .org/booze/fctindex.htm.

soda or fruit juices. The body uses the calories in alcohol in the same manner it uses those found in carbohydrates: for immediate energy or for storage as fat if not immediately needed.

The breakdown of alcohol occurs at a fairly constant rate of 0.5 ounce per hour (approximately equivalent to one standard drink). This amount of alcohol is equivalent to 12 ounces of 5 percent beer, 5 ounces of 12 percent wine, or 1.5 ounces of 40 percent (80 proof) liquor. Unmetabolized alcohol circulates in the bloodstream until enough time passes for the body to break it down.

## Blood Alcohol Concentration

**Blood alcohol concentration (BAC)** is the ratio of alcohol to total blood volume. It is the primary method used to measure the physiological and behavioral effects of alcohol. Despite individual differences, alcohol produces some general behavioral effects, depending on BAC (Figure 11.4).

At a BAC of 0.02 percent, a person feels slightly relaxed and in a

**blood alcohol concentration (BAC)** The ratio of alcohol to total blood volume; the factor used to measure the physiological and behavioral effects of alcohol.

good mood. At 0.05 percent, relaxation increases, there is some motor impairment, and a willingness to talk becomes apparent. At 0.08 percent, the person feels euphoric, and there is further motor impairment. At 0.10 percent, the depressant effects of alcohol become apparent, drowsiness sets in, and motor skills are further impaired, followed by a loss of judgment. Thus, a driver may not be able to estimate distance or speed, and some drinkers lose their ability to make value-related decisions and may do things they would not do when sober. As BAC increases, the drinker suffers increased physiological and psychological effects. All these changes are negative. Alcohol ingestion does not enhance any physical skills or mental functions.

A drinker's BAC depends on weight and body fat, the water content in body tissues, the concentration of alcohol in the beverage consumed, the rate of consumption, and the volume of alcohol consumed. Heavier people have larger body surfaces through which to diffuse alcohol; therefore, they have lower concentrations of alcohol in their blood than do thin people after drinking the same amount. Figure 11.5 compares blood alcohol levels in men and women by weight and consumption.

| Blood Alcohol Concentration (BAC) | Psychological and Physical Effects |
|---|---|
| **Not Impaired** | |
| <0.01% | Negligible |
| **Sometimes Impaired** | |
| 0.01–0.04% | Slight muscle relaxation, mild euphoria, slight body warmth, increased sociability and talkativeness |
| **Usually Impaired** | |
| 0.05–0.07% | Lowered alertness, impaired judgment, lowered inhibitions, exaggerated behavior, loss of small muscle control |
| **Always Impaired** | |
| 0.08–0.14% | Slowed reaction time, poor muscle coordination, short-term memory loss, judgment impaired, inability to focus |
| 0.15–0.24% | Blurred vision, lack of motor skills, sedation, slowed reactions, difficulty standing and walking, passing out |
| 0.25–0.34% | Impaired consciousness, disorientation, loss of motor function, severely impaired or no reflexes, impaired circulation and respiration, uncontrolled urination, slurred speech, possible death |
| 0.35% and up | Unconsciousness, coma, extremely slow heartbeat and respiration, unresponsiveness, probable death |

FIGURE 11.4 **The Psychological and Physical Effects of Alcohol**

Because alcohol does not diffuse as rapidly into body fat as it does into the water content in body tissues, blood alcohol concentration is higher in a person with more body fat. Because a woman is likely to have more body fat and less water in her body tissues than a man of the same weight, she will be more intoxicated than a man after drinking the same amount of alcohol. See the Gender & Health box on page 359 for more on the differences in alcohol's effects on women and men.

Both breath analysis (Breathalyzer tests) and urinalysis are used to determine whether an individual is legally intoxicated, but blood tests are more accurate measures of BAC. An increasing number of states require blood tests for people suspected of driving under the influence of alcohol. In some states, refusal to take the breath or urine test results in immediate revocation of the person's driver's license.

People can develop physical and psychological tolerance of alcohol's effects through regular use. The nervous system adapts over time, so greater amounts of alcohol are required to produce the same physiological and psychological effects. Though BAC may be quite high, the individual has learned to modify his behavior to appear sober. This ability is called **learned behavioral tolerance.**

# Alcohol and Your Health

The immediate and long-term effects of alcohol consumption can vary greatly (see Figure 11.6 on page 358). Whether you experience any consequences as a result of your alcohol use either immediately or long term depends on you as an individual, the amount of alcohol you consume, and your circumstances.

# Immediate and Short-Term Effects of Alcohol

The most dramatic effects produced by ethanol occur within the central nervous system (CNS).

**learned behavioral tolerance** The ability of heavy drinkers to modify behavior so that they appear to be sober even when they have high BAC levels.

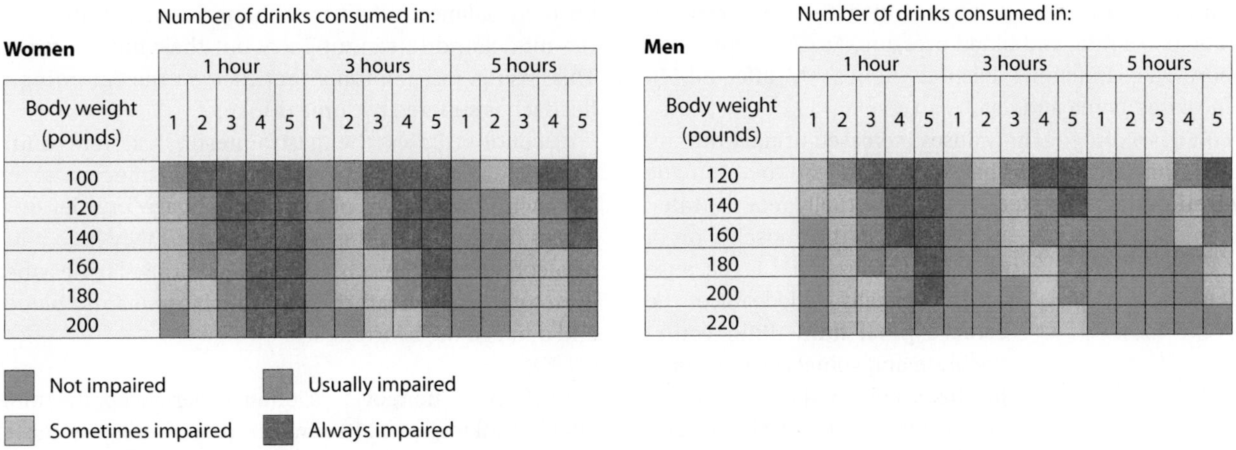

FIGURE 11.5 **Approximate Blood Alcohol Concentration (BAC) Based on Body Weight and Number of Drinks** Remember that there are many variables that can affect BAC, so this is only an estimate of what your BAC would be.

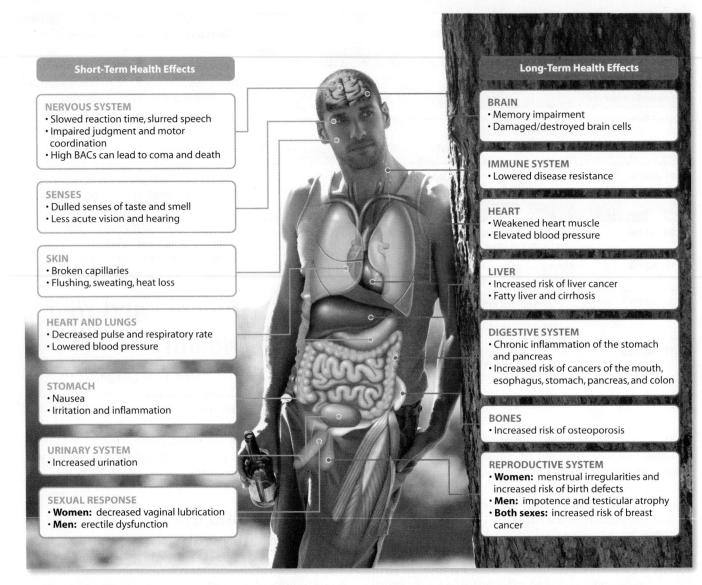

**Short-Term Health Effects**

**NERVOUS SYSTEM**
• Slowed reaction time, slurred speech
• Impaired judgment and motor coordination
• High BACs can lead to coma and death

**SENSES**
• Dulled senses of taste and smell
• Less acute vision and hearing

**SKIN**
• Broken capillaries
• Flushing, sweating, heat loss

**HEART AND LUNGS**
• Decreased pulse and respiratory rate
• Lowered blood pressure

**STOMACH**
• Nausea
• Irritation and inflammation

**URINARY SYSTEM**
• Increased urination

**SEXUAL RESPONSE**
• **Women:** decreased vaginal lubrication
• **Men:** erectile dysfunction

**Long-Term Health Effects**

**BRAIN**
• Memory impairment
• Damaged/destroyed brain cells

**IMMUNE SYSTEM**
• Lowered disease resistance

**HEART**
• Weakened heart muscle
• Elevated blood pressure

**LIVER**
• Increased risk of liver cancer
• Fatty liver and cirrhosis

**DIGESTIVE SYSTEM**
• Chronic inflammation of the stomach and pancreas
• Increased risk of cancers of the mouth, esophagus, stomach, pancreas, and colon

**BONES**
• Increased risk of osteoporosis

**REPRODUCTIVE SYSTEM**
• **Women:** menstrual irregularities and increased risk of birth defects
• **Men:** impotence and testicular atrophy
• **Both sexes:** increased risk of breast cancer

FIGURE 11.6 **Effects of Alcohol on the Body and Health**

Alcohol depresses CNS functions, which decreases respiratory rate, pulse rate, and blood pressure. As CNS depression deepens, vital functions become noticeably affected. In extreme cases, coma and death can result.

Alcohol is a diuretic that causes increased urinary output. Although this effect might be expected to lead to automatic **dehydration** (loss of water), the body actually retains water, most of it in the muscles or in cerebral tissues. This is because water is usually pulled out of the **cerebrospinal fluid** (fluid within the brain and spinal cord), leading to what is known as *mitochondrial dehydration* at the cellular level within the nervous system. Mitochondria are *organelles* within cells that are responsible for cell respiration, and they rely heavily

on fluid balance. When mitochondrial dehydration occurs, the mitochondria cannot carry out their normal functions. This results in symptoms that include the "morning-after" headaches suffered by some drinkers.

Alcohol irritates the gastrointestinal system and may cause indigestion and heartburn if consumed on an empty stomach. In addition, people who engage in brief drinking sprees during which they consume unusually high amounts of alcohol put themselves at risk for irregular heartbeat or even total loss of heart rhythm, which can disrupt blood flow and damage the heart muscle.

**Hangover** A **hangover** is often experienced the morning after a drinking spree. Its symptoms are familiar to most people who drink: headache, muscle aches, upset stomach, anxiety, depression, diarrhea, and thirst. **Congeners,** forms of alcohol that are metabolized more slowly than ethanol and are more toxic, are thought to play a role in the development of a

**dehydration** Loss of fluids from body tissues.
**cerebrospinal fluid** Fluid within and surrounding the brain and spinal cord tissues.
**hangover** The physiological reaction to excessive drinking, including headache, upset stomach, anxiety, depression, diarrhea, and thirst.
**congeners** Forms of alcohol that are metabolized more slowly than ethanol and produce toxic by-products.

# Women and Alcohol

Body fat is not the only contributor to the differences in alcohol's effects on men and women. Compared with men, women have half as much *alcohol dehydrogenase,* the enzyme that breaks down alcohol in the stomach before it reaches the bloodstream and the brain. Therefore, if a man and a woman drink the same amount of alcohol, the woman's blood alcohol concentration (BAC) will be approximately 30 percent higher than the man's, leaving her more vulnerable to slurred speech, careless driving, and other drinking-related impairments.

Cosmopolitans and other drinks popular among women may be sweet and fruity, but the alcohol in them still packs a punch.

Hormonal differences can also affect a woman's BAC. Certain times in the menstrual cycle and the use of oral contraceptives are likely to contribute to longer periods of intoxication. This prolonged peak appears to be related to a woman's estrogen levels.

Women who consume alcohol need to pay close attention to how much they drink. A woman matching her male friend drink for drink could become twice as intoxicated. For example, if a 180-pound college-aged man and a 120-pound college-aged woman each have three drinks within 1 hour, the BAC for the male would be 0.06 percent and for the female 0.11 percent, almost double that of her male friend.

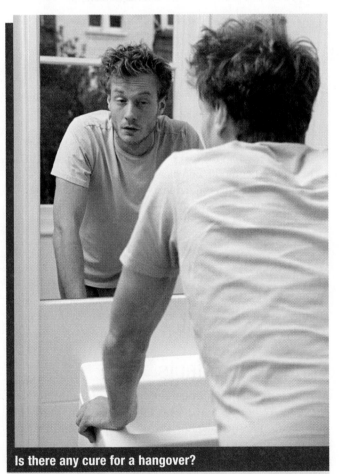

**Is there any cure for a hangover?**

There is no cure for a hangover. Bed rest, solid food, and aspirin may help relieve some of its discomforts—nausea, headache, and thirst—but the only cure for a hangover is abstaining from excessive alcohol use in the first place.

hangover. The body metabolizes the congeners after the ethanol is gone from the system, and their toxic by-products may contribute to the hangover. As previously noted, alcohol also upsets the water balance in the body, resulting in several hangover symptoms, including excess urination, dehydration, and thirst the next day. Increased production of hydrochloric acid can irritate the stomach lining and cause nausea. Recovery from a hangover usually takes 12 hours; once you have consumed enough alcohol to cause a hangover, time is the only cure. Drinking less and drinking slowly, and consuming water or other nonalcoholic beverages between drinks, will also help prevent hangover.

## "Why Should I Care?"

Going drinking with your buddies may be fun at the time, but excessive alcohol consumption can result in a hangover that impairs your functioning the day after you overindulge. Feeling sick with a hangover can lead you to skip class and to miss out on other activities you had planned for the day after drinking.

**Alcohol and Injuries** Alcohol use plays a significant role in the types of injuries people experience. Annually, nearly 524,000 emergency room visits in the United States result from alcohol use alone.[27] Thirteen percent of emergency room visits by undergraduates are related to alcohol; of this total, 34 percent are the result of acute intoxication.[28] A study found that injured patients with a BAC over 0.08 percent who were treated in emergency rooms were 3.2 times more likely to have a violent intentional injury than an unintentional injury.[29] Most people admitted to emergency rooms are men 21 years or older, mostly as the result of accidents or fights in which alcohol was involved.[30] Alcohol use is involved in up to half of fatal injuries during leisure activities such as swimming and boating, and 40 percent of fatal injuries due to house fires.[31] Alcohol use is also a key factor in many suicides and rapes. About two-thirds of all completed suicides involve alcohol and over 30 percent of rape victims reported that their assailant was under the influence of alcohol.[32]

**Alcohol and Sexual Decision Making** Alcohol has a clear influence on one's ability to make good decisions about sex, because it lowers inhibitions, and you may do things you might not do when sober. People who are intoxicated are less likely to use safer sex practices and are more likely to engage in high-risk sexual activity. The chance of acquiring a sexually transmitted infection or an unplanned pregnancy also increases among people who drink more heavily, compared with those who drink moderately or not at all.

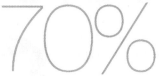 **70%** of college students admit to having engaged in sexual activity primarily as a result of being under the influence of alcohol.

**Alcohol Poisoning** **Alcohol poisoning** (also known as *acute alcohol intoxication*) occurs much more frequently than people realize, and all too often it can be fatal. Drinking large amounts of alcohol in a short period of time can cause the blood alcohol level to quickly reach the lethal range. Alcohol, used either alone or in combination with other drugs, is responsible for more toxic overdose deaths than any other substance.

> **alcohol poisoning** A potentially lethal blood alcohol concentration that inhibits the brain's ability to control consciousness, respiration, and heart rate; usually occurs as a result of drinking a large amount of alcohol in a short period of time. Also known as *acute alcohol intoxication*.

The amount of alcohol that causes a person to lose consciousness is dangerously close to the lethal dose. Death from alcohol poisoning can be caused by either CNS and respiratory depression, or by the inhalation of vomit or fluid into the lungs. Alcohol depresses the nerves that control involuntary actions such as breathing and the gag reflex (which prevents choking). As BAC levels reach higher concentrations, eventually these functions can be completely suppressed. If a drinker becomes unconscious and vomits, there is a danger of asphyxiation, through choking to death on one's own vomit. It is important to realize that blood alcohol concentration can continue rising even after a drinker becomes unconscious, because alcohol in the stomach and intestine continues to empty into the bloodstream.

The **Skills for Behavior Change** box at right describes the signs of alcohol poisoning. If you are with someone who has been drinking heavily and who exhibits these symptoms, or if you

 ## Dealing with an Alcohol Emergency

Being very drunk can be life threatening. People who have passed out from drinking should be watched very closely. If you think someone has alcohol poisoning, call 9-1-1 to get help. Do not take friends who have passed out to their beds and leave them to sleep it off.

Know and recognize the signs of acute alcohol intoxication:

✳ Mental confusion, stupor, or coma, or the person cannot be roused
✳ Vomiting
✳ Seizures
✳ Slow breathing (fewer than eight breaths per minute)
✳ Rapid or irregular pulse (100 beats or more per minute)
✳ Irregular breathing (10 seconds or more between breaths)
✳ Cool, clammy, bluish skin color, paleness
✳ Bluish fingernails or lips.

If you suspect someone has alcohol poisoning:

✳ Do not wait for all the signs to be present.
✳ Be aware that the person passed out could die.
✳ If there is any suspicion of an alcohol overdose, call 9-1-1 for help. Don't try to guess the level of someone's intoxication.
✳ Roll an unconscious drinker onto his side with knees up to minimize the chance of vomit obstructing the airway.
✳ If the drinker vomits, make certain her head is positioned lower than the rest of the body. You may need to reach into her mouth and clear the airway.
✳ Try to determine if the drinker has taken any medications or drugs that may interact with alcohol.
✳ Stay with the drinker until medical help arrives.

are unsure about the person's condition, call your local emergency number (9-1-1 in most areas) for immediate assistance.

# Long-Term Effects

Alcohol is distributed throughout most of the body and may affect many organs and tissues. Problems associated with long-term, habitual alcohol abuse include diseases of the nervous system, cardiovascular system, and liver, as well as some cancers.

**Effects on the Nervous System** The nervous system is especially sensitive to alcohol. Even people who drink moderately experience shrinkage in brain size and weight and a loss of some degree of intellectual ability.

New research suggests that developing brains in adolescents are much more prone to damage than was previously thought. Alcohol appears to damage the frontal areas of the adolescent brain, which are crucial for controlling impulses and thinking through consequences of intended actions.[33] In addition, researchers suggest that people who begin drinking at an early age face enormous risks of becoming alcoholics: 47 percent of those who begin drinking alcohol before age 14 become alcohol dependent at some time in their lives, compared with 9 percent of those who wait until at least age 21.[34]

**Effects on the Cardiovascular System** Alcohol affects the cardiovascular system in many ways. Numerous studies have associated light-to-moderate alcohol consumption (no more than two drinks a day) with a reduced risk of coronary artery disease. Several mechanisms have been proposed to explain how this might happen. The strongest evidence favors an increase in high-density lipoprotein (HDL) cholesterol, which is known as "good" cholesterol. Another factor might be the *antithrombotic effect.* Alcohol consumption is associated with a decrease in clotting factors that contribute to the development of atherosclerosis. However, this does not mean that alcohol consumption is recommended as a preventive measure against heart disease—it causes many more cardiovascular health hazards than it does benefits. Alcohol contributes to high blood pressure and slightly increased heart rate and cardiac output.

**Liver Disease** One of the most common diseases related to alcohol abuse is **cirrhosis** of the liver (Figure 11.7). It is among the top ten causes of death in the United States. One result of heavy drinking is that the liver begins to store fat—a condition known as *fatty liver.* If there is insufficient time between drinking episodes, this fat cannot be transported to storage sites, and the fat-filled liver cells stop functioning. Continued drinking can cause a further stage of liver deterioration called *fibrosis,* in which the damaged area of the liver develops fibrous scar tissue. Cell function can be partially restored at this stage with proper nutrition and abstinence from alcohol. If the person continues to drink, however, cirrhosis results. At this point, the liver cells die and the damage becomes permanent. **Alcoholic hepatitis** is another serious condition resulting from prolonged alcohol use. A chronic inflammation of the liver develops, which may be fatal in itself or progress to cirrhosis.

**Cancer** Alcohol is considered a carcinogen. The repeated irritation caused by its long-term use has been linked to cancers of the esophagus, stomach, mouth, tongue, and liver. In one study, a team of scientists from the NIAAA discovered a possible link between acetaldehyde and DNA damage that could help explain the connection between drinking and certain types of cancer.[35]

There is substantial evidence that women consuming high levels of alcohol (more than three drinks per day) have a higher risk of breast cancer compared with abstainers.[36] Girls and young women who drink alcohol increase their risk of

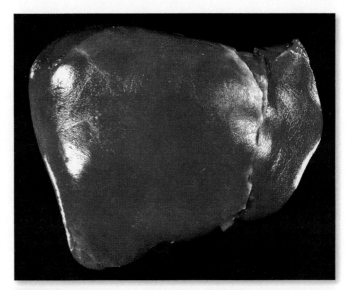

(a) A normal liver

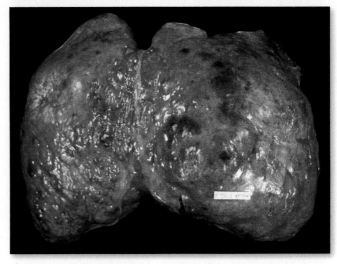

(b) A liver with cirrhosis

FIGURE 11.7 **Comparison of a Healthy Liver with a Cirrhotic Liver**

benign (noncancerous) breast disease. Benign breast disease increases the risk for developing breast cancer. In a recent study, girls and young women who drank 6 or 7 days a week were 5.5 times more likely to have benign breast disease than those who didn't drink or who had less than one drink per week. Those diagnosed with benign breast disease on average drank more often, drank more on each occasion, and had an average daily consumption that was two times that of those who did not have benign breast disease.[37]

**Other Effects** Alcohol abuse is a major cause of chronic inflammation of the pancreas, the organ that produces digestive enzymes and insulin. Chronic alcohol abuse

**cirrhosis** The last stage of liver disease associated with chronic heavy alcohol use, during which liver cells die and damage becomes permanent.
**alcoholic hepatitis** A condition resulting from prolonged use of alcohol in which the liver is inflamed; can be fatal.

inhibits enzyme production, which further inhibits the absorption of nutrients. Evidence also suggests that alcohol impairs the body's ability to recognize and fight foreign bodies such as bacteria and viruses.

Drinking alcohol can block the absorption of calcium, a nutrient that strengthens bones. This should be of particular concern to women because of their risk for osteoporosis; bone thinning and calcium loss increases with age. Heavy consumption of alcohol worsens this condition.

## Alcohol and Pregnancy

Recall from Chapter 6 that *teratogenic* substances cause birth defects. Of the 30 known teratogens in the environment, alcohol is one of the most dangerous and common. If a woman ingests alcohol while pregnant, it will pass through the placenta and enter the growing fetus's bloodstream. A recent study found that more than 12 percent of children have been exposed to alcohol *in utero* and 2 percent of pregnant women reported binge drinking.[38] Consuming four or more drinks a day during pregnancy may significantly increase the risk of childhood mental health and learning problems. However, any use can result in varying degrees of effects, ranging from mild learning disabilities to major physical, mental, and intellectual impairment. Alcohol consumed during the first trimester poses the greatest threat to organ development; exposure during the last trimester, when the brain is developing rapidly, is most likely to affect CNS development.

---

**fetal alcohol syndrome (FAS)** A disorder involving physical and mental impairment that may affect the fetus when the mother consumes alcohol during pregnancy.

---

A disorder called **fetal alcohol syndrome (FAS)** is associated with alcohol consumption during pregnancy. Fetal alcohol syndrome is the third most common birth defect and one of the leading causes of mental retardation in the United States, with an estimated incidence of 1 to 2 in every 1,000 live births.[39] It is the most common preventable cause of mental impairment in the Western world. Among the symptoms of FAS are mental retardation; small head; tremors; and abnormalities of the face, limbs, heart, and brain. Children with FAS may experience problems such as poor memory and impaired learning, reduced attention span, impulsive behavior, and poor problem-solving abilities, among others.

Some children may have fewer than the full physical or behavioral symptoms of FAS, and may be diagnosed with disorders such as partial fetal alcohol syndrome (PFAS) or alcohol-related neurodevelopmental dis-

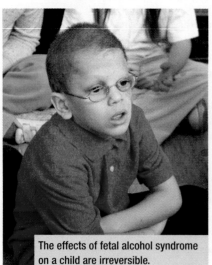

The effects of fetal alcohol syndrome on a child are irreversible.

order (ARND); all of these disorders (including FAS) fall under the umbrella term *fetal alcohol spectrum disorders* (FASD). An estimated 40,000 infants in the United States are affected by FASD each year—more than those affected by spina bifida, Down syndrome, and muscular dystrophy combined.[40] Infants whose mothers habitually consumed more than 3 ounces of alcohol (approximately six drinks) in a short time period when pregnant are at high risk for FASD. Risk levels for babies whose mothers consume smaller amounts are uncertain. To avoid any chance of harming her fetus, any woman of childbearing age who is or may become pregnant should not consume alcohol.

## Drinking and Driving

Traffic accidents are the leading cause of accidental death for all age groups from 5 to 65 years old.[41] Approximately 32 percent of all traffic fatalities in the United States in 2008—11,773 deaths—involved at least one alcohol-impaired driver (having a BAC of 0.08 percent or higher).[42] This number represents an average of one alcohol-related fatality approximately every 45 minutes. Unfortunately, college students are overrepresented in alcohol-related crashes. A recent survey reported that 25 percent of college students have driven after drinking alcohol and 3.7 percent of students said that, in the past 30 days, they had driven after drinking five or more drinks.[43]

Over the past 20 years, the percentage of drivers involved in fatal crashes who were intoxicated (BAC of 0.08 percent or greater) decreased for all age groups (Figure 11.8). Several factors probably contributed to these reductions in fatalities: laws that raised the drinking age to 21; stricter law enforcement; increased emphasis on zero tolerance (laws prohibiting

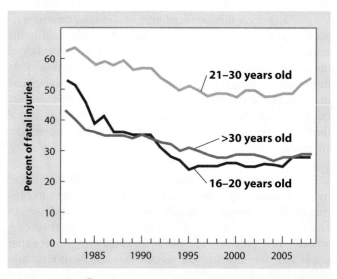

FIGURE 11.8 **Percentage of Fatally Injured Drivers with BACs > 0.08 Percent, by Driver Age, 1982–2008**

**Source:** Insurance Institute for Highway Safety: www.iihs.org, "Fatality Facts 2008: Alcohol," 2010. Used with permission.

# 3 in 10

**Americans will be involved in an alcohol-related accident at some time in their lives.**

anyone under 21 from driving with any detectable BAC); and educational programs designed to discourage drinking and driving. The legal limit for BAC in all states is 0.08 percent. Furthermore, all states have zero-tolerance laws for driving while intoxicated, and the penalty is usually suspension of the driver's license.[44]

Despite all these measures, the risk of being involved in an alcohol-related automobile crash remains substantial. Your ability to control a vehicle is affected when you consume even a small amount of alcohol. Among the predictable effects:[45]

● At 0.02 BAC: Your ability to control eye muscles and to perform two tasks at the same time declines.
● At 0.05 BAC: Your coordination, ability to track moving objects, to respond to emergency situations, and to steer declines.
● At 0.08 BAC: Your ability to concentrate, control speed, perceive traffic hazards, and recognize traffic signals and signs diminishes; your reaction time slows and you experience short-term memory loss.
● At 0.10 BAC: Your ability to maintain lane position and to brake diminishes.
● At 0.15 BAC: Your ability to process information from sight and hearing slows; you experience substantial impairment and the inability to control your vehicle.

Researchers have shown a direct relationship between the amount of alcohol in a driver's bloodstream and the likelihood of a crash. A driver with a BAC level of 0.10 percent is approximately ten times more likely to be involved in a car accident than a driver who has not been drinking.[46]

Alcohol-related fatal car crashes occur more often at night than during the day; the hours between midnight and 3 AM are the most dangerous. Seventy-five percent of fatally injured drivers involved in nighttime single-vehicle crashes had detectable levels

**What are the legal consequences if you are caught drinking and driving?**

Getting behind the wheel if you have consumed alcohol is a dangerous choice, with serious legal consequences if you are caught and convicted of driving under the influence (DUI). If you are under age 21 and have any detectable alcohol in your bloodstream, your license can be revoked. Other penalties for DUI often include restrictions of your driver's license, fines, mandatory counseling, and jail time, even for a first offense. In many states, if you are convicted three times for DUI, you are considered a habitual violator and penalized as a felon, meaning that you lose your right to vote and to own a weapon, among other rights, as well as possibly losing your license permanently. If you are involved in an accident in which someone is injured or killed, the consequences are even more serious. Involvement in such an incident is considered a felony in many states. If a person dies as a result of the accident, the drunk driver may be charged with manslaughter or second-degree murder.

of alcohol in their blood.[47] The risk of being involved in an alcohol-related crash increases not only with the time of day, but also with the day of the week. In 2008, 25 percent of all fatal crashes during the week were alcohol related, compared with 49 percent on weekends.[48] For a driver with a BAC of 0.15 percent on weekend nights, the likelihood of dying in a single-vehicle crash is more than 382 times higher than for a nondrinker.

# Alcohol Abuse and Alcoholism

Alcohol use becomes **alcohol abuse** when it interferes with work, school, or social and family relationships or when it entails any violation of the law, including driving under the influence (DUI). **Alcoholism,** or **alcohol dependency,** results when personal and health problems related to alcohol use are severe, and stopping alcohol use causes withdrawal symptoms.

**alcohol abuse** Use of alcohol that interferes with work, school, or personal relationships or that entails violations of the law.
**alcoholism (alcohol dependency)** Condition in which personal and health problems related to alcohol use are severe and stopping alcohol use results in withdrawal symptoms.

## what do you think?

What do you think the legal BAC for drivers should be? ● What should the penalty be for people arrested for driving under the influence of alcohol for the first offense? ● The second offense? ● The third offense?

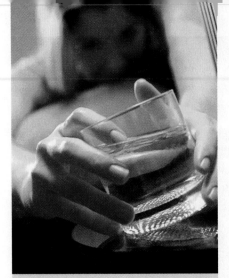

Drinking alone or in secret and using alcohol to cope with stress and emotional problems are all potential signs of alcohol dependency.

# Identifying a Problem Drinker

As with other drug addictions, tolerance, psychological dependence, and withdrawal symptoms must be present to qualify a drinker as an addict (see Chapter 10). Irresponsible and problem drinkers, such as people who get into fights or embarrass themselves or others when they drink, are not necessarily alcoholics. Alcoholics can be found at all socioeconomic levels and in all professions, ethnic groups, geographical locations, religions, and races. Data indicate that about 15 percent of people in the United States are problem drinkers, and about 5 to 10 percent of male drinkers and 3 to 5 percent of females would be diagnosed as alcohol dependent.[49]

Recognizing and admitting the existence of an alcohol problem is often extremely difficult. Alcoholics deny their problem, often making statements such as, "I can stop any time I want to. I just don't want to right now." Their families also tend to deny the problem, saying things like, "He really has been under a lot of stress lately. Besides, he only drinks beer." The fear of being labeled a "problem drinker" often prevents people from seeking help.

Alcoholism is characterized by several symptoms, including craving, loss of control, physical dependence, and tolerance. People who recognize one or more of these behaviors in themselves may wish to seek professional help to determine whether alcohol has become a controlling factor in their lives.

## How to Cut Down on Your Drinking

If you suspect that you drink too much, talk with a counselor or a clinician at your student health center to be sure. Either of these professionals can tell you whether you should cut down or abstain. If you have a severe drinking problem, alcoholism in your family, or other medical problems, you should stop drinking completely. Your counselor or clinician will advise you about what is right for you.

If you need to cut down on your drinking, these steps can help you:

* **Write your reasons for cutting down or stopping.** There are many reasons you may want to cut down or stop drinking. You may want to improve your health, sleep better, or get along better with your family or friends.
* **Set a drinking goal.** Determine a limit for how much you will drink. You may choose to cut down or to not drink at all. If you aren't sure what goal is right for you, talk with your counselor. Once you determine your goal, write it down on a piece of paper. Put it where you can see it, such as on your refrigerator or bathroom mirror.
* **Keep a diary of your drinking.** For 1 week, write down every time you have a drink. Try to keep your diary for 3 or 4 weeks. This will show you how much you drink and when. You may be surprised. How different is your goal from the amount you drink now?
* **Keep little or no alcohol at home.** You don't need the temptation.
* **Drink slowly.** When you drink, sip slowly. Take a break of 1 hour between drinks. Drink a nonalcoholic beverage, such as soda, water, or juice, after every alcoholic drink you consume. Do not drink on an empty stomach! Eat food when you are drinking.
* **Take a break from alcohol.** Pick a day or two each week when you will not drink at all. Then try to stop drinking for 1 week. Think about how you feel physically and emotionally on these days. When you succeed and feel better, you may find it easier to cut down for good.
* **Learn how to say no.** You do not have to drink when other people are, or take a drink when offered one. Practice ways to say no politely. Stay away from people who give you a hard time about not drinking.
* **Stay active.** Use the time and money once spent on drinking to do something fun with your family or friends. Go out to eat, see a movie, or play sports or a game.
* **Get support.** Cutting down on your drinking may be difficult at times. Ask your family and friends for support to help you reach your goal. Talk to your counselor if you are having trouble cutting down. Get the help you need to reach your goal.
* **Avoid temptations.** Watch out for people, places, or times that make you drink, even if you do not want to. Plan ahead of time what you will do to avoid drinking when you are tempted. Do not drink when you are angry, upset, or having a bad day.
* **Remember, don't give up!** Most people don't cut down or give up drinking all at once. Just like a diet, it is not easy to change. That's OK. If you don't reach your goal the first time, try again. Remember, get support from people who care about you and want to help.

The **Skills for Behavior Change** box above gives some common tips for cutting down on drinking, but it is recommended that people wishing to address their problem-drinking habits seek the advice of a professional substance abuse counselor.

One study has shown that 19 percent of college students meet the criteria for a diagnosis of alcohol abuse or dependence (alcoholism).[50] Despite the prevalence of alcohol disorders on campus, only 5 percent of these students sought treatment a year prior to the study and 3 percent thought they should seek help, but did not. The heaviest drinkers are the least likely to seek treatment, yet they experience and are responsible for the most alcohol-related problems on campus.[51]

## Alcohol and Prescription Drug Abuse

Recent studies have shown that men and women with alcohol use disorders are 18 times more likely to report nonmedical use of prescription drugs than people who do not drink at all.[52] Young adults aged 18 to 24 are at most risk for concurrent or simultaneous abuse of both alcohol and drugs. In a study of college students, it was revealed that in the past year, 12 percent had used both alcohol and prescription drugs nonmedically but at different times, and 7 percent had taken them simultaneously.[53] Students who took prescription drugs while drinking were more likely than those who drank without taking drugs to black out, vomit, and engage in other risky behaviors such as drunk driving and unplanned sex. The prescription drugs that are most commonly combined with alcohol include opioids (e.g., Vicodin, Oxy-Contin, Percocet), stimulants (e.g., Ritalin, Adderall, Concerta), sedative/anxiety medications (e.g., Ativan, Xanax), and sleeping medications (e.g., Ambien, Halcion).

## The Causes of Alcohol Abuse and Alcoholism

We know that alcoholism is a disease with biological, social, and environmental components, but we do not yet know what role each component plays in the disease.

**Biological and Family Factors** Everyone with a family history of alcoholism is at risk for developing alcohol abuse disorders. The development of alcoholism among individuals with a family history of alcoholism is about four to eight times more common than it is among individuals with no such family history.[54] Research into the hereditary and environmental causes of alcoholism has found higher rates of alcoholism among children of alcoholics than in the general population.[55]

Despite evidence of heredity's role in alcoholism, scientists do not yet understand the precise role of genes and increased risk for alcoholism, nor have they identified a specific "alco-

## 1 in 4

**Americans is affected by the alcoholism of a friend or family member.**

**"Why Should I Care?"**

Alcohol is not just a beverage—it's a drug that can interact with other drugs you may be using. When alcohol and prescription drugs are taken together, severe medical problems can result, including alcohol poisoning, unconsciousness, respiratory depression, and death.

holism" gene. Adoption studies demonstrate a strong link between biological parents' substance use and their children's risk for addiction.[56] However, there is nothing deterministic about the genetic basis to addiction. No single gene causes addiction, but multiple genes can affect the ability to develop addiction.[57]

**Social and Cultural Factors** Social and cultural factors may trigger the affliction for many people who are not genetically predisposed to alcoholism. Some people begin drinking as a way to dull the pain of an acute loss or an emotional or social problem. For example, college students may drink to escape the stress of college life; disappointment over unfulfilled expectations; difficulties in forming relationships; or loss of the security of home, loved ones, and close friends. Involvement in a painful relationship, death of a family member, and other problems may trigger a search for an anesthetic. Unfortunately, the emotional discomfort that causes many people to turn to alcohol also ultimately causes them to become even more uncomfortable as the drug's depressant effect begins taking its toll. Thus, the person who is already depressed may become even more depressed, antagonizing friends and other social supports. Eventually, the drinker becomes physically dependent on the drug.

Family attitudes toward alcohol also seem to influence whether a person will develop a drinking problem. It has been clearly demonstrated that people who are raised in cultures in which drinking is a part of religious or ceremonial activities or in which alcohol is a traditional part of the family meal are less prone to alcohol dependence. In contrast, in societies in which alcohol purchase is carefully controlled and drinking is regarded as a rite of passage to adulthood, the tendency for abuse appears to be greater. Apparently, then, some combination of heredity and environment plays a decisive role in the development of alcoholism. The **Health in a Diverse World** box on page 366 discusses some of the patterns of alcohol use and abuse among different racial and ethnic groups in the United States.

The amount of alcohol a person consumes seems to be directly related to the drinking habits of that individual's social group. A recent study found that those whose friends and relatives drank heavily were 50 percent more likely to drink heavily themselves.[58] Moreover, even having friends of friends who drank heavily appeared to influence individual alcohol consumption. The opposite is also true, that people who were friends with abstinent individuals or had family members who were abstinent were less likely to drink themselves. This finding has increased importance for individuals who are in treatment or have been in treatment and their need to sever ties with heavy drinkers to successfully maintain their abstinence.

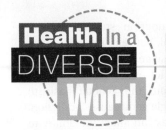
# Alcohol and Ethnic or Racial Differences

Different ethnic and racial minority groups have their own patterns of alcohol consumption and abuse. Social or cultural factors, such as drinking norms and attitudes and, in some cases, genetic factors, may account for those differences. Better understanding of ethnic and racial differences in alcohol-use patterns and factors that influence alcohol use can help guide the development of culturally appropriate prevention and treatment programs.

Among Native American populations, alcohol is the most widely used drug; the rate of alcoholism in this population is two to three times higher than the national average, and the death rate from alcohol-related causes is eight times higher than the national average. Poor economic conditions and the cultural belief that alcoholism is a spiritual problem, not a physical disease, may partially account for high rates of alcoholism in this group.

African American and Latino populations also exhibit distinct patterns of abuse. On average, African Americans drink less than white Americans; however, those who do drink tend to be heavy drinkers. Among Latino populations, men have a higher than average rate of alcohol abuse and alcohol-related health problems. In contrast, many Latinas abstain. Many researchers agree

that a major factor for alcohol problems in this ethnic group is the key role that drinking plays in Latino culture.

Asian Americans have a very low rate of alcoholism. Social and cultural influences, such as strong kinship ties, are thought to discourage heavy drinking in Asian groups. Asians also have a genetic predisposition that might influence their low risk for alcohol abuse: Many possess a variant of the gene coding the enzyme aldehyde dehydrogenase, which plays a key role in the metabolism of alcohol. People with this variant gene experience unpleasant side effects from consuming alcohol, making drinking a less pleasurable experience. Because of

the presence of this gene, Asian populations tend to consume less alcohol and have lower rates of alcoholism than do other ethnic groups.

**Sources:** Substance Abuse and Mental Health Services Administration, "Results from the 2008 National Survey on Drug Use and Health: National Findings," NSDUH Series H-36, DHHS Publication no. SMA 09-4434 (Rockville, MD: Office of Applied Studies, U.S. Department of Health and Human Services, 2009), Available at www.oas.samhsa.gov/nsduh/2k8nsduh/2k8Results.cfm; F. H. Galvan et al., "Alcohol Use and Related Problems among Ethnic Minorities in the United States," *Alcohol and Health Research* 27, no. 1 (2003): 87–94; T. Wall and C. Ehlers, "Genetic Influences Affecting Alcohol Use among Asians," *Alcohol Health and Research World* 19, no. 3 (1995): 184–89.

### Prevalence of Heavy Alcohol Use* by Ethnicity

| Ethnic Group | Percent of Total Population |
| --- | --- |
| Whites | 7.7 |
| African Americans | 5.6 |
| Latino | 5.7 |
| Native Americans/Alaska Natives | 5.7 |
| Asian Americans | 4.7 |
| Persons reporting two or more races | 7.4 |

*"Heavy alcohol use" is defined by the Substance Abuse and Mental Health Services Administration as five or more drinks on at least 5 days within the past month.

# Effects of Alcoholism on Family and Friends

Alcohol abusers and alcoholics hurt more than just themselves. Alcohol abuse and alcoholism can have a tremendous impact on the abuser's family and friends. Everyone close to the addicted person suffers and becomes a part of the dynamics of addiction. Alcoholism is a family disease, and friends, members of a fraternity or sorority, a residence hall floor, and roommates can all be considered a family.

Only recently have people begun to recognize that the alcoholic's entire family can suffer alongside the alcoholic. Although most research focuses on family effects during the

late stages of alcoholism, the family unit actually begins to react early on as the person starts showing symptoms of the disease.

There are an estimated 27.8 million children in the United States affected or exposed to a family alcohol problem. These children are at increased risk for a range of problems, including physical illness, emotional disturbances, behavioral problems, lower educational performance, and susceptibility to alcoholism or other addictions later in life.[59]

In dysfunctional families, children learn certain rules from an early age: Don't talk, don't trust, and don't feel. These unspoken rules allow the family to avoid dealing with real problems and issues as family members unconsciously adapt to the alcoholic's behavior by adjusting their own behavior.

Unfortunately, these behaviors enable the alcoholic to keep drinking. Children in such dysfunctional families generally assume at least one of the following roles:

- **Family hero.** Tries to divert attention from the problem by being too good to be true
- **Scapegoat.** Draws attention away from the family's primary problem through delinquency or misbehavior
- **Lost child.** Becomes passive and quietly withdraws from upsetting situations
- **Mascot.** Disrupts tense situations by providing comic relief

For children in alcoholic homes, life is a struggle. They have to deal with constant stress, anxiety, and embarrassment. Because the alcoholic is the center of attention, the children's wants and needs are often ignored. It is not uncommon for these children to be victims of violence, abuse, neglect, or incest. As we have discussed, when such children grow up, they are much more prone to alcoholic behaviors than are children from nonalcoholic families.

Living with a family member (or friend or roommate) who is an alcoholic can be extremely stressful. As discussed in Chapter 10, people around addicts can find themselves in codependent relationships that enable the alcoholic's addiction. Codependency often affects a spouse, sibling, friend, roommate, or coworker. Codependent relationships can be emotionally destructive or abusive. Characteristics of codependent people include an exaggerated sense of responsibility for the actions of others; a tendency to do more than their

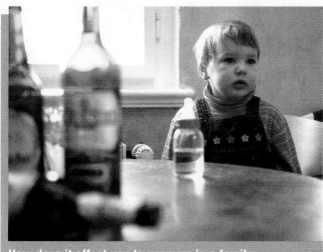

**How does it affect you to grow up in a family with alcoholism?**

Adult children of alcoholics have unique problems stemming from a lack of parental nurturing during childhood: difficulty in developing social attachments, a need to be in control of all emotions and situations, low self-esteem, and depression. Fortunately, not everyone who grows up in an alcoholic family is doomed to have lifelong problems. As they mature, many of them develop resiliency in response to their families' problems. Thus, they enter adulthood armed with positive strengths and valuable career-oriented skills, such as the ability to assume responsibility, strong organizational skills, and realistic expectations of their jobs and others.

share all of the time; and an extreme need for approval and recognition. Codependents try to cover up for the alcoholic: They may take notes in classes, phone a professor to say their friend is sick and can't take an exam, make excuses for the drinker's behavior, or lie to cover for the alcoholic. Eventually, the codependent needs to recognize what that behavior is doing and stop it if she or he is to help the alcoholic move toward recovery. For more information on how addiction can affect families and friends, see Chapter 10.

# Costs to Society

Alcohol-related costs to society are estimated to be well over $185 billion when health insurance, criminal justice costs, treatment costs, and lost productivity are factored in.[60] Reportedly, alcoholism is directly or indirectly responsible for over 25 percent of the nation's medical expenses and lost earnings.[61]

**Workplace Prevalence of Alcohol Dependence and Abuse** Most people with alcohol problems are employed. In fact, employed adults have a 27 percent greater risk of having an alcohol problem compared to adults not in the workforce. Among adults who are currently dependent on alcohol, 75 percent work full-time and 16 percent work part-time.[62] Rates of alcohol problems vary greatly from industry to industry (see Table 11.1).[63] It is estimated that alcohol problems contribute to 500 million lost workdays annually.

| TABLE 11.1 | Prevalence of Alcohol Problems by Industry Sector (%) |
|---|---|
| Industry Sector | Overall Prevalence |
| Leisure, hospitality, arts | 15.0 |
| Construction and mining | 14.7 |
| Wholesale trade | 11.9 |
| Professional | 10.6 |
| Retail trade | 9.7 |
| Finance and real estate | 9.2 |
| Manufacturing | 8.6 |
| Transportation and utilities | 8.2 |
| Information and communication | 8.1 |
| Agriculture, forestry, fishing, and hunting | 7.2 |
| Other services | 6.4 |
| Education, health, and social services | 5.4 |
| Public administration | 5.3 |

**Source:** Adapted from Ensuring Solutions to Alcohol Problems, *Workplace Screening and Brief Intervention: What Employers Can and Should Do about Excessive Alcohol Use* (Washington, DC: George Washington University Medical Center, 2008), 5. Used with permission.

### The Cost of Underage Drinking

A recent study estimated that underage drinking costs society $61.9 billion annually.[64] These costs take into consideration crashes, violence, property crime, suicide, burns, drowning, fetal alcohol syndrome, high-risk sex, poisoning, psychosis, and treatment for alcohol dependence. The largest costs were related to violence ($34.7 billion) and drunk driving accidents ($13.5 billion), followed by high-risk sex (nearly $5 billion), property crime ($3 billion), and addiction treatment programs (nearly $2 billion). By dividing the cost of underage drinking by the estimated number of underage drinkers, the study estimated that every underage drinker costs society an average of $4,680 a year.[65]

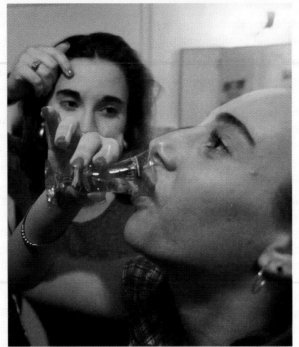

As rates of drinking by women rise, the number of female alcoholics is likely to increase as well.

## Women and Alcoholism

**intervention** A planned confrontation with an alcoholic in which family members, friends, and professional counselors express their concern about the alcoholic's drinking.

Women are the fastest growing population of alcohol abusers. Studies indicate that there are now almost as many female as male alcoholics. Women tend to become alcoholic at a later age and after fewer years of heavy drinking than do male alcoholics. Women get addicted faster with less alcohol use and then suffer the consequences more profoundly. Women alcoholics have death rates 50 to 100 percent higher than male alcoholics, including deaths from suicide, alcohol-related accidents, heart disease and stroke, and cirrhosis.[66]

Women at highest risk are those who are unmarried but living with a partner, are in their twenties or early thirties, or have a husband or partner who drinks heavily. Other risk factors for drinking problems among *all women* include a family history of drinking problems, pressure to drink from a peer or spouse, depression, and stress.

It is estimated that only 14 percent of women who need treatment for alcohol dependency get it.[67] In one study, women cited the following reasons for not seeking treatment: potential loss of income, not wanting others to know they may have a problem, inability to pay for treatment, and fear that treatment would not be confidential.[68]

### what do you think?

Why do you think women appear to be drinking more heavily today than they did in the past? ● Does society look at men's and women's drinking habits in the same way? ● Can you think of ways to increase support for women in their recovery process?

# Treatment and Recovery

Despite growing recognition of our national alcohol problem, only 15 percent of alcoholics in the United States receive any care.[69] Factors contributing to this low figure include inability or unwillingness to admit to an alcohol problem; the social stigma attached to alcoholism; breakdowns in referral and delivery systems (failure of physicians or psychotherapists to follow through with recommended treatments, or failure of rehabilitation facilities to give quality care); and failure of the medical establishment to recognize and diagnose alcoholic symptoms among patients.

Most problem drinkers who seek help have experienced a turning point; for example, a spouse walks out, taking children and possessions; or the boss issues an ultimatum to dry out or ship out. Devoid of hope, physically depleted, and spiritually despairing, the alcoholic finally recognizes that alcohol controls his or her life. The first steps on the road to recovery are to regain that control and assume responsibility for personal actions.

## The Family's Role in Recovery

Members of an alcoholic's family sometimes take action before the alcoholic does. An effective method of helping an alcoholic to confront the disease is a process called **intervention.** Essentially, this is a planned confrontation with the alcoholic that involves family members and friends plus professional counselors. See Chapter 10 for more on intervention, and see the Skills for Behavior Change box at right for additional guidelines.

## Treatment Programs

The alcoholic who is ready for help has several avenues of treatment: psychologists and psychiatrists specializing in the treatment of alcoholism, private treatment centers, hospitals specifically designed to treat alcoholics, community mental health facilities, and support groups.

**Private Treatment Facilities** Private treatment facilities have made concerted efforts to attract patients through radio and television advertising. On admission, the patient receives a complete physical exam to determine whether underlying medical problems will interfere with treatment.

## Talking about Alcohol Use

Are you worried that a friend or relative might have an alcohol problem? Ask yourself:

## HOW DOES IT AFFECT YOU?

Have you ever . . .

* Lost time from classes, studying, or a job because of this person's drinking?
* Felt embarrassed or hurt by something that person said or did while intoxicated?
* Had to take care of that person because of his alcohol use?

## HOW DOES IT AFFECT THEM?

Does this person . . .

* Drink to get drunk?
* Do dangerous things because of alcohol?
* Drink to steady her nerves or get rid of a hangover?
* Get into trouble because of drinking?
* Drink to cope with problems or stress?

The more questions you answer yes to, the more likely it is that there is a problem.

## HOW TO TALK TO YOUR FRIEND

* Talk to the person when she is sober. The sooner you can arrange this after a bad episode, the better.
* Restrict your comments to what you have experienced of the person's behavior.
* Be specific: "Our relationship means a lot to me. I don't like to see what's been happening."
* Openly discuss the negative consequences of your friend or family member's drinking. Use concrete examples.
* Emphasize the difference between sober behavior that you like and drinking behavior that you dislike: "You have the most wonderful sense of humor, but when you drink, it turns into cruel sarcasm."
* Distinguish between the person and the behavior: "I think you're a great person, but the more you drink, the less you seem to care about anything."
* Encourage your friend or family member to consult a professional. Offer to go with him.

## WHAT NOT TO DO

* Don't accuse or argue.
* Don't lecture or moralize. Remain factual and listen.
* Don't give up. Make it clear you're available to talk.

Alcoholics who quit drinking will experience *detoxification,* the process by which addicts end their dependence on a drug. Withdrawal symptoms include hyperexcitability, confusion and agitation, sleep disorders, convulsions, tremors, depression, headaches, and seizures. For a small percentage of people, alcohol withdrawal results in a severe syndrome known as **delirium tremens (DTs),** which is characterized by confusion, delusions, agitated behavior, and hallucinations.

**delirium tremens (DTs)** A state of confusion brought on by withdrawal from alcohol; symptoms include hallucinations, anxiety, and trembling.

Shortly after detoxification, alcoholics begin their treatment for psychological addiction. Most treatment facilities keep their patients from 3 to 6 weeks. Treatment at private treatment centers costs several thousand dollars, but some insurance programs or employers will assume most of this expense.

**Therapy** Several types of therapy, including family therapy, individual therapy, and group therapy, are commonly used in alcoholism recovery programs. In family therapy, the person and family members gradually examine the psychological reasons underlying the addiction. In individual and group therapy with fellow addicts, alcoholics learn positive coping skills for situations that have regularly caused them to turn to alcohol.

On some college campuses, the problems associated with alcohol abuse are so great that student health centers are opening their own treatment programs. For example, the University of Texas offers a new support service called Complete Recovery 101, and at other schools, students in recovery live together in special housing. Programs such as these hope to provide the support and comfortable environment recovering students need.

**Pharmacological Treatment** Disulfiram (trade name Antabuse) is a drug commonly used for treating alcoholism. It is given to deter drinking, as it causes an individual to become acutely ill when he or she consumes alcohol. Disulfiram inhibits the breakdown of acetaldehyde from the liver. If individuals taking this drug drink alcohol or consume any foods with alcohol content, acetaldehyde will build up in the liver and cause nausea and vomiting. Other unpleasant effects, such as headache, bad breath, drowsiness, and temporary impotence, discourage drinking. Because disulfiram does not reduce the cravings for alcohol, this treatment works best with ongoing psychotherapy and support groups.

Naltrexone is another pharmaceutical used to reduce the craving for alcohol and decrease the pleasant reinforcing effects of alcohol without making the user ill. It also works most effectively with counseling and other forms of psychotherapy. The most recent pharmaceutical treatment for alcoholism approved by the U.S. Food and Drug Administration (FDA) is acamprosate (Campral). Acamprosate is thought to restore normal brain balance, which has been disturbed in someone who is alcohol dependent. It also helps reduce the physical distress and emotional discomfort associated with someone staying alcohol free. As with other pharmacological treatments for alcoholism, acamprosate should be used in conjunction with psychotherapy and support groups.

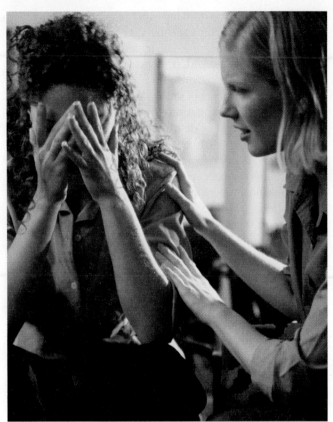
Most alcohol-dependent people need the help of others during their recovery, whether through support groups, family therapy, or group therapy.

**Group Support Treatments** Alcoholics Anonymous (AA) is a private, nonprofit, self-help organization founded in 1935. The organization, which relies on group support to help people stop drinking, currently has branches all over the world and more than 1 million members. At meetings, last names are never used, and no one is forced to speak. Members are taught that their alcoholism is a lifetime problem and that they cannot drink alcohol again. They share their struggles with one another and talk about the devastating effects alcoholism has had on their personal and professional lives. All members are asked to place their faith and control of the habit into the hands of a "higher power." The road to recovery is taken one step at a time. Alcoholics Anonymous offers specialized meetings for Spanish speakers, gays, atheists, people with HIV, and a variety of other people with alcohol problems.

Alcoholics Anonymous also has auxiliary groups to help spouses or partners, friends, and children of alcoholics. *Al-Anon* is the group dedicated to helping adult relatives and friends of alcoholics understand the disease and how they can contribute to the recovery process.

**Alcoholics Anonymous (AA)** An organization whose goal is to help alcoholics stop drinking; includes auxiliary branches such as Al-Anon and Alateen.

*Alateen,* another AA-related organization, helps adolescents living with alcoholic parents. They are taught that they are not at fault for their parents' problems. They develop their self-esteem to overcome their guilt and function better socially.

Other self-help groups include Women for Sobriety and Secular Organizations for Sobriety (SOS). Women for Sobriety addresses the differing needs of female alcoholics, who often have more severe problems than males. Unlike AA meetings, where attendance can be quite large, each group has no more than ten members. These meetings focus on behavioral changes by positive reinforcement (approval and encouragement), cognitive strategies (positive thinking), letting the body help (relaxation techniques, meditation, diet, and physical exercise), and dynamic group involvement. Secular Organizations for Sobriety was founded to help people who are uncomfortable with AA's spiritual emphasis. It is a self-empowerment approach to recovery and maintains that sobriety is a separate issue from all else. Like AA, SOS holds confidential meetings, celebrates sobriety anniversaries, and views recovery as a one-day-at-a-time process.

The support gained from talking with others who have similar problems is one of the greatest benefits derived from self-help groups. Many members learn to exert greater control over their own lives and rid themselves of the guilt they feel about their participation in their loved one's alcoholism.

## Relapse

Success with recovery varies with the individual. The alcoholics most likely to recover completely are those who developed their dependencies after the age of 20, those with intact and supportive family units, and those who have reached a high level of personal disgust coupled with strong motivation to recover. Over half of alcoholics relapse within the first 3 months of treatment. Why is the relapse rate so high? Treating an addiction requires more than getting the addict to stop using a substance; it also requires getting the person to break a pattern of behavior that has dominated his or her life. Many alcoholics refer to themselves as "recovering" throughout their lifetime; they never use the word *cured.*

People who are seeking to regain a healthy lifestyle must not only confront their addiction, but also guard against the tendency to relapse. Drinkers with compulsive personalities must learn to understand themselves and take control. To be effective, a recovery program must offer the alcoholic ways to increase self-esteem and resume personal growth. A comprehensive approach that includes drug therapy, group support, family therapy, and personal counseling designed to improve living and coping skills is usually the most effective course of treatment. A very small number of recovering alcoholics are able to resume drinking on a limited basis without reverting to alcoholic behavior. To prevent returning to the bottle, abstinence is the safest and sanest path.

# What's Your Risk of Alcohol Abuse?

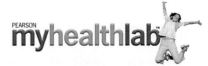

1. **How often do you have a drink containing alcohol?**
   - ⓪ Never
   - ① Monthly or less
   - ② 2 to 4 times a month
   - ③ 2 to 3 times a week
   - ④ 4 or more times a week

2. **How many alcoholic drinks do you have on a typical day when you are drinking?**
   - ⓪ 1 or 2        ① 3 or 4
   - ② 5 or 6        ③ 7 to 9
   - ④ 10 or more

3. **How often do you have six drinks or more on one occasion?**
   - ⓪ Never        ① Less than monthly
   - ② Monthly      ③ Weekly
   - ④ Daily or almost daily

4. **How often during the past year have you been unable to stop drinking once you had started?**
   - ⓪ Never        ① Less than monthly
   - ② Monthly      ③ Weekly
   - ④ Daily or almost daily

5. **How often during the past year have you failed to do what was normally expected from you because of drinking?**
   - ⓪ Never        ① Less than monthly
   - ② Monthly      ③ Weekly
   - ④ Daily or almost daily

6. **How often during the past year have you needed a first drink in the morning to get yourself going after a heavy drinking session?**
   - ⓪ Never        ① Less than monthly
   - ② Monthly      ③ Weekly
   - ④ Daily or almost daily

7. **How often during the past year have you had a feeling of guilt or remorse after drinking?**
   - ⓪ Never
   - ① Less than monthly
   - ② Monthly
   - ③ Weekly
   - ④ Daily or almost daily

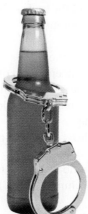

Fill out this assessment online at www.pearsonhighered.com/myhealthlab or www.pearsonhighered.com/donatelle.

8. **How often during the past year have you been unable to remember what happened the night before because you had been drinking?**
   - ⓪ Never
   - ① Less than monthly
   - ② Monthly
   - ③ Weekly
   - ④ Daily or almost daily

9. **Have you or someone else been injured as a result of your drinking?**
   - ⓪ No
   - ① Yes, but not in the past year
   - ② Yes, during the past year

10. **Has a relative, friend, or a doctor or other health care professional been concerned about your drinking or suggested you cut down?**
   - ⓪ No
   - ① Yes, but not in the past year
   - ② Yes, during the past year

## Scoring

**Scores above 8:** Your drinking patterns are putting you at high risk for illness, unsafe sexual situations, or alcohol-related injuries, and may even affect your academic performance.

**Source:** Taken from the AUDIT Manual, box 4, p. 17, World Health Organization, Division of Mental Health and Prevention of Substance Abuse. http://whqlibdoc.who.int/hq/2001/WHO_MSD _MSB_01.6a.pdf. Copyright © 2001 World Health Organization. Used with permission.

# YOUR PLAN FOR CHANGE

The **Assess yourself** activity gave you a chance to evaluate your alcohol use. If some of your answers concerned you, consider taking steps to change your behavior.

### Today, you can:

◯ Start a diary of your drinking habits—how much you drink, how much money you spend on drinks, and how you feel when you are drinking.

◯ Spend some time thinking about the ways your family members use alcohol.

Consider whether your current alcohol use is healthy, or whether it is likely to create problems for you in the future.

### Within the next 2 weeks, you can:

◯ Make your first drink a glass of water or another nonalcoholic beverage the next time you go to a party.

◯ Intersperse alcoholic drinks with nonalcoholic beverages to help you pace your consumption.

### By the end of the semester, you can:

◯ Cultivate friendships and explore activities that do not center on alcohol. If your current group of friends drinks heavily, and it is becoming a problem for you, you may need to step back from the group for a while.

## Summary

✴ Alcohol is a central nervous system (CNS) depressant used by about half of all Americans. About 70 percent of all college students report drinking in the past 30 days. Although consumption trends are slowly creeping downward, college students are under extreme pressure to consume alcohol.

✴ Negative consequences associated with alcohol use among college students are lower grade point averages, academic problems, traffic accidents, dropping out of school, unplanned sex, hangovers, alcohol poisoning, and injury.

✴ Alcohol's effect on the body is measured by the blood alcohol concentration (BAC), the ratio of alcohol to total blood volume: the higher the BAC, the greater the drowsiness and impaired judgment and coordination.

✴ Long-term alcohol overuse can cause damage to the nervous system, cardiovascular damage, liver disease, and increased risk for cancer. Drinking during pregnancy can cause fetal alcohol spectrum disorders (FASDs).

✴ Alcohol use becomes alcoholism when it interferes with school, work, or social and family relationships or entails violations of the law. Causes of alcoholism include biological, family, social, and cultural factors. Alcoholism has far-reaching effects on families, especially on children, who have problematic childhoods and may take those problems into adulthood.

✴ Most alcoholics do not admit to having a problem until reaching a major life crisis, or until their families intervene. Treatment options include detoxification at private medical facilities, therapy (family, individual, or group), and self-help programs such as Alcoholics Anonymous. Most alcoholics relapse (over half within 3 months) because alcoholism is a behavioral addiction as well as a chemical addiction.

## Pop Quiz

1. If a man and a woman drink the same amount of alcohol, the woman's BAC will be approximately
   a. the same as the man's BAC.
   b. 60 percent higher than the man's BAC.
   c. 30 percent higher than the man's BAC.
   d. 30 percent lower than the man's BAC.

2. Which of the following is a *true* statement regarding how one can metabolize alcohol faster to lower one's blood alcohol level?
   a. Drink black coffee.
   b. Take a cold shower.
   c. Engage in vigorous exercise.
   d. Only time can metabolize and rid the body of high alcohol content.

3. BAC is the
   a. concentration of plant sugars in the bloodstream.
   b. percentage of alcohol in a beverage.
   c. level of alcohol content in the blood.
   d. ratio of alcohol to the total blood volume.

4. Which is a strategy you could take to avoid drinking too much alcohol?
   a. Alternate alcoholic beverages with nonalcoholic drinks.
   b. Eat before and during drinking.
   c. Pace your drinks to one or fewer per hour.
   d. All of the above

5. Which of the following statements is *false*?
   a. College students under 21 drink less often than older students but drink more heavily.
   b. College students tend to underestimate the amount that their peers drink.
   c. In the past 10 years, the number of female college students who report being drunk 10 or more times has increased.
   d. Alcohol is involved in at least two-thirds of suicides on campus.

6. Which of the following is *not* typical of a child born with fetal alcohol syndrome?
   a. A small head
   b. Deafness
   c. Impaired learning
   d. Abnormal facial features

7. The fastest-growing population of alcohol abusers is
   a. older adults.
   b. adolescents.
   c. women.
   d. immigrants.

8. When Amanda goes out with her friends on the weekends, she usually has four or five beers in a row. This type of high-risk drinking is called
   a. tolerance.
   b. alcoholic addiction.
   c. alcohol overconsumption.
   d. binge drinking.

9. Drinking large amounts of alcohol in a short period of time that leads to passing out is known as
   a. learned behavioral tolerance.
   b. alcoholic unconsciousness.
   c. alcohol poisoning.
   d. acute metabolism syndrome.

10. Jake was raised in an alcoholic family. To adapt to his father's alcoholic behavior, he played the obedient and good son to his parents. What role did Jake assume?
    a. Family hero
    b. Mascot
    c. Scapegoat
    d. Lost child

*Answers to these questions can be found on page A-1.*

## Think about It!

1. When it comes to drinking alcohol, how much is too much? How can you avoid drinking amounts that will affect your judgment? When you see a friend having too many drinks at a party, what actions do you normally take? What actions could you take?

2. What are some of the most common negative consequences college students experience from drinking? What are secondhand effects of binge drinking? Why do students tolerate the negative behaviors of students who have been drinking?

3. Determine what your BAC would be if you drank four beers in 2 hours (assume they are spaced at equal intervals). What physiological effects will you feel after each drink? Would a person of similar weight show greater effects after having four gin and tonics instead of four beers? Why or why not? At what point in your life should you start worrying about the long-term effects of alcohol abuse?

4. Describe the difference between a problem drinker and an alcoholic. What factors can cause someone to slide from responsibly consuming alcohol to becoming an alcoholic? What effect does alcoholism have on an alcoholic's family?

5. Does anyone ever recover from alcoholism? Why or why not? Do you think society's views on drinking have changed over the years? Explain your answer.

## Accessing Your Health on the Internet

The following websites explore further topics and issues related to personal health. For links to the websites below, visit the Companion Website for *Access to Health,* 12th Edition, at www.pearsonhighered.com/donatelle.

1. *Alcoholics Anonymous (AA).* This website provides general information about AA and the 12-step program. www.aa.org

2. *College Drinking: Changing the Culture.* This online resource center targets three audiences: the student population as a whole, the college and its surrounding environment, and the individual at-risk or alcohol-dependent drinker. www.collegedrinkingprevention.gov

3. *The Alcohol Calculators.* This link allows you to do the following calculations related to alcohol use: the cost of your drinking on a monthly and annual basis, the amount of calories you are regularly consuming from alcohol, and your BAC. www.collegedrinkingprevention.gov/ CollegeStudents/calculator/default.aspx

4. *Had Enough.* This site is designed for college students who have suffered the secondhand effects (babysitting a roommate who has been drinking, having sleep interrupted, and so on) of other students' drinking. http://gbgm-umc.org/mission_programs/ cim/hadenough/home

5. *Higher Education Center for Alcohol, Drug Abuse, and Violence Prevention.* This website is funded through the U.S. Department of Education and provides information relevant to colleges and universities. A specific site exists for students who are seeking information regarding alcohol. www.higheredcenter.org

## References

1. A. Klatsky, "Alcohol and Cardiovascular Health," *Physiology and Behavior* 100, no. 1 (2010): 76–81; K. Tucker et al., "Effects of Beer, Wine and Liquor Intakes on Bone Mineral Density in Older Men and Women," *American Journal of Clinical Nutrition* 89, no. 4 (2009): 1188–96; H. Macdonald, "Alcohol and Recommendations for Bone Health: Should We Still Exercise Caution?" *American Journal of Clinical Nutrition* 89, no. 4 (2009): 999–1000; W. Snow et al., "Alcohol Use and Cardiovascular Health Outcomes: A Comparison across Age and Gender in the Winnipeg Health and Drinking Survey Cohort," *Age and Ageing* 38, no. 2 (2009): 206–12.

2. Centers for Disease Control and Prevention, National Center for Health Statistics, *Health, United States, 2008, with Special Feature on the Health of Young Adults* (Hyattsville, MD: National Center for Health Statistics, 2009); J. R. Pleis, J. W. Lucas, and B. W. Ward, "Summary Health Statistics for U.S. Adults: National Health Interview Survey, 2008, National Center for Health Statistics," *Vital and Health Statistics* 10, no. 242 (2009), Available at www.cdc.gov/nchs/products/series.htm.

3. Ibid.

4. R. LaVallee et al., "Apparent Per Capita Alcohol Consumption: National, State, and Regional Trends, 1977–2007," Surveillance Report #87 (Bethesda, MD: National Institute on Alcohol Abuse and Alcoholism, 2009), Available at http://pubs.niaaa.nih .gov/publications/surveillance87/ CONS07.htm.

5. American College Health Association, *American College Health Association— National College Health Assessment II: Reference Group Executive Summary Fall 2009* (Linthicum, MD: American College Health Association, 2010), Available at www.acha -ncha.org/reports_ACHA-NCHAII.html.

6. U.S. Department of Health and Human Services, National Institute on Alcohol Abuse and Alcoholism, "What Colleges Need to Know: An Update on College Drinking Research," NIH Publication no. 07-5010, November 2007, Available at www.collegedrinkingprevention.gov.

7. American College Health Association, *American College Health Association— National College Health Assessment II,* 2010.

8. Ibid.

9. R. Hingson et al., "Magnitude of Alcohol-Related Mortality and Morbidity among U.S. College Students Ages 18–24: Changes from 1998 to 2005," *Journal of Studies on Alcohol and Drugs* (2009): 12–20.

10. R. R. Wetherill et al., "Perceived Awareness and Caring Influences Alcohol Use by High School and College Students," *Psychology of Addictive Behaviors* 21, no. 2 (2007): 147–54.

11. L. D. Johnston, *Monitoring the Future National Survey Results on Drug Use, 1975–2008: Volume II, College Students and Adults Ages 19–50,* NIH Publication no. 09-7403 (Bethesda, MD: National Institute on Drug Abuse, 2009), Available at www.monitoringthefuture.org.

12. Ibid.

13. J. W. Labrie et al., "What Men Want: The Role of Reflective Opposite-Sex Normative Preferences in Alcohol Use among College Women," *Psychology of Addictive Behavior* 23, no. 1 (2009): 157–62.

14. J. Reingle et al., "An Exploratory Study of Bar and Nightclub Expectancies," *Journal of American College Health* 57, no. 6 (2009): 629–38.

15. E. Allen and M. Madden, *Hazing in View: College Students at Risk* (Orono, ME: National Collaborative for Hazing Research and Prevention, 2008), Available at www.hazingstudy.org.

16. R. J. O'Mara et al., "Alcohol Price and Intoxication in College Bars," *Journal on Studies of Alcohol* 33, no. 11 (2009): 1973–80.

17. National Center on Addiction and Substance Abuse at Columbia University, *Wasting the Best and the Brightest: Substance Abuse at America's Colleges and Universities,* March 2007, Available at www.casacolumbia.org/templates/publications_reports.aspx.

18. L. D. Johnston, *Monitoring the Future National Survey Results on Drug Use, 1975–2008,* 2009; S. Wells et al., "Policy Implications of the Widespread Practice of 'Pre-drinking' or 'Pre-gaming' before Going to Public Drinking Establishments—Are Current Prevention Strategies Backfiring?" *Addiction* 104 (2008): 4–9.

19. R. Hingson et al., "Magnitude of Alcohol-Related Mortality and Morbidity," 2008.

20. The Higher Education Center for Alcohol, Drug Abuse, and Violence Prevention, *Sexual Violence and Alcohol and Other Drug Use on Campus* (Newton, MA: The Higher Education Center for Alcohol, Drug Abuse, and Violence Prevention, 2008), available at www.higheredcenter.org/services/publications/sexual-violence-and-alcohol-and-other-drug-use-campus.

21. National Institute on Alcohol Abuse and Alcoholism, "College Drinking: A Snapshot of Annual High-Risk College Drinking Consequences," Reviewed July 2010, www.collegedrinkingprevention.gov/StatsSummaries/snapshot.aspx.

22. Higher Education Center for Alcohol, Drug Abuse and Violence Prevention, "Academic Performance," Accessed April 12, 2010, www.higheredcenter.org/high-risk/alcohol/consequences/academic-performance.

23. U.S. Department of Health and Human Services, National Institute on Alcohol Abuse and Alcoholism, "What Colleges Need to Know," 2007.

24. C. Elliott et al., "Computer-based Interventions for College Drinking: A Qualitative Review," *Addictive Behaviors*, 33, no. 8 (2008): 994–1005.

25. J. Labrie et al., "A Night to Remember: A Harm-Reduction Birthday Card Intervention Reduces High Risk Drinking During 21st Birthday Celebrations," *Journal of American College Health* 57 no. 6 (2009): 659–63.

26. American College Health Association, *American College Health Association—National College Health Assessment II,* 2010.

27. Substance Abuse and Mental Health Services Administration (SAMHSA), *Drug Abuse Warning Network, 2008: Selected Tables of National Estimates of Drug-Related Emergency Department Visits* (Rockville, MD: Office of Applied Studies, SAMHSA, 2009), Available at https://dawninfo.samhsa.gov/data.

28. J. Turner et al., "Serious Health Consequences Associated with Alcohol Use among College Students: Demographic and Clinical Characteristics of Patients Seen in the Emergency Department," *Journal of Studies on Alcohol* 65, no. 2 (2004): 179.

29. S. MacDonald, "The Criteria for Causation of Alcohol in Violent Injuries in Six Countries," *Addictive Behaviors* 30, no. 1 (2005): 103–13.

30. J. Turner et al., "Serious Health Consequences Associated with Alcohol Use among College Students," 2004.

31. Centers for Disease Control and Prevention, "Injury Prevention and Control: Home and Recreational Safety: Unintentional Drowning: Fact Sheet," Updated June 2010, www.cdc.gov/HomeandRecreationalSafety/Water-Safety/waterinjuries-factsheet.html; Centers for Disease Control and Prevention, "Injury Prevention and Control: Home and Recreational Safety: Fire Deaths and Injuries: Fact Sheet," Updated October 2009, www.cdc.gov/HomeandRecreationalSafety/Fire-Prevention/fires-factsheet.html.

32. L. Sher, "Alcohol Consumption and Suicide," *QJM: An International Journal of Medicine* 99, no. 1 (2006): 57–61; Bureau of Justice Statistics, "Criminal Victimization in the United States, Table 32, Percent Distribution of victimizations by perceived drug or alcohol use by offender, 2007," Accessed June 2010, http://bjs.ojp.usdoj.gov/content/pub/html/cvus/alcohol.cfm.

33. K. Butler, "The Grim Neurology of Teenage Drinking," *New York Times* (July 4, 2006).

34. R. W. Hingson et al., "Age at Drinking Onset and Alcohol Dependence," *Archives of Pediatric and Adolescent Medicine* 160 (2006): 739–46.

35. J. Theruvathu et al., "Polyamines Stimulate the Formation of Mutagenic 1, N2-Propanodeoxyguanosine Adducts from Acetaldehyde," *Nucleic Acids Research* 33, no. 11 (2005): 3513–20.

36. American Association for Cancer Research, "Excessive Alcohol Drinking Can Lead to Increased Risk of Breast Cancer, Study Suggests," *ScienceDaily*, April 14, 2008, www.sciencedaily.com/releases/2008/04/080413173510.htm; National

Institute on Alcohol Abuse and Alcoholism, *Alcohol: A Women's Health Issue,* NIH Publication no. 03-4956 (Bethesda, MD: National Institutes of Health, revised 2008), Available at www.niaaa.nih.gov/Publications/PamphletsBrochuresPosters/English/Pages/default.aspx.

37. C. S. Berkey et al., "Prospective Study of Adolescent Alcohol Consumption and Risk of Benign Breast Disease in Young Women," *Pediatrics* 125, no. 5 (2010): e1081–e1087.

38. Centers for Disease Control and Prevention, "Alcohol Use among Pregnant and Nonpregnant Women of Childbearing Age—United States, 1991–2005," *Morbidity and Mortality Weekly* 58, no. 19 (2009): 529–32.

39. Centers for Disease Control and Prevention, "Fetal Alcohol Spectrum Disorders (FASDs) Data and Statistics," Updated May 2010, www.cdc.gov/ncbddd/fasd/data.html.

40. National Organization on Fetal Alcohol Syndrome, "FASD: What Everyone Should Know," 2006, Available at www.nofas.org/resource/factsheet.aspx.

41. Centers for Disease Control and Prevention, "Injury Mortality: Unintentional Injury: US 2001–2006," 2009, http://205.207.175.93/HDI/TableViewer/tableView.aspx?ReportId=71.

42. National Highway Traffic Safety Administration, "Traffic Safety Facts Research Note: 2008 Traffic Safety Annual Assessment—Highlights," DOT HS 811 172, 2009, http://www-nrd.nhtsa.dot.gov/pubs/811016.pdf.

43. American College Health Association, *American College Health Association,* 2010.

44. Ibid.

45. A. Quinn-Zobeck, *Screening and Brief Intervention Tool Kit for College and University Campuse,* (U.S. Department of Transportation, National Highway Traffic Safety Administration [NHTSA] with The BACCHUS Network: Washington, DC, 2007) DOT HS 810 751, page 14, Available at www.stopimpaireddriving.org/3672Toolkit/index.htm.

46. Insurance Institute for Highway Safety, "Fatality Facts 2008: Alcohol," 2009, www.iihs.org/research/fatality_facts_2008/alcohol.html.

47. Ibid.

48. Ibid.

49. National Institutes of Health, Medline Plus, "Alcoholism and Alcohol Abuse," Updated May 2010, www.nlm.nih.gov/medlineplus/ency/article/000944.htm.

50. J. Knight et al., "Alcohol Abuse and Dependence among U.S. College Students," *Journal of Studies on Alcohol* 63, no. 3 (2002): 263–70.

51. C. A. Presley et al., "The Introduction of the Heavy and Frequent Drinker:

A Proposed Classification to Increase Accuracy of Alcohol Assessments in Post-secondary Education Settings," *Journal of Alcohol Studies on Alcohol* 67 (2006): 324–31.

52. National Institute on Drug Abuse, "Alcohol Abuse Makes Prescription Drug Abuse More Likely," *NIDA Notes* 21, no. 5 (2008), Available at www.drugabuse.gov/NIDA_notes/NNvol21N5/alcohol.html.

53. Ibid.

54. W. R. Lovallo et al., "Working Memory and Decision-Making Biases in Young Adults with a Family History of Alcoholism: Studies from the Oklahoma Family Health Patterns Project," *Alcoholism: Clinical & Experimental Research* 30, no. 5 (2006): 763–73; National Institute on Alcohol Abuse and Alcoholism, U.S. Department of Health and Human Services, *A Family History of Alcoholism: Are You at Risk?* NIH Publication no. 03–5340 (Bethesda, MD: National Institute on Alcohol Abuse and Alcoholism, 2007), Available at www.niaaa.nih.gov/Publications/PamphletsBrochuresPosters/English/Pages/default.aspx.

55. C. Wilson and J. Knight, "When Parents Have a Drinking Problem," *Contemporary Pediatrics* 18, no. 1 (January 2001): 67.

56. A. Agrawal and M. T. Lynskey, "Are There Genetic Influences on Addiction? Evidence from Family, Adoption and Twin Studies," *Addiction* 103 (2008): 1069–81.

57. C. Wilson and J. Knight, "When Parents Have a Drinking Problem," 2001.

58. J. Niels Rosenquist et al., "The Spread of Alcohol Consumption Behavior in a Large Social Network," *Annals of Internal Medicine* 152, no. 7 (2010): 426–33.

59. Claudia Black, "Children of Addiction," The Many Faces of Addiction Blog, *Psychology Today*, February 8, 2010, www.psychologytoday.com/blog/the-many-faces-addiction/201002/children-addiction.

60. Ensuring Solutions to Alcohol Problems, *Workplace Screening & Brief Intervention: What Employers Can and Should Do about Excessive Alcohol Use* (The George Washington University Medical Center: Washington, DC, March 2008), Available at www.jointogether.org/resources/2008/workplace-sbi.html.

61. Ibid.

62. Ibid.

63. Ibid.

64. T. R. Miller et al., "Societal Costs of Underage Drinking," *Journal of Studies on Alcohol* 67, no. 4 (2006): 519–28.

65. Ibid.

66. National Institute on Alcohol Abuse and Alcoholism, *Alcohol: A Women's Health Issue*, revised 2008.

67. National Institute on Drug Abuse, "Info Facts: Treatment Methods for Women," Updated 2009, www.drugabuse.gov/infofacts/treatwomen.html.

68. Ibid.

69. E. Cohen et al., "Alcohol Treatment Utilization: Findings from the National Epidemiologic Survey on Alcohol and Related Conditions," *Drug and Alcohol Dependence* 86, nos. 2–3 (2007): 214–21.

# 12

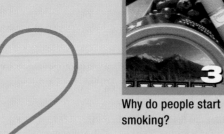
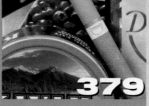
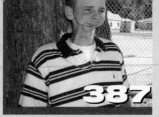

**379** Why do people start smoking?

**383** Is social smoking really that bad for me?

**387** Is chewing tobacco as harmful as smoking cigarettes?

# Ending Tobacco Use

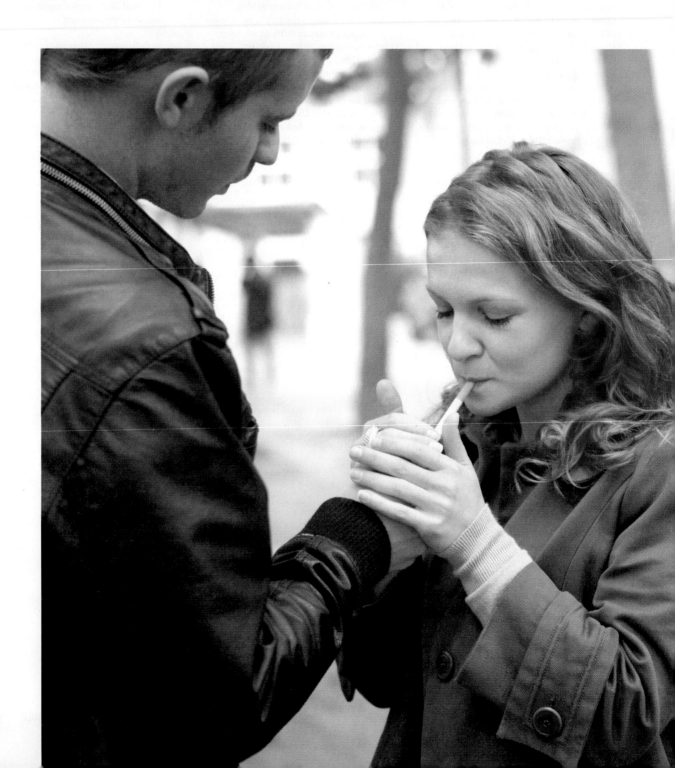

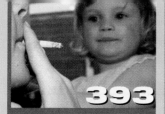

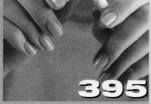

What are the health risks of secondhand smoke?

Will quitting smoking reverse the damage that's already done?

## Objectives

✳ Discuss tobacco use in the United States and on college campuses, and the social and political issues involved in tobacco use.

✳ Describe how the chemicals in tobacco products affect the body.

✳ Discuss the health risks of smoking and using smokeless tobacco, and the dangers of environmental tobacco smoke.

✳ Describe quitting strategies, including strategies aimed at breaking the nicotine addiction and smoking habit.

The substantial decline (58.2%) in the prevalence of smoking among adults since 1964 has been characterized as one of the ten greatest achievements in public health in the twentieth century.[1] However, in 2010, tobacco use is still the single most preventable cause of death in the United States.[2] Smoking affects the health of people at all stages of their life. The health hazards of tobacco use are well documented, and yet 20 percent of Americans are smokers. Each year, nearly 443,000, or 1 in 5, American deaths are from tobacco-related diseases.[3] Most of these deaths are due to three major diseases: lung cancer (129,000 deaths), ischemic heart disease (126,000 deaths), and chronic obstructive pulmonary disease (COPD, 93,000 deaths).[4] For every person who dies from tobacco use, another 20 suffer from at least one serious tobacco-related illness.[5] Smoking cigarettes kills more Americans than alcohol, car accidents, suicide, AIDS, homicide, and illegal drugs combined.[6] Any contention by the tobacco industry that tobacco use is not dangerous is irresponsible and ignores the scientific evidence. This

## 30%
of all cancer deaths have smoking as a primary causal factor.

chapter provides information about tobacco use in the United States and on college campuses, about tobacco and its effects, the health hazards associated with using it, and facts about quitting.

# Tobacco Use in the United States

Approximately 71 million Americans report using tobacco products (cigarettes, cigars, smokeless tobacco, and pipe tobacco) at least once in the past month. Following the Surgeon General's report on smoking in 1964, cigarette smoking declined sharply for men and at a slower pace for women, thus narrowing the gap between smoking rates for men and women. Declines in current cigarette smoking over the past two decades have slowed compared with earlier periods. In 2008, 23 percent of men and 18 percent of women were current cigarette smokers. Men aged 25 to 44 were most likely to smoke cigarettes (26% in 2008), and this percentage decreased with increasing age. Among women aged 18 to 64, 21 percent were current cigarette smokers, and the percentage of current cigarette smoking declined substantially among women aged 65 and over (8%).[7] Every day 1,000 people under 18 become regular smokers and 1,800 over 18 become daily smokers.[8]

Education is closely linked to cigarette use: Adults with a bachelor of arts degree or higher education are three times *less* likely to smoke than are those with less than a high school education. Cigarette smoking also varies by ethnicity and gender, with the highest rates of smoking found among non-Hispanic black men and American Indian and Alaska

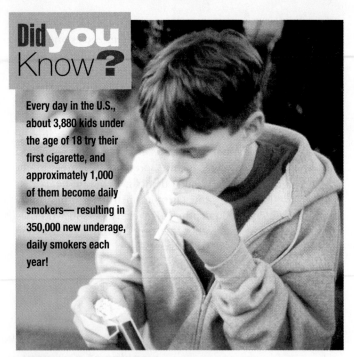
Native men.[9] Table 12.1 shows the percentage of Americans who smoke, by demographic group.

More than 20 percent of Americans are former smokers, and about 60 percent have never smoked. The most commonly used tobacco product is cigarettes, followed by cigars and smokeless tobacco. Approximately 6 percent of Americans smoke cigars and 7 percent of men and less than 1 percent of women use smokeless tobacco.[10]

The production and distribution of tobacco products in the United States and abroad involve many political and economic issues. Tobacco-growing states derive substantial income from tobacco production, and federal, state, and local governments benefit enormously from cigarette taxes.

# Why Do People Smoke?

Somewhere between 60 and 80 percent of people have tried a cigarette. They might try one out of curiosity, because their parents smoke, or because they are under peer pressure. Why do some walk away from cigarettes while others get hooked? This is a complicated question, but there are several possible reasons. First, nicotine is a very addictive drug; second, people can become hooked on the habit of picking up a cigarette; third, weight control can motivate smokers to continue smoking; and finally, people in the United States are bombarded with powerful cigarette advertising messages every day.

**nicotine poisoning** Symptoms often experienced by beginning smokers, including dizziness, diarrhea, light-headedness, rapid and erratic pulse, clammy skin, nausea, and vomiting.

| TABLE 12.1 | Percentage of Population That Smokes (Aged 18 and Older) among Select Groups in the United States | |
|---|---|---|
| | | **Percentage** |
| United States overall | | 20.6 |
| **Race** | | |
| Asian | | 9.9 |
| Black, non-Hispanic | | 21.3 |
| Hispanic | | 15.8 |
| Native American | | 32.4 |
| White, non-Hispanic | | 22.0 |
| **Age** | | |
| 18–24 | | 21.4 |
| 25–44 | | 23.7 |
| 45–64 | | 22.6 |
| 65+ | | 9.3 |
| **Sex** | | |
| Male | | 23.1 |
| Female | | 18.3 |
| **Education** | | |
| Undergraduate | | 10.6 |
| Some college | | 22.7 |
| High school | | 25.5 |
| 9–11 years | | 35.7 |
| **Income Level** | | |
| Below poverty level | | 31.5 |
| At or above poverty level | | 19.6 |

**Source:** Centers for Disease Control and Prevention, "Cigarette Smoking among Adults and Trends in Smoking Cessation—United States 2008," *Morbidity and Mortality Weekly Report* 58, no. 44 (2009): 1227–32.

**Nicotine Addiction** Beginning smokers usually feel the effects of nicotine with their first puff. These symptoms, called **nicotine poisoning,** can include dizziness, light-headedness, rapid and erratic pulse, clammy skin, nausea, vomiting, and diarrhea. These symptoms cease as tolerance to the chemical develops, which happens almost immediately in new users, perhaps after the second or third cigarette. In contrast, tolerance to most other drugs, such as alcohol, develops over a period of months or years. Regular smokers often do not experience the "buzz" of smoking. They continue to smoke simply because stopping is too difficult.

Two different studies on twins found genetic factors to be more influential than environmental factors in smoking initiation and nicotine dependence.[11] Two specific genes may influence smoking behavior by affecting the action of the brain chemical dopamine.[12] Understanding the influence of genetics on nicotine addiction could be crucial to developing more effective treatments for smoking cessation.[13]

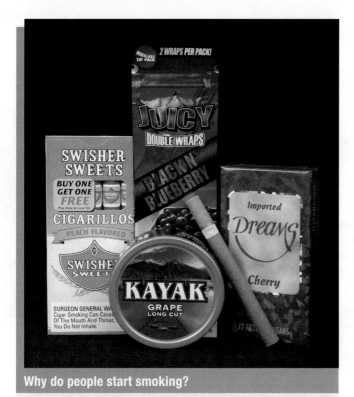

## Why do people start smoking?

Most people smoke because they have a physical and psychological addiction to nicotine. But they wouldn't be addicted if they didn't smoke, so why did they start in the first place? Peer pressure plays a large role, as do advertising and the portrayal of smoking in films and on TV. Tobacco companies know that once a person starts smoking, chances are good that he or she will get hooked and become a long-term customer, so they make a concerted effort to attract kids and teens by using bright, colorful packaging and candy-, fruit-, and alcohol-flavored products that mask the harshness of tobacco.

**Behavioral Dependence** People who smoke are not just physically dependent on nicotine; they are also psychologically dependent. Did you ever wonder why friends or family who are former smokers miss lighting up a cigarette at a bar, after a meal, or while driving a car? Nicotine "tricks" the brain into creating pleasurable memory associations between sensory stimuli or environmental cues that may trigger the urge for a cigarette.[14] Even those who occasionally smoke might find it hard to quit because of paired associations between smoking and a particular behavior such as having a drink or a morning cup of coffee.

Many smokers have a difficult time imagining not being a smoker. They often describe their cigarette as their friend. For some smokers, simply holding a cigarette provides comfort and can have a calming effect. Some former smokers remain vulnerable to sensory and environmental cues, such as smelling tobacco, driving in their car, or seeing a cigarette ad, for many years after they quit smoking.

**Weight Control** Nicotine is an appetite suppressant and slightly increases the smoker's basal metabolic rate. People who start smoking often lose weight. After smoking a cigarette a smoker's metabolism increases right away and then returns to a normal level. But "pack-a-day" smokers have surges in metabolism throughout the day. As a result, heavy smokers experience less of an appetite than those who smoke less or not at all. When a smoker quits, the metabolic rate slows down and appetite returns. People tend to eat more foods, in particular sweets, when they stop smoking. Fear of gaining weight is one of the biggest reasons smokers are reluctant to quit. The average weight gain is between 5 to 8 pounds. Ways to avoid weight gain after quitting smoking include avoiding crash diets, keeping low-calorie treats handy, and drinking plenty of water.

**Advertising** The tobacco industry spends an estimated $36 million per day on advertising and promotional material.[15] With the number of smokers declining by about 1 million each year, the industry must actively recruit new smokers. Campaigns are directed at all age, social, and ethnic groups, but because children and teenagers constitute 90 percent of all new smokers, much of the advertising has been directed toward them. Evidence of product recognition among under-age smokers is clear: 86 percent of underage smokers prefer one of the three most heavily advertised brands—Marlboro, Newport, or Camel.[16]

One of the most blatant advertisements aimed at young people was the popular Joe Camel ad campaign. After R. J. Reynolds introduced the cartoon figure, Camel's market share among underage smokers jumped from 3 to 13.3 percent in 3 years.[17] Tobacco companies have also targeted children and teens with tobacco products that have candy, fruit, or alcohol flavorings that mask the harshness of the tobacco, thus making these items more appealing and palatable to young people.[18] In addition, novel products for creating and sustaining nicotine addiction—including teabag-like pouches and dissolvable candy-like tablets—particularly appeal to young people.

Cigarette advertisements in women's magazines imply that smoking is the key to financial success, independence, and social acceptance. In the past several years, the tobacco industry has launched aggressive campaigns aimed at women that depict cigarette smoking as feminine and fashionable. Camel No. 9 cigarettes packaged in shiny black boxes with hot pink and teal borders that evoke images of Chanel perfumes have been heavily advertised. The advertisement slogans "Light and Luscious" and "Now Available in Stiletto" for a thin version of the cigarette were pitched to "the most fashion forward women." Many brands also have

# Catching Up to the Men: Women and Smoking

Although smoking rates among women have historically been lower than among men, by 1965 over 50 percent of American women smoked regularly. What led to this increase? Part of the answer lies in the marketing efforts of the tobacco industry. Beginning during World War II and continuing to this day, tobacco marketers have used themes of social desirability, independence, and weight control to attract women smokers.

Today, slightly more than 1 in 6 women in America smoke, and men's and women's smoking rates are nearly equal: 18.3 percent for women, 23.1 percent for men. Accordingly, women have assumed a much larger burden of smoking-related diseases than they did in the past. However, not all women are equally likely to smoke. For example:

✱ Smoking among women differs by race and ethnicity: non-Hispanic white women—20.6 percent; African-American women—17.8 percent; Hispanic women—10.7 percent; Asian-American women—4.7 percent; and Native American/Alaskan Native women—22.4 percent.

✱ Smoking among women varies with education level. Among U.S. women who earned a general equivalency diploma (GED), 37.5 percent are smokers. Among college graduates, 9.7 percent are smokers, whereas only 5.9 percent of those who completed graduate work smoke.

✱ Affluent women are less likely to smoke than women are who are poor. Thirty-two percent of women with incomes below the poverty line smoke.

Despite recent declines in smoking overall, the prevalence of tobacco-related disease continues to increase, especially among women. Consider the following:

✱ Every year, tobacco-related disease kills an estimated 174,000 women, making it the largest preventable cause of death among women in the United States.

✱ Women who die of a smoking-related disease lose, on average, 14.5 years of potential life. Men who die of a smoking-related disease lose 13 years of life, on average.

✱ Women who begin smoking at an early age (within 5 years of their first menstrual period) are at higher risk of developing breast cancer.

✱ Evidence suggests that breast cancer is more likely to spread to the lungs in women who smoke than it is in women who do not smoke.

✱ Recent data from the Centers for Disease Control and Prevention indicate that smoking-related cancer deaths are decreasing among men but are increasing among women.

✱ Some studies suggest that smoking cigarettes dramatically increases the risk of heart disease among younger women who are also taking birth control pills.

> Cigarette companies have become adept at marketing to women using "glamorous" packaging and ad campaigns borrowed from cosmetics, perfume (such as the famous Chanel scents evoked by this Camel No. 9 brand), and the fashion industry.

✱ Postmenopausal women who smoke have lower bone density than do women who never smoked, putting these women at increased risk for osteoporosis.

**Sources:** American Cancer Society, "Women and Smoking: An Epidemic of Smoking-Related Cancer and Disease in Women," Revised November 2009, www.cancer.org/Cancer/Cancer Causes/TobaccoCancer/WomenandSmoking/ women-and-smoking-intro; American Heart Association, "Women, Heart Disease, and Stroke," 2009, www.americanheart.org/presenter .jhtml?identifier=4786; Office on Smoking and Health, Centers for Disease Control and Prevention, "Cigarette Smoking among Adults— United States, 2007," *Morbidity and Mortality Weekly Report* 57, no. 45 (2008): 1221–26; Centers for Disease Control and Prevention, "Smoking-Attributable Mortality, Years of Potential Life Lost, and Productivity Losses— United States, 2000–2004," *Morbidity and Mortality Weekly Report* 57, no. 45 (2008): 1226–28; Centers for Disease Control and Prevention, "Cigarette Smoking Among Adults and Trends in Smoking Cessastion—United States, 2008," *Morbidity and Mortality Weekly Report* 58, no. 44 (2009): 1227–32.

thin spokeswomen pushing "slim" and "light" cigarettes to cash in on women's fear of gaining weight. These ads have apparently been working. From the mid-1970s through the early 2000s, cigarette sales to women increased dramatically. Not coincidentally, by 1987, cigarette-induced lung cancer had surpassed breast cancer as the leading cancer killer among women.[19] Although lung cancer rates are decreasing for men, lung cancer rates have yet to decline for

women. See the **Gender & Health** box above for more on the smoking and smoking-related disease trends among women in the United States.

But women are not the only targets of gender-based cigarette advertisements. Men in cigarette ads are depicted in locker rooms, charging over rugged terrain in off-road vehicles, or riding stallions into the sunset in blatant appeals to a need to feel and appear masculine. Minorities are also often targeted. Recent studies have shown a higher concentration of tobacco advertising in magazines aimed at African Americans, such as *Jet* and *Ebony*, than in similar magazines aimed at broader audiences, such as *Time* and *People*. Billboards and posters aiming the cigarette message at Hispanics have spotted the landscape in Hispanic communities for many years, especially in low-income areas. Recent innovations by tobacco companies have included sponsorship of community-based events such as festivals and annual fairs.

## Financial Costs to Society

The use of tobacco products is costly to all of us in terms of lost productivity and lost lives. Estimates show that tobacco use causes over $193 billion in annual health-related economic losses. The economic burden of tobacco use totals more than $96 billion in medical expenditures (costs include hospital, physician, and nursing home expenses; prescription drugs; and home health care expenditures) and $97 billion in indirect costs (absenteeism, added cost of fire insurance, training costs to replace employees who die prematurely, disability payments, and so on). The economic costs of smoking are estimated to be about $3,391 per smoker per year.[20] These costs far exceed the tax revenues on the sale of tobacco products, even though the average cigarette tax in 2010 was $1.34 per pack and is rising in some states.[21]

14 percent of college students reported having smoked cigarettes in the past 30 days, down from about 30 percent in 1999.[22] About 11 percent of college students meet the criteria for tobacco dependence. Many who report smoking in college (80%) started doing so before age 18. Those who began smoking before age 18 report smoking four times as many cigarettes in the past month and on twice as many days as those who began smoking after age 18.[23] College men and women have nearly identical rates of cigarette smoking, but men use more cigars and smokeless tobacco.[24]

## Gender and Tobacco Use on Campus

It is during the transition from high school to college that the most significant increase in smoking is seen among women, roughly the time when many turn 18. On college campuses, female students who smoke are viewed in a more negative light than male students who smoke. Some students describe smoking among females as "trashy," "unladylike," "uncontrolled," and "a big turn off."[25] In contrast, male smokers are described as "masculine or manly," "cool," "relaxed," and "in control." Despite the negative perception of female smokers, some college women smoke, particularly at parties, to change their image (e.g., to appear less uptight and more fun, intriguing, and outgoing); a cigarette essentially serves as a prop.

## College Students and Tobacco Use

College students are the targets of heavy tobacco marketing and advertising campaigns. The tobacco industry has set up aggressive marketing promotions at bars, music festivals, and the like, specifically targeted at the 18- to 24-year-old age group (see the **Student Health Today** box on page 382). Being placed in a new, often stressful, social and academic environment makes college students especially vulnerable to advertising. For many, the college years are their initial taste of freedom from parental supervision. Peer influence and the desire to emulate peers can prompt fellow students to start smoking, and many colleges and universities still sell tobacco products in campus stores.

However, in spite of these influences, cigarette smoking among U.S. college students has decreased in recent years (see **Figure 12.1**). In a 2009 study, about

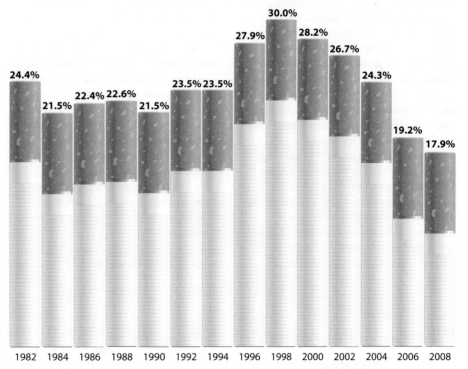

FIGURE 12.1 **Trends in Prevalence of Cigarette Smoking in the Past Month among College Students**

**Source:** Data are from L. D. Johnston, P. M. O'Malley, J. G. Bachman, and J. E. Schulenberg, *Monitoring the Future National Survey Results on Drug Use, 1975–2008, Volume II: College Students and Adults Ages 19–50*, NIH Publication no. 09-7403 (Bethesda, MD: National Institute on Drug Abuse, 2009).

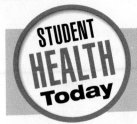

# PITCHING TOBACCO PRODUCTS ON COLLEGE CAMPUSES

The tobacco industry is very interested in convincing college-aged people to smoke, according to Stanton A. Glantz, director of the Center for Tobacco Control Research at the University of California, San Francisco: "Historically, if you go far enough back to the '30s, '40s, '50s and even '60s, a lot of smoking initiation occurred in that age group."

Tobacco companies turned to even younger potential smokers in the 1970s and 1980s, Glantz says, but they remained interested in college-aged people, because many develop permanent smoking habits during that stage of their lives. About one-third of people who experiment with cigarettes as young adults go on to become smokers.

According to a recent Harvard University survey, tobacco companies often give away cigarettes at college bars and campus social events. The survey found that free cigarettes were handed out on 109 of 119 campuses. The research suggests that tobacco companies are targeting college students, according to the study's coauthor Henry Wechsler, director of the College Alcohol Studies Program at the Harvard School of Public Health. "These are very important years," says Wechsler. "They're also the earliest years that the tobacco industry can legally try to get new customers."

The researchers found that the students exposed to the giveaways were three times more likely to start smoking or use smokeless tobacco by age 19. Wechsler said the study's design made it impossible to confirm that there's a cause-and-effect relationship. However, he added, "from my perspective, people

wouldn't be giving all this stuff away if they didn't think it had some effect."

Of the students surveyed, 8.5 percent said they had attended a bar or social event during the previous 6 months where free cigarettes were given out. Most of those students said they ran into the giveaways off campus. But 3.2 percent said the promotions took place at campus bars (many colleges have pubs designed for faculty, staff, and students of drinking age) or social events. The events reinforce brand visibility, allow the industry to reach specific target groups, and generate names for future marketing efforts. Promotions at social events have the potential to increase tobacco use by encouraging nonsmokers to try cigarettes, by encouraging experimental smokers to use regularly, and by discouraging current smokers from quitting.

Dana Bolden, a spokesman for Philip Morris, the largest tobacco company in the world, said not all tobacco companies distribute free cigarettes. Philip Morris, he added, doesn't engage in giveaways and wants the federal government to ban the practice. Bolden added that his company does hold invitation-only music events for customers who sign up to receive information about its products. As for the charge that tobacco companies are trying to entice college students to smoke, Bolden said his company only markets to adults aged 21 and older, even though it could legally pursue potential customers as young as 18.

**Sources:** R. Dotinga, "Tobacco Promotions Woo College Crowd," *Lifespan Health News* (December

College students and young adults are the targets of heavy tobacco marketing and advertising campaigns. The tobacco industry has set up aggressive marketing promotions at bars, sponsored concerts, music festivals, and the like, specifically targeted at the 18- to 24-year-old age group.

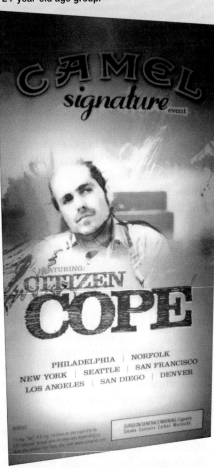

28, 2004); N. Rigotti et al., "U.S. College Students' Exposure to Tobacco Promotions: Prevalence and Association with Tobacco Use," *American Journal of Public Health* 94, no. 12 (2004): 1–7.

## Why Do College Students Smoke?

So why do college students become smokers? In a recent survey, the main reason students gave for their smoking was to relax or to reduce stress (38%).[26] According to this study, smokers are more likely to have higher levels of perceived stress than nonsmokers. Other key reasons provided by students were to fit in, or because of social pressure

(16%) and because they cannot stop or are addicted (12%; see Figure 12.2).

For some students weight control is an important motivator and fear of weight gain is a common reason for smoking relapse among those who quit. Other research finds that students diagnosed or treated for depression are 7.5 times more likely to use tobacco compared to students who were never diagnosed or treated for depression.[27]

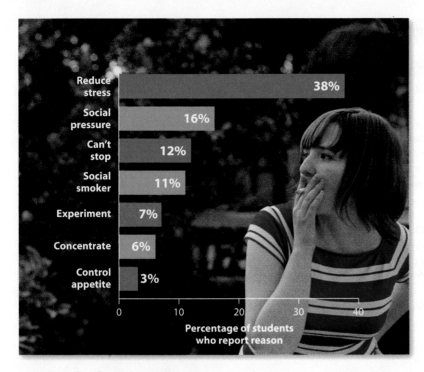

FIGURE 12.2 **Reasons for Tobacco Use among College Student Smokers**

**Source:** National Center on Addiction and Substance Abuse at Columbia University, *Wasting the Best and the Brightest: Substance Abuse at America's Colleges and Universities* (New York: National Center on Addiction and Substance Abuse at Columbia University, March 2007), 48. Copyright © 2007. Used with permission.

hood of heart disease, blood clots, stroke, liver cancer, and gallbladder disease.[30] Pregnant women who smoke only occasionally still run a risk of giving birth to unhealthy babies.

## Most Student Smokers Want to Quit

Unlike social smokers, most students who smoke regularly and are nicotine dependent do want to stop smoking. In one study, over the course of 4 years of college, about half of students who smoked every few days, every few weeks, or every few months quit, as did 13 percent of daily smokers.[31] More than a quarter cut back. Unfortunately, in spite of their efforts or desire to quit, almost all daily smokers continue to smoke throughout college.[32] To reduce the incidence of smoking among students, colleges and universities need to engage in antismoking efforts, strictly control tobacco advertising, provide smoke-free residence halls, and offer greater access to smoking-cessation programs. See the **Points of View** box on page 384 for a discussion of banning smoking on campuses.

## Occasional or Social Smoking

Many college smokers identify themselves as "social smokers"—those who smoke when they are with people, rather than alone. What differentiates a social smoker from a smoker? Social smokers smoke less often and less intensely, and they are less dependent on nicotine. They also do not view themselves as being addicted to cigarettes but are less likely to quit or have any intention to quit. However, even occasional smoking is not without risks. Social smoking in college or anytime can lead to a complete dependence on nicotine and, thus, to all the same health risks as smoking regularly.

## what do you think?

Have you noticed a change in the number of your friends who are regular or occasional smokers? ● How many of them smoked prior to coming to college, and how many picked up the habit at school? ● What are their reasons for smoking? ● What barriers keep your friends from quitting?

In research studies, smoking less than a pack of cigarettes a week has been shown to damage blood vessels and to increase the risk of heart disease and cancer.[28] Occasional or social smokers also experience an increased occurrence of colds, sore throats, shortness of breath, and fatigue.[29] In women taking birth control pills, even a few cigarettes a week can increase the likeli-

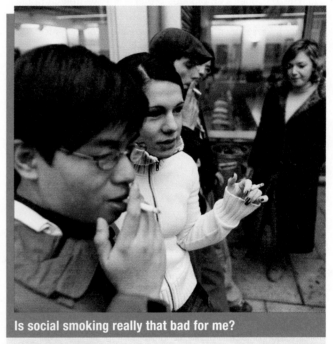

**Is social smoking really that bad for me?**

An occasional puff once in a while when you are out with friends can't hurt, right? Wrong! There is no "safe" amount of tobacco use—any smoking or exposure to smoke increases your risks for negative health effects such as heart disease and lung cancer. And even if you smoke only once or twice a week and consider yourself a "social smoker," chances are you're on the road to dependence and a more frequent smoking habit.

<br>

# POINTS OF VIEW

# Smoking on College & University Campuses:
## SHOULD IT BE BANNED?

Approximately 20 percent of students begin smoking in college and another 50 percent intensify their smoking behavior. In a recent study, 83 percent of students reported having been exposed to environmental tobacco smoke (ETS) at least once in the 7 days preceding the survey. Most of those exposures (65%) happened at a restaurant or bar, followed by exposure at home or in the same room as a smoker (55%) and in a car (38%).

Daily and occasional smokers were more likely than nonsmokers to report exposure, perhaps not surprising given that they are more likely than other students to have friends who smoke and to frequent or live in locations where smoking occurs, according to the study. Similarly, students who binge drink were more likely than other students to report exposure to ETS or sidestream smoke. This is not surprising given there is a well-established link between smoking and drinking behaviors. Other factors that appeared to be associated with increased exposure to ETS included living in residence locations where smoking is allowed or locations associated with smoking, such as Greek houses and off-campus housing; being female; being of white race; having parents with higher education levels; and attending a public versus private school. Nearly all nonsmokers (93.9%) and the majority of smokers (57.8%) reported that ETS was somewhat or very annoying.

As a result, at least 381 campuses have all-out prohibitions or significant restrictions on tobacco use, with many more campuses pursuing becoming smoke free. The debate regarding tobacco-free campuses is contentious at many schools. Below are some of the major points for both sides of the question.

### Arguments for Banning Tobacco on Campuses

○ The majority of college students—4 out of 5—do not smoke.

○ Two-thirds of students prefer to attend classes held on a smoke-free campus.

○ Most college employees prefer a smoke-free campus.

○ Three-quarters of students (both smokers and nonsmokers) say it is OK for colleges to prohibit smoking on campus to keep secondhand smoke away from students and staff.

○ One in five students say they have experienced some immediate health impact from exposure to ETS.

○ Nonsmokers are 40 percent less likely to become smokers if they live in smoke-free dorms.

### Arguments against Banning Tobacco on Campuses

○ There are so many other causes of potentially harmful fumes on campus—from diesel trucks, for example—that banning smoking wouldn't really affect the overall health and air quality on campus.

○ Smoking is not illegal, so students should be able to do it somewhere on campus; it would be a violation of individual rights to not let adults do something that is legally allowed.

○ The policy would be difficult if not impossible to enforce. For example, when visitors come to campus for athletic or community events, it would be unenforceable.

○ Where can students go to smoke that is safe if they live in residence halls?

○ Smoking bans in public and private places violate the rights of smokers and encourage discriminatory treatment of people addicted to nicotine.

○ Colleges should focus more money and effort on smoking-cessation programs, not on implementing and enforcing smoking bans.

### Where Do You Stand?

○ Is smoking on a college campus a threat to public health?

○ Do you think that someone has the right to smoke in dorms, in campus buildings, in adjacent parks, or in other public places on campus? Why or why not?

○ How do you feel when you are walking across campus and someone is smoking close to you? Do you feel as though you could ask or should ask smokers to put out their cigarettes?

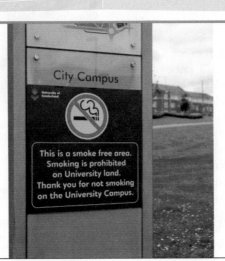

○ Would banning smoking be discriminatory? A violation of individual rights? Should student smokers be singled out for exclusion on college campuses?

**Sources:** American Cancer Society, "Smoke-Free College Campus Initiative," 2010, http://ww2.cancer.org/docroot/com/content/div_northwest/com_5_1x_smoke-free_college_campus_initiative.asp; Tobacco-Free Oregon, *Making Your College Campus Tobacco-Free*, 2010, http://smokefree oregon.com/college/resources; M. Wolfson, T. McCoy, and E. Sutfin, "College Students' Exposure to Secondhand Smoke," *Nicotine and Tobacco Research* 11, no. 8 (2009): 977–84.

# Tobacco: Its Components and Effects

Smoking, the most common form of tobacco use, delivers a strong dose of nicotine directly to the lungs, as well as 4,000 other chemical substances, including 250 that are harmful or toxic and 50 known carcinogens (cancer-causing agents).[33] You might be surprised to learn that some of the chemicals contained in tobacco smoke can also be found in chemical weapons, household cleaners, car exhaust, and embalming fluid (see Table 12.2). Inhaling hot toxic gases exposes sensitive mucous membranes to irritating chemicals that weaken the tissues and contribute to cancers of the mouth, larynx, and throat. The heat from tobacco smoke, which can reach 1,616°F, is also harmful.

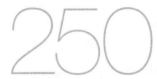

**250** of the 4,000 chemical components found in tobacco smoke are known to be harmful.

## Nicotine

The highly addictive chemical stimulant **nicotine** is the major psychoactive substance in all tobacco products. In its natural form, nicotine is a colorless liquid that turns brown on exposure to air. When tobacco leaves are burned in a cigarette, pipe, or cigar, nicotine is released and inhaled into the lungs. Sucking or chewing tobacco releases nicotine into the saliva, and the nicotine is then absorbed through the mucous membranes in the mouth.

Nicotine is a powerful central nervous system stimulant that produces a variety of physiological effects. In the cerebral cortex, it produces an aroused, alert mental state. Nicotine stimulates the adrenal glands, which increases the production of adrenaline. It also increases heart and respiratory rates, constricts blood vessels, and, in turn, increases blood pressure because the heart must work harder to pump blood through the narrowed vessels.

## Tar and Carbon Monoxide

Cigarette smoke is a complex mixture of chemicals and gases produced by the burning of tobacco and its additives. Particulate matter condenses in the lungs to form a thick, brownish sludge called **tar,** which contains various carcinogenic agents, such as benzopyrene, and chemical irritants, such as phenol. Phenol has the potential to combine with other chemicals that contribute to developing lung cancer.

In healthy lungs, millions of tiny hairlike projections (*cilia*) on the surfaces lining the upper respiratory passages sweep away foreign matter, which is expelled from the lungs by coughing. However, the cilia's cleansing function is impaired in smokers' lungs by nicotine, which paralyzes the cilia for up to 1 hour following a single cigarette. This allows tars and other solids in tobacco smoke to accumulate and irritate sensitive lung tissue. Figure 12.3 illustrates how tobacco smoke damages the lungs.

| T A B L E 12.2 | What Exactly Are You Inhaling? |
|---|---|
| **Chemical in Tobacco Smoke** | **Where Else Can You Find It?** |
| Acetic acid | Vinegar |
| Acetone | Nail polish remover |
| Ammonia | Floor/toilet cleaner |
| Arsenic | Rat poison |
| Benzene | Gasoline |
| Beryllium | Industrial alloy |
| Butane | Lighter fluid |
| Cadmium | Rechargeable batteries |
| Carbon monoxide | Car exhaust |
| Chromium | Steel manufacture |
| DDT/dieldrin | Insecticides |
| Ethanol | Alcohol |
| Ethylene oxide | Sterilizer of medical devices |
| Formaldehyde | Embalming fluid, fabric preservative |
| Hexamine | Barbecue lighter |
| Hydrogen cyanide | Gas chamber poison, chemical weapons |
| Lead | Motor vehicle batteries, formerly in paint and gasoline |
| Mercury | Fluorescent lamps, electronics |
| Methane | Swamp gas, cow flatulence |
| Methanol | Rocket fuel |
| Naphthalene | Mothballs |
| Nickel | Steel manufacture and industrial alloys |
| Nicotine | Insecticide/addictive drug |
| Nitrobenzene | Gasoline additive |
| Nitrous oxide phenols | Disinfectant |
| Polonium-210 | Radioactive element |
| Polycyclic aromatic hydrocarbons | Coal tar |
| Stearic acid | Candle wax |
| Toluene | Industrial solvent, paint thinner |
| Vinyl chloride | Plastics manufacture |

**nicotine** The primary stimulant chemical in tobacco products; nicotine is highly addictive.

**tar** A thick, brownish substance condensed from particulate matter in smoked tobacco.

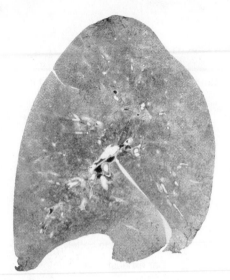

(a) A healthy lung

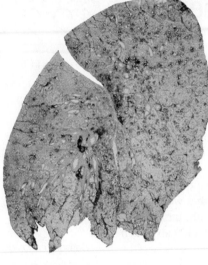

(b) A smoker's lung permeated with deposits of tar

FIGURE 12.3 **Lung Damage from Chemicals in Tobacco Smoke**
Smoke particles irritate lung pathways, causing extra production of mucus, and nicotine paralyzes the cilia that normally function to keep the lungs clear of excess mucus. The result is difficulty breathing, "smoker's cough," and chronic bronchitis. At the same time, tar collects within the alveoli (air sacs), ultimately causing their walls to break, leading to emphysema. Tar and other carcinogens in tobacco smoke also cause cellular mutations that lead to cancer.

Cigarette smoke also contains poisonous gases, the most dangerous of which is **carbon monoxide,** the deadly gas that comes out of exhaust pipes in cars. In the human body, carbon monoxide reduces the oxygen-carrying capacity of the red blood cells by binding with the receptor sites for oxygen; this causes oxygen deprivation in many body tissues. It is at least partly responsible for increased risk of heart attacks and strokes in smokers.

# what do you think?
Because nicotine is highly addictive, should it be regulated? ● How could tobacco be regulated effectively? ● Should more resources be used for research into nicotine addiction? Why or why not?

## Tobacco Products

Tobacco comes in several forms. Cigarettes, cigars, pipes and water pipes, and bidis are used for burning and inhaling tobacco. Smokeless tobacco is sniffed or placed in the mouth.

**Cigarettes** Cigarettes are the most common form of tobacco available today. Some people purchase loose tobacco and rolling papers to roll their own cigarettes, but most people buy manufactured cigarettes. Almost all manufactured cigarettes have filters that are designed to reduce levels of gases such as hydrogen cyanide and carbon monoxide. However, these filtered products may not be much better than their nonfiltered

**carbon monoxide** A gas found in cigarette smoke that binds at oxygen receptor sites in the blood.

counterparts. Filters themselves have chemical substances in them that may be inhaled. People who smoke filtered products may think they are protected and, therefore, take deeper "drags" or inhale more often, as may smokers using low-tar or low-nicotine products. Some even smoke more cigarettes, thinking they are "healthier." The truth is, no cigarette is healthy. How deeply you inhale, how close you smoke the cigarette down to the burning end, the ambient air in the room where you smoke, and a host of other factors may compound your risks.

*Clove cigarettes* contain about 40 percent ground cloves and 60 percent tobacco. Many users mistakenly believe that these products are made entirely of ground cloves and that smoking them eliminates the risks associated with tobacco. In fact, clove cigarettes contain higher levels of tar, nicotine, and carbon monoxide than do regular cigarettes—and the numbing effect of eugenol, an ingredient in cloves, allows smokers to inhale more deeply. The same effect is true of *menthol cigarettes:* The throat-numbing effect of the menthol allows for deeper inhalation. Menthol cigarettes also have higher carbon monoxide concentrations than do regular cigarettes.

**Cigars** Those big stogies that we see celebrities and government figures smoking are nothing more than tobacco fillers wrapped in more tobacco. Since 1993, cigar sales in the United States have increased dramatically, up nearly 124 percent between 1993 and 2007.[34] The fad, especially popular among young men and women, is fueled in part by the willingness of celebrities to be photographed puffing on a cigar. It's also fueled by the fact that cigars cost much less than cigarettes in most states. Also, among some women, cigar smoking symbolizes being slightly outrageous and liberated. According to a recent national survey, about 11 percent of Americans aged 18 to 25 had smoked a cigar in the past month.[35]

Many people believe that cigars are safer than cigarettes, when in fact the opposite is true. Cigar smoke contains 23 poisons and 43 carcinogens. Most cigars contain as much nicotine as several cigarettes, and when cigar smokers inhale, nicotine is absorbed as rapidly as it is with cigarettes. For those who don't inhale, nicotine is still absorbed through the mucous membranes in the mouth.

**Pipes and Hookahs** Pipes have had a long history of use throughout the world, including ritualistic and ceremonial usage for many cultures. Often thought to be safer than cigarettes or cigars, pipes are not risk-free options for those wanting to smoke. According to cumulative research by the

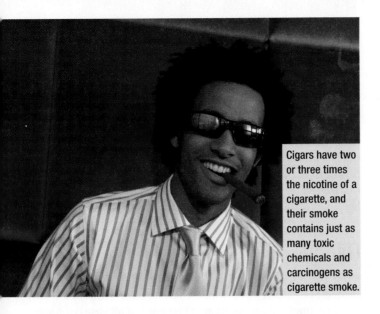

Cigars have two or three times the nicotine of a cigarette, and their smoke contains just as many toxic chemicals and carcinogens as cigarette smoke.

National Cancer Institute and the American Cancer Society, pipe smoking carries similar risks to cigar smoking. Of concern in recent years is the increasing prevalence, particularly among college students, of the use of "hookahs," or water pipes, as a newer, cooler way of smoking. Hookah smoking originated in the Middle East and involves burning flavored tobacco in a water pipe and inhaling the smoke through a long hose. Hookahs are marketed as a safe alternative to cigarettes because they reduce your risks from hazardous chemicals by filtering the smoke through water before you inhale. In fact, water pipes may cool the smoke; however, they do not eliminate or filter out harmful substances such as nicotine, carbon monoxide, or tar.[36] In addition to the health risks associated with all tobacco products, unique risks associated with hookah use include hygiene and sanitation concerns from sharing the pipe, and the possibility of infectious disease transmission.

**Bidis** Generally made in India or Southeast Asia, **bidis** are small, hand-rolled cigarettes that come in a variety of flavors, such as vanilla, chocolate, and cherry, and resemble a marijuana joint or a clove cigarette. They have become increasingly popular with college students, because they are viewed to be safer and cheaper than cigarettes. However, they are far more toxic than cigarettes. Smoke from a bidi contains three times more carbon monoxide and nicotine and five times more tar than cigarettes.[37] The leaf wrappers are nonporous, which means that smokers must suck harder to inhale and must inhale more to keep the bidi lit. This results in much more exposure to the higher amounts of tar, nicotine, and carbon monoxide. Bidis also lack any sort of filter. Bidi smoking increases the risk for oral cancer, lung cancer, stomach cancer, and esophageal cancer. It is also associated with emphysema and chronic bronchitis.[38]

**Smokeless Tobacco** An estimated 3 percent of adults in the United States use smokeless tobacco products.[39] In the most recent National College Health Assessment, about 8 per-

cent of college men and 1 percent of college women reported having used smokeless tobacco in the past 30 days.[40] Use of chewing tobacco by teenage boys, especially in rural areas, has increased by 30 percent in the past 10 years.[41] There are two types of smokeless tobacco: chewing tobacco and snuff.

**Chewing tobacco** comes in three forms—loose leaf, plug, or in a pouch—and contains tobacco leaves treated with molasses and other flavorings. The user "dips" the tobacco by placing a small amount between the lower lip and teeth to stimulate the flow of saliva and release the nicotine. **Dipping** rapidly releases nicotine into the bloodstream.

**Snuff** is a finely ground form of tobacco that can be inhaled, chewed, or placed against the gums. It comes in dry or moist powdered form or sachets (tea bag–like pouches). In 2009, "snus" became the latest form of smokeless tobacco to hit the market in the United States. Popular for more than 100 years in Sweden, these small sachets of tobacco are placed inside the cheek and sucked. Some people prefer snus to chewing tobacco because it doesn't require the user to spit frequently.

**bidis** Hand-rolled flavored cigarettes.
**chewing tobacco** A stringy type of tobacco that is placed in the mouth and then sucked or chewed.
**dipping** Placing a small amount of chewing tobacco between the front lip and teeth for rapid nicotine absorption.
**snuff** A powdered form of tobacco that is sniffed or absorbed through the mucous membranes in the nose or placed inside the cheek and sucked.

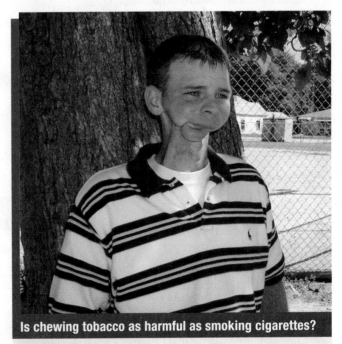

**Is chewing tobacco as harmful as smoking cigarettes?**

No matter in what form you use it—cigar, pipe, bidi, dip, snuff, or cigarette—tobacco is hazardous to your health. Chewing tobacco and snuff actually contain more nicotine than cigarettes and just as many toxic and carcinogenic chemicals. This young cancer survivor began using smokeless tobacco at age 13; by age 17, he was diagnosed with squamous cell carcinoma. He has undergone surgery to remove neck muscles, lymph nodes, and his tongue, and he now educates others about the dangers of chewing tobacco.

Smokeless tobacco is just as addictive as cigarettes and actually contains more nicotine—holding an average-sized dip or chew in the mouth for 30 minutes delivers as much nicotine as smoking four cigarettes. A two-can-a-week snuff user gets as much nicotine as a ten-pack-a-week smoker.

It is time to banish the notion the idea that smokeless tobacco is safe. All forms of oral tobacco have chemicals known to cause cancer. A pinch of smokeless tobacco exposes users to the same amount of dangerous chemicals as the smoke of five cigarettes. Smokeless tobacco causes an increase in heart rate, blood pressure, and epinephrine. There are also strong carcinogens in smokeless tobacco including nitrosamines, polycyclic aromatic hydrocarbons (PAHs), and radiation-emitting polonium.

## what do you think?

Should smokeless tobacco be banned in all venues that also ban smoking? ● What is attractive about using smokeless tobacco? ● Why do you think it is popular with many athletes and young men?

# Health Hazards of Tobacco Products

Cigarette smoking adversely affects the health of every person who smokes, as well as the health of everyone nearby. Each day, cigarettes contribute to more than 1,200 deaths from cancer, cardiovascular disease, and respiratory disorders.[42] In addition, tobacco use can negatively affect the health of almost every system in your body. Figure 12.4 summarizes some of the short-term physiological and long-term health effects of smoking.

## Cancer

Lung cancer is the leading cause of cancer deaths in the United States. The American Cancer Society estimates that tobacco smoking causes 85 to 90 percent of all cases of lung cancer and 87 percent of lung cancer deaths; fewer than 10 percent of cases occur among nonsmokers.[43] Figure 12.5

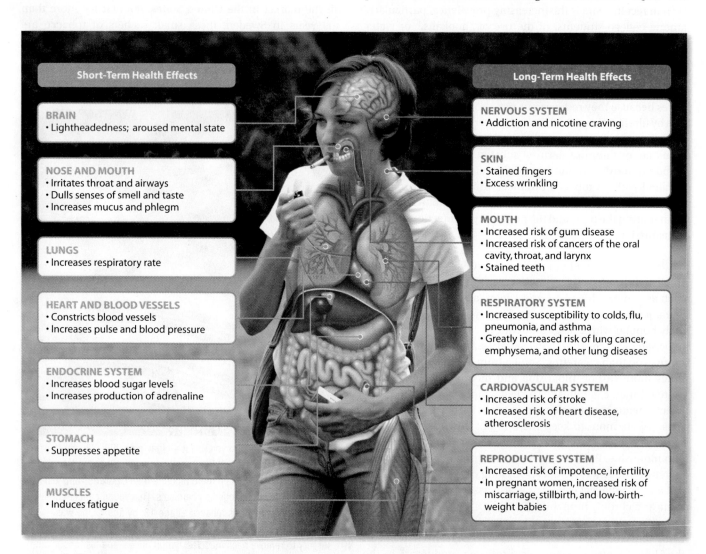

**Short-Term Health Effects**

**BRAIN**
• Lightheadedness; aroused mental state

**NOSE AND MOUTH**
• Irritates throat and airways
• Dulls senses of smell and taste
• Increases mucus and phlegm

**LUNGS**
• Increases respiratory rate

**HEART AND BLOOD VESSELS**
• Constricts blood vessels
• Increases pulse and blood pressure

**ENDOCRINE SYSTEM**
• Increases blood sugar levels
• Increases production of adrenaline

**STOMACH**
• Suppresses appetite

**MUSCLES**
• Induces fatigue

**Long-Term Health Effects**

**NERVOUS SYSTEM**
• Addiction and nicotine craving

**SKIN**
• Stained fingers
• Excess wrinkling

**MOUTH**
• Increased risk of gum disease
• Increased risk of cancers of the oral cavity, throat, and larynx
• Stained teeth

**RESPIRATORY SYSTEM**
• Increased susceptibility to colds, flu, pneumonia, and asthma
• Greatly increased risk of lung cancer, emphysema, and other lung diseases

**CARDIOVASCULAR SYSTEM**
• Increased risk of stroke
• Increased risk of heart disease, atherosclerosis

**REPRODUCTIVE SYSTEM**
• Increased risk of impotence, infertility
• In pregnant women, increased risk of miscarriage, stillbirth, and low-birth-weight babies

FIGURE 12.4 **Effects of Smoking on the Body and Health**

shows a correspondence between tobacco consumption rates in the United States and lung cancer death rates. There were an estimated 222,520 *new* cases of lung cancer in the United States in 2010 alone, and an estimated 157,300 Americans died from the disease in 2010.[44]

Lung cancer can take 10 to 30 years to develop, and the outlook for its victims is poor. Most lung cancer is not diagnosed until it is fairly widespread in the body; at that point, the 5-year survival rate is only 16 percent. When a malignancy is diagnosed and recognized while still localized, the 5-year survival rate rises to 53 percent.[45]

If you are a smoker, your risk of developing lung cancer depends on several factors. First, the amount you smoke per day is important. Someone who smokes two packs a day is 15 to 25 times more likely to develop lung cancer than a nonsmoker. Smoking as little as one cigar per day can double the risk of several cancers, including that of the oral cavity (lip, tongue, mouth, and throat), esophagus, larynx, and lungs. The risks increase with the number of cigars smoked per day.

## "Why Should I Care?"

If the life-threatening health consequences aren't enough to make you give up smoking, consider the negative impact smoking can have on your social (and romantic!) life. Popular media may make smoking seem glamorous and sexy, but in reality, smoking makes your breath, hair, and clothing smell bad; it causes your skin to age prematurely; it yellows your teeth; and it can interfere with a man's ability to achieve and maintain an erection.

A second factor is when you started smoking; if you started in your teens, you have a greater chance of developing lung cancer than people who start later. And a third risk factor is whether you inhale deeply when you smoke. Smokers are also more susceptible to the cancer-causing effects of exposure to other irritants, such as asbestos and radon, than are nonsmokers.

A major risk of chewing tobacco is **leukoplakia,** a condition characterized by leathery white patches inside the mouth that are produced by contact with irritants in tobacco juice. Three to 17 percent of diagnosed leukoplakia cases develop into oral cancer.[46]

An estimated 75 percent of the 36,540 new oral cancer cases in 2010 resulted from either smokeless tobacco or cigarettes.[47] Users of smokeless tobacco are 50 times more likely to develop oral cancers than are nonusers. Warning signs include lumps in the jaw or neck; color changes or lumps inside the lips; white, smooth, or scaly patches in the mouth or on the neck, lips, or tongue; a red spot or sore on the lips or gums or inside the mouth that does not heal in 2 weeks; repeated bleeding in the mouth; and difficulty or abnormality in speaking or swallowing.

The lag time between first use and contracting cancer is shorter for smokeless tobacco users than for smokers, because absorption through the gums is the most efficient route of nicotine administration. Many smokeless tobacco users eventually "graduate" to cigarettes and increase their risk for developing additional problems.

Tobacco is linked to other cancers as well. The rate of pancreatic cancer is more than twice as high for smokers as it is for nonsmokers. Typically, people diagnosed with pancreatic cancer live about 3 months after their diagnosis. Cancers of the lip, tongue, salivary glands, and esophagus are five times more likely to occur among smokers than among nonsmokers. Smokers are also more likely to develop kidney, bladder, and larynx cancers. A growing body of evidence suggests that long-term use of smokeless tobacco also increases the risk of cancer of the larynx, esophagus, nasal cavity, pancreas, kidney, and bladder.

**leukoplakia** A condition characterized by leathery white patches inside the mouth; produced by contact with irritants in tobacco juice.

**FIGURE** 12.5 **Tobacco Use in the United States, 1900–2006**
A dramatic rise in lung cancer death rates echoed the rise in popularity of cigarettes and other tobacco products in the last century. After tobacco use and smoking rates began to decline in the 1980s, the lung cancer death rates began to decline as well.

**Sources:** Death rates data from U.S. Mortality Files, National Center for Health Statistics, Centers for Disease Control and Prevention, 2010; Cigarette consumption data from U.S. Department of Agriculture, 1900–2006.

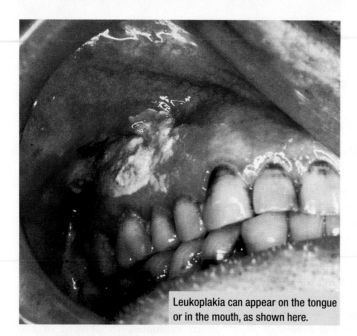
Leukoplakia can appear on the tongue or in the mouth, as shown here.

## Cardiovascular Disease

Over a third of all tobacco-related deaths occur from heart disease.[48] Smokers have a 70 percent higher death rate from heart disease than nonsmokers, and heavy smokers have a 200 percent higher death rate than moderate smokers. In fact, smoking cigarettes poses as great a risk for developing heart disease as high blood pressure and high cholesterol levels do. Daily cigar smoking, especially for people who inhale, also increases the risk of heart disease (cigar smokers double their risk of heart attack and stroke compared to nonsmokers) and chronic obstructive pulmonary disease (COPD; see Chapter 17).[49] Smoking contributes to heart disease by adding the equivalent of 10 years of aging to the arteries.[50] One explanation is that smoking and exposure to environmental tobacco smoke (ETS) encourages and accelerates the buildup of fatty deposits (plaque) in the heart and major blood vessels (*atherosclerosis*). Smokers can experience a 50 percent increase in plaque accumulation in the arteries, compared with ex-smokers. People regularly exposed to ETS can have a 20 percent increase in plaque buildup.[51] For unknown reasons, smoking decreases blood levels of high-density lipoproteins, the "good" cholesterol that helps protect against heart attacks.

**platelet adhesiveness** Stickiness of red blood cells associated with blood clots.

**emphysema** A chronic lung disease in which the tiny air sacs in the lungs are destroyed, making breathing difficult.

Smoking also contributes to **platelet adhesiveness,** where red blood cells stick together, and is associated with blood clots. The oxygen deprivation associated with smoking decreases the oxygen supplied to the heart and can weaken tissues. Smoking also contributes to irregular heart rhythms, which can trigger a heart attack. Both carbon monoxide and nicotine can precipitate angina attacks (pain spasms in the chest when the heart muscle does not get the blood supply it needs).

Smokers are twice as likely to suffer strokes as nonsmokers.[52] A stroke occurs when a small blood vessel in the brain bursts or is blocked by a blood clot, denying oxygen and nourishment to vital portions of the brain. Depending on the area of the brain affected, stroke can result in paralysis, loss of mental functioning, or death. Smoking contributes to strokes by raising blood pressure, which increases the stress on vessel walls. Platelet adhesiveness contributes to blood clot formation.

The number of years a person has smoked does not seem to bear much relation to cardiovascular risk. If a person quits smoking, the risk of dying from a heart attack falls by half after only 1 year without smoking and declines steadily thereafter. After about 15 years without smoking, the ex-smoker's risk of cardiovascular disease and stroke is similar to that of people who have never smoked.[53]

## Respiratory Disorders

Smoking quickly impairs the respiratory system. Smokers can feel its impact in a relatively short period of time—they are more prone to breathlessness, chronic cough, and excess phlegm production than are nonsmokers their age. Also, smokers tend to miss work one-third more often than nonsmokers do, primarily because of respiratory diseases. Over time, cumulative lung damage can lead to COPD, including chronic bronchitis and emphysema. Ultimately, smokers are up to 18 times more likely to die of lung disease than are nonsmokers.[54]

*Chronic bronchitis* may develop in smokers, because their inflamed lungs produce more mucus, which they constantly try to expel along with foreign particles. This results in the persistent cough known as "smoker's hack." Smokers are also more prone than nonsmokers to respiratory ailments such as influenza, pneumonia, and colds.

**Emphysema** is a chronic disease in which the alveoli (the tiny air sacs in the lungs) are destroyed, impairing the lungs' ability to obtain oxygen and remove carbon dioxide. As a result, breathing becomes difficult. Whereas healthy people expend only about 5 percent of their energy in breathing, people with advanced emphysema expend nearly 80 percent. Because the heart has to work harder to do even the simplest tasks, it may become enlarged and death from heart damage may result. There is no known cure for emphysema, and the damage is irreversible. Approximately 80 percent of all cases of emphysema are related to cigarette smoking.[55]

## Sexual Dysfunction and Fertility Problems

Despite tobacco advertisers' attempts to make smoking appear sexy, research shows just the opposite: It can cause impotence in men. Several studies have found that male smokers are about two times more likely than nonsmokers to suffer from some form of impotence.[56] Toxins in cigarette smoke damage blood vessels, reducing blood flow to the penis and leading to an inadequate erection. Impotence may indicate oncoming cardiovascular disease.

In women, smoking can lead to infertility and problems with pregnancy. Women who smoke increase their risk for infertility, ectopic pregnancy, spontaneous abortion, and stillbirth. They also increase their baby's risk of sudden infant death syndrome and its chances of being born with a cleft lip or cleft palate.[57] Smoking during pregnancy accounts for approximately 30 percent of premature births, and increases the risk of low birth weight (less than 5.5 pounds), which in turn increases babies' likelihood of illness or death.[58]

## what do you think?

Most smokers are very aware of the long-term hazards of tobacco use, yet they continue to smoke. Why do you think this is? ● What strategies might be effective to reduce the number of people who begin smoking?

## Other Health Effects

Dental problems are common among users of both smokeless tobacco and cigarettes. Contact with tobacco juice causes receding gums, tooth decay, bad breath, and discolored teeth. Damage to both the teeth and jawbone can contribute to early loss of teeth among smokeless tobacco users. Gum disease is three times more common among smokers than among nonsmokers, and smokers lose significantly more teeth.[59]

Nicotine and other ingredients in tobacco smoke can interfere with the body's metabolism of certain drugs. In particular, nicotine speeds up the process by which the body uses and eliminates drugs, making medications less effective for smokers. In addition, recent research suggests that heavy smokers might be accelerating damage to the brain, which could lead to Alzheimer's disease.[60]

# Environmental Tobacco Smoke

Although fewer than 30 percent of Americans smoke, air pollution from smoking in public places continues to be a problem. **Environmental tobacco smoke (ETS),** also known as *secondhand smoke,* is divided into two categories: **mainstream smoke** (smoke exhaled by a smoker) and **sidestream smoke** (smoke from a burning cigarette, pipe, or cigar).[61] People who breathe smoke from someone else's smoking product are said to be *involuntary,* or *passive,* smokers. Since the 1986 Surgeon General's report, *The Health Consequences of Involuntary Smoking,* detectable levels of nicotine exposure in nonsmoking Americans has decreased 44 percent. The decrease in exposure to secondhand smoke is due to the growing number of laws that ban smoking in work and public places.[62]

Children are more heavily exposed to ETS than adults. Almost 60 percent of U.S. children aged 3 to 11 years—or 22 million children—are exposed to ETS.[63] Disparities in ETS also occur along ethnic and racial lines and according to income level. African Americans have been found to have higher levels of exposure to ETS than whites and Hispanics. Environmental tobacco smoke exposure is also higher for low-income persons.[64]

## Risks from Environmental Tobacco Smoke

Although involuntary smokers breathe less tobacco than active smokers do, they still face risks from exposure. Secondhand smoke actually contains more carcinogenic substances than the smoke that a smoker inhales; it has about 2 times more tar and nicotine, 5 times more carbon monoxide, and 50 times more ammonia than mainstream smoke. Every year, ETS is estimated to be responsible for approximately 3,400 lung cancer deaths in nonsmoking adults, 46,000 coronary and heart disease deaths in nonsmoking adults who live with smokers, and 430 deaths in newborns from sudden infant death syndrome.[65]

The Environmental Protection Agency (EPA) has designated secondhand smoke as a known carcinogen (group A carcinogen). According to the Surgeon General's *The Health Consequences of Involuntary Exposure to Tobacco Smoke,* there are more than 50 cancer-causing agents found in secondhand smoke.[66] The most likely mechanism whereby secondhand smoke causes lung cancer is continuous exposure to the carcinogens over time. There is also strong evidence that secondhand smoke interferes with normal functioning of the heart, blood, and vascular systems, significantly increasing the risk for heart disease and having immediate effects on the cardiovascular system. Studies indicate that nonsmokers exposed to secondhand smoke were 20 to 30 percent more likely to have coronary heart disease than nonsmokers not exposed to smoke.[67] The **Be Healthy, Be Green** box on page 392 discusses some of the measures being taken to address the problem of ETS, as well as steps you can take to protect yourself and others from its hazards.

**environmental tobacco smoke (ETS)** Smoke from tobacco products, including sidestream and mainstream smoke; commonly called *secondhand smoke.*
**mainstream smoke** Smoke that is drawn through tobacco while inhaling.
**sidestream smoke** The cigarette, pipe, or cigar smoke breathed by nonsmokers.

**Children and ETS** Exposure to ETS increases children's risk of lower respiratory tract infections. Consequently, there are an estimated 150,000 to 300,000 new cases of bronchitis and pneumonia diagnosed in children each year.[68] In addition, children exposed to secondhand smoke have a greater chance of developing other respiratory problems such as coughing, wheezing, asthma, and chest colds, along with a decrease in lung function. The greatest effects of secondhand smoke are seen in children under the age of 5. Children exposed to secondhand smoke daily in the home miss 33 percent more school days and have 10 percent more

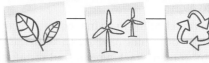
## Clear the Air!

What's the primary cause of indoor air pollution? Environmental tobacco smoke, or secondhand smoke. From irritating allergies to contributing to heart disease, tobacco smoke in the environment causes problems for all who encounter it, in effect making everyone who comes in contact with it an involuntary or passive smoker. Efforts to reduce the hazards associated with secondhand smoke have gained momentum in recent years. The Surgeon General has concluded that smoke-free policies are the only effective way to eliminate secondhand smoke exposure in the workplace—separating smokers from nonsmokers, cleaning the air, and ventilating buildings are not enough to eliminate exposure. Groups such as Action on Smoking and Health (ASH) and Americans for Nonsmokers' Rights (ANR) have been working since the early 1970s to reduce smoking in public places, both indoors and out. As a result of their efforts, 17,628 municipalities across the United States are covered by a 100 percent smoke-free provision in workplaces, and/or restaurants, and/or bars, by either a state, commonwealth, or local law, representing 74.2 percent of the U.S. population. To break this down further:

✱ 38 states, along with the District of Columbia, have laws in effect that require 100 percent smoke-free workplaces and/or restaurants and/or bars.
✱ 25 states, Puerto Rico, and the District of Columbia have a law in effect that requires restaurants and bars to be 100 percent smoke free. These laws, along with local laws, protect 57.1 percent of the U.S. population.
✱ 19 states, Puerto Rico, and the District of Columbia have a law in effect that requires workplaces, restaurants, and bars to be 100 percent smoke free. These laws, along with local laws, protect 41 percent of the U.S. population.

In addition to government bans on smoking, the hospitality industry has also taken steps to protect the health of nonsmokers. Hotels and motels set aside rooms for nonsmokers, and many hotels are now 100 percent smoke free. Car rental agencies designate certain vehicles for nonsmokers. Smoking is banned on all U.S. airlines, and many other countries ban smoking on their airlines as well. Many other organizations and facilities, including colleges and universities, have rules in effect banning smoking in all public places.

Do you know the smoke-free policies of your school, your town, and your state? You can take steps to protect yourself and your loved ones from secondhand smoke by finding out about these policies and advocating for change. The ANR provides information about smoking-free communities across the United States on its website, www.no-smoke.org, as well as tips for taking action to ban smoking in your home, workplace, or in other public places you frequent.

If you are a smoker, the single best way to protect your family and others from secondhand smoke is to quit smoking. In the meantime, you can protect your family and friends by making your home and vehicles smoke free and smoking only outside. A smoke-free home rule can also help you quit smoking.

If you live in a multiunit building and you are encountering secondhand smoke in your home, speak to the management about enacting smoke-free policies. Property owners, be they landlords, corporations, or educational institutions, have the right to ban smoking on their property. Smokers are not a protected class: It is not discrimination to prohibit smoking; there is no legal "right to smoke."

Business owners have the right to ban smoking on their premises as well, so talk to your boss about enacting a smoke-free policy if you are encountering secondhand smoke in your workplace. Make sure that

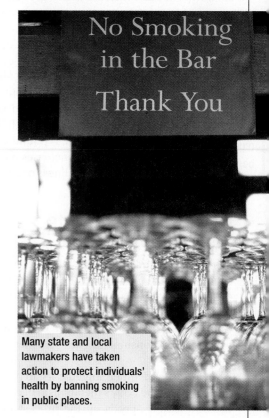

No Smoking in the Bar Thank You

Many state and local lawmakers have taken action to protect individuals' health by banning smoking in public places.

your children's day care center or school is also smoke free and teach your children to avoid secondhand smoke in general. Let business owners who allow smoking know that secondhand smoke is harmful to your health and the health of others, and that the presence of smoke on their premises is preventing you from patronizing them. Even if you are uncomfortable approaching business owners about their policies, you can encourage change simply by choosing to patronize only smoke-free businesses, and by thanking them for being smoke free.

**Sources:** American Nonsmokers' Rights Foundation, "Overview List: How Many Smokefree Laws?" 2010, www.no-smoke.org/pdf/mediaordlist.pdf; Office on Smoking and Health, *The Health Consequences of Involuntary Exposure to Tobacco Smoke: A Report of the Surgeon General—Executive Summary* (Washington, DC: U.S. Department of Health and Human Services, 2006).

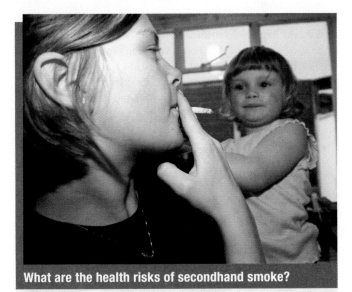

**What are the health risks of secondhand smoke?**

Every year, ETS is estimated to be responsible for approximately 3,400 lung cancer deaths in nonsmoking adults, 46,000 coronary and heart disease deaths in nonsmoking adults who live with smokers, and 430 deaths in newborns from sudden infant death syndrome. Because their bodies and brains are still developing, babies and children are particularly vulnerable to the toxins in secondhand smoke: It can cause respiratory problems, including lower respiratory infections and increased frequency and severity of asthma attacks, as well as other health concerns, such as greater risk of ear infections.

colds and acute respiratory infections than those not exposed.[69]

Secondhand smoke affects not only children's physical health, but also their cognitive abilities and academic success. One study found that children exposed to high levels of secondhand smoke had lower standardized test scores in reading, math, and problem solving.[70] In addition, children exposed to secondhand smoke are twice as likely to become smokers during adolescence than children who are not exposed.[71]

## what do you think?

What rights, if any, should smokers have regarding smoking in public places? ● Does your campus allow smoking in residence halls? ● Does your community have completely nonsmoking restaurants or does it have only designated nonsmoking sections in restaurants? ● Do you think your community would support smoke-free restaurants and bars? Why or why not?

**ETS and Additional Health Problems** Cigarette, cigar, and pipe smoke in enclosed areas presents other hazards. Environmental tobacco smoke can cause allergic reactions such as itchy eyes, difficulty in breathing, painful headaches, nausea, and dizziness in response to minute amounts of smoke. Environmental tobacco smoke may also increase the risk of breast cancer in women; cancer of the nasal sinus cavity and of the pharynx in adults; and leukemia, lymphoma, and

brain tumors in children.[72] The level of carbon monoxide in cigarette smoke contained in enclosed places is 4,000 times higher than that allowed in the clean-air standard recommended by the EPA.

# Tobacco Use Prevention Policies

It has been more than 40 years since the government began warning that tobacco use was hazardous to the nation's health. In an effort to recoup state expenditures on health care costs related to treating smokers, 46 states sued the tobacco industry.[73] In 1998, the tobacco industry reached a master's settlement agreement with 40 states. The agreement requires tobacco companies to pay approximately $206 billion over 25 years nationwide. The agreement also includes a variety of measures to support antismoking education and advertising and to fund research to determine effective smoking-cessation strategies. The agreement also curbs tobacco industry billboard advertising and promotions and advertising that appeal to youth (including

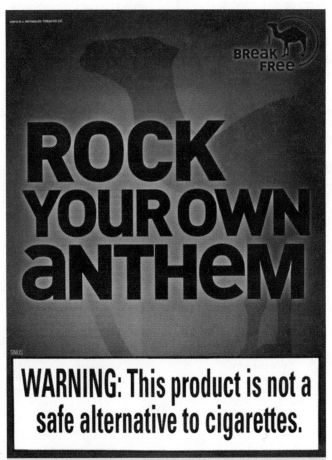

The Family Smoking Prevention and Tobacco Control Act requires that smokeless tobacco ads, such as this full-page magazine ad for Snus, now must contain a warning that fills 20 percent of the advertising space.

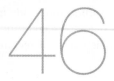**46** states have sued tobacco companies to recover health care costs related to treating smokers.

merchandise samples and using cartoon characters in ads). Faced with the settlement restrictions and strong opposition from antismoking organizations, the tobacco companies have been struggling to improve their image.

Unfortunately, most of the money designated for tobacco control and prevention at the state level has not been used for this purpose. Facing budget woes, many states have drastically cut spending on antismoking programs. In the few states that have spent the settlement money on smoking-cessation programs, there has been some reported success in decreasing cigarette use.[74] The Family Smoking Prevention and Tobacco Control Act signed into law in 2009 allows the U.S. Food and Drug Administration (FDA) to forbid advertising geared toward children, to lower the amount of nicotine in tobacco products, to ban sweetened cigarettes that appeal to young people, and to prohibit labels such as "light" and "low tar."[75] One of the most significant impacts of the law is that it requires more prominent health warnings on advertising of tobacco products. Beginning June 22, 2010, smokeless tobacco ads now must contain a warning that

fills 20 percent of the advertising space. Cigarette packages and advertising are required to have bigger, stronger warnings as of June 22, 2011. These warnings must cover the top half of the front and back of each package and include "color graphics depicting the negative health consequences of smoking." The graphics are to be modeled on ads in Canada, Australia, and New Zealand, showing cancers, lung disease, and other damaging effects of using these products.

# Quitting

Approximately 70 percent of adult smokers in the United States want to quit smoking, and up to 44 percent make a serious attempt to quit each year. However, only somewhere between 4 and 7 percent succeed.[76] Quitting smoking isn't easy. Smokers must break the physical addiction to nicotine and the psychological habit of lighting up at certain times of the day. (See the **Assess Yourself** box on page 400 to determine whether you are dependent on tobacco.) From what we know about successful quitters, quitting is often a lengthy process involving several unsuccessful attempts before success is finally achieved. Even successful quitters suffer occasional slips, which emphasizes the fact that quitting is a dynamic process that occurs over time.

## Benefits of Quitting

According to the American Cancer Society, many tissues damaged by smoking can repair themselves. As soon as smokers stop, the body begins the repair process (see Figure 12.6). Within 8 hours, carbon monoxide and oxygen levels return to normal, and "smoker's breath" disappears. Often,

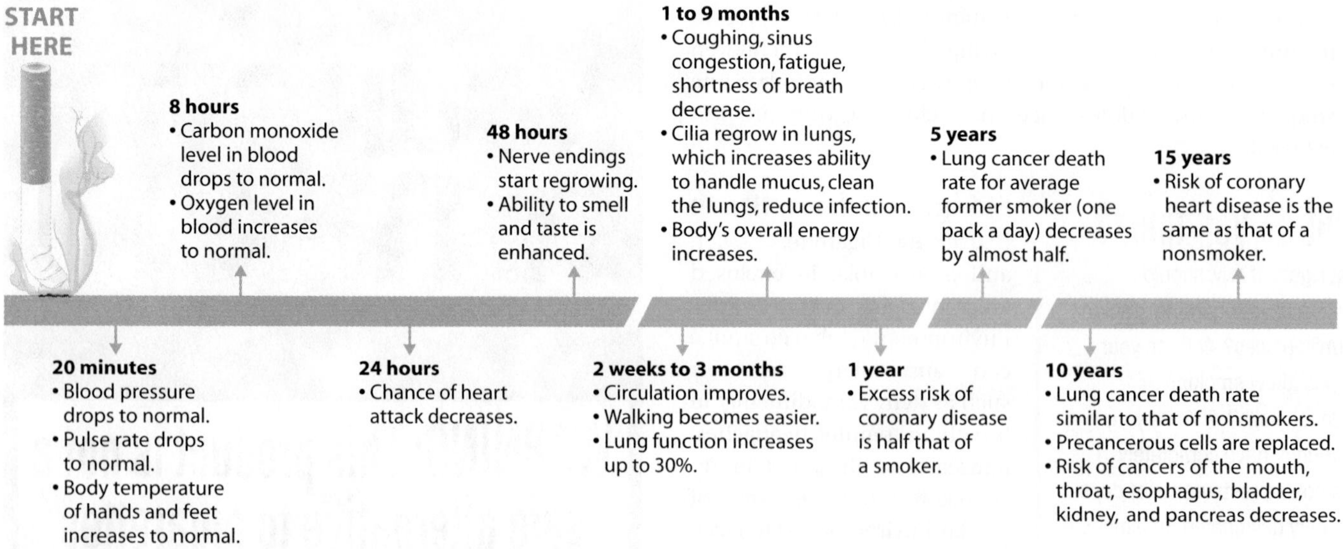

**what do you think?**

Consider that smokers make their own choice to start smoking. Is it fair to blame tobacco companies if smokers develop tobacco-related health problems? ● What is a tobacco company's ethical obligation to society? ● Should it be different from the ethical obligations of companies in other industries?

**START HERE**

**8 hours**
• Carbon monoxide level in blood drops to normal.
• Oxygen level in blood increases to normal.

**48 hours**
• Nerve endings start regrowing.
• Ability to smell and taste is enhanced.

**1 to 9 months**
• Coughing, sinus congestion, fatigue, shortness of breath decrease.
• Cilia regrow in lungs, which increases ability to handle mucus, clean the lungs, reduce infection.
• Body's overall energy increases.

**5 years**
• Lung cancer death rate for average former smoker (one pack a day) decreases by almost half.

**15 years**
• Risk of coronary heart disease is the same as that of a nonsmoker.

**20 minutes**
• Blood pressure drops to normal.
• Pulse rate drops to normal.
• Body temperature of hands and feet increases to normal.

**24 hours**
• Chance of heart attack decreases.

**2 weeks to 3 months**
• Circulation improves.
• Walking becomes easier.
• Lung function increases up to 30%.

**1 year**
• Excess risk of coronary disease is half that of a smoker.

**10 years**
• Lung cancer death rate similar to that of nonsmokers.
• Precancerous cells are replaced.
• Risk of cancers of the mouth, throat, esophagus, bladder, kidney, and pancreas decreases.

FIGURE 12.6 **When Smokers Quit**
Within 20 minutes of smoking that last cigarette, the body begins a series of changes that continues for years. However, by smoking just one cigarette a day, the smoker loses all of these benefits of quitting smoking, according to the American Cancer Society.

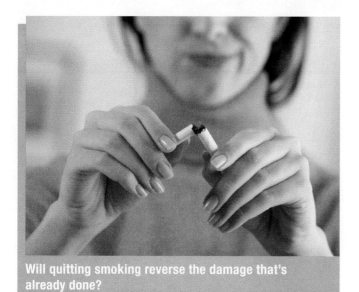

**Will quitting smoking reverse the damage that's already done?**

Quitting smoking is a challenging task to undertake, and you may be wondering whether the effort to quit will result in long-term health benefits. The answer is a definite yes. Tobacco causes serious injury to your heart and lungs, but when you quit using it, your body immediately starts to recover and to repair the damage. Over time, the body's repair processes reduce the former smoker's risks of heart disease and cancer; after 10 years, heart disease and lung cancer risks are comparable to those of nonsmokers.

within a month of quitting, the mucus that clogs airways is broken up and eliminated. Circulation and the senses of taste and smell improve within weeks. Many ex-smokers say they have more energy, sleep better, and feel more alert.

After 1 year of not smoking, the risk for lung cancer and stroke decreases. Ex-smokers considerably reduce their chances of developing cancers of the mouth, throat, esophagus, larynx, pancreas, bladder, and cervix. They also cut their risk of peripheral artery disease, COPD, coronary heart disease, and ulcers. Women are less likely to bear babies of low birth weight. Within 2 years, the risk for heart attack drops to near normal. At the end of 10 smoke-free years, ex-smokers can expect to live out their normal life span.

Another significant benefit of quitting smoking is the money saved. A pack of cigarettes averages $5.28, including taxes. Using this number, a pack-a-day smoker burns through about $36.96 per week, or $1,921.92 per year. That is money that could otherwise have gone toward a car payment or a much-earned vacation over spring break. It is estimated that a 40-year-old who quits smoking and puts the savings into a 401(k) earning 9 percent a year would have approximately $250,000 by age 70.

## How Can You Quit?

Those who wish to quit smoking have several options. Many people who are successful at quitting do so "cold turkey"—that is, they simply decide not to smoke again. Others choose

short-term programs, such as those offered by the American Cancer Society, which are based on behavior modification and a system of self-rewards. Still others turn to treatment centers that are part of large franchises, to a community outreach plan sponsored by a local medical clinic, or to a telephone quit line. Finally, some people work privately with their physicians to reach their goal.

Prospective quitters must decide which method or combination of methods will work best for them. Programs that combine several approaches have shown the most promise. Financial considerations, personality characteristics, and level of addiction are all factors to consider.

## Breaking the Nicotine Addiction

Nicotine addiction may be one of the toughest addictions to overcome. Symptoms of **nicotine withdrawal** include irritability, restlessness, nausea, vomiting, and intense cravings for tobacco (see Table 12.3 on page 396). The evidence is strong that consistent pharmacological treatments can help a smoker quit: An estimated 25 to 33 percent of people who have used nicotine replacement therapy or smoking-cessation medications continue to abstain from cigarettes for over 6 months.[77]

> **nicotine withdrawal** Symptoms, including nausea, headaches, irritability, and intense tobacco cravings, suffered by addicted smokers who stop using tobacco.

**Nicotine Replacement Products** Nontobacco products that replace depleted levels of nicotine in the bloodstream have helped some people stop using tobacco. The two most common are nicotine chewing gum and the nicotine patch, both of which are available over the counter. The FDA has also approved nicotine lozenges, a nicotine nasal spray, and a nicotine inhaler.

Nicotine gum is available without a prescription. The user chews up to 20 pieces of gum a day for 1 to 3 months. Nicotine gum delivers about as much nicotine as a cigarette does, but because it is absorbed through the mucous membrane of the mouth, it doesn't produce the same rush. Users experience no withdrawal symptoms and fewer cravings for nicotine as the dosage is reduced until they are completely weaned.

Nicotine-containing lozenges are the newest form of nicotine-replacement therapy on the market. Lozenges are available over the counter and, as with nicotine gum, come in two strengths: 2 mg and 4 mg. The manufacturer recommends a 12-week program of lozenge use that allows the user to taper off the drug.

The nicotine patch is generally used in conjunction with a comprehensive smoking-behavior cessation program. A small, thin patch placed on the smoker's upper body delivers a continuous flow of nicotine through the skin, helping to relieve cravings. Patches can be bought with or without a prescription and are available in different dosages. The FDA recommends using the patch for a total of 3 to 5 months. During this time, the dose of nicotine is gradually reduced until the smoker is fully weaned from the drug. Occasional side effects include mild skin irritation, insomnia, dry mouth, and

| Symptom | Reason | Duration | Relief |
|---|---|---|---|
| Coughing, dry throat, nasal drip | Body is getting rid of mucus. | A few days to several weeks | Drink plenty of fluids; use cough drops. |
| Bad breath | Nicotine absorption in tissues. | 1–2 weeks | Brush teeth frequently; use mouthwash; drink plenty of water. |
| Stomach pain, nausea, constipation | Intestinal movement decreases. | 1–2 weeks | Drink fluids; add fiber to the diet (fruits, vegetables, and whole grains). |
| Inability to concentrate | Nicotine increases concentration. | 1–2 weeks | Get enough sleep; exercise and eat well. |
| Headaches | Brain is getting more oxygen. | 1–2 weeks | Drink plenty of water. |
| Dizziness | Brain is getting more oxygen. | 1–2 days | Move slowly; be intentional with your movements. |
| Irritability | Body craves nicotine. | 2–4 weeks | Take walks; practice relaxation techniques; take hot baths. |
| Trouble sleeping | Nicotine is a powerful stimulant. | 2–4 weeks | Don't consume caffeine after 6 PM. Take a warm bath. Listen to soothing music. |
| Hunger | Nicotine craving can feel like hunger. | Several weeks | Drink water or low-calorie drinks; eat low-calorie snacks. |
| Craving for a cigarette | Withdrawal from nicotine. | Several months | Distract yourself; exercise; use relaxation techniques. |

**Source:** Healthways' Quitnet, www.quitnet.com. Used with permission.

nervousness. The patch costs less than a pack of cigarettes—about $4—and some insurance plans will pay for it.

The nasal spray, which requires a prescription, is much more powerful and delivers nicotine to the bloodstream faster than gum or the patch. Patients are warned to be careful not to overdose; as little as 40 mg of nicotine taken at once could be lethal. The FDA has advised that it should be used for no more than 3 months and never for more than 6 months, so that smokers don't find themselves as dependent on nicotine in spray form as they were on cigarettes. The FDA also advises that no one who experiences nasal or sinus problems, allergies, or asthma should use it.

The nicotine inhaler, which also requires a prescription, consists of a mouthpiece and cartridge. By puffing on the mouthpiece, the smoker inhales air saturated with nicotine, which is absorbed through the lining of the mouth, not the lungs. This nicotine enters the body much more slowly than the nicotine in cigarettes does. Using the inhaler mimics the hand-to-mouth actions used in smoking and causes the back of the throat to feel as it would when inhaling tobacco smoke.

**Smoking-Cessation Medications** Although the patch, gum, lozenges, nasal spray, and inhaler all serve to replace nicotine in the system, some smoking-cessation aids are aimed at reducing withdrawal symptoms and decreasing craving for nicotine. In 1997, the FDA approved buproprion, an antidepressant, for use as a smoking-cessation aid. The drug, sold under the brand name Zyban, is thought to work on dopamine and norepinephrine receptors in the brain to decrease craving and withdrawal symptoms. Because of the way this prescription medication works, it is important to start the pills 1 to 2 weeks before the targeted quit date; it requires planning ahead.

Chantix (generic name varenicline) is the newest prescription smoking-cessation drug on the market. Approved by the FDA in March 2006, this drug works in two specific ways: It reduces nicotine cravings and the urge to smoke, and it blocks the effects of nicotine at nicotine receptor sites in the brain.

A radical new way to help smokers quit is NicVAX, an antismoking vaccine due out on the market soon. The vaccination is intended to prevent nicotine from reaching the brain, making smoking less pleasurable and therefore easier to give up. A small amount that may reach the brain eases the discomfort of withdrawal. One of the advantages of the vaccine over other cessation methods is that it will reduce relapses by making the cigarette much less enjoyable when the quitter tries one again. Early clinical trial results report that twice as many people given the vaccine had quit smoking as those given the placebo.[78] See Table 12.4 for a summary

TABLE

12.4

## Recommended Therapies for Smoking Cessation

| Therapy | Duration |
|---|---|
| **Buproprion (Zyban)**<br><br>A non-nicotine-based antidepressant that helps reduce nicotine withdrawal symptoms and the urge to smoke. Common side effects are dry mouth, difficulty sleeping, dizziness, and skin rash. Contraindicated if smoker has a history of seizures.<br><br>*Availability:* Prescription only with a doctor consultation | 7–12 weeks; maintenance up to 6 months; start 1–2 weeks before the quit date  |
| **Varenicline (Chantix)**<br><br>A non-nicotine-based prescription medicine developed for the sole purpose of helping people stop smoking. Interferes with nicotine receptors in the brain to lessen the pleasurable physical effects from smoking and to reduce symptoms of nicotine withdrawal. Usually well tolerated, but reported side effects have included headaches, nausea, vomiting, difficulty sleeping, flatulence, changes in taste, and depressed mood.<br><br>*Availability:* Prescription only with a doctor consultation | 12 weeks; maintenance of 12 weeks after successfully quitting; start 1–2 weeks in advance 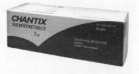 |
| **Nicotine Gum**<br><br>A chewing gum that releases nicotine into the bloodstream through the lining of the mouth; might not be appropriate for people with temporomandibular joint disease or those with dentures or other dental work. Up to 2 mg dose if less than 25 cigarettes/day; 4 mg dose if more than 25 cigarettes/day.<br><br>*Availability:* Over the counter (OTC) | Up to 12 weeks 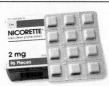 |
| **Nicotine Lozenges**<br><br>The lozenges are available in 2 strengths as part of a 12-week program. Doses can be regularly lowered as treatment progresses. Users should not eat or drink 15 minutes before using lozenges.<br><br>*Availability:* OTC | The recommended dose is one lozenge every 1–2 hours for 6 weeks, then one lozenge every 2–4 hours for weeks 7–9, and one lozenge every 4–8 hours for weeks 10–12 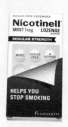 |
| **Nicotine Patch**<br><br>Patch supplies a steady amount of nicotine to the body through the skin. Is sold in varying strengths as an 8-week smoking-cessation treatment. Doses can be regularly lowered as treatment progresses or given as a steady dose during treatment. May not be a good choice for people with skin problems or allergies to adhesive tape.<br><br>*Availability:* Either OTC or by prescription with a doctor consultation | 4 weeks; then 2 weeks; then 2 weeks (8 weeks total)  |
| **Nicotine Nasal Spray**<br><br>Comes in a pump bottle containing nicotine that tobacco users can inhale when they have an urge to smoke. Not recommended for people with nasal or sinus conditions, allergies, or asthma, or for young tobacco users.<br><br>*Availability:* Prescription only with a doctor consultation | 3–6 months  |
| **Nicotine Inhaler**<br><br>This device delivers a vaporized form of nicotine to the mouth through a mouthpiece attached to a plastic cartridge. Nicotine travels to the mouth and throat and is absorbed through the mucous membranes. Common side effects include throat and mouth irritation and coughing. Anyone with bronchial problems should use caution.<br><br>*Availability:* Prescription only with a doctor consultation | Up to 6 months 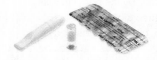 |

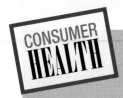
# ALTERNATIVE TOBACCO-USE CESSATION METHODS: ARE THEY EFFECTIVE?

In addition to nicotine-replacement therapies and other smoking-cessation drugs, there are many complementary and alternative methods that may also help some people stop smoking. Although there is no strong scientific evidence that the following can improve your chances of quitting, they are worth mentioning for people seeking alternative cessation methods.

**✱ Hypnosis.** Hypnosis methods vary a great deal, which makes hypnosis hard to study as a smoking-cessation method. For the most part, reviews that looked at studies of hypnosis to help people quit smoking have not supported it as a quitting method that works. Still, some people find it useful to work with a hypnotherapist.

**✱ Acupuncture.** Acupuncture, the traditional Chinese medical practice of stimulating anatomical points through the precise placement of needles, has been used by people to quit smoking, but there is little evidence to show that it works. Acupuncture for smoking cessation is usually done on certain parts of the ears.

**✱ Low-level laser therapy.** This technique, also called cold laser therapy, is related to acupuncture. The laser beams are used instead of needles to stimulate the body's acupuncture points. The treatment is supposed to relax the smoker and release endorphins (pain-relief substances that are made naturally by the body) to mimic the effects of nicotine in the brain, or balance the body's energy to relieve the addiction.

Despite claims of success by some cold laser therapy providers, there is no scientific evidence that shows this helps people to stop smoking. In addition, the lasers used for this therapy vary in intensity and output, so it's difficult to know whether you are receiving the intended treatment.

**✱ Filters.** Filters that reduce tar and nicotine in cigarettes do not work in helping people quit smoking. In fact, studies have shown that smokers who use filters tend to smoke more.

**✱ Herbs and supplements.** There is little scientific evidence to support the use of homeopathic aids and herbal or dietary supplements as stop-smoking methods. Because they are marketed as dietary supplements (not drugs), they don't need approval by the U.S. Food and Drug Administration (FDA) to be sold. The manufacturers don't have to prove they work, or even that they're safe. Be sure to look closely at the label of any product that claims it can help you stop smoking. These products usually contain a combination of herbs, but not nicotine.

**✱ Atropine and scopolamine combination therapy.** A few smoking-cessation clinics offer a program using shots of the drugs atropine and scopolamine, sometimes along with other drugs, to help reduce nicotine withdrawal symptoms. These drugs block the action of acetylcholine, a signal transmitter in the nervous system. Called anticholinergics, these drugs are FDA-approved for

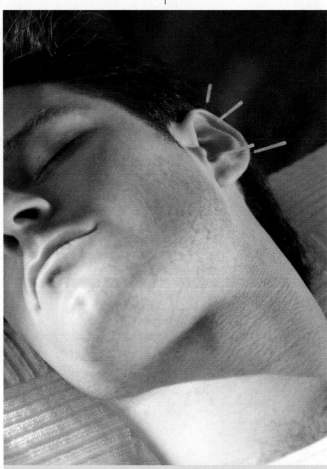

Acupuncture is one of several alternative therapies sometimes used to aid in smoking cessation.

other uses, such as digestive problems, motion sickness, or Parkinson's disease, and have not been formally studied or approved for help in quitting smoking. Smoking-cessation treatment with these drugs usually involves shots given in the clinic on one day, then a few weeks of taking pills and wearing a patch behind the ear. (People who are pregnant, or have heart problems, glaucoma, or uncontrolled high blood pressure are not allowed to take part in these programs.) Other drugs may

be needed to help with side effects. Side effects of this treatment can include dizziness, constipation, dry mouth, changes in the sense of taste and smell, problems urinating, and blurry vision. Some clinics claim high success rates, but the available published scientific research does not back up these claims.

**Source:** Adapted from "Guide to Quitting Smoking: Other Methods of Quitting." Reprinted by the permission of the American Cancer Society, Inc. from www.cancer.org. All rights reserved.

of information about recommended smoking-cessation therapies.

In addition to the medications and methods described above, there are numerous alternative methods for quitting smoking. Unlike the strategies previously discussed, these alternative tobacco-use cessation methods have not been scientifically proven to be effective. However, anything that may help a smoker to quit is beneficial, so some of these methods are discussed in the **Consumer Health** box at left.

## Breaking the Smoking Habit

For some smokers, the road to quitting includes antismoking therapy. Two common techniques are operant conditioning and self-control therapy. Pairing the act of smoking with an external stimulus is a typical example of an operant strategy. For example, one technique requires smokers to carry a timer that sounds a buzzer at different intervals. When the buzzer sounds, the patient is required to smoke a cigarette right away. Once the smoker is conditioned to associate the sound of the buzzer with smoking, the buzzer is eliminated, and, one hopes, so is the smoking.

## what do you think?

Do you know people who have tried to quit smoking? ● What were their motivations for trying to quit? ● What was the experience like for them? ● Were they successful? ● If not, what factors contributed to relapse? ● What will they do differently the next time that they try?

Self-control strategies view smoking as a learned habit associated with specific situations, such as driving, studying, drinking, or watching TV. Therapy is aimed at identifying these situations and teaching smokers the skills necessary to resist smoking.

The **Skills for Behavior Change** box at right presents one of the American Cancer Society's approaches to quitting smoking.

## Tips for Quitting Smoking

If you're a smoker and you're ready to quit, try these tips to help kick the habit:

✳ Use the four Ds to fight the urge to smoke:
  ✳ Delay—put off smoking for 10 minutes; when the 10 minutes are up, put it off for another 10 minutes.
  ✳ Deep breathing
  ✳ Drink water
  ✳ Do something else
✳ Keep "mouth toys" handy: hard candy, gum, toothpicks, and carrot sticks can help.
✳ If you've had trouble stopping before, ask your doctor about nicotine chewing gum, patches, nasal sprays, inhalers, or lozenges.
✳ Make an appointment with your dental hygenist to have your teeth cleaned.
✳ Examine those associations that trigger your urge to smoke.
✳ Tell your family and friends that you've stopped smoking so they won't offer you a cigarette.
✳ Aim to spend your time in places that don't allow smoking.
✳ Take up a new sport, exercise program, hobby, or organizational commitment. This will help shake up your routine and distract you from smoking.
✳ Throw out your cigarettes or keep them in a place that's harder to get to or that makes smoking inconvenient, such as in the freezer, in your car's glove compartment, or at a friend's house.

# Assess yourself

## Are You Nicotine Dependent?

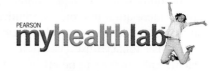

Many social smokers (who often consider themselves nonsmokers) may be more addicted to nicotine than they think. Do you have a dependence on nicotine? Take the following quiz to see.

Fill out this assessment online at www.pearsonhighered.com/myhealthlab or www.pearsonhighered.com/donatelle.

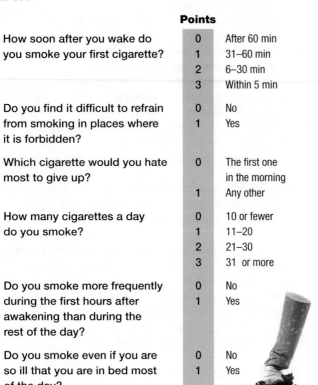

**Points**

**1** How soon after you wake do you smoke your first cigarette?
- 0 After 60 min
- 1 31–60 min
- 2 6–30 min
- 3 Within 5 min

**2** Do you find it difficult to refrain from smoking in places where it is forbidden?
- 0 No
- 1 Yes

**3** Which cigarette would you hate most to give up?
- 0 The first one in the morning
- 1 Any other

**4** How many cigarettes a day do you smoke?
- 0 10 or fewer
- 1 11–20
- 2 21–30
- 3 31 or more

**5** Do you smoke more frequently during the first hours after awakening than during the rest of the day?
- 0 No
- 1 Yes

**6** Do you smoke even if you are so ill that you are in bed most of the day?
- 0 No
- 1 Yes

### Interpreting Your Score

**0–1 points (20% of smokers):** You have a very low dependence, and are likely to experience few and light withdrawal symptoms. You should be able to quit without assistance.

**2–3 points (30% of smokers):** You have a certain degree of dependence and may experience difficult withdrawal symptoms. Many smokers in this group are able to quit by themselves, but medicines can be of help.

**4–5 points (30% of smokers):** You have above average dependence and you have a real risk for smoking-related disorders. Smokers in this group commonly experience withdrawal symptoms and often find medicines very helpful in quitting.

**6–7 points (15% of smokers):** You have a strong dependence and will likely experience strong withdrawal symptoms. Your risk for smoking-related disorders is high. Both support treatment and medicines (possibly in higher doses and for longer durations) will be important in helping you quit.

**8–10 points (5% of smokers):** You have extreme dependence and are likely to experience handicapping withdrawal symptoms. Most smokers within this group will already have smoking-related disorders. Support treatment and medications (preferably long term and in high doses) are essential in helping people in this group quit.

**Source:** T. F. Heatherton, L. T. Kozlowski, R. C. Frecker, and K. O. Fagerstrom, "The Fagerstrom Test for Nicotine Dependence: A Revision of the Fagerstrom Tolerance Questionnaire," *British Journal of Addictions* 86 (1991): 1119–27. Reprinted by permission of Dr. Karl Fagerstrom.

# YOUR PLAN FOR CHANGE

The **Assess yourself** activity gave you the chance to evaluate your current smoking habits. Regardless of your current level of nicotine addiction, now is the time to take steps toward kicking the habit.

### Today, you can:

◯ Develop a plan to kick the tobacco habit. The first step in quitting smoking is to identify why you want to quit. Write your reasons down on a sheet of paper.

◯ Think about the times and places you usually smoke. What could you do instead of smoking at those times? Make a list of positive tobacco alternatives.

### Within the next 2 weeks, you can:

◯ Say good-bye to your cigarettes. Pick a day to stop smoking, fill out a behavior change contract, and have a family member or friend sign it.

◯ Throw away all your cigarettes, lighters, and ashtrays.

### By the end of the semester, you can:

◯ Make a list of the good things about not smoking. Carry a copy with you, and look at it whenever you have the urge to smoke.

◯ If you are experiencing difficulty quitting, contact your campus health center or consult with your personal physician to discuss medications or other therapies that may help you quit.

## Summary

* Tobacco use is widespread in the United States and involves many social and political issues. Smoking costs the nation as much as $193 billion per year. Tobacco companies target college students in their marketing campaigns.
* Tobacco is available in smoking and smokeless forms, both of which contain nicotine, an addictive psychoactive substance. Smoking delivers 4,000 additional chemicals to the lungs of smokers.
* Health hazards of smoking include markedly higher rates of cancer, heart and circulatory disorders, respiratory diseases, and gum diseases. Smoking during pregnancy presents risks for the fetus. Smokeless tobacco dramatically increases risks for oral cancer and other oral problems.
* Environmental tobacco smoke (secondhand smoke) puts non-smokers at risk for cancer and heart disease.
* In a landmark legal settlement, the tobacco industry agreed to reimburse states for health care costs related to smoking and to finance various antismoking initiatives.
* To quit, smokers must kick a chemical addiction and a behavioral habit. Nicotine replacement products or drugs can help wean smokers off nicotine. A nicotine vaccine in development, NicVAX, makes tobacco less pleasurable. Therapy methods can also help.

## Pop Quiz

1. What are bidis?
   a. A type of clove cigarette
   b. An Indian-made sweet, flavored cigarette
   c. A type of cigar made in India
   d. Tobacco rolled with marijuana

2. What is sidestream smoke?
   a. The smoke that is inhaled by the smoker
   b. The smoke released from the burning end of the cigarette
   c. The smoke from a lower tar cigarette
   d. None of the above

3. What does carbon monoxide do to smokers?
   a. It makes it difficult for a smoker to breathe.
   b. It causes dizzy spells and light-headedness.
   c. It interferes with the ability of hemoglobin in the blood to adequately carry oxygen.
   d. It impairs the cleaning function of the lung's cilia.

4. What age group is most targeted by tobacco advertisers?
   a. Teenagers aged 14 to 17
   b. College students aged 18 to 24
   c. Young adults aged 25 to 30
   d. Married men aged 31 to 35

5. What is the major psychoactive ingredient in tobacco products?
   a. Carbon monoxide
   b. Tar
   c. Formaldehyde
   d. Nicotine

6. What does nicotine do to cilia?
   a. Instantly destroys them
   b. Thickens them
   c. Paralyzes them
   d. Accumulates on them

7. Which type of tobacco product contains eugenol, which allows smokers to inhale the smoke more deeply?
   a. Bidis
   b. Cigars
   c. Snuff
   d. Clove cigarettes

8. Why do college students smoke?
   a. Stress reduction
   b. Social pressure
   c. Addiction
   d. All of the above

9. A major health risk of chewing tobacco is
   a. lung cancer.
   b. leukoplakia.
   c. heart disease.
   d. emphysema.

10. Quitting smoking
    a. usually results in minor withdrawal symptoms.
    b. will do little to reverse damage to the lungs.
    c. can be aided by nicotine replacement.
    d. is best done by transitioning first to "light" cigarettes.

*Answers to these questions can be found on page A-1.*

## Think about It!

1. Discuss the varied ways in which tobacco is used. Is any method less addictive or hazardous to health than another?
2. Discuss short- and long-term health hazards associated with tobacco. Who should be responsible for the medical expenses of smokers?
3. Do you think restrictions on smoking are fair? Do they infringe on people's rights? Are the restrictions too strict or not strict enough?
4. Describe the pros and cons of several different methods of tobacco cessation.

## Accessing Your Health on the Internet

The following websites explore further topics and issues related to personal health. For link to the websites below, visit the Companion Website for *Access to Health,* 12th Edition, at www.pearsonhighered.com/donatelle.

1. *American Lung Association.* This site offers a wealth of information regarding smoking trends, environmental smoke, and advice on smoking cessation. www.lungusa.org
2. *ASH (Action on Smoking and Health).* The nation's oldest and largest antismoking organization, ASH works to fight smoking and protect the rights of nonsmokers. www.ash.org
3. *TIPS (Tobacco Information and Prevention Source).* This site provides information regarding tobacco use in the United States, with specific information for and about young people. www.cdc.gov/tobacco

# References

1. Committee on Reducing Tobacco Use: Strategies, Barriers, and Consequences, R. Bonnie, K. Stratton, and R. Wallace, eds., *Ending the Tobacco Problem, A Blueprint for the Nation* (Washington, DC: The National Academies of Press, 2007), Available at www.nap.edu/catalog.php?record _id=11795.
2. Centers for Disease Control and Prevention, *Tobacco Control State Highlights, 2010* (Atlanta: U.S. Department of Health and Human Services, Centers for Disease Control and Prevention, National Center for Chronic Disease Prevention and Health Promotion, Office on Smoking and Health, 2010), Available at www.cdc.gov/tobacco/ data_statistics/state_data/state_highlights/ 2010/index.htm.
3. Centers for Disease Control and Prevention, "Smoking-Attributable Mortality, Years of Potential Life Lost, and Productivity Losses, 2000–2004," *Morbidity and Mortality Weekly Report* 57, no. 45 (2008): 1226–28.
4. Ibid.
5. Ibid.
6. American Cancer Society, "Cigarette Smoking," Revised November 2009, www .cancer.org/docroot/ped/content/ped _10_2x_cigarette_smoking.asp.
7. National Center for Health Statistics, *Health, United States, 2009: With Special Feature on Medical Technology* (Hyattsville, MD: National Center for Health Statistics, 2010), Available at www .cdc.gov/nchs/hus.htm; Centers for Disease Control and Prevention, "Cigarette Smoking among Adults and Trends in Smoking Cessation—United States 2008,"
*Morbidity and Mortality Weekly Report* 58, no. 44 (2009): 1227–32.
8. Substance Abuse and Mental Health Administration, *Results from the 2008 National Survey on Drug Use and Health: Detailed Tables* (Rockville, MD: Office of Applied Studies, 2009), Available at www .oas.samhsa.gov/nsduh/reports.htm#2k8.
9. Centers for Disease Control and Prevention, "Cigarette Smoking among Adults," 2009.
10. Centers for Disease Control and Prevention, *Tobacco Control State Highlights, 2010,* 2010.
11. A. Agrawal et al., "Are There Genetic Influences on Addiction? Evidence from Family, Adoption and Twin Studies," *Addiction* 103, no. 7 (2008): 1069–81.
12. W. Hall, "Will Nicotine Genetics and a Nicotine Vaccine Prevent Cigarette Smoking and Smoking-Related Diseases?" *PLoS Med* 2, no. 9 (2005): e266.
13. National Institute on Drug Abuse, "Topics in Brief: Tobacco and Nicotine Research," Updated August 2008, www.drugabuse. gov/tib/tobnico.html.
14. G. Gutierrez, "Nicotine Creates Stronger Memories, Cues to Drug Use," Modified September 2009, www.bcm.edu/news/ packages/nicotine.cfm.
15. Campaign for Tobacco-Free Kids, "Tobacco Company Marketing to Kids," 2010, Available at www.tobaccofreekids. org/research/factsheets.
16. Centers for Disease Control and Prevention, "Cigarette Brand Preference among Middle and High School Students Who Are Established Smokers—United States, 2004 and 2006," *Morbidity and Mortality Weekly* 58, no. 5 (2009): 112–15.
17. Campaign for Tobacco-Free Kids, "Toll of Tobacco in the United States of America," January 2010, Available at www.tobac cofreekids.org/research/factsheets.
18. Campaign for Tobacco-Free Kids, *Big Tobacco's Guinea Pigs: How an Unregulated Industry Experiments on America's Kids and Consumers* (Washington, DC: Campaign for Tobacco-Free Kids, 2008), Available at www.tobaccofreekids.org/reports/ products.
19. American Cancer Society, *Cancer Facts & Figures 2010* (Atlanta: American Cancer Society, 2010), Available at www.cancer .org/Research/CancerFactsFigures/ CancerFactsFigures/cancer-facts-and- figures-2010.
20. Centers for Disease Control and Prevention, *Tobacco Control State Highlights, 2010,* 2010; Centers for Disease Control and Prevention, "Smoking-Attributable Mortality, Years of Potential Life Lost, and Productivity Losses, 2000–2004," 2008.
21. Reuters, "U.S. Would Reap Billions from $1 Cigarette Tax Hike," February 10, 2010, www.reuters.com/article/idUSTRE6194 SD20100210.
22. American College Health Association, *American College Health Association– National College Health Assessment II: Reference Group Data Report, Fall 2009* (Baltimore, American College Health Association, 2010), Available at www .achancha.org/reports_ACHA-NCHAII .html.
23. National Center on Addiction and Substance Abuse at Columbia University, *Wasting the Best and the Brightest: Substance Abuse at America's Colleges and Universities* (New York: National Center on Addiction and Substance Abuse at Columbia University, March 2007), Available at www.casacolumbia.org/templates/ publications_reports.aspx.
24. American College Health Association, *American College Health Association– National College Health Assessment II,* 2010.
25. National Center on Addiction and Substance Abuse at Columbia University, *Wasting the Best and the Brightest,* 2007.
26. Ibid.
27. Ibid.
28. L. Stoner et al., "Occasional Cigarette Smoking Chronically Affects Arterial Function," *Ultrasound in Medicine and Biology* 34, no. 12 (2008): 1885–92.
29. L. An et al., "Symptoms of Cough and Shortness of Breath among Occasional Young Adult Smokers," *Nicotine & Tobacco Research* 11, no. 2 (2009): 126–33.
30. Stop Smoking! "Smoking and Birth Control Pills Are Not Made for Each Other," Retrieved May 8, 2010, www.stop-smoking -updates.com/quitsmoking/smoking -factsheet/facts/smoking-and-birth -control-pills-are-not-made-for-each -other.htm.
31. National Center on Addiction and Substance Abuse at Columbia University, *Wasting the Best and the Brightest,* 2007.
32. Ibid.
33. U.S. Department of Health and Human Services, *The Health Consequences of Involuntary Exposure to Tobacco Smoke: A Report of the Surgeon General* (Atlanta, GA: U.S. Department of Health and Human Services, Centers for Disease Control and Prevention, Coordinating Center for Health Promotion, National Center for Chronic Disease Prevention and Health Promotion, Office on Smoking and Health, 2006), Available at www.surgeongeneral .gov/library/secondhandsmoke; National Toxicology Program. *Report on Carcinogens,* 11th ed. (Rockville, MD: U.S. Department of Health and Human Services,

Public Health Service, National Toxicology Program, 2005).

34. American Cancer Society, "Cigar Smoking: Who Smokes Cigars?" Revised July 2010, www.cancer.org/Cancer/CancerCauses/TobaccoCancer/CigarSmoking/cigar-smoking-who-smokes-cigars.

35. Ibid.

36. American Cancer Society, "Questions about Smoking, Tobacco, and Health: What about More Exotic Forms of Smoking Tobacco, Such as Clove Cigarettes, Bidis, and Hookahs?" Revised July 2010, www.cancer.org/Cancer/CancerCauses/TobaccoCancer/QuestionsaboutSmokingTobaccoandHealth/questions-about-smoking-tobacco-and-health-other-forms-of-smoking.

37. Centers for Disease Control and Prevention, "Smoking and Tobacco Use: Bidis and Kreteks," Updated May 2009, www.cdc.gov/tobacco/data_statistics/fact_sheets/tobacco_industry/bidis_kreteks.

38. Ibid.

39. Centers for Disease Control and Prevention, "Smoking and Tobacco Use: Smokeless Tobacco Facts," September 2009, www.cdc.gov/tobacco/data_statistics/fact_sheets/smokeless/smokeless_facts/index.htm.

40. American College Health Association, *American College Health Association–National College Health Assessment II*, 2010.

41. W. Dunham, "Chewing Tobacco Use Surges among Boys," Reuters, March 25, 2009. www.reuters.com/article/idUSTRE5240WJ20090305.

42. Centers for Disease Control and Prevention, "Smoking-Attributable Mortality, Years of Potential Life Lost, and Productivity Losses, 2000–2004," 2008.

43. American Cancer Society, *Cancer Facts & Figures 2010*, 2010.

44. Ibid.

45. Ibid.

46. Ibid.

47. Ibid.

48. American Heart Association, *Heart Disease and Stroke Statistics—2010 Update* (Dallas: American Heart Association, 2010), Available at www.americanheart.org/presenter.jhtml?identifier=3000090.

49. Ibid.

50. Ibid.

51. Ibid.

52. American Heart Association, "Stroke Risk Factors," 2010, www.americanheart.org/presenter.jhtml?identifier=4716.

53. American Lung Association, "Benefits of Quitting," Accessed June 2010, www.lungusa.org/stop-smoking/how-to-quit/why-quit/benefits-of-quitting.

54. American Cancer Society, *Cancer Facts & Figures, 2010*, 2010.

55. John Hopkins Health Alerts, "Emphysema: Symptoms and Remedies," Accessed April 2010, www.johnshopkinshealthalerts.com/symptoms_remedies/emphysema/96-1.html.

56. National Kidney and Neurological Diseases Information Clearing House, "Erectile Dysfunction," NIH Publication no. 06–3923, December 2005, http://kidney.niddk.nih.gov/kudiseases/pubs/impotence.

57. Centers for Disease Control and Prevention, "Pregnant? Don't Smoke! Learn How and Why to Quit for Good," Updated November 2009, www.cdc.gov/Features/PregnantDontSmoke.

58. Centers for Disease Control and Prevention, "Tobacco Use and Pregnancy," Modified May 2009, www.cdc.gov/reproductivehealth/TobaccoUsePregnancy/index.htm.

59. American Academy of Periodontology, "Tobacco Use and Periodontal Disease," 2010, www.perio.org/consumer/smoking.htm.

60. American Academy of Neurology, "Alzheimer's Starts Earlier for Heavy Drinkers, Smokers," Press Release, April 16, 2008, www.aan.com/press/index.cfm?fuseaction=release.view&release=594.

61. American Cancer Society, "Secondhand Smoke," Revised October 2009, www.cancer.org/docroot/ped/content/ped_10_2x_secondhand_smoke-clean_indoor_air.asp.

62. Centers for Disease Control and Prevention, "Smoking and Tobacco Use Fact Sheet: Secondhand Smoke," Updated January 2010, www.cdc.gov/tobacco/data_statistics/fact_sheets/secondhand_smoke/general_facts/index.htm.

63. Ibid.

64. Ibid.

65. U.S. Department of Health and Human Services, *The Health Consequences of Involuntary Exposure to Tobacco Smoke*, 2006; American Cancer Society, "Secondhand Smoke," Revised October 2009, www.cancer.org/docroot/ped/content/ped_10_2x_secondhand_smoke-clean_indoor_air.asp.

66. U.S. Department of Health and Human Services, *The Health Consequences of Involuntary Exposure to Tobacco Smoke*, 2006.

67. U.S. Department of Health and Human Services, *The Health Consequences of Involuntary Exposure to Tobacco Smoke*, 2006; Centers for Disease Control and Prevention, "Smoking and Tobacco Use Fact Sheet," 2010.

68. U.S. Department of Health and Human Services, *The Health Consequences of Involuntary Exposure to Tobacco Smoke*, 2006.

69. S. Leatherdale et al., "Second-Hand Exposure in Homes and in Cars among Canadian Youth: Current Prevalence, Beliefs about Exposure, and Changes between 2004–2006," *Cancer Causes & Control* 20, no. 6 (2009): 1573–1625.

70. K. Yolton et al., "Exposure to Environmental Tobacco Smoke and Cognitive Abilities among U.S. Children and Adolescents," *Environmental Health Perspectives* 113, no. 1 (2005): 9–103.

71. M. R. Becklake et al., "Childhood Predictors of Smoking in Adolescence: A Follow-Up Study of Montreal School Children," *Canadian Medical Association Journal* 173, no. 4 (2005): 377–79.

72. O. Shafey, M. Eriksen, H. Ross, and J. Mackay, "Secondhand Smoking," chap. 9 in *The Tobacco Atlas*, 3d ed. (Atlanta: American Cancer Society, 2009), Available at www.cancer.org/aboutus/GlobalHealth/CancerandTobaccoControlResources/the-tobacco-atlas-3rd-edition.

73. Centers for Disease Control and Prevention, *Tobacco Control State Highlights, 2010*, 2010.

74. M. Fogarty, "Public Health and Smoking Cessation," *Scientist* 17, no. 6 (2003): 23.

75. *Family Smoking Prevention and Tobacco Control Act of 2009*, HR 1256, 111th Congress of the United States of America, Available at www.govtrack.us/congress/billtext.xpd?bill=h111-1256.

76. M. C. Fiore et al., *Treating Tobacco Use and Dependence: 2008 Update. Clinical Practice Guideline* (Rockville, MD: U.S. Department of Health and Human Services. Public Health Service, May 2008), Available at www.surgeongeneral.gov/tobacco; U.S. Department of Health and Human Services, "Effective Strategies for Tobacco Cessation Underused, Panel Says" National Institutes of Health News Press Release, June 2006, www.nih.gov/news/pr/jun2006/od-14.htm.

77. American Cancer Society, "Guide to Quitting Smoking: A Word about Quitting Success Rates," Revised July 2010, www.cancer.org/Healthy/StayAwayfromTobacco/GuidetoQuittingSmoking/guide-to-quitting-smoking-success-rates.

78. V. Willingham, "Nicotine Vaccine Effective in Early Tests," CNN Health, April 22, 2010, www.cnn.com/2010/HEALTH/04/21/nicotine.vaccine.nicvax/index.html.

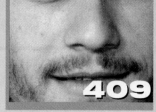

**409**

Why is prescription drug abuse on the rise?

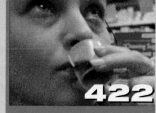

**422**

Why is it so hard to quit using heroin?

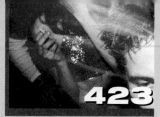

**423**

Just how risky are "club drugs"?

# Avoiding Drug Misuse and Abuse

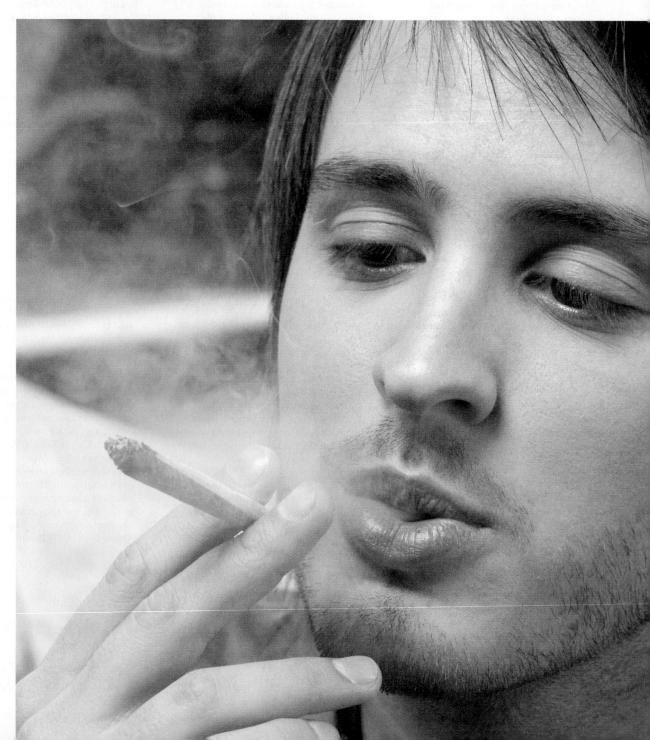

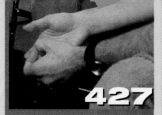

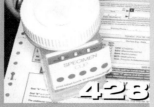

**What works in helping people recover from drug addiction?**

**Is it legal for employers to require employees to take a drug test?**

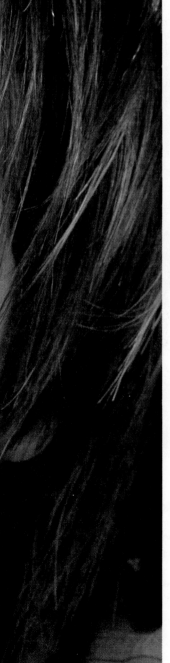

## Objectives

* Discuss the six categories of drugs and their routes of administration.

* Discuss the use of illicit drugs among college students.

* Review problems relating to the misuse and abuse of prescription drugs.

* Discuss the use and abuse of controlled substances, including cocaine, amphetamines, marijuana, opioids, hallucinogens, club drugs, inhalants, and steroids.

* Profile illicit drug use in the United States, including who uses illicit drugs, financial impact, and impact on college campuses and the workplace.

Drug misuse and abuse are enormous problems in our society. Whether it is the meth addict who has lost everything in a harrowing fall into dependence and crime, or the high functioning executive who gets hooked on prescription drugs like OxyContin or Vicodin to help ease excruciating back pain, drug addiction wreaks havoc on individuals, families, businesses, and society. The use and abuse of drugs occurs at all income levels, among all ethnic groups and at all ages. In 2008, an estimated 20 million Americans aged 12 or older were current users of illicit (illegal) drugs: This represents 8 percent of the population.[1] Some 14 percent of people aged 12 or older report having used illicit drugs in the past year, and the 2009 Youth Risk Behavior Survey found that over 20 percent of high school students have taken prescription drugs without a doctor's permission.[2] Drug misuse and abuse can be incredibly damaging to people's lives, causing problems ranging from deterioration of relationships, to loss of employment, to death. It's impossible to put a dollar amount on the pain, suffering, and dysfunction that drugs cause in our everyday lives.

Why do people use drugs? Human beings appear to have a need to alter their consciousness, or mental state. We like to feel good, to escape, and to feel different. Sometimes we like to reduce pain or dull our senses. Consciousness can be altered in many ways: Children spinning until they become dizzy and adults enjoying the thrill of extreme sports are two examples. To change our awareness, some of us listen to music, skydive, ski, read, daydream, meditate, pray, or have sexual relations. Others turn to drugs to alter consciousness.

# Drug Dynamics

Drugs work because they physically resemble the chemicals produced naturally within the body. Most bodily processes result from chemical reactions or from changes in electrical charge. Because drugs possess an electrical charge and chemical structure similar to those of chemicals that occur naturally in the body, they can affect physical functions in many different ways.

## How Drugs Affect the Brain

Pleasure, which scientists call *reward,* is a very powerful biological force for survival. If you do something that you experience as pleasurable, the brain is wired in such a way that you tend to do it again. Life-sustaining activities, such as eating, activate a circuit of specialized nerve cells devoted to producing and regulating pleasure. One important set of these nerve cells, which uses a chemical **neurotransmitter** called *dopamine,* sits at the very top of the brainstem in the *ventral tegmental area* (*VTA*). These dopamine-containing neurons relay messages about pleasure through their nerve fibers to nerve cells in the limbic system,

**neurotransmitter** One of many chemical substances, such as acetylcholine or dopamine, that transmit nerve impulses between nerve fibers.

**405**

structures in the brain regulating emotions. Still other fibers connect to a related part of the frontal region of the cerebral cortex, the area of the brain that plays a key role in memory, perception, thought, and consciousness. So, this "pleasure circuit," known as the *mesolimbic dopamine* system, spans the survival-oriented brainstem, the emotional limbic system, and the thinking frontal cerebral cortex.

All drugs that are addicting can activate the brain's pleasure circuit. Drug addiction is a biological, pathological process that alters the way in which the pleasure center, as well as other parts of the brain, functions. Almost all **psychoactive drugs** (those that change the way the brain works) do so by affecting chemical neurotransmission, either enhancing it, suppressing it, or interfering with it. Some drugs, such as heroin and lysergic acid diethylamide (LSD), mimic the effects of a natural neurotransmitter. Others, such as phencyclidine (PCP), block receptors and thereby prevent neuronal messages from getting through. Still others, such as cocaine, block the *reuptake* of neurotransmitters by neurons, thus producing an increased concentration of the neurotransmitters in the synaptic gap, the space between individual neurons (Figure 13.1). Finally, some drugs, such as methamphetamine, act by causing neurotransmitters to be released in greater amounts than is normal.

**psychoactive drugs** Drugs that have the potential to alter mood or behavior.

## Types of Drugs

Scientists divide drugs into 6 categories: prescription, over-the-counter (OTC), recreational, herbal, illicit, and commercial drugs. Each category includes some drugs that stimulate the body, some that depress body functions, and others that produce hallucinations (images, auditory or visual, that are perceived but are not real). Each category also includes psychoactive drugs.

- **Prescription drugs.** These can be obtained only with a prescription from a licensed health practitioner. More than 10,000 types of prescription drugs are sold in the United States.
- **Over-the-counter drugs.** These can be purchased without a prescription. More than 300,000 OTC products are available, and an estimated 3 out of 4 people routinely self-medicate with them.[3] Although prescription drugs are available at approximately 58,000 pharmacies nationwide, OTC medicines are available for consumers at over 750,000 retailers in the United States. Studies show that Americans are making more use of widely available OTC medicines each year.[4] (See Chapter 18 for a discussion of the OTC label and common types of OTC drugs.)
- **Recreational drugs.** These belong to a somewhat vague category whose boundaries depend upon how the term *recreation*

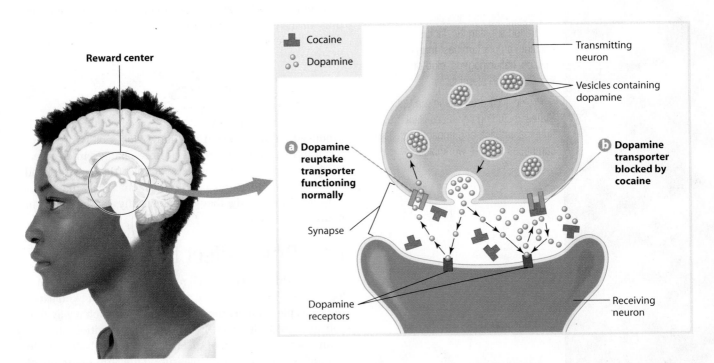

FIGURE 13.1 **The Action of Cocaine at Dopamine Receptors in the Brain, an Example of Psychoactive Drug Action**
In normal neural communication, dopamine is released into the synapse between neurons. It binds temporarily to dopamine receptors on the receiving neuron, and then is recycled back into the transmitting neuron by a transporter. When cocaine molecules are present, they attach to the dopamine transporter and block the recycling process. Too much dopamine remains active in the synaptic gaps between neurons, creating feelings of excitement and euphoria.

**Source:** Adapted from *NIDA Research Report—Cocaine Abuse and Addiction* (NIH Publication no. 09-4166, printed May 1999, revised May 2009), www.nida .nih.gov/PDF/RRCocaine.pdf.

is defined. Generally, recreational drugs contain chemicals used to help people relax or socialize. Most of them are legal even though they are psychoactive. Alcohol, tobacco, and caffeine products are included in this category.

● **Herbal preparations.** These encompass approximately 750 substances, including herbal teas and other products of botanical (plant) origin that are believed to have medicinal properties. (See Chapter 18 for more on herbal preparations.)

● **Illicit (illegal) drugs.** These are the most notorious type of drug. Although laws governing their use, possession, cultivation, manufacture, and sale differ from state to state, illicit drugs are generally recognized as harmful. All of them are psychoactive.

● **Commercial preparations.** These are the most universally used yet least commonly recognized chemical substances. More than 1,000 of them exist, including seemingly benign items such as perfumes, cosmetics, household cleansers, paints, glues, inks, dyes, and pesticides.

*Using a needle to inject drugs poses health threats beyond the effects of the drug.*

# Routes of Drug Administration

*Route of administration* refers to the way in which a given drug is taken into the body. The route largely determines the rapidity of the drug's effect on the body (Figure 13.2). The most common route is **oral ingestion**—swallowing a tablet, capsule, or liquid. Drugs taken by mouth don't reach the bloodstream as quickly as drugs introduced to the body by other means. A drug taken orally may not reach the bloodstream for 30 minutes.

Drugs can also enter the body through the respiratory tract via sniffing, smoking, or inhaling (**inhalation**). Drugs that are inhaled and absorbed by the lungs travel the most rapidly of all the routes of drug administration. Another rapid form of drug administration is by **injection** directly into the bloodstream (intravenously), muscles (intramuscularly), or just under the skin (subcutaneously). Intravenous

**oral ingestion** Intake of drugs through the mouth.
**inhalation** The introduction of drugs through breathing into the lungs.
**injection** The introduction of drugs into the body via a hypodermic needle.

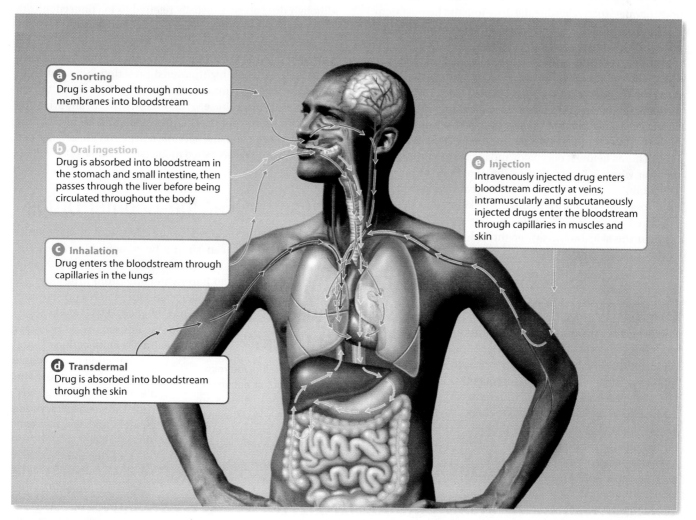

**a Snorting**
Drug is absorbed through mucous membranes into bloodstream

**b Oral ingestion**
Drug is absorbed into bloodstream in the stomach and small intestine, then passes through the liver before being circulated throughout the body

**c Inhalation**
Drug enters the bloodstream through capillaries in the lungs

**d Transdermal**
Drug is absorbed into bloodstream through the skin

**e Injection**
Intravenously injected drug enters bloodstream directly at veins; intramuscularly and subcutaneously injected drugs enter the bloodstream through capillaries in muscles and skin

FIGURE 13.2 **Routes of Drug Administration**
Drugs are most commonly swallowed, inhaled, or injected. They can also be absorbed through the skin or mucous membranes (as in snorting and suppository use, not shown here).

**transdermal** The introduction of drugs through the skin.
**suppositories** Mixtures of drugs and a waxy medium (designed to melt at body temperature) that are inserted into the anus or vagina.
**receptor sites** Specialized areas of cells and organs where chemicals, enzymes, and other substances interact.
**polydrug use** Taking several medications, vitamins, recreational drugs, or illegal drugs simultaneously.
**synergism** The interaction of two or more drugs that produces more profound effects than would be expected if the drugs were taken separately; also called *potentiation*.
**antagonism** A drug interaction in which two drugs compete for the same available receptors, potentially blocking each other's actions.

injection, which involves inserting a hypodermic needle directly into a vein, is the most common method of injection for drug users, due to the rapid speed (within seconds in most cases) in which a drug's effect is felt. It is also the most dangerous method of administration due to the risk of damaging blood vessels and contracting HIV (human immunodeficiency virus) and hepatitis (a severe liver disease). Drugs can also be absorbed through the skin or tissue lining (**transdermal**)—the nicotine patch is a common example of a drug that is administered in this manner—or through the mucous membranes, such as those in the nose (snorting) or in the vagina or anus (**suppositories**). Suppositories are typically mixed with a waxy medium that melts at body temperature, releasing the drug into the bloodstream.

However the drug enters the system, it eventually finds its way to the bloodstream and is circulated throughout the body to various **receptor sites** where chemicals, enzymes, and other substances interact. Psychoactive drugs are able to cross the blood–brain barrier in order to reach receptor sites in the brain, where they can affect cognition, emotions, and physiological functioning. Once a drug reaches receptor sites in the brain and other body organs, it may remain active for several hours before it dissipates and is carried by the blood to the liver where it is metabolized (broken down by enzymes). The products of enzymatic breakdown, called *metabolites*, are then excreted, primarily through the kidneys (in urine) or the bowels (in feces), but also through the skin (in sweat), or through the lungs (in expired air).

## Drug Interactions

**Polydrug use**—taking several medications, vitamins, recreational drugs, or illegal drugs simultaneously—can lead to dangerous health problems. Alcohol in particular frequently has dangerous interactions with other drugs. The most hazardous interactions are synergism, antagonism, inhibition, intolerance, and cross-tolerance.

**Synergism,** also called *potentiation*, is an interaction of two or more drugs in which the effects of the individual drugs are multiplied beyond what would normally be expected if they were taken alone. You might think of synergism as 2 + 2 = 10. A synergistic reaction can be very dangerous and even deadly.

**Antagonism,** although usually less serious than synergism, can also produce unwanted and unpleasant effects. In an antagonistic reaction, drugs work at the same receptor site so that one drug blocks the action of the other. The blocking drug occupies the receptor site and prevents the other drug from attaching, thus altering its absorption and action.

With **inhibition,** the effects of one drug are eliminated or reduced by the presence of another drug at the receptor site. **Intolerance** occurs when drugs combine in the body to produce extremely uncomfortable reactions. The drug Antabuse (disulfiram), used to help alcoholics give up alcohol, works by producing this type of interaction. A final type of interaction, **cross-tolerance,** occurs when a person develops a physiological tolerance to one drug and shows a similar tolerance to certain other drugs as a result.

## Using, Misusing, and Abusing Drugs

Although drug abuse is usually referred to in connection with illicit psychoactive drugs, many people also abuse and misuse prescription and OTC medications. **Drug misuse** involves using a drug for a purpose for which it was not intended. For example, taking a friend's high-powered prescription painkiller for your headache is a misuse of that drug. This is not too far removed from **drug abuse,** or the excessive use of any drug, and may cause serious harm. The misuse and abuse of any drug may lead to addiction, the habitual reliance on a substance or a behavior to produce a desired mood (see Chapter 10).

## Abuse of Over-the-Counter Drugs

Over-the-counter medications are drugs that do not require a prescription and can simply be bought in drug stores, supermarkets, and the like. Although many people assume that no harm can come from drugs that are not illegal and for which a prescription is not needed, OTC medications can be abused, with resultant health complications and potential addiction. People who appear to be most vulnerable to abusing OTC drugs are teenagers, young adults, and people over the age of 65.

Over-the-counter drugs are abused when the drug is taken in more than the recommended dosage, combined with other drugs, or taken over a longer period of time than is recommended. Abuse of and addiction to OTC drugs can be

### "Why Should I Care?"

You may think drugs are helping you relax, improving your concentration, or enhancing your social enjoyment, but those effects are transient—and often illusory—and they are nothing compared to the many negative effects those same drugs can have on your life and health. Sooner or later, drug misuse and abuse is likely to catch up with you and cause problems—be they academic, social, career, legal, financial, or health-related. Are a few moments of excitement really worth a lifetime of trouble?

accidental. A person may develop tolerance from continued use, creating an unintended dependence. Teenagers and young adults sometimes intentionally abuse OTC medications in search of a cheap high—by drinking large amounts of cough medicine, for instance. The following are a few types of OTC drugs that are subject to misuse and abuse:

- **Sleep aids.** These drugs may be harmful in excess as they can cause problems with the sleep cycle, weaken areas of the body, or induce narcolepsy (a condition of excessive, intrusive sleepiness). Continued use of these products can lead to tolerance and dependence.
- **Cold medicines (cough syrups and tablets).** There are many different ingredients in cough and cold medicines, but one of particular concern is dextromethorphan (DXM), which is present in about 125 different types of OTC medications. As many as 6 percent of high school seniors report taking drugs containing DXM in order to get high.[5] Large doses of products containing DXM can cause hallucinations, loss of motor control, and "out-of-body" (disassociative) sensations. Other possible side effects of DXM abuse include confusion, impaired judgment, blurred vision, dizziness, paranoia, excessive sweating, slurred speech, nausea, vomiting, abdominal pain, irregular heartbeat, high blood pressure, headache, lethargy, numbness of fingers and toes, facial redness, and dry and itchy skin. In extreme cases, abuse of DXM can lead to loss of consciousness, seizures, brain damage, and even death. Some states have passed laws limiting the amount of products containing DXM a person can purchase, or prohibiting sale to individuals under age 18.[6]

Pseudoephedrine is another cold and allergy medication ingredient that is frequently abused, most commonly in the illegal manufacture of methamphetamine (discussed later). United States law limits the amount of products containing this drug that an individual may purchase in a month, and requires that it be sold "behind the counter" (i.e., without a prescription, but only through a pharmacist), and that photo identification be presented and recorded. Pharmacists are required to keep a record of purchasers for at least 2 years.[7]

> Over-the-counter cough syrup is frequently abused by young people seeking a high from the ingredient DXM.

- **Diet pills.** Some teens use diet pills as a way of getting high, whereas other people use these drugs in an attempt to lose weight. Diet pills often contain a stimulant such as caffeine (discussed later in the chapter) or an herbal ingredient claimed to promote weight loss, such as *Hoodia gordonii*. Many diet pills are marketed as "dietary supplements" and so are regulated by the U.S. Food and Drug Administration (FDA) as "food," not as "drugs." This means their manufacturers may make unsubstantiated claims of effectiveness or use untested and unsafe ingredients.

## Nonmedical Use or Abuse of Prescription Drugs

In the United States today, the abuse of prescription medications is at an all-time high. Only marijuana is more widely abused.[8] Individuals abuse these drugs because they are an easily accessible and

**inhibition** A drug interaction in which the effects of one drug are eliminated or reduced by the presence of another drug at the same receptor site.

**intolerance** A drug interaction in which the combination of two or more drugs in the body produces extremely uncomfortable symptoms.

**cross-tolerance** Development of a physiological tolerance to one drug that reduces the effects of another, similar drug.

**drug misuse** Use of a drug for a purpose for which it was not intended.

**drug abuse** Excessive use of a drug.

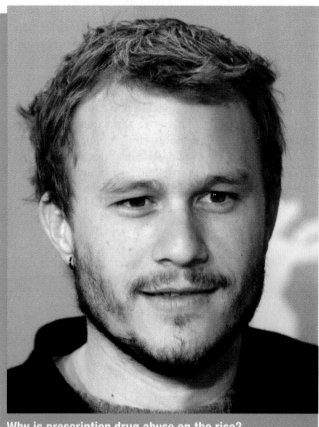

**Why is prescription drug abuse on the rise?**

Because there are legitimate, legal applications of prescription drugs, they are more readily available and easier to obtain than illicit drugs. As more and more people—especially students—turn to these medications to help them study or to get high, the more socially acceptable their usage becomes and the rate of use continues to rise. In addition, the fact that prescription drugs are regulated and approved by the FDA leads to the impression that they are safer than illicit drugs. This is a fallacy, as was tragically demonstrated by the 2008 death of actor Heath Ledger from an accidental overdose of prescription painkillers, sleeping pills, and anti-anxiety medication.

# 55.9%

of people who use pain relievers nonmedically get the drug from a friend or relative.

inexpensive means of altering a user's mental and physical state. Some people also have the mistaken idea that prescription drugs are a "safer high."

The latest data available indicate that over 48 million Americans aged 12 and older have used prescription drugs for nonmedical reasons in their lifetimes.[9] Of these, 15.2 million people over the age of 12 (7%) report abusing controlled prescription drugs in the past year.[10] Prescription drug abuse is particularly common among teenagers and young adults. In 2008, 2.9 percent of teenagers 12 to 17 reported abusing prescription drugs; in 2009 it was reported that 6 percent of people aged 18 to 25 reported nonmedical use of prescription drugs in the previous month.[11] Recent research indicates that the problem may be getting worse, particularly among the youngest segments of society, with nearly one-quarter of 12th graders reporting abuse of prescription drugs by the time they graduate from high school.[12]

The prescription drugs that are most commonly abused in the United States fall under three major categories: opioids/narcotics, depressants, and stimulants, each with associated risks. Abuse of opioids, narcotics, and pain relievers can result in life-threatening respiratory depression (reduced breathing). Individuals who abuse depressants place themselves at risk of seizures, respiratory depression, and decreased heart rate. Stimulant abuse can cause elevated body temperature, irregular heart rate, cardiovascular system failure, and fatal seizures. It can also result in hostility or feelings of paranoia. Individuals who abuse prescription drugs by injecting them expose themselves to additional risks, including contracting HIV, hepatitis B and C, and other bloodborne viruses.

Unfortunately, prescription drugs are often easier to obtain than illegal ones. In some cases, unscrupulous pharmacists or other medical professionals either steal the drugs or sell fraudulent prescriptions. In a process called *doctor shopping*, abusers visit several doctors to obtain multiple prescriptions. Some may fake or exaggerate symptoms in order to persuade physicians to write prescriptions. Individuals may also call pharmacies with fraudulent prescriptions. Young people typically obtain prescription drugs from peers, friends, or family members. Some teenagers and college students who have legitimate prescriptions sell or give away their medications to other students, or trade them for others. Some abusers order from Internet pharmacies where prescriptions are not always required.

**College Students and Prescription Drug Abuse** Like the rest of the U.S. population, college student prescription drug abuse has increased dramatically over the past decade. Many college students seem to think prescription drugs are safer than illicit drugs because they are prescribed by doctors and approved by the FDA. However, when these drugs are misused, they can be even more unsafe than illegal drugs.

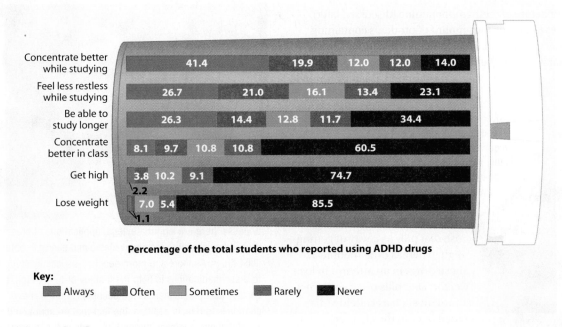

**Concentrate better while studying:** 41.4 | 19.9 | 12.0 | 12.0 | 14.0
**Feel less restless while studying:** 26.7 | 21.0 | 16.1 | 13.4 | 23.1
**Be able to study longer:** 26.3 | 14.4 | 12.8 | 11.7 | 34.4
**Concentrate better in class:** 8.1 | 9.7 | 10.8 | 10.8 | 60.5
**Get high:** 3.8 | 10.2 | 9.1 | 2.2 | 74.7
**Lose weight:** 7.0 | 5.4 | 1.1 | | 85.5

Percentage of the total students who reported using ADHD drugs

**Key:** Always | Often | Sometimes | Rarely | Never

FIGURE 13.3 **College Students' Stated Reasons for Nonmedical Use of ADHD Drugs**
Although a small percentage of students in this study used ADHD drugs to get high or to lose weight, the majority of students reported using the drugs to enhance their academic performance.
**Source:** Data are from D. L. Rabiner et al., "Motives and Perceived Consequences of Nonmedical ADHD Medication Use by College Students: Are Students Treating Themselves for Attention Problems?" *Journal of Attention Disorders*, 13, no. 3 (2009): 259–70.

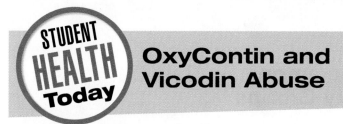

## OxyContin and Vicodin Abuse

Since the mid-1990s there has been a sharp increase in prescription drug abuse among youth and college students. Among college students, the results of the 2009 Monitoring the Future (MTF) study found that approximately 7 percent of college students had used Vicodin and 4 percent used OxyContin, both prescription painkillers, without a doctor's prescription in the past year.

As with most other drugs, some of the reasons college students use OxyContin and Vicodin are that they feel young and often invincible; they need to express their new-found independence; they like the excitement of risk-taking; or they feel pressure from their peers. Often, there is the perception that prescription drugs are safer than illicit drugs.

Because abuse of prescription medicines is a growing and not highly recognized problem, many do not realize the dangers. Painkillers such as OxyContin, Percocet, Percodan, Vicodin, and others are highly addictive if taken for prolonged periods of time. OxyContin, in particular, can be a highly addictive and dangerous narcotic when abused. The "rush" is similar to that of heroin. In fact, it's common for

people who are addicted to OxyContin to turn to heroin when they can't afford to buy OxyContin. Chronic use can also result in increasing tolerance, and more of the drug is needed to achieve the desired effect.

Studies find that many who are abusing prescription medications are simultaneously abusing illegal drugs. According to the MTF study, students who obtained prescription painkillers from peers reported higher levels of binge drinking and marijuana abuse than nonabusers or those who received painkillers from family. This poses another set of problems, as alcohol in combination with any one of these medications can make a dangerous cocktail. If a friend or someone you know seems unusually drunk, drowsy, slurs speech, has trouble moving, or passes out, call for help immediately.

**Sources:** L. D. Johnston et al., *Monitoring the Future: National Survey Results on Drug Use, 1975–2008, Volume II, College Students and Adults Ages 19–50*, NIH Publication no. 09-7403 (Bethesda, MD: National Institute on Drug Abuse, 2009), Available at http://monitoringthefuture.org/new.html; Higher Education Center for Alcohol, Drug Abuse and Violence Prevention, "OxyContin & Oxycodone," 2010, www.higheredcenter.org/high-risk/drugs/prescription-drugs/oxycontin.

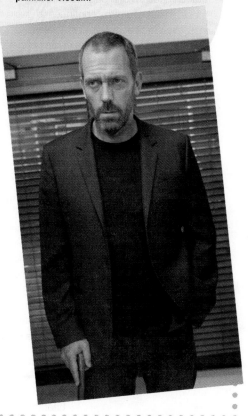

Dr. Gregory House, Hugh Laurie's character on the popular TV show *House, M.D.*, is well-known for his addiction to the painkiller Vicodin.

---

Many students also perceive the misuse of prescription drugs to be more socially acceptable than other forms of drug use.

From 1993 to 2005, the rate of student abuse of prescription painkillers rose 343 percent. This number equals approximately 240,000 full-time students. Students who abuse prescription painkillers such as Vicodin, OxyContin, or Percocet say they do so to relax or get high (see the **Student Health Today** box above for more on the abuse of these painkillers).[13] Over the same period, abuse of prescription stimulants rose 93 percent, abuse of prescription tranquilizers rose 450 percent, and abuse of sedatives 225 percent.[14]

Of particular concern on college campuses is the increased abuse of stimulant drugs such as Adderall and Ritalin, which are intended to treat attention-deficit/hyperactivity disorder (ADHD). Students primarily report using ADHD drugs for academic gain (Figure 13.3). A recent study on two university campuses revealed that 9 percent of students had used ADHD drugs without a prescription at some point in their college careers, whereas 5.4 percent had done so in the past 6 months.[15] An analysis of several studies found

that between 16 and 29 percent of students with prescribed stimulant medications for ADHD reported having sold, traded, or been asked for their medications.[16]

## Illicit Drugs

Like the nonmedical use of prescription drugs, the problem of illicit drug use touches us all. We may use illicit substances ourselves, watch someone we love struggle with drug abuse, or become the victim of a drug-related crime. At the very least, we are forced to pay increasing taxes for law enforcement and drug rehabilitation. When our coworkers use drugs, the effectiveness of our own work is diminished. If the car we drive was assembled by

### What's Working for You?

You may already have come up with healthy ways to handle the use and abuse of drugs that may be happening around you. Which of these statements are true for you?

☐ I have a few ways to say no to drugs.

☐ I am busy with lots of different activities—I don't have time for drugs!

☐ I know how to get in touch with counselors on campus if a friend of mine needs help with a drug problem.

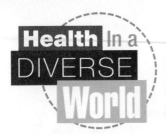
# Trends in Drug Use among Racial and Ethnic Minority Groups

The percentage of the U.S. population that is made up of members of racial/ethnic minority groups continues to increase. Socioeconomic disparities among racial/ethnic groups in the United States, combined with the association between low socioeconomic status and substance abuse, mean that an increasing number of members of racial/ethnic minorities may be at risk of substance abuse. The accompanying table shows drug use in various population groups. Each number is the percentage in that population group.

Sociodemographic differences among racial/ethnic groups explain, at least in part, the different rates of substance use. For example, we know that individuals in households with low family income tend to have a high rate of past-year use of any illicit drug, and the percentage of the population with low family income is higher among Mexicans, non-Hispanic blacks, and Puerto Ricans than in the total

U.S. population. Thus, family income differences partially explain the relatively high rates of illicit drug use among Mexicans, Puerto Ricans, and non-Hispanic blacks.

Interestingly, regardless of the racial/ethnic group, relatively high rates of illicit drug use are found among individuals who reside in the West; reside in metropolitan areas with populations greater than 1 million; lack health insurance coverage; are unemployed; have 9 to 11 years of schooling; or have never been married. Moreover, regardless of racial/ethnic group, adolescents who dropped out of school or who reside in households with fewer than two biological parents have relatively high rates of past-year use of illicit drugs.

Although numerous groups have called for increased funding to help meet the challenges of drug abuse in diverse populations, funding for such programs is limited. Additionally, a wide

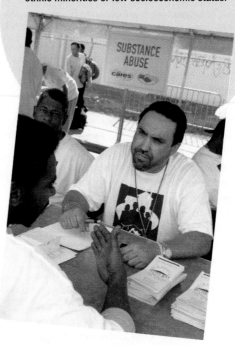

Substance abuse counseling outreach programs are aimed at addressing the high rates of substance abuse among people of ethnic minorities or low socioeconomic status.

range of socioeconomic, cultural, environmental, religious, and other differences pose unique challenges in trying to tailor programs to work with different populations. Research examining factors that influence prevention, intervention, and treatment effectiveness in diverse populations is needed and funding for improvements in programming is essential.

**Source:** Substance Abuse and Mental Health Services Administration, *Results from the 2008 National Survey on Drug Use and Health: National Findings,* NSDUH Series H-36, HHS Publication no. SMA 09-4434 (Rockville, MD: Office of Applied Studies, 2009), Available at www.oas .samhsa.gov/nsduh/2k8nsduh/2k8Results.cfm.

### Illicit Drug Use among Persons Aged 12 or Older, 2008 (%)

| | Lifetime Use | Past-Year Use | Past-Month Use | Past-Year Illicit Drug Dependence |
|---|---|---|---|---|
| Hispanic or Latino | 36.4 | 12.3 | 3.6 | 9.5 |
| White | 50.7 | 14.4 | 8.2 | 9.0 |
| Black or African American | 46.1 | 16.9 | 10.1 | 8.8 |
| American Indian or Alaska Native | 57.6 | 19.5 | 9.5 | 11.1 |
| Native Hawaiian or Other Pacific Islander | * | * | 7.3 | * |
| Asian | 21.2 | 7.4 | 3.6 | 4.2 |
| Two or more races | 56.1 | 21.2 | 14.7 | 9.8 |

*Low precision; no estimate reported.

drug-using workers at the plant, we are in danger. A drug-using bus driver, train engineer, or pilot jeopardizes our safety.

Many of us have stereotyped notions of illicit drug users but it is difficult to generalize. Illicit drug users span all age groups, genders, ethnicities, occupations, and socioeconomic groups (see the **Health in a Diverse World** box above).

No matter the group, illicit drug use has a devastating effect on users and their families in the United States and in many other countries.

The good news is that the use of illicit drugs in the United States has leveled off and is not increasing for most groups of people. Use of most drugs increased from the early 1970s to

## 13.1 30-Day Drug Use Prevalence, Full-Time College Students vs. Respondents 1–4 Years beyond High School

| | Full-Time College (%) | Others (%) | | Full-Time College (%) | Others (%) |
|---|---|---|---|---|---|
| Any illicit drug | 18.9 | 22.8 | Heroin | * | 0.3 |
| Any illicit drug other than marijuana | 7.3 | 12.0 | Narcotics other than heroin | 2.3 | 5.5 |
| Marijuana | 17.0 | 19.2 | Amphetamines, adjusted | 2.8 | 2.7 |
| Inhalants | 0.4 | 0.6 | Crystal methamphetamine | * | 0.1 |
| Hallucinogens | 1.7 | 1.1 | Sedatives (barbiturates) | 1.4 | 2.8 |
| LSD | 0.8 | 0.4 | Tranquilizers | 1.6 | 4.6 |
| Hallucinogens other than LSD | 1.3 | 0.9 | Alcohol | 69.0 | 55.0 |
| Ecstasy (methylene-dioxymethamphetamine, MDMA) | 0.6 | 1.8 | Been drunk | 45.3 | 30.8 |
| | | | Flavored alcoholic beverage | 35.8 | 28.1 |
| Cocaine | 1.2 | 3.0 | Cigarettes | 17.9 | 31.4 |
| Crack | 0.1 | 0.8 | *Approximate weighted N =* | 1,270 | 780 |
| Other cocaine | 1.1 | 3.1 | | | |

*Indicates prevalence less than 0.05%.

**Source:** L. D. Johnston et al., *Monitoring the Future National Survey Results on Drug Use, 1975–2008*, Volume 2, *College Students and Adults Ages 19–50*, NIH Publication no. 09-7403 (Bethesda, MD: National Institute on Drug Abuse, 2009), Available at http://monitoringthefuture.org/new.html.

the late 1970s, peaked between 1979 and 1986, and declined until 1992, from which point it has not changed. In 2007, an estimated 20.4 million Americans were illicit drug users, compared to the 1979 peak level of 25 million users.[17] Among youth, however, illicit drug use, notably of marijuana, has been rising in recent years.

### Illicit Drug Use on Campus

After more than a decade of declining use on American college campuses, illicit drugs have reappeared. In 2008, the number of college students nationwide who had tried any drug stood at almost 50 percent; over a third had smoked marijuana in the past year, and 20 percent had done so in the past month (see Table 13.1). Daily use of marijuana is at its highest point since 1989.[18] Cocaine use is down sharply, but LSD use has more than doubled.

For many students, their college environment coupled with our culture's societal mores regarding substance use and abuse on college campuses may make substance use and abuse seem like the norm. On most campuses, drugs have a presence, although perhaps not as much as students perceive. While 9 out of 10 college students do not abuse drugs, the percentage of those who do has increased dramatically in the past decade. For example, the proportion of students who use illicit drugs other than marijuana, such as cocaine, heroin, and Ecstasy, increased 52 percent—from 5 percent to 8 percent of all students—in the past decade.[19] College administrators, staff, and faculty are concerned about the link between substance abuse and poor academic performance, depression, anxiety, suicide, property damage, vandalism, fights, serious medical problems, and death.[20]

### Why Do Some College Students Use Drugs?

Research has identified the following factors in a student's life that increase the risk of substance abuse. The more factors there are, the greater the risk will be:

- **Positive expectations.** The most common reason students give to explain why they drink, smoke, or use drugs is to relax, reduce stress, or forget about problems (Figure 13.4 on page 414). As noted previously, some students take drugs, most notably prescription ADHD drugs and caffeine, in the belief that the drugs will aid their concentration and help them study.
- **Genetics and family history.** Genetics and family history play a significant role in the risk for developing an addiction.
- **Substance use in high school.** Two-thirds of college students who use illicit drugs began doing so in high school.
- **Mental health problems.** Students who report being diagnosed with depression are more likely to have abused prescription drugs, or to have used marijuana or other illicit drugs.
- **Sorority and fraternity membership.** Being a member of a sorority or fraternity increases the likelihood of using alcohol, marijuana, or cocaine and makes one twice as likely to abuse prescription drugs.
- **Stress.** For some students under academic and social stress, seemingly easy relief comes in the form of drugs or alcohol. Taking a pill to calm oneself, to relax and be more social in an uncomfortable situation, or just to "fit in" may push many otherwise non–drug-using students to begin to use or abuse drugs they otherwise might avoid.

### Why *Don't* Some College Students Use Drugs?

There can be many factors influencing a student to avoid drugs; some of the most commonly reported include the following:[21]

- **Parental attitudes and behavior.** Those students who say they are more influenced by their parents' concerns or

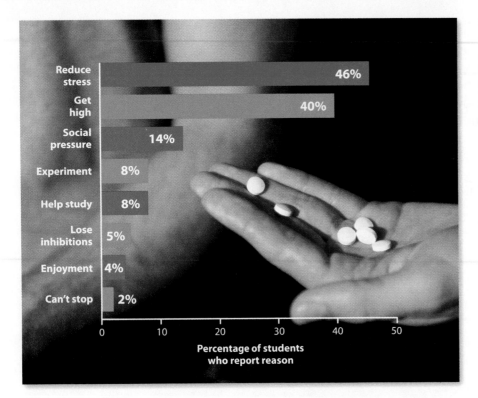

FIGURE 13.4 **Reasons College Students Use Illicit Drugs or Controlled Prescription Drugs**

**Source:** Adapted from *Wasting the Best and the Brightest: Substance Abuse at America's Colleges and Universities.* New York: National Center on Addiction and Substance Abuse at Columbia University, March 2007, page 47. Copyright © 2007. Used with permission. www.casacolumbia.org/templates/publications_reports.aspx.

expectations drink, use marijuana, and smoke significantly less than those students less influenced by parents.

- **Religion and spirituality.** The greater the students' level of religiosity (hours in prayer, attendance at services), the less likely they are to drink, smoke, or use other drugs.
- **Student engagement.** The more a student is involved in learning and in extracurricular activities, the less likely he or she is to binge drink, use marijuana, or abuse prescription drugs.
- **College athletics.** College athletes drink at higher rates than nonathletes but are less likely to use illicit drugs.
- **Healthy social network.** Having a wide range of friends and supports to help cope with the challenges of life is a well known protective factor for many negative behaviors, including drug use.

To prepare yourself for a possible offer of drugs on campus, and to be ready to make the decision that is best for *you*, see the **Skills for Behavior Change** box on the next page.

# Common Drugs of Abuse

Hundreds of drugs are subject to abuse—some are legal, such as recreational drugs and prescription medications, whereas many others are illegal and classified as "controlled substances." For general purposes, drugs can be divided into the following categories: *stimulants, mar-*

**stimulants** Drugs that increase activity of the central nervous system.

*ijuana and other cannabinoids, depressants, hallucinogens, inhalants,* and *steroids.* These categories are discussed in subsequent sections; Table 13.2 on pages 416 and 417 summarizes the categorization, uses, and effects of various drugs of abuse, both legal and illicit.

## Stimulants

A **stimulant** is a drug that increases activity of the central nervous system. Its effects usually involve increased activity, anxiety, and agitation; users often seem jittery or nervous while high. Commonly used stimulants include cocaine, amphetamines, methamphetamine, and caffeine. See Chapter 12 for a discussion of nicotine, the addictive substance in tobacco products, which is another common stimulant.

**Cocaine** A white crystalline powder derived from the leaves of the South American coca shrub (not related to cocoa plants), *cocaine* ("coke") has been described as one of the most powerful naturally occurring stimulants. It binds at receptor sites in the central nervous system, producing an intense high that usually disappears quickly, leaving a powerful craving for more.

**Methods of Use and Physical Effects** Cocaine can be taken in several ways, including snorting, smoking, and injecting. The powdered form is snorted through the nose, which can damage mucous membranes and cause sinusitis. It can destroy the user's sense of smell, and occasionally it even eats a hole through the septum. When snorted, the drug enters the bloodstream through the lungs in less than 1 minute and reaches the brain in less than 3 minutes.

Cocaine alkaloid, or *freebase*, is obtained by removing the hydrochloride salt from cocaine powder. *Freebasing* refers to the smoking of freebase by placing it at the end of a pipe and holding a flame near it to produce a vapor, which is then inhaled. *Crack* is identical pharmacologically to freebase, but the hydrochloride salt is still present and is processed with baking soda and water. It is a cheap, widely available drug that is smokable and very potent. Crack is commonly smoked in the same manner as freebase. Because crack is such a pure drug, it takes little time to achieve the desired high, and a crack user can become addicted quickly.

Some cocaine users inject the drug intravenously, which introduces large amounts into the body rapidly, creating a brief, intense high, and subsequent crash. Injecting users place themselves at risk not only for contracting HIV and hepatitis through shared needles, but also for skin infections, vein damage, inflamed arteries, and infection of the heart lining.

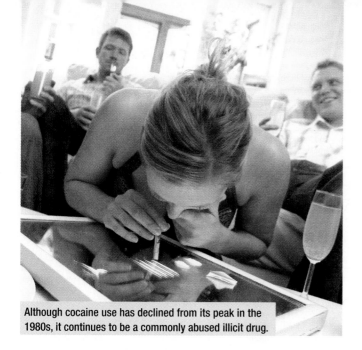

Although cocaine use has declined from its peak in the 1980s, it continues to be a commonly abused illicit drug.

## Responding to an Offer of Drugs

No matter what your experience has been up until now, it is likely that you will be invited to use drugs at some point in your life. Here are some questions to consider *before* you find yourself in a situation in which you have the opportunity or feel pressure to use illicit drugs:

✳ Why am I considering trying drugs? Am I trying to fit in or impress my friends? What does this say about my friends if I need to take drugs to impress them? Are my friends really looking out for what is best for me?
✳ Am I using this drug to cope or feel different? Am I depressed?
✳ What could taking drugs cost me? Will this cost me my career if I am caught using? Could using drugs prevent me from getting a job?
✳ What are the long-term consequences of using this drug?
✳ What will this cost me in terms of my friendships and family? How would my close family and friends respond if they knew I was using drugs?

Even when you make the decision not to use drugs, it can be difficult to say no gracefully. Some good ways to turn down an offer:

✳ "Thanks, but I've got a big test (game, meeting) tomorrow morning."
✳ "I've already got a great buzz right now. I really don't need anything more."
✳ "I don't like how (insert drug name here) makes me feel."
✳ "I'm driving tonight. So I'm not using."
✳ "I want to go for a run in the morning."
✳ "No."

Cocaine is both an anesthetic and a central nervous system stimulant. In tiny doses, it can slow the heart rate. In larger doses, the physical effects are dramatic: increased heart rate and blood pressure, loss of appetite that can lead to dramatic weight loss, convulsions, muscle twitching, irregular heartbeat, and even death resulting from an overdose. Other effects of cocaine include temporary relief of depression, decreased fatigue, talkativeness, increased alertness, and heightened self-confidence. However, as the dose increases, users become irritable and apprehensive, and their behavior may turn paranoid or violent.

### Amphetamines
The **amphetamines** include a large and varied group of synthetic agents that stimulate the central nervous system. Small doses of amphetamines improve alertness, lessen fatigue, and generally elevate mood. With repeated use, however, physical and psychological dependencies develop. Sleep patterns are affected (insomnia); heart rate, breathing rate, and blood pressure increase; and restlessness, anxiety, appetite suppression, and vision problems are common. High doses over long time periods can produce hallucinations, delusions, and disorganized behavior.

Certain types of amphetamines or amphetamine-like drugs are used for medicinal purposes. As discussed earlier, drugs prescribed to treat ADHD are stimulants, and are increasingly abused on campus.

### Methamphetamine
An increasingly common form of amphetamine, *methamphetamine* (commonly called simply "meth") is a potent, long-acting, addictive drug that strongly activates the brain's reward center by producing a sense of euphoria. Methamphetamine can be snorted, smoked, injected, or orally ingested. When snorted, the effects can be felt in 3 to 5 minutes; if orally ingested, effects occur within 15 to 20 minutes. The pleasurable effects of methamphetamine are typically an intense rush lasting only a few minutes when snorted; in contrast, smoking the drug can produce a high lasting more than 8 hours.

In the short term, methamphetamine produces increased physical activity, alertness, euphoria, rapid breathing, increased body temperature, insomnia, tremors, anxiety, confusion, and decreased appetite; however, the drug's effects quickly wear off, leaving the user seeking more. Users often experience tolerance after the first use, making methamphetamine a highly addictive drug.

**amphetamines** A large and varied group of synthetic agents that stimulate the central nervous system.

The long-term effects of methamphetamine can include severe weight loss, cardiovascular damage, increased risk of heart attack and stroke, hallucinations, extensive tooth decay and tooth loss, violence, paranoia, psychotic behavior, and even death. Brain damage similar to Parkinson's disease and Alzheimer's disease has been reported in long-term meth users.

TABLE

13.2
**Drugs of Abuse: Uses and Effects**

| Category | Drugs | Trade or Street Names | Dependence | Usual Method | Possible Effects | Effects of Overdose | Withdrawal Syndrome |
|---|---|---|---|---|---|---|---|
| **Stimulants** | Cocaine | Coke, Flake, Snow, Crack, *Coca, Blanca, Perico* | *Physical:* Possible *Psychological:* High *Tolerance:* Yes | Snorted, smoked, injected | Increased alertness, excitation, euphoria, increased pulse rate and blood pressure, insomnia, loss of appetite | Agitation, increased body temperature, hallucinations, convulsions, possible death | Apathy, long periods of sleep, irritability, depression, disorientation |
| | Amphetamine, methamphetamine | Crank, Ice, Cristal, Crystal Meth, Speed, Adderall, Dexedrine | *Physical:* Possible *Psychological:* High *Tolerance:* Yes | Oral, injected, smoked | | | |
| | Methylphenidate | Ritalin (Illys), Concerta, Focalin, Metadate | *Physical:* Possible *Psychological:* High *Tolerance:* Yes | Oral, injected, snorted, smoked | | | |
| **Cannabis** | Marijuana | Pot, Grass, Sinsemilla, Blunts, *Mota, Yerba, Grifa* | *Physical:* Possible *Psychological:* High *Tolerance:* Yes | Oral, smoked | Euphoria, relaxed inhibitions, increased appetite, disorientation | Fatigue, paranoia, possible psychosis | Occasional reports of insomnia, hyperactivity, decreased appetite |
| | Hashish, hashish oil | Hash, Hash oil | *Physical:* Unknown *Psychological:* Moderate *Tolerance:* Yes | Smoked, oral | | | |
| **Narcotics** | Heroin | Diamorphine, Horse, Smack, Black tar, *Chiva* | *Physical:* High *Psychological:* High *Tolerance:* Yes | Injected, snorted, smoked | Euphoria, drowsiness, respiratory depression, constricted pupils, nausea | Slow and shallow breathing, clammy skin, convulsions, coma, possible death | Watery eyes, runny nose, yawning, loss of appetite, irritability, tremors, panic, cramps, nausea, chills and sweating |
| | Morphine | MS-Contin, Roxanol | *Physical:* High *Psychological:* High *Tolerance:* Yes | Oral, injected | | | |
| | Hydrocodone, oxycodone | Vicodin, OxyContin, Percocet, Percodan | *Physical:* High *Psychological:* High *Tolerance:* Yes | Oral | | | |
| | Codeine | Acetaminophen w/Codeine, Tylenol w/Codeine | *Physical:* Moderate *Psychological:* Moderate *Tolerance:* Yes | Oral, injected | | | |
| **Depressants** | Gamma-hydroxybutrate | GHB, Liquid Ecstasy, Liquid X | *Physical:* Moderate *Psychological:* Moderate *Tolerance:* Yes | *Oral* | Slurred speech, disorientation, drunken behavior without odor of alcohol, impaired memory of events, interacts with alcohol | Shallow respiration, clammy skin, dilated pupils, weak and rapid pulse, coma, possible death | Anxiety, insomnia, tremors, delirium, convulsions, possible death |
| | Benzodiazepines | Valium, Xanax, Halcion, Ativan, Rohypnol (Roofies, R-2), Klonopin | *Physical:* Moderate *Psychological:* Moderate *Tolerance:* Yes | Oral, injected | | | |
| | Other depressants | Ambien, Sonata, Barbiturates, Methaqualone (Quaalude) | *Physical:* Moderate *Psychological:* Moderate *Tolerance:* Yes | Oral | | | |
| **Hallucinogens** | Methylene-dioxymethamphetamine (MDMA), analogs | Ecstasy, XTC, Adam, MDA (Love Drug), MDEA (Eve) | *Physical:* None *Psychological:* Moderate *Tolerance:* Yes | Oral, snorted, smoked | Heightened senses, teeth grinding, dehydration | Increased body temperature, electrolyte imbalance, cardiac arrest | Muscle aches, drowsiness, depression, acne |
| | LSD | Acid, Microdot, Sunshine, Boomers | *Physical:* None *Psychological:* Unknown *Tolerance:* Yes | Oral | Illusions and hallucinations, altered perception of time and distance | Longer, more intense "trips" | None |
| | Phencyclidine, analogs | PCP, Angel Dust, Hog, Ketamine (Special K) | *Physical:* Possible *Psychological:* High *Tolerance:* Yes | Smoked, oral, injected, snorted | | Unable to direct movement, feel pain, or remember | Drug-seeking behavior |
| | Other hallucinogens | Psilocybe mushrooms, Mescaline, Peyote, Dextromethorphan | *Physical:* None *Psychological:* None *Tolerance:* Possible | Oral | | | |

*Continued on next page*

| Category | Drugs | Trade or Street Names | Dependence | Usual Method | Possible Effects | Effects of Overdose | Withdrawal Syndrome |
|---|---|---|---|---|---|---|---|
| Inhalants | Amyl and butyl nitrite | Pearls, Poppers, Rush, Locker Room | *Physical:* Unknown<br>*Psychological:* Unknown<br>*Tolerance:* No | Inhaled | Flushing, hypotension, headache | Methemo-globinemia | Agitation |
| | Nitrous oxide | Laughing gas, balloons, Whippets | *Physical:* Unknown<br>*Psychological:* Low<br>*Tolerance:* No | Inhaled | Impaired memory, slurred speech, drunken behavior, slow-onset vitamin deficiency, organ damage | Vomiting, respiratory depression, loss of consciousness, possible death | Trembling, anxiety, insomnia, vitamin deficiency, confusion, hallucinations, convulsions |
| | Other inhalants | Adhesives, spray paint, hairspray, lighter fluid | *Physical:* Unknown<br>*Psychological:* High<br>*Tolerance:* No | Inhaled | | | |
| Anabolic Steroids | Testosterone | Depo Testosterone, Sustanon, Sten, Cypt | *Physical:* Unknown<br>*Psychological:* Unknown<br>*Tolerance:* Unknown | Injected | Virilization, edema, testicular atrophy, gynecomastia, acne, aggressive behavior | Unknown | Possible depression |
| | Other anabolic steroids | Parabolan, Winstrol, Equipose, Anadrol, Dianabol | *Physical:* Unknown<br>*Psychological:* Yes<br>*Tolerance:* Unknown | Oral, injected | | | |

**Source:** Adapted from U.S. Department of Justice Drug Enforcement Administration, "Drugs of Abuse/Uses and Effects," 2004, www.usdoj.gov/dea/pubs/abuse/chart.htm.

*Ice* is a potent form of methamphetamine that is imported primarily from Asia, particularly South Korea and Taiwan. It is purer and more crystalline than the version manufactured in the United States, and it is odorless when smoked. Its effects can last for more than 12 hours.

Like other amphetamines, the downside of methamphetamine is devastating. Prolonged use can cause fatal lung and kidney damage as well as long-lasting psychological damage. In some instances, major psychological dysfunction can persist as long as 2.5 years after last use. Methamphetamine can cause psychosis, increased risk for heart attack and stroke, and brain damage that results in impaired motor skills and cognitive functions.

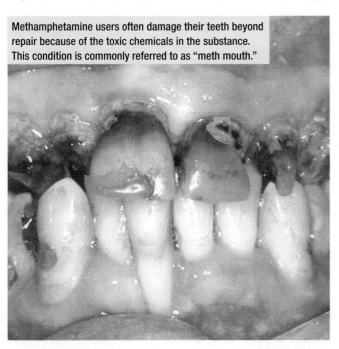

Methamphetamine users often damage their teeth beyond repair because of the toxic chemicals in the substance. This condition is commonly referred to as "meth mouth."

Methamphetamine abuse is an increasingly serious problem, especially in rural areas of the United States. In 2008, 2.8 percent of high school seniors reported using methamphetamine in their lifetime. Rates among adults are difficult to determine, but it is believed that more than 12 million Americans have tried methamphetamine.[22] A possible contributing factor to the increasing rate of methamphetamine use is that it is relatively easy to make using recipes that often include common OTC ingredients such as ephedrine and pseudoephedrine.

**Caffeine** What is the most popular and widely consumed drug in the United States? Caffeine. Almost half of all Americans drink coffee every day, and many others consume caffeine in some other form, mainly for its well-known "wake-up" effect. Drinking coffee, tea, soft drinks, and other caffeine-containing products is legal, even socially encouraged. Caffeine may seem harmless, but excessive consumption is associated with addiction and certain health problems.

*Caffeine* is derived from the chemical family called *xanthines,* which are found in plant products from which coffee, tea, and chocolate are made. The xanthines are mild, central nervous system stimulants that enhance mental alertness and reduce feelings of fatigue. Other stimulant effects include increased heart muscle contractions, oxygen consumption, metabolism, and urinary output. A person feels these effects within 15 to 45 minutes of ingesting a caffeinated product. It takes 4 to 6 hours for the body to metabolize half of the caffeine ingested, so, depending on the amount of caffeine taken in, it may continue to exert effects for a day or longer. Figure 13.5 on page 418 compares the caffeine content of various products.

Side effects of the xanthines include wakefulness, insomnia, irregular heartbeat, dizziness, nausea, indigestion, and

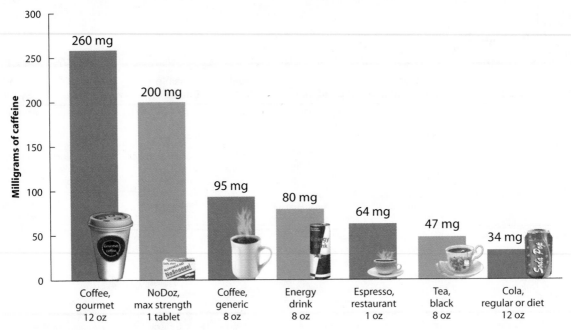

FIGURE 13.5 **Caffeine Content Comparison**

**Source:** Data are from *USDA National Nutrient Database for Standard Reference*, Release 22 (2009), www.ars.usda.gov/ba/bhnrc/ndl.

sometimes mild delirium. Some people also experience heartburn. As the effects of caffeine wear off, frequent users may feel let down—mentally or physically depressed, exhausted, and weak. To counteract this, they commonly choose to drink another cup of coffee. Habitually engaging in this practice leads to tolerance and psychological dependence. Symptoms of excessive caffeine consumption include chronic insomnia, jitters, irritability, nervousness, anxiety, and involuntary muscle twitches. Withdrawing from caffeine may compound the effects and produce severe headaches, fatigue, and nausea. Because caffeine meets the requirements for addiction—tolerance, psychological dependence, and withdrawal symptoms—it can be classified as addictive.

> **marijuana** Chopped leaves and flowers of *Cannabis indica* or *Cannabis sativa* plants (hemp); a psychoactive stimulant.
>
> **tetrahydrocannabinol (THC)** The chemical name for the active ingredient in marijuana.

Long-term caffeine use has been suspected of being linked to several serious health problems. However, no strong evidence exists to suggest that moderate caffeine use (less than 300 mg daily, approximately 3 cups of regular coffee) produces harmful effects in healthy, nonpregnant people. Caffeine does not appear to cause long-term high blood pressure, has not been linked to strokes, nor is there any evidence of a relationship between caffeine and heart disease.[23] However, people who suffer from irregular heartbeat are cautioned against using caffeine, because the resultant increase in heart rate might be life threatening.

**what do you think?**

How much caffeine do you consume regularly, and why? ● What is your pattern of caffeine consumption? ● Have you ever experienced any ill effects after going without caffeine for a period of time?

## Marijuana and Other Cannabinoids

Although archaeological evidence indicates that **marijuana** ("grass," "weed," "pot") was used as long as 6,000 years ago, the drug did not become popular in the United States until the 1960s. Today, marijuana is the most commonly used illicit drug in the country. Approximately 41 percent of Americans over the age of 12 has tried marijuana at least once.[24] Some 26 million have used marijuana in the past year, and more than 15.2 million have done so in the past month. Marijuana use is also on the rise on college campuses, following the trend of increased use in the general population.[25]

**Methods of Use and Physical Effects** Marijuana is derived from either the *Cannabis sativa* or *Cannabis indica* (hemp) plant. Most of the time, marijuana is smoked, although it can also be ingested, as in brownies baked with marijuana in them. When marijuana is smoked, it is usually rolled into cigarettes (joints) or placed in a pipe or water pipe (bong).

**Tetrahydrocannabinol (THC)** is the psychoactive substance in marijuana and the key to determining how powerful a high it will produce. More potent forms of the drug can contain up to 27 percent THC, but most average 7 percent.[26] *Hashish*, a potent cannabis preparation derived mainly from the plant's thick, sticky resin, contains high THC concentrations. Hash oil, a substance produced by percolating a solvent such as ether through dried marijuana to extract the THC, is a tarlike liquid that may contain up to 300 mg of THC in a dose.

The effects of smoking marijuana are generally felt within 10 to 30 minutes and usually wear off within 3 hours. The most noticeable visible effect of THC is the dilation of the eyes' blood vessels, which gives the smoker bloodshot eyes. Marijuana smokers also exhibit coughing; dry mouth and throat ("cotton mouth"); increased thirst and appetite; lowered blood pressure; and mild muscular weakness, primarily exhibited in drooping eyelids. Users can also experience severe anxiety, panic, paranoia, and psychosis, and may have intensified reactions to various stimuli—colors, sounds, and the speed at which things move may seem altered. High doses of hashish may produce vivid visual hallucinations.

One common way of smoking marijuana is to use a pipe.

**Marijuana and Driving** Marijuana use presents clear hazards for drivers of motor vehicles and others on the road with them. The drug substantially reduces a driver's ability to react and make quick decisions. Perceptual and other performance deficits resulting from marijuana use may persist for some time after the high subsides. Users who attempt to drive, fly, or operate heavy machinery often fail to recognize their impairment. Overall, marijuana is the most prevalent illegal drug detected in impaired drivers, fatally injured drivers, and motor vehicle crash victims.[27] In many of these cases, alcohol is detected as well. Research by the National Highway Traffic Safety Administration indicates that a moderate dose of marijuana alone impairs driving performance; however, the effects of even a low dose of marijuana combined with alcohol are markedly greater than for either drug alone.[28]

**Effects of Chronic Marijuana Use** Because marijuana is illegal in most parts of the United States and has been widely used only since the 1960s, long-term studies of its effects have been difficult to conduct. Also, studies conducted in the 1960s involved marijuana with THC levels only a fraction of today's levels, so their results may not apply to the stronger forms available today.

Numerous studies have shown that marijuana smoke contains 50 to 70 percent more carcinogenic hydrocarbons than does tobacco smoke. Because marijuana smokers typically inhale more deeply and hold their breath longer than tobacco smokers, the lungs are exposed to more carcinogens. As well, effects from irritation (e.g., cough, excessive phlegm, and increased lung infections) similar to those experienced by tobacco smokers can occur.[29] Lung conditions such as chronic bronchitis, emphysema, and other lung disorders are also associated with smoking marijuana.

Inhaling marijuana smoke introduces carbon monoxide to the bloodstream. Because the blood has a greater affinity for carbon monoxide than it does for oxygen, its oxygen-carrying capacity is diminished, and the heart must work harder to pump oxygen to oxygen-starved tissues. Furthermore, the tar from cannabis contains higher levels of carcinogens than does tobacco smoke.

Recent research has found that frequent and/or long-term marijuana use may significantly increase a man's risk of developing testicular cancer. The researchers found that being a marijuana smoker at the time of diagnosis was associated with a 70 percent increased risk of testicular cancer.[30] The risk was particularly elevated (about twice that of those who never smoked marijuana) for those who used marijuana at least weekly or who had long-term exposure to the substance beginning in adolescence. The results also suggested that the association with marijuana use might be limited to *nonseminoma*, an aggressive, fast-growing testicular malignancy that tends to strike early, between ages 20 and 35, and accounts for about 40 percent of all testicular cancer cases.[31]

According to the National Survey on Drug Use and Health, teens and young adults who use marijuana are more likely to develop serious mental health problems. A number of studies have shown an association between marijuana use and increased rates of anxiety, depression, suicidal ideation, and schizophrenia.[32] Some of these studies have shown age at first use as an indicator of vulnerability to later problems. Among individuals 18 and older, those who used marijuana before the age of 12 were twice as likely to have a serious mental illness as those who first used marijuana at age 18 or older.[33]

Other risks associated with marijuana use include suppression of the immune system, blood pressure changes, and impaired memory function. Recent studies suggest that pregnant women who smoke marijuana are at a higher risk for stillbirth or miscarriage and for delivering low-birth-weight babies and babies with abnormalities of the nervous system.[34]

**Marijuana as Medicine** Although recognized as a dangerous drug by the U.S. government, marijuana has several medical purposes. It helps control the severe nausea and vomiting produced by chemotherapy. It improves appetite

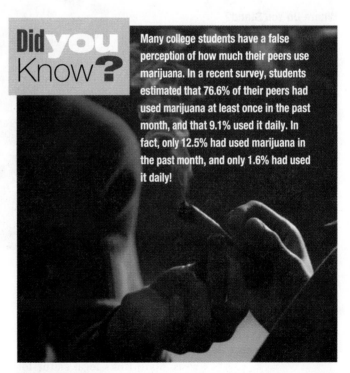

**Did you Know?**

Many college students have a false perception of how much their peers use marijuana. In a recent survey, students estimated that 76.6% of their peers had used marijuana at least once in the past month, and that 9.1% used it daily. In fact, only 12.5% had used marijuana in the past month, and only 1.6% had used it daily!

**Source:** Data are from American College Health Association, *American College Health Association—National College Health Assessment II (ACHA-NCHA II): Reference Group Data Report Fall 2009* (Baltimore: American College Health Association, 2010).

# Medical Marijuana:
## TOO LEGAL OR NOT LEGAL ENOUGH?

For years, the use of medical marijuana has been hotly debated. Currently, 31 states and the District of Columbia have laws that recognize marijuana's medical value. Eight states have symbolic laws that recognize marijuana's medical value but fail to protect patients from arrest for possession of an illegal drug. Voters in 14 states (Alaska, California, Colorado, Hawaii, Maine, Michigan, Montana, New Mexico, New Jersey, Nevada, Oregon, Rhode Island, Vermont, and Washington) have chosen to legalize marijuana for medicinal use. These new state laws, however, conflict with federal laws against the possession of marijuana and have led to new, yet unresolved, battles in court.

The arguments for and against the legalization of marijuana have been very strong over the past few decades. Below are some of the major points from both sides of the issue.

### Arguments for Legalization

○ Marijuana is a safe and effective treatment for certain complications of dozens of conditions, such as cancer, AIDS, multiple sclerosis, pain, migraines, glaucoma, and epilepsy.

○ Legalizing marijuana and taxing its sale would bring in revenue for the government.

○ Legal government and U.S. Food and Drug Administration (FDA) oversight would allow for standardization of marijuana growth and production and could promote more responsible cultivation methods.

### Arguments against Legalization

○ It is not necessary to legalize marijuana for medical use because there are already FDA-approved drugs that are just as effective in treating the same conditions.

○ Marijuana use poses dangerous side effects including lung injury, immune system damage, and interference with fertility that make it inappropriate for FDA approval.

○ Marijuana is known to be addictive and may lead to harder drug use.

### Where Do You Stand?

○ Do you think medical marijuana should be legalized by the federal government? What potential problems do you think this would create or solve?

○ Do you think marijuana use in general should be legalized?

○ What criteria do you think should be used to determine the legality of a particular substance? Who should make those determinations?

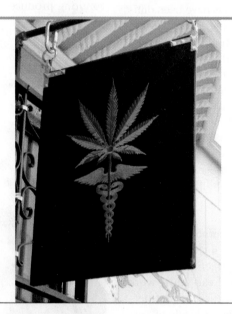

○ What are your feelings on drug laws in general—do you think they should be more or less prohibitive? What sort of policies would you propose to protect individuals and their rights?

**Sources:** Marijuana Policy Project, *State by State Medical Marijuana Laws: How to Remove the Threat of Arrest* (Washington, DC: 2008); Marijuana Policy Project, "Medical Marijuana Overview," 2009, www.mpp.org/library/research/medical-marijuana-overview.html; ProCon.org, "Medical Marijuana," 2009, http://medicalmarijuana.procon.org.

and forestalls the loss of lean muscle mass associated with AIDS-wasting syndrome. Marijuana also reduces the muscle pain and spasticity caused by diseases such as multiple sclerosis. Marijuana's legal status for medicinal purposes continues to be hotly debated (see the **Points of View** box above).

**depressants** Drugs that slow down the activity of the central nervous system.

## Depressants

Whereas central nervous system stimulants increase muscular and nervous system activity, **depressants** have the opposite effect. These drugs slow down neuromuscular activity and cause sleepiness or calmness. If the dose is high enough, brain function can be stopped, causing death. Alcohol is the most widely used central nervous system depressant (see Chapter 11). Other forms include opioids, benzodiazepines, and barbiturates.

## Opioids

**Opioids** cause drowsiness, relieve pain, and produce euphoria. Also called *narcotics,* opioids are derived from the parent drug **opium,** a dark, resinous substance made from the milky juice of the opium poppy seedpod, and they are all highly addictive. Opium and heroin are both illegal in the United States, but some opioids are available by prescription for medical purposes: Morphine is sometimes prescribed for severe pain, and codeine is found in prescription cough syrups and other painkillers. Several prescription drugs, including Vicodin, Percodan, OxyContin, Demerol, and Dilaudid, contain synthetic opioids.

**Physical Effects of Opioids** Opioids are powerful depressants of the central nervous system. In addition to relieving pain, these drugs lower heart rate, respiration, and blood pressure. Side effects include weakness, dizziness, nausea, vomiting, euphoria, decreased sex drive, visual disturbances, and lack of coordination.

The human body's physiology could be said to encourage opioid addiction. Opioid-like hormones called **endorphins** are manufactured in the body and have multiple receptor sites, particularly in the central nervous system. When endorphins attach themselves at these points, they create feelings of painless well-being; medical researchers refer to them as "the body's own opioids." When endorphin levels are high, people feel euphoric. The same euphoria occurs when opioids or related chemicals are active at the endorphin receptor sites. Of all the opioids, heroin has the greatest notoriety as an addictive drug. The following section discusses the progression of heroin addiction; addiction to any opioid follows a similar path.

**Heroin Use** *Heroin* is a white powder derived from morphine. *Black tar heroin* is a sticky, dark brown, foul-smelling form of heroin that is relatively pure and inexpensive. Once considered a cure for morphine dependence, heroin was later discovered to be even more addictive and potent than morphine. Today, heroin has no medical use.

Heroin is a depressant that produces drowsiness and a dreamy, mentally slow feeling. It can cause drastic mood swings, with euphoric highs followed by depressive lows. Heroin slows respiration and urinary output and constricts the pupils of the eyes. Symptoms of tolerance and withdrawal can appear within 3 weeks of first use.

Opium is extracted from opium poppy seedpods like this one.

It is estimated that more than 4 million people have used heroin at one time in their lives. The most common route of administration for heroin addicts is "mainlining"—intravenous injection of powdered heroin mixed in a solution. Many users describe the "rush" they feel when injecting themselves as intensely pleasurable, whereas others report unpredictable and unpleasant side effects. The temporary nature of the rush contributes to the drug's high potential for addiction—many addicts shoot up four or five times a day. Mainlining can cause veins to scar and eventually collapse. Once a vein has collapsed, it can no longer be used to introduce heroin into the bloodstream. Addicts become expert at locating new veins to use: in the feet, the legs, the temples, under the tongue, or in the groin. While heroin is usually injected, the contemporary version of heroin is so potent that users can get high by snorting or smoking the drug. This has attracted a more affluent group of users who may not want to inject, for reasons such as the increased risk of contracting diseases such as HIV.

**Treatment for Heroin Addiction** Heroin addicts experience a distinct pattern of withdrawal. Symptoms of withdrawal include intense desire for the drug, sleep disturbance, dilated pupils, loss of appetite, irritability, goose bumps, and muscle tremors. The most difficult time in the withdrawal process occurs 24 to 72 hours following last use. All of the preceding symptoms continue, along with nausea, abdominal cramps, restlessness, insomnia, vomiting, diarrhea, extreme anxiety, hot and cold flashes, elevated blood pressure, and rapid heartbeat and respiration. Once the peak of withdrawal has passed, all these symptoms begin to subside. Still, the recovering addict has many hurdles to jump.

Methadone maintenance is one treatment available for people addicted to heroin or other opioids. Methadone is chemically similar enough to opioids to control the tremors, chills, vomiting, diarrhea, and severe abdominal pains of withdrawal. However, methadone maintenance is controversial because of the drug's own potential for addiction. Critics contend that the program merely substitutes one addiction for another. Proponents argue that people on methadone maintenance are less likely to engage in criminal activities to support their habits than heroin addicts are. For this reason, many methadone maintenance programs are financed by state or federal government and are available free of charge or at reduced cost.

A number of new drug therapies for opioid dependence are emerging. Naltrexone (Trexan), an opioid antagonist, has been approved as a treatment. While on naltrexone, recovering addicts do not have the compulsion to use heroin, and if they do use it, they don't get high, so there is no point in using the drug. More recently, researchers have reported promising results with buprenorphine (Temgesic), a mild,

**opioids** Drugs that induce sleep and relieve pain; includes derivatives of opium and synthetics with similar chemical properties; also called *narcotics.*

**opium** The parent drug of the opioids; made from the seedpod resin of the opium poppy.

**endorphins** Opioid-like hormones that are manufactured in the human body and contribute to natural feelings of well-being.

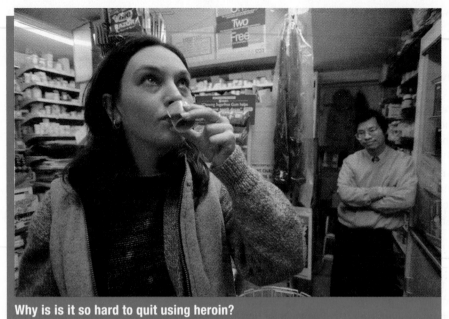

**Why is is it so hard to quit using heroin?**

Heroin's effect on the body is similar to the painless well-being created by endorphins. Stopping heroin use causes withdrawal symptoms that can be very difficult to manage, which keeps many addicts from attempting to quit. Methadone is a synthetic narcotic that blocks the effects of withdrawal. Although it is still a narcotic and must be administered under the supervision of clinic or pharmacy staff, methadone allows many heroin addicts to lead somewhat normal lives.

for one sedative or become dependent on it and develop tolerance for others as well. Withdrawal from sedative or hypnotic drugs may range from mild discomfort to severe symptoms, depending on the degree of dependence.

**Rohypnol** One benzodiazepine of concern is Rohypnol, a potent tranquilizer similar in nature to Valium but many times stronger. The drug produces a sedative effect, amnesia, muscle relaxation, and slowed psychomotor responses. The most publicized "date rape" drug, Rohypnol has gained notoriety as a growing problem on college campuses. The drug has been added to punch and other drinks at parties, where it is reportedly given to women in hopes of lowering their inhibitions and facilitating potential sexual conquests. See Chapter 19 for more information about drug-facilitated rape.

**GHB** *Gamma-hydroxybutyrate (GHB)* is a central nervous system depressant known to have euphoric, sedative, and anabolic (bodybuilding) effects. It was originally sold over the counter to bodybuilders to help reduce body fat and build muscle. Concerns about GHB led the FDA to ban OTC sales in 1992, and GHB is now a Schedule I controlled substance.[35] Gamma-hydroxybutyrate is an odorless, tasteless fluid that can be made easily at home or in a chemistry lab. Like Rohypnol, GHB has been slipped into drinks without being detected, resulting in loss of memory, unconsciousness, amnesia, and even death. Other dangerous side effects include nausea, vomiting, seizures, hallucinations, coma, and respiratory distress.

nonaddicting synthetic opioid that, like heroin and methadone, bonds to certain receptors in the brain, blocks pain messages, and persuades the brain that its cravings for heroin have been satisfied.

**Benzodiazepines and Barbiturates** A *sedative* drug promotes mental calmness and reduces anxiety, whereas a *hypnotic* drug promotes sleep or drowsiness. The most common sedative-hypnotic drugs are **benzodiazepines,** more commonly known as *tranquilizers*. These include prescription drugs such as Valium, Ativan, and Xanax. Benzodiazepines are most commonly prescribed for tension, muscular strain, sleep problems, anxiety, panic attacks, and alcohol withdrawal. **Barbiturates** are sedative-hypnotic drugs that include Amytal and Seconal. Today, benzodiazepines have largely replaced barbiturates, which were used medically in the past for relieving tension and inducing relaxation and sleep.

Sedative-hypnotics have a synergistic effect when combined with alcohol, another central nervous system depressant. Taken together, these drugs can lead to respiratory failure and death. All sedative or hypnotic drugs can produce physical and psychological dependence in several weeks. A complication specific to sedatives is cross-tolerance, which occurs when users develop tolerance

**benzodiazepines** A class of central nervous system depressant drugs with sedative, hypnotic, and muscle relaxant effects.

**barbiturates** Drugs that depress the central nervous system and have sedating, hypnotic, and anesthetic effects.

**hallucinogens** Substances capable of creating auditory or visual distortions and heightened states.

# Hallucinogens

**Hallucinogens,** or *psychedelics,* are substances that are capable of creating auditory or visual hallucinations and unusual changes in mood, thoughts, and feelings. The major receptor sites for most of these drugs are in the reticular formation (located in the brainstem at the upper end of the spinal cord), which is responsible for interpreting outside stimuli before allowing these signals to travel to other parts of the brain. When a hallucinogen is present at a reticular formation site, messages become scrambled, and the user may see wavy walls instead of straight ones or may "smell" colors and "hear" tastes. This mixing of sensory messages is known as *synesthesia.* Users may also become less inhibited or recall events long buried in the subconscious mind. The most widely recognized hallucinogens are LSD, Ecstasy,

**4.6%** of college students report having tried hallucinogens.

mescaline, psilocybin, PCP, and ketamine. All are illegal and carry severe penalties for manufacture, possession, transportation, or sale.

## LSD

Of all the psychedelics, *lysergic acid diethylamide* (*LSD*) is the most notorious. First synthesized in the late 1930s by Swiss chemist Albert Hoffman, LSD received media attention in the 1960s when young people used the drug to "turn on and tune out." In 1970, federal authorities placed LSD on the list of controlled substances (Schedule I). The drug's popularity peaked in 1972 then tapered off, primarily because of users' inability to control dosages accurately.

Today this dangerous psychedelic drug, known on the street as "acid," has been making a comeback. LSD especially attracts younger users. Over 9 percent of Americans, most of them under age 35, have tried LSD at least once.[36] A national survey of college students showed that 1.5 percent had used the drug in the past year.[37]

The most common and popular form of LSD is blotter acid—small squares of blotter-like paper that have been impregnated with a liquid LSD mixture. The blotter is swallowed or chewed briefly. LSD also comes in tiny thin squares of gelatin called *windowpane* and in tablets called *microdots*, which are less than an eighth of an inch across (it would take ten or more to equal the size of an aspirin tablet).

One of the most powerful drugs known to science, LSD can produce strong effects in doses as low as 20 micrograms (μg). (To give you an idea of how small a dose this is, the average postage stamp weighs approximately 60,000 μg.) The potency of a typical dose currently ranges from 20 to 80 μg, compared to 150 to 300 μg commonly used in the 1960s.

The psychological effects of LSD vary. Euphoria is the common psychological state produced by the drug, but dysphoria (a sense of evil and foreboding) may also be experienced. LSD also causes distortions of ordinary perceptions, such as the movement of stationary objects, as well as auditory or visual hallucinations. In addition, the drug shortens attention span, causing the mind to wander. Thoughts may be interposed and juxtaposed, so the user experiences several different thoughts simultaneously. Users become introspective, and suppressed memories may surface, often taking on bizarre symbolism. Many more effects are possible, including decreased aggressiveness and enhanced sensory experiences.

In addition to its psychedelic effects, LSD produces several physical effects, including increased heart rate, elevated blood pressure and temperature, goose-flesh (roughened skin), increased reflex speeds, muscle tremors and twitches, perspiration, increased salivation, chills, headaches, and mild nausea. Because the drug also stimulates uterine muscle contractions, it can lead to premature labor and miscarriage in pregnant women. Research into long-term effects has been inconclusive.

Although there is no evidence that LSD creates physical dependency, it may well create psychological dependence. Many LSD users become depressed for 1 or 2 days following a trip and turn to the drug to relieve this depression. The result is a cycle of LSD use to relieve post–LSD depression, which can lead to psychological addiction.

## Ecstasy

*Ecstasy* is the most common street name for the drug *methylene-dioxymethamphetamine* (*MDMA*), a synthetic compound with both stimulant and mildly hallucinogenic effects. It is one of the most well-known **club drugs** or "designer drugs," terms applied to synthetic analogs of existing illicit drugs that tend to be popular among teens and young adults at nightclubs, bars, raves, and other all-night parties. Ecstasy creates feelings of extreme euphoria, openness and warmth,

**club drugs** Synthetic analogs (drugs that produce similar effects) of existing illicit drugs.

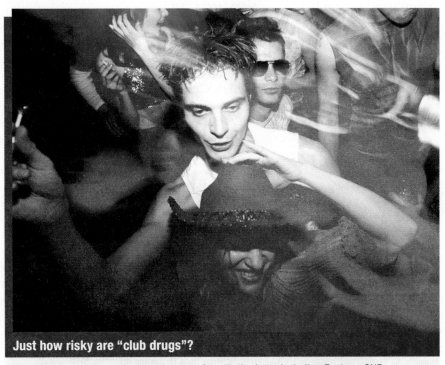

**Just how risky are "club drugs"?**

So-called club drugs are a varied group of synthetic drugs including Ecstasy, GHB, ketamine, Rohypnol, and meth that are often abused by teens and young adults at nightclubs, bars, or all-night dances. The sources and chemicals used to make these drugs vary, so dosages are unpredictable and drugs may not be "pure." Although users may think them relatively harmless, research has shown that club drugs can produce hallucinations, paranoia, amnesia, dangerous increases in heart rate and blood pressure, coma, and, in some cases, death. Some club drugs work on the same brain mechanisms as alcohol and can be particularly dangerous when used in combination with alcohol. In addition, some club drugs can be easily slipped into unsuspecting partygoers' drinks, thus facilitating sexual assault and other crimes.

an increased willingness to communicate, feelings of love and empathy, increased awareness, and heightened appreciation for music. Like other hallucinogenic drugs, Ecstasy can enhance the sensory experience and distort perceptions, but it does not create visual hallucinations. Effects begin within 20 to 90 minutes and can last for 3 to 5 hours.

Psilocybe mushrooms produce hallucinogenic effects when ingested.

Some of the risks associated with Ecstasy use are similar to those of other stimulants. Because of the nature of the drug, Ecstasy users are at greater risk of inappropriate and/or unintended emotional bonding and have a tendency to say things they might feel uncomfortable about later. More physical consequences of Ecstasy use may include such things as mild to extreme jaw clenching, tongue and cheek chewing, short-term memory loss or confusion, increased body temperature as a result of dehydration and heat stroke, and increased heart rate and blood pressure. Individuals with high blood pressure, heart disease, or liver trouble are at greatest danger when using this drug. Combined with alcohol, Ecstasy can be extremely dangerous and sometimes fatal. As the effects of Ecstasy begin to wear off, the user can experience mild depression, fatigue, and a hangover that can last from days to weeks. Chronic use appears to damage the brain's ability to think and to regulate emotion, memory, sleep, and pain. Some studies indicate that the drug may cause long-lasting neurotoxic effects by damaging brain cells that produce serotonin.[38]

**Mescaline** *Mescaline* is one of hundreds of chemicals derived from the peyote cactus, a small, button-like plant that grows in the southwestern United States and in Latin America. Natives of these regions have long used the dried peyote "buttons" for religious purposes. It is both a powerful hallucinogen and a central nervous system stimulant. Products sold on the street as mescaline are likely to be synthetic chemical relatives of the true drug.

Mescaline comes from "buttons" of the peyote cactus, like this one.

Users typically swallow 10 to 12 buttons. They taste bitter and generally induce immediate nausea or vomiting. Longtime users claim that the nausea becomes less noticeable with frequent use. Those who are able to keep the drug down begin to feel the effects within 30 to 90 minutes, when mescaline reaches maximum concentration in the brain. It may persist for up to 9 or 10 hours.

**Psilocybin** *Psilocybin* and *psilocin* are the active chemicals in a group of mushrooms sometimes called "magic mushrooms." Psilocybe mushrooms, which grow throughout the world, can be cultivated from spores or harvested wild. When consumed, these mushrooms can cause hallucinations. Because many mushrooms resemble the psilocybe variety, people who harvest wild mushrooms for any purpose should be certain of what they are doing. Mushroom varieties can be easily misidentified, and mistakes can be fatal. Psilocybin is similar to LSD in its physical effects, which generally wear off in 4 to 6 hours.

**PCP** *Phencyclidine* (*PCP*) is a synthetic substance that became a black-market drug in the early 1970s. It was originally developed as a dissociative anesthetic, which means that patients administered this drug could keep their eyes open, apparently remain conscious, and feel no pain during a medical procedure. Afterward, they would experience amnesia for the time that the drug was in their system. Such a drug had obvious advantages as an anesthetic, but its unpredictability and drastic effects (postoperative delirium, confusion, and agitation) made doctors abandon it, and it was withdrawn from the legal market.

On the illegal market, PCP is a white, crystalline powder that users often sprinkle onto marijuana cigarettes. It is dangerous and unpredictable regardless of the method of administration. The effects of PCP depend on the dosage. A dose as small as 5 mg will produce effects similar to those of strong central nervous system depressants—slurred speech, impaired coordination, reduced sensitivity to pain, and reduced heart and respiratory rate. Doses between 5 and 10 mg cause fever, salivation, nausea, vomiting, and total loss of sensitivity to pain. Doses greater than 10 mg result in a drastic drop in blood pressure, coma, muscular rigidity, violent outbursts, and possible convulsions and death.

Psychologically, PCP may produce either euphoria or dysphoria. It is also known to produce hallucinations as well as delusions and overall delirium. Some users experience a prolonged state of "nothingness." The long-term effects of PCP use are unknown.

**Ketamine** The liquid form of *ketamine,* or Special K, as it is commonly called, is used as an anesthetic in some hospital and veterinary clinics. After stealing it from hospitals or medical suppliers, dealers typically dry the liquid (usually by cooking it) and grind the residue into powder. Special K causes hallucinations, as it inhibits the relay of sensory input; the brain fills the resulting void with visions, dreams, memories, and sensory distortions. The effects of ketamine are similar to those of PCP—confusion, agitation, aggression, and lack of coordination—and less predictable. The aftereffects of

Special K are less severe than those of Ecstasy, so it has grown in popularity as a club drug among people who must go to work or school the next day after a night of partying.

## Inhalants

**Inhalants** are chemicals whose vapors, when inhaled, can cause hallucinations and create intoxicating and euphoric effects. Not commonly recognized as drugs, inhalants are legal to purchase and universally available but dangerous. They generally appeal to young people who can't afford or obtain illicit substances. Some misused products include rubber cement, model glue, paint thinner, aerosol sprays, lighter fluid, varnish, wax, spot removers, and gasoline. Most of these substances are sniffed or "huffed" by users in search of a quick, cheap high.

Because they are inhaled, the volatile chemicals in these products reach the bloodstream and then the brain within seconds. This characteristic, along with the fact that dosages are extremely difficult to control because everyone has unique lung and breathing capacities, makes inhalants particularly dangerous. The effects of inhalants usually last for fewer than 15 minutes and resemble those of central nervous system depressants. Users may experience dizziness, disorientation, impaired coordination, reduced judgment, and slowed reaction times. Combining inhalants with alcohol produces a synergistic effect and can cause severe and sometimes fatal liver damage. An overdose of fumes from inhalants can cause unconsciousness. If the user's oxygen intake is reduced during the inhaling process, death can result within 5 minutes. Sudden sniffing death (SSD) syndrome can be a fatal consequence, whether it's the user's first time or not. This syndrome can occur if a user inhales deeply and then participates in physical activity or is startled.

**Amyl Nitrite** Sometimes called "poppers" or "rush," *amyl nitrite* is packaged in small, cloth-covered glass capsules that can be crushed to release the active chemical for the user to inhale. The drug is often prescribed to alleviate chest pain in heart patients, because it dilates small blood vessels and reduces blood pressure. Dilation of blood vessels in the genital area is thought to enhance sensations or perceptions of orgasm. It also produces fainting, dizziness, warmth, and skin flushing.

**Nitrous Oxide** *Nitrous oxide* is sometimes used as an adjunct to dental anesthesia or minor surgical anesthesia. It is also a propellant chemical in aerosol products such as whipped toppings. Users who inhale nitrous oxide experience a state of euphoria, floating sensations, and illusions. Effects also include pain relief and a silly feeling, demonstrated by

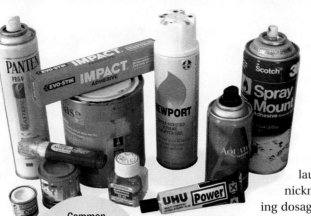

Common household products, such as aerosol sprays, solvents, or glues, can be inhaled for a quick high.

**70%** of first-time users of inhalants in 2008 were under age 18.

laughing and giggling (hence its nickname "laughing gas"). Regulating dosages of this drug can be difficult. Sustained inhalation can lead to unconsciousness, coma, and death.

## Anabolic Steroids

**Anabolic steroids** are artificial forms of the male hormone testosterone that promote muscle growth and strength. Steroids are available in two forms: injectable solutions and pills. These **ergogenic drugs** are used primarily by people who believe the drugs will increase their strength, power, bulk (weight), speed, and athletic performance.

It was once estimated that approximately 17 to 20 percent of college athletes used steroids. Now that stricter drug-testing policies have been instituted by the National Collegiate Athletic Association (NCAA), reported use of anabolic steroids among intercollegiate athletes has decreased.[39] However, a recent survey among high school students found that there has been a significant increase in the use of anabolic steroids since 1991.[40] Few data exist on the extent of steroid abuse by adults. It has been estimated that approximately 1 million adults have used anabolic steroids.[41] Among both adolescents and adults, steroid abuse is higher among men than it is among women. However, steroid abuse is growing most rapidly among young women.[42]

**inhalants** Products that are sniffed or inhaled in order to produce highs.
**anabolic steroids** Artificial forms of the hormone testosterone that promote muscle growth and strength.
**ergogenic drug** Substance believed to enhance athletic performance.

**Physical Effects of Steroids** Anabolic steroids produce a state of euphoria, diminished fatigue, and increased bulk and power in both sexes. These characteristics give steroids an addictive quality. When users stop, they can experience psychological withdrawal and sometimes severe depression, in some cases leading to suicide attempts. If untreated, depression associated with steroid withdrawal has been known to last for a year or more after steroid use stops.

Men and women who use steroids experience a variety of adverse effects, including mood swings (aggression and violence, sometimes known as "'roid rage"); acne; liver tumors; elevated cholesterol levels; hypertension; kidney disease; and immune system disturbances. There is also a danger of transmitting HIV and hepatitis through shared needles. In women, large doses of anabolic steroids may trigger the development of masculine attributes such as lowered voice, increased facial and body hair, and male pattern baldness; they may also result in an enlarged clitoris, smaller breasts, and changes in or absence of menstruation. When taken by healthy males, anabolic steroids shut down the body's production of testosterone, causing men's breasts to grow and testicles to atrophy.

**Steroid Use and Society** To combat the growing problem of steroid use, Congress passed the Anabolic Steroids Control Act (ASCA) of 1990. This law makes it a crime to possess, prescribe, or distribute anabolic steroids for any use other than the treatment of specific diseases. Penalties for their illegal use include up to 5 years' imprisonment and a $250,000 fine for the first offense and up to 10 years' imprisonment and a $500,000 fine for subsequent offenses.

The use of steroids and related substances among professional athletes periodically makes the news. In recent years, high-profile athletes in sports such as cycling, track and field, swimming, and baseball have all garnered media attention for suspected use of steroids or other banned performance-enhancing drugs. The Mitchell Report released in December 2007 was an investigation into the history of steroid and human growth hormone use by Major League Baseball players, 89 of whom are alleged by the report to have used steroids or other ergogenic drugs.

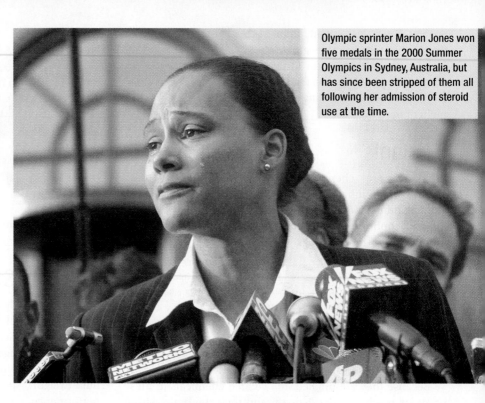

Olympic sprinter Marion Jones won five medals in the 2000 Summer Olympics in Sydney, Australia, but has since been stripped of them all following her admission of steroid use at the time.

**what do you think?**

Do you believe an athlete's admission of steroid use invalidates his or her athletic achievements? ● How do you think professional athletes who have used steroids or other performance enhancers should be disciplined? ● If you are an athlete, have you ever considered using some type of ergogenic aid to improve your performance?

# Treatment and Recovery

An estimated 23.1 million Americans aged 12 or older needed treatment for an illicit drug or alcohol use problem in 2008. Of these, only 2.3 million—approximately 10 percent—received treatment.[43] The most difficult step in the recovery process is for the substance abuser to admit that he or she is an addict. This can be difficult because of the power of *denial*—the inability to see the truth. Denial is the hallmark of addiction. It can be so powerful that a planned intervention is sometimes necessary to break down the addict's defenses against recognizing the problem.

**detoxification** The early abstinence period during which an addict adjusts physically and cognitively to being free from the substance's influence.

Recovery from drug addiction is a long-term process and frequently requires multiple episodes of treatment. The first step generally begins with abstinence—refraining from using. **Detoxification** refers to the early abstinence period during which an addict adjusts physically and cognitively to being free from the substance's influence. It occurs in virtually every recovering addict. Although it is uncomfortable for most addicts, it can be dangerous for some. For these people, early abstinence may involve profound withdrawal that requires medical supervision. Because of this, most inpatient treatment programs provide a pretreatment component of supervised detoxification to achieve abstinence safely before further treatment begins.

## Treatment Approaches

*Outpatient behavioral treatment* encompasses a variety of programs for addicts who visit a clinic at regular intervals. Most of the programs involve individual or group drug counseling. *Residential treatment programs* can also be very effective, especially for those with more severe problems. For example, therapeutic communities (TCs) are highly structured programs in which addicts remain at a residence, typically for 6 to 12 months. The focus of the TC is on the resocialization of the addict to a drug-free lifestyle.

**12-Step Programs** The first 12-step program was Alcoholics Anonymous (AA), begun in 1935 in Akron, Ohio. The 12-step program has since become the most widely used approach to dealing not only with alcoholism, but also drug abuse and various other addictive or dysfunctional behaviors. There are more than 200 different recovery programs based

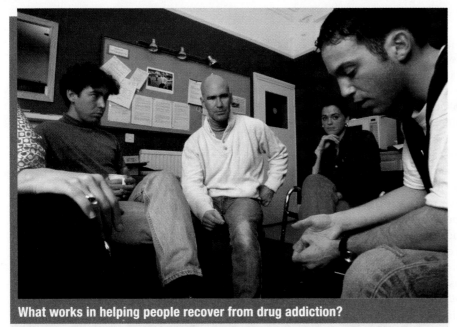

**What works in helping people recover from drug addiction?**

For most addicts, recovery is a long, difficult progress—for some people it can be a lifelong journey. Treatment and recovery for drug addiction usually begins with a period of detoxification, which may involve intense physical and psychological withdrawal symptoms. Once his or her body has adjusted to being without the drug, the addict usually enters behavioral or cognitive therapy to learn how to cope without the drug and avoid relapse. Therapy often takes the form of group meetings, such as those held by 12-step programs, for example Narcotics Anonymous.

tion (rehab) inpatient facility. The needs of college students seeking drug treatment in rehab do not differ greatly from other adult recovering addicts, but for best results, the community of addicts should include others of a similar age and educational background. Private therapy, group therapy, cognitive training, nutrition counseling, and health therapies can all be used to help with recovery.

A growing number of colleges and universities offer special services to students who are recovering from alcohol and other drug addiction and want to stay in school without being exposed to excessive drinking or drug use. For example, the University of Texas at Austin opened its Center for Students in Recovery, which provides students with a support system and a for-credit academic course called "Principles of Recovery and Relapse Prevention." Another campus, Texas Tech University, recently received a $250,000 federal grant to create a national model of its students-in-recovery program. The program offers scholarships to students in recovery, as well as on-campus 12-step meetings and academic support.

on the program, including Narcotics Anonymous, Cocaine Anonymous, Crystal Meth Anonymous, Gamblers Anonymous, and Pills Anonymous.

The 12-step program is nonjudgmental and based on the idea that a program's only purpose is to work on personal recovery. Working the 12 steps involves admitting to having a serious problem, recognizing there is an outside power that could help, consciously relying on that power, admitting and listing character defects, seeking deliverance from defects, apologizing to those individuals one has harmed in the past, and helping others with the same problem. The 12-step meetings are held at a variety of times and locations in almost every city. There is no membership cost and the meetings are open to anyone who wishes to attend.

## College Students' Treatment and Recovery

For college students who have developed substance or behavioral addictions, early intervention increases the likelihood of successful treatment, successful sobriety, and completion of a college education. Depending on the severity of the abuse or dependence, college students undergoing drug treatment may be required to spend time away from school in a residential drug rehabilita-

## Addressing Drug Misuse and Abuse in the United States

Stories of people who have tried illegal drugs, enjoyed them, and suffered no consequences may tempt you to try them yourself. You may convince yourself that one-time use is harmless. Given the dangers surrounding these substances, however, you should think twice. The risks associated with drug use extend beyond the personal. The decision to try any illicit substance supports illicit drug manufacture and transport, thus contributing to the national drug problem.

Illegal drug use in the United States costs about $215 billion per year.[44] This estimate includes costs associated with substance abuse treatment and prevention, health care, reduced job productivity and lost earnings, and social consequences such as crime and social welfare. In addition, roughly half of all expenditures to combat crime are related to illegal drugs. The burden of these costs is absorbed primarily by the government (46%), followed by people who abuse drugs and members of their households (44%).[45]

10 million people reported driving under the influence of illicit drugs in the past year.

## Drugs in the Workplace

According to the National Survey on Drug Use and Health, 73 percent of all U.S. workers who use illicit drugs are employed full- or part-time.[46] With such a large segment of drug users employed to some degree, the cost to American businesses soars into the billions of dollars. These costs reflect reduced work performance and efficiency, lost productivity, absenteeism, and turnover. Not surprisingly, it is estimated that the annual economic impact of illicit drug use is $128.6 billion in lost productivity alone.[47]

Many companies have instituted drug testing for their employees. Mandatory drug urinalysis is controversial. Critics argue that such testing violates Fourth Amendment rights of protection from unreasonable search and seizure. Proponents believe the personal inconvenience entailed in testing pales in comparison to the problems caused by drug use in the workplace.

Drug testing is expensive, with costs running as high as $100 per test. Moreover, some critics question the accuracy and reliability of the results. Both false positives and false negatives can occur. As drug testing becomes more common in the work environment, it is gaining greater acceptance by employees, who see testing as a step toward improving safety and productivity.

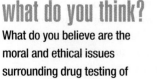

**what do you think?**

What do you believe are the moral and ethical issues surrounding drug testing of employees? ● Are you in favor of drug testing? ● Should employers have the right to conduct drug testing at the worksite?

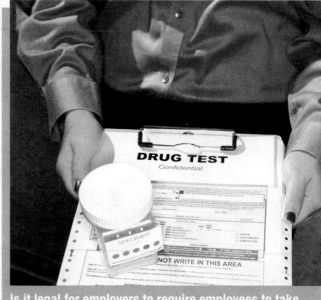

**Is it legal for employers to require employees to take a drug test?**

Several court decisions have affirmed the right of employers to test their employees for drug use. They contend that Fourth Amendment rights pertain only to employees of government agencies, not to those of private businesses. Most Americans apparently support drug testing for certain types of jobs.

## Preventing Drug Use and Abuse on Campus

Strategies that college and university campuses should consider to reduce the number of students who become involved in substance use include the following:

● Changing student expectations that college is a time to party and experiment with drugs
● Engaging parents about substance use on campus and encouraging them to continue open communication with their children
● Identifying high-risk students through early detection screening programs
● Providing services such as treatment programs specifically tailored for students needing treatment and recovery support services

Most anti-drug programs have not been effective, because they have focused on only one aspect of drug abuse rather than examining all factors that contribute to the problem. The pressure to take drugs is often tremendous, and the reasons for using them are complex. People who develop drug problems generally believe they can control their drug use when they start out. Initially, they often view taking drugs as a fun and manageable pastime. In addition, peer influence is a strong motivator, especially among adolescents, who greatly fear not being accepted as part of the group. Since most illegal drugs and many prescription drugs produce physical and psychological dependency, it is unrealistic to think that a person can use them regularly without becoming addicted.

**what do you think?**

What is the attitude toward drug use on your campus? ● Are some substances considered more acceptable than others? ● Is drug use considered more acceptable at certain times or occasions?

## Possible Solutions to the Drug Problem

Americans are alarmed by the increasing use of illegal drugs. Respondents in public opinion polls feel that the most important strategy for fighting drug abuse is educating young people. They also endorse strategies such as the following:

● Stricter border surveillance to reduce drug trafficking
● Longer prison sentences for drug dealers
● Increased government spending on prevention
● Enforcing anti-drug laws
● Greater cooperation between government agencies and private groups and individuals providing treatment assistance

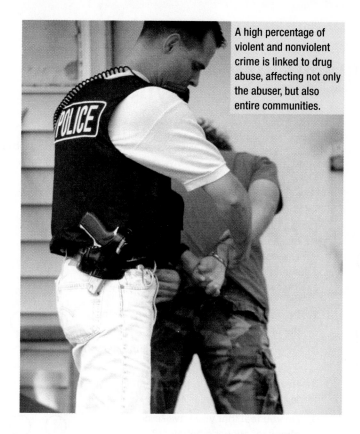

A high percentage of violent and nonviolent crime is linked to drug abuse, affecting not only the abuser, but also entire communities.

All of these approaches will probably help up to a point, but they do not offer a total solution to the problem. Drug abuse has been a part of human behavior for thousands of years, and it is not likely to disappear in the near future. For this reason, it is necessary to educate ourselves and to develop the self-discipline necessary to avoid dangerous drug dependence.

For many years, the most popular anti-drug strategy has been total prohibition. This approach has proved to be ineffective. Prohibition of alcohol during the 1920s created more problems than it solved, as did prohibition of opioids in 1914. A more recent campaign is commonly referred to as the "War on Drugs," undertaken by the U.S. government with the assistance of participating countries. This campaign includes laws and policies that are intended to reduce the illegal drug trade and to diminish and discourage the production, distribution, and consumption of illicit substances.

In general, researchers in the field of drug education agree that a multimodal approach is best. Students should be taught the difference between drug use, misuse, and abuse. Factual information that is free of scare tactics must be presented; lecturing and moralizing have proved not to work.

**Harm Reduction Strategies** Harm reduction is a set of practical approaches to reducing negative consequences of drug use, incorporating a spectrum of strategies from safer use to managed use to abstinence. Harm reduction approaches have been widely used in needle exchange programs, where injection drug users receive clean needles and syringes and bleach for cleaning needles; these efforts help reduce the number of cases of HIV and hepatitis B. Harm reduction may involve changing the legal sanctions associated with drug use, increasing the availability of treatment services to drug abusers, and/or attempting to change drug users' behavior through education. Harm reduction strategies meet drug users "where they're at," addressing conditions of use along with the use itself. This strategy recognizes that people always have and always will use drugs and, therefore, attempts to minimize the potential hazards associated with drug use rather than the use itself.

# Assess yourself

## Do You Have a Problem with Drugs?

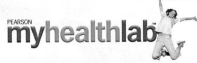

### 1 Are You Controlled by Drugs?

A dependent person can't stop using drugs. This abuse hurts the user and everyone around him or her. The more "yes" checks you make below, the more likely it is that you have a problem.

Fill out this assessment online at www.pearsonhighered.com/myhealthlab or www.pearsonhighered.com/donatelle.

|  | Yes | No |
|---|---|---|
| 1. Do you use drugs to handle stress or escape from life's problems? | ○ | ○ |
| 2. Have you unsuccessfully tried to cut down on or quit using your drug? | ○ | ○ |
| 3. Have you ever been in trouble with the law or been arrested because of your drug use? | ○ | ○ |
| 4. Do you think a party or social gathering isn't fun unless drugs are available? | ○ | ○ |
| 5. Do you avoid people or places that do not support your usage? | ○ | ○ |
| 6. Do you neglect your responsibilities because you'd rather use your drug? | ○ | ○ |
| 7. Have your friends, family, or employer expressed concern about your drug use? | ○ | ○ |
| 8. Do you do things under the influence of drugs that you would not normally do? | ○ | ○ |
| 9. Have you seriously thought that you might have a chemical dependency problem? | ○ | ○ |

Source: Reprinted by permission of Krames Communications, 1100 Grundy Lane, San Bruno, CA 94066-3030, www.krames.com.

### 2 Are You Controlled by a Drug User?

Your love and care may actually be enabling another person to continue chemical abuse, hurting you and others. The more "yes" checks you make below, the more likely there's a problem.

|  | Yes | No |
|---|---|---|
| 1. Do you often have to lie or cover up for the chemical abuser? | ○ | ○ |
| 2. Do you spend time counseling the person about the problem? | ○ | ○ |
| 3. Have you taken on additional financial or family responsibilities? | ○ | ○ |
| 4. Do you feel that you have to control the chemical abuser's behavior? | ○ | ○ |
| 5. At the office, have you done work or attended meetings for the abuser? | ○ | ○ |
| 6. Do you often put your own needs and desires after the user's? | ○ | ○ |
| 7. Do you spend time each day worrying about your situation? | ○ | ○ |
| 8. Do you analyze your behavior to find clues to how it might affect the chemical abuser? | ○ | ○ |
| 9. Do you feel powerless and at your wit's end about the abuser's problem? | ○ | ○ |

## YOUR PLAN FOR CHANGE

The **Assess yourself** activity describes signs of being controlled by drugs or by a drug user. Depending on your results, you may need to change certain behaviors that may be detrimental to your health.

### Today, you can:

○ Imagine a situation in which someone offers you a drug and think of several different ways of refusing. Rehearse these scenarios in your head.

○ Stop by your campus health center to find out about any drug treatment programs or support groups they may have.

### Within the next 2 weeks, you can:

○ Think about the drug use patterns among your social group. Are you ever uncomfortable with these people because of their drug use? Is it difficult to avoid using drugs when you are with them? If the answers are yes, begin exploring ways to expand your social circle.

○ If you are concerned about your own drug use or the drug use of a close friend, make an appointment with a counselor to talk about the issue.

### By the end of the semester, you can:

○ Participate in clubs, activities, and social groups that do not rely on substance abuse for their amusement.

○ If you have a drug problem, make a commitment to enter a treatment program. Acknowledge that you have a problem and that you need the assistance of others to help you overcome it.

# Summary

* Mood-altering substances and experiences produce biochemical reactions that make the body feel good; when absent, the person feels the effects of withdrawal.
* The six categories of drugs are prescription drugs, over-the-counter (OTC) drugs, recreational drugs, herbal preparations, illicit drugs, and commercial preparations. Routes of administration include oral ingestion, inhalation, injection (intravenous, intramuscular, and subcutaneous), transdermal, and insertion of suppositories.
* Over-the-counter medications are drugs that do not require a prescription. Some OTC medications, including sleep aids, cold medicines, and diet pills, can be addictive.
* Prescription drug abuse is at an all-time high, particularly among college students. Only marijuana is more commonly abused. The most commonly abused prescription drugs are opioids/narcotics, depressants, and stimulants.
* People from all walks of life use illicit drugs, although college students report higher usage rates than do the general population. Drug use declined from the mid-1980s to the early 1990s but has remained steady since then. However, among young people, use of drugs has been rising in recent years.
* Controlled substances include cocaine and its derivatives, amphetamines, methamphetamine, marijuana, opioids, depressants, hallucinogens/psychedelics, inhalants, and steroids. Each has its own set of risks and effects.
* Treatment begins with abstinence from the drug or addictive behavior, usually instituted through intervention by close family, friends, or other loved ones. Treatment programs may include individual, group, or family therapy, as well as 12-step programs.
* The drug problem reaches everyone through crime and elevated health care costs. Public health and governmental approaches to the problem involve regulation, enforcement, education, and harm reduction.

# Pop Quiz

1. Cross-tolerance occurs when
   a. drugs work at the same receptor site so that one blocks the action of the other.
   b. the effects of one drug are eliminated or reduced by the presence of another drug at the receptor site.
   c. a person develops a physiological tolerance to one drug and shows a similar tolerance to selected other drugs as a result.
   d. two or more drugs interact and the effects of the individual drugs are multiplied beyond what normally would be expected if they were taken alone.

2. Rebecca takes a number of medications for various conditions, including Prinivil (an antihypertensive drug), insulin (a diabetic medication), and Claritin (an antihistamine). This is an example of
   a. synergism.
   b. illegal drug use.
   c. polydrug use.
   d. antagonism.

3. Which of the following is not an example of drug misuse?
   a. Excessive use of and dependency on a drug
   b. Taking a friend's prescription medicine
   c. Taking medicine more than is recommended
   d. Not following the instructions when taking a medicine

4. The most common method of injection among drug abusers is
   a. intramuscular.
   b. intravenous.
   c. subcutaneous.
   d. all of the above.

5. The most common method for taking drugs is
   a. injection.
   b. inhalation.
   c. oral ingestion.
   d. transdermal.

6. The most widely used illegal drug in the United States is
   a. alcohol.
   b. heroin.
   c. marijuana.
   d. methamphetamine.

7. Which of the following is classified as a stimulant drug?
   a. Amphetamines
   b. Alcohol
   c. Marijuana
   d. LSD

8. *Freebasing* is
   a. mixing cocaine with heroin.
   b. burning heroin and inhaling the vapor.
   c. injecting a drug into the veins.
   d. burning cocaine and inhaling the vapor.

9. Drugs that depress the central nervous system are called
   a. narcotics.
   b. sedatives.
   c. depressants.
   d. psychedelics.

10. The psychoactive drug mescaline is found in what plant?
    a. Mushrooms
    b. Peyote cactus
    c. Marijuana
    d. Belladona

*Answers to these questions can be found on page A-1.*

## Think about It!

1. Explain the terms *synergism, antagonism,* and *inhibition.*
2. Do you think there is such a thing as responsible use of illicit drugs? Would you change any of the current laws governing drugs? How would you determine what is legitimate and illegitimate use?
3. What are the arguments for and against drug testing in the workplace? Would you apply for a job that had drug testing as an interview requirement? Why or why not?
4. Why do you think so many young people today are abusing prescription drugs? Do you perceive prescription drug abuse as being less dangerous or illegal than illicit drug use? Why? Do you think this is an accurate or biased perception?
5. What types of programs do you think would be effective in preventing drug abuse among high school and college students? How might programs for high school students differ from those for college students?
6. What could you do to help a friend who is fighting a substance abuse problem? What resources on your campus could help you?

## Accessing Your Health on the Internet

The following websites explore further topics and issues related to personal health. For links to the websites below, visit the Companion Website for *Access to Health,* 12th Edition, at www.pearsonhighered.com/donatelle.

1. *Club Drugs.* This website disseminates science-based information about club drugs. www.clubdrugs.org
2. *Join Together.* This is an excellent site for the most current information related to substance abuse. This site also includes information on alcohol and drug policy and provides advice on organizing and taking political action. www.jointogether.org
3. *National Institute on Drug Abuse (NIDA).* The home page of this U.S. government agency has information on the latest statistics and findings in drug research. www.nida.nih.gov
4. *Substance Abuse and Mental Health Services Administration (SAMHSA).* SAMHSA's site is an outstanding resource for information about national surveys, ongoing research, and national drug interventions. www.samhsa.gov

## References

1. Substance Abuse and Mental Health Services Administration, *Results from the 2008 National Survey on Drug Use and Health: National Findings,* NSDUH Series H-36, HHS Publication no. SMA 09-4434, (Rockville, MD: Office of Applied Studies, 2009), Available at www.oas.samhsa.gov/nsduh/2k8nsduh/2k8Results.cfm.
2. National Drug Intelligence Center, "National Drug Threat Assessment 2010," 2010, www.justice.gov/ndic/pubs38/38661/drugImpact.htm; Centers for Disease Control and Prevention, "CDC Statement Regarding the Misuse of Prescription Drugs," June 2010, www.cdc.gov/media/pressrel/2010/s100603.htm.
3. P. Kittenger and D. Herrick, "Patient Power: Over-the-Counter Drugs," National Center for Policy Analysis, *Brief Analysis,* no. 524, August 2005, Available at www.ncpa.org/pub/ba/ba524.
4. Consumer Healthcare Products Association, *OTC Medicines Serve an Important Health Care Need,* 2009, www.chpa-info.org/media/resources/r_4862.pdf.
5. L. D. Johnston et al., *Monitoring the Future: National Survey Results on Drug Use, 1975–2008, Volume I, Secondary School Students,* NIH Publication no. 09-7402 (Bethesda, MD: National Institute on Drug Abuse, 2009), Available at http://monitoringthefuture.org/pubs.html.
6. The U.S. Department of Justice's National Drug Intelligence Center, *Intelligence Bulletin: DXM (Dextromethorphan),* DOJ Publication no. 2004-L0424-029 (Johnstown, PA: National Drug Intelligence Center, 2004), Available at www.justice.gov/ndic/pubs11/11563/index.htm.
7. U.S. Food and Drug Administration, "Legal Requirements for the Sale and Purchase of Drug Products Containing Pseudoephedrine, Ephedrine, and Phenylpropanolamine," Updated July 2009, www.fda.gov/Drugs/DrugSafety/InformationbyDrugClass/ucm072423.htm.
8. National Youth Anti-Drug Media Campaign, "Prescription Drug (Rx) Abuse," 2010, www.theantidrug.com/drug-information/otc-prescription-drug-abuse/prescription-drug-rx-abuse/default.aspx.
9. National Institute on Drug Abuse, *Research Report Series: Prescription Drugs: Abuse and Addiction,* NIH Publication no. 05-4881 (Bethesda, MD: National Institute on Drug Abuse, 2005), Available at www.nida.nih.gov/researchreports/prescription/prescription.html.
10. Substance Abuse and Mental Health Services Administration, *Results from the 2008 National Survey on Drug Use and Health,* 2009; Office of National Drug Control Policy, "Prescription Opioid-Related Deaths Increased 114 Percent from 2001 to 2005," 2009, www.ondcp.gov/news/press09/052009.html.
11. Ibid.
12. National Association of School Nurses, "Educational Campaigns: Drugs of Abuse," 2010, www.nasn.org/Default.aspx?tabid=506.
13. National Center on Addiction and Substance Abuse at Columbia University, *Wasting the Best and the Brightest: Substance Abuse at America's Colleges and Universities* (New York: National Center on Addiction and Substance Abuse at Columbia University, 2007), Available at www.casacolumbia.org/templates/publications_reports.aspx.
14. Ibid.
15. D. L. Rabiner et al., "Motives and Perceived Consequences of Nonmedical ADHD Medication Use by College Students: Are Students Treating Themselves for Attention Problems?" *Journal of Attention Disorders* 13, no. 3 (2009): 259–70.
16. T. E. Wilens et al. "Misuse and Diversion of Stimulants Prescribed for ADHD: A Systematic Review of the Literature," *Journal of the American Academy of Child and Adolescent Psychiatry* 47, no. 1, (2008): 21–31.
17. Substance Abuse and Mental Health Services Administration, *Results from the 2008 National Survey on Drug Use and Health,* 2009.
18. L. D. Johnston et al., *Monitoring the Future National Survey Results on Drug Use, 1975–2008, Volume II, College Students and Adults Ages 19–50,* NIH Publication no. 09-7403 (Bethesda, MD: National Institute on Drug Abuse, 2009), Available at http://monitoringthefuture.org/pubs.html.
19. National Center on Addiction and Substance Abuse at Columbia University, *Wasting the Best and the Brightest,* 2007.
20. Ibid.
21. Ibid.

22. L. D. Johnston et al., *Monitoring the Future National Survey Results on Drug Use, 1975–2008, Volume I*, 2009.

23. D. Schardt, "Caffeine: The Good, the Bad, and the Maybe," *Nutrition Action Healthletter* (March 2008): 1–7, Available at http://cspinet.org/nah/archives.html.

24. Office of National Drug Control Policy, "Marijuana Facts and Figures," 2009, www.whitehousedrugpolicy.gov/drugfact/marijuana/marijuana_ff.html.

25. W. Compton et al., "Prevalence of Marijuana Use Disorders in the United States 1991–1992 and 2001–2002," *Journal of the American Medical Association* 291, no. 17 (2004): 2114–21.

26. National Institute on Drug Abuse, *Marijuana: Facts for Teens*, NIH Publication no. 04-4037, (Rockville, MD: Office of Applied Studies, 2009), Revised March 2008, Available at www.nida.nih.gov/marijbroch/marijteens.html.

27. National Institute on Drug Abuse, *Research Report: Marijuana Abuse*, NIH Publication no. 05-3859, 2005, Available at www.drugabuse.gov/ResearchReports/Marijuana; National Institute on Drug Abuse, "NIDA InfoFacts: Drugged Driving," 2009, www.nida.nih.gov/infofacts/driving.html.

28. National Highway Traffic Safety Administration, "Drugs and Human Performance Fact Sheets: Cannabis/Marijuana," 2004, www.nhtsa.gov/people/injury/research/job185drugs/cannabis.htm.

29. National Institute on Drug Abuse, "NIDA InfoFacts: Marijuana," Revised July 2009, http://drugabuse.gov/infofacts/marijuana.html.

30. J. R. Daling et al., "Association of Marijuana Use and the Incidence of Testicular Germ Cell Tumors," *Cancer* 115, no. 6 (2009): 1215–23.

31. Ibid.

32. W. Hall and L. Degenhardt, "Adverse Health Effects of Non-Medical Cannabis Use," *The Lancet* 374, no. 9698 (2009): 1383–91.

33. Substance Abuse and Mental Health Services Administration, *Results from the 2008 National Survey on Drug Use and Health: National Findings*, 2009.

34. National Institute on Drug Abuse, *Marijuana: Facts Parents Need to Know*, NIH Publication no. 07-4036 (Rockville, MD: National Institutes of Health, 2007), Revised August 2007, Available at www.nida.nih.gov/marijbroch/marijparentsN.html.

35. National Institute on Drug Abuse, "NIDA InfoFacts: Club Drugs (GHB, Ketamine, and Rohypnol)," Revised July 2010, www.drugabuse.gov/infofacts/clubdrugs.html.

36. Substance Abuse and Mental Health Services Administration, *Results from the 2008 National Survey on Drug Use and Health: National Findings*, 2009.

37. L. D. Johnston et al., *Monitoring the Future National Survey Results on Drug Use, 1975–2008, Volume II*, 2009.

38. National Institute on Drug Abuse, "NIDA InfoFacts: MDMA (Ecstasy)," Revised March 2010, www.drugabuse.gov/infofacts/ecstasy.html.

39. National Collegiate Athletic Association, *NCAA Study of Substance Use of College Student-Athletes* (Indianapolis, IN: National College Athletic Association, 2006), Available at www.ncaa.org/wps/portal/ncaahome?WCM_GLOBAL_CONTEXT=/ncaa/ncaa/research/student-athlete+well-being/sa_substance_use.html.

40. L. D. Johnston et al., *Monitoring the Future National Survey Results on Drug Use, 1975–2008, Volume I*, 2009.

41. Office of National Drug Control Policy, "Steroids Facts & Figures," 2010, www.whitehousedrugpolicy.gov/drugfact/steroids/steroids_ff.html.

42. National Institute on Drug Abuse, NIDA for Teens, "Anabolic Steroids," 2010, http://teens.drugabuse.gov/drnida/drnida_ster1.php.

43. Substance Abuse and Mental Health Services Administration, *Results from the 2008 National Survey on Drug Use and Health: National Findings*, 2009.

44. National Drug Intelligence Center, *National Drug Threat Assessment 2010*, DOJ 2010-Q0317-001 (Washington, DC: National Drug Intelligence Center, 2010), Available at www.justice.gov/ndic/pubs38/38661/index.htm.

45. Ibid.

46. Substance Abuse and Mental Health Services Administration, *Results from the 2008 National Survey on Drug Use and Health: National Findings*, 2009.

47. Butler Center for Research, *Research Update: Substance Use in the Workplace* (Center City, MN: Hazelden Foundation, 2009), Available at www.hazelden.org/web/public/researchupdates.page.

# 14

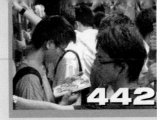

**442**

Why are vaccinations important?

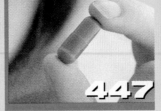

**447**

Can echinacea prevent me from catching a cold?

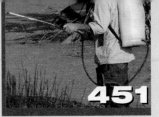

**451**

What can be done to prevent new diseases from emerging and spreading?

# Protecting against Infectious Diseases and Sexually Transmitted Infections

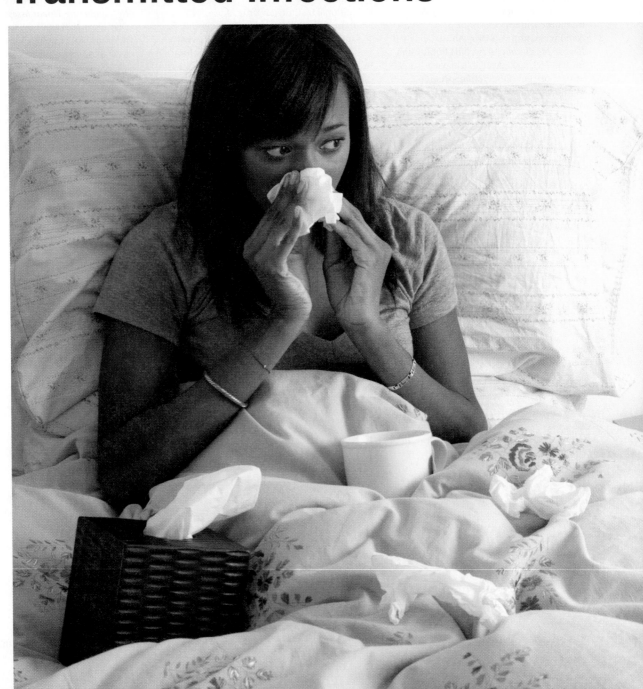

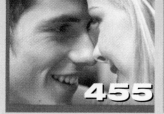
**455**

How can I tell if someone I'm dating has an STI?

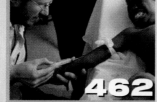
**462**

Is HIV/AIDS still an epidemic?

## Objectives

✳ Explain how your immune system works to protect you, and what you can do to boost its effectiveness.

✳ Discuss actions that you can take to protect yourself from the most common infectious diseases today.

✳ Describe the most common pathogens infecting humans today and the typical diseases caused by each.

✳ Explain the major emerging and resurgent diseases affecting humans nationally and internationally; discuss why they are increasing in incidence and what actions are being taken to reduce risks.

✳ Discuss antimicrobial resistance, why it occurs, and what we can do to reduce the prevalence of resistant pathogens.

✳ Discuss the various sexually transmitted infections, their means of transmission, and actions that can be taken to prevent their spread.

✳ Discuss human immunodeficiency virus (HIV) and acquired immunodeficiency syndrome (AIDS), trends in infection and treatment, and the impact of HIV/AIDS on special populations.

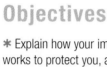

Every moment of every day, you are in contact with microscopic organisms that have the ability to cause illness or even death. In otherwise healthy individuals, most of these microorganisms, or microbes, pose little threat. However, in 2009, when a new strain of killer flu, *H1N1*, became a global threat, healthy young adults seemed to be at greatest risk. Schools were closed, church services were canceled, and people feared the slightest cough or sneeze from others. At the same time that rumors of a potentially deadly flu were swirling, media reports of tens of thousands dying in hospitals from a potent form of staph infection (methicillin-resistant *Staphylococcus aureus,* or MRSA) emerged. The combined effect of this media blitz of information about infectious disease caused people to fear for their safety in hospitals, wear masks in public, and avoid selected community settings.

Having lived in a cocoon of vaccine and antibiotic safety for several decades, we find it hard to believe that there isn't "something" that the pharmaceutical and medical community can do to "fix" threats from infectious diseases. Today, virtually every segment of the population, rich or poor, young or old, seems at risk for yet another outbreak of a disease. Are we facing a microbial battle that we are powerless against? Or, are there actions that we can take to reduce risks from infection without hiding in our homes or wearing masks and "gloving up" when we go out to protect us from "germy" others?

Disease-causing agents, called **pathogens,** are found in air and food and on nearly every object or person. We inhale them, swallow them, rub them in our eyes, and are constantly in a hidden, high-stakes battle with them, even as we sleep. New varieties of pathogens arise all the time, and scientific evidence indicates that many have existed for as long as there has been life on this planet. At times, infectious diseases wiped out whole groups of people through **epidemics** such as the Black Death, or bubonic plague, which killed up to one-third of the population of Europe in the 1300s. A **pandemic,** or global epidemic, of influenza killed more than 20 million people in 1918, and strains of tuberculosis and cholera continue to cause premature death throughout the world even today. New, resistant forms of older organisms defy even our most advanced pharmacological weapons aimed at eradication, leaving many to wonder about the very future of human life.

**pathogen** A disease-causing agent.
**epidemic** Disease outbreak that affects many people in a community or region at the same time.
**pandemic** Global epidemic of a disease.

Despite constant bombardment by pathogens, our immune systems are adept at protecting us. Exposure to invading microorganisms actually helps us build resistance to various pathogens. Millions of *endogenous microorganisms* live in and on our bodies all the time, usually in a symbiotic, peaceful coexistence. These are generally harmless to someone in good health; but in sick people or those with weakened immune systems, these organisms can cause serious health problems.

*Exogenous microorganisms* are those that do not normally inhabit the body. When they do, they are apt to produce an infection or illness. The more easily these pathogens can gain a foothold in the body and sustain themselves, the more **virulent,** or aggressive, they may be in causing disease. By keeping your immune system strong, you increase your ability to resist and fight off even the most virulent pathogen.

# The Process of Infection

Most diseases are **multifactorial:** they are caused by the interaction of several factors inside and outside the person. For a disease to occur, the person, or *host,* must be *susceptible,* which means that the immune system must be in a weakened condition (**immunocompromised**); an *agent* capable of *transmitting* a disease must be present; and the *environment* must be *hospitable* to the pathogen in terms of temperature, light, moisture, and other requirements. Although all pathogens pose a threat if they gain entry and begin to grow in your body, the chances that they will do so are actually quite small.

---

**virulent** Strong enough to overcome host resistance and cause disease.
**multifactorial disease** Disease caused by interactions of several factors.
**immunocompromised** Having an immune system that is impaired.
**autoinoculate** Transmit a pathogen from one part of your body to another part.

---

## Routes of Transmission

Pathogens enter the body in several ways. They may be transmitted by *direct contact* between infected persons, such as during sexual relations, kissing, or touching, or by *indirect contact,* such as by touching an object the infected person has had contact with. Table 14.1 lists common routes of transmission. You may also **autoinoculate** yourself, or

T A B L E
## 14.1 | Routes of Disease Transmission

| Mode of Transmission | Aspects of Transmission |
|---|---|
| Contact | Either *direct* (e.g., skin or sexual contact) or *indirect* (e.g., infected blood or body fluid) |
| Food- or waterborne | Eating or coming in contact with contaminated food or water, or products passed through them |
| Airborne | Inhalation; droplet-spread as through sneezing, coughing, or talking |
| Vectorborne | Vector-transmitted via secretions, biting, egg laying, as done by mosquitoes, ticks, snails, or birds |
| Perinatal | Similar to contact infection; happens in the uterus or as the baby passes through the birth canal, or through breast-feeding |

transmit a pathogen from one part of your body to another. For example, you may touch a herpes sore on your lip and transmit the virus to your eye when you scratch your itchy eyelid.

Your best friend may be the source of *animalborne pathogens.* Dogs, cats, livestock, and wild animals can spread numerous diseases through their bites or feces or by carrying infected insects into living areas and transmitting diseases either directly or indirectly. Although *interspecies transmission* of diseases (diseases passed from humans to animals and vice versa) is rare, it does occur.

# Risk Factors You Can Control

With all these pathogens floating around, how can you be sure you don't get sick? Fortunately, there are some things you can avoid in order to take care of yourself. Too much stress, inadequate nutrition, a low fitness level, lack of sleep,

## Reduce Your Risk of Infectious Disease

* **Limit your exposure to pathogens.** Stay home if you are not feeling well and encourage others to do the same. Don't drag yourself to classes or work and infect others. Don't share utensils or drinking glasses, keep your toothbrush away from those of other people, and wash your hands often. Sneeze or cough into your arm or sleeve rather than your hands. Keep hands away from your mouth, nose, eyes, and other body orifices. Use disposable tissues rather than cloth, reusable "hankies."

* **Exercise regularly.** Regular exercise raises core body temperature and kills pathogens. Sweat and oil make the skin a hostile environment for many bacteria. Avoid excessive exercise that could overtax the immune system.

* **Get enough sleep.** Sleep allows the body time to refresh itself, produce necessary cells, and reduce inflammation. Even a single night without sleep can increase inflammatory processes and delay wound healing.

* **Stress less.** Rest and relaxation, stress management practices, laughter, and calming music have all been shown to promote healthy cellular activity and bolster immune functioning.

* **Optimize eating.** Enjoy a healthy diet, including adequate amounts of water, protein, and complex carbohydrates. Eat more omega-3 fatty acids to reduce inflammation, and restrict saturated fats, replacing them with good fats such as olive oil. Antioxidants are believed to be important in immune functioning, so make sure you get your daily fruits and vegetables.

**Skills for Behavior Change**

misuse or abuse of legal and illegal drugs, poor personal hygiene, and high-risk behavior significantly increase the risk for many diseases. College students, in particular, often are at higher risk because of many of the above, in addition to the fact that alcohol and other drugs, increasing numbers of sexual experiences, and close living conditions, all create higher risk for exposure to pathogens. There are things you can do to eliminate, reduce, or change your susceptibility to various pathogens. The **Skills for Behavior Change** box lists some actions

you can take to keep your body's defenses in top form. There are also changes you can make in your community to clean up toxins, set policies on contaminant levels, and reduce the likelihood of being exposed to pathogens or toxins that could harm the immune system. The chain of infection between pathogen, environment, and host presents multiple opportunities for individuals and communities to intercede and "break the chain," preventing and controlling disease transmission; see **Figure 14.1**.

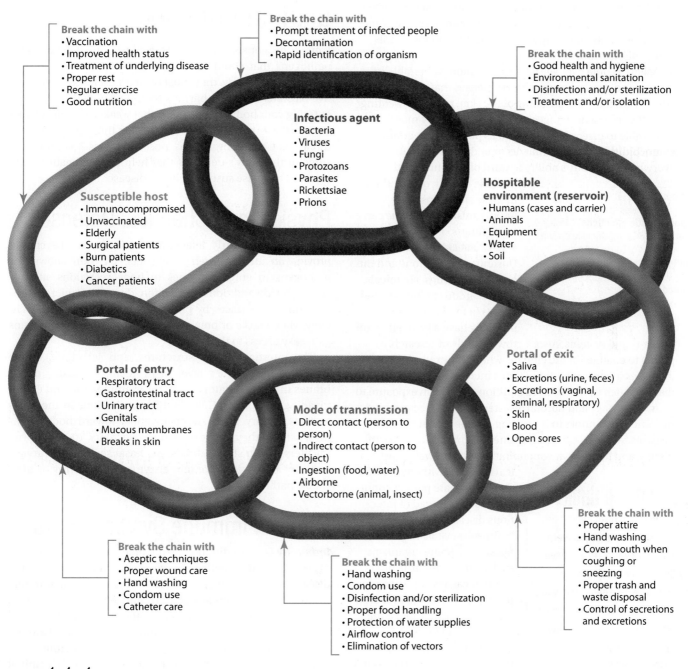

**Break the chain with**
• Vaccination
• Improved health status
• Treatment of underlying disease
• Proper rest
• Regular exercise
• Good nutrition

**Break the chain with**
• Prompt treatment of infected people
• Decontamination
• Rapid identification of organism

**Break the chain with**
• Good health and hygiene
• Environmental sanitation
• Disinfection and/or sterilization
• Treatment and/or isolation

**Infectious agent**
• Bacteria
• Viruses
• Fungi
• Protozoans
• Parasites
• Rickettsiae
• Prions

**Susceptible host**
• Immunocompromised
• Unvaccinated
• Elderly
• Surgical patients
• Burn patients
• Diabetics
• Cancer patients

**Hospitable environment (reservoir)**
• Humans (cases and carrier)
• Animals
• Equipment
• Water
• Soil

**Portal of entry**
• Respiratory tract
• Gastrointestinal tract
• Urinary tract
• Genitals
• Mucous membranes
• Breaks in skin

**Mode of transmission**
• Direct contact (person to person)
• Indirect contact (person to object)
• Ingestion (food, water)
• Airborne
• Vectorborne (animal, insect)

**Portal of exit**
• Saliva
• Excretions (urine, feces)
• Secretions (vaginal, seminal, respiratory)
• Skin
• Blood
• Open sores

**Break the chain with**
• Aseptic techniques
• Proper wound care
• Hand washing
• Condom use
• Catheter care

**Break the chain with**
• Hand washing
• Condom use
• Disinfection and/or sterilization
• Proper food handling
• Protection of water supplies
• Airflow control
• Elimination of vectors

**Break the chain with**
• Proper attire
• Hand washing
• Cover mouth when coughing or sneezing
• Proper trash and waste disposal
• Control of secretions and excretions

**FIGURE 14.1 The Chain of Infection**
The three key factors in transmission of an infectious disease are a susceptible host, an infectious agent, and a hospitable environment. Connecting these three factors are the portal of entry, mode of transmission, and portal of exit. Interfering with any of the links in the chain can prevent the transmission of infectious disease.

## Risk Factors You Typically Cannot Control

Unfortunately, some of the factors that make you susceptible to a certain disease are either hard to control or completely beyond your control. The following are the most common:

- **Heredity.** Perhaps the single greatest factor influencing disease risk is genetics. It is often unclear whether hereditary diseases are due to inherited genetic traits or to inherited insufficiencies in the immune system. Some believe that we may inherit the quality of our immune system, so that some people are naturally "tougher" than others and more resistant to disease and infection.
- **Aging.** People over age 65 are often more vulnerable to infectious diseases because body defenses that we take for granted are reduced. Thinning of the skin, reduced sweating and other physical changes can make the elderly more vulnerable to disease. In addition, as people age, certain **comorbidities** (diseases that occur at the same time), overwhelm the body's ability to ward off enemies, and increase the risk of infection. In these situations, **opportunistic infections** can cause illness.
- **Environmental conditions.** Unsanitary conditions and the presence of drugs, chemicals, and hazardous pollutants and wastes in food and water probably have a great effect on our immune systems. Also, a growing body of research points to changes in the climate, where, for example, increases in mosquito populations increase the spread of diseases such as malaria.[1] In addition, long-term exposure to toxic chemicals, and natural disasters are believed to be significant contributors to increasing numbers of infectious diseases.[2] Catastrophic environmental crises such as earthquakes and floods that contaminate food and water and leave victims without medical care also create perfect conditions for the spread of infectious disease.
- **Organism virulence and resistance.** Some organisms, such as the foodborne organism that causes *botulism,* are particularly virulent, and even tiny amounts may make the most hardy of us ill. Other organisms have mutated and become resistant to the body's defenses and to medical treatments. Multidrug-resistant strains of tuberculosis, *Staphylococcus,* and other

**comorbidities** The presence of one or more diseases at the same time.
**opportunistic infections** Infections that occur when the immune system is weakened or compromised.
**antigen** Substance capable of triggering an immune response.
**antibodies** Substances produced by the body that are individually matched to specific antigens.

**what do you think?**

Do you have any risks for infectious disease that you were probably born with? Do you have any that are the result of your lifestyle? ● What actions can you take to reduce your risks? ● What behaviors do you or your friends engage in that might make you more susceptible to various infections? ● Are your risks greater today than before you entered college? Why or why not?

organisms are emerging in many parts of the world. See the **Be Healthy, Be Green** box on page 440 for more on this topic.

- **College environment.** The living conditions in which many college students find themselves are often conducive to the spread of infectious diseases. Living and studying in close quarters, lack of sleep, and poor cleaning habits all can contribute to increased susceptibility to disease.

# Your Body's Defenses against Infection

Your body constantly protects against and defends from pathogens that could make you ill. For pathogens to gain entry into your body, they must overcome a number of effective barriers: There are barriers that prevent pathogens from entering your body, mechanisms that weaken organisms that breach these barriers, and substances that counteract the threat that these organisms pose. Figure 14.2 summarizes some of the body's defenses that help protect against invasion and decrease susceptibility to disease.

## Physical and Chemical Defenses

Our most critical early defense system is the skin. Layered to provide an intricate web of barriers, the skin allows few pathogens to enter. Enzymes in body secretions such as sweat provide additional protection, destroying microorganisms on skin surfaces by producing inhospitable pH levels. Only when cracks or breaks occur in the skin can pathogens gain easy access to the body.

The internal linings, structures, and secretions of the body provide another layer of protection. Mucous membranes in the respiratory tract, for example, trap and engulf invading organisms. Cilia, hairlike projections in the lungs and respiratory tract, sweep invaders toward body openings, where they are expelled. Nose hairs trap airborne invaders with a sticky film. Tears, nasal secretions, earwax, and other secretions contain enzymes that destroy or neutralize pathogens.

## How the Immune System Works

*Immunity* is a condition of being able to resist a particular disease by counteracting the substance that produces the disease. Any substance capable of triggering an immune response is called an **antigen.** An antigen can be a virus, a bacterium, a fungus, a parasite, a toxin, or a tissue or cell from another organism. The immune system has elaborate mechanisms for protecting you from invading microbes.

As soon as an antigen breaches the body's initial defenses, the body responds by forming substances called **antibodies** that are matched to that specific antigen, much as a key is matched to a lock. The body analyzes the antigen, considering the size and shape of the invader, verifies that

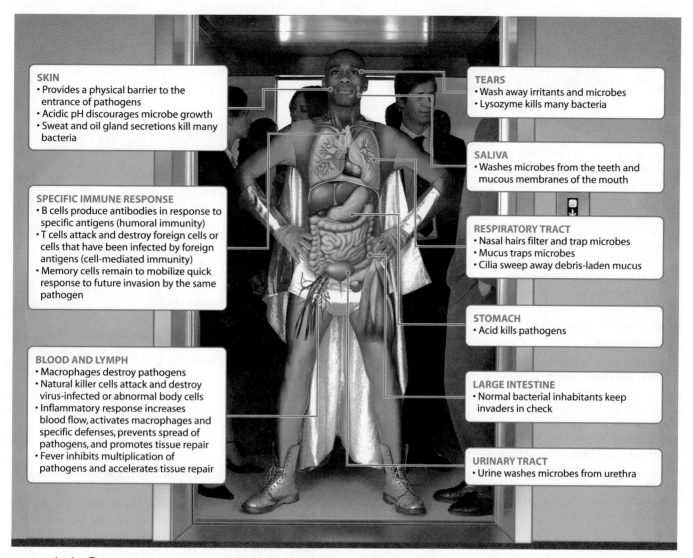

**SKIN**
- Provides a physical barrier to the entrance of pathogens
- Acidic pH discourages microbe growth
- Sweat and oil gland secretions kill many bacteria

**SPECIFIC IMMUNE RESPONSE**
- B cells produce antibodies in response to specific antigens (humoral immunity)
- T cells attack and destroy foreign cells or cells that have been infected by foreign antigens (cell-mediated immunity)
- Memory cells remain to mobilize quick response to future invasion by the same pathogen

**BLOOD AND LYMPH**
- Macrophages destroy pathogens
- Natural killer cells attack and destroy virus-infected or abnormal body cells
- Inflammatory response increases blood flow, activates macrophages and specific defenses, prevents spread of pathogens, and promotes tissue repair
- Fever inhibits multiplication of pathogens and accelerates tissue repair

**TEARS**
- Wash away irritants and microbes
- Lysozyme kills many bacteria

**SALIVA**
- Washes microbes from the teeth and mucous membranes of the mouth

**RESPIRATORY TRACT**
- Nasal hairs filter and trap microbes
- Mucus traps microbes
- Cilia sweep away debris-laden mucus

**STOMACH**
- Acid kills pathogens

**LARGE INTESTINE**
- Normal bacterial inhabitants keep invaders in check

**URINARY TRACT**
- Urine washes microbes from urethra

FIGURE 14.2 **The Body's Defenses against Disease-Causing Pathogens**
In addition to the defenses listed, many of the body's defensive secretions and fluids, such as earwax, tears, mucus, and blood, contain enzymes and other proteins that can kill some invading pathogens or prevent or slow their reproduction.

the antigen is not part of the body itself, and then produces a specific antibody to destroy or weaken the antigen. This process, which is much more complex than described here, is part of a system called *humoral immune responses*. **Humoral immunity** is the body's major defense against many bacteria and the poisonous substances, called **toxins,** that they produce.

In **cell-mediated immunity,** specialized white blood cells called **lymphocytes** attack and destroy the foreign invader. Lymphocytes constitute the body's main defense against viruses, fungi, parasites, and some bacteria, and they are found in the blood, lymph nodes, bone marrow, and certain glands. Other key players in this immune response are **macrophages** (a type of phagocytic, or cell-eating, white blood cell).

Two forms of lymphocytes in particular, the *B lymphocytes* (B cells) and *T lymphocytes* (T cells), are involved in the

immune response. *Helper T cells* are essential for activating B cells to produce antibodies. They also activate other T cells and macrophages. Another form of T cell, known as the *killer T cell,* directly attacks infected or malignant cells. *Suppressor T cells* turn off or suppress the activity of B cells, killer T cells, and macrophages. After a successful attack on a pathogen, some of the attacker T and B cells are preserved as *memory T* and *B cells,* enabling the body to recognize and respond quickly to subsequent attacks by the same kind of organism at a later time.

Once people have survived certain infectious diseases, they become immune to those diseases,

**humoral immunity** Aspect of immunity that is mediated by antibodies secreted by white blood cells.
**toxins** Poisonous substances produced by certain microorganisms that cause various diseases.
**cell-mediated immunity** Aspect of immunity that is mediated by specialized white blood cells that attack pathogens and antigens directly.
**lymphocyte** A type of white blood cell involved in the immune response.
**macrophage** A type of white blood cell that ingests foreign material.

## Antibiotic Resistance: Bugs versus Drugs

Antibiotics are supposed to wipe out bacteria that are susceptible to them. However, many of our antibiotics are becoming ineffective against resistant strains. Bacteria and other microorganisms that cause infections and diseases evolve and develop ways to survive drugs that should kill or weaken them. This means that some of the bacteria and microorganisms are becoming "superbugs" that cannot be stopped with existing medications.

### WHY IS ANTIBIOTIC RESISTANCE ON THE RISE?

✱ **Improper use of antibiotics and resulting growth of superbugs.** When used improperly, antibiotics kill only the weak bacteria and leave the strongest versions to thrive and replicate. Because bacteria can swap genes with one another under the right conditions, hardy drug-resistant germs can share their resistance mechanisms with other germs. They adapt and mutate, and eventually an entire colony of resistant bugs grows and passes on its resistance traits to new generations of bacteria. Over time, most pathogens evolve anyway. Human negligence just speeds the resistant ones on their journey.

If patients begin an antibiotic regimen, and stop taking the drug as soon as they start to feel better, rather than finishing the course of antibiotics, then the surviving bacteria build immunity to the drugs used to treat them. Doctors also overprescribe antibiotics: The Centers for Disease Control and Prevention (CDC) estimates that one-third of the 150 million prescriptions written each year are unnecessary, resulting in bacterial strains that are tougher than the drugs used to fight them.

✱ **Overuse of antibiotics in food production.** About 70 percent of antibiotic production today is used to treat sick animals living in crowded feedlots and to encourage growth in livestock and poultry. Farmed fish may be given antibiotics to fight off disease in controlled water areas. Although research in this area is only in its infancy, many believe that ingesting meats, animal products, and fish full of antibiotics may contribute to antibiotic resistance in humans. In addition, water runoff and sewage from feedlots can contaminate the water in rivers and streams with antibiotics.

✱ **Misuse and overuse of antibacterial soaps and other cleaning products.** Preying on the public's fear of germs and disease, the cleaning industry adds antibacterial ingredients to many of its dish soaps, hand cleaners, shower scrubs, surface scrubs, and most household products. Just how much these products contribute to overall resistance is difficult to assess; as with antibiotics, the germs these products do not kill may become stronger than before.

### WHAT CAN YOU DO?

✱ **Be responsible with medications.** To help prevent antibiotic resistance, use antimicrobial drugs only for bacterial, not viral, infections. Take medications as prescribed and finish the full course. Consult with your health care provider if you feel it is necessary to stop your medication.

✱ **Use regular soap—not antibacterial soap—when washing your hands.** Some experts say that antibacterial cleaning products do more harm than good. Research suggests that antibacterial agents contained in soaps actually may kill normal bacteria, thus creating an environment for resistant, mutated bacteria that are impervious to antibacterial cleaners and antibiotics.

✱ **Avoid food treated with antibiotics.** Buy meat from animals that were not unnecessarily dosed with antibiotics. (Look for that information on the label of meat products.)

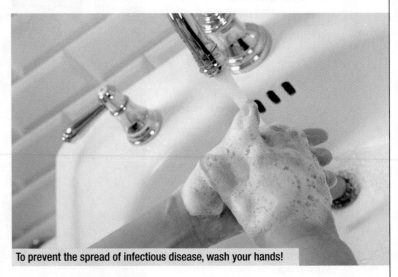

To prevent the spread of infectious disease, wash your hands!

**Sources:** Centers for Disease Control and Prevention, National Center for Emerging and Zoonotic Infectious Diseases, Division of Healthcare Quality Promotion, "Diseases/Pathogens Associated with Antimicrobial Resistance," Updated July 2010, www.cdc.gov/drugresistance/DiseasesConnectedAR.html; Centers for Disease Control and Prevention, National Center for Immunization and Respiratory Diseases, Division of Bacterial Diseases, "Antibiotic Resistance Questions & Answers," Updated June 2009, www.cdc.gov/getsmart/antibiotic-use/anitbiotic-resistance-faqs.html; H. Boucher et al., "Bad Bugs, No Drugs: No ESKAPE! An Update from the Infectious Diseases Society of America," *Clinical Infectious Diseases* 48, no. 1 (2009): 1–12; Global Health Council, "The Impact of Infectious Diseases," 2010, www.globalhealth.org/infectious_diseases.

meaning that in all probability they will not develop them again. Upon subsequent attack by the same disease-causing microorganisms, their memory T and B cells are quickly activated to come to their defense. Figure 14.3 provides a summary of the cell-mediated immune response.

## When the Immune System Misfires: Autoimmune Diseases

Although the immune response generally works in our favor, the body sometimes makes a mistake and targets its own tissue as the enemy, builds up antibodies against that tissue, and attempts to destroy it. This is known as **autoimmune disease** (*auto* means "self"). The National Institutes of Health estimates that over 24 million Americans suffer from some form of autoimmune disease and that the numbers are increasing. Researchers estimate that there are between 80 and 140 different types of autoimmune disease, many of which are chronic, debilitating, and life threatening. Common autoimmune disorders include *rheumatoid arthritis, systemic lupus erythematosus (SLE), type 1 diabetes,* and *multiple sclerosis.* (See Chapter 17 and Focus On: Minimizing Your Risk for Diabetes beginning on

### "Why Should I Care?"

An increasing number of chronic diseases are being linked to the inflammation that occurs when certain pathogens invade. Avoiding infections and their inflammatory side effects now has the added benefit that it may help you avoid certain chronic diseases later.

page 514 for more on these diseases.) Many people do not realize that autoimmune diseases are among the leading causes of death in female children and women under the age of 65.[3]

### Inflammatory Response, Pain, and Fever

If an infection is localized, pus formation, redness, swelling, and irritation often occur. These symptoms are components of the body's inflammatory response, and they indicate that the invading organisms are being fought systemically. The four cardinal signs of inflammation are redness, swelling, pain, and heat.

Pain is often one of the earliest signs that an injury or infection has occurred. Pathogens can kill or injure tissue at the site of infection, causing swelling that puts pressure on nerve endings in the area, causing pain. Although pain does not feel good, it plays a valuable role in the body's response to injury or invasion. For example, it can cause a person to avoid activity that may aggravate the injury or site of infection, thereby protecting against further damage.

**autoimmune disease** Disease caused by an overactive immune response against the body's own cells.

In addition to inflammation, another frequent indicator of infection is *fever,* or a body temperature above the average norm of 98.6°F. Fever is frequently caused by toxins secreted by pathogens that interfere with the control of body temperature. Although extremely elevated temperatures are harmful to the body, a mild fever is protective: Raising body temperature by one or two degrees provides an environment that destroys some disease-causing organisms. A fever also stimulates the body to produce more white blood cells, which destroy more invaders. Of course, as fevers increase beyond 101 or 102°F, risks to the patient outweigh any fever benefits. In these cases, medical treatment should be obtained.

## Vaccines: Bolstering Your Immunity

Recall that once people have been exposed to a specific pathogen, subsequent attacks will activate their memory T and B cells, thus giving them

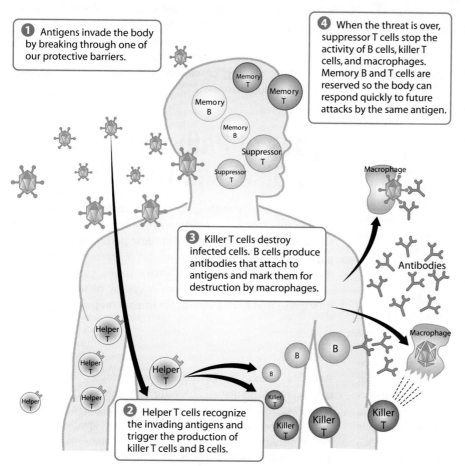

❶ Antigens invade the body by breaking through one of our protective barriers.

❹ When the threat is over, suppressor T cells stop the activity of B cells, killer T cells, and macrophages. Memory B and T cells are reserved so the body can respond quickly to future attacks by the same antigen.

❸ Killer T cells destroy infected cells. B cells produce antibodies that attach to antigens and mark them for destruction by macrophages.

❷ Helper T cells recognize the invading antigens and trigger the production of killer T cells and B cells.

Macrophage

Antibodies

Macrophage

FIGURE 14.3 **The Cell-Mediated Immune Response**

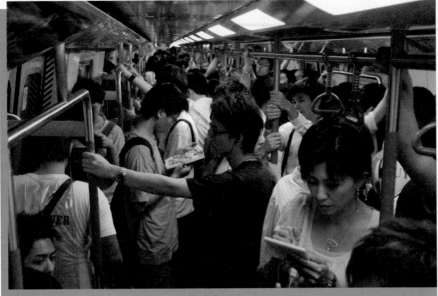

**Why are vaccinations important?**

Vaccinations can protect an individual from certain infectious diseases, and they are also important in controlling the prevalence of diseases in society at large. Certain diseases such as polio and diphtheria have become very rare as a result of immunizations, but until a disease is completely eradicated, it is important to keep vaccinating people against it. Otherwise, there is nothing to stop the disease from making a comeback and causing an epidemic. People who spend time in crowded places, such as commuters or frequent air travelers, and people at particular risk, such as hospital workers or college students who often live in close quarters, should be especially certain to stay up to date on their vaccinations.

| TABLE 14.2 | Recommended Vaccinations for Teens and College Students |
|---|---|

- Tetanus-diphtheria-pertussis vaccine (Td/Tdap)
- Meningococcal vaccine*
- HPV vaccine series
- Hepatitis B vaccine series
- Polio vaccine series
- Measles-mumps-rubella (MMR) vaccine series
- Varicella (chickenpox) vaccine series
- Influenza vaccine
- Pneumococcal polysaccharide (PPV) vaccine
- Hepatitis A vaccine series

*Recommended for previously unvaccinated college first-year students living in dormitories.
**Source:** Centers for Disease Control and Prevention, "Recommendations and Guidelines: Vaccines Needed by Teens and College Students," Modified January 2010, www.cdc.gov/vaccines/recs/schedules/teen-schedule.htm.

**vaccination** Inoculation with killed or weakened pathogens or similar, less dangerous antigens in order to prevent or lessen the effects of some disease.
**bacteria** (singular: *bacterium*) Simple, single-celled microscopic organisms; about 100 known species of bacteria cause disease in humans.

immunity. This is the principle on which **vaccination** is based.

A vaccine consists of killed or weakened versions of a disease-causing microorganism or an antigen that is similar to but less dangerous than the disease antigen. It is administered to stimulate the person's immune system to produce antibodies against future attacks—without actually causing the disease (or by causing a very minor case of it). Vaccines typically are given orally or by injection, and this form of immunity is termed *artificially acquired active immunity,* in contrast to *naturally acquired active immunity* (which is obtained by exposure to antigens in the normal course of daily life) or *naturally acquired passive immunity* (as occurs when a mother passes immunity to her fetus via their shared blood supply or to an infant via breast milk).

Specific schedules have been established for various population groups. See Table 14.2 for recommended vaccines for one such group, teens and college students. Figure 14.4 shows the recommended vaccination schedule for the general adult population. Childhood vaccine schedules are available at the Centers for Disease Control and Prevention (CDC) website. Concern about the safety of vaccines has caused an increase in the number of parents who refuse to vaccinate their children (see the **Health Headlines** box on page 444).

Because of their close living quarters and frequent interactions with people, college students face a higher than average risk of infection from diseases that are largely preventable. Vaccines that should be a high priority among 20-somethings include tetanus-diphtheria-pertussis vaccine (Tdap), meningococcal conjugate vaccine (MCV4), and human papillomavirus (HPV).

# Types of Pathogens and the Diseases They Cause

We can categorize pathogens into six major types: bacteria, viruses, fungi, protozoans, parasitic worms, and prions. Figure 14.5 shows examples of several of these pathogens. Each has a particular route of transmission and characteristic elements that make it unique. In the following pages, we discuss each of these categories and give an overview of some diseases they cause that have a significant impact on public health.

## Bacteria

**Bacteria** (singular: *bacterium*) are simple, single-celled microscopic organisms. There are three major types of bacteria, classified by their shape: cocci, bacilli, and spirilla. Although there are several thousand known species of bacteria (and many thousands more that are unknown), just over 100 cause disease in humans. In many cases, it is not the bacteria themselves that cause disease but rather the toxins that they produce.

| Vaccine | Age group | | | | |
|---|---|---|---|---|---|
| | 19–26 years | 27–49 years | 50–59 years | 60–64 years | ≥65 years |
| Tetanus, diphtheria, pertussis (Td/Tdap)* | Substitute 1-time dose of Tdap for Td booster; then boost with Td every 10 years | | | | Td booster every 10 years |
| Human papillomavirus (HPV)* | 3 doses (females) | | | | |
| Varicella* | 2 doses | | | | |
| Zoster | | | | 1 dose | |
| Measles, mumps, rubella (MMR)* | 1 or 2 doses | | 1 dose | | |
| Influenza* | 1 dose annually | | | | |
| Pneumococcal (polysaccharide) | 1 or 2 doses | | | | 1 dose |
| Hepatitis A* | 2 doses | | | | |
| Hepatitis B* | 3 doses | | | | |
| Meningococcal* | 1 or more doses | | | | |

*Covered by the Vaccine Injury Compensation Program

For all persons in this category who meet the age requirements and who lack evidence of immunity (e.g., lack documentation of vaccination or have no evidence of prior infection)

Recommended if some other risk factor is present (e.g., on the basis of medical, occupational, lifestyle, or other indications)

No recommendation

FIGURE 14.4 **Recommended Adult Immunization Schedule, by Vaccine and Age Group, 2010**
Note that there are important explanations and additions to these recommendations that should be consulted by checking the latest schedule at www.cdc.gov/vaccines/recs/schedules/adult-schedule.htm.

**Source:** Centers for Disease Control and Prevention, "Recommended Adult Immunization Schedule—United States, 2010," *MMWR Weekly* 59, no. 1 (2010): 1–4.

Diseases caused by bacteria can be treated with **antibiotics;** penicillin is one of the oldest and historically most well-known antibiotics. However, today's arsenal of antibiotics is becoming less effective, as strains of bacteria with **antibiotic resistance** become more common. Such "superbugs" can result when successive generations of bacteria mutate to develop an ability to withstand the effects of specific drugs. Refer back to the Be Healthy, Be Green box on page 440 for more on the issues and concerns relating to superbugs and antibiotic resistance.

**antibiotics** Medicines used to kill microorganisms, such as bacteria.
**antibiotic resistance** The ability of bacteria or other microbes to withstand the effects of an antibiotic.

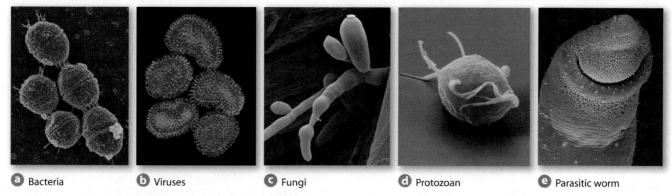

ⓐ Bacteria  ⓑ Viruses  ⓒ Fungi  ⓓ Protozoan  ⓔ Parasitic worm

FIGURE 14.5 **Examples of Five Major Types of Pathogens**
(a) Color-enhanced scanning electron micrograph (SEM) of *Streptococcus* bacteria, magnified 40,000×. (b) Colored transmission electron micrograph (TEM) of influenza (flu) viruses, magnified 32,000×. (c) Color SEM of *Candida albicans,* a yeast fungus, magnified 50,000×. (d) Color TEM of *Trichomonas vaginalis,* a protozoan, magnified 9,000×. (e) Color-enhanced SEM of a female blood fluke, magnified 350×.

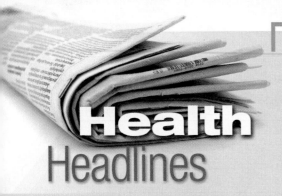

# Health
# Headlines

## VACCINE BACKLASH: ARE THEY SAFE? ARE THEY NECESSARY?

Immunizations against widespread infectious diseases are one of the greatest public health success stories of all time—so successful, in fact, that most people have never seen or heard of anyone having the diseases that once wiped out entire populations. Today, fear of the old "killer" diseases has waned, and many question whether they really need to get vaccinated. Add in the costs of vaccines and a growing distrust of health care, the government, and drug companies, and it's no wonder that there is growing anti-vaccine sentiment in some segments of the public.

How serious a problem is this? In some communities, such as Ashland, Oregon, up to 25 percent of kindergartners' parents opted their children out of at least one vaccine last year. In other U.S. school districts and counties, these rates are even higher, and a general trend of avoiding vaccinations is growing.

Undervaccination rates are particularly high in non-Hispanic, college-educated white families with incomes above

$75,000 a year. Religious tenets, fear of vaccine safety, and worry about vaccine overload are among some of the more common reasons for parents' refusal to vaccinate their children. Others object to mandatory vaccinations because they consider them to be a government intrusion into their individual rights.

The vaccine concerns receiving the most attention include fear that the measles, mumps, rubella (MMR) vaccine can lead to autism; fear that the hepatitis B vaccine is related to multiple sclerosis (MS); and fear that the combined tetanus-diphtheria-pertussis (Tdap) vaccine can cause sudden infant death syndrome (SIDS). Are these concerns valid? Research is ongoing, but the Centers for Disease Control and Prevention (CDC) has found no clear evidence that the MMR vaccine causes autism, that hepatitis B shots are the culprit behind MS, or that the Tdap vaccine leads to SIDS. Virtually all medical and public health organizations support vaccinations, pointing to stringent safety controls in the manufacturing and testing of vaccines, as well as ongoing safety monitoring, the long history of vaccines in wiping out killer diseases across the globe, and the fact that risks from the diseases themselves are almost always much greater than any risks associated with a vaccine. If large numbers of people were to avoid vaccinations, old killers would be likely to reemerge, and those people who were already sick or weak from other conditions would be extremely vulnerable.

The reasons for vaccination far outweigh any arguments against. That said, it's important to note that, despite extensive testing, no vaccine is completely safe and effective and that

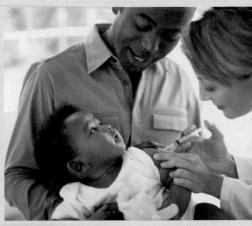

Some parents have expressed concern over the safety of vaccinations.

there are often risks from temporary, minor side effects from any given vaccine. Local rashes and reactions at injection sites, low-grade fever, discomfort, and even allergic reactions can occur. Major risks from getting vaccinations are extremely rare and studies supporting the "anti-vaccine" rhetoric are unsubstantiated.

**Sources:** Centers for Disease Control and Prevention, "Vaccine Safety: Concerns about Autism," Modified January 2010, www.cdc.gov/vaccinesafety/Concerns/Autism/Index.html; E. J. Gangarosa et al., "Impact of Anti-Vaccine Movements on Pertussis Control: The Untold Story," *Lancet* 351, no. 9099 (1998): 356–61; Institute of Medicine of the National Academies, *Immunization Safety Review: Vaccines and Autism* (Washington, DC: National Academy of Sciences, 2004), Available at www.iom.edu/Reports/2004/Immunization-Safety-Review-Vaccines-and-Autism.aspx; Institute of Medicine of the National Academies, *Immunization Safety Review: Vaccinations and Sudden Unexpected Death in Infancy* (Washington, DC: National Academy of Sciences, 2003), Available at www.iom.edu/Reports/2003/Immunization-Safety-Review-Vaccinations-and-Sudden-Unexpected-Death-in-Infancy.aspx.

---

**staphylococci** A group of round bacteria, usually found in clusters, that cause a variety of diseases in humans and other animals.

**colonization** The process of bacteria or some other infectious organisms establishing themselves in a host without causing infection.

**infection** The state of pathogens being established in or on a host and causing disease.

### Staphylococcal Infections

**Staphylococci** are normally present on the skin or in the nostrils of 20 to 30 percent of us at any given time. Usually they cause no problems for otherwise healthy persons. The presence of bacteria on or in a person without infection is called **colonization.** A person can be colonized and then spread the

infection to others, yet never develop the disease. In contrast, when the pathogen is present and there is a cut or break in the *epidermis,* or outer layer of the skin, staphylococci may enter the system and cause an **infection.** If you have ever suffered from acne, boils, styes (infections of the eyelids), or infected wounds, you have probably had a "staph" infection.

Although most of these infections are readily defeated by the immune system, resistant forms of staph bacteria are on the rise. One of these resistant forms of staph, **methicillin-resistant *Staphylococcus aureus* (MRSA),** has come under intense international scrutiny as numerous cases have arisen around the world, especially in the United States.[4] Symptoms of MRSA infection often start with a rash or pimplelike skin irritation. Within hours, these early symptoms may progress to redness, inflammation, pain, and deeper wounds. If untreated, MRSA may invade the blood, bones, joints, surgical wounds, heart valves, and lungs, and can be fatal.[5]

Most cases of MRSA are contracted in health care facilities such as hospitals, nursing homes, or clinics. These cases, referred to as *health care associated* or *health care acquired MRSA (HA-MRSA)* arise in settings where invasive treatments, infectious pathogens, and weakened immune systems converge. Cases of MRSA are also on the rise among those who return home from treatment and are infected by family members or surfaces in the home. Others who have never seen a doctor are becoming infected during their normal daily activities, from surfaces at home, at work, at the gym, or in other public places. Known as *community acquired MRSA (CA-MRSA)*, this form is on the increase.

Finally, *linezolid-resistant* Staphylococcus aureus, or LRSA, is a particularly potent bacterium that has evolved among patients using the antibiotic linezolid to treat MRSA. Dubbed the "new MRSA," this resistant superbug has killed hundreds in Europe and is spreading rapidly in other countries. LRSA infections are prevalent among those recovering from surgical treatment, those with weakened immune systems, and those who have underlying respiratory problems. Because linezolid was one of the few remaining effective treatments for the most severe forms of MRSA, many wonder whether the antibiotic "well" may finally be running dry. LRSA organisms seem to be unfazed by any of the latest antibiotics we can throw at them.

## Streptococcal Infections

At least five types of the *Streptococcus* microorganism are known to cause bacterial infections. Group A streptococci (GAS) cause the most common diseases, such as streptococcal pharyngitis ("strep throat") and scarlet fever, which is often preceded by a sore throat.[6] One particularly virulent group of GAS can lead to a rare but serious disease called *necrotizing fasciitis* (often referred to as "flesh-eating strep").[7] Group B streptococci can cause illness in newborn babies, pregnant women, older adults, and adults with other illnesses such as diabetes or liver disease.[8]

The species *Streptococcus pneumoniae* causes thousands of cases of meningitis and pneumonia and 7 million cases of ear infections in the United States each year. Currently, about 30 percent of these cases are resistant to penicillin, the primary drug for treatment. Many penicillin-resistant strains are also resistant to other antibiotics.

## Meningitis

Meningitis is an infection and inflammation of the *meninges,* the membranes that surround the brain and spinal cord. Some forms of bacterial meningitis are contagious and can be spread through contact with saliva, nasal discharge, feces, or respiratory and throat secretions. *Pneumococcal meningitis,* the most common form of menin-

gitis, is also the most dangerous form of bacterial meningitis. Several thousand cases of meningitis are reported in the United States each year. *Meningococcal meningitis,* a virulent form of meningitis, has risen dramatically on college campuses in recent years.[9] College students living in dormitories have a higher risk of contracting this disease than those who live off campus.

The signs of meningitis are sudden fever, severe headache, and a stiff neck, particularly causing difficulty touching your chin to your chest. Persons who are suspected of having meningitis should receive immediate, aggressive medical treatment. Vaccines are available for some types of meningitis; talk to the medical or health education staff at your local student health center to see if they have the vaccine most likely to protect you in your area.

## Pneumonia

Pneumonia is a general term for a wide range of conditions that result in inflammation of the lungs and difficulty in breathing. It is characterized by chronic cough, chest pain, chills, high fever, fluid accumulation, and eventual respiratory failure. Although bacterial and viral pathogens are the most common cause of pneumonia, it can also be caused by fungi, yeast infections, occupational exposure, or trauma.

Bacterial pneumonia responds readily to antibiotic treatment in the early stages, but can be deadly in more advanced stages. Other forms of pneumonia caused by viruses, fungi, chemicals, or other substances in the lungs are more difficult to treat. Although medical advances have reduced the overall incidence of pneumonia, it continues to be a major threat in the United States and throughout the world. Vulnerable populations include children; the poor; those

**methicillin-resistant *Staphylococcus aureus* (MRSA)** Highly resistant form of staph infection that is growing in international prevalence.
***Streptococcus*** A round bacterium, usually found in chain formation.
**meningitis** An infection of the meninges, the membranes that surround the brain and spinal cord.
**pneumonia** Inflammatory disease of the lungs characterized by chronic cough, chest pain, chills, high fever, and fluid accumulation; may be caused by bacteria, viruses, fungi, chemicals, or other substances.

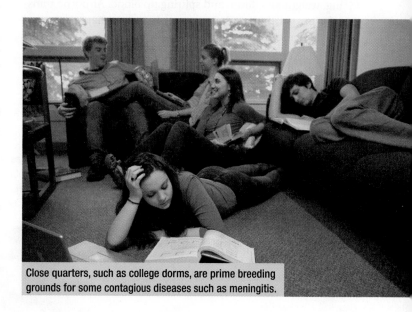

Close quarters, such as college dorms, are prime breeding grounds for some contagious diseases such as meningitis.

displaced by war, famine, and natural disasters; older adults; those who have been occupationally exposed to chemicals and particulates that damage the lungs; and those already suffering from other illnesses.

## Tuberculosis (TB)

A major killer in the United States in the early twentieth century, **tuberculosis (TB)** was largely controlled by 1950 as a result of improved sanitation, isolation of infected persons, and treatment with drugs such as *rifampin* or *isoniazid*. Many health professionals assumed that TB was conquered, but that appears not to be the case. During the past 20 years, several factors have led to an epidemic rise in the disease: deteriorating social conditions, including overcrowding and poor sanitation; failure to isolate active cases of TB; a weakening of public health infrastructure, which has led to less funding for screening; and migration of TB to the United States through immigration and international travel. In 2008, the most recent year for which data are available, there were 12,904 active cases of TB in the United States, compared to 85,000 in 1950.[10]

tuberculosis (TB) A disease caused by bacterial infiltration of the respiratory system.

multidrug resistant TB (MDR-TB) Form of TB that is resistant to at least two of the best antibiotics available.

extensively drug resistant TB (XDR-TB) Form of TB that is resistant to nearly all existing antibiotics.

rickettsia A small form of bacteria that live inside other living cells.

peptic ulcer Damage to the stomach or intestinal lining, usually caused by digestive juices; most ulcers result from infection by the bacterium *Helicobacter pylori*.

The World Health Organization (WHO) reports that almost 2 billion people (a third of the world's entire population) have been exposed to TB. Some 80 percent of tuberculosis-related deaths occur in developing countries, where it accounts for 26 percent of preventable deaths.[11] TB is the number one infectious killer of women of reproductive age worldwide, as well as the leading cause of death among HIV-positive patients.

Referred to as "consumption" in many parts of the world, this bacterial respiratory disease leads to wasting, chronic cough, fluid- and blood-filled lungs, and eventual spread throughout the body. Symptoms include persistent coughing, weight loss, fever, and spitting up blood. Airborne transmission via the respiratory tract is the primary and most efficient mode of transmitting TB. Infected people can be contagious without actually showing any symptoms themselves and can transmit the disease while talking, coughing, sneezing, or singing. Those at highest risk for TB include the poor, especially children, and the chronically ill. People residing in crowded prisons and homeless shelters with poor ventilation who continuously inhale the same contaminated air are at higher risk. Persons with compromised immune systems are also at high risk, as are those in situations where comorbidity (suffering from more than one disease) exists.

As with many bacterial diseases, resistant forms of TB are increasing in the global population. **Multidrug resistant TB (MDR-TB)** is a form of TB that is currently resistant to at least two of the best anti-TB drugs in use today. An even more dangerous form, **extensively drug resistant TB**

**(XDR-TB),** is resistant to nearly all first- and second-line drug defenses against it and is extremely difficult to treat. These newer strains of tuberculosis are reaching epidemic proportions in many regions of the world, particularly among those whose immune systems are already compromised by HIV and other diseases.

## Tickborne Bacterial Diseases

In the past few decades, certain tickborne diseases have become major health threats in the United States. Those that are most noteworthy include two bacterially caused diseases, *Lyme disease* and *ehrlichiosis,* both of which spike in the summer months in many states and which can cause significant disability and threats to humans and animals.

Once believed to be closely related to viruses, **rickettsia** are now considered a small form of bacteria. They produce toxins and multiply within small blood vessels, causing vascular blockage and tissue death. Rickettsia require an insect vector (carrier) for transmission to humans. Two common forms of human rickettsial disease are *Rocky Mountain spotted fever* (*RMSF*), carried by a tick; and *typhus,* carried by a louse, flea, or tick. These diseases produce similar symptoms, including high fever, weakness, rash, and coma, and both can be life threatening.

For all insect-borne diseases, the best protection is to stay indoors at dusk and early morning to avoid hours of high insect activity. If you must go out, wear protective clothing or use bug sprays containing natural oils, pyrethrins, or DEET (diethyl toluamide), all products regarded as generally safe. If you are traveling in areas where insect-borne diseases are prevalent, bed nets and other protective measures may be necessary.

## Peptic Ulcers

A **peptic ulcer** is a chronic ulcer or lesion that occurs in the lining of the stomach (gastric ulcer) or in the *duodenum* (duodenal ulcer), a section of the small intestine, usually as a result of an irritant. For decades, nobody thought that ulcers had anything to do with infectious diseases. However, research now indicates that more than 60 percent of peptic ulcers result from infection by a common bacterium, *Helicobacter pylori*.[12] Although bacteria are responsible for most peptic ulcers, other factors do increase risk, including smoking, caffeine consumption, stress, excess levels of digestive enzymes and stomach acids, and regular use of nonsteroidal anti-inflammatory drugs (NSAIDs) such as aspirin, ibuprofen, and naproxen sodium. The disorder, which affects more than 4.5 million Americans every year, generally responds to antibiotics and/or avoidance of NSAIDs, along with appropriate use of anti-secretory therapy.[13]

Ticks are a vector for several devastating bacterial diseases.

# Viruses

**Viruses** are the smallest known pathogens, approximately 1/500th the size of bacteria. Essentially, a virus consists of a protein structure that contains either *ribonucleic acid* (*RNA*) or *deoxyribonucleic acid* (*DNA*). Viruses are incapable of carrying out any life processes on their own. To reproduce, they must invade and inject their own DNA and RNA into a host cell, take it over, and force it to make copies of themselves. The new viruses then erupt out of the host cell and seek other cells to invade. Hundreds of viruses are known to cause diseases in humans.

Because viruses cannot reproduce outside living cells, they are especially difficult to culture in a laboratory, making their detection and study extremely time consuming. Viral diseases can be difficult to treat, because many viruses can withstand heat, formaldehyde, and large doses of radiation with little effect on their structure. Some viruses have **incubation periods** (the length of time required to develop fully and cause symptoms in their hosts) that last for years, which delays diagnosis. Drug treatment for viral infections is also limited. Drugs powerful enough to kill viruses generally kill the host cells, too, although some medications block stages in viral reproduction without damaging the host cells.

**The Common Cold** Caused by any number of viruses (some experts claim there may be over 200 different viruses responsible), any given cold's most likely cause is the rhinovirus, which is responsible for up to 40 percent of all colds, followed by the coronavirus, which causes about 20 percent of all colds.[14] Colds are **endemic** (always present to some degree) throughout the world, with increasing prevalence as the weather turns colder and people spend more time indoors. Otherwise healthy people carry cold viruses in their noses and throats most of the time. These viruses are held in check until the host's resistance is lowered. It is possible to "catch" a cold—from the airborne droplets of another person's sneeze or from skin-to-skin or mucous membrane contact—though the hands are the greatest avenue for transmitting colds and other viruses. Obviously, then, covering your nose and mouth with a tissue, handkerchief, or even the crook of your elbow when sneezing is better than using your bare hand. Contrary to popular belief, you cannot catch a cold from getting a chill, but the chill may lower your immune system's resistance to a pathogenic virus if one is present.

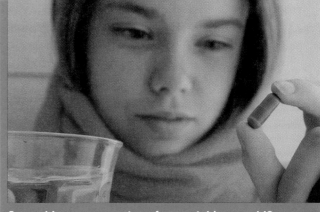

**Can echinacea prevent me from catching a cold?**

Research to date indicates that taking echinacea cannot prevent you from catching a cold if you are exposed to a virus. Study continues, however, into the use of echinacea to treat upper respiratory infections once they are contracted. Your best strategy is to keep your resistance level high and do your best to avoid exposure to the virus in the first place.

Although numerous theories exist concerning how to "cure" the common cold, including taking vitamin C, zinc, or echinacea, there is little proof of their efficacy to date.[15] The best rule of thumb is to keep your resistance level high. A nutritious diet, adequate rest, reduced stress levels, and regular exercise appear to be the best bets in fighting off infection. Avoid people with newly developed colds (colds appear to be most contagious during the first 24 hours of onset). Wash your hands often around people with colds, and keep your hands away from your nose, mouth, and eyes in order to avoid infection. The Skills for Behavior Change box on page 436 provides useful reminders on avoiding all infectious diseases, including colds.

If you contract a cold, getting plenty of rest and fluids and eating a healthy diet are the best ways to help you recover quickly. Children should not be given aspirin for colds or the flu, because this could lead to development of *Reye's syndrome,* a potentially fatal disease. Several nonaspirin over-the-counter preparations are effective for alleviating certain symptoms.

**Influenza** In otherwise healthy people, **influenza,** or flu, is usually not life threatening (see **Figure 14.6** on page 448). However, for certain vulnerable populations, such as individuals with respiratory problems or heart disease, older adults (over age 65), or young children (under age 5), the flu can be very serious. Five to 20 percent of Americans get the flu each year, and of these, 200,000 will need hospitalization.[16] Once a person gets the flu, treatment is *palliative,* meaning that it is focused on relief of symptoms, rather than cure.

**viruses** Minute microbes consisting of DNA or RNA that invade a host cell and use the cell's resources to reproduce themselves.
**incubation period** The time between exposure to a disease and the appearance of symptoms.
**endemic** Describing a disease that is always present to some degree.
**influenza** A common viral disease of the respiratory tract.

| SYMPTOMS | COLD | FLU |
|---|---|---|
| **Fever** | Rare | Usual; high (100–102°F, occasionally higher, especially in children); lasts 3–4 days |
| **Headache** | Rare | Common |
| **General aches and pains** | Slight | Usual; often severe |
| **Fatigue, weakness** | Sometimes | Usual; can last up to 2–3 weeks |
| **Extreme exhaustion** | Never | Usual; at the beginning of the illness |
| **Stuffy nose** | Common | Sometimes |
| **Sneezing** | Usual | Sometimes |
| **Sore throat** | Common | Sometimes |
| **Chest discomfort, cough** | Common; mild to moderate, hacking cough | Common; can become severe |
| **TREATMENT** | Antihistamines, decongestants, nonsteroidal anti-inflammatory medicines | Antiviral medicines—see your doctor |
| **PREVENTION** | Wash your hands often with soap and water; avoid close contact with anyone with a cold | Annual vaccination; antiviral medicines—see your doctor |
| **COMPLICATIONS** | Sinus congestion, middle ear infection, asthma | Bronchitis, pneumonia; can worsen chronic conditions; can be life threatening |

**FIGURE 14.6 Is It a Cold or the Flu?**

**Source:** Adapted from the National Institute of Allergy and Infectious Diseases, "Is It a Cold or the Flu?", 2008, www.niaid.nih.gov/topics/flu/documents/sick.pdf.

at risk should get these shots in the fall before the flu season begins.

**Infectious Mononucleosis** Initial symptoms of **mononucleosis,** or "mono," include sore throat, fever, headache, nausea, chills, and pervasive weakness or fatigue. As the disease progresses, lymph nodes may enlarge and other signs may appear such as spleen enlargement, body rashes, aching joints, and jaundice (yellowing of the whites of the eyes and the skin). College students who are under high stress levels, don't get enough sleep, and may not eat healthfully may be at increased risk for mono, particularly if their immune systems are compromised.

Caused by the Epstein-Barr virus, mononucleosis is readily detected through a blood test. Because many viruses are caused by transmission of body fluids, many people once believed that young people contracted mono through kissing (hence its nickname, "the kissing disease"). However, mono is not highly contagious and does not appear to be easily contracted through normal, everyday personal contact; kissing is actually not a common mode of transmission. Treatment of mononucleosis is often a lengthy process that involves bed rest, balanced nutrition, and medications.

To date, three major varieties of flu virus have been discovered, with many different strains existing within each variety. The A form of the virus is generally the most virulent, followed by the B and C varieties. If you contract one form of influenza, you may develop immunity to it, but you will not necessarily be immune to other forms of the disease. New strains of influenza appear all the time. In 2009, one flu in particular, H1N1, the so-called swine flu, captured world attention and rose to pandemic levels.

**mononucleosis** A viral disease that causes pervasive fatigue and other long-lasting symptoms.

Some vaccines have proven effective against certain strains of flu virus, but they are totally ineffective against others. In spite of minor risks, people over age 65, pregnant women, people with heart or lung disease, and people with certain other illnesses should be vaccinated. Flu shots take 2 to 3 weeks to become effective, so people

## 36,000
**Americans die of the flu each year.**

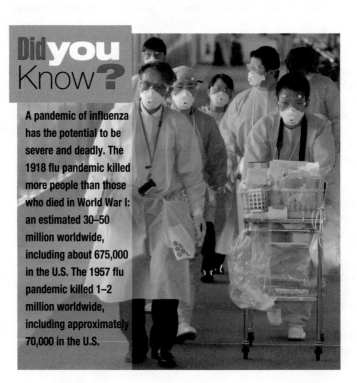

**Did you Know?**

A pandemic of influenza has the potential to be severe and deadly. The 1918 flu pandemic killed more people than those who died in World War I: an estimated 30–50 million worldwide, including about 675,000 in the U.S. The 1957 flu pandemic killed 1–2 million worldwide, including approximately 70,000 in the U.S.

**Hepatitis** One of the most highly publicized viral diseases is **hepatitis,** a virally caused inflammation of the liver. Hepatitis symptoms include fever, headache, nausea, loss of appetite, skin rashes, pain in the upper right abdomen, dark yellow (with brownish tinge) urine, and jaundice. Internationally, viral hepatitis is a major contributor to liver disease and accounts for high morbidity and mortality. Currently, there are several known forms (A, B, C, D, and E), with hepatitis A, B, and C having the highest rates of incidence.

Hepatitis A (HAV) is contracted by eating food or drinking water contaminated with human feces. Since vaccinations became available, HAV rates have declined by nearly 90 percent in the United States. However, over 25,000 people per year are still infected.[17] Handlers of infected food, children at day care centers, those who have sexual contact with HAV-positive individuals, or those who travel to regions where HAV is endemic are at higher risk. In addition, those who ingest seafood from contaminated water and people who use contaminated needles are also at risk. Fortunately, individuals infected with hepatitis A do not become chronic carriers, and vaccines for the disease are available. Many who contract HAV are asymptomatic (symptom-free).

Hepatitis B (HBV) is spread through body fluid exchange during unprotected sex, sharing needles when injecting drugs; through needlesticks on the job; or, in the case of a newborn baby, from an infected mother. Hepatitis B can lead to chronic liver disease or liver cancer. In spite of vaccine availability since 1982, there are currently over 1.2 million people in the United States who are chronically infected with HBV, with over 43,000 new cases each year.[18] Needle exchange programs have helped reduce risks of HBV infection in some populations. Globally, HBV infections are on the decline, but they continue to be a major health problem, with over 350 million chronic carriers and over 1 million deaths each year. Three-quarters of the world's population live in areas where there are high rates of infection.[19]

Hepatitis C (HCV) infections are on an epidemic rise in many regions of the world as resistant forms of the virus are emerging. Some cases can be traced to blood transfusions or organ transplants. Currently, an estimated 17,000 new cases of HCV are diagnosed in the United States each year, with over 3.2 million people chronically infected.[20] Over 85 percent of those infected develop chronic infections; if the infection is left untreated, the person may develop cirrhosis of the liver, liver cancer, or liver failure. Liver failure resulting from chronic hepatitis C is the leading reason for liver transplants in the United States.[21] Currently, there is no vaccine for HCV.

To prevent the spread of HBV and HCV, follow these precautions: use latex condoms correctly every time you have sex; don't share personal-care items that might have blood on them, such as razors or toothbrushes; get a blood test for HBV so you know your status; never share needles; if you are having body art done, go only to reputable artists or piercers who follow established sterilization and infection-control protocols.

**Mumps** In 1968, a vaccine became available for mumps, a common viral disorder among children, and the disease seemed to be largely under control, with reported cases declining from 80 per 100,000 people in 1968 to less than 2 per 100,000 people in 1984. This example of the benefits of vaccinations is one that is often cited when people question the efficacy of vaccines. However, an epidemic in 2006 among college students, primarily those living in dorms, infected thousands of people, mainly in Iowa and the central United States.[22] No one knows how this outbreak started, but it is suspected that many did not receive their second mumps vaccination, making them susceptible. An outbreak of over 1,500 cases in 2009, triggered by an 11-year-old boy who had just returned from the United Kingdom, was a grim reminder that even though mumps is largely controlled in the United States, many countries of the world have continued problems and outbreaks here may be just a plane ride away.[23]

Approximately one-half of all mumps infections are not apparent, because they produce only minor symptoms. Many cases are never reported, so the actual incidence may be higher than indicated. Typically, there is an incubation period of 16 to 18 days, followed by symptoms caused by the lodging of the virus in the neck glands. The most common symptom is the swelling of the parotid (salivary) glands; however, about one-third of all infected people never have this symptom. One of the greatest dangers associated with mumps is the potential for sterility in men who contract the disease in young adulthood. Some victims suffer hearing loss.

### Herpes Viruses: Chickenpox (HVZV), Shingles, and Herpes Gladiatorum

Herpes viruses are among the more common forms of viruses infecting humans. From the annoying cold sore that is highly contagious, to chickenpox, shingles, herpes gladiatorum, and other herpes-caused diseases, painful, blistering rashes are hallmarks of these infections. These diseases are easily transmitted via physical contact and can become chronic problems for the person infected.

Caused by the *herpes varicella zoster virus* (*HVZV*), **chickenpox** produces characteristic symptoms of fever and fatigue 13 to 17 days after exposure, followed by skin eruptions that itch, blister, and produce a clear fluid. The virus is present in these blisters for approximately 1 week. Although a vaccine for chickenpox is available, and all children should receive it, many parents incorrectly assume that the vaccine is not necessary and that if a child gets the disease, it will ensure lifelong immunity. The failure to vaccinate means that many children still contract the disease.

For a small segment of the population, the chickenpox virus becomes reactivated later in life during times of high stress or when the immune system is taxed by other diseases. This painful, blistering rash with other possible complications is called **shingles.** Shingles

**hepatitis** A viral disease in which the liver becomes inflamed, producing symptoms such as fever, headache, and possibly jaundice.
**chickenpox** A highly infectious disease caused by the herpes varicella zoster virus
**shingles** A disease characterized by a painful rash that occurs when the chickenpox virus is reactivated.

affects over 1 million people in the United States; most of whom are over the age of 60. A vaccine for those over 60 is now recommended.[24]

Another form of herpes-caused disease that is increasing on college campuses is **herpes gladiatorum (Figure 14.7)**, caused by the herpes simplex type 1 virus. It is prevalent particularly among those who engage in contact sports, such as wrestling. Highly contagious via mats used by many people, for example, in a yoga studio or a gym, or body-to-body contact, herpes gladiatorum is also referred to as "mat pox" or "wrestler's herpes." Symptoms of blistering rash and pain are common, particularly on the face, neck, and torso.

**herpes gladiatorum** A skin infection caused by the herpes simplex type 1 virus and seen among athletes participating in contact sports.

**measles** A viral disease that produces symptoms such as an itchy rash and a high fever.

**rubella (German measles)** A milder form of measles that causes a rash and mild fever in children and may damage a fetus or a newborn baby.

**rabies** A viral disease of the central nervous system; often transmitted through animal bites.

**fungi** A group of multicellular and unicellular organisms that obtain their food by infiltrating the bodies of other organisms, both living and dead; several microscopic varieties are pathogenic.

### Measles and Rubella

Measles is a viral disorder that often affects young children but is increasing among young adults today, particularly on college campuses where vaccinations are not required or monitored. Many young adults today may not have been vaccinated in their youth, as their parents may not have thought the disease was a problem anymore in the United States. Symptoms, appearing about 10 days after exposure, include an itchy rash and a high fever.

**Rubella (German measles)** is a milder viral infection that is believed to be transmitted by inhalation, after which it multiplies in the upper respiratory tract and passes into the bloodstream. It causes a rash, especially on the upper extremities. It usually runs its course in 3 to 4 days. The major exceptions to this rule are among newborns and pregnant women. Rubella can damage a fetus, particularly during the first trimester, by creating a condition called *congenital rubella,* in which the infant may be born blind, deaf, cognitively impaired, or with heart defects. Immunization has reduced the incidence of both measles and rubella. Infections in children not immunized against measles can lead to fever-induced problems such as rheumatic heart disease, kidney damage, and neurological disorders.

### Rabies

The **rabies** virus infects many warm-blooded animals. Bats are believed to be asymptomatic carriers. Their urine, which they spray when flying, contains the virus, and even the air of densely populated bat caves may be infectious. In most other hosts, the disease is extremely virulent and usually fatal. A characteristic behavior of rabid animals is excessive salivating and frenzied biting of other animals and people. Not only does this behavior cause injury, but it also spreads the virus through the infected animal's saliva. The most obvious symptoms of the disease are extreme activity in the cerebral region of the brain, rage,

Bats infected with rabies do not exhibit symptoms of the disease and easily spread it.

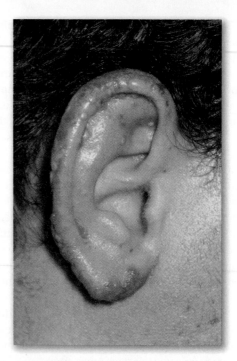

**FIGURE** 14.7 **Herpes Gladiatorum**
A series of fluid-filled blisters on the face, neck, or torso can be a sign of this form of herpes, which is easily spread, especially among athletes.

increased salivation, spasms in the throat muscles, extreme drive to find water, and the inability to swallow.

The incubation period for rabies is usually 1 to 3 months, although it may range from 1 week to 1 year. The disease may be fatal if not treated immediately with the rabies vaccine. Anyone bitten by an animal that might be carrying rabies should seek immediate medical attention and try to bring the animal along for testing. If you are wondering whether you should spring for the cost of rabies shots for your pets, do it. Pets that bite and are not current on their rabies vaccinations are routinely euthanized.

## Other Pathogens

Bacteria and viruses account for many, but not all, of the common diseases in both adults and children. Other very small or microscopic organisms can also infect and cause disease symptoms in a host. Among these are fungi, protozoans, parasitic worms, and prions.

**Fungi** Our environment is inhabited by hundreds of species of **fungi,** multi- or unicellular organisms that obtain their food by infiltrating the bodies of other organisms, both living and dead. Many fungi, such as edible mushrooms, penicillin, and the yeast used in making bread, are useful to humans, but some species can produce infections. *Candidiasis* (as in a vaginal yeast infection, discussed later), ringworm, jock itch, and toenail fungus are examples of some of the most common fungal diseases. With most fungal diseases, keeping the affected area clean and dry, and treating it promptly with appropriate medications will generally bring relief. Fungal diseases are transmitted via physical contact, so avoid going barefoot in public showers, hotel rooms, and other areas where fungus may be present.

**Protozoans** **Protozoans** are microscopic single-celled organisms that are generally associated with tropical diseases such as African sleeping sickness and malaria. Although these pathogens are prevalent in nonindustrialized countries, they are largely controlled in the United States. The most common protozoan disease in the United States is *trichomoniasis* (discussed in this chapter's section on sexually transmitted infections). A common waterborne protozoan disease in many regions of the country is *giardiasis*. Persons who are exposed to the *giardia* pathogen may suffer intestinal pain and discomfort weeks after infection. Protection of water supplies is the key to prevention.

**Parasitic Worms** **Parasitic worms** are the largest of the pathogens. Ranging in size from small pinworms typically found in children to the large tapeworms found in warm-blooded animals, including humans, most parasitic worms are more a nuisance than they are a threat. Of special note today are the worm infestations associated with eating raw fish (as in sushi). You can prevent worm infestations by cooking fish and other foods to temperatures sufficient to kill the worms and their eggs. Other preventive measures you can take include getting your pets checked for worms and wearing shoes in parks or public places where animal feces are present.

**Prions** A **prion** is a self-replicating, protein-based agent that can infect humans and other animals. One such prion is believed to be the underlying cause of spongiform diseases such as *bovine spongiform encephalopathy* (*BSE*, or "mad cow disease"). Evidence indicates that there is a relationship between outbreaks of BSE in Europe and a disease in humans called *variant Creutzfeldt-Jakob disease* (*vCJD*).[25] Both disorders are fatal brain diseases with unusually long incubation periods (measured in years), and both are caused by prions. To date, there have been no confirmed human infections from U.S. beef; however, infected cattle have been found.

# Emerging and Resurgent Diseases

Although our immune systems are adept at responding to challenges, microbes and other pathogens appear to be gaining ground. Within the past decade, rates for infectious diseases have rapidly increased. This trend can be attributed to a combination of overpopulation, inadequate health care systems, increasing poverty, extreme environmental degradation, and drug resistance.[26] At the same time that world travel has become increasingly fast and easy, drug-resistant pathogens—those that are not killed or inhibited by antibiotics and antimicrobial compounds—have been on the rise globally.

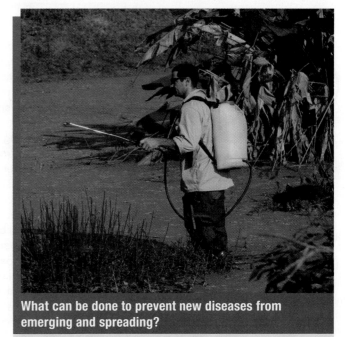

**What can be done to prevent new diseases from emerging and spreading?**

Many factors contribute to the emergence and spreading of new diseases, such as the recent West Nile virus and avian (bird) flu outbreaks. Poor control of pests, such as mosquitoes, is a symptom of larger problems such as infrastructure overload, pesticide misuse, lack of government funding, poverty, and environmental degradation. Attention to these issues is essential in preventing new and more virulent forms of disease from emerging and spreading.

**Dengue** Transmitted by mosquitoes, *dengue* viruses are the most widespread mosquito-borne viruses in the world. Dengue is endemic in at least 100 countries in Asia, the Pacific, the Americas, Africa, and the Caribbean. It is estimated that 50 to 100 million infections occur yearly with over 22,000 deaths, mostly among children.[27] There are several thousand cases in U.S. citizens each year, mostly from island communities such as Puerto Rico, the Virgin Islands, and Guam.[28] Dengue symptoms include nausea, aches, and chronic fatigue and weakness. *Dengue hemorrhagic fever,* a more serious form of the disease, can kill children in 6 to 12 hours, as the virus causes capillaries to leak and spill fluid and blood into surrounding tissue. Dengue is on the rise in the United States, largely due to increased international travel.

**protozoans** Microscopic single-celled organisms that can be pathogenic.
**parasitic worms** The largest of the pathogens, most of which are more a nuisance than they are a threat.
**prion** A recently identified self-replicating, protein-based pathogen.

**West Nile Virus** Until 1999, few Americans had heard of *West Nile virus* (*WNV*), which is spread by infected mosquitoes. Several thousand active cases of WNV surface in the United States every year, resulting in chronic disability or even death for some victims. The elderly and those with impaired immune systems bear the brunt of the disease burden.[29] Today, only Alaska and Hawaii remain free of the disease.

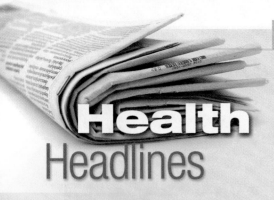

# PANDEMIC FLU: SCI-FI WORRY OR GLOBAL THREAT?

Imagine a world in which millions were sick or dying, hospitals and morgues were overflowing, bodies were stacked outside of buildings, and there were riots in the streets over who would get the last few vials of vaccine to ensure survival. Sound like the stuff of the latest sci-fi thriller? It may be more realistic than you realize.

Less than 100 years ago, in 1918, a pandemic flu swept the globe, wiping out over one-third of Europe's population. Throughout human history, there have been pandemics, plagues, and pestilence that have quickly killed millions. Think this could never happen today? Think again. In many regions of the world, scientists are quietly focusing on a grim scenario in which a form of pandemic again sweeps the planet, leaving death and destruction in its path. They are asking, "What if?" "When?" and "Which?" of several pathogens that may emerge to cause such a catastrophe.

Among the leading worries is Avian influenza, a form of "mutated type A" influenza that is currently killing birds by the millions and has sickened a few people. The concern is that the pathogen will mutate until it becomes transmissible via human-to-human contact, perhaps through coughing or sneezing. If this were to happen, the next pandemic flu could wipe out millions in a matter of days, thanks to airplanes and the global distribution of people and products.

To date, there are no vaccines available for avian influenza. Fearing the worst, nations throughout the world have begun making plans, including accelerating research and production of vaccines, prioritizing vaccines that might be available, ensuring fair and rational distribution of medicines, planning for quarantines and mandatory work by public service workers, and a host of other tactics designed to save as many people as possible.

What do you think are the most pressing issues for a planet facing a potential pandemic flu disaster? Who

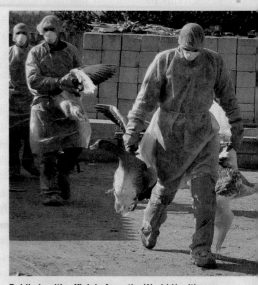

Public health officials from the World Health Organization (WHO) have warned that a worldwide pandemic of the H5N1 bird flu strain could easily kill millions of people and cost the global economy more than $800 billion.

should be given any available vaccines? How would you determine this? What ethical issues would need to be resolved? If hospital beds were in short supply, who should be treated first? Who should make these decisions? These and other emotionally charged questions must be considered if we are to weather the threat of another pandemic.

---

Most people who become infected with WNV will have either mild symptoms or none at all. Rarely, WNV infection can result in severe and sometimes fatal illness. Symptoms include fever, headache, and body aches, often with skin rash and swollen lymph glands, and a form of encephalitis (inflammation of the brain). There is no vaccine or specific treatment for WNV, but avoiding mosquito bites is the best way to prevent it: using EPA-registered insect repellents such as those with DEET or eucalyptus; wearing long-sleeved clothing and long pants when outdoors; staying indoors during dawn, dusk, and other peak mosquito feeding times; and removing any standing water sources around the home.[30]

**Avian (Bird) Flu** Avian influenza is an infectious disease of birds. There has been considerable media flurry in the past few years over a strain of avian (bird) flu, H5N1, which is highly pathogenic and is capable of crossing the species barrier and causing severe illness in humans. This virulent flu strain began to emerge in bird populations throughout Asia, including domestic birds such as chickens and ducks, as early as 1997. By 2007, bird flu had spread to birds in parts of western Europe, eastern Europe, Russia, and northern Africa.[31] Although the virus has yet to mutate into a form highly infectious to humans, outbreaks in which people contract the disease from birds in rural areas of the world (where people often live in close proximity to poultry and other animals) have occurred. As of August 2010, the WHO had recorded 503 cases of bird flu in humans, with 299 deaths.[32]

Many health experts suggest that if this virus becomes transmissible between humans, it is virulent enough to surpass the lethality of the influenza epidemics of 1918 and 1919, which swept the global community, causing millions of deaths. This type of pandemic flu or global epidemic could decimate the world's population (see the **Health Headlines** box).

**Escherichia coli O157:H7** *Escherichia coli* O157:H7 is one of over 170 types of *E. coli* bacteria that can infect humans. Most *E. coli* organisms are harmless and live in the intestines of healthy animals and humans. *E. coli* O157:H7, however, produces a lethal toxin and can cause severe illness or death. It can live in the intestines of healthy cattle and then contaminate food products at slaughterhouses. Eating ground beef that is rare or undercooked, drinking unpasteurized milk or juice, or swimming in sewage-contaminated water or public pools can also cause infection via ingestion of infected fecal matter.

A symptom of infection is nonbloody diarrhea, usually 2 to 8 days after exposure; however, asymptomatic cases have been noted. Children, older adults, and people with weakened immune systems are particularly vulnerable to serious side effects such as kidney failure.

Although *E. coli* continues to pose threats to public health, strengthened regulations on the cooking of meat and regulation of chlorine levels in pools have helped. However, the 2006 *E. coli* outbreak linked to contaminated raw spinach and other outbreaks in recent years have caused the U.S. Department of Agriculture (USDA) and others in the agriculture industry to review regulations and consider new safety measures.

**Listeriosis** Foods that are improperly cooked or that don't require cooking (such as luncheon meats or deli foods) are particularly susceptible to transmitting the bacterium responsible for listeriosis, a disease that has proved fatal in many cases in recent years. Early symptoms begin with mild fever and progress to headache and inflammation of the brain. Those who are immunocompromised and pregnant women are at greatest risk. New regulations that require strict monitoring of food-processing plants should help reduce the risk of listeria infection. When in doubt as to the safety of food, remember the old adage, "When in doubt, throw it out!"

**Malaria** After massive international efforts at eradication in the 1960s, malaria, a disease caused by a parasite and transmitted by the *Anopheles* mosquito, seemed to be on the decline. Today, however, approximately 40 percent of the world's population, mostly those living in the poorest countries, are at risk for malaria. Every year, more than 500 million people become severely ill, and 1 million die, with most cases and deaths occurring in sub-Saharan Africa, Latin America, the Middle East, and parts of Europe.[33]

Travelers from malaria-free regions entering areas where there is malaria transmission are highly vulnerable, as they have little or no immunity and often receive a delayed or wrong malaria diagnosis when they return home.[34] Mosquito nets and use of insect repellents are particularly important to prevention, as is removal of standing water in yards. Natural disasters that leave standing water in which mosquitoes can flourish pose increased risks. Resistance to chloroquine, once a widely used and highly effective treatment, is now found in most regions of the world, and other treatments are losing their effectiveness at alarming rates.

# Sexually Transmitted Infections (STIs)

**Sexually transmitted infections (STIs)** have been with us since our earliest recorded days on Earth. Today, there are more than 20 known types of STIs. Once referred to as *venereal diseases* and then *sexually transmitted diseases,* the current terminology is more reflective of the number and

> **sexually transmitted infections (STIs)** Infections transmitted through some form of intimate, usually sexual, contact.

types of these communicable diseases, and also of the fact that they are caused by infecting pathogens. More virulent strains and antibiotic-resistant forms spell trouble in the days ahead.

## 65 million

**people are currently living with an incurable STI.**

If you live in the United States, you have a 1 in 2 chance of getting an STI by age 25. Every year, there are at least 19 million new cases of STIs, only some of which are curable.[35] Sexually transmitted infections affect men and women of all backgrounds and socioeconomic levels. However, they disproportionately affect women, minorities, and infants. In addition, STIs are most prevalent in teens and young adults.[36]

Early symptoms of an STI are often mild and unrecognizable (see **Figure 14.8** on page 454). Left untreated, some of these infections can have grave consequences, such as sterility, blindness, central nervous system destruction, disfigurement, and even death. Infants born to mothers carrying the organisms for these infections are at risk for a variety of health problems.

As with many communicable diseases, much of the pain and suffering associated with STIs can be eliminated through education, responsible action, simple preventive strategies, and prompt treatment. Anyone can contract a sexually transmitted infection, but you can avoid them if you take appropriate precautions when you decide to engage in a sexual relationship.

## What's Your Risk?

Several reasons have been proposed to explain the present high rates of STIs. The first relates to the moral and social stigmas associated with these infections. Shame and embarrassment often keep infected people from seeking treatment. Unfortunately, they usually continue to be sexually active, thereby infecting unsuspecting partners. People who are uncomfortable discussing sexual issues may also be less likely to use and ask their partners to use condoms to protect against STIs and pregnancy.

Another reason proposed for the STI epidemic is our casual attitude about sex. Bombarded by a media that

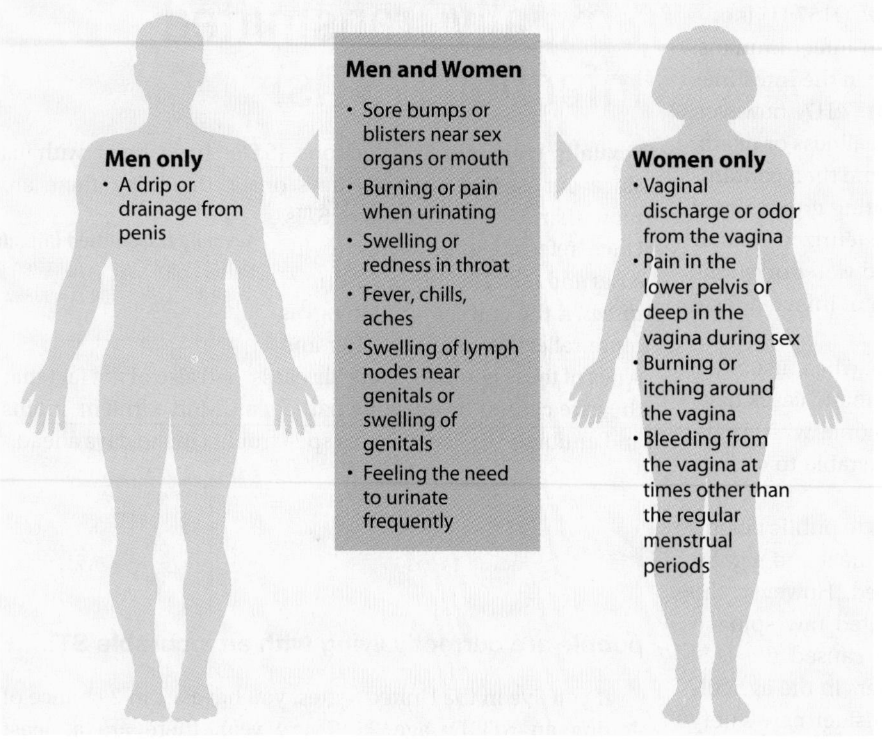

**Men only**
- A drip or drainage from penis

**Men and Women**
- Sore bumps or blisters near sex organs or mouth
- Burning or pain when urinating
- Swelling or redness in throat
- Fever, chills, aches
- Swelling of lymph nodes near genitals or swelling of genitals
- Feeling the need to urinate frequently

**Women only**
- Vaginal discharge or odor from the vagina
- Pain in the lower pelvis or deep in the vagina during sex
- Burning or itching around the vagina
- Bleeding from the vagina at times other than the regular menstrual periods

**FIGURE 14.8 Signs or Symptoms of Sexually Transmitted Infections (STIs)**
In their early stages, many STIs may be asymptomatic or have such mild symptoms that they are easy to overlook.

glamorizes sex, many people take sexual partners without considering the consequences. Others are pressured into sexual relationships they don't really want. Generally, the more sexual partners a person has, the greater the risk for contracting an STI. Evaluate your own attitude and beliefs about STIs by completing the **Assess Yourself** box on page 467.

Ignorance—about the infections, their symptoms, and the fact that someone can be asymptomatic but still infected—is also a factor. A person who is infected but asymptomatic can unknowingly spread an STI to an unsuspecting partner, who may in turn ignore or misinterpret any symptoms. By the time either partner seeks medical help, he or she may have infected several others. In addition, many people mistakenly believe that certain sexual practices—oral sex, for example—carry no risk for STIs. In fact, oral sex practices among young adults may be responsible for increases in herpes and other STIs. Figure 14.9 shows the continuum of risk for various sexual behaviors, and the **Skills for Behavior Change** box offers tips for ways to practice safer sex.

## Routes of Transmission

Sexually transmitted infections are generally spread through some form of intimate sexual contact. Sexual intercourse, oral–genital contact, hand–genital contact, and anal intercourse are the most common modes of transmission. Less likely, but still possible, modes of transmission include mouth-to-mouth contact, or contact with fluids from body sores that may be spread by the hands. Although each STI is a different infection caused by a different pathogen, all STI pathogens prefer dark, moist places, especially the mucous membranes lining the reproductive organs. Most of them are susceptible to light and excess heat, cold, and dryness, and many die quickly on exposure to air. Like other communicable infections, STIs have both pathogen-specific incubation periods and periods of time during which transmission is most likely, called *periods of communicability*.

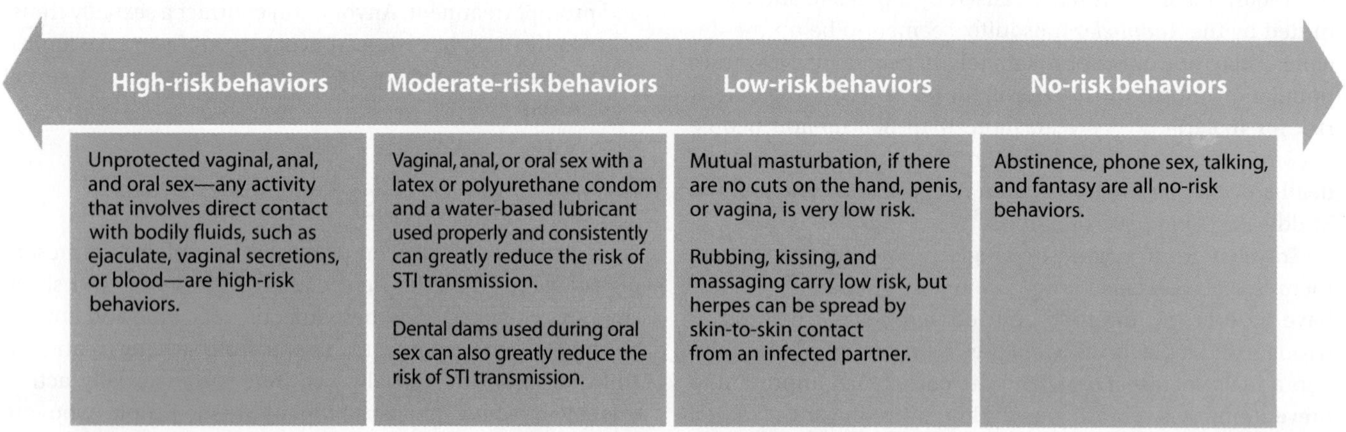

| High-risk behaviors | Moderate-risk behaviors | Low-risk behaviors | No-risk behaviors |
|---|---|---|---|
| Unprotected vaginal, anal, and oral sex—any activity that involves direct contact with bodily fluids, such as ejaculate, vaginal secretions, or blood—are high-risk behaviors. | Vaginal, anal, or oral sex with a latex or polyurethane condom and a water-based lubricant used properly and consistently can greatly reduce the risk of STI transmission.<br><br>Dental dams used during oral sex can also greatly reduce the risk of STI transmission. | Mutual masturbation, if there are no cuts on the hand, penis, or vagina, is very low risk.<br><br>Rubbing, kissing, and massaging carry low risk, but herpes can be spread by skin-to-skin contact from an infected partner. | Abstinence, phone sex, talking, and fantasy are all no-risk behaviors. |

**FIGURE 14.9 Continuum of Risk for Various Sexual Behaviors**
There are different levels of risk for various behaviors and various sexually transmitted infections (STIs); however, no matter what, any sexual activity involving direct contact with blood, semen, or vaginal secretions is high risk.

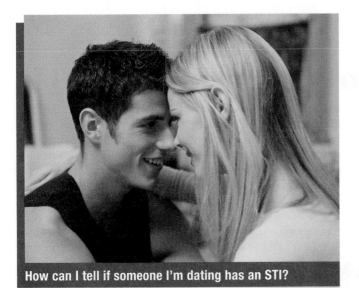

**How can I tell if someone I'm dating has an STI?**

You can't tell if someone has an STI just by looking at them; it isn't something broadcast on a person's face, and many people with STIs are themselves unaware of the infection because it could be asymptomatic. The only way to know for sure is to go to a clinic and get tested. In addition, partners need to be open and honest with each other about their sexual histories, and practice safer sex.

# Chlamydia

**Chlamydia,** an infection caused by the bacterium *Chlamydia trachomatis* that often presents no symptoms, is the most commonly reported STI in the United States. Chlamydia infects an estimated 2.8 million Americans annually, the majority of them women.[37] Public health officials believe that this estimate could be higher, because many cases go unreported.

**chlamydia** Bacterially caused STI of the urogenital tract.

**pelvic inflammatory disease (PID)** Term used to describe various infections of the female reproductive tract.

**Signs and Symptoms** In men, early symptoms may include painful and difficult urination; frequent urination; and a watery, puslike discharge from the penis. Symptoms in women may include a yellowish discharge, spotting between periods, and occasional spotting after intercourse. However, many chlamydia victims display no symptoms and therefore do not seek help until the disease has done secondary damage. Women are especially likely to be asymptomatic; over 70 percent do not realize they have the disease, which can put them at risk for secondary damage.[38]

**Complications** The secondary damage resulting from chlamydia is serious in both men and women. Men can suffer injury to the prostate gland, seminal vesicles, and bulbourethral glands, and they can suffer from arthritis-like symptoms and inflammatory damage to the blood vessels and heart. Men can also experience epididymitis, inflammation of the area near the testicles. In women, chlamydia-related inflammation can injure the cervix or fallopian tubes, causing sterility, and it can damage the inner pelvic structure, leading to

**pelvic inflammatory disease (PID)** (see the **Gender & Health** box on page 456). If an infected woman becomes pregnant, she has a high risk for miscarriage and stillbirth. Chlamydia may also be responsible for one type of *conjunctivitis,* an eye infection that

# Complications of STIs in Women: PID and UTIs

Women disproportionately experience the long-term consequences of sexually transmitted infections (STIs). If not treated, up to 40 percent of women who are infected with *Neisseria gonorrhoeae* or *Chlamydia trachomatis* may develop pelvic inflammatory disease (PID). Pelvic inflammatory disease is a catchall term for a number of infections of the uterus, fallopian tubes, and ovaries that are complications resulting from an untreated STI.

Symptoms of PID vary but generally include lower abdominal pain, fever, unusual vaginal discharge, painful intercourse, painful urination, and irregular menstrual bleeding. The vague symptoms associated with chlamydial and gonococcal PID cause 85 percent of women to delay seeking medical care, thereby increasing the risk of permanent damage and scarring that can lead to infertility and ectopic pregnancy. Among women with PID, ectopic pregnancy (in which an embryo begins to develop outside of the uterus, usually in a fallopian tube) occurs in 9 percent, and chronic pelvic pain in 18 percent.

Women are also at greater risk than men for developing a general urinary tract infection (UTI). Urinary tract infections can be caused by various factors, including untreated STIs. Women are disproportionately affected by UTIs because a woman's urethra is much shorter than a man's, making it easier for bacteria to enter the bladder. In addition, a woman's urethra is

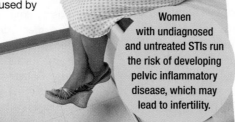

closer to her anus than is a man's, allowing bacteria to spread into her urethra and cause an infection. Symptoms of a UTI in women include a burning sensation during urination and lower abdominal pain. A UTI can be diagnosed through a urine test and treated by antibiotics. If left untreated, UTIs can cause kidney damage.

Note that men can also get UTIs, although they are rarer than UTIs in women. One form is nongonoccocol urethritis, which is most commonly caused by *Chlamydia trachomatis.* Infections should be taken seriously—if you have a milky penile discharge and/or burning during urination, contact your health care provider.

The serious complications that can result from untreated STIs in women further illustrate the need for early diagnosis and treatment. Regular screening is particularly important, because women are often asymptomatic, increasing their risk of complications such as PID and UTIs. Data from a randomized trial of chlamydia screening in a managed care setting suggested that screening programs can reduce the incidence of PID by as much as 60 percent.

**Women with undiagnosed and untreated STIs run the risk of developing pelvic inflammatory disease, which may lead to infertility.**

**Sources:** MedlinePlus, "Pelvic Inflammatory Disease (PID)," Updated September 2009, www.nlm.nih.gov/medlineplus/ency/article/000888.htm; Mayo Clinic Staff, "Urinary Tract Infection: Risk Factors," 2010, www.mayoclinic.com/health/urinary-tract-infection/DS00286/DSECTION=risk-factors; Centers for Disease Control and Prevention, Division of STD Prevention, National Center for HIV/AIDS, Viral Hepatitis, STD, and TB Prevention, "Sexually Transmitted Diseases Surveillance, 2008: STDs in Women and Infants," Updated November 2009, www.cdc.gov/std/stats08/womenandinf.htm.

affects not only adults but also infants, who can contract the disease from an infected mother during delivery (Figure 14.10). Untreated conjunctivitis can cause blindness.[39]

**Diagnosis and Treatment** Diagnosis of chlamydia is determined through a laboratory test. A sample of urine or fluid from the vagina or penis is collected to identify the presence of the bacteria. Unfortunately, chlamydia tests are not a routine part of many health clinics' testing procedures. Usually a person must specifically request it. If detected early, chlamydia is easily treatable with antibiotics such as tetracycline, doxycycline, or erythromycin.

**gonorrhea** Second most common bacterial STI in the United States; if untreated, may cause sterility.

## Gonorrhea

**Gonorrhea** is one of the most common STIs in the United States, surpassed only by chlamydia in number of cases. The CDC estimates that there are over 700,000 cases per year, plus numbers that go unreported.[40] Caused by the bacterial

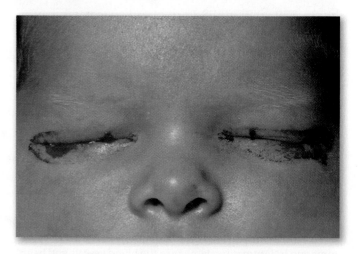

FIGURE 14.10 **Conjunctivitis in a Newborn's Eyes** Untreated chlamydia and gonorrhea in a pregnant woman can be passed to her child during delivery, causing the eye infection conjunctivitis.

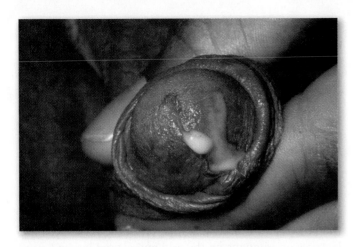

FIGURE 14.11 **Gonorrhea**
One common symptom of gonorrhea in men is a milky discharge from the penis, accompanied by burning sensations during urination. Whereas these symptoms will cause most men to seek diagnosis and treatment, women with gonorrhea are often asymptomatic, so they may not be aware they are infected.

pathogen *Neisseria gonorrhoeae,* gonorrhea primarily infects the linings of the urethra, genital tract, pharynx, and rectum. It may spread to the eyes or other body regions by the hands or through body fluids, typically during vaginal, oral, or anal sex. Most cases occur in individuals between the ages of 20 and 24.[41]

### Signs and Symptoms

In men, a typical symptom is a white, milky discharge from the penis accompanied by painful, burning urination 2 to 9 days after contact (Figure 14.11). Epididymitis can also occur as a symptom of infection. However, some men with gonorrhea are asymptomatic.

In women, the situation is just the opposite: Most women do not experience any symptoms, but if a woman does experience symptoms, it can include vaginal discharge, or a burning sensation on urinating.[42] The organism can remain in the woman's vagina, cervix, uterus, or fallopian tubes for long periods with no apparent symptoms other than an occasional slight fever. Thus a woman can be unaware that she has been infected and that she is infecting her sexual partners.

### Complications

In a man, untreated gonorrhea may spread to the prostate, testicles, urinary tract, kidney, and bladder. Blockage of the vasa deferentia due to scar tissue may cause sterility. In some cases, the penis develops a painful curvature during erection. If the infection goes undetected in a woman, it can spread to the fallopian tubes and ovaries, causing sterility or, at the very least, severe inflammation and PID. The bacteria can also spread up the reproductive tract or, more rarely, through the blood and infect the joints, heart valves, or brain. If an infected woman becomes pregnant, the infection can be transmitted to her baby during delivery, potentially causing blindness, joint infection, or a life-threatening blood infection.

### Diagnosis and Treatment

Diagnosis of gonorrhea is similar to that of chlamydia, requiring a sample of either urine or fluid from the vagina or penis to detect the presence of the bacteria. If detected early, gonorrhea is treatable with antibiotics, but the *Neisseria gonorrhoeae* bacterium has begun to develop resistance to some antibiotics. It is also important to recognize that chlamydia and gonorrhea often occur at the same time, but different antibiotics are needed to treat each infection separately.[43]

## Syphilis

**Syphilis** is caused by a bacterium, the spirochete called *Treponema pallidum.* The incidence of syphilis is highest in women aged 20 to 24 and men aged 35 to 39. The incidence of syphilis in newborns has continued to increase in the United States.[44] Because it is extremely delicate and dies readily on exposure to air, dryness, or cold, the organism is generally transferred only through direct sexual contact or from mother to fetus.

> **syphilis** One of the most widespread bacterial STIs; characterized by distinct phases and potentially serious results.
>
> **chancre** Sore often found at the site of syphilis infection.

### Signs and Symptoms

Syphilis is known as the "great imitator," because its symptoms resemble those of several other infections. It should be noted, however, that some people experience no symptoms at all. Syphilis can occur in four distinct stages:[45]

- **Primary syphilis.** The first stage of syphilis, particularly for men, is often characterized by the development of a **chancre** (pronounced "shank-er"), a sore located most frequently at the site of initial infection that usually appears 3 to 4 weeks after initial infection (see Figure 14.12 on page 458). In men, the site of the chancre tends to be the penis or scrotum; in women, the site of infection is often internal, on the vaginal wall or high on the cervix where the chancre is not readily apparent and the likelihood of detection is not great. Whether or not it is detected, the chancre is oozing with bacteria, ready to infect an unsuspecting partner. In both men and women, the chancre will disappear in 3 to 6 weeks.
- **Secondary syphilis.** If the infection is left untreated, a month to a year after the chancre disappears, secondary symptoms may appear, including a rash or white patches on the skin or on the mucous membranes of the mouth, throat, or genitals. Hair loss may occur, lymph nodes may enlarge, and the victim may develop a slight fever or headache. In rare cases, sores develop around the mouth or genitals. As during the active chancre phase, these sores contain infectious bacteria, and contact with them can spread the infection.
- **Latent syphilis.** After the secondary stage, if the infection is left untreated, the syphilis spirochetes begin to invade body organs, causing lesions called *gummas.* The infection now is rarely transmitted to others, except during pregnancy, when it can be passed to the fetus.
- **Tertiary/late syphilis.** Years after syphilis has entered the body, its effects become all too evident if still untreated. Late-stage syphilis indications include heart and central nervous system damage, blindness, deafness, paralysis, premature senility, and, ultimately, dementia.

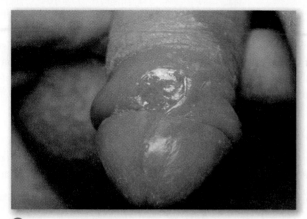

**a** Primary syphilis

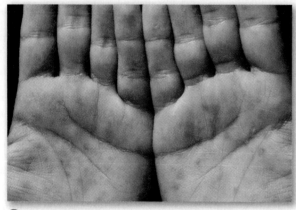

**b** Secondary syphilis

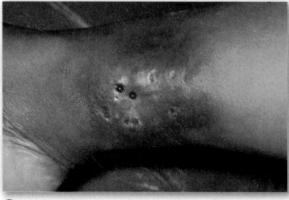

**c** Latent syphilis

FIGURE 14.12 **Syphilis**
A chancre on the site of the initial infection is a symptom of primary syphilis (a). A rash is characteristic of secondary syphilis (b). Lesions called "gummas" are often present in latent syphilis (c).

**Complications** Pregnant women with syphilis can experience complications including premature births, miscarriages, and stillbirths. An infected pregnant woman may transmit the

**genital herpes** STI caused by the herpes simplex virus.

syphilis to her unborn child. The infant will then be born with *congenital syphilis,* which can cause death; severe birth defects such as blindness, deafness, or disfigurement; developmental delays; seizures; and other health problems. Because in most cases the fetus does not become infected until after the first trimester, treatment of the mother during this time will usually prevent infection of the fetus.

**Diagnosis and Treatment** There are two methods that can be used to diagnose syphilis. In the primary stage, a sample from the chancre is collected to identify the bacteria. Another method of diagnosing syphilis is through a blood test. Syphilis can easily be treated with antibiotics, usually penicillin, for all stages except the late stage.

## Herpes

*Herpes* is a general term for a family of infections characterized by sores or eruptions on the skin and caused by the herpes simplex virus. The herpes family of diseases is not transmitted exclusively by sexual contact. Kissing or sharing eating utensils can also exchange saliva and transmit the infection. Herpes infections range from mildly uncomfortable to extremely serious. **Genital herpes** affects approximately 16.2 percent of the population aged 14 to 49 in the United States.[46]

There are two types of herpes simplex virus. Only about 1 in 6 Americans currently has HSV-2; however, 50 to 80 percent of adults have HSV-1, usually appearing as cold sores on their mouths.[47] Both herpes simplex types 1 and 2 can infect any area of the body, producing lesions (sores) in and around the vaginal area; on the penis; and around the anal opening, buttocks, thighs, or mouth (see **Figure 14.13**). Whether you contract HSV-1 or HSV-2 on your genitals, the net results may be just as painful, just as long term, and just as infectious for future partners. Herpes simplex virus remains in certain nerve cells for life and can flare up when the body's ability to maintain itself is weakened.

**"Why Should I Care?"**

Getting an STI can be painful, and you can infect your current partner with it. In the long term it could affect the health of your children or your ability to have children.

**Signs and Symptoms** The precursor phase of a herpes infection is characterized by a burning sensation and redness at the site of infection. During this time, prescription medicines such as acyclovir and over-the-counter medications such as Abreva will often keep the disease from spreading. However, this phase of the disease is quickly followed by the second phase, in which a blister filled with a clear fluid containing the virus forms. If you pick at this blister or otherwise touch the site and spread this fluid with fingers, lipstick, lip balm, or other products, you can autoinoculate other body parts. Particularly dangerous is the possibility of spreading the infection to your eyes, for a herpes lesion on the eye can cause blindness.

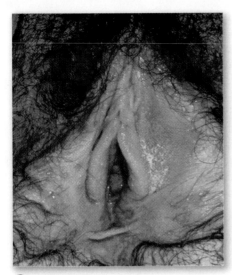

(a) Genital herpes is a highly contagious and incurable STI. It is characterized by recurring cycles of painful blisters on the genitalia.

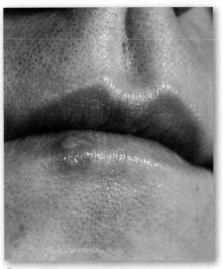

(b) Oral herpes, caused by the same virus as genital herpes, is extremely contagious and can cause painful sores and blisters around the mouth.

FIGURE 14.13 **Herpes**
Both genital and oral herpes can be caused by either herpes simplex virus type 1 or 2.

Over a period of days, the unsightly blister will crust over, dry up, and disappear, and the virus will travel to the base of an affected nerve supplying the area and become dormant. Only when the victim becomes overly stressed, when diet and sleep are inadequate, when the immune system is overworked, or when excessive exposure to sunlight or other stressors occur will the virus become reactivated (at the same site every time) and begin the blistering cycle all over again. Each time a sore develops, it casts off (sheds) viruses that can be highly infectious. However, it is important to note that a herpes site can shed the virus even when no overt sore is present, particularly during the interval between the earliest symptoms and blistering. People may get genital herpes by having sexual contact with others who don't know they are infected or who are having outbreaks of herpes without any sores. A person with genital herpes can also infect a sexual partner during oral sex. The virus is spread only rarely, if at all, by touching objects such as a toilet seat or hot tub seat.

**Complications** Genital herpes is especially serious in pregnant women because the baby can be infected as it passes through the vagina during birth. Many physicians recommend cesarean deliveries for infected women. Additionally, women with a history of genital herpes appear to have a greater risk of developing cervical cancer.

**Diagnosis and Treatment** Diagnosis of herpes can be determined by collecting a sample from the suspected sore or by performing a blood test to identify an HSV-1 or HSV-2 infection. Although there is no cure for herpes at present, certain drugs can be used to treat symptoms. Unfortunately, they seem to work only if the infection is confirmed during the first few

hours after contact. The effectiveness of other treatments, such as L-lysine, is largely unsubstantiated. Over-the-counter medications may reduce the length of time you have sores/symptoms. Other drugs, such as famciclovir (FAMVIR), may reduce viral shedding between outbreaks. This means that if you have outbreaks, you may reduce risks to your sexual partners.[48]

# Human Papillomavirus (HPV) and Genital Warts

**Genital warts** (also known as *venereal warts* or *condylomas*) are caused by a group of viruses known as **human papillomavirus (HPV)**. There are over 100 different types of HPV; more than 30 types are sexually transmitted and are classified as either low risk or high risk. A person becomes infected when certain types of HPV penetrate the skin and mucous membranes of the genitals or anus. This is among the most common forms of STI, with 20 million Americans currently infected with genital HPV and approximately 6 million new cases each year.[49]

**Signs and Symptoms** Genital HPV appears to be relatively easy to catch. The typical incubation period is 6 to 8 weeks after contact. People infected with low-risk types of HPV may develop genital warts, a series of bumps or growths on the genitals, ranging in size from small pinheads to large cauliflower-like growths (see **Figure 14.14** on page 460).

**Complications** Infection with high-risk types of HPV poses a significant risk for cervical cancer in women. It may lead to *dysplasia,* or changes in cells that may lead to a precancerous condition. Exactly how high-risk HPV infection leads to cervical cancer is uncertain. It is known that 6 out of 10 cervical cancers occur in women who have never received a Pap test or have not been tested for HPV in the past 5 years.[50]

Of those cases that become precancerous and are left untreated, 70 percent will eventually result in actual cancer. In addition, HPV may pose a threat to a fetus that is exposed to the virus during birth. Cesarean deliveries may be considered in serious cases. New research has also implicated HPV as a possible risk factor for coronary artery disease. It is hypothesized that HPV causes an inflammatory response in the artery walls, which leads to cholesterol and plaque buildup (see Chapter 15).

**genital warts** Warts that appear in the genital area or the anus; caused by the human papillomavirus (HPV).

**human papillomavirus (HPV)** A group of viruses, many of which are transmitted sexually; some types of HPV can cause genital warts or cervical cancer.

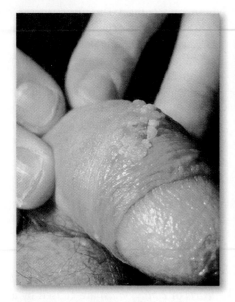
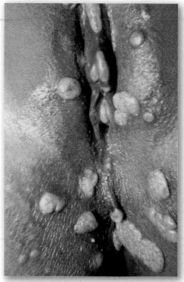

FIGURE 14.14 **Genital Warts**
Genital warts are caused by certain types of the human papillomavirus.

**Diagnosis and Treatment** Diagnosis of genital warts from low-risk types of HPV is determined through a visual examination by a health care provider. High-risk types can be diagnosed in women through microscopic analysis of cells from a Pap smear or by collecting a sample from the cervix to test for HPV DNA. There is currently no HPV DNA test for men.

Treatment is available only for the low-risk forms of HPV that cause genital warts. The warts can be treated with topical medication or can be frozen with liquid nitrogen and then removed. Large warts may require surgical removal. There are currently two HPV vaccines that are licensed by the U.S. Food and Drug Administration (FDA) and recommended by the CDC. See the **Student Health Today** box on the next page for more information about these vaccines.

## Candidiasis (Moniliasis)

Most STIs are caused by pathogens that come from outside the body; however, the yeastlike fungus *Candida albicans* is a normal inhabitant of the vaginal tract in most women. (See Figure 14.5c on page 443 for a micrograph of this fungus.) Only when the normal chemical balance of the vagina is disturbed will these organisms multiply and cause the fungal disease **candidiasis**, also sometimes called *moniliasis* or a *yeast infection*.

**candidiasis** Yeastlike fungal infection often transmitted sexually; also called *moniliasis* or *yeast infection*.
**trichomoniasis** Protozoan STI characterized by foamy, yellowish discharge and unpleasant odor.
**pubic lice** Parasitic insects that can inhabit various body areas, especially the genitals.

**Signs and Symptoms** Symptoms of candidiasis include severe itching and burning of the vagina and vulva, and a white, cheesy vaginal discharge.[51] When this microbe infects the mouth, whitish patches form, and the condition is referred to as *thrush*. Thrush infection can also occur in men

and is easily transmitted between sexual partners. Symptoms of candidiasis can be aggravated by contact with soaps, douches, perfumed toilet paper, chlorinated water, and spermicides.

**Diagnosis and Treatment** Diagnosis of candidiasis is usually made by collecting a vaginal sample and analyzing it to identify the pathogen. Antifungal drugs applied on the surface or by suppository usually cure candidiasis in just a few days.

## Trichomoniasis

Unlike many STIs, **trichomoniasis** is caused by a protozoan, *Trichomonas vaginalis*. (See Figure 14.5d on page 443 for a micrograph of this organism.) An estimated 7.4 million new cases occur in the United States each year, although most people who contract it remain free of symptoms.[52]

**Signs and Symptoms** Symptoms among women include a foamy, yellowish, unpleasant-smelling discharge accompanied by a burning sensation, itching, and painful urination. Most men with trichomoniasis do not have any symptoms, though some men experience irritation inside the penis, mild discharge, and a slight burning after urinating.[53] Although usually transmitted by sexual contact, the "trich" organism can also be spread by toilet seats, wet towels, or other items that have discharged fluids on them.

**Diagnosis and Treatment** Diagnosis of trichomoniasis is determined by collecting fluid samples from the penis or vagina to test for the presence of the protozoan. Treatment includes oral metronidazole, usually given to both sexual partners to avoid the possible "ping-pong" effect of repeated cross-infection typical of STIs.

## Pubic Lice

**Pubic lice,** often called "crabs," are small parasitic insects that are usually transmitted during sexual contact (see **Figure 14.15** on page 462). More annoying than dangerous, they move easily from partner to partner during sex. They have an affinity for pubic hair and attach themselves to the base of these hairs, where they deposit their eggs (nits). One to 2 weeks later, these nits develop into adults that lay eggs and migrate to other body parts, thus perpetuating the cycle.

**Signs and Symptoms** Symptoms of pubic lice infestation include itchiness in the area covered by pubic hair, bluish-gray skin color in the pubic region, and sores in the genital area.

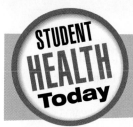

# Q&A ON HPV VACCINES

Most sexually active people will contract some form of human papillomarvirus (HPV) at some time in their lives, though they may never even know it. There are about 40 types of sexually transmitted HPV, most of which cause no symptoms and go away on their own. Low-risk types can cause genital warts, but some high-risk types can cause cervical cancer in women and other less common genital cancers—such as cancers of the anus, vagina, and vulva (area around the opening of the vagina). Every year in the United States, about 12,000 women are diagnosed with cervical cancer, and almost 4,000 die from this disease. There are currently two HPV vaccines that can help prevent women from becoming infected with HPV and subsequently developing cervical cancer.

❉ **Who should get the HPV vaccine?** HPV vaccines are recommended for 11- and 12-year-old girls and can also be given to girls 9 or 10 years of age. It is also recommended for girls and women aged 13 through 26 who have not yet been vaccinated or completed the vaccine series. Ideally, females should get a vaccine before they become sexually active. Females who are sexually active may get less benefit from it, because they may have already gotten an HPV type targeted by the vaccines. However, they would still get protection from those types they have not yet contracted.

One of the HPV vaccines, Gardasil, is also licensed, safe, and effective for males aged 9 through 26 years. Boys and young men may choose to get this vaccine to prevent genital warts.

❉ **Why are HPV vaccines recommended only through the age of 26?** The vaccines have been widely tested in girls and women

aged 9 through 26. New research is being done on the vaccines' safety and efficacy in women older than 26. The U.S. Food and Drug Administration (FDA) will consider licensing the vaccines for these women when there is enough research to show that it is safe and effective for them.

❉ **What HPV vaccines are available in the United States?** Two HPV vaccines are licensed by the FDA and recommended by the Centers for Disease Control and Prevention (CDC): Cervarix and Gardasil.

❉ **How are the two HPV vaccines, Cervarix and Gardasil, similar?** Both vaccines are very effective against high-risk HPV types 16 and 18, which cause 70 percent of cervical cancer cases. Although both vaccines are made with very small parts of the human papillomavirus, they cannot cause infection with HPV. Finally, both vaccines are given as shots and require three doses.

❉ **How are the two HPV vaccines, Cervarix and Gardasil, different?** Only Gardasil protects against low-risk HPV types 6 and 11. These HPV types cause 90 percent of cases of genital warts in females and males, so Gardasil is approved for use with males as well as females.

❉ **What do the two vaccines, Cervarix and Gardasil, _not_ protect against?** The vaccines do not protect against all types of HPV, so they will not prevent all cases of cervical cancer. About 30 percent of cervical cancers will not be prevented by the vaccines, so it will be important for women to continue getting screened for cervical cancer (through regular Pap tests). Also, the vaccines do not prevent other sexually transmitted infections (STIs), so it is still important for sexually active persons to lower their risk for other STIs.

Because the HPV vaccine is relatively new, some first-year college students who are eligible for vaccination have not yet received it. Many state health departments and college campuses offer free or low-cost vaccines for those whose insurance does not cover the cost.

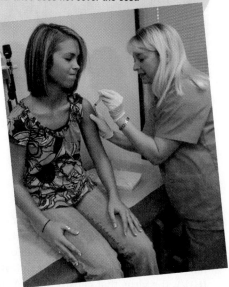

❉ **How safe are the HPV vaccines Cervarix and Gardasil?** The vaccines are licensed by the FDA and approved by the CDC as safe and effective. They have been studied in thousands of females (aged 9 through 26) around the world and their safety continues to be monitored by the CDC and the FDA. Studies have found no serious side effects.

**Sources:** Centers for Disease Control and Prevention, "Vaccines and Preventable Diseases: HPV Vaccine—Questions & Answers," Reviewed January 2010, www.cdc.gov/vaccines/vpd-vac/hpv/vac-faqs.htm; American Cancer Society, 2009, "Human Papillomavirus (HPV), Cancer and HPV Vaccines—Frequently Asked Questions," Revised October 2009, www.cancer.org/Cancer/CancerCauses/OtherCarcinogens/InfectiousAgents/HPV/HumanPapillomaVirusandHPVVaccinesFAQ/hpv-faq.

**Diagnosis and Treatment** Diagnosis of pubic lice involves an examination by a health care provider to identify the eggs in the genital area. Treatment includes washing clothing, furniture, and linens that may harbor the eggs. It usually takes 2 to 3 weeks to kill all larval forms. Although sexual contact is the most common mode of transmission, you can "catch" pubic lice from lying on sheets or sitting on a toilet seat that an infected person has used.

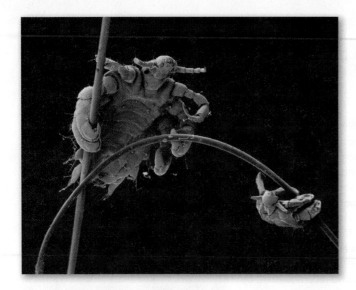

FIGURE 14.15 **Pubic Lice**
Pubic lice, also known as "crabs," are small, parasitic insects that attach themselves to pubic hair.

# HIV/AIDS

**Acquired immunodeficiency syndrome (AIDS)** is a significant global health threat. Since 1981, when AIDS was first recognized, approximately 65 million people in the world have become infected with **human immunodeficiency virus (HIV),** the virus that causes AIDS. At the end of 2008, there were approximately 33.4 million people worldwide living with HIV.[54]

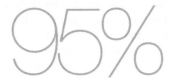

95%
of people with HIV worldwide live in developing nations.

In the United States, there have been approximately 1.1 million people infected with HIV and at least 576,384 have died.[55] In their most recent incidence reports, the CDC estimated that in 2008, there were approximately 37,151 new HIV/AIDS cases diagnosed in the United States.[56]

**acquired immunodeficiency syndrome (AIDS)** A disease caused by a retrovirus, the human immunodeficiency virus (HIV), that attacks the immune system, reducing the number of helper T cells and leaving the victim vulnerable to infections, malignancies, and neurological disorders.
**human immunodeficiency virus (HIV)** The virus that causes AIDS by infecting helper T cells.

Initially, people with HIV were diagnosed as having AIDS only when they developed blood infections, the cancer known as Kaposi's sarcoma, or any of 21 other indicator diseases, most of which were common in male AIDS patients. The CDC has expanded the indicator list to include pulmonary tuberculosis, recurrent pneumonia, and invasive cervical cancer. Perhaps the most significant indicator today is a drop in the level of the body's master immune cells, CD4 cells (also called helper T cells), to one-fifth the level in a healthy person.

AIDS cases have been reported state by state throughout the United States since the early 1980s. Today, the CDC recommends that all states report HIV infections as well as AIDS. Because of medical advances in treatment and increasing

**what do you think?**
Do you think we have grown too apathetic about HIV/AIDS in the United States? ● Is HIV/AIDS prevention discussed on your campus? ● Are people as concerned with HIV as they are with other STIs?

numbers of HIV-infected persons who do not progress to AIDS, it is believed that AIDS incidence statistics may not provide a true picture of the epidemic, the long-term costs of treating HIV-infected individuals, and other key information.

## How HIV Is Transmitted

HIV typically enters one person's body when another person's infected body fluids (e.g., semen, vaginal secretions, blood) gain entry through a breach in body defenses. Mucous membranes of the genital organs and the anus provide the easiest route of entry. If there is a break in the mucous membranes (as can occur during sexual intercourse, particularly anal intercourse), the virus enters and begins to multiply. After initial infection, HIV multiplies rapidly, invading the bloodstream

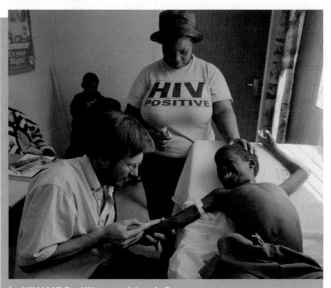

**Is HIV/AIDS still an epidemic?**
Yes! With swine flu and other emerging diseases dominating the news, it may seem as if HIV/AIDS is no longer a problem; however, nothing could be further from the truth. In North America, 1.4 million people are living with HIV, and HIV and AIDS are still at epidemic levels all over the world, especially in developing nations. Sub-Saharan Africa has been hit hardest: 22.4 million people in the region are living with the disease. Another 3.8 million in south/southeast Asia are infected and 2 million in Latin America. The epidemic is spreading most rapidly in eastern Europe and central Asia, where 1.5 million people currently have HIV.

and cerebrospinal fluid. It progressively destroys helper T cells (recall that these cells call the rest of the immune response to action), weakening the body's resistance to disease.

It is important to know that HIV/AIDS is not highly contagious. HIV cannot reproduce outside its living host, except in a controlled laboratory environment, and does not survive well in open air. As a result, HIV cannot be transmitted through casual contact including sharing glasses, cutlery, or musical instruments. Transmission also cannot occur through swimming pools, showers, or by sharing washing facilities or toilet seats.[57] Research also provides overwhelming evidence that insect bites do not transmit HIV.[58]

**Engaging in High-Risk Behaviors** AIDS is not a disease of gay people or minority groups. Although during the early days of the epidemic it appeared that HIV infected only homosexuals, it quickly became apparent that the disease was not confined to groups of people, but rather was related to high-risk behaviors such as having unprotected sexual intercourse and sharing needles.

People who engage in high-risk behaviors increase their risk for the disease; people who do not engage in these behaviors have minimal risk. Figure 14.16 shows the breakdown of sources of HIV infection among U.S. men and women.

The majority of HIV infections arise from the following high-risk behaviors:

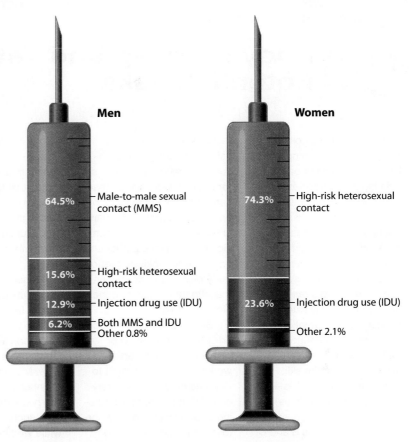

**Men**

- 64.5% — Male-to-male sexual contact (MMS)
- 15.6% — High-risk heterosexual contact
- 12.9% — Injection drug use (IDU)
- 6.2% — Both MMS and IDU
- Other 0.8%

**Women**

- 74.3% — High-risk heterosexual contact
- 23.6% — Injection drug use (IDU)
- Other 2.1%

FIGURE 14.16 **Sources of HIV Infection in Men and Women in the United States, 2008**

**Source:** Data are from Centers for Disease Control and Prevention, *HIV Surveillance Report, 2008,* vol. 20, June 2010, www.cdc.gov/hiv/surveillance/resources/reports/2008report.

- **Exchange of body fluids.** The greatest risk factor is the exchange of HIV-infected body fluids during vaginal or anal intercourse. Substantial research indicates that blood, semen, and vaginal secretions are the major fluids of concern. In rare instances, the virus has been found in saliva, but most health officials state that saliva is a less significant risk than other shared body fluids.
- **Injecting drugs.** A significant percentage of AIDS cases in the United States result from sharing or using HIV-contaminated needles and syringes. Although users of illegal drugs are commonly considered the only members of this category, others may also share needles—for example, people with diabetes who inject insulin or athletes who inject steroids. People who share needles and also engage in sexual activities with members of high-risk groups, such as those who exchange sex for drugs, increase their risks dramatically. Tattooing and piercing can also be risky (see the **Consumer Health** box on page 464).

**Blood Transfusion Prior to 1985** A small group of people have become infected after receiving blood transfusions. In 1985, the Red Cross and other blood donation programs implemented a stringent testing program for all donated blood. Today, because of these massive screening efforts, the risk of receiving HIV-infected blood is almost nonexistent in developed countries, including the United States.

**Mother-to-Child (Perinatal) Transmission** Mother-to-child transmission occurs when an HIV-positive woman passes the virus to her baby. This can occur during pregnancy, during labor and delivery, or through breast-feeding. Without antiretroviral treatment, approximately 25 percent of HIV-positive pregnant women will transmit the virus to their infant.[59]

## Symptoms of HIV/AIDS

A person may go for months or years after infection by HIV before any significant symptoms appear. The incubation time varies greatly from person to person. For adults who receive no medical treatment, it takes an average of 8 to 10 years for the virus to cause the slow, degenerative changes in the immune system that are characteristic of AIDS. During this time, the person may experience *opportunistic infections* (infections that gain a foothold when the immune system is not functioning effectively). Colds, sore throats, fever,

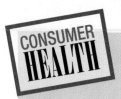

A look around any college campus reveals examples of body art, the use of body piercing and tattoos as a form of self-expression. The practice can be done safely, but health professionals cite several health concerns. The most common problems include skin reactions, infections, allergic reactions, and scarring. Of greater concern is the potential transmission of dangerous pathogens that can occur with any puncture of the skin. The use of unsterile needles—which can cause serious infections and can transmit staph, HIV, hepatitis B and C, tetanus, and other diseases—poses a very real risk.

Laws and policies regulating body piercing and tattooing vary greatly by state. Standards for safety usually include minimum age of clientele, standards of sanitation, use of aseptic techniques, sterilization of equipment, record keeping, informed risks, instructions for skin care, and recommendations for dealing with adverse reactions. Because of the lack of universal regulatory standards and the potential for transmission of dangerous pathogens, anyone who receives a tattoo, body piercing, or permanent makeup tattoo cannot donate blood for 1 year.

Before deciding on a body artist to do your tattoo or piercing, watch the artist working on another client to evaluate the person's safety and skill. If you opt for tattooing or body piercing, take the following safety precautions:

* Look for clean, well-lighted work areas, and inquire about sterilization procedures. Be wary of establishments that won't answer questions or show you their sterilization equipment.
* Packaged, sterilized needles should be used only once and then discarded. A piercing gun should not be used, because it cannot be sterilized properly. Watch that the artist uses new needles and tubes from a sterile package before your procedure begins. Ask to see the sterile confirmation logo on the bag itself.
* Immediately before piercing or tattooing, the body area should be carefully sterilized. The artist should wash his or her hands and put on new latex gloves for each procedure. Make sure the artist changes those gloves if he or she needs to touch anything else, such as the telephone, while working.
* Leftover tattoo ink should be discarded after each procedure. Do not allow the artist to reuse ink that has been used for other customers. Used needles should be disposed of in a "sharps" container, a plastic container with the biohazard symbol clearly marked on it.

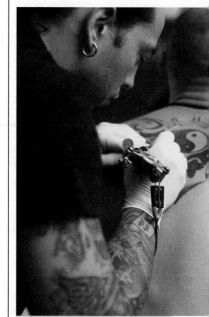

Like any activity that involves bodily fluids, tattooing carries some risk of disease transmission.

**Source:** Mayo Clinic Staff, "Tattoos: Understand Risks and Precautions," February 2010, www.mayoclinic.com/health/tattoos-and-piercings/MC00020.

tiredness, nausea, night sweats, and other generally non–life-threatening conditions commonly appear and are described as pre-AIDS symptoms. Other symptoms of progressing HIV infection include wasting syndrome, swollen lymph nodes, and neurological problems. As the immune system continues to decline, the body becomes more vulnerable to infection. A diagnosis of AIDS, the final stage of HIV infection, is made when the infected person has either a dangerously low CD4 (helper T) cell count (below 200 cells per cubic milliliter of blood) or has contracted one or more opportunistic infections characteristic of the disease (such as Kaposi's sarcoma or *Pneumocystis carinii* pneumonia).

## Testing for HIV Antibodies

Once antibodies have formed in reaction to HIV, a blood test known as the *ELISA* (enzyme-linked immunosorbent assay) may detect their presence. It can take 3 to 6 months after initial infection for sufficient antibodies to develop in the body to show a positive test result. Therefore, individuals with negative test results should be retested within 6 months. If sufficient antibodies are present, the test will be positive. When a person who previously tested *negative* (no HIV antibodies present) has a subsequent test that is *positive,* seroconversion is said to have occurred. In such a situation, the person would typically take another ELISA test, followed by a more precise test known as the *Western blot,* to confirm the presence of HIV antibodies.

It should be noted that these tests are not AIDS tests per se. Rather, they detect antibodies for HIV, indicating the presence of the virus in the person's system. Whether the person will develop AIDS depends to some extent on the strength of the immune system.

Health officials distinguish between *reported* and *actual* cases of HIV infection because it is believed that many HIV-positive people avoid being tested. One reason is fear of

# HIV Testing:
## SHOULD IT BE MANDATORY?

Should there be mandatory testing and reporting of HIV status? The debate concerning this issue is heated and complicated. In a nutshell, the idea is that in order to combat the epidemic of HIV, health care providers need to know who carries the virus. For multiple reasons, however, people in all populations in the United States don't want to be tested. The epidemic continues in part because people who don't know they are infected continue to spread the disease.

### Arguments for Mandatory Testing and Reporting
○ If health care providers know who is infected, they can treat those who are ill.
○ If governments know the true scope of the problem, they can allocate resources to respond to it properly.
○ Studies show that if those who have HIV know that they have it, they are more likely to use protection in order to avoid spreading it.
○ Given that HIV/AIDS is life threatening, mandatory testing and reporting is a matter of protecting society from disease and death.

### Arguments against Mandatory Testing and Reporting
○ Mandatory testing and reporting constitute an invasion of privacy.
○ Once mandatory testing and reporting are in place, forced treatment may follow.
○ Testing is expensive. Funding for HIV/AIDS should focus on prevention efforts instead.
○ Some fear violence at home or discrimination in the workplace as a result of a positive test.

### Where Do You Stand?
○ Should governments gather this information and use it to help combat the epidemic, or is that an invasion of privacy?
○ What sort of limits, if any, might you put on mandatory testing? Should anyone be exempt?
○ If the information is gathered, what limits should there be on how it can be used and who has access to it?

**Sources:** Centers for Disease Control and Prevention, "HIV Testing among Adolescents,"

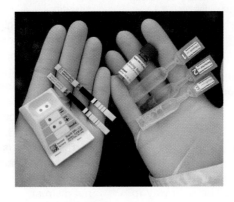

2009, Available at www.cdc.gov/healthyyouth/ sexualbehaviors; G. Marks et al., "Meta-Analysis of High-Risk Sexual Behavior in Persons Aware and Unaware They Are Infected with HIV in the United States: Implications for HIV Prevention Programs," *Journal of Acquired Immune Deficiency Syndromes* 39, no. 4 (2005): 446–53; American Civil Liberties Union, "Increasing Access to Voluntary HIV Testing: The Continuing Relevance of Stigma and Discrimination," March 2007, Available at www.aclu.org/lgbt-rights_hiv-aids/ increasing-access-voluntary-hiv-testing- continuing-relevance-stigma-and-discrim.

knowing the truth. Another is the fear of recrimination from employers, insurance companies, and medical staff. However, early detection and reporting are important, because immediate treatment for someone in the early stages of HIV disease is critical. See the **Points of View** box for more on the issue of HIV testing.

## New Hope and Treatments

New drugs have slowed the progression from HIV to AIDS and have prolonged life expectancies for most AIDS patients. Current treatments combine selected drugs, especially protease inhibitors and reverse transcriptase inhibitors. *Protease inhibitors* (e.g., amprenavir, ritonavir, and saquinavir) act to prevent the production of the virus in chronically infected cells that HIV has already invaded. Other drugs, such as AZT, ddI, ddC, d4T, and 3TC, inhibit the HIV enzyme *reverse transcriptase* before the virus has invaded the cell, thereby preventing the virus from infecting new cells. All of the protease drugs seem to work best in combination with other therapies. These combination treatments are still quite experimental, and no combination has proven to be absolute for all people.

Although these drugs provide new hope and longer survival rates for people living with HIV, it is important to maintain caution. We are still a long way from a cure. Apathy and carelessness may abound if too much confidence is placed in these treatments. Newer drugs that held much promise are becoming less effective as HIV develops resistance to them. Costs of taking multiple drugs are prohibitive, and side effects common. Furthermore, the number of people

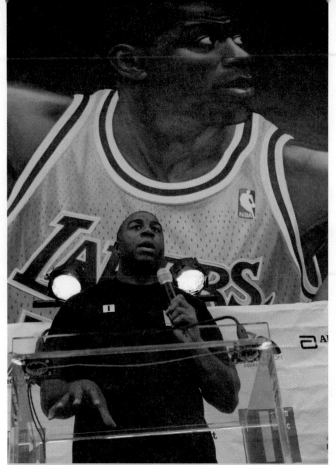

After publicly disclosing his HIV-positive status in 1991, former L.A. Laker star Earvin "Magic" Johnson became the first openly HIV-positive basketball player in the NBA.

becoming HIV-infected each year has increased in some communities, meaning that we are still a long way from beating this disease.

# Preventing HIV Infection

Although scientists have been working on a variety of HIV vaccine trials, none is currently available. The only way to prevent HIV infection is through the choices you make in sexual behaviors and drug use and by taking responsibility for your own health and the health of your loved ones. You can't determine the presence of HIV by looking at a person; you can't tell by questioning the person, unless he or she has been tested recently, is HIV-negative, and is giving an honest answer. So what should you do?

Of course, the simplest answer is abstinence. If you don't exchange body fluids, you won't get the disease. As a second line of defense, if you decide to be intimate, the next best option is to use a condom. However, in spite of all the educational campaigns, surveys consistently indicate that most college students throw caution to the wind if they think they "know" someone—and they have unprotected sex. The **Skills for Behavior Change** box below presents ways to talk to your sexual partner about protecting yourselves from HIV and other STIs.

**Where to Go for Help** If you are concerned about your own risk or that of a close friend, arrange a confidential meeting with the health educator or other health professional at your college health service. He or she will provide you with the information that you need to decide whether you should be tested for HIV antibodies. If the student health service is not an option for you, seek assistance through your local public health department or community STI clinic.

## Communicating about Safer Sex

At no time in your life is it more important to communicate openly than when you are starting an intimate relationship. The following will help you communicate with your partner about potential risks:

✳ Plan to talk before you find yourself in an awkward situation.
✳ Select the right moment and place for both of you to discuss safer sex; choose a relaxing environment in a neutral location, free of distractions.
✳ Remember that you have a responsibility to your partner to disclose your own health status. You also have a responsibility to yourself to stay healthy.
✳ Be direct, honest, and determined in talking about sex before you become involved.
✳ Discuss the issues without sounding defensive or accusatory. Reassure your partner that your reasons for desiring abstinence or safer sex arise from respect and not distrust.
✳ Analyze your own beliefs and values ahead of time. Know where you will draw the line on certain actions, and be very clear with your partner about what you expect.
✳ Decide what you will do if your partner does not agree with you. Anticipate potential objections or excuses, and prepare your responses accordingly.

**Source:** Adapted from Queensland Health, "Talking to Your Partner about Sex," Accessed August 2010, www.health.qld.gov.au/istaysafe/content/letsTalk/talkingToYourPartner.html.

Skills for Behavior Change

# Assess yourself

## STIs: Do You Really Know What You Think You Know?

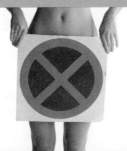

**PEARSON myhealthlab**

Fill out this assessment online at www.pearsonhighered.com/myhealthlab or www.pearsonhighered.com/donatelle.

The following quiz will help you evaluate whether your beliefs and attitudes about sexually transmitted infections (STIs) lead you to behaviors that increase your risk of infection. Indicate whether you believe the following items are true or false, then consult the answer key that follows.

|  | | TRUE | FALSE |
|---|---|---|---|
| 1. | You can always tell when you've got an STI because the symptoms are so obvious. | ○ | ○ |
| 2. | Some STIs can be passed on by skin-to-skin contact in the genital area. | ○ | ○ |
| 3. | Herpes can be transmitted only when a person has visible sores on his or her genitals. | ○ | ○ |
| 4. | Oral sex is safe sex. | ○ | ○ |
| 5. | Condoms reduce your risk of both pregnancy and STIs. | ○ | ○ |
| 6. | As long as you don't have anal intercourse, you can't get HIV. | ○ | ○ |
| 7. | All sexually active females should have a regular Pap smear. | ○ | ○ |
| 8. | Once genital warts have been removed, there is no risk of passing on the virus. | ○ | ○ |
| 9. | You can get several STIs at one time. | ○ | ○ |
| 10. | If the signs of an STI go away, you are cured. | ○ | ○ |
| 11. | People who get an STI have a lot of sex partners. | ○ | ○ |
| 12. | All STIs can be cured. | ○ | ○ |
| 13. | You can get an STI more than once. | ○ | ○ |

### Answer Key

1. **False.** The unfortunate fact is that many STIs show no symptoms. This has serious implications: (a) you can be passing on the infection without knowing it, and (b) the pathogen may be damaging your reproductive organs without you knowing it.

2. **True.** Some viruses are present on the skin around the genital area. Herpes and genital warts are the main culprits.

3. **False.** Herpes is most easily passed on when the sores and blisters are present, because the fluid in the lesions carries the virus. But the virus is also found on the skin around the genital area. Most people contract herpes this way, unaware that the virus is present.

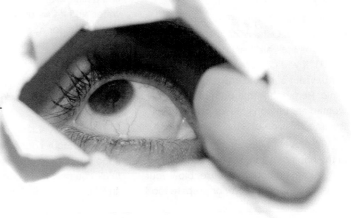

4. **False.** Oral sex is not safe sex. Herpes, genital warts, and chlamydia can all be passed on through oral sex. Condoms should be used on the penis. Dental dams should be placed over the female genitals during oral sex.

5. **True.** Condoms significantly reduce the risk of pregnancy when used correctly. They also reduce the risk of STIs. It is important to point out that abstinence is the only behavior that provides complete protection against pregnancy and STIs.

6. **False.** HIV is present in blood, semen, and vaginal fluid. Any activity that allows for the transfer of these fluids is risky. Anal intercourse is a high-risk activity, especially for the receptive (passive) partner, but other sexual activity is also a risk. When you don't know your partner's sexual history and you're not in a long-term monogamous relationship, condoms are a must.

7. **True.** A Pap smear is a simple procedure involving the scraping of a small amount of tissue from the surface of the cervix (at the upper end of the vagina). The sample is tested for abnormal cells that may indicate cancer. All sexually active women should have regular Pap smears.

8. **False.** Genital warts, which may be present on the penis,

the anus, and inside and outside the vagina, can be removed. However, the virus that caused the warts will always be present in the body and can be passed on to a sexual partner.

9. **True.** It is possible to have many STIs at one time. In fact, having one STI may make it more likely that a person will acquire more STIs. For example, the open sore from herpes creates a place for HIV to be transmitted.

10. **False.** The symptoms may go away, but your body is still infected. For example, syphilis is characterized by various stages. In the first stage, a painless sore called a *chancre* appears for about a week and then goes away.

11. **False.** If you have sex once with an infected partner, you are at risk for an STI.

12. **False.** Some STIs are viruses and therefore cannot be cured. There is no cure at present for herpes, HIV/AIDS, or genital warts. These STIs are treatable (to lessen the pain and irritation of symptoms), but not curable.

13. **True.** Experiencing one infection with an STI does not mean that you can never be infected again. A person can be reinfected many times with the same STI. This is especially true if a person does not get treated for the STI and thus keeps reinfecting his or her partner with the same STI.

**Sources:** Adapted from Jefferson County Public Health, "STD Quiz," Modified March 2009, www.co.jefferson.co.us/health/health_T111_R69.htm. Used with permission; Adapted from Family Planning Victoria, "Play Safe," Updated July 2005, www.fpv.org.au/1_2_2.html. © Family Planning Victoria. Used by permission.

# YOUR PLAN FOR CHANGE

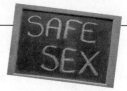

The **Assess yourself** activity let you consider your beliefs and attitudes about STIs and identify possible risks you may be facing. Now that you have considered these results, you can begin to change behaviors that may be putting you at risk for STIs and for infection in general.

### Today, you can:

○ Put together an "emergency" supply of condoms. Outside of abstinence, condoms are your best protection against an STI. If you don't have a supply on hand, visit your local drugstore or health clinic. Remember that both men and women are responsible for preventing the transmission of STIs.

○ To prevent infections in general, get in the habit of washing your hands regularly. After you cough, sneeze, blow your nose, use the bathroom, or prepare food,

find a sink, wet your hands with warm water, and lather up with soap. Scrub your hands for about 20 seconds (count to 20 or recite the alphabet), rinse well, and dry your hands.

### Within the next 2 weeks, you can:

○ Talk with your significant other honestly about your sexual history. Make appointments to get tested if either of you think you may have been exposed to an STI.

○ Adjust your sleep schedule so that you're getting an adequate amount of rest every night. Being well rested is one key aspect of maintaining a healthy immune system.

### By the end of the semester, you can:

○ Check your immunization schedule and make sure you're current with all recommended vaccinations. Make an appointment with your health care provider if you need a booster or vaccine.

○ If you are due for an annual pelvic exam, make an appointment. Ask your partner if he or she has had an annual exam and encourage him or her to make an appointment if not.

## Summary

* Your body uses several defense systems to keep pathogens from invading. The skin is the body's major protection, helped by enzymes. The immune system creates antibodies to destroy antigens. Fever and pain play a role in defending the body. Vaccines bolster the body's immune system against specific diseases.

* The major classes of pathogens are bacteria, viruses, fungi, protozoans, parasitic worms, and prions. Bacterial infections include staphylococcal infections, streptococcal infections, meningitis, pneumonia, tuberculosis, tickborne diseases, and peptic ulcers. Major viral infections include the common cold; influenza; mononucleosis; hepatitis; mumps; the herpes viruses, including chickenpox, shingles, and herpes gladiatorum; measles and rubella; and rabies.

* Emerging and resurgent diseases such as avian flu, West Nile virus, and dengue pose significant threats for future generations. Many factors contribute to these risks. Possible solutions focus on a public health approach to prevention.

* Sexually transmitted infections (STIs) are spread through sexual intercourse, oral–genital contact, anal sex, hand–genital contact, and sometimes through mouth-to-mouth contact. Major STIs include chlamydia, gonorrhea, syphilis, herpes, human papillomavirus (HPV) and genital warts, candidiasis, trichomoniasis, and pubic lice. Sexual transmission may also be involved in some general urinary tract infections (UTIs).

* Acquired immunodeficiency syndrome (AIDS) is caused by the human immunodeficiency virus (HIV). Globally, HIV/AIDS has become a major threat to the world's population. Anyone can get HIV by engaging in high-risk sexual activities that include exchange of body fluids, by having received a blood transfusion before 1985, and by injecting drugs (or by having sex with someone who does). You can reduce your risk for contracting HIV significantly by not engaging in risky sexual activities or IV drug use.

## Pop Quiz

1. Which of the following do not assist the body in fighting disease?
   a. Antigens
   b. Antibodies
   c. Lymphocytes
   d. Macrophages

2. Which of the following diseases is caused by a prion?
   a. Shingles
   b. Listeria
   c. Mad cow disease
   d. Trichomoniasis

3. An example of passive immunity is
   a. inoculation with a vaccine containing weakened antigens.
   b. when the body makes its own antibodies to a pathogen.
   c. the antibody-containing part of the vaccine that came from someone else.
   d. None of the above

4. One of the best ways to prevent contagious viruses from spreading is to
   a. wash your hands frequently.
   b. cover your mouth when sneezing, and dispose of your tissues.
   c. keep your hands away from your mouth and eyes.
   d. All of the above

5. Which of the following is a *viral* disease?
   a. Measles
   b. Pneumonia
   c. Malaria
   d. Streptococcal infection

6. Which of the following STIs cannot be treated with antibiotics?
   a. Chlamydia
   b. Gonorrhea
   c. Syphilis
   d. Herpes

7. Pelvic inflammatory disease (PID) is
   a. a sexually transmitted infection.
   b. a type of urinary tract infection.
   c. an infection of a woman's fallopian tubes or uterus.
   d. a disease that both men and women can get.

8. The most widespread sexually transmitted bacterium is
   a. gonorrhea.
   b. chlamydia.
   c. syphilis.
   d. chancroid.

9. Jennifer touched her viral herpes sore on her lip and then touched her eye. She ended up with the herpes virus in her eye as well. This is an example of
   a. acquired immunity.
   b. passive spread.
   c. autoinoculation.
   d. self-vaccination.

10. Which of the following is *not* a true statement about HIV?
    a. You can tell if a potential sex partner has the virus by looking at him or her.
    b. The virus can be spread through semen or vaginal fluids.
    c. You cannot get HIV from a public restroom toilet seat.
    d. Unprotected anal sex increases risk of exposure to HIV.

*Answers to these questions can be found on page A-1.*

## Think about It!

1. What are three lifestyle changes you could make right now that would reduce your risk of developing an infectious disease? What could you

do to help protect your friends and family members? Partner? How can you help reduce antibiotic resistance in the world today?

2. What is a pathogen? What does it mean if someone says a pathogen is particularly *virulent*? What are *antigens*? *Antibodies*? Discuss uncontrollable and controllable risk factors that can make you more or less susceptible to infectious pathogens in your immediate surroundings.

3. What is the difference between active and passive immunity? How do they compare to natural and acquired immunity? Explain why it is important to wash your hands often when you have a cold.

4. Discuss the importance of vaccinations in reducing societal risks for infectious diseases.

5. Identify five STIs and their symptoms. How do they develop? What are their potential long-term effects?

6. Why are women more susceptible to HIV infection than men? What implication does this have for prevention, treatment, and research?

# Accessing Your Health on the Internet

The following websites explore further topics and issues related to personal health. For links to the websites below, visit the Companion Website for *Access to Health*, 12th Edition, at www.pearsonhighered.com/donatelle.

1. *Centers for Disease Control and Prevention (CDC)*. This is the home page for the government agency dedicated to disease intervention and prevention, with links to all the latest data and publications put out by the CDC—including the *Morbidity and Mortality Weekly Report* (*MMWR*), *HIV/AIDS Surveillance Report*, and the *Journal of Emerging Infectious Diseases*—and access to the CDC research database, Wonder. www.cdc.gov

2. *American Social Health Association*. This site provides facts, support, resources, and referrals about sexually transmitted infections and diseases. www.ashastd.org

3. *San Francisco AIDS Foundation*. This community-based AIDS service organization focuses on ending the HIV/AIDS pandemic through education, services for AIDS patients, advocacy and public policy efforts, and global programs. www.sfaf.org

4. *World Health Organization (WHO)*. You'll gain access to the latest information on world health issues and direct access to publications and fact sheets at WHO's site. www.who.int

5. *Specialized CDC sites*. These sites focus on infectious diseases:

   • National Center for Immunization and Respiratory Diseases. www.cdc.gov/ncird/index.html
   • National Center for Preparedness, Detection and Control of Infectious Diseases. www.cdc.gov/ncpdcid
   • National Center for HIV/AIDS, Viral Hepatitis, STD and TB Prevention. www.cdc.gov/nchhstp

6. *AVERT*. This is an international site with information on HIV/AIDS, global STI statistics, interactive quizzes, and graphics displaying current statistics for vulnerable populations. www.avert.org

# References

1. Environmental Protection Agency, "Climate Change—Health and Environmental Effects," Updated April 2010, www.epa.gov/climatechange/effects/health.html; A. Greer et al., "Climate Change and Infectious Diseases in North America: The Road Ahead," *Canadian Medical Association Journal* 178, no. 6 (2008): 715–22.

2. B. Feingold et al., "A Niche for Infectious Disease in Environmental Health: Rethinking the Toxicological Paradigm, *Environmental Health Perspectives* 118, no. 8 (2010): 1165–72; L. Martin et al., "The Effects of Anthropogenic Global Changes on Immune Functions and Disease Resistance," *Annals of the New York Academy of Sciences* 1195, no. 1 (2010): 129–48.

3. American Autoimmune Related Diseases Association, "Autoimmune Statistics," 2010, www.aarda.org/autoimmune _statistics.php.

4. M. R. Klevens et al., "Invasive Methicillin-Resistant *Staphylococcus aureus* Infections in the United States," *Journal of the American Medical Association* 298, no. 15 (2007): 1763–71.

5. W. Jarvis, "Prevention and Control of Methicillin-Resistant *Staphylococcus aureus*: Dealing with Reality, Resistance, and Resistance to Reality," *Clinical Infectious Diseases* 50, no. 2 (2010): 218–20.

6. Centers for Disease Control and Prevention, "Group A Streptococcal (GAS) Disease," April 2008, www.cdc.gov/ncidod/dbmd/diseaseinfo/groupastreptococcal_g.htm.

7. Ibid.

8. Centers for Disease Control and Prevention, "Group B Strep Prevention (GBS, Baby Strep, Group B Streptococcal Bacteria): Frequently Asked Questions," Modified April 2008, www.cdc.gov/groupbstrep/general/gen _public_faq.htm.

9. Centers for Disease Control and Prevention, "Meningitis Questions and Answers," Updated February 2010, www.cdc.gov/meningitis/about/faq.html; J. Tully et al., "Risk and Protective Factors for Meningococcal Disease in Adolescents: Matched Cohort Study," *British Medical Journal* 332, no. 7539 (2006): 445–50.

10. Centers for Disease Control and Prevention, *Reported Tuberculosis in the United States, 2008* (Atlanta, GA: U.S. Department of Health and Human Services, 2009), Available at www.cdc.gov/tb/statistics/reports/2008/default.htm.

11. World Health Organization, *WHO Report 2009—Global Tuberculosis Control: Epidemiology, Strategy, Financing* (Geneva: World Health Organization, 2009), Available at www.who.int/tb/publications/global _report/2009/en.

12. T. H. Le and G. T. Fantry, eMedicine from WebMD, "Peptic Ulcer Disease," Updated December 2009, http://emedicine.medscape.com/article/181753-overview.

13. Ibid.

14. WebMD, "Cold Guide: Understanding Common Cold—Basics," 2009, www.webmd.com/cold-and-flu/cold-guide/understanding-common-cold-basics.

15. Linus Pauling Institute Micronutrient Information Center, "Micronutrient Center: Vitamin C: Common Cold," Updated November 2009, http://lpi.oregonstate.edu/infocenter/vitamins/vitaminC/index.html#cold; National Center for Complementary and Alternative Medicine, "Herbs at a Glance: Echinacea," NCCAM

Publication no. D271, Updated July 2010, http://nccam.nih.gov/health/echinacea/ataglance.htm.

16. Centers for Disease Control and Prevention, "Seasonal Influenza: Key Facts about Influenza (Flu) and Flu Vaccine," Updated June 2010, www.cdc.gov/flu/keyfacts.htm.

17. Centers for Disease Control and Prevention, "Hepatitis A FAQs for Health Professionals," Updated June 2009, www.cdc.gov/hepatitis/HAV/HAVfaq.htm.

18. A. Wasley et al., "The Prevalence of Hepatitis B Virus in the United States in the Era of Vaccination," *Journal of Infectious Diseases* 202, no. 2 (2010): 192–201; Centers for Disease Control and Prevention, "Hepatitis A FAQs for Health Professionals," 2009.

19. World Health Organization, "Global Alert and Response: Hepatitis B," 2002, www.who.int/csr/disease/hepatitis/whocdscsrlyo20022/en/index.html.

20. Centers for Disease Control and Prevention, "Hepatitis C FAQs for Health Professionals," Updated June 2009, www.cdc.gov/hepatitis/HCV/HCVfaq.htm.

21. S. Rajaguru and M. Nettleman, "Hepatitis C," MedicineNet.com, 2010, www.medicinenet.com/hepatitis_c/article.htm.

22. Centers for Disease Control and Prevention, "Mumps Outbreaks," Updated May 2010, www.cdc.gov/mumps/outbreaks.html.

23. A. E. Barskey et al., "Mumps Resurgences in the United States: A Historical Perspective on Unexpected Elements," *Vaccine* 27, no. 44 (2009): 6186–95.

24. Centers for Disease Control and Prevention, "Prevention of Herpes Zoster: Recommendations of the Advisory Committee on Immunization Practices (ACIP)," *MMWR Recommendations and Reports* 57, no. 5 (2008) 1–30.

25. Centers for Disease Control and Prevention, "vCJD (Variant Creutzfeldt-Jakob Disease)," June 2007, www.cdc.gov/ncidod/dvrd/vcjd/index.htm.

26. Centers for Disease Control and Prevention, "Get Smart: Know When Antibiotics Work: Fast Facts," Updated March 2010, www.cdc.gov/getsmart/antibiotic-use/fast-facts.html; J. Ritterman, "Preventing Antibiotic Resistance: The Next Step," *Permanente Journal* 10, no. 3 (2006): 22–24.

27. Centers for Disease Control and Prevention, "Dengue: Epidemiology," Updated July 2010, www.cdc.gov/Dengue/epidemiology.

28. Ibid.

29. Centers for Disease Control and Prevention, "Final 2009 West Nile Virus Activity in the United States," Modified April 2010, www.cdc.gov/ncidod/dvbid/westnile/surv&controlCaseCount09_detailed.htm.

30. Centers for Disease Control and Prevention, "West Nile Virus: Updated Information Regarding Insect Repellents," Modified October 2009, www.cdc.gov/ncidod/dvbid/westnile/RepellentUpdates.htm.

31. World Health Organization, "Confirmed Human Cases of Avian Influenza A (H5N1)," 2010, www.who.int/csr/disease/avian_influenza/country/en.

32. World Health Organization, "Cumulative Number of Confirmed Human Cases of Avian Influenza A/(H5N1) Reported to WHO," Updated August 2010, www.who.int/csr/disease/avian_influenza/country/cases_table_2010_08_03/en/index.html.

33. R. Snow et al., "International Funding for Malaria Control in Relation to Populations at Risk of Stable *Plasmodium falciparum* Transmission," *PLoS Medicine* 5, no. 7 (2008): e142; World Health Organization, "Malaria," Fact Sheet no. 94, April 2010, www.who.int/mediacentre/factsheets/fs094/en.

34. World Health Organization, "Malaria," 2010.

35. Centers for Disease Control and Prevention, *Sexually Transmitted Diseases Surveillance, 2008* (Atlanta: U.S. Department of Health and Human Services, 2009), Available at www.cdc.gov/std/stats08/main.htm.

36. Ibid.

37. Ibid.

38. Center for Young Women's Health, "Chlamydia," Updated January 2010, www.youngwomenshealth.org/chlamydia.html.

39. National Institute of Allergy and Infectious Diseases, "Chlamydia: Complications," Updated March 2009, www.niaid.nih.gov/topics/chlamydia/understanding/pages/complications.aspx.

40. Centers for Disease Control and Prevention, *Sexually Transmitted Diseases Surveillance, 2008*, 2009.

41. MedlinePlus, U.S. National Library of Medicine, "Gonorrhea," Updated May 2009, www.nlm.nih.gov/medlineplus/ency/article/007267.htm.

42. Centers for Disease Control and Prevention, "Gonorrhea: CDC Fact Sheet," Modified February 2008, www.cdc.gov/std/gonorrhea/stdfact-gonorrhea.htm.

43. National Institute of Allergy and Infectious Diseases, "Gonorrhea: Treatment," Updated June 2007, www.niaid.nih.gov/topics/gonorrhea/understanding/pages/treatment.aspx.

44. Centers for Disease Control and Prevention, *Sexually Transmitted Diseases Surveillance, 2008*, 2009.

45. National Institute of Allergy and Infectious Diseases, "Syphilis: Symptoms," Updated April 2009, www.niaid.nih.gov/topics/syphilis/understanding/Pages/symptoms.aspx.

46. Centers for Disease Control and Prevention, "Genital Herpes—CDC Fact Sheet," Modified March 2010, www.cdc.gov/std/herpes/stdfact-herpes.htm.

47. Centers for Disease Control and Prevention, "Genital Herpes—CDC Fact Sheet," 2010; American Social Health Association, "Learn about Herpes: Fast Facts," 2010, www.ashastd.org/herpes/herpes_learn.cfm.

48. Centers for Disease Control and Prevention, "Genital Herpes—CDC Fact Sheet," 2010.

49. Centers for Disease Control and Prevention, "Genital HPV Infection—CDC Fact Sheet" Modified November 2009, www.cdc.gov/std/HPV/STDFact-HPV.htm.

50. Centers for Disease Control and Prevention, "Cervical Cancer," Updated May 2010, www.cdc.gov/cancer/cervical.

51. National Institute of Allergy and Infectious Diseases, "Vaginal Yeast Infection: Symptoms," Updated August 2008, www.niaid.nih.gov/topics/vaginalYeast/Pages/symptoms.aspx.

52. Centers for Disease Control and Prevention, "Trichomoniasis: CDC Fact Sheet," Modified December 2007, www.cdc.gov/std/trichomonas/STDFact-Trichomoniasis.htm.

53. National Institute of Allergy and Infectious Diseases, "Trichomoniasis: Symptoms," Updated March 2009, www.niaid.nih.gov/TOPICS/TRICHOMONIASIS/UNDERSTANDING/Pages/symptoms.aspx.

54. Joint United Nations Programme on HIV/AIDS (UNAIDS) and World Health Organization (WHO), *AIDS Epidemic Update December 2009* (Geneva: UNAIDS, 2009), Available at www.unaids.org/en/KnowledgeCentre/HIVData/EpiUpdate/EpiUpdArchive/2009.

55. Centers for Disease Control and Prevention, *HIV Surveillance Report, 2008*, vol. 20, June 2010, www.cdc.gov/hiv/surveillance/resources/reports/2008report.

56. Centers for Disease Control and Prevention, *HIV Surveillance Report, 2008*, 2010; H. I. Hall et al., "Estimation of HIV Incidence in the United States," *Journal of the American Medical Association* 300, no. 5 (2008): 520–29.

57. AVERT, "Can You Get HIV From . . . ?" Updated July 2010, www.avert.org/can-you-get-hiv-aids.htm.

58. Ibid.

59. Centers for Disease Control and Prevention, "Mother-to-Child (Perinatal) HIV Transmission and Prevention," October 2007, www.cdc.gov/hiv/topics/perinatal/resources/factsheets/perinatal.htm; AVERT, "Preventing Mother-to-Child Transmission of HIV (PMTCT)," Updated July 2010, www.avert.org/motherchild.htm.

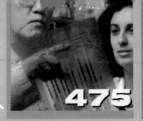
**475**
What makes genes so important to health?

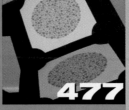
**477**
Why is color blindness common in males—and rare in females?

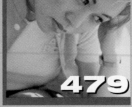
**479**
Do genes play a role in any psychiatric disorders?

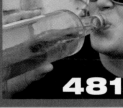
**481**
Are certain addictive tendencies predetermined by heredity?

# FOCUS ON Understanding Your Health Inheritance

It was spring break, and most of Ben's classmates were off to the beach to hang out with friends. Although Ben had tickets to fly to Cancun, he had to make a quick change of plans and head to Minneapolis to be with his family. His older brother Nathan, aged 29, had just had a major heart attack.

As Ben arrived at the hospital, he had memories of being there just 5 years earlier when he had witnessed his father die at age 46 of a major coronary event. Fear, anxiety, and flashbacks to the discussions with his father's doctors all kept Ben in a near panic as he watched the minutes tick by on his 3-hour flight. He remembered his doctor talking about how some aspects of heart disease risks were hereditary and how in a long-term study of coronary risks, some families had had no males live into their forties. It had all been just mumbo jumbo to him at the time. However, terms such as *high cholesterol, stroke,* and *increased risk for family members* now flashed before him. The doctor had also spoken of the need for Ben and his brothers to get regular checkups and watch the amount of saturated fat in their diet. He knew that, like his father, his grandfather had also died young of heart disease.

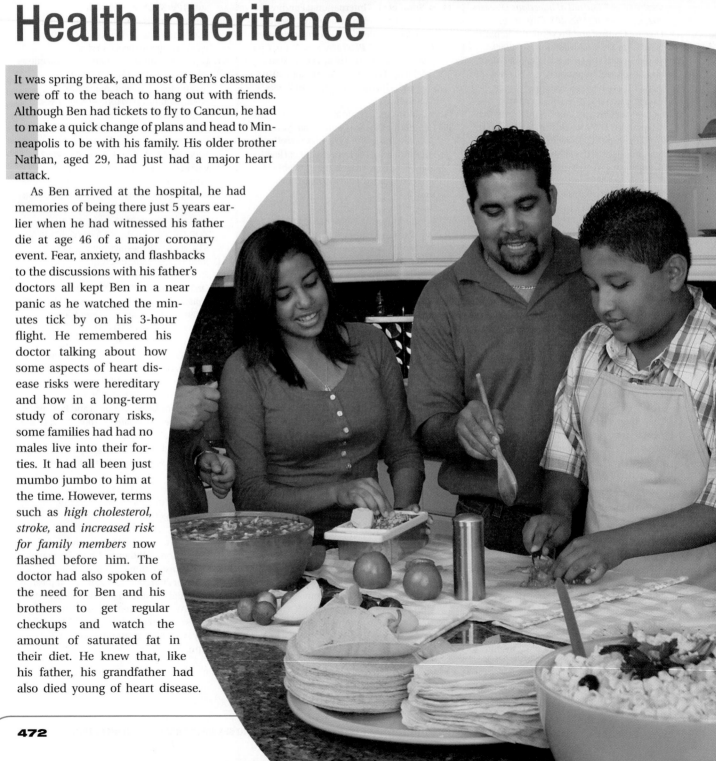

But who worries about developing heart disease when you are in your early twenties?

Ben's hereditary risk profile may be more dramatic than the norm. We seldom think of young adults dying of heart disease or other chronic illnesses, and statistically such situations are rare. However, research such as the study that Ben's doctor described points to a clear hereditary risk for certain conditions in some families.[1] Not only do we inherit our tendency to be short or tall, or have blue or brown eyes, we also inherit a tendency for increased risk for certain conditions. Are we "doomed" by our genetic predispositions? Are

> Your family influences everything that defines you, from the foods you like to eat, to the way you interact with others. Through the genes you inherit, your family also plays a significant role in your present and future health.

some conditions inevitable? If so, why do we hear so much about prevention and risk reduction? What about all those other determinants we talked about in Chapter 1: our personal behaviors, aspects of our social and physical environment, public policies and interventions, and access to health care? Where do they fit in?

### "Why Should I Care?"

You may have inherited traits or characteristics that affect your health every day, such as color blindness or a tendency toward depression. Knowing your family's health history, and sharing it with your health care provider, may help you treat symptoms or head off conditions that you might otherwise overlook or ignore.

We do have an increased risk of developing inherited diseases that have been experienced by other members of our family. However, inheritance is just one determinant of health—it doesn't dictate anyone's destiny! Throughout this book we have shown you how your health choices and behaviors—from what you eat and how much you exercise to whether you smoke or misuse alcohol—can affect your quality of life and your risk of major disease and disability. If that's the case, then why should you bother to find out your family health history? There are three reasons. First, if you know that certain diseases run in your family, you can change your behaviors to reduce your risk. Second, you can share your family health portrait with your health care providers so that they can provide better care, for instance, by looking for early warning signs of a condition in your family. Third, compiling a family health history is important if you are planning to have children. That's because a handful of disorders are indeed controlled by inheritance. These are known collectively as *genetic disorders,* and we'll discuss them later in this chapter. If your research were to

reveal a family history of any of these genetic disorders, you could then talk to your health care provider about genetic testing and counseling.

If you're adopted, or your parents and grandparents are already deceased, it may be more challenging for you to determine your family health history. But undertaking the investigation is important, because it has become increasingly evident that your genetic background plays a role in your future health. Before you set out to gather your family health history, you need to understand the basic substances, structures, and processes involved in human inheritance.

## What Role Do Genes Play in Inheritance?

**Inheritance** is the process by which physical and biological characteristics—called *traits*—are transmitted from parents to their offspring. For instance, you may have inherited your dad's curly hair, but your mom's blood type. To appreciate how this transmission of traits occurs, let's look at the key players in the process.

## Genes Are Coding Regions of DNA

You probably know that all of the structures of your body—from your skin to your bones—are composed of functional units called *cells*. Within each cell is a small, dark sac called the *nucleus:* It's dark because it's densely packed with **DNA (deoxyribonucleic acid)**, a complex molecule that stores

**inheritance** Process by which physical and biological characteristics—called traits—are transmitted from parents to their offspring.
**DNA (deoxyribonucleic acid)** Acid molecule that resides in the nucleus of a cell and stores in its sequence of chemical subunits the instructions for assembling body proteins.

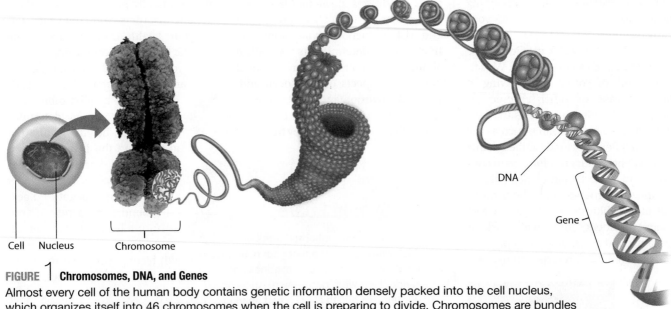

Cell  Nucleus  Chromosome

DNA

Gene

**FIGURE 1  Chromosomes, DNA, and Genes**
Almost every cell of the human body contains genetic information densely packed into the cell nucleus, which organizes itself into 46 chromosomes when the cell is preparing to divide. Chromosomes are bundles composed of DNA, a weak acid that forms long strands of a characteristic double helix shape. DNA consists of noncoding regions as well as regions called *genes* that code for the assembly of body proteins.

**Source:** Adapted from JOHNSON, MICHAEL D., HUMAN BIOLOGY: CONCEPTS AND CURRENT ISSUES, 5th, © 2010. Printed and Electronically reproduced by permission of Pearson Education, Inc., Upper Saddle River, New Jersey.

all of the programming code that your body uses for its initial assembly, growth from infancy to adulthood, and functioning throughout life **(Figure 1)**. DNA is an extraordinarily long molecule that's shaped like a twisted rope ladder (commonly known as a *double helix*) with two long side strands connected by short "rungs." For much of the life of a cell, its DNA exists as tangled masses dispersed within the nucleus. But when a cell gets ready to divide, its DNA becomes organized into 46 distinct bundles called **chromosomes** (see Figure 1). These 46 chromosomes exist as two sets of 23; you get one full set of 23 chromosomes from each parent.

The long rope ladder of DNA that makes up each chromosome contains hundreds of unique regions called **genes** that store the code for assem-

bling particular body proteins. Genes occupy less than 2 percent of the total DNA in human chromosomes.[2] The rest of your DNA has non-coding functions, such as assisting in regulating the quantity of proteins made, or maintaining the structure of the chromosome.[3] Your full complement of DNA—including genes and noncoding regions—is your **genome.** The branch of human biology that studies the human genome, genetic variation, and inheritance is known as *genetics.*

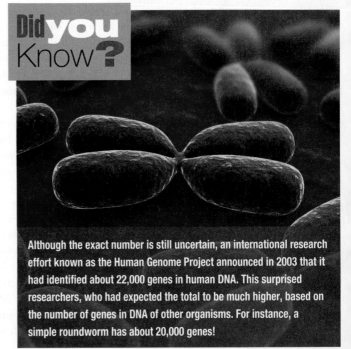

Although the exact number is still uncertain, an international research effort known as the Human Genome Project announced in 2003 that it had identified about 22,000 genes in human DNA. This surprised researchers, who had expected the total to be much higher, based on the number of genes in DNA of other organisms. For instance, a simple roundworm has about 20,000 genes!

**chromosome** Discrete bundle of DNA, 46 of which are present in the nucleus of almost all cells of the human body.
**gene** Discrete segment of DNA in a chromosome that stores the code for assembling a particular body protein.
**genome** All of the genetic information an organism possesses.

## Genes Are Expressed as Proteins

Genes can be likened to particular "pages" in the code book of DNA, in that they contain the instructions for assembling—or *expressing*—specific body proteins. But what makes pro-

teins so important? Essentially all cells and tissues of the human body are composed of proteins. In addition, proteins include a vast array of molecules that participate in the physiological processes that enable you to function. Therefore, by controlling the expression of proteins, genes control

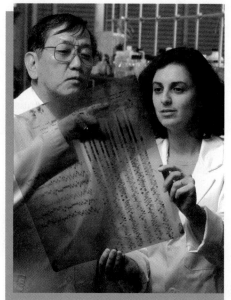

your body's appearance and structure as well as its functioning.

To understand how genes express proteins, it's important to recall that proteins are made up of subunits called *amino acids.* Just as a vast quantity of 20 different Lego parts could be assembled in various combinations into thousands of different toys, a vast quantity of the 20 amino acids in your body can be assembled into an estimated 10,000 to 50,000 unique body proteins.[4] For the instructions indicating how to make each of these proteins, the cell turns to DNA: Each gene on the DNA is a sequence of chemical instructions for combining amino acids into a specific protein.

## Proteins Express Traits

Minute differences in proteins from one person to another result in the unique physical and physiological characteristics each of us possesses. For instance, pigments are proteins, and they account for variations in the color of people's skin, hair, and eyes. But proteins also account for traits that are not visible, such as aspects of our functioning. For example, certain proteins contribute to three different types of cone cells in the eye. Cone cells allow us to distinguish colors, and if we don't have the genes to code for all three types of cone cells, we will have some form of color blindness.

## How Are Traits Inherited?

You may have inherited your father's height or your mother's hazel eyes, or even a grandparent's jawline or big nose. Just as people can inherit aspects of their appearance from family members, people can inherit genetic disorders or susceptibility to chronic diseases experienced by others in their family. But precisely how are such traits passed down?

## Traits Are Inherited via Chromosomes

We said earlier that your body cells have two sets of 23 chromosomes, one set from each parent. In other words, chromosomes exist as pairs that are alike in size and appearance. Geneticists can arrange chromosomes by pair in a configuration called a *karyotype* (Figure 2), with pair 1 being the largest and pair 22 the smallest. These are the 22 pairs of body chromosomes, called *autosomes.*

Pair 23 is your solitary pair of *sex chromosomes,* called XX or XY, which determines whether you are female or male, respectively. That is, every female gets one X chromosome from each parent to make up her twenty-third pair. The one she gets from her mother is one of the two Xs that make up her mother's twenty-third pair. The one she gets from her father is the only X he has to give—

of the DNA sequence in humans is identical; the remaining 0.1% is what makes each person unique.

because the other chromosome in his twenty-third pair is a Y. Every male gets his father's only Y chromosome, but he could get either one of his mother's two Xs. Notice that, for this reason, it is the father's genetic contribution that determines the baby's sex.

Because you have two copies of each chromosome you have two copies of each gene. Again, one copy comes from your father, and one from your mother. Your two gene copies may be similar, or they may be different. Different forms of the same gene are known as **alleles.**

For example, do you have freckles? Researchers believe that the presence or absence of freckles is coded by just one gene. However, that gene has two alleles—two forms. If you have freckles, you may have inherited the allele for freckles from both of your parents. But even if you inherited the freckle allele from just one parent, you'll still have

**allele** One of potentially several variants of the same gene.

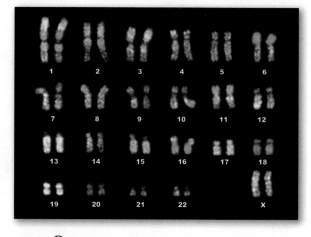

FIGURE 2 | **Human Karyotype**
A karyotype is a complete set of chromosomes arranged into pairs by size. This karyotype is from a female. You can tell because the chromosomes making up the last pair (pair 23) look almost identical (XX). In contrast, the male's XY chromosomes look different (the Y chromosome is shorter).

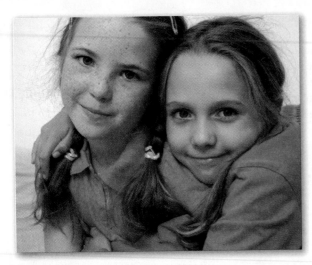

FIGURE 3 **Effect of Dominant versus Recessive Alleles**
Freckles are coded for by a single gene with two forms, or alleles. The allele that codes for freckles is dominant, whereas the allele that results in absence of freckles is recessive. If you inherit the dominant allele from both parents, or even from just one parent, you'll have freckles (*left*). If you inherit the recessive gene from both parents, you won't have freckles (*right*).

**dominant** Term describing an allele that is expressed even if there is only one copy in the pair.
**recessive** Term describing an allele that is expressed only in the absence of a dominant allele, that is, if both alleles are recessive, or if the recessive gene is on the X chromosome of the twenty-third pair.
**single-gene disorder** A disorder characterized by structural and/or functional impairments resulting from a defect involving only one gene.

freckles! Why? Because the allele for freckles is **dominant,** whereas the allele for absence of freckles is **recessive.** A dominant allele always "dominates"; that is, it always expresses the trait it codes for. In contrast, a recessive allele "recedes" in the presence of a dominant allele. When there is no dominant allele around, for instance, when you inherit two recessive alleles, then you express that recessive trait (Figure 3).

So if you *don't* have freckles, you must have inherited the recessive allele from both of your parents. Is it possible for you to have freckle-free skin even if both of your parents have freckles? The answer is yes. If both parents have one dominant and one recessive allele, they will both have freckles. Yet they could both have transmitted to you their recessive allele, in which case you would not have freckles.

Just as humans can pass on physical traits—like freckles—that are the ex-pressions of proteins, they can also pass on genetic disorders. That's because any genetic defect, at its most fundamental level, is either the pro-duction of a defective form of a body protein, or a failure to produce a body protein at all. *Geneticists*—scientists who specialize in genetics—recognize three types of genetic disease: single-gene disorders, multifactorial disor-ders, and chromosome disorders.

## Some Genetic Disorders Are Caused by Mutations in a Single Gene

**Single-gene disorders** occur as a result of a defect, called a *mutation,* involving just one gene. For example, the disease *cystic fibrosis* occurs because of a defect on the *CFTR* gene on chromo-some 7. Without the protein normally coded by this gene, a person with cystic fibrosis develops thick, sticky mucus that clogs his or her lungs and airways, making breathing difficult. Although many single-gene disorders, like cystic fibrosis, show up in childhood, a few manifest only in adulthood.

There are four common types of single-gene disorders (Figure 4). These

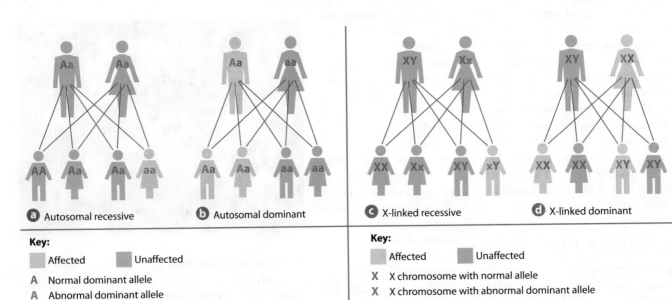

ⓐ Autosomal recessive    ⓑ Autosomal dominant    ⓒ X-linked recessive    ⓓ X-linked dominant

**Key:**

▮ Affected    ▮ Unaffected

A   Normal dominant allele
A   Abnormal dominant allele
a   Normal recessive allele
a   Abnormal recessive allele

**Key:**

▮ Affected    ▮ Unaffected

X   X chromosome with normal allele
X   X chromosome with abnormal dominant allele
x   X chromosome with abnormal recessive allele
Y   Y chromosome

FIGURE 4 **Inheritance Patterns of Single-Gene Disorders**

are classified according to the type of chromosome affected (autosome or sex chromosome) and type of allele (recessive or dominant).

## Autosomal Recessive Disorders

Cystic fibrosis is classified as an **autosomal recessive disorder,** that is, it occurs on an autosome (recall that all body chromosomes, 1 through 22, are autosomes) and the allele responsible is recessive (see Figure 4a). Autosomal recessive disorders are rare because very few people inherit the recessive allele for the disorder from both parents. However, many more people are "silent carriers" of the responsible recessive gene. A **carrier** is a person who has one dominant normal allele and one recessive abnormal allele. Carriers thus do not develop the disorder and may have no idea that they carry the recessive gene. In fact, grandparents and even great-grandparents may unknowingly also be carriers.

Common autosomal recessive disorders include the following:

- *Albinism* is a partial or complete lack of pigmentation of the skin, hair, and eyes.
- *Tay-Sachs disease* is a neurological disorder that causes a progressive deterioration of mental and physical abilities that begins around 6 months of age and is typically fatal before age 4.

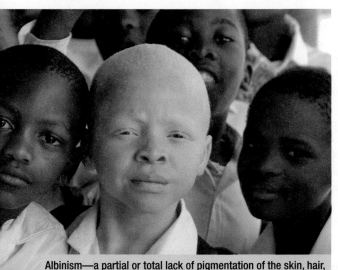

Albinism—a partial or total lack of pigmentation of the skin, hair, and eyes—is an autosomal recessive disorder: It is inherited only if the defective allele is passed on from both parents.

## Autosomal Dominant Disorders

An **autosomal dominant disorder** will occur even if an individual inherits just one defective allele, because the defective allele is dominant (see Figure 4b). This is the case, for example, with *Huntington's disease,* in which a defective gene on chromosome 4 causes cells to synthesize a flawed protein. This flaw eventually causes nerve cells in the brain and spinal cord to deteriorate, so the person begins to experience involuntary movements, memory loss, and changes in personality. The disease typically begins around middle age and, although its progression varies according to the extent of the genetic defect, most patients die within 20 years of initial symptoms.

Recall that with autosomal recessive disorders, it's entirely possible that neither parent of the affected child has the disease—both may be "silent carriers" of the recessive gene. In contrast, in autosomal dominant disorders, a parent does manifest the disease, and offspring have a 50/50 chance of inheriting it. Thus, affected families are more likely to be aware of their health history and seek genetic counseling.

## X-Linked Recessive Disorders

Some single-gene disorders are carried on the twenty-third chromosome pair—the sex chromosomes. The most common are **X-linked recessive disorders** (see Figure 4c). An example of X-linked inheritance is color blindness, which we mentioned earlier is a failure of normal assembly of proteins involving the cone cells of the eye.

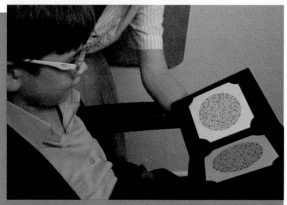

### Why is color blindness common in males—and rare in females?

One out of every 10 American males is color blind, most commonly being unable to distinguish between red and green. Color blindness is more common in males because the trait is carried by a gene on the X chromosome. Although it is a recessive trait, there is no comparable gene on the male's Y chromosome; thus, a man needs only one copy of the recessive allele to be color blind. Females inherit two X chromosomes and so will only be color blind if they inherit two copies of the recessive allele.

This condition is coded by a recessive allele, so if a dominant, normal gene is present, the child will not be color blind. However, it is carried on the X chromosome of pair 23—the sex chromosomes, which determine gender. Recall that, whereas females inherit an X chromosome each from their father and their mother, males inherit an X chromosome from their mother, but a Y chromosome from their father. The Y chromosome has different genes from those of the X chromosome. So if the X chromosome a male inherits from his mother has a defective gene, even if it's recessive, it won't have any competition from a dominant, normal gene from his father. Thus, the male child will inherit the disorder.

---

**autosomal recessive disorder** Single-gene disorder that occurs in individuals who have inherited two copies of an autosome with the affected recessive allele.
**carrier** Individual who has one copy of an autosome with a recessive allele for a particular trait, but is unaffected by it.
**autosomal dominant disorder** Single-gene disorder that occurs in individuals who have inherited at least one copy of an autosome with the affected dominant allele.
**X-linked recessive disorder** Single-gene disorder that occurs in individuals who have inherited only one copy of an X chromosome with the affected recessive allele.

Notice, too, that a man who is color blind will never pass on the problem to his son, since the son will get his Y gene. However, he will always pass on the trait to his daughter, who will be a carrier. The only instance in which a female will be color blind is when she inherits the recessive allele from both her father and her mother.

Other commonly known X-linked recessive disorders include the following:

- *Hemophilia* is a rare bleeding disorder caused by a genetic defect that results in the absence of a protein that assists blood to clot (called a clotting factor). Fortunately, the missing clotting factor is now produced in laboratories and can be injected into the bloodstream.
- *Duchenne muscular dystrophy* is a disorder that causes muscle weakness that progresses throughout childhood until, by about age 12, the child is usually unable to walk. It is caused by a defective gene for dystrophin, a muscle protein.

**X-Linked Dominant Disorders** X-**linked dominant disorders** are extremely rare (see Figure 4d). The most common affect the bones or the kidneys, and in males are often fatal. Even though the responsible allele is dominant, when females inherit it, the single copy of the recessive, normal allele can mitigate somewhat the disorder's effects.

## In Multifactorial Disorders, Genes Interact with Other Factors

Genes operate in a complex network, interacting and overlapping with one another in ways that can promote health or lead to disease. Moreover,

**X-linked dominant disorder** Single-gene disorder that occurs in individuals who have inherited at least one copy of an X chromosome with the affected dominant allele.
**multifactorial disorder** A disorder attributable to more than one of a variety of factors.

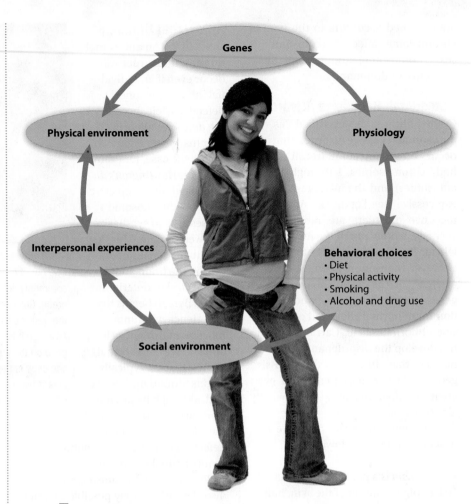

FIGURE 5 **Multifactorial Disorders**
Whereas single-gene disorders are determined entirely by genes, multifactorial disorders result from the influence of multiple genes on a vast number of physiological processes, all interacting with behavioral choices, interpersonal experiences, and a variety of factors in the social and physical environment.

genes interact with aspects of the environment, including diet, exposure to cigarette smoke and other toxins, viruses, radiation, and probably many other factors. These factors can act like a switch, turning on or off genes so that the proteins they code for are, or are not, assembled. Disorders in which genes play a role—but not the only role—are called **multifactorial disorders** (Figure 5). They are known to include obesity, heart disease, type 2 diabetes, Alzheimer's disease, and certain types of cancer; however, some researchers contend that nearly all conditions and diseases have a genetic component.[5]

In addition, genes are known to play at least some role in certain psychiatric disorders. These include the following:

- *Schizophrenia* is a complex disorder in which the person interprets reality in an abnormal way. In addition to genetic factors, exposure to malnutrition or viruses during fetal development is linked to schizophrenia, as are stress and the use of certain psychoactive drugs.
- *Bipolar disorder*, which formerly was known as manic-depression, is characterized by periods of excitability and exuberance alternating with periods of depression. Although researchers have not identified specific genes involved, bipolar disorder is more common in people who have a family member with the disorder. In addition, structural differences in the brain, imbalances in certain hormones and neurotransmitters, and

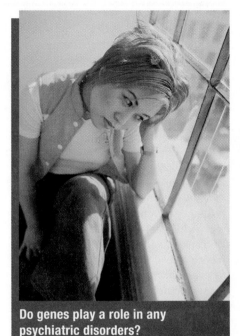

**Do genes play a role in any psychiatric disorders?**

Genetic factors probably play some role in the development of psychiatric disorders such as depression, schizophrenia, and bipolar disorder. However, other aspects of the individual's environment and development are also critical. Factors such as stress, use of psychoactive drugs, imbalances in hormones and neurotransmitters, and childhood trauma are all implicated in the risk of certain psychiatric disorders.

stress and drug or alcohol abuse may contribute.

● *Clinical depression* (also called *major depression*) is characterized by persistent feelings of sadness, hopelessness, and/or irritability. As with bipolar disorder, no specific "depression" genes have yet been identified; however, the disorder is more common in people whose family members have also had the condition. Biological differences in the brain, imbalances in hormones and neurotransmitters, stress, and childhood trauma such as abuse or the loss of a parent are also thought to be involved.

In short, although genes do play a role in multifactorial disorders, they are just one determinant of anyone's health. If a multifactorial disorder runs in your family, you should learn about the other factors influencing development of the disorder and make healthy choices to reduce your risk.

## Some Disorders Involve Missing, Extra, or Damaged Chromosomes

**Chromosome disorders** are caused by errors in an entire chromosome or part of a chromosome, rather than in one or a few genes.[6] For example, an entire chromosome may be missing, or an extra chromosome may be present, or a chromosome may be broken. Such problems sometimes arise while the mother's egg or the father's sperm is developing. After the egg and sperm unite at conception, the chromosomal defect is repeated with every cell division as the embryo grows to become a fetus and then an infant. The additional or missing genetic code can then be expressed as a wide range of abnormalities, including heart defects, kidney disorders, and mental retardation. With severe defects, the child may not survive.

One of the most common chromosome disorders is *Down syndrome*, a pattern of mental retardation and physical abnormalities, including heart defects and characteristic facial features such as a somewhat flattened profile. Down syndrome occurs when the child inherits an extra copy of chromosome 21, a defect that occurs at conception. Although researchers do not understand why, the chance of having a child with Down syndrome increases significantly as the mother ages: In their twenties, women have about a 1 in 1,230 chance of having a child with Down syndrome. By age 35, the risk increases to 1 in 270, and at age 45, the risk is 1 in 22.[7]

## Ethnicity Plays a Role in Many Genetic Disorders

Some genetic disorders tend to occur more frequently among people who trace their ancestry to a particular geographic area.[8] People in an ethnic group often share certain versions of their genes, which have been passed down from common ancestors. If one of these genes contains a disease-causing mutation, a particular genetic disorder may be more frequently seen in this group.

For example, Tay-Sachs disease, mentioned earlier, is more common among Jewish people of eastern and central Europe, and French Canadians. About 1 in 27 American Jews carries the recessive allele for Tay-Sachs disease, whereas only about 1 in 250 are carriers in the population at large.[9] In addition, both cystic fibrosis and Huntington's disease are more common among Americans of European descent.[10]

Ethnicity is also believed to play at least some role in many multifactorial diseases. For example, hypertension, heart attack, and stroke are all more common among African Americans.

---

**chromosome disorder** A disorder arising from a missing or extra chromosome, or damage to part of a chromosome.

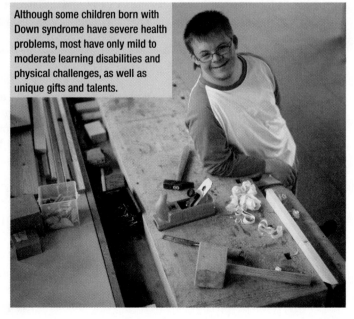

Although some children born with Down syndrome have severe health problems, most have only mild to moderate learning disabilities and physical challenges, as well as unique gifts and talents.

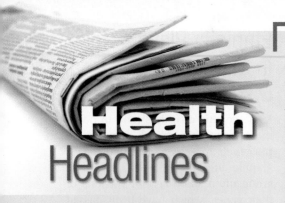

## THE ETHICS OF GENETIC TESTING

If you sprained your ankle last year, or had food poisoning, or got the flu, chances are you wouldn't mind discussing the incident with friends or family members, and you wouldn't worry about it having an effect on your job prospects or your health insurance coverage. But genetic information is different: It has long-term implications for you and for your family members. As more Americans seek genetic testing, concerns regarding the ethical implications involving the information gathered have surfaced. They include the following:

✳ **Who has access to genetic information?** The American Society of Human Genetics (ASHG) recommends that results be communicated only to the patient receiving the test and any individuals for whom the patient has given consent. Test results should never be provided without consent to outside parties. A new federal law, the Genetic Information Nondiscrimination Act of 2008, prohibits discrimination from health insurers and employers because

of differences in a person's DNA that may affect their health. However, what happens if the results of a genetic test reveal that the patient's family members—such as siblings—are at risk and the patient refuses to disclose the test results to the at-risk family members? When disease is preventable, or medical treatment or screening is available, the ASHG suggests that disclosure by health care providers to at-risk family members is permissible. However, such cases may end up in court: The duty to inform varies by state, and courts have ruled on both sides.

✳ **What are the benefits—and costs—of genetic testing for disorders for which there is no treatment?** Genetic testing for some disorders for which there is no treatment has the potential to cause psychological harm. Genetic testing for Huntington's disease is an example. Recall that the disorder is autosomal dominant. A person who is found to have the responsible gene will typically begin to experience symptoms by middle age. There are no effective treatments or preventive measures currently available. Thus, many people at risk choose not to undergo testing. Extensive psychological counseling is recommended prior to testing, and follow-up support is critical. Although knowledge that one has the disease helps some people to make informed choices about marrying, having children, and planning their career and other life goals, other people suffer from depression and are at increased risk for suicide.

✳ **What about reproductive issues?** Prenatal genetic screening is commonly used to

identify pregnancies at high risk for genetic conditions such as Down syndrome. A positive screening result is usually followed by more definitive tests to verify if the condition is actually present in the fetus. If the follow-up tests are also positive, the couple may face the question of whether to terminate the pregnancy. Many couples, at least initially, feel overwhelmed and incapable of making such a decision. They can be helped by psychological counseling as well as by meeting with other couples who have faced the decision or who are raising a child with the given disorder. Conversely, if couples choose not to pursue prenatal screening at all, their health care providers may be concerned about the possibility of a malpractice case if the baby is born with an unexpected birth defect.

Many other ethical issues surround genetic testing for medical conditions—from whether consumers should be able to purchase "home test kits" over the counter, to what level of accuracy a test should have before it can be marketed. As the integration of medicine and genetics continues, more such questions are sure to arise.

**Sources:** New England Public Health Genetics Education Collaborative, *Understanding Genetics*, 2010, www.geneticalliance.org/understanding .genetics; National Human Genome Research Institute, "Genetic Information Nondiscrimination Act of 2008," 2009, www.nhgri.nih.gov/10002328; D. H. Lea et al., "Ethical Issues in Genetic Testing: Why Genetic Testing May Lead to Ethical Dilemmas," *Journal of Midwifery & Women's Health* 50, no. 3 (2005): 234–40.

---

Type 2 diabetes is more common among African Americans, Hispanic Americans, Native Americans, and Asian Americans than among Caucasian Americans. Whether developing type 2 diabetes is due to ethnic background, lifestyle, or environmental factors or it is caused by a combination of these factors remains in question. Also, although it's not clear why, African Americans are more likely to develop cancer than are Caucasian Americans, whereas Hispanic and Asian Americans are less likely to develop most

cancers.[11] Still to be determined is how large a role genetics plays in these trends, and how much is a result of environmental factors shared by people of a certain ethnicity.

## Genetic Counseling Helps Families Evaluate Options

If you were to discover a family history of a genetic or multifactorial disease, one smart response would be to see a

genetic counselor. Most genetic counselors have graduate degrees and experience in medical genetics, and work within health care organizations to provide information and support to families. For instance, they help couples identify their risk for giving birth to a baby with a genetic disorder, investigate disorders already present within a family, review available options, and provide supportive counseling.[12]

Some people who consult a genetic counselor decide to undergo testing. A DNA sample can be obtained from any tissue. Gene tests can tell you whether or not you are a carrier of a genetic disorder. They can also be used for prenatal diagnosis, newborn screening, or to predict the presence of an adult-onset genetic disorder prior to symptom development. Testing is also available to estimate the risk of a very rare form of breast cancer associated with certain genes, as well as a particularly severe form of Alzheimer's disease linked to certain genes. Genetic testing can also confirm a diagnosis of specific disorders in individuals with symptoms.[13] There are significant ethical issues connected with genetic testing; see the **Health Headlines** box at left.

# Do Genes Influence Behavior?

Animal breeders have long recognized that certain species of domestic and farm animals have a higher prevalence of certain desirable behavioral traits than others. For instance, border collies are famous for their herding behavior and belted Galloways (a Scottish breed of cattle) are known for their docility. Recently a relatively new field of **behavioral genetics** has begun to study how genetic factors might contribute to variations in human behaviors as well. One tool commonly used in behavioral genetics is *twin studies* involving identical twins. Because identical twins have the same DNA, differences between them are assigned to variations in their environment—whether during fetal life, growing up in the same family, or growing up apart.

Even in studies involving twins, teasing out genetics from environment is not an easy task for several reasons:[14] First, in order to study a behavior, researchers have to be able to define and measure it precisely. It's easy to

## 1,200

**genetic tests are currently available.**

define, say, short stature in a child as being below the fifth percentile for height, and then measure each child in the study. But what would constitute a valid scientific definition of shyness? And how would you measure it? Finally, because behaviors, like most disorders, involve multiple genes and many factors within the environment, any claim we make about the hereditary nature of a behavior tells us only about the precise population studied. We can't readily extrapolate from there to the general population.

With these limitations in mind, let's look at what the research has to say about the heritability of the following behaviors.

- **Personality.** Human personality traits that can be reliably measured by rating scales do show a considerable heritable component.[15] In some cases, the effect of genes is expressed as variations in the production of certain neurotransmitters. Researchers have asserted claims for a genetic basis of impulsivity, novelty seeking, aggression, and nurturing. However, environmental factors significantly modify gene effects.
- **Intelligence.** The controversy over the relative contributions of "nature versus nurture" to human intelligence has raged for over a century. Although twin studies suggest that intelligence is influenced by genetics, other studies show that nutrient status, socioeconomic status, and aspects of the fetal environment play critical roles. Moreover, both genetics and environment appear to influence your ability to develop your intellectual potential.[16]

- **Addictive behaviors.** Genetic variation may underlie a substantial proportion of people's vulnerability to addictive behaviors.[17] For example, research over many decades has identified at least a dozen genes that influence susceptibility to alcohol dependence.[18] Still, alcohol dependence is not entirely genetic: Genes affect processes in the body, including the brain, that interact with one another and with an individual's life experiences to produce either protection or susceptibility.[19] Similar gene–environment interactions may be at work in addictions to tobacco, illegal drugs, and even prescription drugs.[20]

**behavioral genetics** The science that studies the role of inheritance in human behavior.

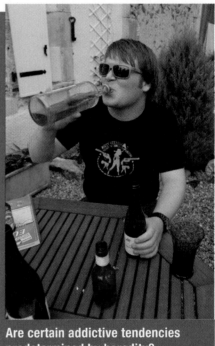

**Are certain addictive tendencies predetermined by heredity?**

No one is destined to engage in addictive behaviors. Genes only affect body processes that interact with one another and with your life experiences to influence your susceptibility. Many other factors, including environment, physiology, and behavioral choices contribute to the development of an addiction.

# What's Your Family Health History?

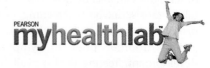

A family health history is a record of health information about a person and his or her close relatives. Creating your own family health history can help you identify whether you have higher risk for certain diseases. It can also help your health care practitioner provide better care for you and recommend actions for reducing your personal risk of disease.

**Gather information on at least three generations of your family: (1) your grandparents; (2) your parents, aunts, and uncles; and (3) you, your siblings, and your cousins. If possible, include your great-grandparents, and if you have children, include them as well.**

For each person, identify the following:

**1.** Person's name

**2.** Current age if the person is still living, or the age at which the person died

**3.** Any major diseases that the person experienced, is currently experiencing, or from which the person died, including chronic diseases, mental disorders, learning disabilities, and reproductive problems (miscarriage, stillbirth, birth defects, and infertility)

**4.** Any detrimental health habits such as alcohol or drug abuse, smoking or other tobacco use, or significant environmental factors such as exposure to asbestos, chemicals, radiation leaks, and so on

In gathering this information, you may need to ask your parents or other family members for assistance. Be sensitive to the fact that some of your relatives may not be comfortable sharing information about themselves, their parents and siblings, or their children. Respect any requests for privacy and confidentiality.

If you're adopted, ask your adoptive parents for any medical information they might have received about your biological parents.

**Once you've gathered the information, assemble it into a diagram that depicts the relationships and conditions. Refer to the key below and the sample diagram at right to help you fill in the blank chart on page 484. Alternatively, you could use an online tool, such as the U.S. Department of Health and Human Services My Family Health Portrait** (http://familyhistory.hhs.gov/fhh-web/home.action), **to complete your health history online.**

## Standard symbols used in family health trees

| INDIVIDUALS | | RELATIONSHIPS | |
|---|---|---|---|
| Males  Females | | I, II, III | Generation number |
| □  ○ | Individual | □—○ | Marriage/defacto |
| ■  ● | Individual with condition | □—#—○ | Marriage/relationship has ended |
| ⊙ | Carrier status in females (X-linked condition) | ○—#—□—○ | Second marriage or relationship |
| ⊘  ⊘ | Deceased | | Twins (identical) |
| □ OR ○ | Index person (yourself or individual through whom family is ascertained) | | Twins (non-identical) |
| □  ○ | Individual without children | □—○ | Consanguinity (closely related partners) |
| ◨  ◑ | Recessive gene carrier | | Adoption out of a family |
| **Others** | | | Adoption into a family |
| ◇ | Sex unknown | | A father and mother with one son and two daughters |
| ⊤ | Miscarriage | | |

▶ Begin with yourself and any siblings, then proceed to fill in the information for the rest of your family in the spaces indicated. Remember to record all categories of information identified above.

▶ Identify females with circles, and males with squares.

▶ Draw a diagonal line through the circle or square if the person has died.

▶ Note that a horizontal line indicates a marriage or sibling relationship, and vertical lines link parents and children.

▶ Try to identify siblings in order of age, with the oldest at the left and the youngest at the right.

▶ If you don't have complete information about a certain family member, leave the circle or square blank. Missing information is preferable to guesswork.

Now that you've assembled your family health history, answer the following questions:

1. Does your family health history include any single-gene disorders?  Y  N

2. Does your family health history reveal a pattern indicating a possible increased risk of:

|  | Yes | No |  | Yes | No |
|---|---|---|---|---|---|
| ▶ Heart disease | ○ | ○ | ▶ Reproductive disorders | ○ | ○ |
| ▶ Type 2 diabetes | ○ | ○ | ▶ Use of tobacco | ○ | ○ |
| ▶ Cancer | ○ | ○ | ▶ Alcohol or drug abuse | ○ | ○ |
| ▶ Asthma | ○ | ○ | ▶ Other disorders | ○ | ○ |
| ▶ Mental disorders | ○ | ○ |  |  |  |

**Sample completed family health tree**

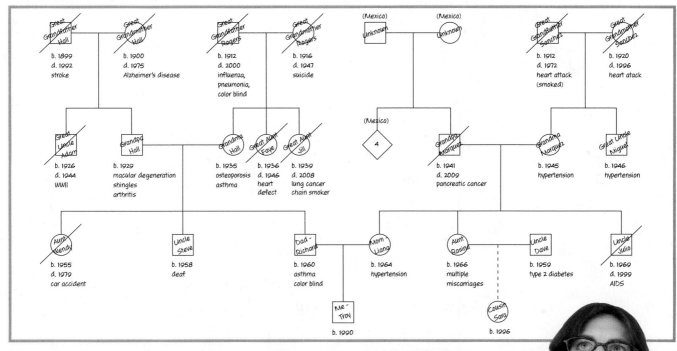

# YOUR PLAN FOR CHANGE

The **Assess yourself** activity gave you the chance to create your own family health history and identify the health risks present in your family. Now you can take steps to make sure you stay in control of your destiny!

**Today, you can:**

○ List the disorders that occur within your family. For each, identify the environmental factors and/or lifestyle choices most strongly associated with development of the disorder.

○ Jot down one small step you can take to positively influence your risk. For example, let's say that two close relatives have experienced lung cancer. You identify smoking as a lifestyle factor in each case. Maybe you don't smoke—but your roommate does. Today, you can share with your roommate your family history of lung cancer and ask your roommate to smoke outside from now on.

**Within the next 2 weeks, you can:**

○ Share your health history—and the patterns it reveals—with other members of your family. Invite them to fill in any gaps, and talk to them about the healthy choices you're making.

**By the end of the semester, you can:**

○ Share your health history with your primary health care provider. Ask him or her for more advice about choices you can make to take charge of your health.

○ If there is a multifactorial disorder in your family history, commit to behavior changes that reduce your risk of developing the disorder, such as getting your cholesterol checked or beginning an exercise program.

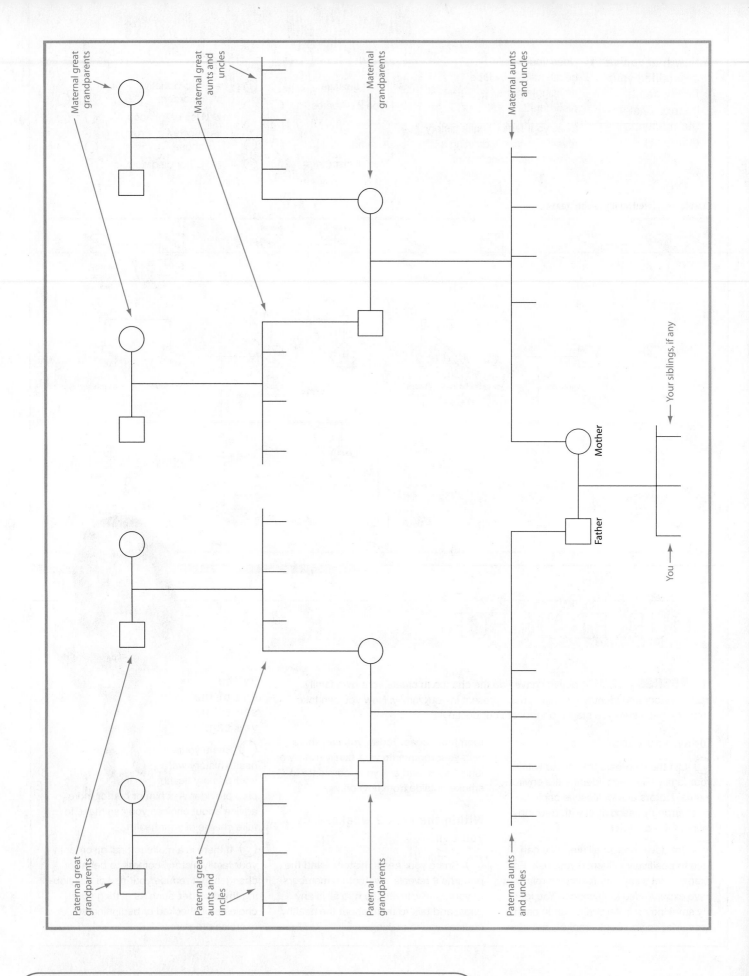

# References

1. Framingham Heart Study, "About the Framingham Heart Study," 2010, www .framinghamheartstudy.org/about/index .html.
2. G. Elgar and T. Vavouri, "Tuning In to the Signals: Noncoding Sequence Conservation in Vertebrate Genomes," *Trends in Genetics* 24, no. 7 (2008): 344–52.
3. Genetic Alliance and the New England Public Health Genetics Education Collaborative, *Understanding Genetics: A New England Guide for Patients and Health Professionals* (Washington, DC: Genetic Alliance, 2010), Available at www.geneticalliance.org/understanding .genetics.
4. J. L. Thompson and M. M. Manore, *Nutrition: An Applied Approach,* 3rd ed. (San Francisco: Benjamin Cummings, 2011).
5. Genetics Home Reference, "Mutations and Health," 2010, http://ghr.nlm.nih .gov/handbook/mutationsanddisorders.
6. March of Dimes, "Birth Defects: Chromosomal Abnormalities," December 2009, www.marchofdimes.com/Baby/ birthdefects_chromosomal.html.
7. Ibid.
8. Genetics Home Reference, "Inheriting Genetic Conditions," 2010, http://ghr .nlm.nih.gov/handbook/inheritance.
9. National Human Genome Research Institute, "Learning about Tay-Sachs Disease," 2010, www.genome.gov/ page.cfm?pageID=10001220.
10. Genetics Home Reference, "Genetic Conditions," 2010, http://ghr.nlm.nih .gov/condition.
11. American Cancer Society, *Cancer Facts & Figures 2010* (Atlanta: American Cancer Society, 2010), Available at www.cancer .org/Research/CancerFactsFigures.
12. Human Genome Project, "Genetic Counseling," 2008, www.ornl.gov/sci/ techresources/Human_Genome/ medicine/genecounseling.shtml.
13. Human Genome Project, "Gene Testing," 2008, www.ornl.gov/sci/techresources/ Human_Genome/medicine/genetest .shtml.
14. Human Genome Project, "Behavioral Genetics," 2008, www.ornl.gov/sci/ techresources/Human_Genome/else/ behavior.shtml.
15. V. McKusick et al., "Novelty Seeking Personality Trait," 2010, www.ncbi.nlm .nih.gov/omim/601696.
16. F. Grasso, "I.Q.—Genetics or Environment," 2004, http://allpsych.com/ journal/iq.html.
17. M. J. Kreek et al., "Genetic Influences on Impulsivity, Risk Taking, Stress Responsivity, and Vulnerability to Drug Abuse and Addiction," *Nature Neuroscience* 8, no. 11 (2005): 1450–57.
18. V. McKusick et al., "Alcohol Dependence," 2010, Available at www.ncbi.nlm.nih.gov/ omim/103780.
19. J. I. Nurnberger Jr. and L. J. Bierut, "Seeking the Connections: Alcoholism and

15

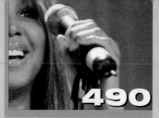

**490**

Why should I worry about cardiovascular disease?

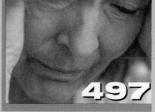

**497**

Can you die from a broken heart?

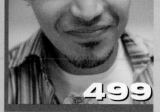

**499**

Is there anything I can do to improve my cholesterol level?

# Preventing Cardiovascular Disease

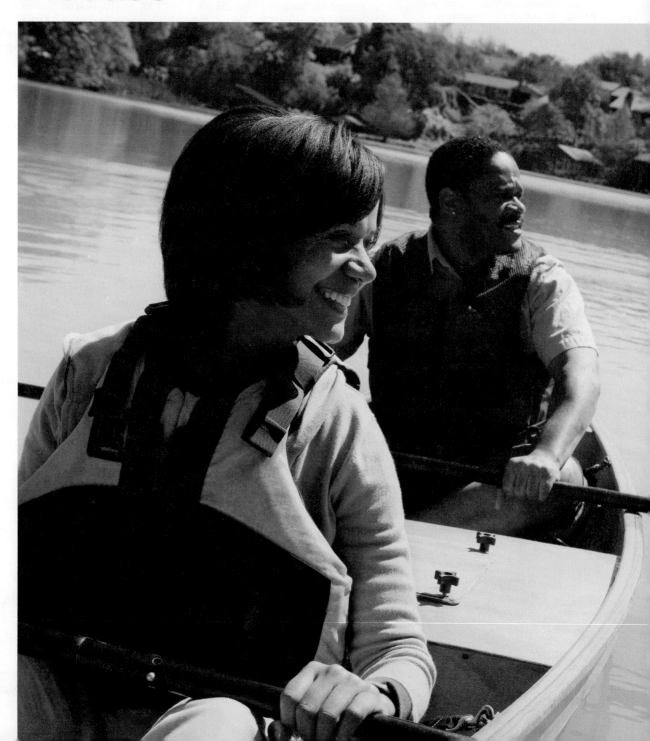

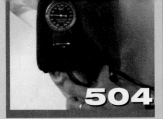

**504** Is heart disease hereditary?

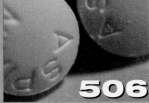

**506** Can aspirin really help prevent heart disease?

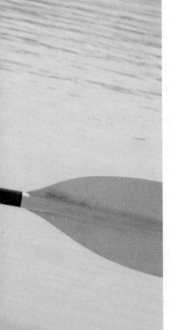

## Objectives

* Describe the anatomy and physiology of the heart and circulatory system and the importance of healthy heart function.

* Discuss the incidence, prevalence, and outcomes of cardiovascular disease in the United States, including its impact on society.

* Review major types of cardiovascular disease.

* Discuss modifiable and nonmodifiable risk factors, methods of prevention, and current strategies for diagnosis and treatment of cardiovascular disease.

Over 81 million Americans—1 out of every 3 adults—suffer from one or more types of **cardiovascular disease (CVD),** the broad term used to describe diseases of the heart and blood vessels.[1] Cardiovascular disease is not a new problem. It has been the leading killer of U.S. adults every year since 1900, except in 1918, when a pandemic flu killed more people. We spend billions on research for prevention strategies, treatments, and cures, and we have the most sophisticated media warnings and educational programs telling us how to avoid risks. Nevertheless, growing rates of obesity, hypertension, and diabetes continue to contribute to the high incidence of CVD both in the United States and worldwide. This chapter describes a healthy cardiovascular system and what happens when various diseases occur. It provides an epidemiological overview of CVD in the United States and why it's important for you to understand it, regardless of your age. It concludes with information critical to you, including things you can do today to reduce your own long-term risks for CVD and optimize your cardiovascular health.

# Understanding the Cardiovascular System

Before we can talk about cardiovascular disease, it's helpful to understand how the system normally functions. The **cardiovascular system** is the network of organs and vessels through which blood flows as it carries oxygen and nutrients to all parts of the body. It includes the heart, arteries, arterioles (small arteries), veins, venules (small veins), and capillaries (minute blood vessels).

## The Heart: A Mighty Machine

The heart is a muscular, four-chambered pump, roughly the size of your fist. It is a highly efficient, extremely flexible organ that contracts 100,000 times each day and pumps the equivalent of 2,000 gallons of blood to all areas of the body. In a 70-year lifetime, an average human heart beats 2.5 billion times.

Under normal circumstances, the human body contains approximately 6 quarts of blood, which transports nutrients, oxygen, waste products, hormones, and enzymes throughout the body. Blood also aids in regulating body temperature, cellular water levels, and acidity levels of body components, and it helps defend the body against toxins and harmful microorganisms. An adequate blood supply is essential to health and well-being.

The heart's four chambers work together to circulate blood constantly throughout the body. The two upper chambers of the heart, called **atria,** are large collecting chambers that receive blood from the rest of the body. The two lower

**cardiovascular disease (CVD)** Diseases of the heart and blood vessels.

**cardiovascular system** Organ system, consisting of the heart and blood vessels, that transports nutrients, oxygen, hormones, metabolic wastes, and enzymes throughout the body.

**atria** (singular: *atrium*) The heart's two upper chambers, which receive blood.

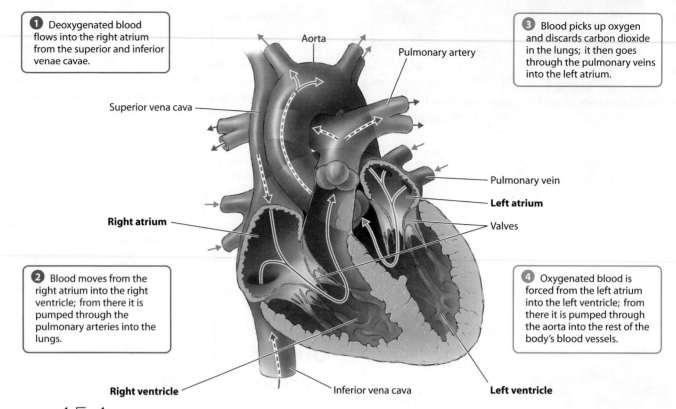

① Deoxygenated blood flows into the right atrium from the superior and inferior venae cavae.

③ Blood picks up oxygen and discards carbon dioxide in the lungs; it then goes through the pulmonary veins into the left atrium.

Aorta

Pulmonary artery

Superior vena cava

Pulmonary vein

**Left atrium**

**Right atrium**

Valves

② Blood moves from the right atrium into the right ventricle; from there it is pumped through the pulmonary arteries into the lungs.

④ Oxygenated blood is forced from the left atrium into the left ventricle; from there it is pumped through the aorta into the rest of the body's blood vessels.

**Right ventricle**

Inferior vena cava

**Left ventricle**

FIGURE 15.1 **Blood Flow within the Heart**

chambers, known as **ventricles,** pump the blood out again. Small valves regulate the steady, rhythmic flow of blood between chambers and prevent leakage or backflow between chambers.

**Heart Function** Heart activity depends on a complex interaction of biochemical, physical, and neurological signals. To understand blood flow through the heart, follow the steps in **Figure 15.1,** from deoxygenated blood entering the heart to oxygenated blood being pumped into the blood vessels. Various types of blood vessels are required for different parts of this process.

**ventricles** The heart's two lower chambers, which pump blood through the blood vessels.
**arteries** Vessels that carry blood away from the heart to other regions of the body.
**arterioles** Branches of the arteries.
**capillaries** Minute blood vessels that branch out from the arterioles and venules; their thin walls permit exchange of oxygen, carbon dioxide, nutrients, and waste products among body cells.
**veins** Vessels that transport waste and carry blood back to the heart from other regions of the body.
**venules** Branches of the veins.
**sinoatrial node (SA node)** Cluster of electric pulse-generating cells that serves as a natural pacemaker for the heart.

**Arteries** carry blood away from the heart; all arteries carry oxygenated blood, *except* for pulmonary arteries, which carry deoxygenated blood to the lungs, where the blood picks up oxygen and gives up carbon dioxide. After the arteries branch off from the heart, they branch into smaller blood vessels called **arterioles,** and then into even smaller blood vessels known as **capillaries.** Capillaries have thin walls that permit the exchange of oxygen, carbon dioxide, nutrients, and waste products with body cells. Carbon dioxide and other waste products are transported to the lungs and kidneys through **veins** and **venules** (small veins).

For the heart to function properly, the four chambers must beat in an organized manner. Your heartbeat is governed by an electrical impulse that directs the heart muscle to move when the impulse travels across it, which results in a sequential contraction of the chambers. This signal starts in a small bundle of highly specialized cells in the right atrium, called the **sinoatrial node (SA node).** The SA node serves as a natural pacemaker for the heart. People with a damaged SA node must often have a mechanical pacemaker implanted to make the heart beat.

The average adult heart at rest beats 70 to 80 times per minute, although a well-conditioned heart may beat only 50 to 60 times per minute to achieve the same results. If your resting heart rate is routinely in the high 80s or 90s, it may indicate that you are out of shape, carrying too much weight, or suffering from some underlying illness. When overly stressed, a heart may beat more than 200 times per minute. A healthy heart functions more efficiently and is less likely to suffer damage from overwork.

# Cardiovascular Disease: An Epidemiological Overview

Cardiovascular disease claims more lives each year than the next three leading causes of death combined (cancer, chronic lower respiratory diseases, and accidents), accounting for 34.3 percent of all deaths in the United States.[2] Consider the following facts:[3]

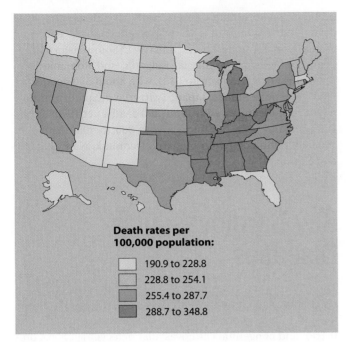

FIGURE 15.2 **Total Cardiovascular Disease Death Rates by State, Age Adjusted**

**Death rates per 100,000 population:**

- 190.9 to 228.8
- 228.8 to 254.1
- 255.4 to 287.7
- 288.7 to 348.8

**Source:** American Heart Association, *Heart Disease and Stroke Statistics, 2010 Update At-a-Glance* (Dallas: American Heart Association, 2010). Reprinted with permission. www.americanheart.org. © 2009, American Heart Association, Inc. All requests to use or reproduce this information must come through the AHA.

- More than 2,300 Americans die each day from CVD—an average of 1 death every 38 seconds (Figure 15.2). This totals nearly 1.4 million CVD-related deaths annually, nearly 56 percent of all deaths in the United States, for which CVD is listed as an underlying or contributing cause. Many of these fatalities are **sudden cardiac deaths,** meaning an abrupt, profound loss of heart function (cardiac arrest) that causes death either instantly or shortly after symptoms occur.
- One in 2.6 women each year dies from CVD. It may surprise you to know that in terms of total deaths, CVD has claimed the lives of more women than men every year since 1984. Only among those people aged 20 to 39 is CVD significantly more prevalent among men than it is among women (Figure 15.3).
- African American adults have the highest rates of hypertension in the world, at greater than 43 percent. Forty-nine percent of African American adults have two or more CVD risks; 38 percent of men and 36 percent of women have multiple risks.
- Over 10 percent of 12- to 19-year-olds already have metabolic syndrome (MetS), a major grouping of key risk factors for CVD.
- Twenty-six percent of college graduates have multiple risk factors compared to more than 53 percent among those having only a high school diploma. The more education you have, the lower your risks will be for CVD.

Of the millions of Americans who currently live with one of the major categories of CVD, many lack health insurance

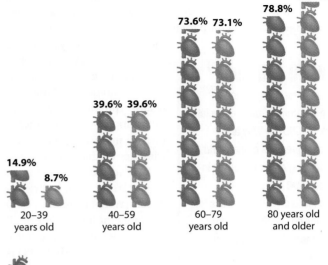

 Men with CVD; each heart = 10% of the population

Women with CVD; each heart = 10% of the population

FIGURE 15.3 **Prevalence of Cardiovascular Disease (CVD) in U.S. Adults Aged 20 and Older by Age and Sex**

**Source:** Adapted from American Heart Association, *Heart Disease and Stroke Statistics—2010 Update* (Dallas: American Heart Association, 2010).

and fail to receive appropriate screening and diagnostic tests. Others fail to recognize subtle symptoms until they result in a major cardiovascular event. Still others live in rural or remote areas where emergency transportation and care are not available. In spite of major improvements in medication, surgery, and other health care procedures, the prognosis for many of these individuals is not good:[4]

- Twenty-five percent of men and 38 percent of women will die within 1 year after having an initial heart attack. The older the age is at first heart attack, the greater the risk of dying will be.
- Within 6 years of a recognized heart attack, 18 percent of men and 35 percent of women will have another, 7 percent of men and 6 percent of women will experience sudden death, and about 22 percent of men and 46 percent of women will be disabled with heart failure.
- After surviving an initial heart attack, approximately 19 percent of the U.S. labor force is left with some form of disability.

> **sudden cardiac death** Death that occurs as a result of abrupt, profound loss of heart function.

Although it is impossible to place a monetary value on human life, the economic burden of cardiovascular disease on our society is huge—more than $503.2 billion estimated for 2010.[5] This figure includes the direct cost of physician and nursing services, hospital and nursing home services, medications, and home health care, as well as the indirect costs of lost productivity resulting from illness, disability, and death. As Americans live longer with chronic diseases, costs will continue to increase, resulting in a tremendous burden on the health care system. While economic concerns are huge, the effects of CVD on patients, their families, communities, the health care system and society may be even greater.

Cardiovascular disease is not a uniquely American health problem. With an international trend toward obesity, more and more countries face epidemic CVD rates. In fact, according to the most recent World Health Organization (WHO) estimates, CVD accounts for 30 percent of all deaths globally. Many have the mistaken idea that CVD is only a "developed" nation problem. Unfortunately, even some of the poorer, less-developed regions of the world are noting epidemic increases in obesity, diabetes, and CVD.[6] Some eastern European nations such as Russia, Bulgaria, and Romania have the highest death rates from CVD, with about 500 deaths per 100,000 people. France, Japan, Switzerland, Spain, and Italy have the lowest rates, with about 200 deaths per 100,000. The United States is in the middle, with 300 to 400 deaths per 100,000, right along with England, Denmark, New Zealand, and Germany.[7]

## what do you think?

Why are certain populations within the United States especially at risk for CVD? ● Why are developing regions of the world experiencing major increases in CVD rates? ● With all of the media focus on reducing risks for CVD, why do you think we aren't seeing more dramatic reductions in CVD deaths?

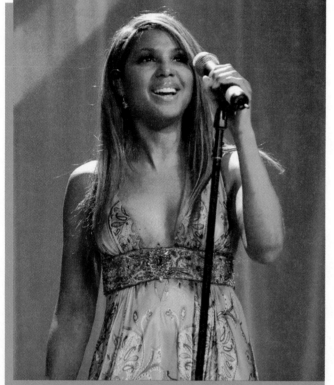

**Why should I worry about cardiovascular disease?**

Cardiovascular disease can affect even the youngest and most fit people. Award-winning singer Toni Braxton was first diagnosed with heart disease in 2003, at the age of 34. At that time she had pericarditis (an inflammation of the lining of the heart) and since then she has been diagnosed with high blood pressure, and was briefly hospitalized for microvascular angina. In recent years, Braxton has been a vocal spokesperson for the American Heart Association, urging women not to ignore signs of possible heart disease or to assume that it won't affect them because they are too young and because it is a "men's disease." In fact, heart disease is the number one killer for both men and women.

# Key Cardiovascular Diseases

There are several types of cardiovascular disease, including atherosclerosis, coronary heart disease (CHD), stroke, hypertension, angina pectoris, arrhythmia, congestive heart failure (CHF), and congenital cardiovascular defects. Figure 15.4 presents a breakdown of deaths from these different diseases in the United States.

Many of these forms of CVD are potentially fatal; many can also cause significant physical and psycholological disability. Although death rates are relatively easy to calculate, the short- and long-term psychological problems that occur after a person has a heart attack are harder to measure. Imagine wondering each time you exercise if your heart will fail you, or fearing you might have another heart attack during a particularly passionate sexual encounter. Getting a grip on the fears that follow a cardiac event can be challenging. Knowing more about your specific CVD risks and what you can do about them is key to taking healthy action.

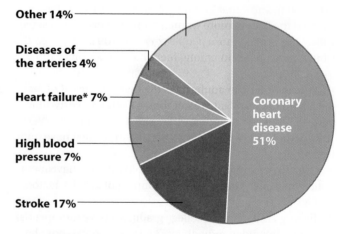

Other 14%
Diseases of the arteries 4%
Heart failure* 7%
High blood pressure 7%
Stroke 17%
Coronary heart disease 51%

FIGURE 15.4 **Percentage Breakdown of Deaths from Cardiovascular Disease in the United States**
Totals may not add up to 100% due to rounding.
*Not a true underlying cause.
**Source:** Adapted from *Heart Disease and Stroke Statistics—2010 Update.* (Dallas: American Heart Association, 2010).

# Atherosclerosis and Coronary Artery Disease

**Atherosclerosis** comes from the Greek words *athero* (meaning gruel or paste) and *sclerosis* (hardness). In this condition, fatty substances, cholesterol, cellular waste products, calcium, and fibrin (a clotting material in the blood) build up in the inner lining of an artery. *Hyperlipidemia* (an abnormally high blood lipid level) is a key factor in this process, and the resulting buildup is called **plaque.**

As plaque accumulates, vessel walls become narrow and may eventually block blood flow or cause vessels to rupture (Figure 15.5). The pressure buildup is similar to putting your thumb over the end of a hose while water is on. Pressure builds within arteries just as pressure builds in the hose. If vessels are weakened and pressure persists, they may burst or the plaque itself may break away from the walls of the vessels, and obstruct blood flow. In addition, fluctuation in the blood pressure levels within arteries can damage their internal walls, making it even more likely that plaque will stick to injured wall surfaces and accumulate.

Atherosclerosis is often called **coronary artery disease (CAD)** because of the damage to the body's main coronary arteries on the outer surface of the heart. These are the arteries that provide blood supply to the heart muscle itself. Most heart attacks result from blockage of these arteries. Athero-

## 80—90%

of the two main arteries were blocked in Daryl Kile's heart when the 33-year-old professional baseball player died suddenly in 2002 from atherosclerosis.

sclerosis and other circulatory impairments also often reduce blood flow and limit the heart's blood and oxygen supply, a condition known as **ischemia.**

When atherosclerosis occurs in the lower extremities, such as in the feet, calves, or legs, or in the arms, it is called **peripheral artery disease (PAD).** In recent years, increased attention has been drawn to PAD's role in subsequent blood clots and resultant heart attacks. In June 2008, when Tim Russert, a well-known NBC news correspondent, died suddenly of a heart attack after a long flight to Italy, there was speculation that he might have had a blood clot form

**atherosclerosis** Condition characterized by deposits of fatty substances (plaque) on the inner lining of an artery.
**plaque** Buildup of deposits in the arteries.
**coronary artery disease (CAD)** A narrowing or blockage of coronary arteries, usually caused by atherosclerotic plaque build up.
**ischemia** Reduced oxygen supply to a body part or organ.
**peripheral artery disease (PAD)** Atherosclerosis occurring in the lower extremities, such as in the feet, calves, or legs, or in the arms.

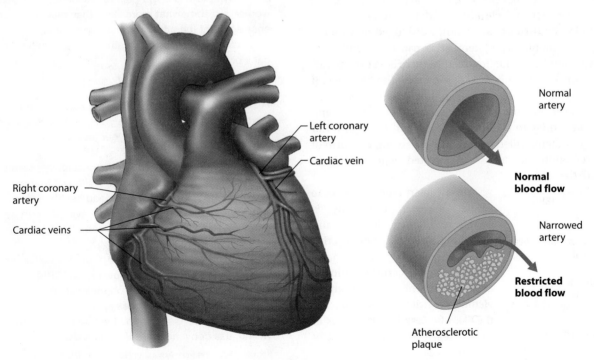

FIGURE 15.5 **Atherosclerosis and Coronary Artery Disease**
The coronary arteries are located on the exterior of the heart and supply blood and oxygen to the heart muscle itself. In atherosclerosis, arteries become clogged by a buildup of plaque. When atherosclerosis occurs in coronary arteries, blood flow to the heart muscle is restricted and a heart attack may occur.
**Sources:** Adapted from JOHNSON, MICHAEL D., HUMAN BIOLOGY: CONCEPTS AND CURRENT ISSUES, 4th, © 2008 (left image) and BLAKE, JOAN SALGE, NUTRITION AND YOU, 1st, © 2008 (right image). Both Printed and Electronically reproduced by permission of Pearson Education, Inc., Upper Saddle River, New Jersey.

in his legs from sitting for a prolonged period. This theory has not been confirmed; however, people are routinely advised to get up and walk around and flex or extend their legs to keep blood from pooling during long airplane flights or when sitting at a desk for long periods.

Whether from CAD or PAD, damage to vessels and the resulting threats to health can be severe. According to current thinking, five factors are responsible for this damage: inflammation, elevated levels of cholesterol and triglycerides in the blood, high blood pressure, heredity, and tobacco smoke. These factors are considered later in the chapter.

## Coronary Heart Disease

Of all the major cardiovascular diseases, **coronary heart disease (CHD)** is the greatest killer, accounting for nearly 1 in 6 deaths in the United States. Approximately 610,000 new heart attacks and 325,000 recurrent attacks occur each year. Another 200,000 people have silent heart attacks.[8] A **myocardial infarction (MI),** or **heart attack,** involves an area of the heart that suffers permanent damage because its normal blood supply has been blocked. This condition is often brought on by a **coronary thrombosis** (clot) or an atherosclerotic narrowing that blocks a coronary artery (an artery supplying the heart muscle with blood; refer to Figure 15.5). When a clot, or **thrombus,** becomes dislodged and moves through the circulatory system, it is called an **embolus.** Whenever blood does not flow readily, there is a corresponding decrease in oxygen flow to tissue below the blockage. If the blockage is extremely minor, an otherwise healthy heart will adapt over time by enlarging existing blood vessels and growing new ones to reroute needed blood through other areas. This system, called **collateral circulation,** is a form of self-preservation that allows an affected heart muscle to cope with damage.

# 40%

**of heart attack victims die within the first hour following the heart attack.**

When a heart blockage is more severe, however, the body is unable to adapt on its own, and outside lifesaving support is critical. The hour following a heart attack is the most crucial period— over 40 percent of heart attack victims die within this time. See the Skills for Behavior Change box at right to learn what to do in case of a heart attack.

**coronary heart disease (CHD)** A narrowing of the small blood vessels that supply blood to the heart.

**myocardial infarction (MI)** or **heart attack** A blockage of normal blood supply to an area in the heart.

**coronary thrombosis** A blood clot occurring in a coronary artery.

**thrombus** Blood clot attached to a blood vessel's wall.

**embolus** A blood clot that becomes dislodged from a blood vessel wall and moves through the circulatory system.

**collateral circulation** Adaptation of the heart to partial damage accomplished by rerouting needed blood through unused or underused blood vessels while the damaged heart muscle heals.

## Stroke

Like heart muscle cells, brain cells must have a continuous and adequate supply of oxygen in order to

## What to Do in the Event of a Heart Attack

People often miss the signs of a heart attack, or they wait too long to seek help, which can have deadly consequences. Knowing what to do in an emergency could save your life or somebody else's.

### KNOW THE WARNING SIGNS

Symptoms of a heart attack can begin a few minutes or a few hours before the actual attack, and all warning signs do not necessarily occur with every episode.

The following are common heart attack symptoms:

\* Discomfort (including uncomfortable pressure, squeezing, fullness, or pain) in the center of the chest lasting more than a few minutes, or going away and coming back

\* Pain or discomfort in one or both arms, the back, neck, jaw or stomach

\* Shortness of breath with or without chest discomfort

\* Breaking out in a cold sweat

\* Nausea or feelings of indigestion

\* Lightheadedness or dizziness

For both men and women, the most common heart attack symptom is chest pain or discomfort. However, women are somewhat more likely than men to experience some of the other common symptoms, particularly shortness of breath, nausea/vomiting, and back or jaw pain.

### BE PREPARED

\* Keep a list of emergency rescue service numbers next to your telephone and in your pocket, wallet, or purse. Be aware of whether your local area has a 9-1-1 emergency service.

\* Expect the person to deny the possibility of anything as serious as a heart attack, particularly if that person is young and appears to be in good health. If you're with someone who appears to be having a heart attack, don't take no for an answer; insist on taking prompt action.

\* If you are with someone who suddenly collapses, perform cardiopulmonary resuscitation (CPR). See www.heart.org for information on the new chest-compression-only techniques recommended by the American Heart Association. If you're trained and willing, use conventional CPR methods.

**Sources:** Adapted from American Heart Association, "Heart Attack, Stroke, and Cardiac Arrest Warning Signs," 2010, www.americanheart.org/presenter.jhtml?identifier=3053.

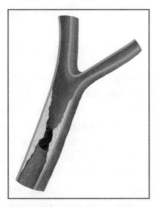

**a** A thrombus is a blood clot that forms inside a blood vessel and blocks the flow of blood at its origin. A thrombus in a cerebral artery can lead to an ischemic stroke.

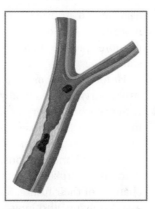

**b** An embolus is a blood clot that breaks off from its point of formation and travels in the bloodstream until it lodges in a narrowed vessel and blocks blood flow. Emboli in brain blood vessels can cause ischemic strokes.

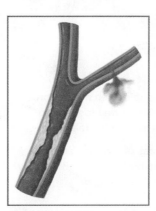

**c** A hemorrhage occurs when a blood vessel bursts allowing blood to flow into the surrounding tissue or between tissues. There are two types of hemorrhagic strokes: subarachnoid, in which a vessel on the brain's surface bursts, and intracerebral, in which a vessel within the brain bursts.

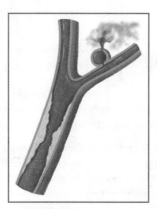

**d** An aneurysm is the bulging of a weakened blood vessel wall. Aneurysms in the brain can cause hemorrhagic strokes if they burst.

FIGURE 15.6 **Blood Vessel Disorders That Can Lead to Stroke**

survive. A **stroke** (also called a *cerebrovascular accident*) occurs when the blood supply to the brain is interrupted. Strokes may be either *ischemic* (caused by plaque formation or a clot that reduces blood flow) or *hemorrhagic* (due to a weakening of a blood vessel that causes it to bulge or rupture). Figure 15.6 illustrates some of the blood vessel disorders that can lead to a stroke. An **aneurysm** is the most well known and most life-threatening of the hemorrhagic strokes. When any

of these events occur, oxygen deprivation kills brain cells, which do not have the capacity to heal or regenerate.

Some strokes are mild and cause only temporary dizziness or slight weakness or numbness. More serious interruptions in blood flow may impair speech, memory, or motor control. Other strokes affect the parts of the brain that regulate heart and lung function and kill within minutes. According to the American Heart Association's latest statistics, every year more than 6.4 million Americans suffer strokes, 137,000 of whom die as a result. Hypertension is a leading risk factor for stroke. Men have more strokes in their younger years; women suffer more strokes in their later years, accounting for over 60 percent of stroke cases in the United States. Strokes cause much disability and suffering, and account for 1 in 18 deaths each year, surpassed only by CHD and cancer.[9]

Many strokes are preceded days, weeks, or months earlier by **transient ischemic attacks (TIAs),** brief interruptions of the blood supply to the brain that cause temporary impairment. Symptoms of TIAs include dizziness, particularly when first rising in the morning, weakness, temporary paralysis or numbness in the face or other regions, temporary memory loss, blurred vision, nausea, headache, slurred speech or difficulty in speaking, or other unusual physiological reactions. Some people may actually experience unexpected falls or have blackouts; others may have no obvious symptoms. Transient ischemic attacks often indicate an impending major stroke. The earlier a stroke is recognized and treatment

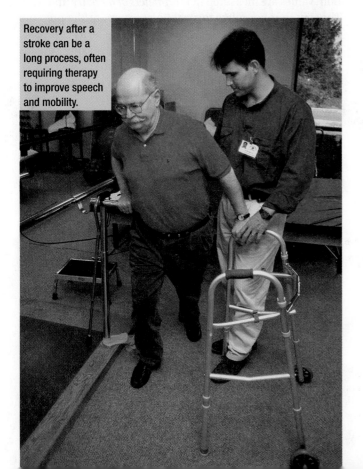

Recovery after a stroke can be a long process, often requiring therapy to improve speech and mobility.

**stroke** A condition occurring when the brain is damaged by disrupted blood supply; also called *cerebrovascular accident.*

**aneurysm** A weakened blood vessel that may bulge under pressure and, in severe cases, burst.

**transient ischemic attack (TIA)** Brief interruption of the blood supply to the brain that causes only temporary impairment; often an indicator of impending major stroke.

## Stroke Warning Signs

As they do with heart attacks, people often misinterpret the early warning signs of a stroke, or wait too long to seek help. Stroke warning signs include the following:

* Sudden numbness or weakness of the face, arm, or leg, especially on one side of the body
* Sudden loss of speech or trouble talking or understanding speech
* Sudden dimness or loss of vision in one or both eyes
* Sudden trouble walking, dizziness, or loss of balance or coordination
* Sudden, severe headache with no known cause

If you suspect someone you are with is having a stroke, use the 60-second test:

1. Ask the person to smile.
2. Ask the person to raise both arms.
3. Ask him or her to repeat a simple sentence such as "It is sunny out today."

If you or someone with you has one or more of the signs above or has difficulty performing any of the tasks in the 60-second test, don't delay! Immediately call 9-1-1 or the emergency medical service (EMS) number so an ambulance (ideally with advanced life support) can be dispatched. Also, note the time so that you'll know when the first symptoms appeared. If given within 3 hours of the start of symptoms, a clot-busting drug called *tissue plasminogen activator (tPA)* can reduce long-term disability from ischemic strokes, the most common type of stroke.

**Source:** Adapted from American Heart Association, "Heart Attack, Stroke, and Cardiac Arrest Warning Signs," 2010, www.americanheart.org/presenter.jhtml?identifier=3053.

also helped improve stroke statistics. It is estimated that more than half of all remaining strokes could be avoided if more people followed the recommended preventive standards.

Unfortunately, like many victims of other forms of CVD, stroke survivors do not always make a full recovery. Problems with speech, memory, swallowing, and activities of daily living and other consequences can persist, even though remarkable improvements have been noted with physical therapy and medications. Depression is also an issue for many post-stroke survivors as they face the challenges and changes of their future. Shortages of rehabilitation facilities, assisted living, and long-term care facilities pose additional challenges for families and communities as more and more individuals survive strokes and need assistance in their recovery and treatment.

# Hypertension

**Hypertension** refers to sustained high blood pressure. In general, the higher your blood pressure is, the greater your risk will be for CVD. Hypertension is known as the silent killer because it often has few overt symptoms and people don't know that they have it. Its prevalence has increased by over 30 percent in the past 10 years; today 1 in 3 adults in the United States has blood pressure above the recommended level.[11] The prevalence of high blood pressure (HBP) in African Americans in the United States is among the highest in the world and it's increasing. More than 44 percent of African American women have HBP, compared to 28 percent of white women.

Blood pressure is measured in two parts and is expressed as a fraction—for example, 110/80, stated as "110 over 80." Both values are measured in *millimeters of mercury* (mm Hg). The first number refers to **systolic pressure,** or the pressure applied to the walls of the arteries when the heart contracts, pumping blood to the rest of the body. The second value is **diastolic pressure,** or the pressure applied to the walls of the arteries during the heart's relaxation phase. During this phase, blood is reentering the chambers of the heart, preparing for the next heartbeat.

Normal blood pressure varies depending on weight; age; physical condition; and for different groups of people, such as women and minorities. Systolic blood pressure tends to increase with age, whereas diastolic blood pressure increases until age 55 and then declines. As a

started, the more effective that treatment will be. See the **Skills for Behavior Change** box for tips on recognizing a stroke.

One of the great medical successes in recent years has been the decline in the death rate from strokes, which has dropped by one-third in the United States since the 1980s and continues to fall.[10] Improved diagnostic procedures, better surgical options, clot-busting drugs injected soon after a stroke has occurred, and acute care centers specializing in stroke treatment and rehabilitation have all been factors. Increased awareness of risk factors for stroke, especially high blood pressure, diabetes, and sodium consumption, as well as knowledge of warning signals and an emphasis on prevention have

**hypertension** Sustained elevated blood pressure.

**systolic pressure** The upper number in the fraction that measures blood pressure, indicating pressure on arterial walls when the heart contracts.

**diastolic pressure** The lower number in the fraction that measures blood pressure, indicating pressure on arterial walls during the relaxation phase of heart activity.

## "Why Should I Care?"

Hypertension is becoming more common among college students. You can't tell whether you have it by how you feel or how you look in the mirror, but it poses a major potential threat to your quality of life. Get your blood pressure checked. It's easy to do, and it could save your life!

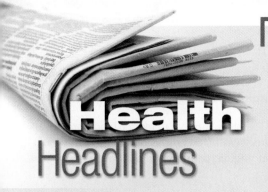

# Health Headlines

## YOUNG ADULTS AND HYPERTENSION

"College Students Face Obesity, High Blood Pressure, Metabolic Syndrome"— this recent headline in *ScienceDaily* shocked many. The article described a study of 800 University of New Hampshire students in a general-education nutrition course in which "one-third of UNH students were overweight or obese, 8 percent of men had metabolic syndrome, 60 percent of men had high blood pressure and more than two-thirds of women did not meet nutritional needs for iron, calcium or folate."

Those findings shouldn't come as any surprise. With epidemic rates of obesity and sedentary lifestyles, the numbers of children and young adults afflicted with diseases continue to rise. According to recent reports, the percentage of adults aged 20 to 44 who take anticholesterol medications increased from 2.5 percent in 2001 to over 4 percent (4.2 million young adults) in 2006. During that same period, the percentage of young adults who took hypertension medications reached 8 percent, meaning that 8.5 million young adults were on hypertension medications.

Young men, particularly young African American men, seem to be at highest risk,

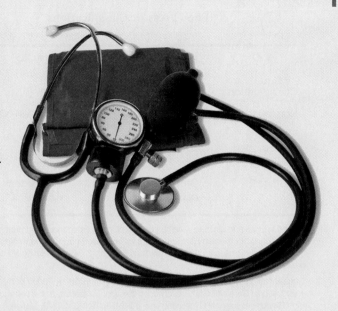

although young adults of all races and both genders are at increased risk. Men under the age of 35 are more likely to ignore early symptoms and delay return visits to doctors after a preliminary discussion about their high blood pressure. Interestingly, younger men with high blood pressure typically have high diastolic pressure (the lower number of the fraction) as compared to older men who are more likely to have higher systolic pressure. Two factors that increase risks for hypertension are depression and high consumption of alcohol, both of which are major problems among college-aged adults. In fact, new onset hypertension is almost twice as likely to be present among those diagnosed with depression.

The good news is that young adults seem to have better control of their high blood pressure once they are treated and taking antihypertension medicines as compared to older individuals. Hypertension can have devastating long-term effects on nearly every organ of the body. Among the many health problems that they may encounter, men with prehypertension and hypertension are nearly three times as likely to experience erectile dysfunction as men without these cardiac problems. Reducing sodium consumption, losing weight, and exercising, among other measures, can make a huge difference in risk reduction and help you avoid medical intervention.

**Sources:** University of New Hampshire, "College Students Face Obesity, High Blood Pressure, Metabolic Syndrome," *ScienceDaily,* June 18, 2007, www.sciencedaily.com/releases/2007/06/070614113310.htm; J. Flynn, "Pediatric Hypertension Update," *Current Opinion in Nephrology and Hypertension.* 19, no. 3 (2010): 292–97; *Washington Times,* "Heart Patients Getting Younger," October 30, 2007, www.washingtontimes.com/news/2007/oct/30/heart-patients-getting-younger; B. Rosner et al., "Blood Pressure Differences by Ethnic Group among United States Children and Adolescents," *Hypertension* 54, no. 3 (2009): 502–08; D. Lackland, "High Blood Pressure: A Lifetime Issue," *Hypertension* 54, no. 3 (2009): 457–58; L. Skarnulis, "High Blood Pressure in Young Men," WebMD, 2005, www.webmd.com/hypertension-high-blood-pressure/guide/hypertension-serious-in-young-men; S. Pattenet et al., "Major Depression as a Risk Factor for High Blood Pressure: Epidemiologic Evidence from a National Longitudinal Study," *Psychosomatic Medicine* 71, no. 3 (2009): 273–79; J. Flynn, "Hypertension in the Young: Epidemiology, Sequelae, and Therapy," *Nephrology, Dialysis, Transplantation* 24, no. 2 (2009): 370–75.

rule, men have a greater risk for high blood pressure than do women until age 55, when their risks become about equal. After age 75, women are more likely to have high blood pressure than men are.[12] The **Health Headlines** box has more information on hypertension among college students in particular.

For the average person, 110/80 is a healthy blood pressure level. High blood pressure is usually diagnosed when systolic pressure is 140 or above. When only systolic pressure is high, the condition is known as *isolated systolic hypertension (ISH)*, the most common form of high blood pressure in older

Americans. Diastolic pressure does not have to be high to indicate high blood pressure. See Table 15.1 on page 496 for a summary of blood pressure values and what they mean.

Treatment of hypertension can involve dietary changes (reducing sodium and calorie intake), weight loss (when appropriate), the use of diuretics and other medications (when prescribed by a physician), regular exercise, treatment of sleep disorders such as sleep apnea, and the practice of relaxation techniques and effective coping and communication skills.

TABLE

15.1 | **Blood Pressure Classifications**

| Classification | Systolic Reading (mm Hg) | | Diastolic Reading (mm Hg) |
|---|---|---|---|
| Normal | Less than 120 | and | Less than 80 |
| Prehypertension | 120–139 | or | 80–89 |
| Hypertension | | | |
| Stage 1 | 140–159 | or | 90–99 |
| Stage 2 | Greater than or equal to 160 | or | Greater than or equal to 100 |

**Note:** If systolic and diastolic readings fall into different categories, treatment is determined by the highest category. Readings are based on the average of two or more properly measured, seated readings on each of two or more health care provider visits.

**Source:** National Heart, Lung, and Blood Institute, *The Seventh Report of the Joint National Committee on Prevention, Detection, Evaluation, and Treatment of High Blood Pressure* (NIH Publication no. 03-5233), Bethesda, MD: National Institutes of Health, 2003.

## Angina Pectoris

People with ischemia often suffer from varying degrees of **angina** (pronounced "an-JY-nuh") **pectoris,** a condition that often feels like pressure or squeezing in the chest or pain in the shoulders, arms, neck, jaw, or even the back. The pain is caused by reduced oxygen flow to the heart. Over 7 million men and women suffer mild to crushing forms of chest pain each day, and many take powerful medications to control their symptoms.[13] Although someone experiencing angina symptoms may think he or she is having a heart attack, it's not an actual attack. It does, however, usually provide an early warning of heart problems that should be checked out by trained medical personnel. It is important to remember that not all chest pain or discomfort is angina. An actual heart attack, lung problems (such as an infection or a clot), heartburn, or acute anxiety can trigger these symptoms.

Currently, there are several methods of treating angina. In mild cases, rest is critical. The most common treatments for more severe cases involve drugs that affect either the supply of blood to the heart muscle or the heart's demand for oxygen. Pain and discomfort are often relieved with *nitroglycerin,* a drug used to relax (dilate) veins, thereby reducing the amount of blood returning to the heart and thus lessening its workload. Patients whose angina is caused by spasms of the coronary arteries are often given drugs called *calcium channel blockers,* which prevent calcium atoms from passing through coronary arteries and causing

**angina pectoris** Chest pain occurring as a result of reduced oxygen flow to the heart.

**arrhythmia** An irregularity in heartbeat.

**fibrillation** A sporadic, quivering pattern of heartbeat that results in extreme inefficiency in moving blood through the cardiovascular system.

**congestive heart failure (CHF)** An abnormal cardiovascular condition that reflects impaired cardiac pumping and blood flow; pooling blood leads to congestion in body tissues.

# 400,000
new cases of angina are diagnosed each year.

heart contractions. They also appear to reduce blood pressure and slow heart rate. *Beta-blockers,* the other major type of drugs used to treat angina, control potential overactivity of the heart muscle.

## Arrhythmias

Millions of Americans experience some type of **arrhythmia,** an irregularity in heart rhythm that may result in symptoms of heart fluttering, palpitations, or racing, dizziness or fainting. It can be severe enough to result in death.[14] A person who complains of a racing heart in the absence of exercise or anxiety may be experiencing *tachycardia,* the medical term for abnormally fast heartbeat. On the other end of the continuum is *bradycardia,* or abnormally slow heartbeat. When a heart goes into **fibrillation,** it beats in a sporadic, quivering pattern that causes extreme inefficiency in moving blood through the cardiovascular system. If untreated, fibrillation may be fatal.

Not all arrhythmias are life threatening. In many instances, excessive caffeine or nicotine consumption or panic attacks and other anxiety disorders can trigger an arrhythmia episode. However, severe cases may require drug therapy or external electrical stimulus to prevent serious complications.

## Congestive Heart Failure

When the heart muscle is damaged or overworked and lacks the strength to keep blood circulating normally through the body, **congestive heart failure (CHF)** can occur. Congestive heart failure affects millions of Americans, particularly those over the age of 65 who have a history of heart disease or heart attack.[15] The heart muscle may be injured by numerous health conditions, atherosclerosis, past heart attacks, high blood pressure, or congenital heart defects. The weakened heart muscle performs poorly, reducing blood flow out of the heart through the arteries. The return flow of blood through the veins begins to back up, causing congestion in body tissues. The pooling of blood enlarges the heart, makes it less efficient, and decreases the amount of blood that can be circulated. Fluid begins to accumulate in other areas of the body, such as the vessels in the legs, ankles, or lungs, causing swelling or difficulty in breathing.

Today, CHF is a major cause of hospitalization in those with recurrent heart problems. If untreated, it can be fatal. However, most cases respond well to treatment, which includes *diuretics* (water pills) to relieve fluid accumulation; drugs such as *digitalis* that increase the heart's pumping action; and *vasodilators,* drugs that expand blood vessels and decrease resistance, allowing blood to flow more easily and making the heart's work easier.

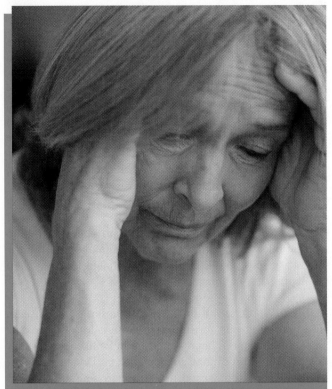

**Can you die from a broken heart?**

Songs and stories abound of spurned lovers dying from a broken heart. Can this really happen? In a limited sense, it appears the answer is yes. As first reported in a 2005 article in the *New England Journal of Medicine,* researchers have noticed a phenomenon in which the heart is so stressed, it apparently receives a form of "concussion"—a type of heart attack triggered by extreme, overwhelming stress, grief, horror, or anger. Formally known as *stress-induced cardiomyopathy,* this strikes mostly women after the age of menopause and is believed to affect about 6 percent of women who have an apparent heart attack. Victims show no evidence of obstructed arteries or severe tissue damage; instead, the heart muscle seems to be temporarily overwhelmed by an intense surge of adrenaline that interferes with the heart's pumping ability. Almost all victims recover without permanent damage, but in a few instances, the patient's heart loses so much pumping capacity that the result is fatal.

## Congenital Cardiovascular Defects

Approximately 36,000 children are born in the United States each year with some form of **congenital cardiovascular defect** (*congenital* means the problem is present at birth).[16] These forms may be relatively minor, such as slight *murmurs* (low-pitched sounds caused by turbulent blood flow through the heart) caused by valve irregularities that some children outgrow. Other congenital problems involve serious complications in heart function that can be corrected only with surgery. Their underlying causes are unknown but may be related to hereditary factors; maternal diseases, such as rubella, that occurred during fetal development; or the mother's chemical intake (particularly alcohol or methamphetamine) during pregnancy. Because of advances in pediatric cardiology, the prognosis for children with congenital heart defects is better than ever before.

**Rheumatic heart disease** can cause similar heart problems in children. It is attributed to rheumatic fever, an inflammatory disease caused by an unresolved *streptococcal infection* of the throat (strep throat). Over time, this strep infection can affect many connective tissues of the body, especially those of the heart, joints, brain, or skin. In some cases, this infection can lead to an immune response in which antibodies attack the heart as well as the bacteria. Many of the thousands of annual operations on heart valves in the United States are related to rheumatic heart disease.

# Reducing Your Risks

Scientific evidence has shown a large cluster of factors related to a person's being at a higher risk for developing cardiovascular diseases over the life span. Obesity, lack of physical activity, high cholesterol, and high blood pressure have all shown strong associations with subsequent CVD problems.[17] Interestingly, although selected factors increase risks specific to CVD, the combination of these and other risk factors appears also to increase risks for insulin resistance and type 2 diabetes.[18] The term **cardiometabolic risks** refers to these combined risks, which indicate physical and biochemical changes that can lead to these major diseases. Some of these risks result from choices and behaviors, and so are modifiable, whereas others are inherited or are intrinsic to you (such as your age and gender) and therefore cannot be modified.

## Metabolic Syndrome

Over the past decade, different health professionals have attempted to establish diagnostic cutoff points for a cluster of combined cardiometabolic risks, variably labeled as *syndrome X, insulin resistance syndrome,* and, most recently, **metabolic syndrome (MetS).** Historically, MetS is believed to increase the risk for atherosclerotic heart disease by as much as three times the normal rates. It has captured international attention, as an estimated 47 million people potentially meet the criteria for it.[19] The more risk factors there are in the cluster, the greater the risk of CVD becomes. Typically, for a diagnosis of MetS, a person would have three or more of the following:

- Abdominal obesity (waist measurement of more than 40 inches in men or 35 inches in women)
- Elevated blood fat (triglycerides greater than 150 mg/dL)

**congenital cardiovascular defect** Cardiovascular problem that is present at birth.
**rheumatic heart disease** A heart disease caused by untreated streptococcal infection of the throat.
**cardiometabolic risks** Physical and biochemical changes that are risk factors for the development of cardiovascular disease and type 2 diabetes.
**metabolic syndrome (MetS)** A group of metabolic conditions occurring together that increase a person's risk of heart disease, stroke, and diabetes.

- Low levels of high-density lipoprotein (HDL; "good" cholesterol) (less than 40 mg/dL in men and less than 50 mg/dL in women)
- Blood pressure greater than 130/85 mm Hg
- Fasting glucose greater than 100 mg/dL (a sign of insulin resistance or glucose intolerance)
- Levels of C-reactive proteins greater than 10 mg/L, indicating inflammation is present.

The use of the MetS classification and other, similar terms has been important in highlighting the relationship between the number of risks a person possesses and that person's likelihood of developing CVD and diabetes. In this case, more appears to mean "worse." However, critics have questioned the usefulness of this risk profile, saying that the way data are collected makes it impossible to determine whether additional and compounded risk factors really contribute more to total risk. In addition, these classifications have not been as useful in telling patients and health care providers which risk factors might be more important and which ones should be given the highest priority when taking action to reduce risks. Research continues in this area and on other factors that may contribute to MetS and/or CVD risks. Potential newer risks include a constant low-grade inflammation in the body, a fatty liver, polycystic ovarian syndrome (a tendency to develop cysts on the ovaries), gallstones, and sleep apnea.[20]

Although the link between MetS and the risks of CVD is still being researched, it is clear that having several of the characteristics of MetS can affect your daily life even without a diagnosis of CVD (see Figure 15.7).

# Modifiable Risks

Although younger adults often think heart attacks and strokes are things that happen to "old" people, the reality is that you may already be on course to having significant risks. In fact, hypertension, pre-diabetes, high cholesterol, and other risks have increased significantly among elementary, high school, and college students in the United States and globally. African Americans, Mexican American males, and white females are among the highest risk groups for both obesity and hypertension, while male college students have higher rates of obesity, hypertension, and triglycerides than do female students.[21] Behaviors you choose today and over the coming decades can actively reduce or increase your risk for CVD. Among the most important behaviors you can adopt are choosing not to smoke, following a healthy diet and maintaining a healthy weight, staying physically active, controlling diabetes and blood pressure, and managing stress.

### Avoid Tobacco Smoke

The risk of cardiovascular disease is 70 percent greater for smokers than it is for nonsmokers. Smokers who have a heart attack are more likely to die suddenly (within 1 hour) than are nonsmokers. Evidence also indicates that chronic exposure to environmental tobacco smoke (ETS, or secondhand smoke) increases the risk of heart disease by as much as 30 percent, with over 35,000 nonsmokers dying from ETS exposure each year.[22]

How does smoking damage the heart? There are two plausible explanations. One is that nicotine increases heart rate, heart output, blood pressure, and thus oxygen use by heart muscles. The heart is forced to work harder to obtain sufficient

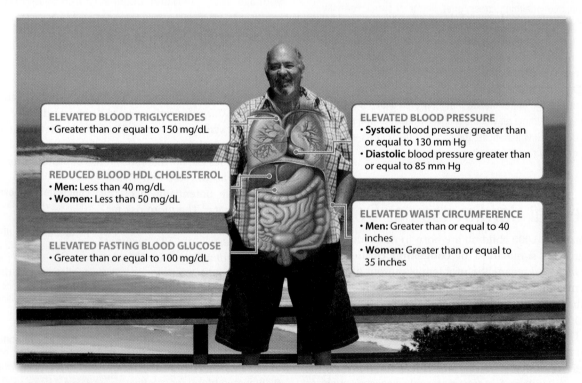

**ELEVATED BLOOD TRIGLYCERIDES**
- Greater than or equal to 150 mg/dL

**REDUCED BLOOD HDL CHOLESTEROL**
- **Men:** Less than 40 mg/dL
- **Women:** Less than 50 mg/dL

**ELEVATED FASTING BLOOD GLUCOSE**
- Greater than or equal to 100 mg/dL

**ELEVATED BLOOD PRESSURE**
- **Systolic** blood pressure greater than or equal to 130 mm Hg
- **Diastolic** blood pressure greater than or equal to 85 mm Hg

**ELEVATED WAIST CIRCUMFERENCE**
- **Men:** Greater than or equal to 40 inches
- **Women:** Greater than or equal to 35 inches

FIGURE 15.7 **Risk Factors Associated with Metabolic Syndrome**

oxygen. The other explanation is that chemicals in smoke damage and inflame the lining of the coronary arteries, allowing cholesterol and plaque to accumulate more easily, increasing blood pressure and forcing the heart to work harder.

The good news is, if you stop smoking, your heart appears to be able to mend itself. After one year, the former smoker's risk of heart disease drops by 50 percent. After 15 years, the risk drops to approximately equal that of nonsmokers. Between 5 years and 15 years, the risk of stroke is similar to that of nonsmokers.[23]

### Cut Back on Saturated Fat and Cholesterol

Cholesterol is a type of soft, waxy fat-like substance found in your bloodstream and in your body cells. Your body produces it at a rate of about 2 grams per day and thus accounts for about 75 percent of your blood cholesterol levels. The remaining 25 percent comes from your diet, usually from oils and fats. Cholesterol is carried in the blood by lipoproteins, LDL and HDL (defined below), and serves many important functions. Cholesterol plays an important role in the production of cell membranes and hormones (estrogen and testosterone), and it helps process vitamin D. However, when levels of it in the blood get too high, your risk for CVD increases.

Diets high in saturated fat and *trans* fats are known to raise cholesterol levels, send the body's blood-clotting system into high gear, and make the blood more viscous in just a few hours, increasing the risk of heart attack or stroke. Increased levels of cholesterol in the blood also contribute to atherosclerosis. Switching to a low-fat diet lowers the risk of clotting; even a 10 percent decrease in total cholesterol levels may result in an estimated 30 percent reduction in the incidence of heart disease.[24] If you have a hereditary predisposition to high cholesterol, it's even more important that you control it.

The *type* of cholesterol is just as important as total cholesterol. **Low-density lipoprotein (LDL),** often referred to as "bad" cholesterol, is believed to build up on artery walls. In contrast, **high-density lipoprotein (HDL),** or "good" cholesterol, appears to remove cholesterol from artery walls. In theory, if LDL levels get too high or HDL levels too low, cholesterol will accumulate inside arteries and lead to cardiovascular problems. Scientists now believe that there are other blood lipid factors that may also increase CVD risk, such as *lipoprotein-associated phospholipase $A_2$ (Lp-PLA$_2$)*, an enzyme that circulates in the blood and attaches to LDL. Lp-PLA$_2$ plays an important role in plaque accumulation and increased risk for stroke and coronary events, particularly in men. Studies suggest that the higher the Lp-PLA$_2$ level, the higher the risk of developing CVD.[25] Another relatively new consideration is the presence of apolipoprotein B (apo B), a primary component of LDL that is essential for cholesterol delivery to cells. Although the mechanism is unclear, some researchers believe that apo B levels may be more important to heart disease risk than total cholesterol or LDL levels.[26]

**Triglycerides** are also gaining increasing attention as a key factor in CVD risk. When you consume extra calories, the body converts the extra to triglycerides, which are stored in fat cells. Hormones release triglyercides throughout the day to provide energy. High counts of blood triglycerides are often found in people who are obese and overweight, have high cholesterol levels, heart problems, or diabetes. As they get older, heavier, or both, people's triglyceride and cholesterol levels tend to rise. It is recommended that a baseline cholesterol test (known as a lipid panel or lipid profile) be taken at age 20, with follow-ups every 5 years. The test measures triglyceride levels, HDL, LDL, and total cholesterol levels. Men over the age of 35 and women over the age of 45 should have their lipid profile checked annually, with more frequent tests for those at high risk. See Table 15.2 on page 500 for recommended levels of cholesterol and trigylcerides.

Most authorities agree that looking only at LDL ignores the positive effects of HDL. Perhaps the best method of evaluating risk is to examine the ratio of HDL to total cholesterol, or the percentage of HDL in total cholesterol. If the level of HDL is lower than 35 mg/dL, the risk increases. To reduce risk, the goal is to manage the ratio of HDL to total cholesterol by lowering LDL levels, raising HDL, or both. Regular exercise and a healthy diet low in saturated fat continue to be the best methods for maintaining healthy ratios.

Almost half of the more than 100 million Americans who have high cholesterol levels should be able to reach their LDL and HDL goals through lifestyle changes alone. People who are at higher risk or those for whom lifestyle modifications are not effective may need to take

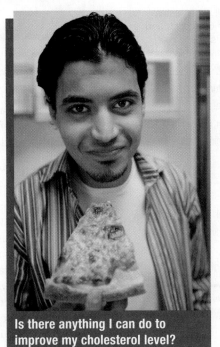

**Is there anything I can do to improve my cholesterol level?**

You get cholesterol from two primary sources: from your body (which involves genetic predisposition) and from food. Much of your cholesterol level is predetermined: 75 percent of blood cholesterol is produced by your liver and other cells, and the other 25 percent comes from the foods you eat. The good news is that the 25 percent you get from foods is the part where you can make real improvements in overall cholesterol profiles, even if you have a high genetic risk. Controlling your intake of saturated fats and *trans* fats will help you keep your cholesterol level in check.

**low-density lipoproteins (LDLs)** Compounds that facilitate the transport of cholesterol in the blood to the body's cells and cause the cholesterol to build up on artery walls.

**high-density lipoproteins (HDLs)** Compounds that facilitate the transport of cholesterol in the blood to the liver for metabolism and elimination from the body.

**triglycerides** The most common form of lipid in the body; excess calories are converted into triglycerides and stored as body fat.

TABLE

15.2 | Recommended Cholesterol Levels for Adults

| Total Cholesterol Level (lower numbers are better) | |
|---|---|
| Less than 200 mg/dL | Desirable level that puts you at lower risk for coronary heart disease. |
| 200 to 239 mg/dL | Borderline high. |
| 240 mg/dL and above | High blood cholesterol. A person with this level has more than twice the risk of coronary heart disease as someone whose cholesterol is below 200 mg/dL. |

| HDL Cholesterol Level (higher numbers are better) | |
|---|---|
| Less than 40 mg/dL (for men) Less than 50 mg/dL (for women) | Low HDL cholesterol. A major risk factor for heart disease. |
| 60 mg/dL and above | High HDL cholesterol. An HDL of 60 mg/dL and above is considered to be protective against heart disease. |

| LDL Cholesterol Level (lower numbers are better) | |
|---|---|
| Less than 100 mg/dL | Optimal |
| 100 to 129 mg/dL | Near or above optimal |
| 130 to 159 mg/dL | Borderline high |
| 160 to 189 mg/dL | High |
| 190 mg/dL and above | Very high |

| Triglyceride Level (lower numbers are better) | |
|---|---|
| Less than 150 mg/dL | Normal |
| 150–199 mg/dL | Borderline high |
| 200–499 mg/dL | High |
| 500 mg/dL and above | Very high |

**Source:** Adapted from American Heart Association, "Cholesterol Levels: AHA Recommendations," 2010, www.americanheart.org/presenter.jhtml?identifier=4500.

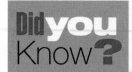

Research suggests that the cocoa flavonols in chocolate may reduce the risk of blood clots and improve blood flow in the brain!

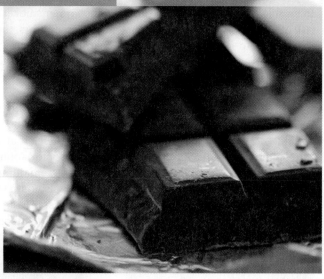

cholesterol-lowering drugs while they continue modifying their lifestyle.

## Modify Other Dietary Habits
According to recent research, over 37 percent of all Americans have added fish oil/omega 3 to their diet and another 15.9 percent have added flaxseed or flaxseed oil to their diets in an effort to reduce their risks of high cholesterol and cardiovascular disease.[27] Others routinely gulp down gallons of tea, gobble up soy in meat substitutes or drink it in soy drinks, add garlic to everything possible, and consume coenzyme Q10 to ward off heart attacks. Are these foods really helpful in reducing CVD risks? Dietary modifications such as these continue to be investigated to find real proof of their efficacy (see the **Consumer Health** box on page 502).

**plant sterols** Essential components of plant membranes that, when consumed in the diet, appear to help lower cholesterol levels.

An overall approach, such as the DASH eating plan from the National Heart, Lung, and Blood Institute (Figure 15.8), has strong evidence to back up its recommendations. The guidelines include the following dietary changes to reduce CVD risk:

- Consume 5 to 10 milligrams per day of soluble fiber from sources such as oat bran, fruits, vegetables, legumes, and psyllium seeds. Even this small dietary modification may result in a 5 percent drop in LDL levels.
- Consume about 2 grams per day of **plant sterols.**[28] Sterols are present naturally in small quantities in many fruits, vegetables, nuts, seeds, cereals, legumes, vegetable oils, and other plant sources. You can also get them from sterol derivatives in substances such as Benecol or Take Control margarine. This amount of plant sterols has the potential to reduce LDL by another 5 percent.
- Eat less sodium. Excess sodium has been linked to high blood pressure, which can in turn affect CVD risk.

See the **Skills for Behavior Change** box on page 503 for more tips on eating to maintain your heart health.

## Maintain a Healthy Weight
Overweight people are more likely to develop heart disease and stroke even if they have no other risk factors. If you're heavy, losing even 5 to 10 pounds can make a significant difference. This is especially true if you're an "apple" (thicker around your upper body and waist) rather than a "pear" (thicker around your hips and thighs). See Chapter 8 to learn how to determine if you are at a healthy weight and for more tips on weight management.

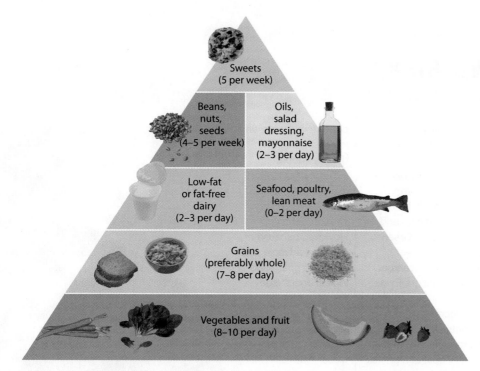

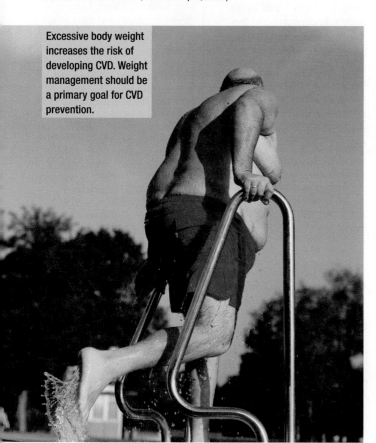

Excessive body weight increases the risk of developing CVD. Weight management should be a primary goal for CVD prevention.

FIGURE 15.8 **The DASH Eating Plan**

DASH (Dietary Approaches to Stop Hypertension) is a set of nutritional guidelines designed to reduce blood pressure. Recommended by the National Heart, Lung, and Blood Institute (NHLBI) and the American Heart Association (AHA), the plan is rich in whole grains, fruits, vegetables, and low-fat dairy products; reduces consumption of fats, red meat, sodium, sweets, and added sugars; and specifies recommended levels of potassium, magnesium, calcium, protein, and fiber.

**Source:** Data adapted from U.S. Department of Health and Human Services, National Institutes of Health, National Heart, Lung, and Blood Institute, *Your Guide to Lowering Your Blood Pressure with DASH* (NIH Publication no. 06-4082, Revised April, 2006).

**Exercise Regularly** Inactivity is a definite risk factor for CVD.[29] The good news is that you do not have to be an exercise fanatic to reduce your risk. Even modest levels of low-intensity physical activity—walking, gardening, housework, dancing—are beneficial if done regularly and over the long term. Exercise can increase HDL, lower triglycerides, and reduce coronary risks in several ways. For more information on the many health benefits of exercise, see Chapter 9.

**Control Diabetes** People with diabetes have clear risks for a wide range of CVD problems, including problems with blood flow to the extremities, retina of the eye, and the gastrointestinal (GI) tract, increased levels of inflammation, and many other concerns.[30] People with diabetes who have taken insulin for many years have a greater chance of developing CVD. In fact, CVD is the leading cause of death among diabetic patients. Because overweight people have a higher risk for diabetes, distinguishing between the effects of the two conditions is difficult. Diabetics also tend to have elevated blood fat levels, and increased atherosclerosis. However, through a prescribed regimen of diet, exercise, and medication, diabetics can control much of their increased risk for CVD. See Focus On: Minimizing Your Risk for Diabetes beginning on page 514 for more on preventing and controlling diabetes.

**Control Your Blood Pressure** Although blood pressure typically creeps up with aging, lifestyle changes can make a dramatic difference in reducing your risks. Among the most beneficial actions you can take are losing the extra pounds, cutting back sodium in your diet, exercising more, reducing alcohol intake, quitting smoking, and reducing your caffeine intake.

**Manage Psychological Factors and Stress Levels** High stress levels, chronic anxiety, depression, and high levels of anger or hostility can all impact the cardiovascular system over time. Some scientists have noted a relationship between CVD risk and a person's stress level, behaviors, and socioeconomic status. These factors may influence established risk factors. For example, people under stress may start smoking or smoke more than they otherwise would. A large study funded by the National Heart, Lung, and Blood Institute found that impatience and hostility, two key components of the Type A behavior pattern, increase young adults' risk of developing high blood pressure.[31] This research was the first to study stress and

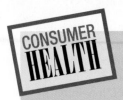

# CAN A SINGLE FOOD REDUCE CVD RISK?

Most dietary approaches to reducing cardiovascular disease (CVD) risk involve changes to your overall diet. Are there any single foods that, if you eat the right amount of them, can reduce your CVD risk? Researchers investigating garlic, tea, soy, niacin, and coenzyme Q10 report the following:

✳ **Garlic.** Despite promising results in animal studies, evidence of effectiveness is inconsistent in humans, both for raw and pill forms of garlic. When taken daily for 3 months, very large doses of garlic may inhibit platelet aggregation and modestly improve serum lipid levels. However, it is not known if this would be sufficient to reduce CVD or heart attack risk over time and there is no evidence to support garlic's use for blood pressure reduction.

✳ **Tea.** Results from a recent large meta-analysis (summary of studies) indicate that 24 ounces of tea per day resulted in an 11 percent decrease in heart attacks among high-risk individuals. If tea consumption increased to 5 cups a day, there was a 26 percent reduction in heart attack rates. It's important to note, though, that over time, studies have shown inconsistent and variable results for both black tea and

green tea. Overall, tea shows more benefits and is more protective for women; studies must be conducted to examine whether benefits are realized in all ages, in healthy and at-risk populations, and what concentrations. Green tea in particular requires considerably more research. One important caution: Excessive green tea consumption appears to decrease effects of anticoagulants such as warfarin (brand name Coumadin). People at high risk for CVD who are on these medications should consult their doctors before drinking large amounts of green tea.

✳ **Soy.** In studies in which 50 milligrams of soy were substituted for animal protein, only a 3 percent reduction in low-density lipoprotein (LDL) cholesterol was noted. Soy may not have the potent effect on CVD risk that scientists had hoped, but it is still lower in calcium and fat, and higher in protein, than many animal-based products.

✳ **Niacin.** Also known as vitamin $B_3$ or nicotinic acid, niacin has been recommended for reducing high lipid levels. Several major studies have shown significant benefits in reducing heart attack, stroke, and transient ischemic attacks (TIAs); lowering triglyceride and

cholesterol levels; and increasing high-density lipoprotein (HDL) levels. In short, it has been widely accepted as being *cardioprotective.* However, because of potential adverse side effects in pharmacological doses (see Chapter 7 for Recommended Daily Allowances), patients are advised to work closely with a physician, take lower doses of niacin, and combine those doses with other, cholesterol-lowering medications.

✳ **Coenzyme Q10.** Preliminary research has shown that coenzyme Q10 (CoQ10), a fat-soluble compound produced by the body and consumed in the diet or via supplements, may be useful in helping patients undergoing treatment for congestive heart failure. Although initial results are promising, much more research is needed before CoQ10 is widely recommended for persons with severe heart problems.

For the best advice about supplements, rely on professional groups such as the

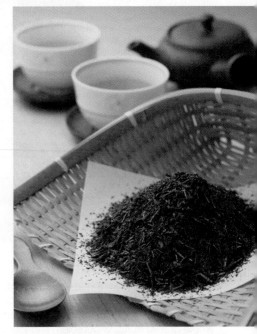

Green tea is one of several foods popular for their possible heart-healthy properties.

American Heart Association; U.S. Department of Agriculture; National Heart, Lung and Blood Institute; and the Linus Pauling Institute; and talk with your doctor.

**Sources:** The Linus Pauling Institute, "Micronutrient Information Center," 2010, http://lpi.oregonstate.edu/infocenter; Office of Dietary Supplements, Annual Bibliography of Significant Advances in Dietary Supplement Research 2007 (Bethesda, MD: U.S. Department of Health and Human Services, National Institutes of Health, 2008), NIH Publication no. 08-6456, Available at http://ods.od.nih.gov/Research/Annual_Bibliographies.aspx.

other behavioral risks together, rather than as isolated conditions and has clear implications for prevention. In recent years, scientists tend to agree that unresolved stress—whether real or perceived, personal, work-related, or from a combination of factors—appears to increase risk for hypertension, heart disease, and stroke.[32] While the exact mechanism is unknown, scientists are closer to discovering why stress can affect us so negatively. Newer studies indicate that chronic stress may

result in three times the risk of hypertension, CHD, and sudden cardiac death and that there is a link between anxiety, depression, and negative cardiovascular effects.[33]

Researcher-physician Robert S. Eliot first demonstrated over 20 years ago that approximately 1 in 5 people has an extreme cardiovascular reaction to stressful stimulation.[34] These people—called *hot reactors*—experienced alarm and resistance so strongly that, when under stress, their bodies

## Choosing Foods for Heart-Healthy Eating

Several foods have been shown to reduce the chances that cholesterol will be absorbed in the cells, reduce levels of low-density lipoprotein (LDL) cholesterol, or enhance the protective effects of high-density lipoprotein (HDL) cholesterol. To protect your heart, include the following in your diet:

✳ **Fish high in omega-3 fatty acids.** If you can't afford fresh or frozen fish, look for canned versions. Canned salmon, tuna, and many lower-cost fish pack a big dose of fish oil in an inexpensive can. Add a tablespoon of cod liver oil or other fish oil to your oil-and-vinegar salad dressings, chili, or other places where you can hide the taste!

✳ **Get your omega-3 the easy way.** Add a tablespoon of crushed flaxseed to your salad or cereal, bake it in your banana breads or muffins, or spread it on toast with peanut butter.

✳ **Use monounsaturated fats in cooking.** Extra virgin olive oil is one of the best oils for lowering cholesterol and raising your HDL levels. Use it on salads, in cooking, and in dips. "Butter" your bread with small amounts of fresh olive oil and satisfy your cravings. Canola oil; margarine labeled "*trans* fat free"; and cholesterol-lowering margarines such as Benecol, Promise Activ, or Smart Balance are also excellent choices.

✳ **Eat whole grains and fiber.** Make sure to buy products labeled "100% whole wheat." Avoid products labeled "multi-grain" or that include ingredients that sound only vaguely healthy, such as "wheat flour" or "enriched flour."

✳ **Plant sterols.** Look for juices and yogurts that are fortified with sterols. Eat more vegetables, particularly those that grow on stalks, such as broccoli and Brussels sprouts.

✳ **Nuts.** Buy nuts in bulk. Keep them refrigerated or in airtight containers. Pack a small plastic bag of 20 almonds or walnuts and have 5 or so as a snack with a glass of water or good quality juice. Use nuts in pancakes and cookies. Sprinkle chopped nuts in your oatmeal or other cereal for an added protein benefit each day.

✳ **Chocolate and red wine.** If you drink wine, make it red. Remember, more isn't more beneficial: One glass is best. If you like chocolate, go dark. Red wine and dark chocolate might be an excellent treat—in moderation—for achieving your health goals for 1 month.

**Sources:** A. Mente et al., "A Systematic Review of the Evidence Supporting a Causal Link between Dietary Factors and Coronary Heart Disease," *Archives of Internal Medicine* 169, no. 7 (2009): 659–69; L. Hooper et al., "Flavonoids, Flavonoid-Rich Foods, and Cardiovascular Risk: A Meta-Analysis of Randomized Controlled Trials," *American Journal of Clinical Nutrition* 88, no. 1 (2008): 38–50; E. Corti et al., "Cocoa and Cardiovascular Health," *Circulation* 119, no. 10 (2009):1433–41; R. Corder, "Red Wine, Chocolate and Vascular Health: Developing the Evidence Base," *Heart* 94, no. 7 (2008): 821–23.

produced large amounts of stress chemicals, which in turn caused tremendous changes in the cardiovascular system, including remarkable increases in blood pressure. Although their blood pressure may be normal when they are not under stress—for example, in a doctor's office—it increased dramatically in response to even small amounts of everyday tension. *Cold reactors* (even those with Type A personalities) were those who could experience stress without showing harmful cardiovascular responses. Cold reactors may internalize stress, but their self-talk and perceptions about the stressful events lead them to a nonresponse state in which their cardiovascular system remains virtually unaffected.

More recent studies suggest that personality does play a role in coping, both positively and negatively. Some research indicates that people who are chronically hostile may be at greatest risk for CVD. A new study points out that it may be that optimism is most important in lowering CVD risk, particularly for women. In a study of nearly 100,000 women over the age of 50, researchers found that optimistic women, compared to pessimistic women, had a 9 percent lower risk of developing heart disease and a 14 percent lower risk of dying from any cause. Pessimistic African-American women, in particular, had a higher risk of dying in the study.[35]

### What's Working for You?

Maybe you're already managing the modifiable risks to your heart's health. Which of the things below are you already incorporating into your life?

☐ I don't smoke.

☐ I eat a balanced diet.

☐ My family has a history of hypertension, so I monitor my blood pressure and control salt in my diet.

☐ I'm trying to get organized to reduce my stress levels.

## Nonmodifiable Risks

There are, unfortunately, some risk factors for CVD that we cannot prevent or control. The most important are the following:

● **Race and ethnicity.** Health disparities in CVD death rates continue to decline; however, significant differences persist. White Americans have the highest overall rate of heart disease in the United States, followed closely by African Americans. In contrast, Asian American/Pacific Islanders have the highest rates of hypertension, followed by African Americans. See Figure 15.9 on page 504 for a summary of the percentages of total deaths for various races by heart disease and stroke.

● **Heredity.** A family history of heart disease appears to increase the risk of CVD significantly. As stated previously, the amount of cholesterol you produce, tendencies to form plaque, and a host of other factors seem to have genetic links. If you have close relatives with CVD, your risk may be double that of others. Clearly, those who have identified genetic risks may need to work harder to reduce future risks, whether it means dietary changes, exercise increases, or new medications designed to reduce risks.

● **Age.** Although cardiovascular disease can affect people of any age, 75 percent of all heart attacks occur in people over

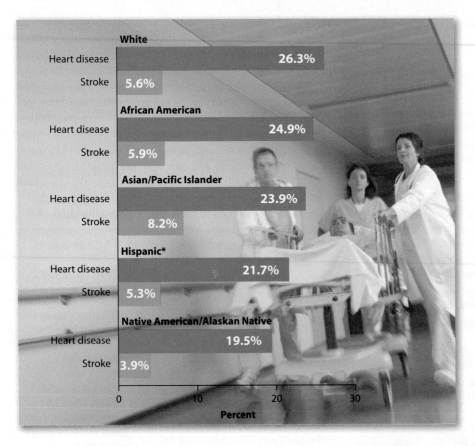

FIGURE 15.9 **Deaths from Heart Disease and Stroke in the United States by Ethnicity**

*Persons of Hispanic origin may be of any race.

**Source:** Data are from M. Heron, "Deaths: Leading Causes for 2006,"*National Vital Statistics Reports* 58, no. 14 (Hyattsville, MD: National Center for Health Statistics, 2010): 1–100.

---

date, several factors, including cigarette smoke, high blood pressure, high LDL cholesterol, diabetes mellitus, certain forms of arthritis, and exposure to toxic substances, have all been linked to increased risk of inflammation. However, the greatest risk appears to be from certain infectious disease pathogens, most notably *Chlamydia pneumoniae*, a common cause of respiratory infections; *Helicobacter pylori* (a bacterium that causes ulcers); herpes simplex virus (a virus that most of us have been exposed to); and *cytomegalovirus* (another herpes virus infecting most Americans before the age of 40). During an inflammatory reaction, C-reactive proteins (CRPs) tend to be present at high levels. Many scientists believe the presence of these proteins in the blood may signal elevated risk for angina and heart attack even though evidence that you can prevent CHD by reducing inflammatory processes is lacking.[37] Doctors can test patients

age 65. Increasing rates of obesity, diabetes, hypertension, and CVD risk factors among the young are reasons for concern.

● **Gender.** Men are at greater risk for CVD until about age 60, when women catch up and then surpass them. Women under age 35 have a fairly low risk unless they have high blood pressure, kidney problems, or diabetes. Using oral contraceptives and smoking also increase the risk. Hormonal factors appear to reduce risk for women, although after menopause or after estrogen levels are otherwise reduced (for example, because of hysterectomy), women's LDL levels tend to go up, which increases their chances for CVD.

## Other Risk Factors

Several other factors and indicators have been linked to CVD risk, including inflammation and homocysteine levels.

**Inflammation and C-Reactive Protein** Recent research has prompted many experts to believe that inflammation may play a major role in atherosclerosis development.[36] Inflammation occurs when tissues are injured, for example by bacteria, trauma, toxins, or heat. Injured vessel walls are more prone to plaque formation. To

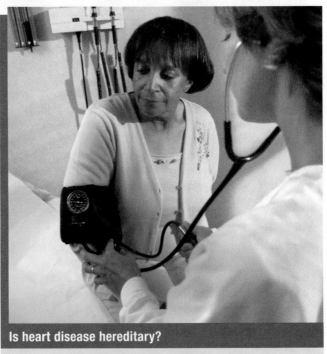

**Is heart disease hereditary?**

Many behavioral and environmental factors contribute to a person's risk for cardiovascular diseases, but research suggests that there are hereditary aspects as well. If there is a history of CVD in your family or your racial or ethnic background indicates a propensity for CVD, it is all the more important for you to have regular blood pressure and blood cholesterol screenings, and for you to avoid lifestyle risks including tobacco use, physical inactivity, and poor nutrition.

using a highly sensitive assay called hs-CRP; if levels are high, action could be taken to prevent progression to a heart attack or other coronary event.[38]

**Homocysteine** Homocysteine, an amino acid normally present in the blood, also appears to increase risk for coronary heart disease, stroke, and peripheral vascular disease as levels increase in the blood. Although research is still in its infancy in this area, scientists hypothesize that homocysteine works in much the same way as CRP, inflaming the inner lining of the arterial walls and promoting fat deposits on the damaged walls and development of blood clots.[39] Folic acid and other B vitamins may help break down homocysteine in the body; however, conclusive evidence of risk reduction from folic acid is not available, and authorities such as the American Heart Association do not currently recommend taking folic acid supplements to lower homocysteine levels and prevent CVD.[40] For now, a healthy, balanced diet that includes at least five servings of fruits and vegetables a day is the best preventive action.

> Tomatoes, citrus fruit, vegetables, and fortified grain products are good sources of the daily recommended 400 micrograms of folic acid, which is believed to help lower blood levels of homocysteine.

# Diagnosing, Treating, and Recovering from Cardiovascular Disease

Today, CVD patients have many diagnostic, treatment, prevention, and rehabilitation options. Medications can strengthen heartbeat, control arrhythmias, remove fluids, reduce blood pressure, and improve heart function. *Statins* can be used to lower blood cholesterol levels, *ace-inhibitors* can lower blood pressure by causing the muscles surrounding blood vessels to contract, and *beta-blockers* can reduce blood pressure by blocking the effects of the hormone epinephrine. Long-standing methods of cardiopulmonary resuscitation (CPR) have also changed recently to focus primarily on chest compressions rather than mouth-to-mouth procedures. The thinking behind this is that people will be more likely to do CPR if the risk for exchange of body fluids is reduced, and any effort to save a person in trouble is better than inaction.

## Techniques for Diagnosing Cardiovascular Disease

Electrocardiogram, angiography, and positron emission tomography scans are some techniques for diagnosing CVD. An **electrocardiogram (ECG)** is a record of the heart's

electrical activity. Patients may undergo a *stress test*—standard exercise on a stationary bike or treadmill with an electrocardiogram and no injections—or a *nuclear stress test,* which involves injecting a radioactive dye and taking images of the heart to reveal problems with blood flow. Although these tests provide a good indicator of potential heart blockage or blood flow abnormalities, a more accurate method of testing for heart disease is **angiography** (also referred to as *cardiac catheterization*), in which a needle-thin tube called a *catheter* is threaded through heart arteries, a dye is injected, and an X ray is taken to discover which areas are blocked. A more recent and even more effective method of measuring heart activity is a **positron emission tomography (PET) scan,** which produces three-dimensional images of the heart as blood flows through it. During a PET scan, a patient receives an intravenous injection of a radioactive tracer at rest and during exercise. As the tracer decays, it emits positrons that are picked up by the scanner and transformed by a computer into color images of the heart. Newer *single-photon emission computed tomography* (*SPECT*) scans provide an even better view. Other tests include the following:

**electrocardiogram (ECG)** A record of the electrical activity of the heart; may be measured during a stress test.
**angiography** A technique for examining blockages in heart arteries.
**positron emission tomography (PET) scan** Method for measuring heart activity by injecting a patient with a radioactive tracer that is scanned electronically to produce a three-dimensional image of the heart and arteries.

- *Radionuclide imaging* procedures involve injecting small nuclear isotopes or *radionuclides* into the bloodstream that aggregate in tissue and aid in imaging.

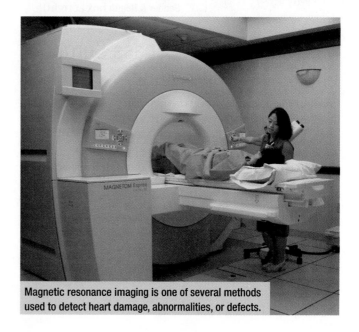

Magnetic resonance imaging is one of several methods used to detect heart damage, abnormalities, or defects.

Computer-generated pictures can then show blockages in the heart and reveal how well the heart muscle is supplied with blood, how well the heart's chambers are functioning, and which part of the heart has been damaged by a heart attack.

● *Magnetic resonance imaging* (*MRI*) involves using powerful magnets to look inside the body. Computer-generated pictures can show the heart muscle and help physicians identify damage from a heart attack, diagnose congenital heart defects, and evaluate disease of larger blood vessels such as the aorta.

● *Ultrafast computed tomography* (*CT*), an especially fast form of heart X ray, can be used to evaluate bypass grafts, diagnose ventricular function, and identify other heart irregularities.

● *Coronary calcium score* is derived from another type of ultrafast CT used to diagnose levels of calcium in heart vessels. Calcium accumulations on vessel walls provide an indication of plaque formation and heart attack risks; however, most people will show some level of calcium accumulation.

● *Digital subtraction angiography* (*DSA*). This modified form of computer-aided imaging records pictures of the heart and its blood vessels.

There may be important differences between men and women in their diagnosis and treatment of CVD (see the **Gender & Health** box at right).

## what do you think?

Do any of your relatives have heart disease? With all the new diagnostic procedures, treatments, and differing philosophies about various prevention and intervention techniques, how do they ensure that they will get the best treatment? ● Where do they go for information?

## Surgical Options: Bypass Surgery, Angioplasty, and Stents

**Coronary bypass surgery** has helped many patients who suffered coronary blockages or heart attacks. In a coronary artery bypass graft (CABG, referred to as a "cabbage"), a blood vessel is taken from another site in the patient's body (usually the saphenous vein in the leg or the internal thoracic artery [ITA] in the chest) and implanted to "bypass" blocked coronary arteries and transport blood to heart tissue.

Another procedure, **angioplasty** (sometimes called *balloon angioplasty*), carries fewer risks and may be more effective than bypass surgery in selected cases. As in angiography, a thin catheter is threaded through blocked heart arteries. The catheter has a balloon at the tip, which is inflated to flatten fatty deposits against the arterial walls, allowing blood to flow more freely.

Today, many people with heart blockage undergo angioplasty and have a **stent** inserted to hold the vessel open after the procedure. A stent is a stainless steel, meshlike tube that is inserted to prop open the artery. Although stents are highly effective, inflammation and tissue growth in the area may actually increase after the procedure, leading to blockage. In 30 to 60 percent of people who receive a stent, the gradual buildup of material around the stent can be large enough to cause the blockage to return to its original (or worse) severity. This buildup occurs over a 6-week to 6-month period and is known as *restenosis*.[41] Newer stents are usually medicated to reduce this risk.

Some patients may undergo the procedure as many as three times within a 5-year period. Some surgeons argue that given this high rate of recurrence, bypass may be a more effective treatment. Today, newer forms of laser angioplasty and *atherectomy,* a procedure that removes plaque, are being done in several clinics.

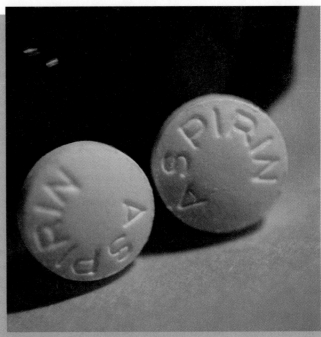

**Can aspirin really help prevent heart disease?**

Americans bought more than 44 million packages of low-dose aspirin marketed for heart protection last year. In 2007, the American Heart Association recommended regular aspirin intake for its blood-thinning qualities, and in 2009, the Agency for Healthcare Research and Quality (AHRQ) recommended that men aged 45 to 79 take low-dose aspirin for heart attack prevention and women aged 55 to 79 take it to prevent stroke risks. Concerns over aspirin's side effects, which can include bleeding ulcers, ringing in the ears, brain bleeding, increased surgical bleeding risks, and other gastrointestinal tract issues, have surfaced. Others argue that people with multiple risk factors, such as diabetes, high blood pressure, and obesity, may benefit more from taking low-dose aspirin than not taking it. Talk to your doctor if you are trying to determine whether to start or stop aspirin therapy.

## Gender&Health

# Key Gender Differences in CVD Detection and Prognosis

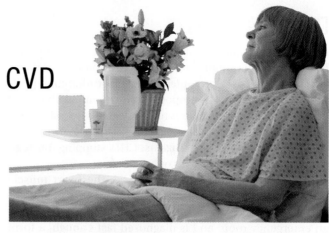

As more research is done concerning diagnosis and treatment of cardiovascular disease (CVD), it is clear that women differ from men in the symptoms they experience and the different treatments they require.

## FEELING PAIN DIFFERENTLY

Several studies have documented that women experience pain more acutely and frequently than men do, indicating that the sexes may detect and react to pain differently, and react differently to pain medications. Women reported worse pain intensity, greater pain-related interference with function, and more disability due to pain. They also had worse depression, anxiety, and more disability days due to pain. This finding suggests that receptors for inhibiting pain may vary by sex. Also, women appear to be less responsive than men to non-steroidal anti-inflammatory drugs (NSAIDs) such as ibuprofen. Finally, women typically need slightly lower doses of aspirin and should be warned that taking 325 milligrams of aspirin per day may result in anticoagulation levels that exceed those of men.

## HEART ATTACK SYMPTOMS CAN VARY BY GENDER

We are taught that the classic symptom of a heart attack is chest-crushing pain. However, this symptom is not that common in women. Women's heart attacks tend to exhibit as shortness of breath, weakness, unusual fatigue, cold sweats, dizziness, and pain or pressure in the back or high chest. Women tend to suffer their first heart attack 10 years later than men do; and, in part because they are older when they have these attacks, they are more likely to die. Overall, women tend not to fare as well, with more adverse outcomes, death, repeat heart attacks, stroke, or re-hospitalization.

## DIFFERENCES IN TREATMENT OF HEART DISEASE IN WOMEN

During the past decade, research has suggested that a combination of lack of awareness among women and less aggressive and sophisticated diagnosis and treatment for women may contribute to their poorer CVD outcomes. Some explanations for diagnostic and therapeutic difficulties that women encounter include the following:

✳ Delay in diagnosing a possible heart attack. Women have historically not been referred as often for diagnostic testing that men would routinely receive.
✳ Among Medicare patients, men are two to three times as likely as women to receive an implantable cardioverter defibrillator for prevention of sudden cardiac death.
✳ When women are given cardiac medications, they do not seem to work as effectively as they do in men. Drugs that are beneficial for men may even be harmful to women. For example, the drug digoxin used to treat patients with heart failure was associated with an increased risk of death among women but not men.

✳ A new study has raised alarms in the health community as it seems to show that long-standing recommendations for women to take calcium supplements may, in fact, prove detrimental to cardiovascular health even though calcium may prevent osteoporosis.
✳ Women's coronary arteries are often smaller than men's, making surgical or diagnostic procedures more difficult.

## GENDER BIAS IN CVD RESEARCH?

The traditional view that heart disease is primarily a male problem has carried over into research as well. Historically, CVD studies and clinical trials have often been done with inadequate numbers of women or no women at all. In fact, women represented just 38 percent or fewer subjects in National Institutes of Health (NIH)–funded cardiovascular research up until 2004. Although rates are improving, they are still not equal to men's study rates. In addition, three-quarters of recent CVD clinical trials have failed to report sex-specific results, making it difficult to determine where differences between the sexes may occur. It wasn't until it became evident that heart disease is also a women's disease, and that women as a rule were understudied in the research, that a national effort to mandate equal research funding and studies was implemented. The NIH has launched the Women's Health Initiative, a 15-year, $625 million study of 140,000 postmenopausal women, focusing on the leading causes of death and disease. This research is largely responsible for what we now know about the unique differences between men and women in CVD outcomes.

**Sources:** American Heart Association, "Heart Disease and Stroke Statistics—2010 Update: A Report from the American Heart Association," *Circulation* 121, no. 7 (2010): e46–e215, Available at http://circ.ahajournals.org/cgi/content/full/121/7/e46; American Heart Association, "Facts: Cardiovascular Disease: Women's No. 1 Health Threat," 2009, www.americanheart.org/presenter.jhtml?identifier=3039317; L. Mosca et al., "Twelve-Year Follow-Up of American Women's Awareness of Cardiovascular Disease Risk and Barriers to Heart Health," *Circulation: Cardiovascular Quality and Outcomes* 3, no. 2 (2010): 120–27; R. Gear et al., "Kappa-opioids Produce Significantly Greater Analgesia in Women Than in Men," *Nature Medicine* 2, no. 11 (1996): 1248–50; L. Stutts et al., "Sex Differences in Prior Pain Experience," *Journal of Pain* 10, no. 12 (2009): 1226–30; D. Stubbs et al., "Sex Differences in Pain and Pain-Related Disability among Primary Care Patients with Chronic Musculoskeletal Pain," *Pain Medicine* 11, no. 2 (2010): 232–39; S. Day et al., "Sex-Related Differences in the Presentation, Treatment and Outcomes among Patients with Acute Coronary Syndromes: The Global Registry of Acute Coronary Events," *Heart* 95 (2009): 20–26; C. Melloni et al., "Representation of Women in Randomized Clinical Trials of Cardiovascular Disease Prevention," *Circulation: Cardiovascular Quality and Outcomes* 3, no. 2 (2010): 135–42; M. Bolland et al., "Effect of Calcium Supplements on Risk of Myocardial Infarction and Cardiovascular Events: Meta-analysis," *BMJ* 341 (2010): c3691.

## Drug Therapies

Research is ongoing into drugs that may offer some hope for heart attack prevention and reduction of harm from heart attack. Aspirin has been touted for its blood-thinning qualities, although even its proponents recommend that only people of certain ages take it regularly, due to possible side effects. Furthermore, once a patient has taken aspirin regularly for possible protection against CHD, stopping this regimen may, in fact, increase his or her risk.[42]

When a coronary artery is blocked, the heart muscle doesn't die immediately. Time determines how much damage occurs, and prompt action is vital. If a victim reaches an emergency room and is diagnosed fast enough, a form of clot-busting therapy called **thrombolysis** can be performed. Thrombolysis involves injecting an agent such as *tissue plasminogen activator* (*tPA*) to dissolve the clot and restore some blood flow, thereby reducing the amount of tissue that dies from ischemia.[43] These drugs must be administered within 1 to 3 hours after a heart attack for best results.

**thrombolysis** Injection of an agent to dissolve clots and restore some blood flow, thereby reducing the amount of tissue that dies from ischemia.

## Cardiac Rehabilitation and Recovery

Every year, more than 1 million Americans survive heart attacks. Over 7 million more have unstable angina, approximately 1.43 million have angioplasty, 448,000 have bypass procedures, 1.2 million have diagnostic angiograms, nearly 100,000 receive implantable defibrillators, and nearly 200,000 have pacemakers implanted to keep their hearts working properly.[44] Many patients leave the hospital with varying degrees of heart failure and fear of future cardiac problems. Although most of these patients are eligible for cardiac rehabilitation (including exercise training and health education classes on good nutrition and CVD risk management), and only need a doctor's prescription for these services, many will not attend these programs. Either they lack insurance, lack transportation, lack facilities close to their home, or face other barriers. Perhaps the biggest deterrent is fear of having another attack due to exercise. The benefits of cardiac rehabilitation (including increased stamina and strength and faster recovery), however, far out-

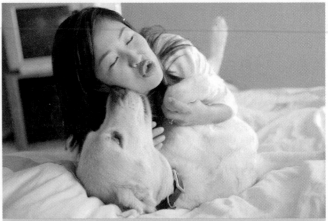

Stress reduction is an important part of recovery from a cardiac event. Having a pet is one way to focus on something other than your medical condition.

weigh the risks when these programs are run by certified health professionals.

People who suspect they have cardiovascular disease are often overwhelmed and frightened. Where should they go for diagnosis? What are the best treatments? Should they stay closer to home for ease of treatment and family assistance, or should they travel to a top-notch facility in another city or state? What are their options? Answering these questions becomes even more difficult if they are upset, scared, or tend to listen unquestioningly to doctors' orders. Usually, it is a son or daughter (particularly those in college and computer savvy) who is called on to be a personal advocate, do the behind-the-scenes research, and help with decision making and follow-up. If you are called on to help, having the information in this chapter will help. In addition, the information in Chapter 18 focused on maneuvering in an increasingly complex health care system will be invaluable.

We still have much to learn about CVD and its causes, treatments, and risk factors. Staying informed is an important part of staying healthy. Good dietary habits, regular exercise, stress management, prompt attention to suspicious symptoms, and other healthy behaviors will greatly enhance your chances of remaining CVD free. Other factors that influence risk include how much emphasis our health care systems place on access to health care for all underserved populations, education about risk, and other community-based interventions. Action on both community and individual levels can help address the challenge of CVD.

# Assess yourself

## What's Your Personal CVD Risk?

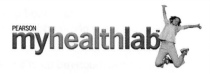

Each of us has a unique level of risk for various diseases, including cardiovascular disease. Answer each of the following questions and total your points in each section.

Fill out this assessment online at
www.pearsonhighered.com/myhealthlab or
www.pearsonhighered.com/donatelle.

## 1 Your Family Risk for CVD

| | Yes (1 point) | No (0 points) | Don't Know |
|---|---|---|---|
| 1. Do any of your primary relatives (parents, grandparents, siblings) have a history of heart disease or stroke? | ○ | ○ | ○ |
| 2. Do any of your primary relatives have diabetes? | ○ | ○ | ○ |
| 3. Do any of your primary relatives have high blood pressure? | ○ | ○ | ○ |
| 4. Do any of your primary relatives have a history of high cholesterol? | ○ | ○ | ○ |
| 5. Would you say that your family consumed a high-fat diet (lots of red meat, whole dairy, butter/margarine) during your time spent at home? | ○ | ○ | ○ |

**Total points:** _____

## 2 Your Lifestyle Risk for CVD

| | Yes (1 point) | No (0 points) | Don't Know |
|---|---|---|---|
| 1. Is your total cholesterol level higher than it should be? | ○ | ○ | ○ |
| 2. Do you have high blood pressure? | ○ | ○ | ○ |
| 3. Have you been diagnosed as pre-diabetic or diabetic? | ○ | ○ | ○ |
| 4. Do you smoke? | ○ | ○ | ○ |
| 5. Would you describe your life as being highly stressful? | ○ | ○ | ○ |

**Total points:** _____

## 3 Your Additional Risks for CVD

1. How would you best describe your current weight?
   a. Lower than what it should be for my height (0 points)
   b. About what it should be for my height (0 points)
   c. Higher than what it should be for my height (1 point)

2. How would you describe the level of exercise that you get each day?
   a. Less than what I should be exercising each day (1 point)
   b. About what I should be exercising each day (0 points)
   c. More than what I should be exercising each day (0 points)

3. How would you describe your dietary behaviors?
   a. Eating only the recommended number of calories each day (0 points)
   b. Eating less than the recommended number of calories each day (0 points)
   c. Eating more than the recommended number of calories each day (1 point)

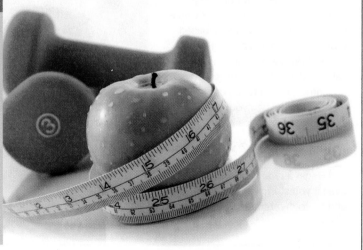

4. Which of the following statements best describes your typical dietary behavior?

    a. I eat from the major food groups, especially trying to get the recommended fruits and vegetables. (0 points)

    b. I eat too much red meat and consume too much saturated and *trans* fats from meat, dairy products, and processed foods each day. (1 point)

    c. Whenever possible, I try to substitute olive oil or canola oil for other forms of dietary fat. (0 points)

5. Which of the following (if any) describes you?

    a. I watch my sodium intake and try to reduce stress in my life. (0 points)

    b. I have a history of chlamydia infection. (1 point)

    c. I try to eat 5 to 10 milligrams of soluble fiber each day and to substitute a soy product for an animal product in my diet at least once each week. (0 points)

**Total points:** _____

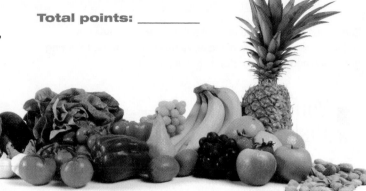

## Scoring

If you score between 1 and 5 in any section, consider your risk. The higher the number you've scored, the greater your risk is. If you answered "don't know" for any question, talk to your parents or other family members as soon as possible to find out if you have any unknown risks.

# YOUR PLAN FOR CHANGE

The **Assessyourself** activity evaluated your risk of heart disease. Based on your results and the advice of your physician, you may need to take steps to reduce your risk of CVD.

## Today, you can:

◯ Get up and move! Take a walk in the evening, use the stairs instead of the escalator, or ride your bike to class. Start thinking of ways you can incorporate more physical activity into your daily routine.

◯ Begin improving your dietary habits by eating a healthier dinner. Replace the meat and processed foods you might normally eat with a serving of fresh fruit or soy-based protein and green leafy vegetables. Think about the amounts of saturated and *trans* fats you consume—which foods contain them, and how can you reduce consumption of these items?

## Within the next 2 weeks, you can:

◯ Begin a regular exercise program, even if you start slowly. Set small goals and try to meet them. See Chapter 9 for ideas.

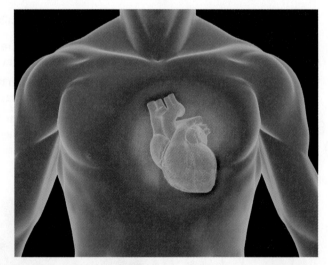

◯ Practice a new stress management technique. For example, learn how to meditate. See Chapter 3 for other ideas for managing stress.

◯ Get enough rest. Make sure you get at least 8 hours of sleep per night.

## By the end of the semester, you can:

◯ Find out your hereditary risk for CVD. Call your parents and find out if your grandparents or aunts or uncles developed CVD. Ask if they know their latest cholesterol LDL/HDL levels. Do you have a family history of diabetes?

◯ Have your own cholesterol and blood pressure levels checked. Once you know your levels, you'll have a better sense of what risk factors to address. If your levels are high, talk to your doctor about how to reduce them.

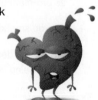

# Summary

* The cardiovascular system consists of the heart and circulatory system and is a carefully regulated, integrated network of vessels that supplies the body with the nutrients and oxygen necessary to perform daily functions.
* Rates of cardiovascular disease vary among different groups in the United States. Cardiovascular diseases include atherosclerosis, coronary artery disease, peripheral artery disease, coronary heart disease, stroke, hypertension, angina pectoris, arrhythmias, congestive heart failure, and congenital and rheumatic heart disease. These combine to make CVD the leading cause of death in the United States today.
* *Cardiometabolic risks* refer to combined factors that increase a person's chances of CVD and diabetes. A person who possesses three or more cardiometabolic risk factors may have metabolic syndrome.
* Many risk factors for cardiovascular disease can be modified, such as cigarette smoking, high blood cholesterol and triglyceride levels, hypertension, lack of exercise, a diet high in saturated fat, obesity, diabetes, and emotional stress. Some risk factors, such as age, gender, and heredity, cannot be modified. Many of these factors have a compounded effect when combined.
* New methods developed for treating heart blockages include coronary bypass surgery and angioplasty with the use of stents. Drug therapies can be used to prevent and treat CVD.

# Pop Quiz

1. The heart's upper chambers are called the
   a. valves.
   b. ventricles.
   c. atria.
   d. sinoatrial node.

2. Which of the following is NOT correct about aspirin?
   a. It can cause gastrointestinal tract bleeding, increased surgical risks, and ulcers.
   b. It is recommended for all college students who are overweight.
   c. It has been shown to reduce risks of stroke in older women.
   d. It seems to reduce risks by "thinning" the blood.

3. What does a person's cholesterol level indicate?
   a. The formation of fatty substances, called *plaque*, which can clog the arteries
   b. The level of triglycerides in the blood, which can increase risk of coronary disease
   c. Hypertension, which leads to thickening and hardening of the arteries
   d. None of the above

4. CVD kills more Americans every year than which of the following?
   a. Breast cancer
   b. Respiratory diseases
   c. Lung cancer
   d. All of the above

5. A stroke results
   a. when a heart stops beating.
   b. when cardiopulmonary resuscitation has failed to revive the stopped heart.
   c. when blood flow in the brain has been compromised, either due to blockage or hemorrhage.
   d. when blood pressure rises above 120/80 mm Hg.

6. An irregularity in the heartbeat is called a(n)
   a. fibrillation.
   b. bradycardia.
   c. tachycardia.
   d. arrhythmia.

7. The "bad" type of cholesterol found in the bloodstream is known as
   a. high-density lipoprotein (HDL).
   b. low-density lipoprotein (LDL).
   c. total cholesterol.
   d. triglyceride.

8. Ken's physician informed him that he has hypertension and must work at lowering it to avoid a possible heart attack. Possible strategies include
   a. decreasing sodium.
   b. increasing levels of exercise.
   c. practicing stress management/control.
   d. All of the above

9. Severe chest pain due to reduced oxygen flow to the heart is called
   a. angina pectoris.
   b. arrhythmias.
   c. myocardial infarction.
   d. congestive heart failure.

10. Which of the following is *correct* about metabolic syndrome?
    a. It is decreasing among the general population both in the United States and globally.
    b. It lowers your risk of cardiovascular disease.
    c. High fasting blood glucose, obesity, high triglyceride levels, hypertension, and other risks are part of the symptoms often experienced.
    d. All of the above

*Answers to these questions can be found on page A-1.*

# Think about It!

1. Which risk factors for CVD are modifiable? Which ones are *not*? What are your risks right now for CVD? How are these affected by your family medical history? How might you lower your risks in the next year?
2. List the different types of CVD. Compare and contrast their symptoms, risk factors, prevention, and treatment.
3. Why do you think hypertension rates are rising among today's college students?

4. Discuss the role that exercise, stress management, dietary changes, medical checkups, sodium reduction, and other factors can play in reducing risk for CVD. What role might chronic infections play in CVD risk?

5. Discuss why age is an important factor in women's risk for CVD. Do men face the same age-related risks? Why or why not? What can be done to decrease women's risk in later life?

6. Describe some of the diagnostic, preventive, and treatment alternatives for CVD. Who should be taking a low-dose aspirin each day? Why? If you had a heart attack today, which treatment would you prefer? Explain why.

# Accessing Your Health on the Internet

The following websites explore further topics and issues related to personal health. For links to the websites below, visit the Companion Website for *Access to Health*, 12th Edition, at www.pearsonhighered.com/donatelle.

1. *American Heart Association.* This is the home page of the leading private organization dedicated to heart health. This site provides information, statistics, and resources regarding cardiovascular care, including an opportunity to test your risk for CVD. www.heart.org

2. *National Heart, Lung, and Blood Institute.* This valuable resource provides information on all aspects of cardiovascular health and wellness. www.nhlbi.nih.gov

3. *Global Cardiovascular Infobase.* This site contains epidemiological data and statistics for cardiovascular diseases for countries throughout the world, with a focus on developing nations. www.cvdinfobase.ca

# References

1. American Heart Association, "Heart Disease and Stroke Statistics—2010 Update: A Report from the American Heart Association," *Circulation* 121, no. 7 (2010): e46–e215, Available at http://circ.ahajournals.org/cgi/content/full/121/7/e46.
2. Ibid.
3. Ibid.
4. Ibid.
5. Ibid.
6. American Heart Association, "Statistical Fact Sheet—Populations 2009 Update: International Cardiovascular Disease Statistics," 2009, Available at www.americanheart.org/presenter.jhtml?identifier=3001008.
7. World Health Organization, "Cardiovascular Disease: Prevention and Control," World Health Organization Global Strategy on Diet, Physical Activity, and Health, 2008, www.who.int/dietphysicalactivity/publications/facts/cvd/en; American Heart Association, "Heart Disease and Stroke Statistics," 2010.
8. American Heart Association, "Heart Disease and Stroke Statistics," 2010.
9. Ibid.
10. Ibid.
11. Ibid.
12. Ibid.
13. National Heart, Lung and Blood Institute. "Angina: What Is Angina?" Revised March 2010, www.nhlbi.nih.gov/health/dci/Diseases/Angina/Angina_WhatIs.html.
14. American Heart Association, "Heart Disease and Stroke Statistics," 2010.
15. Ibid.
16. Ibid.
17. J. Arnlov et al., "Impact of Body Mass Index and the Metabolic Syndrome on the Risks of CVD and Death in Middle-aged Men," *Circulation* 121, no. 2 (2010): 230–36; D. Conen et al., "Metabolic Syndrome, Inflammation, and Risk of Symptomatic Peripheral Artery Disease in Women: A Prospective Study," *Circulation* 120, no. 12 (2009): 1041–47; J. Després et al., "Abdominal Obesity and Metabolic Syndrome: Contribution to Global Cardiometabolic Risk," *Arteriosclerosis, Thrombosis, and Vascular Biology* 28, no. 6 (2008): 1039–49; S. Haffner, "Epidemiology of Cardiometabolic Diseases," *Mechanisms and Syndromes of Cardiometabolic Disease: Emerging Science in Atherosclerosis Hypertension and Diabetes*, 2008, Medscape CME, http://cme.medscape.com/viewprogram/8704; American Heart Association, "Heart Disease and Stroke Statistics," 2010; J. Rosenzwigg et al., "Primary Prevention of Cardiovascular Disease and Type 2 Diabetes in Patients at Metabolic Risk: An Endocrine Society Clinical Practice Guideline," *Journal of Clinical Endocrinology and Metabolism* 93, no. 10 (2008): 3671–89.
18. S. Haffner, "Epidemiology of Cardiometabolic Diseases," 2009; J. Després et al., "Abdominal Obesity and Metabolic Syndrome," 2008; A. Gami et al., "Metabolic Syndrome and Risk of Incident Cardiovascular Events and Death: A Systematic Review and Meta-Analysis of Longitudinal Studies," *Journal of the American College of Cardiology* 49, no. 4 (2007): 403–14; T. Horwich and G. Fonarow, "Glucose, Obesity, Metabolic Syndrome, and Diabetes: Relevance to Incidence of Heart Failure," *Journal of the American College of Cardiology* 55, no. 4 (2010): 283–93.
19. National Heart, Lung, and Blood Institute, "Metabolic Syndrome: What Is Metabolic Syndrome?" Revised January 2010, www.nhlbi.nih.gov/health/dci/Diseases/ms/ms_whatis.html.
20. Ibid.
21. U. R. Ximena et al., "High Blood Pressure in Schoolchildren: Prevalence and Risk Factors," *BMC Pediatrics* 6 (2006): 32; R. Din-Dzietham et al., "High Blood Pressure Trends in Children and Adolescents in National Surveys, 1963 to 2002," *Circulation* 116, no. 13 (2007): 1488–96; T. Huang et al., "Metabolic Syndrome and Related Disorders in College Students: Prevalence and Gender Differences," *Metabolic Syndrome and Related Disorders* 5, no. 4 (2007): 365–72.
22. American Heart Association, "Heart Disease and Stroke Statistics," 2010.
23. U.S. Department of Health and Human Services, *The Health Consequences of Smoking: A Report of the Surgeon General* (Atlanta: U.S. Department of Health and Human Services, Centers for Disease Control and Prevention, National Center for Chronic Disease Prevention and Health Promotion, Office on Smoking and Health, 2004), Available at www.surgeongeneral.gov/library/smokingconsequences/index.html.
24. American Heart Association, "Heart Disease and Stroke Statistics," 2010; B. Howard et al., "Low-Fat Dietary Pattern and Risk of Cardiovascular Disease: The Women's Health Initiative Randomized Controlled Dietary Modification Trial," *Journal of the American Medical Association* 295, no. 6 (2006): 655–66.
25. C. A. Garza et al., "The Association between Lipoprotein-Associated Phospholipase $A_2$ and Cardiovascular Disease: A Systematic Review," *Mayo Clinic Proceedings* 82, no. 2 (2007): 159–65.

26. P. J. Barter et al., "Apo B versus Cholesterol in Estimating Cardiovascular Risk and in Guiding Therapy: Report of the Thirty-Person/Ten-Country Panel," *Journal of Internal Medicine* 259, no. 3 (2006): 247–58; E. Ingelsson et al., "Clinical Utility of Different Lipid Measures for Prediction of Coronary Heart Disease in Men and Women," *JAMA: The Journal of the American Medical Association* 298, no. 7 (2007): 776–85; M. McQueen et al., "Lipids, Lipoproteins and Apolipoproteins as Risk Markers of Myocardial Infarction in 52 Countries (The INTERHEART Study): A Case-Control Study," *Lancet* 372, no. 9634 (2008): 244–33.

27. The Linus Pauling Institute, "Micronutrient Information Center," Accessed June 2010, http://lpi.oregonstate.edu/infocenter; Office of Dietary Supplements, *Annual Bibliography of Significant Advances in Dietary Supplement Research 2007* (Bethesda, MD: U.S. Department of Health and Human Services, National Institutes of Health, 2008), NIH Publication no. 08-6456, Available at http://ods.od.nih.gov/Research/Annual_Bibliographies.aspx.

28. U.S. Food and Drug Administration, "Food Labeling: Health Claims; Plant Sterol/Stanol Esters and Coronary Heart Disease; Interim Final Rule," 2000, www.fda.gov/Food/LabelingNutrition/LabelClaims/HealthClaimsMeeting SignificantScientificAgreementSSA/ucm074747.htm; International Food Information Council Foundation, "Functional Food Fact Sheet: Plant Stanols and Sterols," 2007, www.foodinsight.org/Resources/Detail.aspx?topic=Functional_Foods_Fact_Sheet_Plant_Stanols_and_Sterols.

29. American Heart Association, "Heart Disease and Stroke Statistics," 2010.

30. C. H. Saely, P. Rein, and H. Drexel, "The Metabolic Syndrome and Risk of Cardiovascular Disease and Diabetes: Experiences with the New Diagnostic Criteria from the International Diabetes Federation," *Hormone and Metabolic Research* 39, no. 9 (2007): 642–50; K. Galassi, K. Reynolds, and J. He, "Metabolic Syndrome and Risk of Cardiovascular Disease: A Meta-Analysis," *American Journal of Medicine* 119, no. 10 (2007): 812–19.

31. R. Williams, J. Barefoot, and N. Schneiderman, "Psychosocial Risk Factors in Cardiovascular Disease: More Than One Culprit at Work," *Journal of the American Medical Association*, 290, no. 16 (2003): 2190–92.

32. A. Tsutsumi et al., "Prospective Study on Occupational Stress and Risk of Stroke," *Archives of Internal Medicine* 169, no. 1 (2009): 56–61.

33. W. Lovello, "Cardiovascular Responses to Stress and Disease Outcomes: A Test of the Reactivity Hypothesis," *Hypertension* 55, no. 4 (2010): 842–43; Y. Chida and A. Steptoe, "Greater Cardiovascular Responses to Laboratory Mental Stress Are Associated with Poor Subsequent Cardiovascular Risk Status: A Meta-Analysis of Prospective Evidence," *Hypertension* 55, no. 4 (2010): 1026–32; M. Esler et al., "Chronic Mental Stress Is a Cause of Essential Hypertension: Presence of Biological Markers of Stress," *Clinical and Experimental Pharmacology and Physiology* 35, no. 4 (2008): 498–502; A. Flaa et al., "Sympathoadrenal Stress Reactivity Is a Predictor of Future Blood Pressure: An 18 Year Follow-Up Study," *Hypertension* 52, no. 2 (2008): 336–41; T. Chadola et al., "Work Stress and Coronary Heart Disease: What Are the Mechanisms?" *European Heart Journal* 29, no. 5 (2008): 640–48; P. Surtees et al., "Psychological Distress, Major Depressive Disorder, and Risk of Stroke," *Neurology* 70, no. 10 (2008): 788–94; J. Dimsdale, "Psychological Stress and Cardiovascular Disease," *Journal of the American College of Cardiology* 51, no. 13 (2008): 1237–46.

34. R. Eliot, "Changing Behavior: A New Comprehensive and Quantitative Approach," Keynote address, annual meeting of the American College of Cardiology on Stress and the Heart (Jackson Hole, WY, July 3, 1987).

35. H. Tindle et al., "Optimism, Cynical Hostility, and Incident Coronary Heart Disease and Mortality in the Women's Health Initiative," *Circulation* 120, no. 8 (2009): 656–62.

36. D. Buckley et al., "C-Reactive Protein as a Risk Factor for Coronary Heart Diseases: A Systematic Review and Meta-Analyses for the U.S. Preventive Services Task Force," *Annals of Internal Medicine* 151, no. 7 (2009): 483–95.

37. Ibid.

38. D. Buckley et al., "C-Reactive Protein as a Risk Factor for Coronary Heart Diseases," 2009; O. Ben-Yehuda, "High-Sensitivity C-Reactive Protein in Every Chart? The Use of Biomarkers in Individual Patients," *Journal of the American College of Cardiology* 49, no. 21 (2007): 2139–41; D. D. Sin and S. F. P. Man, "Biomarkers in COPD: Are We There Yet?" *Chest* 133, no. 6 (2008): 1296–98.

39. F. Sofi et al., "Homocysteine-Lowering Therapy and Risk for Venous Thromboembolism: A Randomized Trial," *Annals of Internal Medicine* 146, no. 11 (2007): 761–67.

40. American Heart Association, "Homocysteine, Folic Acid, and Cardiovascular Disease," 2010, www.americanheart.org/presenter.jhtml?identifier=4677; R. Clarke et al., "Effects of B-Vitamins on Plasma Homocysteine Concentrations and on Risk of Cardiovascular Disease and Dementia," *Current Opinion in Clinical Nutrition and Metabolic Care* 10, no. 1 (2007): 32–39.

41. Heartsite, "Coronary Stents," Reviewed April 2010, www.heartsite.com/html/stent.html.

42. C. Cannon et al., "Current Use of Aspirin and Antithrombotic Agents in the United States among Outpatients with Atherothrombotic Disease (from the REduction of Atherothrombosis for Continued Health [REACH] Registry)," *American Journal of Cardiology* 105, no. 4 (2010): 445–52; G. Biondi-Zoccai et al., "A Systematic Review and Meta-Analysis on the Hazards of Discontinuing or Not Adhering to Aspirin among 50,279 Patients at Risk for Coronary Artery Disease," *European Heart Journal* 27, no. 22 (2006): 2667–74; C. Campbell et al., "Aspirin Dose for the Prevention of Cardiovascular Disease: A Systematic Review," *Journal of the American Medical Association* 297, no. 18 (2007): 2018–24; A. Mathews, "The Danger of Daily Aspirin," *Wall Street Journal,* February 23, 2010, http://online.wsj.com/article/SB10001424052748704511304575075701363436686.html.

43. American Heart Association, "Heart Attack Treatments," 2010, www.americanheart.org/presenter.jhtml?identifier=4601.

44. American Heart Association, "Heart Disease and Stroke Statistics," 2010.

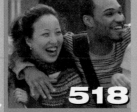 **518**
Do college students really need to be concerned about diabetes?

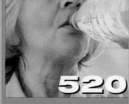 **520**
What does diabetes feel like?

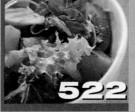 **522**
People with diabetes can't eat sweets—right?

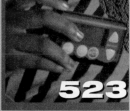 **523**
Do people with diabetes have to give themselves injections?

FOCUS ON

# Minimizing Your Risk for Diabetes

Like many college students, and a majority of American adults, Nora is overweight. She used to figure it was no big deal, and that she'd put herself on a strict diet and exercise program as soon as she graduated with her engineering degree and started to live "a normal life." But last week, her mom called with some bad news. She told Nora that she'd just found out the results of a routine blood test that her doctor had ordered: Nora's mom has type 2 diabetes. Her voice sounded shaky as she told Nora about her own mother's death from kidney failure—a complication of diabetes—at age 52, a few months before Nora was born. When Nora got off the phone, she searched online for information about diabetes. What she discovered made her feel scared, too: Her Hispanic ethnicity, family history, high stress level and lack of sleep, excessive weight, and sedentary lifestyle all increased her own risk for diabetes.

The next morning, Nora stopped off at the campus health center and made an appointment for a diabetes screening. She was instructed to fast the night before, and was scheduled for an appointment first thing in the morning. At her visit, the nurse practitioner took a blood sample. A few days later, she called with the news: Nora has

# 7.8%

of the U.S. population has some form of diabetes.

pre-diabetes, and needs to make changes to reduce her risk for developing type 2 diabetes like her mom.

Worldwide, more than 220 million people have diabetes, and the World Health Organization estimates that the number of diabetes deaths globally will double by the year 2030.[1] In the United States, the National Diabetes Information Clearinghouse estimates that 23.6 million Americans of all ages have dia-

The behaviors you take up in college could lead you on a path to diabetes in the long term—or even in the short term. Do you know whether your lifestyle and family history put you at risk?

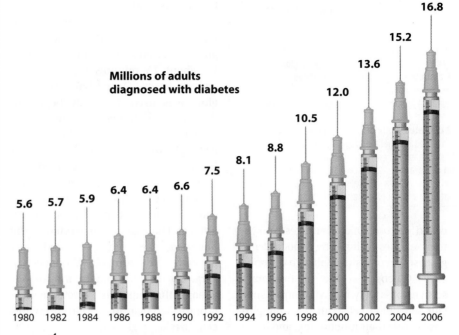

**Millions of adults diagnosed with diabetes**

5.6 — 1980
5.7 — 1982
5.9 — 1984
6.4 — 1986
6.4 — 1988
6.6 — 1990
7.5 — 1992
8.1 — 1994
8.8 — 1996
10.5 — 1998
12.0 — 2000
13.6 — 2002
15.2 — 2004
16.8 — 2006

FIGURE 1 **Percentage of U.S. Adults with Diagnosed Diabetes***

*Includes women with gestational diabetes.

**Source:** Data are from Centers for Disease Control and Prevention, "Diabetes Data and Trends," 2008, http://apps.nccd.cdc.gov/DDTSTRS/default.aspx.

betes.[2] Since 1980, diagnosed diabetes has increased to more than 50 percent of U.S. adults, giving it the dubious distinction of being the fastest growing chronic disease in American history (Figure 1). The rates increase as we age, meaning they aren't as high for college-age adults. The prevalence among Americans aged 20 to 39 is 2.6 percent.[3] Still, one study by the Centers for Disease Control and Prevention (CDC) indicated that diabetes seems to be increasing more dramatically among younger adults than among older Americans—it's up by almost 70 percent among those in their thirties.[4] The risk of diabetes is also increasing in children and adolescents due to the obesity epidemic.[5] Approximately 225,000 people die each year of diabetes-related complications, making diabetes the sixth leading cause of death in America today.[6]

## What Is Diabetes?

**Diabetes mellitus** is a disease characterized by a persistently high level of sugar—technically glucose—in the blood. Another characteristic sign is the production of an unusually high volume of glucose-laden urine, a fact reflected in its name: *Diabetes* is derived from a Greek word meaning "to flow through," and *mellitus* is the Latin word for "sweet." The high blood glucose levels—or **hyperglycemia**—seen in diabetes can lead to a variety of serious health problems and even premature death.

Diabetes is actually a group of diseases, each with its own mechanisms. Before we describe what goes wrong to cause the different types of diabetes, let's look at how the body regulates blood glucose in a healthy person.

## In Healthy People, Glucose Is Taken Up Efficiently by Body Cells

As you learned in Chapter 7, carbohydrates from the foods you eat are broken down into a monosaccharide

**diabetes mellitus** A group of diseases characterized by elevated blood glucose levels.
**hyperglycemia** Elevated blood glucose level.

called *glucose*. Once the digestive system releases it into the bloodstream, glucose becomes available to all body cells. Glucose is one of the main sources of energy for living organisms. Our red blood cells can use only glucose to fuel their functioning, and brain and other nerve cells prefer glucose over other fuels. When glucose levels drop below normal, certain mental functions may be impaired. You may feel "spacey" and unable to concentrate. Many other cells within the body use glucose to fuel metabolism, movement, and other activities. When there is more glucose available then required to meet your body's immediate needs, the excess glucose is stored as glycogen

Singer and pop star Nick Jonas is one of the 5 to 10 percent of diabetics diagnosed with type 1.

in the liver and muscles for later use. The average adult has about 5 to 6 grams of glucose in the blood at any given time, enough to provide energy for about 15 minutes under normal activity levels. Once that circulating glucose is used, the body begins to draw upon its glycogen reserves.

If it's going to power the work of cells, glucose has to be able to get inside them; however, it can't simply cross cell membranes on its own. Instead, cells have structures that transport glucose across in response to a signal. That signal is generated by the **pancreas,** an organ located just beneath the stomach. Whenever a surge of glucose enters the bloodstream, the pancreas secretes a hormone called **insulin.** Insulin stimulates cells to take up glucose from the bloodstream and carry it into the cell, where it's used for immediate energy. Conversion of glucose to glycogen for storage in the liver and muscles is also assisted by insulin. These actions lower the blood level of glucose, and in response, the pancreas stops secreting insulin—until the next influx of glucose arrives.

## Type 1 Diabetes Is an Immune Disorder

The more serious and less prevalent form of diabetes, called **type 1 diabetes** (or insulin-dependent diabetes), is an autoimmune disease; that is, the individual's immune system attacks and destroys normal body cells, in this case the insulin-making cells in the pancreas. Destruction of these cells causes a dramatic reduction, or total cessation, of insulin production. Without insulin, cells cannot take up glucose, and blood glucose levels become permanently elevated.

This form of diabetes used to be called *juvenile diabetes* because it most often appears during childhood or adolescence; however, it can begin at any age. European ancestry, a genetic

predisposition, and an environmental "insult" such as a viral infection all increase the risk.[7]

People with type 1 diabetes require daily insulin injections or infusions and must carefully monitor their diet and exercise levels. Often they face unique challenges as the "lesser known" diabetic type, with fewer funds available for research, fewer community resources, lack of understanding by the public about how the disease differs from type 2 diabetes, and fewer options for treatment.

## Type 2 Diabetes Is a Metabolic Disorder

**Type 2 diabetes** (non-insulin-dependent diabetes) accounts for 90 to 95 percent of all diabetes cases.[8] In type 2, either the pancreas does not make sufficient insulin, or body cells are resistant to its effects and thus don't efficiently use the insulin that is available (Figure 2). This latter condition is generally referred to as **insulin resistance.** Unlike type 1 diabetes, which can appear quite suddenly in someone who had previously seemed entirely healthy, type 2 usually develops slowly.

**Development of the Disease** In early stages of type 2 diabetes, cells throughout the body begin to resist the effects of insulin. One culprit known to contribute to insulin resistance is an overabundance of free fatty acids concentrated in a person's fat cells (as may be the case in an obese individual). These free fatty acids directly inhibit glucose uptake by body cells. They also suppress the liver's sensitivity to insulin, so its ability to self-regulate its conversion of glucose into glycogen begins to fail. As a consequence of both problems, blood levels of glucose gradually rise. Detecting this elevated blood glucose, the pancreas attempts to compensate by producing more insulin.

The pancreas cannot maintain its hyperproduction of insulin indefinitely. As the progression to type 2 diabetes continues, more and more pancreatic insulin-producing cells sustain physical damage and become nonfunctional. As

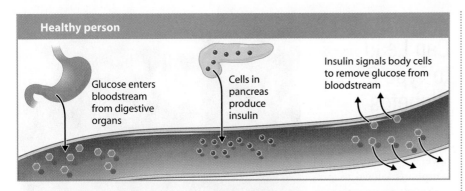

**Healthy person**

Glucose enters bloodstream from digestive organs

Cells in pancreas produce insulin

Insulin signals body cells to remove glucose from bloodstream

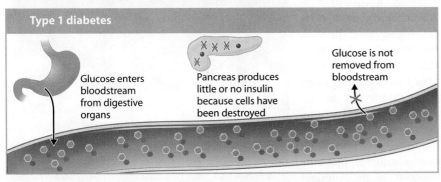

**Type 1 diabetes**

Glucose enters bloodstream from digestive organs

Pancreas produces little or no insulin because cells have been destroyed

Glucose is not removed from bloodstream

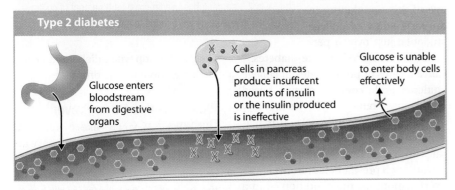

**Type 2 diabetes**

Glucose enters bloodstream from digestive organs

Cells in pancreas produce insufficient amounts of insulin or the insulin produced is ineffective

Glucose is unable to enter body cells effectively

FIGURE 2 **Diabetes: What It Is and How It Develops**
In a healthy person, a sufficient amount of insulin is produced and released by the pancreas and used efficiently by the cells. In type 1 diabetes, the pancreas makes little or no insulin. In type 2 diabetes, either the pancreas does not make sufficient insulin, or cells are resistant to insulin, and are not able to utilize it efficiently.

In addition, certain ethnic groups have higher rates of type 2 diabetes. Among adults aged 20 and older, 14.2 percent of Native Americans and 11.8 percent of non-Hispanic blacks have type 2. This makes them about twice as likely as non-Hispanic whites (6.8%) to have the disease. Persons of Hispanic origin have a diabetes rate of 10.4 percent—almost as high as blacks.[10]

Having a close relative with type 2 diabetes is another significant risk factor. Family history suggests a genetic link, and in fact type 2 has a strong genetic component. A small group of "type 2 diabetes genes" has been identified in a variety of studies so far.[11] But even though genetic susceptibility appears to play a role, given the fact that a population's gene pool shifts quite slowly—over centuries—the current epidemic of type 2 diabetes suggests that lifestyle factors, such as increased caloric intake and decreased physical activity, are more to blame.

**Modifiable Risk Factors** You can't change your age, ethnicity, or genetics, but you can modify lifestyle factors that are considered highly significant in the development of type 2 diabetes. These include your body weight, dietary choices, and your level of physical activity, as well as sleep patterns and your level of stress.

In both children and adults, type 2 diabetes is linked to overweight and obesity. In adults, a body mass index (BMI) of 25 or greater increases the risk. (To determine your own BMI, see Chapter 8.) In particular, excess weight

insulin output declines, blood glucose levels rise high enough to warrant a diagnosis of type 2 diabetes.

**Nonmodifiable Risk Factors** Type 2 diabetes is associated with a cluster of nonmodifiable risk factors, that is, factors over which you have no control. These include increased age, certain ethnicities, genetic factors, and biological factors.

One in five adults over age 65 has the disease. In fact, type 2 diabetes used to be referred to as *adult-onset diabetes*; now, however, it is being diagnosed at younger ages, even among children and teens. In the United States prior to the year 2000, only 1 to 2 percent of patients below age 18 diagnosed with diabetes had type 2. But recent reports indicate that as many as 45 percent of American youth diagnosed with diabetes have type 2.[9]

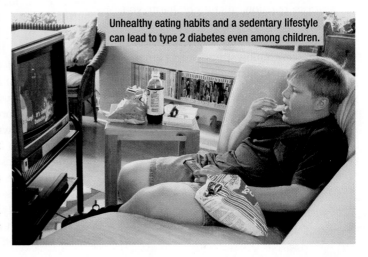

Unhealthy eating habits and a sedentary lifestyle can lead to type 2 diabetes even among children.

**pre-diabetes** Condition in which blood glucose levels are higher than normal, but not high enough to be classified as diabetes.

**gestational diabetes** Form of diabetes mellitus in which women who have never had diabetes before have high blood sugar (glucose) levels during pregnancy.

carried around the waistline—a condition called *central adiposity*—is risky: A waistline measurement of 40 or more inches in males or 35 or more inches in females is highly correlated to the development of type 2 diabetes.[12]

A sedentary lifestyle also increases the risk, not only because inactivity fails to burn calories, but also because activity itself, and buildup of muscle tissue, improves insulin uptake by cells.[13] People with type 2 diabetes who lose weight and increase their physical activity can significantly improve their blood glucose levels.

Several recent studies suggest that sleep contributes to healthy metabolism, including healthy glucose control. In contrast, inadequate sleep may contribute to the development of type 2 diabetes, as well as obesity.[14] For example, people who routinely fail to get enough sleep have been shown to be at higher risk for *metabolic syndrome* (discussed shortly), a cluster of risk factors that include poor glucose metabolism.[15]

Recent data from large epidemiologic studies have provided evidence of a link between diabetes and psychological or physical stress.[16] When the stress response activates the sympathetic nervous system, it can trigger a combination of increased blood glucose and inadequate production and release of insulin.[17] An occasional stress reaction might not harm you, but chronic stress can contribute to the onset or progression of diabetes. That's why controlling stress (see Chapter 3) is critical for diabetes management.

**what do you think?**

Why do you think type 2 diabetes is increasing in the United States? ● Why is it increasing among young people? ● Do you think young people are generally aware of what diabetes is and their own susceptibility for it?

# Pre-Diabetes Can Lead to Type 2 Diabetes

An estimated 57 million Americans age 20 or older have an ominous set of symptoms known as **pre-diabetes,** a condition in which blood glucose levels are higher than normal, but not high enough to be classified as diabetes.[18] This translates into more than 25 percent of the adult population. However, rates of pre-diabetes may not be as high among college students, probably because of the younger age of this population: In an early study of college students, just over 6 percent were found to have pre-diabetes.[19] Current rates of pre-diabetes in college students are unknown; however, based on increased rates of obesity, sedentary lifestyle, and metabolic risks, it is reasonable to assume that pre-diabetic rates on campus are on the rise.

Although pre-diabetes doesn't cause overt symptoms, the condition is, in a sense, like a ticking time bomb: If it's not "defused," diabetes will eventually strike. On the upside, a diagnosis of pre-diabetes represents a tremendous opportunity to take actions that could prevent diabetes or at least delay its onset. We'll identify these actions shortly.

**Pre-Diabetes Plays a Role in Metabolic Syndrome** Often, pre-diabetes is one of the cluster of six conditions linked to overweight and obesity that together constitute a dangerous health risk known as *metabolic syndrome* (*MetS*). In fact, of the six conditions, pre-diabetes and central adiposity appear to be the dominant factors for MetS.[20] As we discussed in Chapter 15, MetS dramatically increases an individual's risk for heart disease. In addition, a person with MetS is five times more

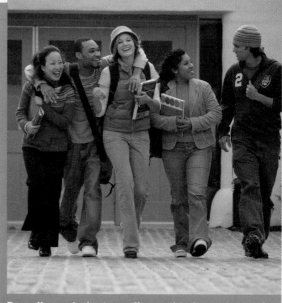

**Do college students really need to be concerned about diabetes?**

The rate of type 1 and type 2 diabetes among people aged 20 to 39 is 2.6 percent; however, more than 6 percent of college students in one study were found to have pre-diabetes.

likely to develop type 2 diabetes than is a person without the syndrome.[21]

**What Can You Do to Prevent Pre-Diabetes?** If you're like Nora, from our chapter-opening story, and have already been diagnosed with pre-diabetes or type 2 diabetes, you can follow the tips in the **Skills for Behavior Change** box to halt or slow the progression of your condition. But what if you've never had your blood glucose tested? Are there steps you could take right now to reduce your risk? Absolutely.

The first step is to consider your risk factors. Use the **Assess Yourself** activity on page 524 to find out whether your risk for diabetes is higher than average. If it is, make an appointment to talk with your heath care provider about diabetes screening.

# Gestational Diabetes Develops during Pregnancy

A third type, **gestational diabetes,** is a state of high blood glucose level that is first recognized in a woman during

## Six Steps to Begin Reducing Your Risk for Diabetes

**Step 1.** Maintain a healthy weight. For tips on sensible weight loss, see Chapter 8.

**Step 2.** Eat right. The following tips are from the National Diabetes Education Program:

✳ Eat less fat (especially saturated fats and *trans* fats) than you currently eat.

✳ Eat smaller portions of high-fat and high-calorie foods than you currently eat.

✳ Make fruits, vegetables, and whole grains the focus of your diet.

✳ Choose fat-free or low-fat milk and milk products.

✳ Include lean meats, poultry, fish, beans, eggs, and nuts in your diet.

✳ Limit your intake of salt, including the sodium in processed foods.

✳ Limit foods and beverages with added sugars.

**Step 3.** Get your body moving. Remember that physical activity not only helps you control your weight, but also improves your cells' response to insulin. At least 30 minutes of moderate activity 5 days a week is a minimum recommendation.

**Step 4.** Quit smoking. You probably know that smoking increases your risk for many types of cancer as well as heart disease, but you might not know that it also increases your blood glucose level. For all these reasons, it's important to quit, and if you don't smoke, don't start.

**Step 5.** Skip the alcohol, or reduce your intake. Alcohol provides 7 calories per gram, and can keep you from achieving or maintaining weight loss. In addition, alcohol can interfere with blood glucose regulation.

**Step 6.** Get enough sleep. Inadequate sleep may contribute to the development of type 2 diabetes.

**Sources:** Adapted from National Diabetes Education Program, *Small Steps, Big Rewards: Your GAME PLAN to Prevent Type 2 Diabetes* (Bethesda, MD: National Institutes of Health, 2006); American Diabetes Association, "Diabetes Basics: Smoking," 2010, www.diabetes.org/diabetes-basics/prevention/checkup-america/smoking.html.

## Did you Know?

Immediately after giving birth, 5 to 10 percent of women with gestational diabetes are found to have diabetes, usually type 2.

Source: Data are from NIDDK, *National Diabetes Statistics, 2007* (Bethesda, MD: National Institutes of Health, 2008) NIH Publication no. 08-3892.

pregnancy. It is thought to be associated with metabolic stresses that occur in response to changing hormonal levels. Gestational diabetes occurs in 4 percent of all pregnancies.[22] Although experts once considered gestational diabetes a transient event that disappeared after pregnancy, they now realize that women with gestational diabetes have a significantly increased risk of progressing to type 2 diabetes within approximately 9 years after giving birth.[23] Studies have shown that up to 70 percent of all women with gestational diabetes later develop type 2 diabetes.[24]

In addition, women with gestational diabetes have an increased risk of birth-related complications such as a difficult labor, high blood pressure, high blood acidity, increased infections, and death. The fetus of a woman with gestational diabetes is also endangered: Risks include malformations of the heart, nervous system, and bones; respiratory distress; and excessive growth that can lead to birth trauma. Gestational diabetes also increases the risk of fetal death.[25]

# What Are the Symptoms of Diabetes?

The symptoms of diabetes are similar for both type 1 and type 2. The following are among the most common:

● **Thirst.** It's the job of the kidneys to filter excessive glucose from the blood. When they do, they dilute it with water so that it can be excreted in urine. This pulls too much water from the body, and leaves the person dehydrated and thirsty.

● **Excessive urination.** For the same reason, the person experiences the need to urinate much more frequently than usual. When tested in a lab, a diabetic's urine has a high concentration of glucose.

● **Weight loss.** Because so many calories are lost in the glucose that passes into urine, the person with diabetes often feels unusually hungry. Despite eating more, he or she typically loses weight.

● **Fatigue.** When glucose cannot enter cells, including brain cells and muscle cells, fatigue and weakness become inevitable.

● **Nerve damage.** A high glucose concentration damages the smallest blood vessels of the body, including those

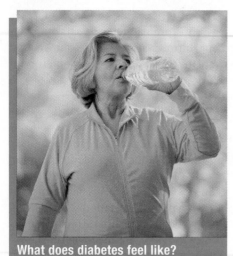

**What does diabetes feel like?**

People with undiagnosed or uncontrolled diabetes may experience blurred vision, tingling in the hands or feet, and fatigue. One of the most common symptoms is unusual thirst.

supplying nerves in the hands and feet. This can cause numbness and tingling.

● **Blurred vision.** Too much glucose causes body tissues to dry out. When this happens to the lens of the eye, vision deteriorates. In addition, high blood glucose levels can damage microvessels in the eye, leading to vision loss.

● **Poor wound healing and increased infections.** High levels of glucose can affect the body's ability to ward off infection, and may affect overall immune system functioning.

## Diabetes Can Have Severe Complications

The high blood glucose levels of poorly controlled diabetes can lead to a variety of significant complications. One of the most frightening is a diabetic coma, which results from a state of high blood acidity known as *diabetic ketoacidosis*. It occurs when, in the absence of glucose, body cells break down stored fat for energy. The process produces acidic mole-

# 65%
**of diabetics die from heart disease or stroke.**

cules called *ketones*. Although essential to provide fuel to the brain in the absence of glucose, ketones released in excessive amounts into the blood raise its acid level dangerously high. In a state of ketoacidosis, normal body functions cannot continue. The diabetic slips into a coma and, without prompt medical intervention, will die.

Other complications of poorly controlled diabetes include the following:[26]

● **Cardiovascular disease.** More than 70 percent of diabetics have hypertension. Blood vessels all over the body become damaged as the glucose-laden blood flows more sluggishly and essential nutrients and other substances are not transported as effectively.

● **Kidney disease.** The kidneys become scarred by their extraordinary workload and the high blood pressure in their vessels. Each year, almost 47,000 diabetics develop kidney failure and more than 175,000 are in treatment for this condition.

● **Amputations.** More than 60 percent of nontraumatic amputations of legs, feet, and toes are due to diabetes (see

Figure 3a). The problem may begin with a minor infection, such as of a toenail; then, an impaired immune response combined with damaged blood vessels enables the infection to spread and resist treatment. Eventually, tissues die and the body part must be amputated.

● **Eye disease and blindness.** Each year, 12,000 to 24,000 people become blind because of diabetic eye disease, making it the leading cause of new blindness in America today (Figure 3b).

● **Flu- and pneumonia-related deaths.** Each year, 10,000 to 30,000 people with diabetes die of complications from flu or pneumonia. They are roughly three times more likely to die of these complications than people without diabetes.

● **Tooth and gum diseases.** Diabetics run an increased risk of periodontal disease.

## Blood Tests Diagnose and Monitor Diabetes

Diabetes and pre-diabetes are diagnosed when a blood test reveals elevated blood glucose levels. But what tests are used, and exactly what do they show?

Generally, a physician orders either of two blood tests to diagnose pre-diabetes or diabetes:

● The *fasting plasma glucose* (*FPG*) *test* requires the patient to fast

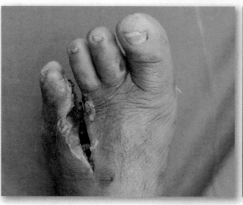

**ⓐ** Infections in the feet and legs are common in people with diabetes, and healing is impaired; thus, amputations are often necessary.

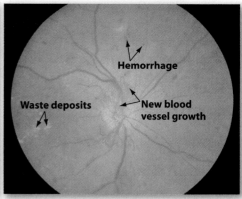

Hemorrhage

Waste deposits

New blood vessel growth

**ⓑ** Uncontrolled diabetes can damage the eye, causing swelling, leaking, and rupture of blood vessels; growth of new blood vessels; deposits of wastes; and scarring. All of these can progress to blindness.

FIGURE 3 **Complications of Uncontrolled Diabetes: Amputation and Eye Disease**

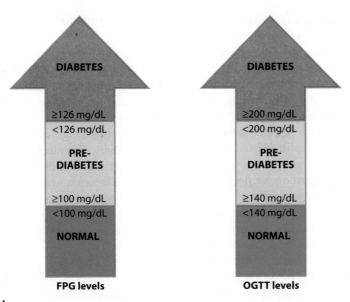

**FIGURE 4 Blood Glucose Levels in Pre-Diabetes and Untreated Diabetes**
The fasting plasma glucose (FPG) test measures levels of blood glucose after a person fasts overnight; the oral glucose tolerance test (OGTT) measures levels of blood glucose after a person consumes a concentrated amount of glucose.

**Source:** American Diabetes Association, "How to Tell If You Have Pre-Diabetes. Copyright © 2010 American Diabetes Association. From www.diabetes.org. Reprinted with permission from *The American Diabetes Association.*

overnight. Then, a small sample of blood is tested for glucose concentration. As you can see in **Figure 4**, an FPG level greater than or equal to 100 mg/dL indicates pre-diabetes, and a level greater than or equal to 126 mg/dL indicates diabetes.

- The *oral glucose tolerance test* (*OGTT*) requires the patient to drink a fluid containing a significant level of concentrated glucose. A sample of blood is drawn for testing 2 hours after the patient drinks the solution. As shown in Figure 4, a reading greater than or equal to 140 mg/dL indicates pre-diabetes, whereas a reading greater than or equal to 200 mg/dL indicates diabetes.

If you have any of the risk factors for type 2 diabetes identified earlier, you should talk with your heath care provider about having your blood glucose levels checked. If they're normal, repeat testing should be done every 3 years.[27]

People with diagnosed diabetes typically have their blood glucose levels monitored by their physicians every 3 to 6 months with the *hemoglobin A1C*

*test*. The A1C test measures the person's average blood glucose levels over the past 2 to 3 months. It is recommended that those diagnosed with diabetes have an A1C test at least twice a year.[28] They also need to check their own blood glucose level several times throughout each day to make sure they stay within their own target range. To check their blood glucose, diabetics must prick their

finger to obtain a drop of blood. A handheld glucose meter is then used to evaluate the blood sample. Each person has individualized instructions from their heath care provider for how to respond when readings are higher or lower than their target level.

# How Is Diabetes Treated?

Treatment options for people with pre-diabetes and types 1 and 2 diabetes vary according to the type that they have and how far the disease has progressed. Numerous pharmaceutical options are available to treat diabetes. In addition, there are several lifestyle changes that can help lower glucose levels and reduce the risks of diabetes complications.

## Lifestyle Changes Can Improve Glucose Levels

For people like Nora who have been diagnosed with pre-diabetes, it's important to initiate lifestyle changes immediately to prevent progression of the condition. In fact, studies have shown that people with pre-diabetes can prevent or delay the development of type 2 diabetes by up to 58 percent through changes to their lifestyle that include modest weight loss and regular exercise.[29] Even for people who have already been diagnosed with type 2 diabetes, lifestyle changes can sometimes prevent or delay the need for medication or insulin injections. As discussed here, weight loss, exercise, and a high-quality diet are all parts of the lifestyle formula.

**"Why Should I Care?"**

You may think you are too young to worry about developing diabetes, but the lifestyle choices you make now have a tremendous impact on your likelihood of developing pre-diabetes or type 2 diabetes 20, 10, or even 5 years from now. Being physically active, maintaining a healthy weight, and eating a diet high in whole grains, fat-free or nonfat milk, and fruits and vegetables can reduce your risk of developing type 2 diabetes, and contribute to a higher quality of life now, and in the future.

**Weight Loss** The key to preventing type 2 diabetes in people with pre-diabetes is weight loss. A Diabetes Prevention Program (DPP) study showed that a loss of as little as 5 to 7 percent of current body weight significantly lowered the risk of progressing to diabetes. Thus, the recommended goal is to lose 5 to 10 percent of current weight.[30] Weight loss is also important for people currently diagnosed with type 2 diabetes.

**Adopting a Healthy Diet** The DPP recommends that people lose weight by adopting a low-fat, reduced-calorie eating plan. In addition, diabetes researchers have studied a variety of specific foods for their effect on blood glucose levels. Here is a brief summary of some intriguing findings:

- **Whole grains.** A recent review of studies over many years suggests that a diet high in whole grains reduces a person's risk of developing type 2 diabetes.[31]
- **High-fiber foods.** Recent research suggests that eating foods high in fiber may reduce the risk of diabetes by improving blood sugar levels.[32] In one study, participants who ate foods high in fiber, including fruits and vegetables, reduced their risk of diabetes by as much as 22 percent.[33] Other high-fiber foods include beans, nuts, and seeds.
- **Fatty fish.** An impressive body of evidence links the consumption of fatty fish such as salmon, which is high in omega-3 fatty acids, with decreased progression of insulin resistance.[34]

It is also important for people with diabetes to pay attention to the glycemic index and glycemic load of the foods they eat to prevent surges in blood sugar. Glycemic index compares the potential of foods containing the same amount of carbohydrate to raise blood glucose. A food's glycemic load is defined as its glycemic index multiplied by the number of grams of carbohydrate it provides, then divided by 100. The concept of glycemic load was developed by scientists to simultaneously describe the quality (glycemic index) and quantity of carbohydrate in a meal.[35] By learning to combine high and low glycemic index foods in order to avoid surges in blood glucose, a diabetic can help control his or her average blood glucose levels throughout the day. Paying attention to the amount of food consumed is also critical.

**Increasing Physical Fitness** The DPP recommends 30 minutes of physical activity 5 days a week to reduce your risk of type 2 diabetes.[36] Brisk walking, swimming, biking, dancing, or any other activity of moderate intensity can be built into your daily schedule. Interestingly, a recent study suggests that improved fitness is even more important than weight loss in improving quality of life for people with diabetes.[37]

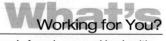

## Oral Medications and Weight Loss Surgery Can Help

When lifestyle changes fail to provide adequate control of type 2 diabetes, oral medications may be prescribed.[38] These include several types, each of which influences blood glucose in a different way. For example, some medications reduce glucose production by the liver, whereas others slow the absorption of carbohydrates from the small intestine. Other medications increase insulin production by the pancreas, whereas still others work to increase the insulin sensitivity of cells.

Of tremendous interest to the scientific community are recent findings that people who have undergone gastric bypass surgery (discussed in Chapter 8) appear to have high rates of diabetes cure, even before their weight has been lost. This has prompted international focus on the role of various regions of the small intestine in insulin regulation. Although gastric bypass comes with its own set of challenges

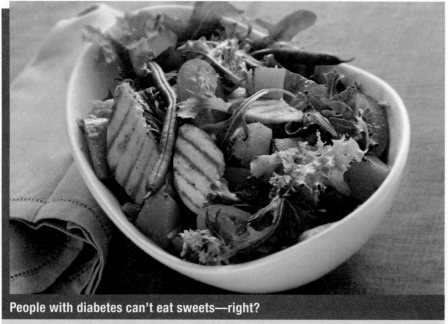

**People with diabetes can't eat sweets—right?**

People with diabetes can occasionally indulge in sweets, but meals low in saturated and *trans* fats and high in fiber, like this salad of salmon and fresh vegetables, are recommended for helping to control blood glucose and body weight.

and risks, other, less drastic methods for achieving these results are under investigation.[39]

## Insulin Injections May Be Necessary

Recall that with type 1 diabetes, the pancreas can no longer produce adequate amounts of insulin. Thus, insulin injections are absolutely essential for those with type 1 diabetes. In addition, people with type 2 diabetes whose blood glucose levels cannot be adequately controlled with other treatment options require insulin injections. Incidentally, insulin cannot be taken in pill form because it's a protein, and would be digested in the gastrointestinal tract. It must therefore be injected into the fat layer under the skin, from which it is absorbed into the bloodstream.

People with diabetes used to have to give themselves two or more insulin injections each day. Now, however, many diabetics use an insulin infusion pump. The external portion is only about the size of an MP3 player and can easily be hidden by clothes. It delivers insulin in minute amounts throughout the day through a thin tube and catheter inserted under the patient's skin. This infusion is more effective than delivering a few larger doses of insulin, and obviously less painful. Insulin inhalers, another form of insulin delivery, although available in the past, were taken off the market due to safety concerns. Ongoing research and advances with the technology may lead to their being available again in the future.

To overcome the limitations of current insulin therapy, researchers are currently working to link glucose monitoring and insulin delivery by developing an artificial pancreas. An artificial pancreas would be a system that would mimic, as closely as possible, the way a healthy pancreas detects changes in blood glucose levels and responds automatically to secrete appropriate amounts of insulin. Although not a cure, an artificial pancreas could significantly improve diabetes care and management and could reduce the burden of monitoring and managing blood glucose.[40]

## Diabetes Care Can Be Expensive

Treatments for diabetes come with a significant price tag. On average, health care costs for diabetics are $15,000 to $25,000 higher per year than they are for healthy patients. The direct and indirect costs of treating diabetes in the United States total $174 billion per year.[41] However, the full burden of diabetes is hard to measure: Death records often do not reflect the role of diabetes in a person's death, for example, from infection, kid-

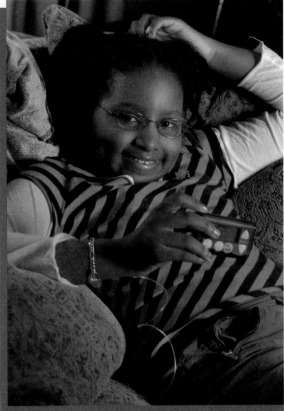

**Do people with diabetes have to give themselves injections?**

Some type 2 diabetics can control their condition with changes in diet and lifestyle habits, or with oral medications. However, some type 2 diabetics and all type 1 diabetics require insulin injections or infusions. Wearing an insulin infusion pump can help many people with diabetes control their blood glucose levels continuously—and avoid painful injections.

ney failure, or a stroke. In addition, the costs related to undiagnosed diabetes are unknown, and the impact of diabetes on quality of life and community resources is difficult to estimate.

## Are You at Risk for Diabetes?

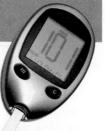

PEARSON
**myhealthlab**

Certain characteristics place people at greater risk for diabetes. Nevertheless, many people remain unaware of the symptoms of diabetes until after the disease has begun to progress. Take the following quiz to help determine your risk for diabetes. If you answer yes to three or more of these questions, consider seeking medical advice.

Fill out this assessment online at www.pearsonhighered.com/myhealthlab or www.pearsonhighered.com/donatelle.

**Yes    No**

1. Is there a history of diabetes in your family?
2. Do any of your primary relatives (parents, siblings, grandparents) have diabetes?
3. Are you overweight or obese?
4. Are you typically sedentary (seldom, if ever, engage in vigorous aerobic exercise)?
5. Have you noticed an increase in your craving for water or other beverages?
6. Have you noticed that you have to urinate more frequently than you used to during a typical day?
7. Have you noticed any tingling or numbness in your hands and feet, which might indicate circulatory problems?
8. Do you often feel a gnawing hunger during the day, even though you usually eat regular meals?

**Yes    No**

9. Are you often so tired that you find it difficult to stay awake?
10. Have you noticed that you are losing weight but don't seem to be doing anything in particular to make this happen?
11. Have you noticed that you have skin irritations more frequently and that minor infections don't heal as quickly as they used to?
12. Have you noticed any unusual changes in your vision (blurring, difficulty in focusing, etc.)?
13. Have you noticed unusual pain or swelling in your joints?
14. Do you often feel weak or nauseated when you wake in the morning, or if you wait too long to eat a meal?
15. If you are a woman, have you had several vaginal yeast infections during the past year?

# YOUR PLAN FOR CHANGE

The **Assess yourself** activity asked you to evaluate whether you are at risk for diabetes. Now that you have considered your results, you may need to take steps to further understand and address your risks.

**Today, you can:**

◯ Call your parents and ask them if there is a history of diabetes mellitus in your family. If there is, ask which type (type 1, 2, or gestational) the family member(s) had.

◯ Take stock of other risk factors you may have for diabetes—do you exercise regularly and watch your weight? Do you eat healthfully? Make a list of small steps

you can take in the immediate future to address any of these potential risk factors.

**Within the next 2 weeks, you can:**

◯ If you are at high risk for diabetes, make an appointment with your health care provider to have your blood glucose levels tested.

◯ If you smoke, begin devising a plan to quit. Look at the suggestions in Chapter 12 to give you ideas about how to go about this. You may want to consult your doctor about medications or nicotine replacement therapies that could help.

**By the end of the semester, you can:**

◯ Make the lifestyle changes that will reduce your risk. Pay attention to what you eat; increase your intake of whole grains, fruits, and vegetables and decrease your consumption of saturated fats, *trans* fats, and sugar.

◯ Make physical activity and exercise part of your daily routine.

# References

1. The World Health Organization, "Diabetes," Fact sheet #312, November 2009, www.who.int/mediacentre/factsheets/fs312/en/index.html.
2. National Diabetes Information Clearinghouse, National Institute of Diabetes and Digestive and Kidney Diseases (NIDDK), *National Diabetes Statistics, 2007* (Bethesda, MD: National Institutes of Health, 2008) NIH Publication no. 08-3892, Available at http://diabetes.niddk.nih.gov/dm/pubs/statistics.
3. Ibid.
4. Centers for Disease Control and Prevention, "Diabetes Data & Trends," 2008, http://apps.nccd.cdc.gov/ddtstrs.
5. Centers for Disease Control and Prevention, "Childhood Overweight and Obesity," Updated March 2010, www.cdc.gov/obesity/childhood/index.html.
6. Centers for Disease Control and Prevention, "Diabetes Data & Trends," 2008.
7. American Diabetes Association, "Diabetes Basics: Type 1," 2010, www.diabetes.org/diabetes-basics/type-1.
8. The World Health Organization, "Diabetes," Fact sheet #312, November 2009.
9. H. Rodbard, "Diabetes Screening, Diagnosis, and Therapy in Pediatric Patients with Type 2 Diabetes," *Medscape Journal of Medicine* 10, no. 8 (2008): 184.
10. American Diabetes Association, "Diabetes Statistics," 2010, www.diabetes.org/diabetes-basics/diabetes-statistics.
11. G. Dedoussis et al., "Genes, Diet, and Type 2 Diabetes Mellitus: A Review," *Review of Diabetic Studies* 4, no. 1 (2007): 13–24; U. Das and A. Rao, "Gene Expression Profile in Obesity and Type 2 Diabetes Mellitus," *Lipids in Health and Disease* 6 (2007): 35.
12. New Mexico Health Care Takes on Diabetes, "Pre-Diabetes Is a Precursor to Diabetes," *Diabetes Resources* 10, no. 2 (2008), Available at http://nmtod.com/diabetesresources.html.
13. American Diabetes Association, "Top 10 Benefits of Being Active," 2010, www.diabetes.org/food-nutrition-lifestyle/fitness/fitness-management/top-10-benefits-being-active.jsp.
14. F. Cappuccio et al., "Quantity and Quality of Sleep and Incidence of Type 2 Diabetes: A Systematic Review and Meta-Analysis," *Diabetes Care* 33, no. 2 (2010): 414–20; R. Aronsohn et al., "Diabetes, Sleep Apnea, and Glucose Control," *American Journal of Respiratory and Critical Care Medicine* 182, no. 2 (2010): 287–89; K. Knutson et al., "The Metabolic Consequences of Sleep Deprivation," *Sleep Medicine Reviews* 11, no. 3 (2007): 163–78.
15. M. H. Hall et al., "Self-Reported Sleep Duration Is Associated with the Metabolic Syndrome in Midlife Adults," *Sleep* 31, no. 5 (2008): 635–43.
16. F. Pouwer et al., "Does Emotional Stress Cause Type 2 Diabetes Mellitus? A Review from the European Depression In Diabetes (EDID) Research Consortium," *Discovery Medicine* 9, no. 45 (2010) 112–18; Y. Fan et al., "Dynamic Changes in Salivary Cortisol and Secretory Immunoglobulin A Response to Acute Stress," *Stress and Health* 25, no. 2 (2009): 189–94.
17. R. Rosmond, "Role of Stress in the Pathogenesis of the Metabolic Syndrome," *Pyschoneuroimmunology* 30 (2005): 1–10.
18. American Diabetes Association, "Diabetes Statistics," 2010.
19. T. Huang et al., "Overweight and Components of the Metabolic Syndrome in College Students," *Diabetes Care* 27 (2004): 3000–01.
20. American Heart Association, "Metabolic Syndrome," 2009, www.americanheart.org/presenter.jhtml?identifier=4756.
21. National Heart Lung and Blood Institute, "What Is Metabolic Syndrome?" Revised January 2010, www.nhlbi.nih.gov/health/dci/Diseases/ms/ms_whatis.html.
22. American Diabetes Association, "Diabetes Basics: What Is Gestational Diabetes?" 2010, www.diabetes.org/diabetes-basics/gestational/what-is-gestational-diabetes.html.
23. American Diabetes Association, "Diabetes Statistics," 2010.
24. C. Kim et al., "Gestational Diabetes and the Incidence of Type 2 Diabetes: A Systematic Review," *Diabetes Care* 25, no. 10 (2002): 1862–68.
25. M. Davidson, M. London, and P. Ladewig, *Olds' Maternal-Newborn Nursing & Women's Health across the Lifespan*, 8th ed. (Upper Saddle River, NJ: Pearson Education, 2008), 450–52.
26. American Diabetes Association, "Diabetes Statistics," 2010.
27. National Diabetes Education Program, *Small Steps, Big Rewards: Your GAME PLAN to Prevent Type 2 Diabetes* (Bethesda, MD: National Institutes of Health, 2006) NIH Publication no. 06-5334, Available at http://ndep.nih.gov/publications/PublicationDetail.aspx?PubId=71.
28. American Diabetes Association, "Living with Diabetes: A1C," 2010, www.diabetes.org/living-with-diabetes/treatment-and-care/blood-glucose-control/a1c.
29. American Diabetes Association, "Diabetes Basics: Pre-Diabetes FAQs," 2010, www.diabetes.org/diabetes-basics/prevention/pre-diabetes/pre-diabetes-faqs.html.
30. National Diabetes Education Program, *Small Steps, Big Rewards*, 2006.
31. J. de Munter et al., "Whole Grain, Bran, and Germ Intake and Risk of Type 2 Diabetes: A Prospective Cohort Study and Systematic Review," *PLoS Medicine* 4, no. 8 (2007): e261.
32. J. Anderson et al., "Health Benefits of Dietary Fiber," *Nutrition Reviews* 67, no. 4 (2009): 188–205.
33. B. Hopping et al., "Dietary Fiber, Magnesium, and Glycemic Load Alter Risk of Type 2 Diabetes in a Multiethnic Cohort in Hawaii," *Journal of Nutrition* 140, no. 1 (2010): 68–74.
34. M. Lankinen et al., "Fatty Fish Intake Decreases Lipids Related to Inflammation and Insulin Signaling—a Lipidomics Approach," *PLoS One* 4, no. 4 (2009): e5258; G. Dedoussis et al., "Genes, Diet, and Type 2 Diabetes Mellitus: A Review," 2007.
35. Linus Pauling Institute, "Glycemic Index and Glycemic Load," Updated April 2010, http://lpi.oregonstate.edu/infocenter/foods/grains/gigl.html.
36. National Diabetes Education Program, *Small Steps, Big Rewards*, 2006.
37. W. Bennett et al., "Fatness and Fitness: How Do They Influence Health-Related Quality of Life in Type 2 Diabetes Mellitus?" *Health and Quality of Life Outcomes* 6 (2008): 110.
38. G. Gillies et al., "Pharmacological and Lifestyle Interventions to Prevent or Delay Type 2 Diabetes in People with Impaired Glucose Tolerance: Systematic Review and Meta-analysis," *British Medical Association Journal* 334 (2007): 299.
39. F. Rubino, "Is Type 2 Diabetes an Operable Intestinal Disease? A Provocative Yet Reasonable Hypothesis," *Diabetes Care* 31 (2008): S290–96.
40. National Diabetes Information Clearinghouse, National Institute of Diabetes and Digestive and Kidney Diseases, "Alternative Devices for Taking Insulin," NIH Publication no. 09–4643. May 2009, Available at http://diabetes.niddk.nih.gov/dm/pubs/insulin/index.htm.
41. American Diabetes Association, "Diabetes Statistics," 2010.

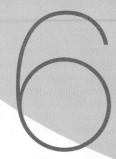

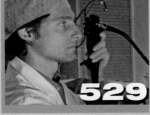

## 16

**529**

What does it mean for a tumor to be malignant?

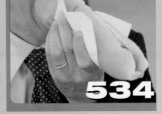

**534**

Are there chemicals in our food that may be linked to cancer?

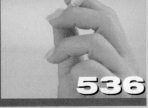

**536**

If my mom quits smoking now, will it reduce her risk of lung cancer or is it too late?

# Reducing Your Cancer Risk

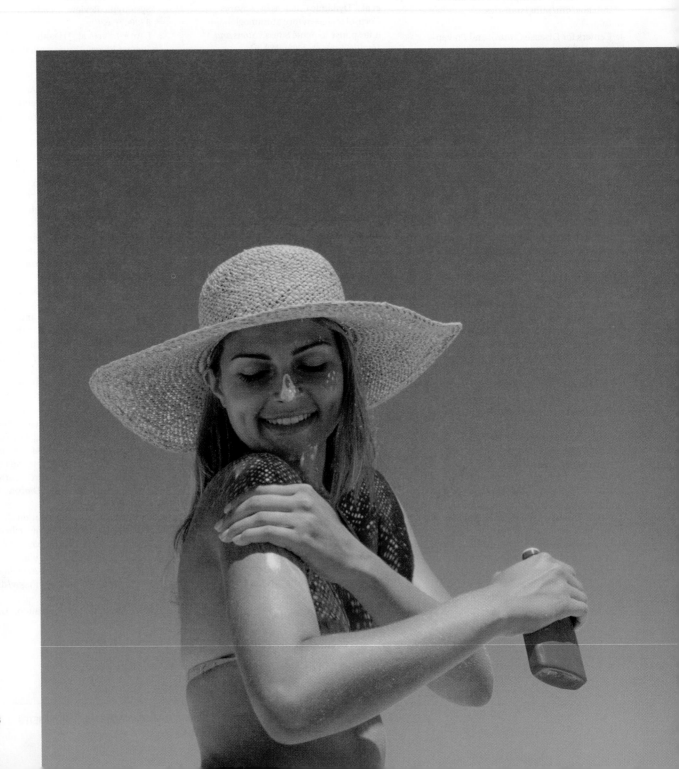

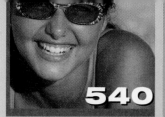

**540**

Is there any safe way to get a tan?

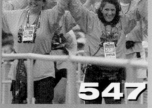

**547**

What are some of the challenges facing cancer survivors?

As recently as 50 years ago, a cancer diagnosis was typically a death sentence. Health professionals could only guess at the cause, and treatments were often as deadly as the disease itself. Because we had no idea how a person "got" cancer, fears about "catching cancer" from those who had it led to ostracism and bigotry—much like people with HIV were treated in the early days of the AIDS epidemic. Fortunately, we've come a long way in our understanding of cancer, our willingness to talk about the disease openly, and our ability to treat cancer successfully.

Although we know that there are multiple causes of cancer and understand that you cannot "catch" cancer from another person, there are some infectious agents that increase your risk. Early detection and significant developments in technology and treatment have dramatically improved the prognosis for most cancer patients, particularly those who are diagnosed in the earliest stages of disease. We also know that there are many actions we can take individually and as a society to prevent cancer. Understanding the facts about cancer, recognizing your own risk, and taking action to reduce your risk are important steps in the battle.

## Objectives

* Understand what cancer is, how it develops, and its causes.

* Discuss ways to prevent cancer and the implications of behavioral risks.

* Describe the different types of cancer and the risks they pose to people at different ages and stages of life.

* Explain the importance of early detection, self-exams, and medical exams, and understand the symptoms related to different types of cancer.

* Discuss cancer diagnosis and treatment, including radiotherapy and chemotherapy, and other common methods of detection and treatment.

## An Overview of Cancer

Although heart disease is the number one cause of death in the United States, cancer continues to be the second leading cause of death for all age groups. Overall, cancer mortality rates are on the decline, decreasing by an average of 2 percent per year over the past decade.[1] Between 1990 and 2005, over 650,000 lives were spared from cancer. Much of this progress is due to advances in diagnosis and treatment of lung, prostate, and colon cancers in men, and dramatic improvements in diagnosis and treatment of breast and colorectal cancer in women. In addition to improved treatment, prevention and early detection are key reasons for these changes.[2]

The **5-year survival rates** (the relative rates for survival in persons who are living 5 years after diagnosis) have increased greatly from the 50 percent survival rates of past generations (Table 16.1). About 68 percent of people diagnosed with cancer each year will still be alive 5 years after their diagnosis.[3] Survival rates for people with cancers caught in their earliest stages approach 100 percent. Of those treated for cancer, many will be considered "cured," meaning that they have no new cancer in their bodies 5 years after their original diagnosis and can expect to live a long and productive life. Among the most amazing improvements in outlook are cancers that were particularly challenging in the past such as acute lymphocytic leukemia in children,

# 25%

**of all deaths that occur on a given day are from some form of cancer.**

**5-year survival rates** The percentage of people in a study or treatment group who are alive 5 years after they were diagnosed with or treated for a disease such as cancer.

**527**

TABLE 16.1

**Trends in 5-Year Relative Survival Rates\* (%) by Year of Diagnosis, United States, 1975–2005**

| Site | 1975–77 | 1984–86 | 1999–2005 |
|------|---------|---------|-----------|
| All sites | 50 | 54 | 68[†] |
| Brain | 24 | 29 | 36[†] |
| Breast (female) | 75 | 79 | 90[†] |
| Colon | 52 | 59 | 66[†] |
| Kidney | 51 | 56 | 69[†] |
| Leukemia | 35 | 42 | 54[†] |
| Liver and bile duct | 4 | 6 | 14[†] |
| Lung and bronchus | 13 | 13 | 16[†] |
| Melanoma of the skin | 82 | 87 | 93[†] |
| Non-Hodgkin lymphoma | 48 | 53 | 69[†] |
| Oral cavity and pharynx | 53 | 55 | 63[†] |
| Ovary | 37 | 40 | 46 |
| Pancreas | 3 | 3 | 6[†] |
| Prostate | 69 | 76 | 100[†] |
| Stomach | 16 | 18 | 27[†] |
| Testis | 83 | 93 | 96[†] |
| Uterine cervix | 70 | 68 | 72[†] |
| Uterine corpus | 88 | 84 | 84[†] |

\*Survival is adjusted for normal life expectancy and is based on cases diagnosed in the Surveillance, Epidemiology and End Results (SEER) Program's "SEER 9"[CA1] areas 1975–1977, 1984–1986, and 1999–2005, and followed through 2006.

[†]The difference in rates between 1975–1977 and 1999–2005 is statistically significant ($p < 0.05$).

**Source:** American Cancer Society, *Cancer Facts & Figures 2010.* Atlanta: American Cancer Society, Inc. Used with permission.

**cancer** A large group of diseases characterized by the uncontrolled growth and spread of abnormal cells.

**neoplasm** A new growth of tissue that serves no physiological function and results from uncontrolled, abnormal cellular development.

**tumor** A neoplasmic mass that grows more rapidly than surrounding tissue.

**malignant** Very dangerous or harmful; refers to a cancerous tumor.

**benign** Harmless; refers to a noncancerous tumor.

**biopsy** Microscopic examination of tissue to determine if a cancer is present.

**metastasis** Process by which cancer spreads from one area to different areas of the body.

**mutant cells** Cells that differ in form, quality, or function from normal cells.

**carcinogens** Cancer-causing agents.

Hodgkin's disease, Burkitt's lymphoma, Ewing's sarcoma (a form of bone cancer), Wilms' tumor (a kidney cancer in children), testicular cancer, and osteogenic (bone) sarcoma.

During 2010, approximately 569,490 Americans died of cancer, and nearly 1.5 million new cases were diagnosed.[4] Of these, one-third of the cancers were related to poor nutrition, physical inactivity, and obesity, which means they could have been prevented. Certain other cancers are related to exposure to infectious organisms such as hepatitis B virus (HBV), human papillomavirus (HPV; also the cause of genital warts), HIV (the virus that causes AIDS), and *Helicobacter pylori* (the bacterium responsible for most peptic ulcers), and could be prevented through behavioral changes, vaccines, or antibiotics.

# What Is Cancer?

**Cancer** is the name given to a large group of diseases characterized by the uncontrolled growth and spread of abnormal cells. If these cells aren't stopped, they can impair vital functions of the body and lead to death. Think of a healthy cell as a small computer, programmed to operate in a particular fashion. When something interrupts normal cell programming, uncontrolled growth and abnormal cellular development result in a **neoplasm,** a new growth of tissue serving no physiological function. This neoplasmic mass often forms a clump of cells known as a **tumor.**

Not all tumors are **malignant** (cancerous); in fact, most are **benign** (noncancerous). Benign tumors are generally harmless unless they grow to obstruct or crowd out normal tissues. A benign tumor of the brain, for instance, becomes life threatening when it grows enough to restrict blood flow and cause a stroke. The only way to determine whether a tumor is malignant is through **biopsy,** or microscopic examination of cell development.

Benign and malignant tumors differ in several key ways. Benign tumors generally consist of ordinary-looking cells enclosed in a fibrous shell or capsule that prevents their spreading to other body areas. Malignant tumors are usually not enclosed in a protective capsule and can therefore spread to other organs (Figure 16.1). This process, known as **metastasis,** makes some forms of cancer particularly aggressive in their ability to overwhelm bodily defenses. By the time they are diagnosed, malignant tumors have frequently metastasized throughout the body, making treatment extremely difficult. Unlike benign tumors, which merely expand to take over a given space, malignant cells invade surrounding tissue, emitting clawlike protrusions that disturb the RNA and DNA within normal cells. Disrupting these substances, which control cellular metabolism and reproduction, produces **mutant cells** that differ in form, quality, and function from normal cells.

# What Causes Cancer?

After decades of research, scientists and epidemiologists believe that most cancers are, at least in theory, preventable. Many specific causes of cancer are well documented, the most important of which are represented by two major classes of factors: hereditary risk and acquired (environmental) risk. Heredity factors cannot be modified. Environmental factors are potentially modifiable. They include the macrophysical environment and personal lifestyle factors and situations, such as tobacco use; poor nutrition; physical inactivity; obesity; certain infectious agents; certain medical treatments; drug and alcohol consumption; excessive sun exposure; and exposures to **carcinogens** (cancer-causing agents), such as chemicals in our foods, the air we breathe, the water we drink, and the homes we live in. Several of these hereditary and environmental factors may interact to make cancer more likely, accelerate cancer progression, or increase individual susceptibility during certain periods of life, but the mechanisms are not fully understood. We do not know why some people have malignant cells in their body and never develop cancer, while others do.

## Lifestyle Risks for Cancer

Anyone can develop cancer; however, most cases affect adults beginning in middle age. In fact, nearly 78 percent of cancers are diagnosed at age 55 and above.[5] Cancer researchers refer to one's cancer risk when they assess risk factors. *Lifetime risk* refers to the probability that an individual, over the course of a lifetime, will develop cancer or die from it. In the United States, men have a lifetime

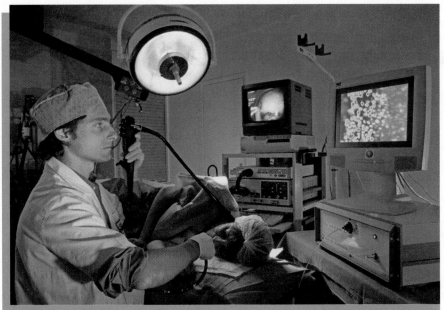

**What does it mean for a tumor to be malignant?**

A malignant tumor is one whose cells are cancerous. Malignant tumors are generally more dangerous than benign tumors because cancer cells divide quickly and can spread, or metastasize, from the original tumor to other parts of the body. Physicians usually order biopsies of tumors, in which sample cells are taken from the tumor and studied under a microscope to determine whether they are cancerous. Newer techniques, such as the minimally invasive "optical biopsy" shown here, allow for the microscopic examination of tissue without doing a physical biopsy.

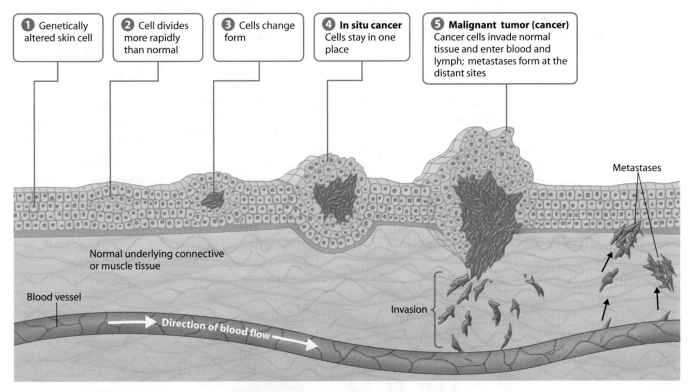

**1** Genetically altered skin cell

**2** Cell divides more rapidly than normal

**3** Cells change form

**4** **In situ cancer** Cells stay in one place

**5** **Malignant tumor (cancer)** Cancer cells invade normal tissue and enter blood and lymph; metastases form at the distant sites

Metastases

Normal underlying connective or muscle tissue

Blood vessel

Direction of blood flow

Invasion

FIGURE 16.1 **Metastasis**
A mutation to the genetic material of a skin cell triggers abnormal cell division and changes cell formation, resulting in a cancerous tumor. If the tumor remains localized, it is considered in situ cancer. If the tumor spreads, it is considered a malignant cancer.

TABLE

16.2

**Probability of Developing Invasive Cancers during Selected Age Intervals by Sex, United States, 2004–2006***

| Site | Sex | Birth to age 39 | Ages 40 to 59 | Lifetime |
|------|-----|-----------------|---------------|----------|
| All types[†] | Male | 1 in 70 | 1 in 12 | 1 in 2 |
|  | Female | 1 in 48 | 1 in 11 | 1 in 3 |
| Breast | Female | 1 in 206 | 1 in 27 | 1 in 8 |
| Colon and rectum | Male | 1 in 1,269 | 1 in 110 | 1 in 19 |
|  | Female | 1 in 1,300 | 1 in 139 | 1 in 20 |
| Lung and bronchus | Male | 1 in 3,461 | 1 in 105 | 1 in 13 |
|  | Female | 1 in 3,066 | 1 in 126 | 1 in 16 |
| Melanoma of the skin[§] | Male | 1 in 638 | 1 in 155 | 1 in 37 |
|  | Female | 1 in 360 | 1 in 183 | 1 in 56 |
| Prostate | Male | 1 in 9,422 | 1 in 41 | 1 in 6 |
| Uterine cervix | Female | 1 in 648 | 1 in 3,743 | 1 in 145 |
| Uterine corpus | Female | 1 in 1,453 | 1 in 136 | 1 in 40 |

*For people free of cancer at beginning of age interval.
[†]Excludes basal and squamous cell skin cancers and in situ cancers except in the urinary bladder.
[§]Statistic is for whites only.

**Sources:** DevCan Statistical Research, "Probability of Developing or Dying of Cancer," 6.3.0. Statistical Research and Applications Branch, National Cancer Institute, 2010, http://srab.cancer.gov/devcan; American Cancer Society, Surveillance and Health Policy Research, 2009.

risk of about 1 in 2; women have a lower risk, at 1 in 3.[6] See Table 16.2 for an overview of the probability of developing cancer by age and sex.

*Relative risk* is a measure of the strength of the relationship between risk factors and a particular cancer. Basically, relative risk compares your risk if you engage in certain known risk behaviors with that of someone who does not engage in such behaviors. For example, if you are a man and smoke, your relative risk of getting lung cancer is about twice that of a male nonsmoker.[7]

Over the years, researchers have found that diet, a sedentary lifestyle (and resultant obesity), overconsumption of alcohol, tobacco use, stress, and other lifestyle factors seem to play a role in the incidence of cancer. Keep in mind that a high relative risk does not guarantee an outcome; it only indicates the likelihood of a particular outcome.

> Of the several lifestyle risk factors for cancer, tobacco use is perhaps the most significant and the most preventable.

**Tobacco Use** Of all the potential risk factors for cancer, smoking is among the greatest. In the United States, tobacco is responsible for nearly 1 in 5 deaths annually, accounting for at least 30 percent of all cancer deaths and 87 percent of all lung cancer

deaths.[8] In fact, by all accounts, smoking is the leading cause of preventable death in the United States and around the world today.[9] Smoking is associated with increased risk of at least 15 different cancers, including nasopharynx, nasal cavity, paranasal sinuses, lip, oral cavity, pharynx, larynx, lung, esophagus, pancreas, uterine cervix, kidney, bladder, stomach, and acute myeloid leukemia. In the past 20 years, British and American lung cancer rates have declined; however, lung cancer rates among men are still increasing in most developing countries and in eastern Europe, where smoking rates remain high and are still increasing in some areas.[10] Although smoking has never been shown to directly cause lung cancer, the evidence showing a direct association between heavy cigarette consumption and increased risk for lung cancer development is strong.

**Alcohol and Cancer Risk** Over the past decade, countless studies have implicated alcohol as a risk factor for development of cancers. One of the earliest comparisons of results from nearly 200 studies found strong and compelling associations between alcohol and various types of cancer, including cancers of the oral cavity, pharynx, esophagus, larynx, stomach, colon, rectum, liver, breast, and ovaries.[11] Although this major study provided some of the first indicators of the potential cancer risks resulting from alcohol, critics argued that the studies did not accurately measure dose and that threshold levels where alcohol significantly increased risk were not established. Today, the evidence linking alcohol and cancer varies considerably by sex, consumption pattern, and other variables. Several recent articles appear to support the following:

- Moderate alcohol intake (above one drink per day) in women appears to increase the risk of cancers of the oral cavity and pharynx, esophagus, larynx, breast, and overall cancer risk. The more women drink, the greater their risk of cancer development.[12]

**what do you think?**

How should we determine whether a behavior or substance is a risk factor for a disease and whether policies and programs should be enacted to reduce the risk or stop a behavior? ● Do you think that a clear, undeniable causal link must be shown between smoking and lung cancer before smoking bans should be enacted in all 50 states?

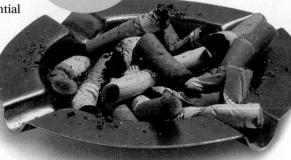

- Heavy alcohol consumption (binge drinking) in men appears to significantly increase the risk of pancreatic cancer.[13]
- In a Canadian study of over 3,500 men aged 35 to 70, regular heavy consumption of alcohol increased the risk of esophageal and liver cancers more than sevenfold. The risk of colon, stomach, and prostate cancers was about 80 percent higher among heavy drinkers, while lung cancer risk rose by almost 60 percent compared to nondrinkers.[14]

## Poor Nutrition, Physical Inactivity, and Obesity

Mounting scientific evidence suggests that about one-third of the cancer deaths that occur in the United States each year may be due to lifestyle factors such as overweight or obesity, physical inactivity, and nutrition—cancers that can be prevented![15] Dietary choices and physical activity are the most important modifiable determinants of cancer risk (besides not smoking). Cancer is more common among people who are overweight, and risk increases as obesity increases. Several studies indicate a relationship between a high body mass index (BMI) and death rates for cancers, particularly cancers of the kidney, pancreas, and colon in both men and women, and cancer of the endometrium in women.[16] A recent study of women in Denmark indicated that women who are overweight or obese tend to have more advanced breast cancer at the time of diagnosis and also have a higher rate of breast cancer mortality.[17] Although obese women appear to have a slightly higher risk of breast cancer and worse long-term outcomes, these poorer outcomes may be related to the fact that obese or morbidly obese women are much less likely to get routine mammograms. More research is necessary to prove this link.[18]

The relative risk of breast cancer in postmenopausal women is 50 percent higher for obese women than for nonobese women, whereas the relative risk of colon cancer in men is 40 percent higher for obese men than for nonobese men. The relative risks of gallbladder and endometrial cancer are five times higher in obese individuals than in individuals of healthy weight. Numerous other studies support the link between cancer and obesity.[19]

## Stress and Psychosocial Risks

Some researchers claim that social and psychological factors play a major role in determining whether a person gets cancer. Stress has been implicated in increased sus-

**"Why Should I Care?"**

Lifestyle, tobacco use, nutrition, and activity are things you control, and areas where you can start good habits now to reduce your chances of developing cancer.

ceptibility to several types of cancers. Although medical personnel are skeptical of overly simplistic solutions, we cannot rule out the possibility that negative emotional states contribute to illness. People who are under chronic, severe stress or who suffer from depression or other persistent emotional problems show higher rates of cancer than their healthy counterparts. Several newer studies appear to support the premise that stress can play a role in cancer development.[20] Sleep disturbances or an unhealthy diet may weaken the body's immune system, increasing susceptibility to cancer.

Another possible contributor to the development of cancer is poverty and the health disparities associated with low socioeconomic status (see the **Health in a Diverse World** box on page 532).

## Genetic and Physiological Risks

If one of your close family members develops cancer, does it mean that you have a genetic predisposition for it? Scientists believe that about 5 percent of all cancers are strongly hereditary. It seems that some people may be more predisposed to the malfunctioning of genes that ultimately cause cancer.[21]

Suspected cancer-causing genes are called **oncogenes.** Although these genes are typically dormant, certain conditions such as age; stress; and exposure to carcinogens, viruses, and radiation may activate them. Once activated, oncogenes cause cells to grow and reproduce uncontrollably. Scientists are uncertain whether only people who develop cancer have oncogenes, or whether we all have genes that can become oncogenes under certain conditions.

Certain cancers, particularly those of the breast, stomach, colon, prostate, uterus, ovaries, and lungs, appear to run in families. For example, a woman runs a much higher risk of breast cancer if her mother or sisters have had the disease, particularly at a young age. Hodgkin's disease and certain leukemias show similar familial patterns. Can we attribute these familial patterns to genetic susceptibility or to the fact that people in the same families experience similar environmental risks? To date, the research in this area is inconclusive. It is possible that we can inherit a tendency toward a cancer-prone, weak immune system or, conversely, that we can inherit a cancer-fighting potential. But the complex interaction of hereditary predisposition, lifestyle, and environment on the development of cancer makes it a challenge to determine a single cause. Even among those predisposed to mutations, avoiding risks may decrease chances of cancer development.

**oncogenes** Suspected cancer-causing genes present on chromosomes.

Some forms of cancer have strong genetic bases; daughters of women with breast cancer have an increased risk of developing the disease.

## Reproductive and Hormonal Factors

The effects of reproductive factors on breast and cervical cancers have been well documented. Increased numbers of fertile or menstrual cycle

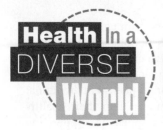
# Disparities in Cancer Rates

There are many factors associated with differences in cancer rates, including work; wealth; income; gender; education; housing; overall standard of living; and the availability of high-quality cancer prevention, early detection, and treatment services. Poverty is widely believed to be the most important factor affecting health and longevity. People from lower socioeconomic levels tend to smoke more, be more obese and sedentary, have less access to fruits and vegetables, drink more alcohol, and carry little or no insurance. Because of the lack of insurance, they tend to lack preventive care and early screenings, which can lead to late-stage diagnosis and they may not be able to afford medications or uncompensated medical charges. They may live in buildings or neighborhoods where there is greater risk of environmental threats. Many of the poorer cancer patients tend to also be from minority populations, many of whom may not be able to speak or write effectively in English. As such they may have difficulty communicating with their health care providers, understanding health recommendations, and/or making informed decisions about their treatment options

How serious are these poverty-related cancer disparities? Consider the following:

✳ People with family annual incomes less than $12,500 have nearly twice the rate of lung cancer and significantly more late-stage breast cancer and late-stage prostate cancer than those with incomes that are $50,000 or higher.

✳ A person living in an affluent census tract has a 5-year survival rate that is 10 percent higher than a person living in a tract below the poverty level. Insured individuals living in the more affluent tracts have the best overall prognosis.

Reducing such disparities is a major initiative of the National Institutes of Health and other professional groups. Planned actions include the following:

✳ **Advocacy.** Including media campaigns; information dissemination; lobbying; coalition formation; and action at the federal, state, and local levels, these efforts are designed to make it easier for those who are subjected to disparities to navigate the health care system.

✳ **Research.** Increased funding for research on the mechanisms of cancer initiation and the factors likely to improve treatment among the poor and disadvantaged will improve health outcomes for cancer patients.

✳ **Education.** Broadening the base for educational materials and multilingual information will increase the number of people who receive key information about signs and symptoms, risk factors, and prevention strategies. In addition, providing at-risk populations with better information about navigating the health care system, accessing health care products and services, and other key information elements will result in earlier diagnosis and better prognosis for treatment.

In the United States, people of lower socioeconomic status and belonging to minority ethnic groups tend to be at increased risk for many types of cancer.

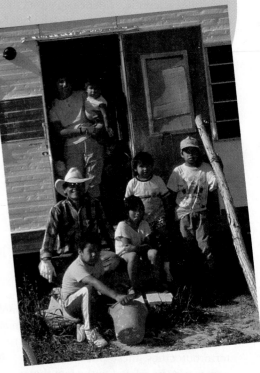

**Sources:** American Cancer Society, *Facts & Figures, 2010* (Atlanta: American Cancer Society, 2008); L. Clegg, M. Reichman, B. Miller et al., "Impact of Socioeconomic Status on Cancer Incidence and Stage of Diagnosis: Selected Findings from the Surveillance, Epidemiology, and End Results: National Longitudinal Mortality Study," *Cancer Causes and Control* 20, no. 4 (2009): 1573–82: American Cancer Society, *Cancer Facts & Figures for Hispanics/Latinos—2009–2011* (Atlanta: American Cancer Society, 2009), Available at www.cancer.org/Research/CancerFactsFigures/CancerFactsFiguresfor HispanicsLatinos/index.

years (early menarche, late menopause), not having children or having them later in life, recent use of birth control pills or hormone replacement therapy, and opting not to breast-feed, all appear to increase risks of breast cancer.[22] However, recent research suggests that while the above factors appear to play a significant role in increased risk for non-Hispanic white women, they do not appear to have as strong of an influence on Hispanic women.[23] Studies also suggest that women on

hormone supplements or hormone replacement therapy have a slightly increased risk of lung cancer.[24]

Breast cancer is much more common in most Western countries than in developing countries. This is partly—and perhaps largely—accounted for by diets high in calories and fat, combined with later first childbirth, bearing fewer children, shorter periods of breast-feeding, higher obesity rates, and a longer life expectancy (people in less developed

# BE HEALTHY, BE GREEN

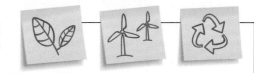

## Go Green against Cancer

We live in an environment that is filled with potential cancer-causing agents. Some of them are natural, but many are created or increased by humans. There are many things you can do to help reduce the number of carcinogens in the environment and to limit your exposure to those that are there. The following are just a few ideas:

**1.** Commute by bicycle or by foot instead of driving a vehicle. This will reduce your carbon footprint and your risk for cancer by increasing your physical activity.

**2.** Choose organic foods when possible to avoid chemicals and pesticides. When we eat these chemicals, our risk for cancer can be elevated.

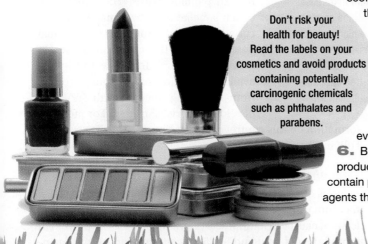

Don't risk your health for beauty! Read the labels on your cosmetics and avoid products containing potentially carcinogenic chemicals such as phthalates and parabens.

**3.** Shop for ecofriendly flooring, carpets, and other products to ensure the best possible indoor air quality and minimize carcinogenic exposures. Such ecofriendly products include bamboo, recycled glass tiles, recycled metal tiles, cork flooring, and flooring made from reclaimed wood products.

**4.** Turn off your lights. According to sleep experts and others, artificial light decreases the production of melatonin, a hormone manufactured in the brain that is produced during sleep cycles. This hormone is being shown to have a protective effect against some forms of cancer.

**5.** Use "green" paper. By purchasing ecofriendly paper products that are bleach free, we reduce the amount of dioxins released into the atmosphere. Dioxins are carcinogenic, and fewer of them in the atmosphere will reduce everyone's risk for cancer.

**6.** Buy ecofriendly hygiene products. Many products contain petroleum and plastics, agents that are not good for

your skin or the environment. Consider avoiding the following:

* Diethanolamine (DEA), commonly found in shampoos, is thought to be carcinogenic.
* Formaldehyde, commonly found in eye shadows, is well known as a carcinogen.
* Phthalates, found in many hygiene and cosmetic products such as nail polish and perfumes, are thought to be carcinogenic.
* Parabens, used as preservatives in food and cosmetic products such as makeup, lotion, shampoo, and soap, have been found in breast tumors and are being researched as potential carcinogens.

**7.** Avoid dry cleaning. Try not to buy clothes that require dry cleaning. Conventional dry cleaning uses a chemical called *perchloroethylene* (*PERC*), an agent known to increase the risk for cancer and harm the environment. If dry cleaning is unavoidable, explore local dry cleaners using ecofriendly alternatives such as "wet cleaning," which includes biodegradable soaps or silicone-based solvents and special machinery used to reduce shrinkage.

---

nations with shorter life expectancy may not live long enough to develop cancer).[25]

## Occupational and Environmental Risks

Overall, workplace hazards account for only a small percentage of all cancers. However, various substances are known to cause cancer when exposure levels are high or prolonged. One is asbestos, a fibrous material once widely used in the construction, insulation, and automobile industries. Nickel; chromate; and chemicals such as benzene, arsenic, and vinyl chloride have been shown definitively to be carcinogens. Also, people who routinely work with certain dyes and radioactive substances may have increased risks for cancer. Working with coal

tars, as in the mining profession, or with inhalants, as in the auto-painting business, is hazardous. So is working with herbicides and pesticides, although the evidence is inconclusive for low-dose exposures. Several federal and state agencies are responsible for monitoring such exposures and ensuring that businesses comply with standards designed to protect workers.

You don't have to work in one of these industries to come in contact with environmental carcinogens. See the **Be Healthy, Be Green** box above to explore some ways you can avoid carcinogens in the products you buy and use every day.

**Radiation** Ionizing radiation (IR)—radiation from X rays, radon, cosmic rays, and ultraviolet radiation (primarily UVB radiation)—is the only form of radiation proven to cause human cancer. Evidence that high-dose IR causes cancer comes from studies of atomic bomb survivors, patients receiving radiotherapy, and certain occupational groups, such as uranium miners. Virtually any part of the body can be affected by IR, but bone marrow and the thyroid are particularly susceptible. Radon exposure in homes can increase lung cancer risk, especially in cigarette smokers. To reduce the risk of harmful effects, diagnostic medical and dental X rays are set at the lowest dose levels possible.

Nonionizing radiation produced by radio waves, cell phones, microwaves, computer screens, televisions, electric blankets, and other products has been a topic of great concern in recent years, but research has not proven excess risk to date. Although highly controversial, some suggest that cell phones beam radio frequency energy that can penetrate the brain, raising concerns about cancers of the head and neck, brain tumors, or leukemia. Most research, including the biggest study of cancer and cell phone risk to date, indicates that having a cell phone glued to your ear for hours causes little more than a sore ear and a hefty bill.[26] See Chapter 20 for more on the potential environmental and health hazards of both ionizing and nonionizing radiation.

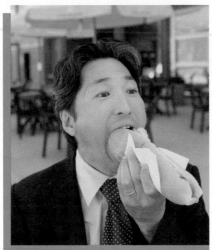

**Are there chemicals in our food that may be linked to cancer?**

Food additives, particularly sodium nitrate, are used to preserve and give color to red meat and to protect against pathogens, particularly *Clostridium botulinum,* the bacterium that causes botulism. Concern about the carcinogenic properties of nitrates, which are often used in hot dogs, hams, and luncheon meats, has led to the introduction of meats that are nitrate-free or contain reduced levels of the substance.

**Chemicals in Foods** Much of the concern about chemicals in food centers on the possible harm caused by pesticide and herbicide residues. Whereas some of these chemicals cause cancer at high doses in experimental animals, the very low concentrations found in some foods are considered by the government to be safe. Continued research regarding pesticide and herbicide use is essential, and scientists and consumer groups stress the importance of a balance between chemical use and the production of high-quality food products.

# Infectious Disease Risks

Infectious diseases can be triggers for cancer. According to the experts, over 25 percent of all malignancies in the United States are caused by viruses, bacteria, and parasites.[27] Worldwide, approximately 20 percent of human cancers have been traced to prior infection by a virus alone.[28] Rates of cancers related to infections are about three times higher in less developed countries than they are in developed countries (26% versus 8%).[29] Although most of us are infected with potential cancer-causing pathogens during our lives, most never get cancer. Those who do, appear to be particularly vulnerable to the genetic errors that oncogenes can trigger at the cellular level. In addition, infections are thought to influence cancer development in several ways, most commonly through chronic inflammation, suppression of the immune

system, or chronic stimulation. Some of the pathogens that are linked to cancers are discussed below.

**Chronic Hepatitis B, Hepatitis C, and Liver Cancer** Viruses such as the ones that cause chronic forms of hepatitis B (HBV) and C (HCV) are believed to stimulate growth of cancer cells in the liver, because they chronically inflame liver tissue. This may prime the liver for cancer or make it more hospitable for cancer development. Global increases in hepatitis B and C rates and concurrent rises in liver cancer rates seem to provide evidence of such an association. Vaccines that prevent hepatitis B may reduce the risk of liver damage as well as cancer.

**Human Papillomavirus and Cervical Cancer** Nearly 100 percent of women with cervical cancer have evidence of human papillomavirus (HPV) infection, which is believed to be a major cause of cervical cancer. Fortunately, only a small percentage of HPV cases progresses to cervical cancer.[30] Today, a vaccine is available to help protect young women from becoming infected with HPV and developing cervical cancer. For more information on this controversial vaccine, see the discussion of HPV in Chapter 14.

*Helicobacter pylori* and Stomach Cancer *Helicobacter pylori* is a potent bacterium that can be found embedded in the stomach lining of approximately 30 to 40 percent of Americans. It causes irritation, scarring, and ulcers for 20 percent of those infected, and another 5 percent develop stomach cancer. *Helicobacter pylori* seems to trigger long-term inflammation and irritation in body tissues. In turn, inflammation triggers faster cell division, which increases the chances of cancer development. Treatment with antibiotics often cures the ulcers; however, it is not known whether such treatment prevents cancer.[31]

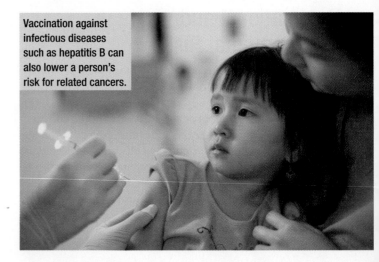

Vaccination against infectious diseases such as hepatitis B can also lower a person's risk for related cancers.

## Medical Factors

Some medical treatments can increase a person's risk for cancer. One example was the use of estrogen and progesterone for relieving women's menopausal symptoms. Estrogen use is now recognized to contribute to multiple cancer risks and to provide fewer benefits than was originally believed. Prescriptions for estrogen therapy have declined dramatically, and many women are trying to reduce or eliminate their use of the hormone. Interestingly, this decrease in hormone therapy is believed to have contributed to the large decline in breast cancer rates among women today.[32] Ironically, medicines used to treat cancers, such as selected chemotherapy drugs, have been shown to increase risks for other cancers. Weighing the benefits versus harms of these treatments is always necessary.

## Types of Cancers

As mentioned earlier, the word *cancer* refers not to a single disease, but to hundreds of different diseases. They are grouped into four broad categories based on the type of tissue from which the cancer arises:

● **Carcinomas.** Epithelial tissues (tissues covering body surfaces and lining most body cavities) are the most common sites for cancers; cancers occurring in epithelial tissue are called *carcinomas.* These cancers affect the outer layer of the skin and mouth as well as the mucous membranes. They metastasize through the circulatory or lymphatic system initially and form solid tumors.

● **Sarcomas.** Sarcomas occur in the mesodermal, or middle, layers of tissue—for example, in bones, muscles, and general connective tissue. They metastasize primarily via the blood in the early stages of disease. These cancers are less common but generally more virulent than carcinomas. They also form solid tumors.

● **Lymphomas.** Lymphomas develop in the lymphatic system—the infection-fighting regions of the body—and metastasize through the lymphatic system. Hodgkin's disease is an example. Lymphomas also form solid tumors.

● **Leukemias.** Cancer of the blood-forming parts of the body, particularly the bone marrow and spleen, is called leukemia. A nonsolid tumor, leukemia is characterized by an abnormal increase in the number of white blood cells that the body produces.

Figure 16.2 shows the most common sites of cancer and the number of new cases and deaths from each type that were estimated to have occurred in 2010. A comprehensive discussion of the many different forms of cancer is beyond the scope of this book, but we will discuss the most common types in the next sections.

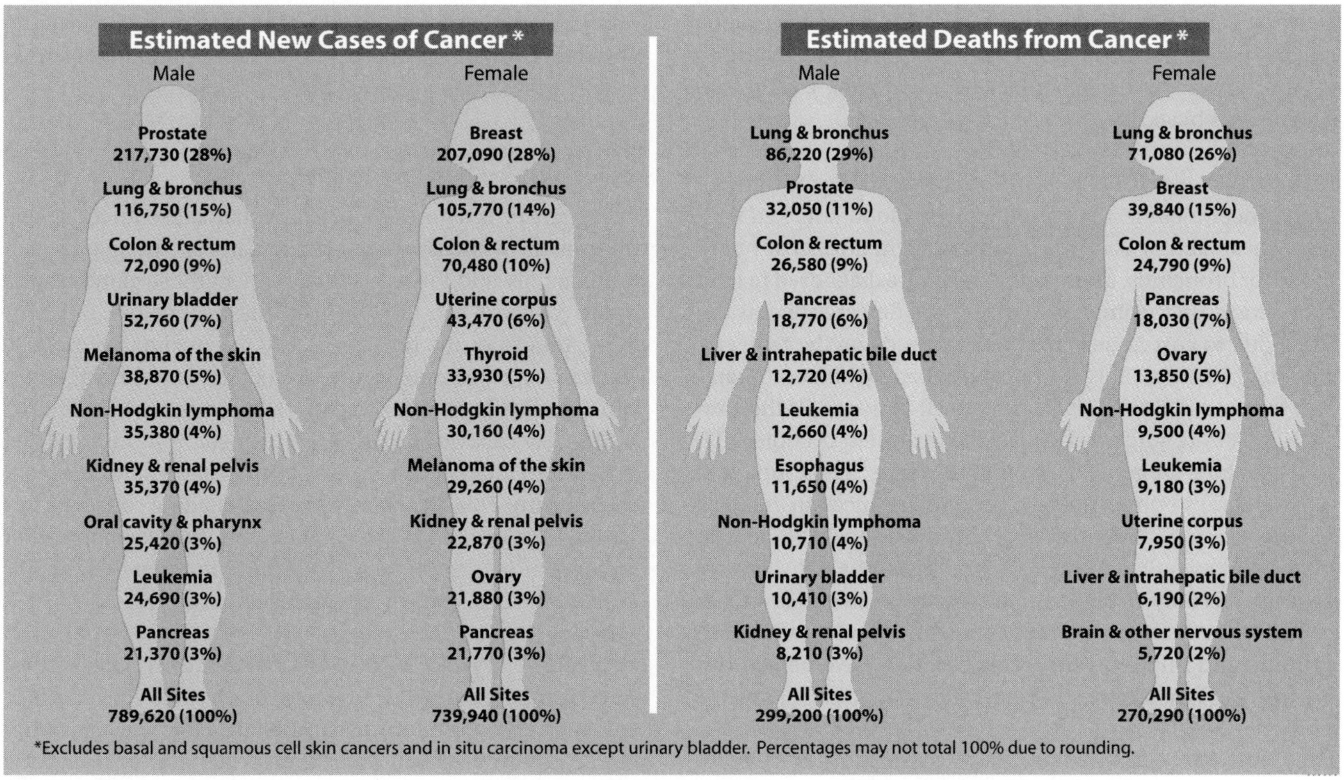

| Estimated New Cases of Cancer * | | Estimated Deaths from Cancer * | |
|---|---|---|---|
| Male | Female | Male | Female |
| Prostate 217,730 (28%) | Breast 207,090 (28%) | Lung & bronchus 86,220 (29%) | Lung & bronchus 71,080 (26%) |
| Lung & bronchus 116,750 (15%) | Lung & bronchus 105,770 (14%) | Prostate 32,050 (11%) | Breast 39,840 (15%) |
| Colon & rectum 72,090 (9%) | Colon & rectum 70,480 (10%) | Colon & rectum 26,580 (9%) | Colon & rectum 24,790 (9%) |
| Urinary bladder 52,760 (7%) | Uterine corpus 43,470 (6%) | Pancreas 18,770 (6%) | Pancreas 18,030 (7%) |
| Melanoma of the skin 38,870 (5%) | Thyroid 33,930 (5%) | Liver & intrahepatic bile duct 12,720 (4%) | Ovary 13,850 (5%) |
| Non-Hodgkin lymphoma 35,380 (4%) | Non-Hodgkin lymphoma 30,160 (4%) | Leukemia 12,660 (4%) | Non-Hodgkin lymphoma 9,500 (4%) |
| Kidney & renal pelvis 35,370 (4%) | Melanoma of the skin 29,260 (4%) | Esophagus 11,650 (4%) | Leukemia 9,180 (3%) |
| Oral cavity & pharynx 25,420 (3%) | Kidney & renal pelvis 22,870 (3%) | Non-Hodgkin lymphoma 10,710 (4%) | Uterine corpus 7,950 (3%) |
| Leukemia 24,690 (3%) | Ovary 21,880 (3%) | Urinary bladder 10,410 (3%) | Liver & intrahepatic bile duct 6,190 (2%) |
| Pancreas 21,370 (3%) | Pancreas 21,770 (3%) | Kidney & renal pelvis 8,210 (3%) | Brain & other nervous system 5,720 (2%) |
| All Sites 789,620 (100%) | All Sites 739,940 (100%) | All Sites 299,200 (100%) | All Sites 270,290 (100%) |

*Excludes basal and squamous cell skin cancers and in situ carcinoma except urinary bladder. Percentages may not total 100% due to rounding.

FIGURE 16.2 **Leading Sites of New Cancer Cases and Deaths, 2010 Estimates**

**Source:** Adapted from American Cancer Society, *Cancer Facts & Figures 2010.* Atlanta: American Cancer Society, Inc. Used with permission.

## Lung Cancer

Nearly 220,000 new cases of lung cancer were diagnosed in 2010. Lung cancer is the leading cause of cancer deaths for both men and women in the United States; it killed an estimated 157,300 in 2010.[33] Since 1987, more women have died each year from lung cancer than from breast cancer, which over the previous 40 years had been the major cause of cancer deaths in women.[34] Although past reductions in smoking rates have boded well for cancer statistics, there is growing concern about the number of young people, particularly young women and persons of low income and low educational levels, who continue to pick up the habit.

## 90%
### of all lung cancers could be avoided if people did not smoke.

There is also growing concern about the increase in lung cancers among lifelong *never smokers*—a group of people who, as the name suggests, have never smoked, but nevertheless now have as many as 15 percent of all lung cancers. Never smokers' lung cancer is believed to be related to exposure to secondhand smoke, radon gas, asbestos, indoor wood-burning stoves, and aerosolized oils caused by cooking with oil and deep fat frying.[35] Because this form of lung cancer seems resistant to traditional lung cancer therapies, some have speculated that it is actually a distinct type of lung cancer. Unfortunately, because doctors often don't think of lung cancer when a never smoker presents with a cough, patients are often put on antibiotics or cough suppressants as therapy. By the time they recognize that it's really lung cancer, the prognosis is bleak.[36]

**Detection, Symptoms, and Treatment** Symptoms of lung cancer include a persistent cough, blood-streaked sputum, chest pain or back pain, and recurrent attacks of pneumonia or bronchitis. Many lung cancers are diagnosed in later stages because the imaging necessary to detect cancer is delayed due to cost issues. Treatment depends on the type and stage of the cancer. Surgery, radiation therapy, chemotherapy, and targeted biological therapies are all options.[37] If the cancer is localized, surgery is usually the treatment of choice. If it has spread, surgery is combined with radiation and chemotherapy. Unfortunately, despite advances in medical technology, survival rates 1 year after diagnosis are low, at 41 percent overall; and the 5-year survival rate for all stages combined is only 16 percent.[38] Newer tests, such as low-dose computerized tomography (CT) scans, molecular markers in sputum, and improved biopsy techniques, have helped improve diagnosis, but we still have a long way to go.

**Risk Factors and Prevention** Risks for cancer increase dramatically based on the quantity of cigarettes smoked and the number of years smoked, often referred to as *pack years*. The greater the number of pack years that a person has smoked, the greater the risk of that person's developing

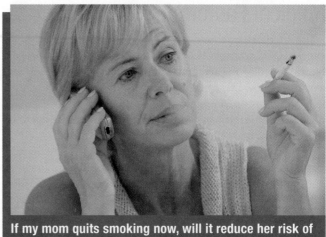

**If my mom quits smoking now, will it reduce her risk of lung cancer or is it too late?**

It's never too late to quit. Stopping smoking at any time will reduce your risk of lung cancer, in addition to the numerous other health benefits that are gained. Studies of women have shown that within 5 years of quitting, their risk of death from lung cancer had decreased by 21 percent, when compared with people who had continued smoking.

cancer. Quitting smoking does reduce the risk of developing lung cancer.[39] People who have been exposed to industrial substances such as arsenic and asbestos or to radiation are at the highest risk for lung cancer. Exposure both to secondhand cigarette smoke and to radon gas (a gas that leaks into houses from naturally occurring uranium in the soil) is believed to play an important role in lung cancer development for smokers, past smokers, and never smokers.[40]

## Breast Cancer

Breast cancer is a group of diseases that cause uncontrolled cell growth in breast tissue, particularly in the glands that produce milk and the ducts that connect those glands to the nipple. Cancers can also form in the connective and lymphatic tissues of the breast. In 2010, approximately 207,090 women and 1,970 men in the United States were diagnosed with invasive breast cancer for the first time. In addition, 54,010 new cases of in situ breast cancer, a more localized cancer, were diagnosed. About 39,840 women (and 390 men) died, making breast cancer the second leading cause of cancer death for women.[41] The good news is that like many other cancers, numbers of new cases and numbers of deaths declined in 2010, each by as much as 2 percent.[42]

**Detection, Symptoms, and Treatment** The earliest signs of breast cancer are usually observable on mammograms, often before lumps can be felt. However, mammograms are not foolproof and there is debate regarding the optimal age at which women should start regularly receiving them (see the **Points of View** box at right). Hence, regular breast self-examination (BSE) is also important (see the **Gender & Health** box on page 538). Mammograms detect between 80

# Mammography for Women under Age 50:
## TO SCREEN OR NOT TO SCREEN?

In November 2009, the U.S. Preventive Services Task Force, made up of experts from across the country, suggested that women in their forties should stop having mammograms until they are 50 and then have an exam every other year. Their rationale was that while accumulated evidence shows that women aged 50 to 74 seem to benefit from mammograms, similar benefits for women under age 40 are much less apparent. Their recommendation caused a furor in the general public and prompted groups such as the National Cancer Institute, American Cancer Society, and Susan G. Komen for the Cure to state to the public that they disagree with the recommendations of the task force.

Consider the following arguments for and against routine mammography screening for women between the ages of 40 and 50.

### Arguments for Mammograms for Women Aged 40 to 50

◯ Early detection offers a woman the best chance for a cure, and mammography is essential for early detection of breast cancer.

◯ Digital mammography significantly improves the detection of cancer in younger women and in women with dense breast tissue.

◯ Women who are screened with mammography between the ages of 39 and 49 experience a 15 percent reduction in breast cancer deaths.

◯ The data supporting elimination of the screenings are unclear.

◯ The United States has one of the highest breast cancer rates in the world. This action would be regressive and is based primarily on cost estimates and financial considerations, not preventive medicine.

### Arguments against Mammograms for Women Aged 40 to 50

◯ There is insufficient evidence indicating that screening mammograms are beneficial in women under the age of 40.

◯ High cumulative doses of low-energy radiation may lead to more cancers in younger women, particularly those with the *BRCA1* or *BRCA2* gene. Although inconclusive, there are studies that show slightly increased risks in eye, lung, and breast cancers in those who have had an annual mammography over many years.

◯ Some studies indicate that there is added anxiety, stress, and other psychological problems that result from mammograms.

◯ Those who receive an abnormal mammogram often have to go back for more screenings, even though there may be a false-positive result. Radiation exposure in these instances may increase overall risks of breast cancer.

◯ Costs for these procedures are high and can vary tremendously between clinics and within regions.

### Where Do You Stand?

◯ What are the implications of the new recommendations regarding mammograms for you? Your family members?

◯ Who should make the decision about whether a woman has a mammogram? Is it appropriate for the government or insurance companies to set policies in these matters?

◯ What are the potential benefits and risks—to individuals or to a society—from such a policy?

◯ When it comes to cancer prevention, do you think more screening is always better? Why or why not?

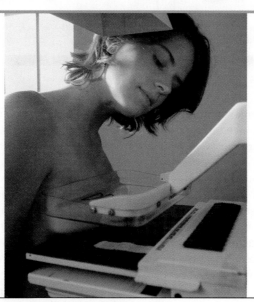

**Sources:** Recommendations of the U.S. Preventive Services Task Force, Agency for Healthcare Research and Quality, "Screening for Breast Cancer: Recommendation Statement," Updated December 2009, www.uspreventiveservicestask force.org/uspstf/uspsbrca.htm; Carol Milgard Breast Center, Breast Screening Guidelines Position Statement, Uploaded March 2010, www .carolmilgardbreastcenter.org/index.php/news/35/ breast_screening_guidelines; American Cancer Society, "Response to Changes to USPSTF Mammography Guidelines," 2009, http://pressroom .cancer.org/index.php?s=43&item=201.

# Breast Awareness and Self-Exam

Combined with annual examinations, and mammography as recommended, monthly breast self-exams can help women 20 and older who want to reduce their risk of a late breast cancer diagnosis. Women should know how their breasts normally look and feel and report any new breast changes to a health professional as soon as these changes are noted. Finding a breast change does not necessarily mean there is a cancer.

The best time for a woman to examine her breasts is when the breasts are not tender or swollen. Women who do self-exams should have their technique reviewed during health check-ups by their health care professional. The American Cancer Society recommends the use of mammography and clinical breast exam in addition to self-examination.

## HOW TO EXAMINE YOUR BREASTS

✳ Lie down and place your right arm behind your head (1). When you are lying down, the breast tissue spreads evenly over the chest wall and is as thin as possible, making it much easier to feel all the breast tissue.

✳ Use the finger pads of the three middle fingers on your left hand to feel for lumps in the right breast (2). Use overlapping dime-sized circular motions of the finger pads to feel the tissue.

✳ Use three different levels of pressure to feel all the breast tissue. Light pressure is needed to feel the tissue closest to the skin; medium pressure to feel a little deeper; and firm pressure to feel the tissue closest to the chest and ribs. A firm ridge in the lower curve of each breast is normal. If you're not sure how hard to press, talk with your doctor or nurse. Use each pressure level to feel the breast tissue before moving on to the next spot.

✳ Move around the breast in an up-and-down pattern starting at an imaginary line drawn straight down your side from the underarm and moving across the breast to the middle of the chest bone (sternum or breastbone) (3). Be sure to check the entire breast area going down until you feel only ribs and up to the neck or collarbone (clavicle).

✳ Repeat the exam on your left breast, using the finger pads of the right hand.

✳ While standing in front of a mirror with your hands pressing firmly down on your hips, look at your breasts for any changes of size, shape, contour, or dimpling, or redness or scaliness of the nipple or breast skin. (The pressing down on the hips position contracts the chest wall muscles and enhances any breast changes.)

✳ Examine each underarm while sitting up or standing and with your arm only slightly raised so you can easily feel in this area. Raising your arm straight up tightens the tissue in this area and makes it harder to examine.

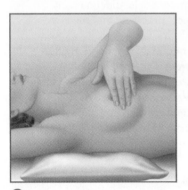

**①** Perform exam lying down.

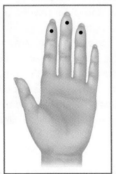

**②** Use pads of the 3 middle fingers.

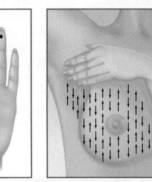

**③** Follow an up-and-down pattern.

**Source:** Adapted from "Breast Awareness and Self-Examination." Reprinted by the permission of the American Cancer Society, Inc., from www.cancer.org. All rights reserved.

and 90 percent of breast cancers in women without symptoms. A newer form of magnetic resonance imaging (MRI) appears to be even more accurate, particularly in women with genetic risks for tumors.[43]

Once breast cancer has grown enough that it can be felt by palpating the area, many women will seek medical care. Symptoms may include persistent breast changes, such as a lump in the breast or surrounding lymph nodes, thickening, dimpling, skin irritation, distortion, retraction or scaliness of the nipple, nipple discharge, or tenderness.

Treatments range from a lumpectomy to radical mastectomy to various combinations of radiation or chemotherapy. Among nonsurgical options, promising results have been noted among women using *selective estrogen-receptor modulators (SERMs)* such as tamoxifen and raloxifene, particularly among women whose cancers appear to grow in response to estrogen. These drugs, as well as new *aromatase inhibitors,* work by blocking estrogen. The 5-year survival rate for people with localized breast cancer (which includes all people living 5 years after diagnosis, whether they are in remission, disease free, or under treatment) has risen from 80 percent in the 1950s to 98 percent today.[44] However, these statistics vary dramatically, based on the stage of the cancer when it is first detected and whether it has spread. If the cancer has spread to the lymph nodes or other organs, the 5-year survival rate drops to as low as 27 percent.[45]

**Risk Factors and Prevention** The incidence of breast cancer increases with age. Although there are many possible risk factors, those that are well supported by research include family history of breast cancer, menstrual periods that started early and ended late in life, obesity after menopause, recent use of oral contraceptives or postmenopausal hormone therapy, never bearing children or bearing a first child after age 30, consuming two or more drinks of alcohol per day, and physical inactivity.[46] Having *BRCA1* and *BRCA2* gene mutations appears to account for approximately 5 to 10 percent of all cases of breast cancer and women who possess these genes have a 60 to 80 percent risk of developing breast cancer by age 70 as compared to a 7 percent risk in women without the mutations. Because these genes are rare, routine screening for them is not recommended unless there is a strong family history of breast cancer.[47]

International differences in breast cancer incidence correlate with variations in diet, especially fat intake, although a causal role for these dietary factors has not been firmly established. Sudden weight gain has also been implicated. Research also shows that regular exercise, even some forms of recreational exercise, can reduce risk.[48] In addition, preliminary studies in China indicate that higher dietary intake of soy may improve breast cancer outcomes. More research with different populations is necessary.[49]

## Colon and Rectal Cancers

Colorectal cancers (cancers of the colon and rectum) continue to be the third most commonly diagnosed cancer in both men and women and the second leading cause of cancer deaths, even though death rates are declining. If current rates of decline continue, experts predict a mortality rate reduction of 50 percent by 2020 due to earlier diagnosis and improved treatments. However, increasing incidence in people under the age of 50 has experts concerned, particularly because early diagnosis is critical and increasing numbers lack the health insurance that would cover necessary screening.[50] In 2010, there were over 142,570 cases diagnosed in the United States and 51,370 deaths.[51]

**Detection, Symptoms, and Treatment** Because colorectal cancer tends to spread slowly, the prognosis is quite good if it is caught in the early stages. However, in its early stages, colorectal cancer typically has no symptoms. As the disease progresses, bleeding from the rectum, blood in the stool, and changes in bowel habits are the major warning signals. A good way to catch the cancer early is through testing. However, only 12.1 percent of all Americans over age 50 have had the most basic screening test—the at-home fecal occult blood test—in the past year, and only 43.1 percent have had an endoscopy test. Although these rates are low, it

should be noted that rates are even lower among people aged 50 to 64 and especially lower among those who are non-white, have fewer years of education, lack health insurance, and are recent immigrants.[52] Colonoscopies and other screening tests should begin at age 50 for most people. Virtual colonoscopies and fecal DNA testing are newer diagnostic techniques that have shown promise. Treatment often consists of radiation or surgery. Chemotherapy, although not used extensively in the past, is today a possibility.

**Risk Factors and Prevention** Anyone can get colorectal cancer, but people who are over age 50, who are obese, who have a family history of colon and rectal cancer, who have a personal or family history of polyps (benign growths) in the colon or rectum, or who have inflammatory bowel problems such as colitis run an increased risk. A history of diabetes also seems to increase risk. Other possible risk factors include diets high in fat or low in fiber, high consumption of red and processed meats, smoking, sedentary lifestyle, high alcohol consumption, and low intake of fruits and vegetables. Regular exercise, a diet with lots of fruits and other plant foods, a healthy weight, and moderation in alcohol consumption appear to be among the most promising prevention strategies. Consumption of milk and calcium also appears to decrease risks. New research suggests that nonsteroidal anti-inflammatory drugs (NSAIDs) such as aspirin, postmenopausal hormones, folic acid, calcium supplements, selenium, and vitamin E may also help.[53]

## Skin Cancer

Skin cancer is the most common form of cancer in the United States today, affecting over 1 million people every year (1 in 5 of all adults). In 2010, an estimated 11,790 people died of skin cancer (8,700 from melanoma and 3,090 from other forms of skin cancer).[54] The two most common types of skin cancer—basal cell and squamous cell carcinomas—are highly curable. **Malignant melanoma,** the third most common form of skin cancer, is the most dangerous, especially for women aged 25 to 29.[55] Between 65 and 90 percent of melanomas are caused by exposure to ultraviolet (UV) light or sunlight.

**malignant melanoma** A virulent cancer of the melanocytes (pigment-producing cells) of the skin.

**Detection, Symptoms, and Treatment** Potentially cancerous growths are often visible as abnormalities on the skin. Basal and squamous cell carcinomas show up most commonly on the face, ears, neck, arms, hands, and legs as warty bumps, colored spots, or scaly patches. Bleeding, itchiness, pain, or oozing are other symptoms that warrant attention. Surgery may be necessary to remove them, but they are seldom life threatening.

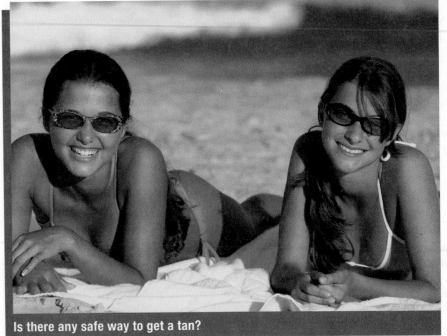

**Is there any safe way to get a tan?**

Unfortunately, no. There is no such thing as a "safe" tan, because a tan is visible evidence of UV-induced skin damage. The injury accumulated through years of tanning contributes to premature aging, as well as increasing your risk for disfiguring forms of skin cancer, eye problems, and possible death from melanoma. Whether the UV rays causing your tan came from the sun or from a tanning bed, the damage—and the cancer risk—is the same. Nor is an existing "base tan" protective against further damage. According to the American Cancer Society, tanned skin can provide only about the equivalent of sun protection factor (SPF) 4 sunscreen—much too weak to be considered protective. It isn't possible or practical to avoid sunlight completely, but wearing sunscreen of SPF 15 or higher every day can prevent further damage and diminish the cumulative effects of sun exposure.

In striking contrast is melanoma, an invasive killer that may appear as a skin lesion. Typically, the lesion's size, shape, or color changes and it spreads to regional organs and throughout the body. Malignant melanomas account for over 75 percent of all skin cancer deaths. Figure 16.3 shows melanoma compared to basal cell and squamous cell carcinomas. The *ABCD* rule can help you remember the warning signs of melanoma:

- **Asymmetry.** One half of the mole or lesion does not match the other half.
- **Border irregularity.** The edges are uneven, notched, or scalloped.
- **Color.** Pigmentation is not uniform. Melanomas may vary in color from tan to deeper brown, reddish black, black, or deep bluish black.
- **Diameter.** Its diameter is greater than 6 millimeters (about the size of a pea).

Treatment of skin cancer depends on the type of cancer, its stage, and its location. Surgery, laser treatments, topical chemical agents, *electrodesiccation* (tissue destruction by heat), and *cryosurgery* (tissue destruction by freezing) are all common forms of treatment. For melanoma, treatment may involve surgical removal of the regional lymph nodes, radiation, or chemotherapy.

**Risk Factors and Prevention** Anyone who overexposes himself or herself to ultraviolet (UV) radiation without adequate protection is at risk for skin cancer. The risk is greatest for people who:

- Have fair skin; blonde, red, or light brown hair; blue, green, or gray eyes
- Always burn before tanning or burn easily and peel readily
- Don't tan easily but spend lots of time outdoors
- Use no or low–sun protection factor (SPF) sunscreens or expired suntan lotions
- Have had skin cancer or have a family history of skin cancer
- Have experienced severe sunburns during childhood

Preventing skin cancer is a matter of limiting exposure to harmful UV rays found in sunlight. What happens when you

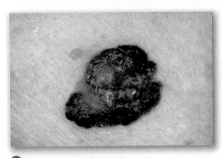
ⓐ Malignant melanoma

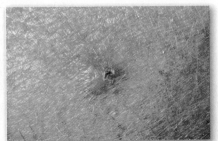
ⓑ Basal cell carcinoma

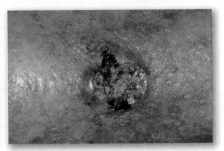
ⓒ Squamous cell carcinoma

FIGURE 16.3 **Types of Skin Cancers**
Preventing skin cancer includes keeping a careful watch for any new, pigmented growths and for changes to any moles. The ABCD warning signs of melanoma (a) include *asymmetrical* shapes, irregular *borders, color* variation, and an increase in *diameter.* Basal cell carcinoma (b) and squamous cell carcinoma (c) should be brought to your physician's attention but are not as deadly as melanoma.

## Tips for Protecting Your Skin in the Sun

✱ Avoid the sun or seek shade from 10 AM to 4 PM, when the sun's rays are strongest. Even on a cloudy day, up to 80 percent of the sun's rays can get through.

✱ Apply an SPF 15 or higher sunscreen evenly to all uncovered skin before going outside. Look for a "broad-spectrum" sunscreen that protects against both UVA and UVB radiation. Check the label for the correct amount of time you should allow between applying the product and going outdoors. If the label does not specify, apply it 15 minutes before going outside.

✱ Check the expiration date on your sunscreen. Sunscreens lose effectiveness over time.

✱ Remember to apply sunscreen to your eyelids, lips, nose, ears, neck, hands, and feet. If you don't have much hair, apply sunscreen to the top of your head, too.

✱ Reapply sunscreen often. The label will tell you how often you need to do this. If it isn't waterproof, reapply it after swimming, or if you are sweating a lot.

✱ Wear loose-fitting, light-colored clothing. You can now purchase clothing that has SPF protection in most sporting goods stores. Wear a wide-brimmed, light-colored hat to protect your head and face.

✱ Use sunglasses with 99 to 100 percent UV protection to protect your eyes. Look for polarization in your shades.

✱ Check your skin for cancer, keeping an eye out for changes in birthmarks, moles, or sunspots.

**Source:** U.S. Food and Drug Administration, "Sun Safety: Save Your Skin!" Updated June 2010, www.fda.gov/ForConsumers/ConsumerUpdates/ucm049090.htm.

expose yourself to sunlight? The skin responds to photodamage by increasing its thickness and the number of pigment cells (melanocytes), which produce the "tan" look. Ultraviolet light damages the skin's immune cells, lowering the normal immune protection of our skin and priming it for cancer. Photodamage also causes wrinkling by impairing the elastic substances (collagens) that keep skin soft and pliable. See the **Skills for Behavior Change** box for tips on staying safe in the sun.

In spite of the risks, over 60 percent of Americans aged 25 and younger report that they are "working on a tan" at some point during the year.[56] Why is this? Recent research suggests a connection between high levels of UV light and endorphins. Those who tan in the sun or by artificial means may experience a short "high" for this reason, and tanning can become a type of addiction. For information on the risks of using tanning booths and salons, see the **Student Health Today** box on page 542.

# Prostate Cancer

Cancer of the prostate is the most frequently diagnosed cancer in American males today, excluding skin cancer, and is the second leading cause of cancer deaths in men after lung cancer. In 2010, about 217,230 new cases of prostate cancer were diagnosed in the United States. About 1 in 6 men will be diagnosed with prostate cancer during his lifetime, but only 1 in 36 will die of it.[57]

**Detection, Symptoms, and Treatment** The prostate is a muscular, walnut-sized gland that surrounds part of a man's urethra, the tube that transports urine and sperm out of the body. A part of the reproductive system, its primary function is to produce seminal fluid. Symptoms of prostate cancer may include weak or interrupted urine flow; difficulty starting or stopping urination; feeling the urge to urinate frequently; pain on urination; blood in the urine; or pain in the low back, pelvis, or thighs. Many men have no symptoms in the early stages.

The American Cancer Society recommends that men aged 50 and over have an annual **prostate-specific antigen (PSA)** test and digital rectal prostate examination. Fortunately, prostate cancers tend to progress slowly and 90 percent of all prostate cancers are detected while they are still in the local or regional stages. Over the past 20 years, the 5-year survival rate for all stages combined has increased from 67 percent to almost 99 percent, and the 15-year survival rate is over 76 percent.[58]

**prostate-specific antigen (PSA)** An antigen found in prostate cancer patients.

**Risk Factors and Prevention** Chances of developing prostate cancer increase dramatically with age. Almost 2 out of every 3 prostate cancers are diagnosed in men over the age

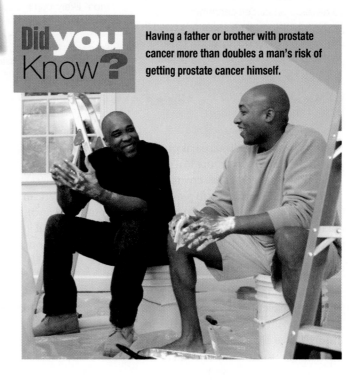

**Did you Know?**

Having a father or brother with prostate cancer more than doubles a man's risk of getting prostate cancer himself.

# ARTIFICIAL TANS: SACRIFICING HEALTH FOR BEAUTY

Tanning is a multibillion-dollar industry that draws almost 30 million Americans into over 25,000 salons each year. The vast majority of them are teens or people in their twenties—usually women. In our culture, being tan is often equated with being healthy, chic, wealthy, and attractive, leading increasing numbers of men and women, but particularly adolescent girls, to seek quick tans in packaged visits to tanning beds.

Most tanning salon patrons incorrectly believe that tanning booths are safer than sitting in the sun. The truth is that there is no such thing as a safe tan from *any* source! Every time you tan, whether in the sun or in a salon, you are exposing your skin to harmful ultraviolet (UV) light rays. All tanning lamps emit UVA rays, and most emit UVB rays as well; both types can cause long-term skin damage and contribute to cancer. Consider the following:

✳ Exposure to tanning beds at a young age increases melanoma risk by 75 percent.
✳ People who use tanning beds are 2.5 times more likely to develop squamous cell carcinoma and 1.5 times more likely to develop basal cell carcinoma.
✳ New high-pressure sunlamps used in some salons emit doses of UV radiation that can be as much as 12 times that of the sun.

✳ Up to 90 percent of visible skin changes commonly blamed on aging are caused by the sun.

Because of the many salons that are springing up across the country, the artificial tanning industry is difficult to monitor and regulate. Dermatologists cite additional factors that make tanning in a salon as bad—or even worse—than sitting in the sun:

✳ Some tanning facilities do not calibrate the UV output of their tanning bulbs or ensure sufficient rotation of newer and older bulbs, which can lead to more or less exposure than you paid for.
✳ Tanning facility patrons often try for a total body tan. The buttocks and genitalia are particularly sensitive to UV radiation and are prone to developing skin cancer.
✳ Shared tanning booths and beds pose significant hygiene risks. Anytime you come in contact with body secretions from others, you run the risk of an infectious disease. Don't assume that those little colored water sprayers used to "clean" the inside of the beds are sufficient to kill organisms. The busier the facility, the more likely you are to come into contact with germs that could make you ill.

**Sources:** S. Danoff-Berg and C. E. Mosher, "Prediction of Tanning Salon Use: Behavioral Alternatives for Enhancing Appearance, Relaxing

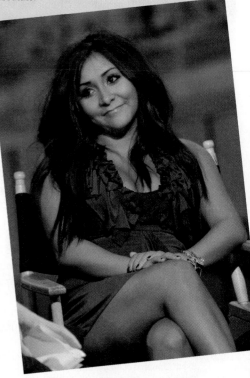

Doctors from the Skin Cancer Foundation staged an "intervention" with Snooki, one of the stars of MTV's *Jersey Shore*. When she saw the evidence of skin damage that indoor tanning can cause, she agreed to use spray-on products as a substitute.

and Socializing," *Journal of Health Psychology* 11, no. 3 (2006): 511–18; Skin Cancer Foundation, "Skin Cancer Facts," 2010, www.skincancer.org/Skin-Cancer/Skin-Cancer-Facts.

---

of 65.[59] Usually the disease has progressed to the point of displaying symptoms, or, more likely, they are seeing a doctor for other problems and get a screening test or PSA test.

Race is also a risk factor in prostate cancer: African American men are 61 percent more likely to develop prostate cancer than white men and are much more likely to be diagnosed at an advanced stage. Prostate cancer is less common among Asian men and occurs at about the same rates among Hispanic men as it does among white men.[60]

Eating more fruits and vegetables, particularly those containing lycopene, a pigment found in tomatoes and other red fruits, may lower the risk of prostate cancer. Some studies have suggested that vitamin E or selenium may be beneficial, but in a major clinical trial of more than 35,000

men conducted over 5 years neither supplement was found to lower prostate cancer risk.[61] The best advice is to follow the dietary recommendations discussed in Chapter 7 and maintain a healthy weight.

## Ovarian Cancer

Ovarian cancer is the fifth leading cause of cancer deaths for women, with about 21,880 being diagnosed with it in 2010 and 13,850 dying from it.[62] Ovarian cancer causes more deaths than any other cancer of the reproductive system because women tend not to discover it until the cancer is at an advanced stage. Overall, 1-year survival rates are 75 percent, and 5-year suvival rates are 46 percent.[63]

**Detection, Symptoms, and Treatment** The most common symptom is enlargement of the abdomen. Women over age 40 may experience persistent digestive disturbances as well. Abnormal vaginal bleeding or discharge is rarely a symptom until the disease is advanced. Other symptoms include vague digestive disturbances (stomach discomfort, gas, pressure, distention), fatigue, pain during intercourse, unexplained weight loss, unexplained changes in bowel or bladder habits, urinary frequency, and incontinence.[64]

Treatment for early stage ovarian cancer typically includes surgery, chemotherapy, and occasionally radiation therapy. Depending on the patient's age and her desire to bear children in the future, one or both ovaries, fallopian tubes, and the uterus may be removed. Chemotherapy and radiation are also sometimes used in addition to surgery.

**Risk Factors and Prevention** Primary relatives (mother, daughter, sister) of a woman who has had ovarian cancer are at increased risk. A family or personal history of breast or colon cancer is also associated with increased risk. Women who have never been pregnant are more likely to develop ovarian cancer than those who have given birth to a child, and the more children a woman has had, the less risk she faces. The use of fertility drugs may also increase a woman's risk.[65]

Research shows that using birth control pills, adhering to a low-fat diet, having multiple children, and breast-feeding can reduce your risk of ovarian cancer.[66] So, should you get pregnant or start taking birth control pills to reduce risk? No. General prevention strategies such as focusing on diet, exercise, sleep, stress management, and weight control are good ideas for combating the risk of ovarian and any of the other cancers discussed in this chapter.

To protect yourself, get a complete annual pelvic examination. Women over 40 should have a cancer-related checkup every year. Uterine ultrasound or a blood test is recommended for those with risk factors or unexplained symptoms.

# Cervical and Endometrial (Uterine) Cancer

Most uterine cancers develop in the body of the uterus, usually in the endometrium. The rest develop in the cervix, located at the base of the uterus. In 2010, an estimated 12,200 new cases of cervical cancer and 43,470 cases of endometrial cancer were diagnosed in the United States.[67] The overall incidence of cervical and uterine cancer has been declining steadily over the past decade. This decline may be due to more regular screenings of younger women using the **Pap test,** a procedure in which cells taken from the cervical region are examined for abnormal cellular activity. Although Pap tests are very effective for detecting early-stage cervical cancer, they are less effective for detecting cancers of the uterine lining. Early warning signs of uterine cancer include bleeding outside the normal menstrual period or after menopause or persistent unusual vaginal discharge.

Risk factors for cervical cancer include early age at first intercourse, multiple sex partners, cigarette smoking, and certain sexually transmitted infections, including HPV (the cause of genital warts) and herpes. For endometrial cancer, age is a risk factor; however, estrogen and obesity are also strong risk factors. In addition, risks are increased by treatment with tamoxifen for breast cancer, metabolic syndrome, late menopause, never bearing children, a history of polyps in the uterus or ovaries, a history of other cancers, and race (white women are at higher risk).[68]

**Pap test** A procedure in which cells taken from the cervical region are examined for abnormal cellular activity.

# Testicular Cancer

Testicular cancer is one of the most common types of solid tumors found in young adult men, affecting nearly 8,400 young men in 2010. Those between the ages of 15 and 35 are at greatest risk. There has been a steady increase in testicular cancer frequency over the past several years in this age group.[69] However, with a 96 percent 5-year survival rate, it is one of the most curable forms of cancer. Although the cause of testicular cancer is unknown, several risk factors have been identified. Men with undescended testicles appear to be at greatest risk, and some studies indicate a genetic influence.

In general, testicular tumors first appear as an enlargement of the testis or thickening in testicular tissue. Because this enlargement is often painless, it is important that young men practice regular testicular self-examination (see the **Gender & Health** box on page 544.

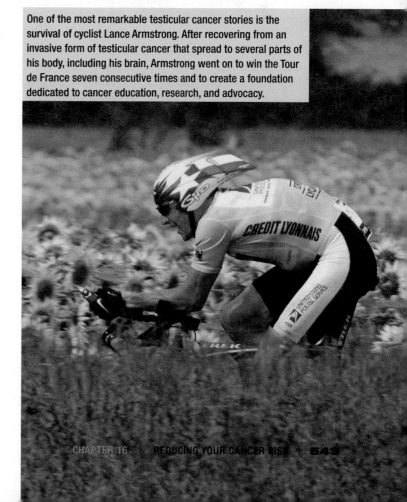

One of the most remarkable testicular cancer stories is the survival of cyclist Lance Armstrong. After recovering from an invasive form of testicular cancer that spread to several parts of his body, including his brain, Armstrong went on to win the Tour de France seven consecutive times and to create a foundation dedicated to cancer education, research, and advocacy.

# Testicular Self-Exam

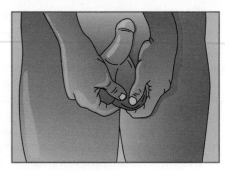

Most testicular cancers can be found at an early stage. The American Cancer Society (ACS) advises men to be aware of testicular cancer and to see a doctor right away if they find a lump in a testicle. Because regular testicular self-exams have not been studied enough to show that they reduce the death rate from this cancer, the ACS does not have a recommendation on regular testicular self-exams for all men. If you have certain risk factors that increase your chance of developing testicular cancer (e.g., an undescended testicle, previous germ cell tumor in one testicle, or a family history), you should seriously consider monthly self-exams and talk about it with your doctor.

## HOW TO EXAMINE YOUR TESTICLES

The best time for you to examine your testicles is during or after a shower, when the skin of the scrotum is relaxed.

✳ Hold the penis out of the way and examine each testicle separately.

✳ Hold the testicle between your thumbs and fingers with both hands and roll it gently between the fingers.

✳ Look and feel for any hard lumps or nodules (smooth, rounded masses) or any change in the size, shape, or consistency of the testes.

You should be aware that each normal testis has an epididymis, which can feel like a small bump on the upper or middle outer side of the testis. Normal testicles also contain blood vessels, supporting tissues, and tubes that conduct sperm. Some men may confuse these with cancer at first. In addition, some non-cancerous problems can sometimes cause swelling or lumps around a testicle. If you have any concerns, ask your doctor. Note that the ACS recommends a testicular exam as part of a routine cancer-related checkup.

**Source:** Adapted from "Do I Have Testicular Cancer? Testicular Self-Exam." Reprinted by the permission of the American Cancer Society, Inc. from www.cancer.org. All rights reserved.

## Leukemia

Leukemia is a cancer of the blood-forming tissues that leads to proliferation of millions of immature white blood cells. These abnormal cells crowd out normal white blood cells (which fight infection), platelets (which control hemorrhaging), and red blood cells (which carry oxygen to body cells). As a result, symptoms such as fatigue, paleness, weight loss, easy bruising, repeated infections, nosebleeds, and other forms of hemorrhaging occur.

Leukemia can be acute or chronic and can strike both sexes and all age groups. An estimated 43,050 new cases were diagnosed in the United States in 2010.[70] Chronic leukemia can develop over several months and have few symptoms. It is usually treated with radiation and chemotherapy. Other methods of treatment include bone marrow and stem cell transplants.

## Lymphoma

Just a few short years ago, not many people had heard much about lymphomas, a group of cancers of the lymphatic system that include Hodgkin's disease and non-Hodgkin lymphoma. Today, however, lymphomas are among the fastest growing cancers, with an estimated 74,030 new cases in 2010.[71] Much of this increase has occurred in women. The cause is unknown; however, a weakened immune system is suspected—particularly one that has been exposed to viruses such as HIV, hepatitis C, Epstein-Barr virus (EBV), and others. Treatment for lymphoma varies by type and stage; however, chemotherapy and radiotherapy are commonly used.

## Facing Cancer

We've made significant progress in preventing cancer, and there is much you can do to help reduce your own risks. Make a realistic assessment of your own risk factors, avoid those behaviors that put you at risk, and increase healthy behaviors. Even if you have significant risks, those are factors you can control. Be sure that you understand and follow the recommendations for self-exams and medical checkups in Table 16.3. The earlier cancer is diagnosed, the better the prognosis will be.

## Detecting Cancer

If you are at high risk for developing cancer, or if you notice potential cancer symptoms, your health care provider might

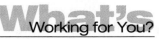

### Working for You?

You may already be taking actions to lessen your cancer risk. Which of the following are true for you?

☐ I don't smoke or I have committed to quitting and joined a group to do this.

☐ I apply sunscreen before I leave the house every day.

☐ I do regular breast or testicular self-exams.

**Screening Guidelines for the Early Detection of Cancer in Average-Risk Asymptomatic People**

| Cancer Site | Population | Test or Procedure | Frequency |
|---|---|---|---|
| **Breast** | Women, aged 20+ | Breast self-examination (BSE) | Beginning in their early 20s, women should be told about the benefits and limitations of BSE. The importance of prompt reporting of any new breast symptoms to a health professional should be emphasized. Women who choose to do BSE should receive instruction and have their technique reviewed during a periodic health examination. It is acceptable for women to choose not to do BSE or to do BSE irregularly. |
| | | Clinical breast examination (CBE) | For women in their 20s and 30s, it is recommended that CBE be part of a periodic health examination, preferably at least every 3 years. Asymptomatic women aged 40 and over should continue to receive a CBE as part of a periodic health examination, preferably annually. |
| | | Mammography | Begin annual mammography at age 40.* |
| **Colon/rectum**[†] | Men and women, aged 50+ | *Tests that find polyps and cancer:* | |
| | | Flexible sigmoidoscopy,[‡] *or* | Every 5 years, starting at age 50 |
| | | Colonoscopy, *or* | Every 10 years, starting at age 50 |
| | | Double-contrast barium enema (DCBE),[‡] *or* | Every 5 years, starting at age 50 |
| | | CT colonography (virtual colonoscopy)[‡] | Every 5 years, starting at age 50 |
| | | *Tests that mainly find cancer:* | |
| | | Fecal occult blood test (FOBT) with at least 50% test sensitivity for cancer, or fecal immuno-chemical test (FIT), with at least 50% test sensitivity for cancer,[‡§] *or* | Annual, starting at age 50 |
| | | Stool DNA test (sDNA)[‡] | Interval uncertain, starting at age 50 |
| **Prostate** | Men, aged 50+ | Prostate-specific antigen (PSA) with or without digital rectal examination (DRE) | Asymptomatic men who have at least a 10-year life expectancy should have an opportunity to make an informed decision with their health care provider about screening for prostate cancer after receiving information about the uncertainties, risks, and potential benefits associated with screening. Men at average risk should receive this information beginning at age 50. Men at higher risk, including African American men and men with a first-degree relative (father or brother) diagnosed with prostate cancer before age 65, should receive this information beginning at age 45. Men at appreciably higher risk (multiple family members diagnosed with prostate cancer before age 65) should receive this information beginning at age 40. |
| **Cervix** | Women, aged 18+ | Pap test | Cervical cancer screening should begin approximately 3 years after a woman begins having vaginal intercourse, but no later than 21 years of age. Screening should be done every year with conventional Pap tests or every 2 years using liquid-based Pap tests. At or after age 30, women who have had three normal test results in a row may get screened every 2 to 3 years with cervical cytology (either conventional or liquid-based Pap test) alone, or every 3 years with an HPV DNA test plus cervical cytology. Women aged 70 and older who have had three or more normal Pap tests and no abnormal Pap tests in the past 10 years and women who have had a total hysterectomy may choose to stop cervical cancer screening. |
| **Endometrium** | Women, at menopause | | At the time of menopause, women at average risk should be informed about risks and symptoms of endometrial cancer and strongly encouraged to report any unexpected bleeding or spotting to their physician. |
| **Cancer-related checkup** | Men and women, aged 20+ | | During a periodic health examination, the cancer-related checkup should include examination for cancers of the thyroid; testicles; ovaries; lymph nodes; oral cavity; and skin; and health counseling about tobacco, sun exposure, diet and nutrition, risk factors, sexual practices, and environmental and occupational exposures. |

*Beginning at age 40, annual CBE should be performed prior to mammography.

[†]Individuals with a personal or family history of colorectal cancer or adenomas, inflammatory bowel disease, or high-risk genetic syndromes should continue to follow the most recent recommendations for individuals at increased or high risk.

[‡]Colonoscopy should be done if test results are positive.

[§]For FOBT or FIT used as a screening test, the take-home multiple sample method should be used. An FOBT or FIT done during a DRE in the doctor's office is not adequate for screening.

**Source:** American Cancer Society, *Cancer Facts & Figures 2010*. Atlanta: American Cancer Society, Inc. Used with permission.

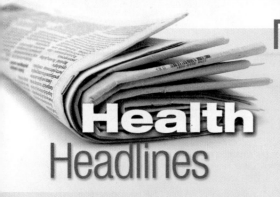

# Health Headlines

## NEW TREATMENTS FOR CANCER

Surgery, chemotherapy, and radiation therapy remain the most commonly used treatments for all types of cancer. However, newer techniques are constantly being investigated that may be more effective for certain cancers or for certain patients. Among the treatments now being investigated or becoming available are the following:

✴ **Immunotherapy.** The goal of immunotherapy is to enhance the body's own disease-fighting systems to help control cancer. Biological response modifiers such as interferon and interleukin-2 are under study. Immunotherapies have been particularly effective against melanomas and certain kidney cancers.

✴ **Biological therapies.** One of the most exciting new approaches for spurring the immune system to ward off cancer is the use of *cancer-fighting vaccines.* These alert the body's immune defenses to good cells that have gone bad. Rather than preventing disease as other vaccines do, they help people who are already ill.

✴ **Gene therapies.** Research on the effectiveness of *gene therapy* has moved into early clinical trials. Scientists have found signs of a virus carrying genetic information that makes the cells it infects (such as cancer cells) susceptible to an antiviral drug. Scientists are also looking at ways to transfer genes that increase the patient's immune response to the cancerous tumor or that confer drug resistance to the bone marrow so that higher doses of chemotherapeutic drugs can be given.

✴ **Angiogenesis inhibitors.** In other studies, researchers are testing compounds that may stop tumors from forming new blood vessels, a process called *angiogenesis.* Without adequate blood supply, tumors either die or grow very slowly, giving other chemotherapeutic agents a better chance to fight them.

✴ **Disruption of cancer pathways.** In recent years, scientists have identified various steps in what is termed the *cancer pathway.* These include oncogene actions, hormone receptors, growth factors, metastasis, and angiogenesis. Preliminary studies are under way to design compounds that inhibit actions at these various steps.

✴ **Smart drugs.** Drugs such as Herceptin, Gleevec, and Avastin are new forms of *targeted smart-drug therapies* that attack only the cancer cells and do not hit the entire body.

✴ **Enzyme inhibitors.** A powerful enzyme inhibitor, *TIMP2,* shows promise for slowing the metastasis of tumor cells. A metastasis suppressor gene, *NM23,* has also been identified. Both of these therapies are aimed at disrupting cancer pathways.

✴ **Neoadjuvant chemotherapy.** This method (which uses chemotherapy to shrink the tumor and then surgically removing it) has been tried against various types of cancers.

✴ **Stem cell research.** Transplants of stem cells from donor bone marrow are used with success to restore blood stem cells (the cells that divide to produce blood cells) when a patient's bone marrow has been destroyed by disease, chemotherapy, or radiation.

---

use one or more tests to diagnose or rule out cancer. **Magnetic resonance imaging (MRI)** uses a huge electromagnet to detect tumors by mapping the vibrations of the atoms in the body on a computer screen. The **computerized axial tomography (CAT) scan** uses X rays to examine parts of the body. In both of these painless, noninvasive procedures, cross-sectioned pictures can reveal a tumor's shape and location more accurately than can conventional X rays. *Prostatic ultrasound* (a rectal probe using ultrasonic waves to produce an image of the prostate) is being investigated as a means to increase the early detection of prostate cancer. Prostatic ultrasound has been combined with the PSA blood test.

## Cancer Treatments

Cancer treatments vary according to the type of cancer and its stage. Surgery, in which the tumor and surrounding tissue are removed, is one common strategy. It may be performed alone or in combination with other treatments. The surgeon may operate using traditional surgical instruments such as a scalpel, or by using a laser, laparoscope, or other tools for less invasive results. Pain and infection are the most common problems after surgery.

**Radiotherapy** (the use of radiation) or **chemotherapy** (the use of drugs) to kill cancerous cells are also used. Radiation destroys malignant cells or stops cell growth. It is most effective in treating localized cancer masses because it can be targeted to a particular area of the body. Over the course of several weeks, patients are treated by a machine that exposes the designated part of the body to high-energy rays. The radiotherapy usually takes place on an out-patient basis. Side effects include fatigue, changes to the skin in the affected area, and a small increase in the chance of developing another type of cancer.

Chemotherapy may be used to shrink a tumor before surgery or radiation therapy, after surgery or radiation therapy to kill remaining cancer cells, or on its own. Powerful drugs are administered, usually in on-and-off cycles so that the body can recover from the effects of the drugs. Side effects may include nausea, hair loss, fatigue, increased chance of bleeding, bruising, infection, and anemia, and go away as the drugs leave the body after treatment. Other possible effects, such as the loss of fertility, may be permanent.

**magnetic resonance imaging (MRI)** A device that uses magnetic fields, radio waves, and computers to generate an image of internal tissues of the body for diagnostic purposes without the use of radiation.
**computerized axial tomography (CAT) scan** A scan by a machine that uses radiation to view internal organs not normally visible in X rays.
**radiotherapy** The use of radiation to kill cancerous cells.
**chemotherapy** The use of drugs to kill cancerous cells.

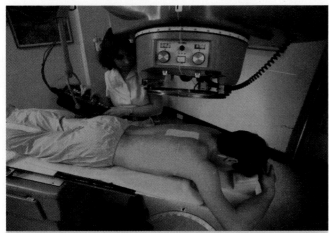

Radiation therapy is often used to target and destroy cancerous tumors. The machine in this photograph emits gamma rays, which are typically used to treat localized secondary cancers and also as pain relief for otherwise untreatable cancer. They are less powerful than the X rays emitted from linear accelerators, the other type of machine most frequently used in radiation therapy.

In the process of killing malignant cells, some healthy cells are also destroyed, and long-term damage to the cardiovascular system and other body systems from radiotherapy and chemotherapy can be significant.

Cancer patient participation in clinical trials (people-based studies of new drugs or procedures) has provided a new source of hope for many undergoing cancer treatment. Because of the many unknown variables, deciding whether to participate in a clinical trial can be a difficult decision. Despite the risks, which should be carefully considered, thousands of clinical trial participants have benefited from treatments that would otherwise be unavailable to them.

Several newer treatments described in the **Health Headlines** box at left are either being used in clinical trials or have become available in selected cancer centers throughout the country. In addition, psychosocial and behavioral research has become increasingly important as health professionals learn more about lifestyle factors that influence risk and survivability. Health care practitioners have become more aware of the psychological needs of patients and families and have begun to tailor treatment programs to meet their diverse needs.

Before beginning any form of cancer therapy, it is imperative to be a vigilant and vocal consumer. Read and seek information from cancer support groups. Check the skills of your surgeon, your radiation therapist, and your doctor in terms of clinical experience and interpersonal interactions. Look at Oncolink and other websites supported by the National Cancer Institute and the American Cancer Society (ACS) and check out clinical trials, reports on effectiveness of various treatments, new experimental therapies, and other options. Also, although you may like and trust your family doctor, it is always a good idea to seek advice or consultation from larger cancer facilities that see many patients and are well equipped to deal with all situations. See the **Consumer Health** box on page 548 for more on being your own advocate or an advocate for someone you love.

## Cancer Survivors

Heightened public awareness and an improved prognosis have made the cancer experience less threatening and isolating than it once was. In fact, assistance for cancer patients—including cancer support groups, cancer information workshops, and low-cost medical consultation—is more widely available than ever. In many cases, however, coping with life after cancer treatment can be difficult.[72]

14%
of the estimated 10.8 million cancer survivors in the U.S. today were diagnosed more than 20 years ago.

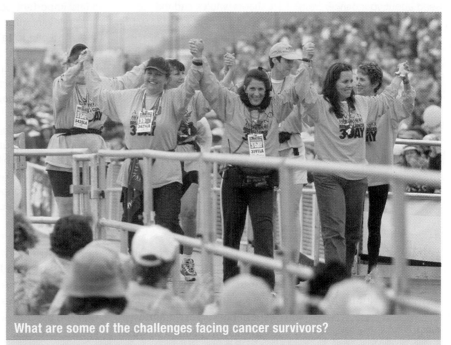

**What are some of the challenges facing cancer survivors?**

The journey through cancer survivorship is not always smooth. Even after the 5-year benchmark is reached, living a full, positive life in cancer's wake can be a major challenge. There may be physical, emotional, and financial issues to cope with for years after diagnosis and treatment. Survivors may find themselves struggling with access to health insurance and life insurance, financial strains, difficulties with employment, and the toll on personal relationships. Survivors also have to live with the possibility of a recurrence. However, cancer survivors can and do live active, productive lives despite these challenges.

# BEING A HEALTH ADVOCATE FOR YOURSELF OR SOMEONE YOU LOVE

Any time cancer is diagnosed, people can react with anxiety, fear, and anger. Emotional distress is sometimes so intense that patients and their loved ones are unable to make critical health care decisions for themselves or for others. Of course you want to remain calm, check out options, and be proactive in making decisions about a treatment plan, but that can be easier said than done. The following actions may help if you or a loved one is diagnosed with cancer:

✱ **Find out as much as possible about the cancer.** Ask the doctor to explain the treatment plan, the other options available, and the potential risks and benefits. Read about your cancer from reliable websites such as the American Cancer Society, the National Cancer Institute, and Susan G. Komen for the Cure. Find out about treatment options in other parts of the country if necessary, or ongoing clinical trials with promising therapies. If your doctor recommends that you participate in a trial, request a copy of the documents outlining potential risks and benefits.

✱ **Get a second opinion.** Request a copy of the diagnostic test results, and get an "out of group" oncologist (someone unaffiliated with your original doctor) to review them. Seek out a cancer specialist at a large teaching hospital where they see a large number of patients with your type of cancer. Don't worry about hurting the original doctor's feelings. It's your life!

✱ **Check out the credentials of the hospital, the surgeon, and the treatment specialist.** If the patient is having surgery, find out about the patient-to-caregiver ratio in the hospital and the plan for aftercare, and ask for recommendations from patients who've had the procedures that are planned for you.

✱ **Find local resources and support groups.** It can be helpful to talk with someone who isn't emotionally involved in the situation. Survivor support groups can provide information you can get only from someone who has lived through cancer. Talking with a counselor is another good way to help the patient focus on getting well.

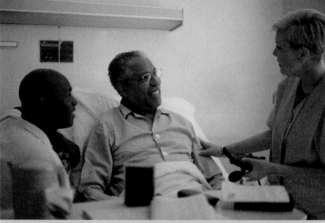

If you or someone you love is diagnosed with cancer, it is important to seek out all the help and information that you can find.

✱ **Get the patient's personal ducks in a row.** Write down financial information, where to find important papers, and other relevant information. Find someone to take care of the person's home while he or she is in the hospital.

✱ **Know what insurance covers and what it doesn't cover.** Call the insurer ahead of time and know what procedures require permission. Find out what percentage of the bill is the patient's responsibility and how this may change if the patient needs to see special-

ists. If the patient doesn't have insurance, talk with social service agencies, your student health center financial director, or others who can help you come up with a plan for payment.

✱ **Mobilize family and friends to help.** If you or your loved one will be bedridden, ask friends to make and deliver dinners, do errands, or help around the house. Don't be afraid to ask for the help you need. Friends and family usually want to have some concrete way to help in times of crisis.

Although survival used to be measured almost exclusively by whether a person had gone 5 years without cancer symptoms, **survivorship** is now viewed much more broadly and is concerned with both years and the quality of life that a person experiences post-diagnosis. Today, survivorship comprises the unique ways in which people survive and thrive after cancer has been diagnosed. The National Cancer Institute defines this term as the "physical, psychological, emotional, and economic issues of cancer from diagnosis until the end of life."[73]

**survivorship** Physical, psychological, emotional, and economic issues of cancer from diagnosis until the end of life.

Accumulating evidence makes clear that breast cancer survivorship, for example, is influenced by a constellation of important factors, including such things as age, socioeconomic status, availability of support services, education level, relationship status, social support, sexual identity, race, stress level, coping styles, spirituality, and depression. Some suggest that the psychosocial factors such as quality of life, including spiritual, social, and emotional well-being, are among the most significant and the most in need of study for understanding their influence in breast cancer survivorship.[74]

Rather than looking only at the number of years people survive, quality of the survival experience is becoming increasingly important. In fact, quality-of-life measures may influence whether a person actually reaches the 5-year survivor milestone. Today, the 5-year survival rate of all people diagnosed with cancer in the years 1999 to 2005 is 68 percent.[75]

## What's Your Personal Risk for Cancer?

**PEARSON**
**myhealthlab**

Fill out this assessment online at www.pearsonhighered.com/myhealthlab or www.pearsonhighered.com/donatelle.

There are many cancer risk factors that you have the power to change. Once you carefully assess your risks, you can make lifestyle changes and pursue risk-reduction strategies that may lessen your susceptibility to various cancers.

Read each question and circle the number corresponding to each Yes or No. Be honest and accurate to get the most complete understanding of your cancer risks. Individual scores for specific questions should not be interpreted as a precise measure of relative risk, but the totals in each section give a general indication.

### 1 Breast Cancer

| | Yes | No |
|---|---|---|
| 1. Do you do a monthly breast self-exam? | 1 | 2 |
| 2. Do you look at your breasts in the mirror regularly, checking for any irregular indentations/lumps, discharge from the nipples, or other noticeable changes? | 1 | 2 |
| 3. Has your mother, sister, or daughter been diagnosed with breast cancer? | 2 | 1 |
| 4. Have you ever been pregnant? | 1 | 2 |
| 5. Have you had lumps or cysts in your breasts or underarm? | 2 | 1 |

Total points: _____

### 2 Skin Cancer

| | Yes | No |
|---|---|---|
| 1. Do you spend a lot of time outdoors, either at work or at play? | 2 | 1 |
| 2. Do you use sunscreens with an SPF rating of 15 or more? | 1 | 2 |
| 3. Do you use tanning beds or sun booths regularly to maintain a tan? | 2 | 1 |
| 4. Do you examine your skin once a month, checking any moles or other irregularities, and using a hand mirror to check hard-to-see areas such as your back, buttocks, genitals, and neck, and under your hair? | 1 | 2 |
| 5. Do you purchase and wear sunglasses that filter out harmful sunrays? | 1 | 2 |

Total points: _____

### 3 Cancers of the Reproductive System

**Men**

| | Yes | No |
|---|---|---|
| 1. Do you examine your penis regularly for unusual bumps or growths? | 1 | 2 |
| 2. Do you perform regular testicular self-exams? | 1 | 2 |
| 3. Do you have a family history of prostate or testicular cancer? | 2 | 1 |
| 4. Do you practice safe sex and wear condoms with every sexual encounter? | 1 | 2 |
| 5. Do you avoid exposure to harmful environmental hazards such as mercury, coal tars, benzene, chromate, and vinyl chloride? | 1 | 2 |

Total points: _____

**Women**

| | Yes | No |
|---|---|---|
| 1. Do you have regularly scheduled Pap tests? | 1 | 2 |
| 2. Have you been infected with the human papillomavirus, Epstein-Barr virus, or other viruses believed to increase cancer risk? | 2 | 1 |
| 3. Has your mother, sister, or daughter been diagnosed with breast, cervical, endometrial, or ovarian cancer (particularly at a young age)? | 2 | 1 |
| 4. Do you practice safe sex and use condoms with every sexual encounter? | 1 | 2 |
| 5. Are you obese, taking estrogen, or consuming a diet that is very high in saturated fats? | 2 | 1 |

Total points: _____

# 4 Cancers in General

|  | | Yes | No |
|---|---|:---:|:---:|
| 1. | Do you smoke cigarettes on most days of the week? | 2 | 1 |
| 2. | Do you consume a diet that is rich in fruits and vegetables? | 1 | 2 |
| 3. | Are you obese, or do you lead a primarily sedentary lifestyle? | 2 | 1 |
| 4. | Do you live in an area with high air pollution levels or work in a job where you are exposed to several chemicals on a regular basis? | 2 | 1 |
| 5. | Are you careful about the amount of animal fat in your diet, substituting olive oil or canola oil for animal fat whenever possible? | 1 | 2 |

|  | | Yes | No |
|---|---|:---:|:---:|
| 6. | Do you limit your overall consumption of alcohol? | 1 | 2 |
| 7. | Do you eat foods rich in lycopenes (such as tomatoes) and antioxidants? | 1 | 2 |
| 8. | Are you "body aware" and alert for changes in your body? | 1 | 2 |
| 9. | Do you have a family history of ulcers or of colorectal, stomach, or other digestive-system cancers? | 2 | 1 |
| 10. | Do you avoid unnecessary exposure to radiation, cell phone emissions, and microwave emissions? | 1 | 2 |

Total points: _____

## Analyzing Your Scores

Look carefully at each question for which you circled a 2. Are there any areas in which you received mostly 2s? Did you receive total points of 6 or higher in parts 1 through 3? Did you receive total points of 11 or higher in part 4? If so, you have at least one identifiable risk. The higher your score is, the more risks you may have.

# YOUR PLAN FOR CHANGE

The **Assess yourself** activity identifies certain behaviors that can contribute to increased cancer risks. If you have identified particular risky behaviors, consider steps you can take to change these behaviors and improve your future health.

### Today, you can:

○ Perform a breast or testicular self-exam (see pages 538 and 544, respectively, for instructions) and commit to doing one every month.

○ Take advantage of the salad bar in your dining hall for lunch or dinner, and load up on greens, or request veggies such as steamed broccoli or sautéed spinach.

### Within the next 2 weeks, you can:

○ Buy a bottle of sunscreen (with SPF 15 or higher) and begin applying it as part of your daily routine. (Be sure to check the expiration date, particularly on sale items!) Also, stay in the shade from 10 AM to 2 PM, as this is when the sun is strongest.

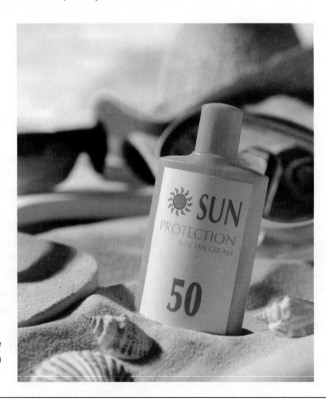

○ Find out your family health history. Talk to your parents, grandparents, or an aunt or uncle to find out if family members have developed cancer. This will help you assess your own genetic risk.

### By the end of the semester, you can:

○ Work toward achieving a healthy weight. If you aren't already engaged in a regular exercise program, begin one now. Maintaining a healthy body weight and exercising regularly will lower your risk for cancer.

○ Stop smoking, avoid secondhand smoke, and limit your alcohol intake.

## Summary

* Cancer is a group of diseases characterized by uncontrolled growth and spread of abnormal cells. These cells may create tumors. Benign (noncancerous) tumors grow in size but do not spread; malignant (cancerous) tumors spread to other parts of the body.
* Lifestyle factors for cancer include smoking and obesity as well as poor diet, lack of exercise, stress, and other factors. Biological factors include inherited genes, age, and gender. Potential environmental carcinogens include asbestos, radiation, preservatives, and pesticides. Infectious agents may increase your risks for cancer; those that appear most likely to cause cancer are chronic hepatitis B and C, human papillomavirus, and genital herpes. Medical factors may elevate the chance of cancer.
* There are many different types of cancer, each of which poses different risks, depending on several factors. Common cancers include that of the lung, breast, colon and rectum, skin, prostate, testis, ovary, and uterus; leukemia; and lymphomas.
* The most common treatments for cancer are surgery, chemotherapy, and radiation; however, newer therapies, including biological, smart drugs, immunotherapy, and others, show promising results and should always be considered.
* Early diagnosis improves survival rate. Self-exams for breast, testicular, and skin cancer aid early diagnosis.

## Pop Quiz

1. When cancer cells have *metastasized*,
   a. they have grown into a malignant tumor.
   b. they have spread to other parts of the body, including vital organs.
   c. the cancer is retreating and cancer cells are dying off.
   d. None of the above

2. A cancerous *neoplasm* is
   a. a type of biopsy.
   b. a form of benign tumor.
   c. a type of treatment for a tumor.
   d. a malignant group of cells or tumor.

3. Who is at a higher risk for developing skin cancer?
   a. People who have fair skin
   b. People who freckle and burn more when in the sun
   c. People who have a history of bad sunburn as a child
   d. All of the above

4. "If you are male and smoke, your chances of getting lung cancer are 23 times greater than those of a nonsmoker." This statement refers to a type of risk assessed statistically, known as
   a. relative risk.
   b. comparable risk.
   c. cancer risk.
   d. genetic predisposition.

5. The leading type of cancer-related deaths for men and women in the United States is
   a. colorectal cancer.
   b. pancreatic cancer.
   c. lung cancer.
   d. stomach cancer.

6. The most common type of cancer in men and women in the United States is
   a. lung.
   b. bladder.
   c. oral.
   d. skin.

7. One of the biggest factors in increased risk for cancer is
   a. increasing age.
   b. presence of another disease.
   c. being of long-lived parents.
   d. increased consumption of fruits and vegetables.

8. One of the best ways to reduce a person's risk of developing cancer is to
   a. quit smoking now if currently smoking.
   b. eat a very healthy diet with more fruits and vegetables.
   c. maintain a healthy weight (avoiding overweight and obesity).
   d. All of the above

9. Which of the following is correct?
   a. Certain infectious diseases can cause inflammation and increase cancer risks.
   b. Carcinoma in situ of the breast is one of the most lethal forms of breast cancer.
   c. Your risk of dying of breast cancer as a 20-year-old female is approximately 1 in 8.
   d. All of the above

10. The more serious and life-threatening type of skin cancer is
    a. basal cell carcinoma.
    b. squamous cell carcinoma.
    c. melanoma.
    d. lymphoma.

*Answers to these questions can be found on page A-1.*

## Think about It!

1. What is cancer? How does it spread? What is the difference between a benign tumor and a malignant tumor?
2. List the likely causes of cancer. Which of these causes would be a risk for you, in particular? What can you do to reduce these risks? What risk factors do you share with family members? Friends?
3. What are the symptoms of lung, breast, prostate, and testicular cancers? How can you reduce your risk of developing these cancers or increase your chances of surviving them?

4. What are the differences between carcinomas, sarcomas, lymphomas, and leukemia? Which is the most common? Least common? Why is it important that you know the stage and level of your cancer?

5. Why are breast and testicular self-exams especially important for college students? What factors keep you from doing your own self-exams? What could you do to make sure you do regular self-exams?

## Accessing Your Health on the Internet

The following websites explore further topics and issues related to personal health. For links to the websites below, visit the Companion Website for *Access to Health*, 12th Edition, at www.pearsonhighered.com/donatelle.

1. *American Cancer Society.* This site provides resources from the leading private organization dedicated to cancer prevention. Here you'll find information, statistics, and resources regarding cancer. www.cancer.org

2. *National Cancer Institute.* Check here for valuable information on cancer facts, results of research, new/ongoing clinical trials, and the Physician Data Query (PDQ), a comprehensive database of cancer treatment information. www.cancer.gov

3. *National Women's Health Information Center (NWHIC).* The NCWHIC provides a wealth of information about cancer in women; the site is cosponsored by the National Cancer Institute. www.4woman.gov

4. *Oncolink.* Sponsored by the University of Pennsylvania Cancer Center, this site seeks to educate cancer patients and their families by offering information on support services, cancer causes, screening, prevention, and common questions. www.oncolink.com

5. *Susan G. Komen for the Cure.* This site provides up-to-date information about breast cancer, issues in treat-

ment, and support groups; there is also a wealth of videos and information. The site is especially useful for those diagnosed patients looking for additional support and advice. ww5.komen.org

6. *National Coalition for Cancer Survivorship.* Cancer survivors share their experiences advocating for themselves during and after cancer treatment. www.canceradvocacy.org/community/survivor-profiles

## References

1. American Cancer Society, *Cancer Facts & Figures 2010* (Atlanta: American Cancer Society, 2010), Available at www.cancer.org/Research/CancerFactsFigures/CancerFactsFigures/cancer-facts-and-figures-2010.

2. A. Jemal et al., "Cancer Statistics," *CA: A Cancer Journal for Clinicians* 2009, 59 (4): 225–49; B. K. Edwards et al., "Annual Report to the Nation on the Status of Cancer, 1975–2006. Featuring Colorectal Cancer Trends and Impact of Interventions (Risk Factors, Screenings, and Treatment) to Reduce Future Rates," *Cancer* 2009, 16(3): 544–73.

3. American Cancer Society, *Cancer Facts & Figures 2010.*

4. Ibid.

5. Ibid.

6. Ibid.

7. Ibid.

8. Ibid.

9. Centers for Disease Control and Prevention, *Tobacco Use: Targeting the Nation's Leading Killer—At-a-Glance 2010* (Atlanta: Centers for Disease Control and Prevention, National Center for Chronic Disease Prevention and Health Promotion, 2010), Available at www.cdc.gov/chronicdisease/resources/publications/AAG/osh.htm.

10. World Health Organization, *WHO Report on Global Tobacco Epidemic, 2008: The MPOWER Package* (Geneva, Switzerland: World Health Organization, 2008), Available at www.who.int/tobacco/mpower/2008/en/index.html.

11. V. Bagnardi et al., "Alcohol Consumption and the Risk of Cancer: A Meta-Analysis," *Alcohol Research and Health* 25, no. 4 (2001): 263–70.

12. N. Allen et al., "Moderate Alcohol Intake and Cancer Incidence in Women," *Journal of the National Cancer Institute* 101, no. 5 (2009): 296–305.

13. S. Gupta et al., "Risk of Pancreatic Cancer by Alcohol Dose, Duration, and Pattern of

Consumption, Including Binge Drinking: A Population-Based Study," *Cancer Causes & Control* 21, no. 7 (2010): 1047–59.

14. A. Benedetti et al., "Lifetime Consumption of Alcoholic Beverages and Risk of 13 Types of Cancer in Men: Results from a Case-Control Study in Montreal," *Cancer Epidemiology* 32, no. 5 (2009): 352–62.

15. American Cancer Society, *Cancer Facts & Figures 2010.*

16. D. Guh et al., "The Incidence of Co-Morbidities Related to Obesity and Overweight: A Systematic Review and Meta-Analysis," *BMC Public Health* 9, no. 88 (2009).

17. M. Ewertz et al., "Effect of Obesity on Prognosis after Early Breast Cancer," *Cancer Research* 69, no. 24 (Suppl, 2009): Abstract nr 18.

18. N. Maurther, S. Bolen, F. Brancat, and J. Clark, "Obesity and Mammography: A Systematic Review and Meta-Analysis," *Journal of General Internal Medicine* 24, no. 5 (2009): 665–77.

19. K. Rapp et al., "Obesity and Incidence of Cancer: A Large Cohort Study of over 145,000 Adults in Austria," *British Journal of Cancer* 93, no. 9 (2005): 1062–67; S. Freedland, "Obesity and Prostate Cancer: A Growing Problem," *Clinical Cancer Research* 11, no. 19 (2005): 6763–66; R. MacInnis et al., "Body Size and Composition and Colon Cancer Risk in Women," *International Cancer Journal* 118 no. 6 (2005): 1496–1500; C. Samanic et al., "Relation of Body Mass Index to Cancer Risk in 362,552 Swedish Men," *Cancer Causes and Control* 17, no. 7 (2005): 901–09; M. McCullough et al., "Risk Factors for Fatal Breast Cancer in African-American Women and White Women in a Large U.S. Prospective Cohort," *American Journal of Epidemiology* 162, no. 8 (2005): 734–42; P. Soliman et al., "Risk Factors for Young Premenopausal Women with Endometrial Cancer," *Obstetrics and Gynecology* 105 no. 3 (2005): 575–80.

20. E. Reiche, H. Morimoto, and S. Nunes, "Stress and Depression-Induced Immune Dysfunction: Implications for the Development and Progression of Cancer," *International Review of Psychiatry* 17, no. 6 (2005): 515–27; K. Ross, "Mapping Pathways from Stress to Cancer Progression," *Journal of the National Cancer Institute* 100, no. 13 (2008): 914–15,17; Tel Aviv University, "Stress and Fear Can Affect Cancer's Recurrence," *Science Daily* (February 29, 2008), www.sciencedaily.com/releases/2008/02/080227142656.htm.

21. American Cancer Society, *Cancer Facts & Figures 2010.*

22. American Cancer Society, "Breast Cancer Overview: What Causes Breast Cancer?" Revised July 2010, www.cancer.org/

Cancer/BreastCancer/OverviewGuide/
breast-cancer-overview-what-causes.

23. L. Hines et al., "Comparative Analysis of Breast Cancer Risk Factors among Hispanic and Non-Hispanic White Women," *Cancer* 116, no. 13 (2010): 3215–23.

24. M. L. McCullough et al., "Body Mass and Endometrial Cancer Risk by Hormone Replacement Therapy and Cancer Subtype," *Cancer Epidemiology Biomarkers & Prevention* 17, no. 1 (2008): 73–79.

25. B. Binukumar and A. Mathew, "Dietary Fat and Risk of Breast Cancer," *World Journal of Surgical Oncology* 3, no. 45 (2005): 1477.

26. J. Schüz et al., "Cellular Telephone Use and Cancer Risk: Update of a Nationwide Danish Cohort," *Journal of the National Cancer Institute* 98, no. 23 (2006): 1707–13.

27. J. Parsonnet, "Infectious Disease: A Surprising Cause of Cancer," *Stanford Medicine News*, (Spring 2008): 4–5, Available at www.stanfordmedicine.org/communitynews/2008spring/infectiousdisease.html.

28. National Institute of Allergy and Infectious Diseases, "Viral Infections: Treating Cancer as an Infectious Disease," Updated March 2009, www.niaid.nih.gov/topics/viral/pages/cancerinfectiousdisease.aspx.

29. American Cancer Society, *Global Cancer Facts and Figures—2007* (Atlanta: American Cancer Society, 2007), Available at www.cancer.org/Research/CancerFactsFigures/GlobalCancerFactsFigures/index.

30. American Cancer Society, *Cancer Facts & Figures 2010*.

31. J. Parsonnet, "Infectious Disease: A Surprising Cause of Cancer," 2008.

32. A. Jemal et al., "Cancer Statistics," 2009.

33. American Cancer Society, *Cancer Facts and Figures 2010*.

34. Ibid.

35. J. Samet et al., "Lung Cancer in Never Smokers: Clinical Epidemiology and Environmental Risk Factors," *Clinical Cancer Research* 15, no. 18 (2009): 5626–45; C. Rudin et al., "Lung Cancer in Never Smokers: A Call to Action," *Clinical Cancer Research* 15, no. 18 (2009): 5622–25.

36. J. Samet et al., "Lung Cancer in Never Smokers," 2009.

37. American Cancer Society, *Cancer Facts & Figures 2010*.

38. Ibid.

39. S. A. Kenfield et al., "Smoking and Smoking Cessation in Relation to Mortality in Women," *Journal of the American Medical Association* 299, no. 17 (2008): 2037–47.

40. American Cancer Society, *Cancer Facts & Figures 2010*.

41. Ibid.

42. B. K. Edwards et al., "Annual Report to the Nation on the Status of Cancer, 1975–2006. Featuring Colorectal Cancer Trends and Impact of Interventions (Risk Factors, Screenings, and Treatment) to Reduce Future Rates," *Cancer* 2009, 16, no. 3 (2009): 544–73

43. American Cancer Society, *Cancer Facts & Figures 2010*.

44. Ibid.

45. Ibid.

46. T. M. Peters et al., "Physical Activity and Postmenopausal Breast Cancer Risk in the NIH-AARP Diet and Health Study," *Cancer Epidemiology, Biomarkers, and Prevention* 18, no. 1 (2009): 289–96; American Cancer Society, *Cancer Facts & Figures 2010*.

47. Susan G. Komen for the Cure, "Table 11: *BRCA1* and *BRCA2* Gene Mutations and Cancer Risk," 2009, ww5.komen.org/BreastCancer/Table11BRCA1or2genemutationsandcancerrisk.html.

48. Susan G. Komen for the Cure, "Table 4: Physical Activity and Breast Cancer Risk," 2009, ww5.komen.org/BreastCancer/Table4Recreationalphysicalactivityandbreastcancerrisk.html; C. M. Dallal et al., "Long-Term Recreational Physical Activity and Risk of Invasive and in situ Breast Cancer: The California Teachers Study," *Archives of Internal Medicine* 167, no. 4 (2007): 408–16.

49. X. Shu et al., "Soy Food Intake and Breast Cancer Survival," *Journal of the American Medical Association* 302, no. 22 (2009): 2437–43; R. Ballard-Barbash and M. Neuhouser, "Challenges in Design and Interpretation of Observational Research on Health Behaviors and Cancer Survival," *Journal of the American Medical Association* 302, no. 22 (2009): 2483–84.

50. B. K. Edwards et al., "Annual Report to the Nation on the Status of Cancer, 1975–2006," 2009.

51. American Cancer Society, *Cancer Facts & Figures 2010*.

52. American Cancer Society, *Colorectal Cancer Facts & Figures 2008–2010* (Atlanta: American Cancer Society, 2010), Available at www.cancer.org/Research/CancerFacts Figures/ColorectalCancerFactsFigures/colorectal-cancer-facts--figures-2008-2010.

53. American Cancer Society, *Colorectal Cancer Facts & Figures 2008–2010*.

54. American Cancer Society, *Cancer Facts & Figures 2010*.

55. Ibid.

56. Ibid.

57. Ibid.

58. Ibid.

59. American Cancer Society, "Prostate Cancer: What Causes Prostate Cancer?" Revised July 2010, www.cancer.org/Cancer/ProstateCancer/OverviewGuide/prostate-cancer-overview-what-causes.

60. American Cancer Society, *Cancer Facts & Figures 2010*.

61. S. M. Lippman et al., "Effect of Selenium and Vitamin E on Risk of Prostate Cancer and Other Cancers: The Selenium and Vitamin E Cancer Prevention Trial (SELECT)," *Journal of the American Medical Association* 301, no. 1 (2009): 39–51.

62. American Cancer Society, *Cancer Facts & Figures 2010*.

63. Ibid.

64. Ibid.

65. National Cancer Institute, "Ovarian Cancer Screening (PDQ)," 2009, www.cancer.gov/cancerinfo/pdq/screening/ovarian/patient.

66. American Cancer Society, *Cancer Facts & Figures 2010*.

67. Ibid.

68. National Cancer Institute, "Endometrial Cancer," 2010, www.cancer.gov/cancertopics/types/endometrial.

69. National Cancer Institute, "Testicular Cancer," 2010, www.cancer.gov/cancertopics/types/testicular.

70. American Cancer Society, *Cancer Facts & Figures 2010*.

71. Ibid.

72. National Cancer Survivors Day Foundation, "Cancer Survivorship Issues," 2010, www.ncsdf.org/Pages/Issues.html.

73. National Cancer Institute, "Dictionary of Cancer Terms," 2010, www.cancer.gov/dictionary.

74. J. Jabson, "Breast Cancer Survivorship: Factors Influencing Ability to Thrive," Doctoral dissertation, Oregon State University, April 2010.

75. American Cancer Society, *Cancer Facts & Figures 2010*.

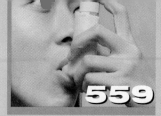
**559**
What causes asthma?

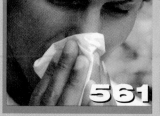
**561**
Why is my hay fever worse at certain times of the year?

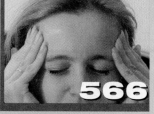
**566**
What triggers a migraine headache?

# 17

# Reducing Risks and Coping with Chronic Conditions

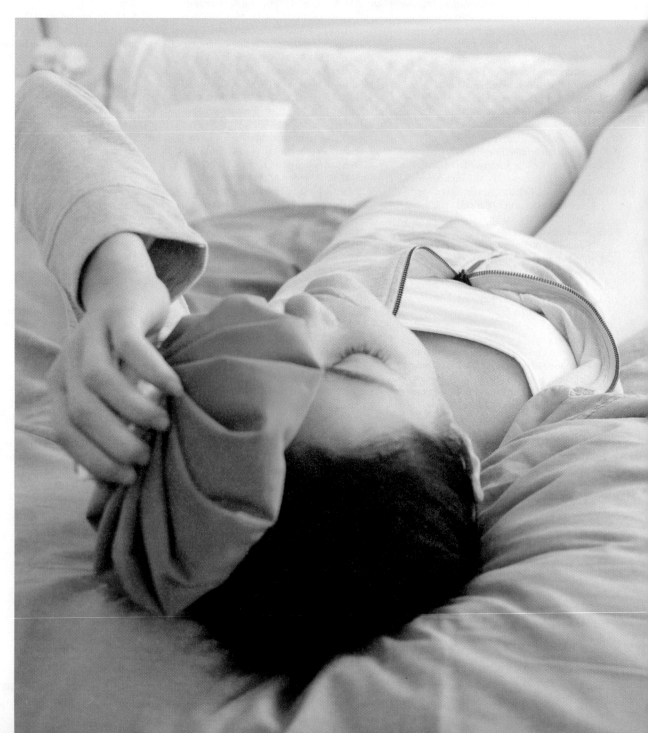

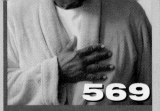

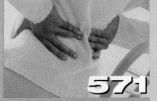

**569**
Is heartburn really a disease?

**571**
What is the major cause of disability among young adults?

## Objectives

✳ Discuss key chronic respiratory diseases, including bronchitis, emphysema, and asthma.

✳ Describe the allergic response and complications associated with allergies.

✳ Explain common neurological disorders, including headaches and seizure disorders.

✳ Understand the major digestive disorders affecting adults in the United States today.

✳ Discuss the effects of various musculoskeletal diseases, including arthritis and low back pain.

Typically, when we think of major noninfectious ailments, we think of "killer" diseases such as cancer and heart disease. Although these diseases do make up the major portion of life-threatening diseases, other chronic conditions can also cause pain, suffering, and long-term disability. Fortunately, many of them can be prevented and their symptoms delayed or relieved.

Chronic diseases and conditions often develop over a long period of time and cause progressive damage to human tissues. Although these conditions normally do not result in death, they do lead to illness and suffering for many people and are often not easily cured. Lifestyle and personal health habits are often implicated as underlying causes; however, a number of "newer" chronic maladies seem to defy conventional wisdom about causation. For those where the underlying cause is known, actions to prevent these causes are presented. For those that are **idiopathic** (of unknown cause), education, reasonable changes in lifestyle, drug therapy, surgery, and public health efforts aimed at research, prevention, and control can minimize their effects. In this chapter, we discuss some of the leading chronic diseases other than CVD and cancer that affect millions of Americans at all ages and stages of life. (The **Health in a Diverse World** box on page 557 describes shortcomings in chronic disease treatment internationally.) Many of the diseases are problems that college students like you may be facing (see **Figure 17.1** on page 556), or you may have family or loved ones that have these problems. Understanding these diseases, knowing the risks and possible avenues for prevention and control is part of a solid strategy for minimizing threats now and in the future.

**idiopathic** Of unknown cause.

**What's Working for You?**

Maybe you're already doing all you can to avoid chronic illness. Which of these are you already incorporating into your life?

☐ I have found out what illnesses I am predisposed to by my family history, so I know what behaviors I particularly need to avoid.

☐ I pay attention to my health: I eat right, exercise, and sleep enough, and I have supportive friends and family.

☐ I get a regular physical checkup, and my doctor and I have discussed my family history and what I can do to avoid chronic illness.

## Coping with Respiratory Problems

Lung disease is the fourth leading cause of death in the United States, behind heart disease, cancer, and stroke. In 2009, lung disease was responsible for 1 in 6 deaths, or over 400,000 people. Today, more than 35 million Americans are living with chronic lung diseases such as asthma, emphysema, and bronchitis.[1]

Virtually any disease or disorder in which lung function is impaired is considered a lung disease. The lungs can be damaged by a single exposure to a toxic chemical or severe heat, or they can be impaired from years of inhaling the tar and chemicals in tobacco smoke. Occupational or home

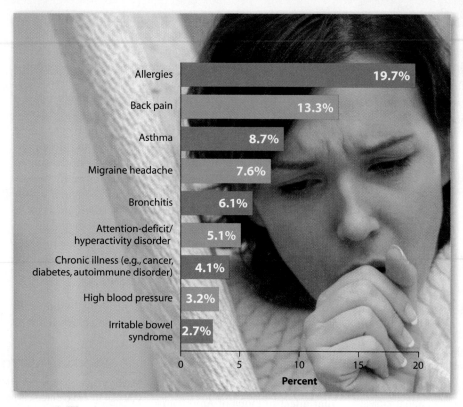

FIGURE 17.1 **Proportion of College Students Diagnosed with or Treated for Chronic Conditions in the Past 12 Months**

Do you think chronic diseases and health problems are a concern only for older Americans? Think again. College students are affected by chronic health issues, too.

**Source:** Data are from American College Health Association, *American College Health Association—National College Health Assessment II (ACHA-NCHA II): Reference Group Data Report Fall 2009* (Baltimore: American College Health Association, 2010).

about 24 million U.S. adults have impaired lung function, with over 12 million believed to have COPD. Eighty-five to 90 percent of persons with COPD have a history of smoking.[2] Occupational exposure to certain industrial fumes or gases and exposure to dusts and other lung irritants increases risks, whether this exposure comes in one big dose or over months and years. There is no cure for COPD; however there is much that can be done, if it's diagnosed early enough, to help people control the illness and lead normal lives for many years. The **Be Healthy, Be Green** box on page 558 describes ways in which exposure to household chemicals can be minimized, to lessen their effect on COPD.

**Bronchitis** **Bronchitis** comes in two forms, *acute* and *chronic*. Regardless of type, the disease involves inflammation and eventual scarring of the lining of the bronchial tubes (*bronchi*) that connect the windpipe to the lungs. When the bronchi become inflamed or infected with bacteria, less air is able to flow from the lungs, and heavy mucus begins to form. Although some mucus is normal and necessary, bronchitis sufferers typically have numerous coughing spasms in a day as they try to rid their bodies of phlegm. Frequent clearing of the throat, a sensation of tightness in the chest, back pain, and shortness of breath are other bronchitis symptoms.

Inhaling certain chemicals, cigarette smoke, and fumes from hairsprays and many other substances can trigger bronchitis. The more common *acute bronchitis* is often caused by other infectious diseases. Symptoms often begin to go away in a week or two once the sources are removed and any inflammation and infections are treated.

When the symptoms of bronchitis last for at least 3 months of the year for 2 consecutive years, the condition is considered *chronic bronchitis*. In some cases, this chronic inflammation and irritation goes undiagnosed for years, particularly in smokers who feel it's a normal part of their lives. By the time these individuals receive medical care, the damage to their lungs is severe and may lead to heart and respiratory failure or to a chronic need to carry oxygen to aid in breathing. Coal miners, grain handlers, metalworkers, painters, and others exposed to fumes, dusts, and hazards are particularly susceptible. Nearly 10 million Americans suffer from chronic bronchitis; 33 percent are under the age of 45.[3]

To prevent bronchitis, stop smoking, avoid particulates that trigger bronchitis attacks, and see a doctor early if you have recurrent, regular symptoms. Prescription drugs can

exposure to toxic environmenal substances like asbestos, silica dust, paint fumes and lacquers, or pesticides can cause lung deterioration. Of course, cancers, infections, and degenerative changes can also wreak havoc with lung function.

When the lungs are impaired, a condition known as **dyspnea,** or a choking type of breathlessness, can occur, even with mild exertion. As the body is deprived of oxygen, the heart is forced to work harder and, over time, cardiovascular problems, suffocation, and death can occur.

**dyspnea** Shortness of breath, usually associated with disease of the heart or lungs.

**chronic obstructive pulmonary diseases (COPDs)** The chronic lung diseases of emphysema and chronic bronchitis.

**bronchitis** Inflammation of the lining of the bronchial tubes.

## Chronic Obstructive Pulmonary Diseases

The term **chronic obstructive pulmonary diseases (COPDs)** refers to two specific lung diseases—chronic bronchitis and emphysema. Because these conditions often occur together, the abbreviation *COPD* is often preferred by health professionals. This term does not include other lung diseases in which breathing is compromised, such as asthma. Currently,

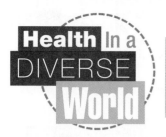

## Health In a DIVERSE World

# CHRONIC DISEASES: AN INCREASING GLOBAL THREAT

*The balance between infectious and non-communicable diseases is shifting. The WHO [World Health Organization] predicts that leading infectious diseases will soon kill fewer people globally, and by 2030, three-quarters of all deaths in the world will be due to chronic non-communicable diseases like heart disease and some cancers.*

*—Colin Mathers, "Better Statistics Key to Tackling Chronic Diseases," 2008*

The statement above may come as a surprise to many. After all, we've long thought of the developing regions of the world as being plagued by killer infectious diseases: polio, smallpox, HIV/AIDS, tuberculosis, and malaria, to name a few. Over the years, these diseases have captured not only the world's attention, but the majority of its financial resources as well. Although these diseases are still present and still cause premature death and disability at alarming rates, the numbers pale in comparison to chronic disease counts.

For example, cancer kills more people annually than HIV/AIDS, malaria, and tuberculosis combined. Yet the WHO spends only $0.50 per person on chronic diseases compared to $7.50 per person for major infectious diseases. Other big philanthropic organizations such as the Bill and Melinda Gates Foundation spend very little on chronic diseases in comparison to their spending for infectious diseases.

Why? Although a full explanation for this lack of attention is hard to find, one reason is that evidence supporting a major chronic disease explosion in the international community is lacking. Only about a third of the world's population is covered by national death registration systems. Although such coverage is over 95 percent in Europe, it is lower than 5 percent in Africa, and when surveillance and death registries exist, they often cover children rather than adults. Statistics about deaths provide rationale of a need for help in controlling certain diseases; without them, progress is slow and priorities change in favor of conditions that garner high levels of media coverage, or in response to political pressures.

Another reason for this seeming neglect is faulty perceptions. Many continue to believe that chronic diseases are primarily diseases of the elderly in wealthy countries. Poorer nations believe they'll have a better chance of getting money for research and treatment through their established networks and are less skilled in seeking chronic disease funds.

Because many international leaders continue to see chronic diseases as "lifestyle choices," they believe that these

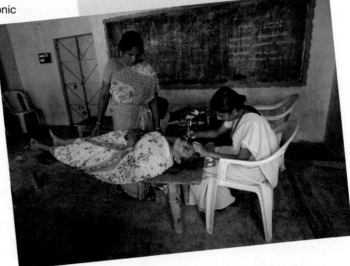

Resources to treat chronic conditions are often lacking in developing countries.

poor outcomes are outside of their range of responsibilities. They are not yet geared up for management of chronic diseases that require long-term and complex treatments. Prevention programs for most chronic diseases are not in place.

What is true is that the growing pandemic of chronic diseases can no longer be ignored. International organizations, leaders, and communities will need to tackle these problems soon.

**Sources:** P. Shetty, "Chronic Disease—a Neglected Priority" 2008, www.scidev.net/en/south-east -asia/editorials/chronic-disease-a-neglected -priority.html; C. Mathers, "Better Statistics Key to Tackling Chronic Diseases," 2008, www.scidev .net/en/middle-east-and-north-africa/opinions/ better-statistics-key-to-tackling-chronic-diseases .html.

---

reduce inflammation, prevent mucus buildup, and stop secondary bacterial infections from setting in. Standard recommendations for a healthy lifestyle should be followed to ensure that you don't become too run down and therefore susceptible to other diseases.

Unfortunately, episodes of bronchitis tend to recur, usually due to continued exposure to irritants. If you suspect bronchitis, see your doctor. Then let your instructors know that you are having a problem, and do your best to avoid trig-

gers, take your medicine, and get enough rest. Avoid smoke-filled bars, or other settings where you could make your situation worse. If the pollution index is high, stay indoors, make sure windows and doors are closed, and use any air filtration systems that you have. Let others know you are having some difficulties and ask for their help if necessary.

**Emphysema** If you have ever seen someone gasping for air for no apparent reason, struggling to breathe after even minor

# BE HEALTHY, BE GREEN

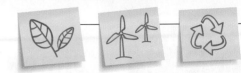

## Be Eco-Clean and Allergen Free

Exposure to household chemicals, dust, and pet dander may exacerbate asthma, allergies, and other respiratory problems. You can reduce exposure to noxious household chemicals and create a clean, comfortable home by using cleaning supplies and household products that are less toxic to the home environment. Because some companies may want you to believe their product is greener than it actually is, read the labels carefully and look for independent certifications such as the Green Seal and the Environmental Protection Agency's (EPA's) Design for the Environment program.

✳ For a handy glass and surface cleaner, mix 1/2 cup of white vinegar with 4 cups of water. Pour the solution into a spray bottle and keep the remainder for a quick and cheap refill.

✳ Combine 2 tablespoons of lemon juice with 4 cups of water for a surface cleaner.

✳ Baking soda works as a great deodorizer and cleaner. Use it to remove carpet odors and to scour sinks, toilets, and bathtubs.

✳ Because chlorine can damage lungs, skin, and eyes, and chlorine production adds toxic chemicals such as carcinogenic dioxins to our environment, use a chlorine bleach alternative. For example, use 1/2 cup of hydrogen peroxide in your laundry or use oxygen-based bleaches.

✳ An all-purpose cleaner can be made of 1/2 cup of borax (found in the laundry aisle) and 1 gallon of hot water.

✳ For green air fresheners, use essential oils, such as lemon or lavender. Many store-bought air fresheners contain phthalates, often called "fragrance," that are related to respiratory problems and other noninfectious conditions. Place a few drops of essential oils on a piece of tissue paper, in a bowl of warm water, or in a store-bought diffuser.

As you transition to green cleaning, do not just throw old products in the trash, as these can wind up polluting landfills and

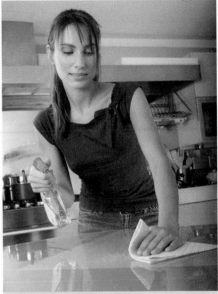

Making your own cleansers ensures that they are not harmful to your health.

leaching into water supplies. Instead, take them to a hazardous chemical recycling facility.

---

exertion, or being hooked up to an oxygen tank and struggling to breathe, you have probably witnessed an emphysemic episode. Over 3.8 million Americans suffer from **emphysema,** with nearly 70 percent of cases occurring in men.[4] Emphysema involves the gradual, irreversible destruction of the **alveoli** (tiny air sacs through which gas exchange occurs) of the lungs. Destruction of the alveoli walls causes impaired transfer of oxygen and carbon dioxide into and out of the blood, and makes the lungs less elastic, which makes it harder to breathe. As the alveoli are destroyed, the affected person finds it more and more difficult to exhale. Persons who have emphysema liken this experience to engaging in heavy exercise while breathing through a straw. What most of us take for granted—the easy, rhythmic flow of air in and out of the lungs—becomes a continuous, anxious, and life-threatening struggle for people with emphysema.

The cause of emphysema is uncertain. There is, however, a strong relationship between emphysema and long-term cigarette smoking and exposure to air pollution. (See Chapter 12 for more on the connection between smoking and emphysema.) To avoid emphysema, don't smoke. If you smoke, quit. If you can't quit, reduce consumption and keep trying to quit. Avoid occupational exposures that involve inhalation of chemicals and fumes. If you must take a job that involves inhaling toxins, use appropriate protection.

Whether you are a person with emphysema, or a family member or loved one caring for such a person, a key to coping is to make sure the patient is complying with doctor's orders. Prescribed medications must actually be taken! Healthy meals, exercise, stress management, and adequate rest are imperative to keep the body functioning at maximum capacity, not to mention keeping depression at bay. Many persons on oxygen supplementation become depressed and irritable. You may need to suggest counseling, or help from social services. Support groups can be very helpful. Also, respite care for the caregiver should be part of planning. Although it is easy to blame the victim, particularly someone

**emphysema** A respiratory disease in which the alveoli become distended or ruptured and are no longer functional.
**alveoli** Tiny air sacs of the lungs where gas exchange occurs (oxygen enters the body and carbon dioxide is removed).

who has smoked for decades, remember that this is not a time for blame. Optimizing living and ensuring quality of life through healthy lifestyle are both imperative.

## Asthma

**Asthma** is a long-term, chronic inflammatory disorder that blocks airflow into and out of the lungs. Asthma causes tiny airways in the lung to overreact with spasms in response to certain triggers (Figure 17.2). Symptoms include wheezing, difficulty breathing, shortness of breath, and coughing spasms. Although most asthma attacks are mild and non–life threatening, severe attacks can trigger bronchospasms (contractions of the bronchial tubes in the lungs) that are so severe that, without rapid treatment, death may occur. Between attacks, most people have few symptoms. Approximately 22 million people in the United States currently have asthma. It is one of the most prevalent respiratory diseases, particularly among children.[5]

Asthma falls into two distinctly different types. The more common form of asthma, known as *extrinsic* or *allergic asthma*, is typically associated with allergic triggers; it tends to run in families and develop in childhood. Often by adulthood, a person has few episodes, or the disorder completely goes away. *Intrinsic* or *nonallergic asthma* may be triggered by anything except an allergy.

Several factors, including genetics, prior infections, and environmental exposure, can increase your risk of develop-

**25%** of all school absences are due to asthma.

ing asthma. If your mom or dad has asthma, if you had infections that damaged your lungs when you were younger, or if you are exposed to environmental allergens and irritants, you are more likely to develop asthma.[6] Asthma attacks can be triggered by exposure to irritants or allergens such as tobacco smoke, occupational chemicals, pollen, cockroaches, feathers, foods, molds, dust, or pet dander. In some individuals, stress, exercise, certain medications, cold air, and sulfites are also potential triggers. Interestingly, 1 in 5 asthmatics can suffer an attack from taking aspirin.[7]

**asthma** A chronic respiratory disease characterized by attacks of wheezing, shortness of breath, and coughing spasms.

Asthma can occur at any age but is most likely to appear between infancy and age 5 and in adults before age 40. In childhood, asthma strikes more boys than girls; in adulthood, it strikes more women than men. The asthma rate is 50 percent higher among African Americans than whites, and four times as many African Americans die of asthma as do whites.[8] In the past few decades, asthma rates have risen dramatically, increasing by more than 65 percent since the 1980s.[9] Asthma has become the most common chronic disease of childhood, affecting more than 1 child in 20. Among

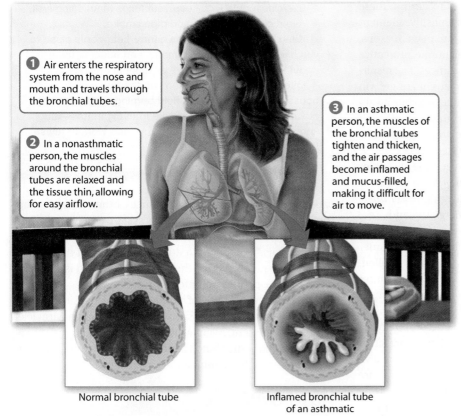

❶ Air enters the respiratory system from the nose and mouth and travels through the bronchial tubes.

❷ In a nonasthmatic person, the muscles around the bronchial tubes are relaxed and the tissue thin, allowing for easy airflow.

❸ In an asthmatic person, the muscles of the bronchial tubes tighten and thicken, and the air passages become inflamed and mucus-filled, making it difficult for air to move.

Normal bronchial tube

Inflamed bronchial tube of an asthmatic

FIGURE 17.2 **Asthma Is an Inflammation of the Airways within the Lungs**

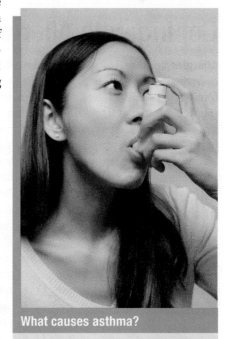

**What causes asthma?**

Asthma is caused by inflammation of the airways in the lungs, restricting them and leading to wheezing, chest tightness, shortness of breath, and coughing. In most people, asthma is brought on by contact with allergens or irritants in the air; some people also have exercise-induced asthma. People with asthma can generally control their symptoms through the use of inhaled medications, and most asthmatics keep a "rescue" inhaler of bronchodilating medication on hand to use in case of a flare-up.

adults, asthma is the fourth leading cause of work absence, resulting in over 10 million lost workdays per year. In 2009, there were over 5,000 asthma-related deaths. Many believe that today's homes contain more triggers (such as dust mites in mattresses, chemicals in carpets and furniture, and airtight structures for efficient cooling and heating).

## what do you think?

Have you or any of your friends or family experienced any of the conditions discussed in this section? ● Why do you think the incidence of COPDs, as a group, is increasing? ● What actions can you or the people in your community take to reduce risks and problems from these diseases on campus? In your homes? In your communities?

Determining whether a specific allergen provokes asthma attacks, taking steps to reduce exposure, and avoiding triggers such as certain types of exercise or stress are important steps in asthma prevention. The **Skills for Behavior Change** box at right offers suggestions for ways to reduce potential asthma and allergy triggers. In addition to avoiding triggers, finding the most effective medications can help asthmatics cope with their condition and avoid severe attacks.

# Coping with Allergies

**Allergies** are diseases of the immune system that cause an overreaction to substances called *allergens* or *antigens*. When foreign pathogens such as bacteria or viruses enter the body, the body responds by producing antibodies to destroy these invaders. Normally, antibody production is a positive element in the body's defense system. However, for unknown reasons, sometimes the body develops an overly elaborate protective mechanism against relatively harmless substances. The resulting *hypersensitivity reaction* to specific allergens or antigens in the environment is fairly common, as anyone who has awakened with a runny nose or itchy eyes can attest. People with severe allergies can suffer much more extreme responses, including hives, vomiting, and anaphylaxis (see below).

Allergies are grouped by the kind of trigger, time of year, or where symptoms appear on the body into *outdoor* or *indoor allergies, food and drug allergies, latex allergies, insect allergies, skin allergies,* and *eye allergies*.[10] Environmental triggers can include molds, animal dander (hair and dead skin), pollen, grasses, ragweed, or dust. Other triggers include foods such as peanuts, shellfish, or milk; insect bites; and medicines (both over-the-counter [OTC] and prescription drugs). Once excessive antibodies to these antigens are produced, they, in turn, trigger the release of **histamine,** a chemical substance that dilates blood vessels, increases mucous secretions,

**allergy** Hypersensitive reaction in which the body produces antibodies to a normally harmless substance in the environment.
**histamine** Chemical substance that dilates blood vessels, increases mucous secretions, and triggers other allergy symptoms.
**immunotherapy** Treatment strategies based on the concept of regulating the immune system, as by administering antibodies or desensitization shots of allergens.
**hay fever** A chronic allergy-related respiratory disorder that is most prevalent when ragweed and flowers bloom.

**Skills for Behavior Change**

## Keys to Asthma Prevention

Although asthma rates continue to increase around the world, there is much that individuals and communities can do to reduce risk:

✳ Purchase a good air filter for your home, and clean furnace filters regularly. If you have a fireplace or wood-burning stove, check it regularly to make sure that it is not spewing smoke and particulate matter.
✳ Wash pillows and sheets regularly. Use pillow protectors and mattress protectors. Don't purchase used mattresses, which may be teeming with mites.
✳ Avoid having cats or dogs that are known for high dander production in the home. If you're a pet lover but animal dander bothers you, try a nonshedding breed. Keep pets off your bed, and wash them and their bedding weekly. Vacuum up their shed hair regularly.
✳ Keep your home clean and pest free; cockroaches and other vermin have enzymes in their saliva or particles on their bodies that may trigger allergic reactions. Use a high-suction vacuum rather than a broom to reduce dust particles suspended in the air.
✳ Use anti-mold cleaners or run a dehumidifier to keep moisture levels down and reduce the growth of mold.
✳ Avoid mowing the lawn or other activities leading to excessive outdoor exposure to pollen during high-pollen times. If you must be outdoors, wear a pollen mask.
✳ Exercise regularly to keep your lungs functioning well.
✳ Avoid cigarette, cigar, and pipe smoke.
✳ Keep asthma medications handy. Let people close to you know that you are asthmatic, and educate them about what to do if you have an asthma attack.
✳ Investigate local regulations on the burning of household and yard trash, field burning, wood-burning stoves, and secondhand smoke from cigarettes—all known triggers for asthma attacks—and work to revise them as necessary.

causes tissues to swell, and produces other allergy symptoms, particularly in the respiratory system (**Figure 17.3**). Many people have found that **immunotherapy** treatment, or "allergy shots," somewhat reduce the severity of their symptoms. In most cases, once the offending antigen is removed, allergy-prone people suffer few symptoms.

More than half (54.9%) of all Americans test positive for one or more allergens and at least 50 percent of homes have at least six allergens present. Allergic disease affects as many as 40 to 50 million people in the United States. If you include asthma as an allergic disease, these numbers are even higher.[11]

## Hay Fever

**Hay fever,** or *pollen allergy,* occurs throughout the world and is one of the most common chronic diseases in the

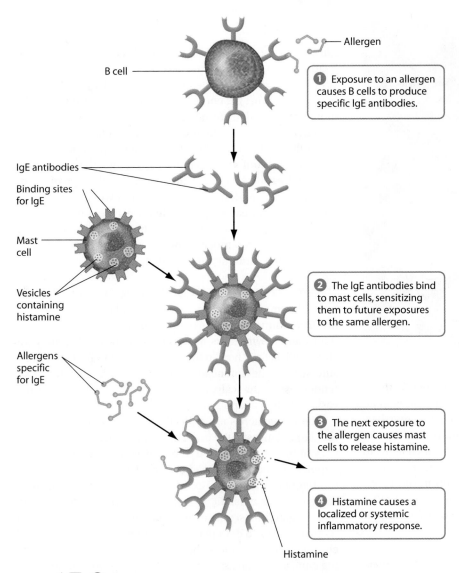

① Exposure to an allergen causes B cells to produce specific IgE antibodies.

② The IgE antibodies bind to mast cells, sensitizing them to future exposures to the same allergen.

③ The next exposure to the allergen causes mast cells to release histamine.

④ Histamine causes a localized or systemic inflammatory response.

B cell

Allergen

IgE antibodies

Binding sites for IgE

Mast cell

Vesicles containing histamine

Allergens specific for IgE

Histamine

**FIGURE 17.3 Steps of an Allergic Response**

Source: Adapted from JOHNSON, MICHAEL D., HUMAN BIOLOGY: CONCEPTS AND CURRENT ISSUES, 5th, © 2010. Printed and Electronically reproduced by permission of Pearson Education, Inc., Upper Saddle River, New Jersey.

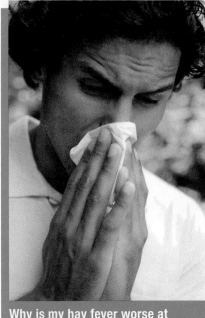

**Why is my hay fever worse at certain times of the year?**

Hay fever is triggered by the pollen from ragweed, a plant most common in the Northeast, Midwest, and South. It produces most of its pollen in the fall, making this the hardest time of year for many allergy sufferers. Steps you can take to minimize your exposure include keeping windows closed, staying indoors when pollen counts are highest (typically 10 AM to 4 PM), and changing clothes after spending time outdoors.

United States, affecting between 10 and 30 percent of all adults and up to 40 percent of all children there.[12] It is usually considered a seasonal disease, because it is most prevalent when ragweed and flowers are blooming. Hay fever attacks are characterized by sneezing and itchy, watery eyes and nose, and they make countless people miserable for weeks at a time every year. As with other allergies, hay fever results from an overzealous immune system that is hypersensitive to certain substances and an inherited tendency to have this hypersensitivity. You are more likely to have hay fever if you have a family history of allergies, are male, were born during pollen season, are a firstborn child, were exposed to cigarette smoke during your first year of life, or are exposed to dust mites.

Avoiding the environmental triggers is the best way to prevent hay fever. If you can't prevent it, shots or antihistamines often provide relief. Decongestants can reduce symptoms, as can air-conditioning and air purifiers. Over-the-counter nose sprays are usually of limited value, and their prolonged use may actually cause symptoms or make them worse. Inhaled steroids are often effective and may be prescribed, as are specific desensitizing injections.[13]

## Food Allergies

A food allergy is an immune response to food. It should not be confused with food intolerance, which is the inability to digest a particular food due to problems with the physical, hormonal, or biochemical systems in your digestive tract. Many people who have an adverse response after eating think they have an allergy, when in fact, they may lack specific enzymes necessary to digest certain foods, such as lactose (see the section on digestion-related disorders later in this chapter). Others may think they have an allergy when they are reacting to specific pathogens found in the food and really have a foodborne illness. True allergies are most often triggered by milk, eggs, peanuts, other nuts, soybeans, wheat, fish, and shellfish.

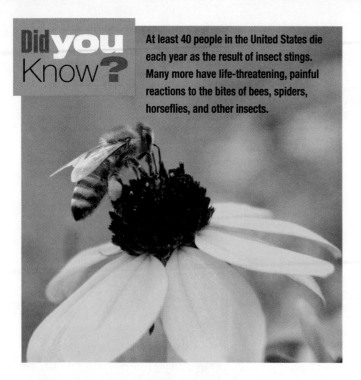
Symptoms of a food allergy are similar to other forms of allergies and may include swelling in the mouth or esophagus, difficulty breathing, itching, stomach pain, diarrhea, dizziness, nausea; the reaction can be so severe that the victim goes into shock, with a rapid heart rate and changes in blood pressure. Over 200 Americans die each year from food allergies, and another 30,000 or more end up in the emergency room because of their symptoms. Millions more suffer from allergies without knowing why they don't feel well or have a bit of itching after eating.[14]

Although some food allergies can be outgrown, there is no cure. If you do have an allergy, you can avoid many reactions by reading labels, asking questions in restaurants, and knowing exactly what you are eating. Wear a medical alert bracelet or necklace that says you have food allergies and let your friends, family members, and instructors know that you react to certain foods. Carry antihistamines or auto-injector devices containing epinephrine (adrenaline) so that you can quickly respond in the event of accidental exposure.

# Coping with Neurological Disorders

There are more than 600 disorders that affect the nervous system, and an estimated 50 million Americans are afflicted with them each year.[15] Some of these disorders, such as migraine headaches and epilepsy, are well known, but there are others known only to those who suffer from them and still others that elude diagnosis (see the **Health Headlines** box at right).

**migraine** A condition characterized by localized headaches that possibly result from alternating dilation and constriction of blood vessels.

# Headaches

Almost all of us have experienced at least one major headache. You party a little too much, you are stressed by your "to do" list, you have an argument with your family or friends, you don't get enough sleep, or you are just one of the millions who suffers from headaches for no apparent reason. Millions of people see their doctors for headaches each year, and millions more silently put up with the pain or take pain relievers to blunt their symptoms. The good news is that most of the time, headaches are usually not the sign of a serious disease or underlying condition and will go away fairly quickly. Most headaches are tension-type headaches or migraines, whereas some are specific to certain underlying causes, such as too much alcohol, or stress; see Table 17.1 on page 564 for a summary of the latter.

**Tension-Type Headaches** Nearly 80 percent of adults have the most common type of headache, *tension-type headache,* during their lives, with women having slightly more than men.[16] Symptoms of tension-type headaches may include dull, aching head pain; a sensation of tightness or pressure across the forehead, sides, and back of your head; tenderness on the scalp, neck, and shoulder muscles; and, occasionally, loss of appetite.[17]

These headaches are typically due to chemical and neuronal imbalances in the brain and/or muscular tension in the back of the neck or scalp that results in pain in the forehead, temples, or back of the head or neck. There is a wide range in the frequency and severity of symptoms, with occurrences categorized as episodic (occurring less than once a month and triggered by stress, anxiety, fatigue, or anger), frequent (occurring 1 to 15 days per month along with migraines), and chronic (occurring more than 15 days per month, with varying pain, and often associated with depression or other emotional problems). Possible triggers include red wine, lack of sleep, fasting, menstruation, or certain food additives or preservatives.

Tension-type headaches are most often prevented by reducing triggers. If stress is a trigger, try to relax with a hot bath, relaxing music, hot compresses, massage, or other relaxation techniques. Exercise can relieve some types of tension headaches, while aspirin, ibuprofen, acetaminophen, and naproxen sodium remain the standby forms of pain relief. If headaches occur more frequently and are difficult to treat with OTC medications, they are probably *chronic tension headaches*—the result of physical or psychological problems or depression. These more difficult forms of tension headaches warrant a visit to the doctor to assess the underlying cause.

**Migraine Headaches** Nearly 30 million Americans suffer from **migraines,** a type of headache that often has severe, debilitating symptoms, including moderate to severe pain on one or both sides of the head, head pain with a pulsating or throbbing quality, pain that worsens with physical activity, or that interferes with regular activity, nausea with or without

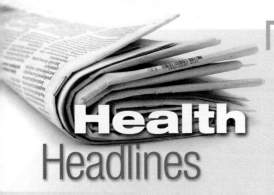

# Health Headlines

## AN EPIDEMIC OF PAIN: WHAT'S IN YOUR FUTURE?

If you're like 80 percent of Americans, you probably have experienced pain in your body at some point in your life. Chronic pain is listed as the most costly health problem in America, estimated at over $90 billion per year.

What *is* pain? According to the International Association for the Study of Pain, pain is "an unpleasant sensory and emotional experience associated with actual or potential tissue damage or described by the patient in terms of such damage." In more simple terms, it is something that hurts, often by degrees ranging from mild to intolerable. Why some people can tolerate high levels of pain while others cringe at the thought remains a mystery.

Although we hate it when we have it, pain isn't all bad. In fact, it can warn you that you have strained a body part too far and need to stop (as in overexercising muscles or joints); it can let you know that you have something wrong (that you have an abscess forming in your tooth or an appendix ready to burst); or it can be the odd sensation that sends you to the doctor to be checked for diseases such as cancer.

*Acute pain* is pain that is intense, may be localized, and may be generated by a variety of things, including inflammation, tissue damage, injury, surgery, or other body assaults. Usually, acute pain resolves with time. In contrast, *chronic pain,* the kind that is most typical of many of the ailments listed in this chapter, persists for weeks, months, or years and can result in major physical disability and emotional suffering. Chronic pain sufferers may be unable to work, eat, sleep, or carry on even the most basic activities of daily living. For them, life may become unbearable.

Often, pain is triggered by some form of assault on the nervous system, an injury; inflammation; reaction to toxins; or exposure to external heat, cold, or pressure. It can be dull, sharp, or "referred," meaning that it originates in one part of the body but is perceived to be in another. There is "phantom pain" that may occur in cases in which a limb has been amputated but the person still feels pain there. It can be *vascular,* as in cases in which there is reduced blood flow, such as in varicose veins, or it can actually be *psychogenic,* meaning that it stems from complex emotional or other psychological factors. The brain and our emotions can play a major role in how we experience pain.

Each year, more than 76 million Americans report pain lasting more than 24 hours. Women report slightly more pain than men (27.1% vs. 24.4%, respectively). Persistent pain is reported by 25 percent of adults aged 20 to 44, 30 percent of adults aged 45 to 64, and 21 percent of adults aged 65 and older. Many pain sufferers become so preoccupied with pain that they can't function. They fear activity because they fear pain. They fear going out, because they might experience pain. As a result, they may become depressed or irritable, or develop insomnia. When they can't sleep, they become more depressed and experience more pain as part of a vicious cycle.

Chronic pain sufferers have a variety of treatment options today and may choose from any of the following, either alone or in combination:

* **Over-the-counter (OTC) medications.** Acetaminophen (Tylenol) and nonsteroidal anti-inflammatory drugs (NSAIDs), such as ibuprofen (Advil, Motrin), aspirin, and naproxen (Aleve).
* **Prescription medications.** A variety of these are available. Compared to OTCs, they may give faster results, but they also present increased risks for patients in terms of addiction and drug interactions.
* **Heat and cold treatments.** Cold packs are used to numb areas, reduce swelling, and ease joint aches. Hot packs are used to relax muscles, bring blood to an area, and aid healing.
* **Acupuncture, acupressure, and massage.** All are designed to reduce pain, relax the patient, and speed healing. See Chapter 18

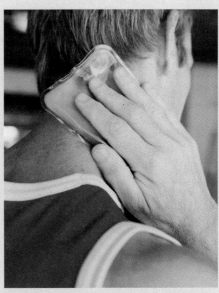

Cold packs are one of many options for pain treatment.

for more on these options and their rates of effectiveness.
* **Local electrical stimulation.** Transcutaneous electrical nerve stimulation (TENS) blocks pain messages to the brain and modifies perceptions of pain. Brief electrical pulses to nerve endings provide pain relief.
* **Psychological treatment.** Among a small percentage of pain sufferers, pain appears to be precipitated by emotional or psychological trauma or suffering. In these cases, counseling, relaxation training, water therapy, meditation, biofeedback, aromatherapy, light therapy, dietary changes, yoga, and other mind–body techniques can reduce the severity of pain or eventually make it go away.
* **Surgery.** If you've tried everything else and nothing seems to work, surgery may be a last option.

**Sources:** International Association for the Study of Pain, Stanford University, Patient Education Section of Pain Center, Accessed September 2010, http://paincenter.stanford.edu/patient_care/pain.html; National Institute of Neurological Disorders and Stroke (NINDS), "Chronic Pain Information Page," Updated June 2010, www.ninds.nih.gov/disorders/chronic_pain/chronic_pain.htm; American Pain Foundation, "Pain Facts and Figures" Updated July 2009, www.painfoundation.org/newsroom/reporter-resources/pain-facts-figures.html; K. Woznicki, "What's Your Pain Tolerance?" 2010, www.webmd.com/pain-management/features/whats-your-pain-tolerance.

TABLE

17.1    **Types of Headaches**

| Type | Symptoms | Precipitating Factors | Treatment | Prevention |
|---|---|---|---|---|
| **Allergy** | Generalized headache. Nasal congestion, watery eyes. | Seasonal allergens such as pollen, molds. Allergies to food are not usually a factor. | Antihistamine medication; topical, nasal cortisone-related sprays, or desensitization injections. | None. |
| **Caffeine-withdrawal** | Throbbing headache caused by rebound dilation of the blood vessels, occurring multiple days after consumption of large quantities of caffeine. | Caffeine. | In extreme cases, treat by terminating caffeine consumption. | Avoid excess caffeine. |
| **Cluster** | Excruciating pain in vicinity of eye. Tearing of eye, nose congestion, flushing of face. Pain frequently develops during sleep and may last for several hours. Attacks occur every day for weeks/months, then disappear for up to a year. 80% of cluster patients are male, most ages 20–50. | Alcoholic beverages, excessive smoking. | Oxygen, ergotamine, sumatriptan, or intranasal application of local anesthetic agent. | Use of steroids, ergotamine, calcium channel blockers, and lithium. |
| **Exertion** | Generalized head pain of short duration (minutes to 1 hour) during or following physical exertion (running, jumping, or sexual intercourse), or passive exertion (sneezing, coughing, moving one's bowels, etc.). | 10% caused by organic diseases (aneurysms, tumors, or blood vessel malformation). 90% are related to migraine or cluster headaches. | Cause must be accurately determined. Most commonly treated with aspirin, indomethacin, or propranolol. Extensive testing is necessary to determine the headache cause. Surgery to correct organic disease is occasionally indicated. | Alternative forms of exercise. Avoid jarring exercises. |
| **Eyestrain** | Usually frontal, bilateral pain, directly related to eyestrain. Rare cause of headache. | Muscle imbalance. Uncorrected vision, astigmatism. | Correction of vision. | Same as treatment. |
| **Hangover** | Migraine-like symptoms of throbbing pain and nausea not localized to one side. | Alcohol, which causes dilation and irritation of the blood vessels of the brain and surrounding tissue. | Liquids (including broth). Consumption of fructose (honey, tomato juice are good sources) to help burn alcohol. | Drink alcohol only in moderation. |
| **Hunger** | Pain strikes just before mealtime. Caused by muscle tension, low blood sugar, and rebound dilation of the blood vessels, oversleeping, or missing a meal. | Strenuous dieting or skipping meals. | Regular, nourishing meals containing adequate protein and complex carbohydrates. | Same as treatment. |
| **New daily persistent headache (NDPH)** | This headache can best be described as the rapid development (less than 3 days) of unrelenting headache, and typically presents in a person with no past history of a headache. | Typically NDPH does not evolve from migraine or episodic tension-type headache. NDPH begins as a new headache. It may be the result of a viral infection. | In some cases, NPDH can resolve on its own within several months. Other cases persist and are more refractory. | Does not respond to traditional options. However, antiseizure medications, topiramate, or gabapentin can be used. |
| **Sinus** | Gnawing pain over nasal area, often increasing in severity throughout the day. Caused by acute infection, usually with fever, producing blockage of sinus ducts and preventing normal drainage. Sinus headaches are rare. Migraine and cluster headaches are often misdiagnosed as sinus in origin. | Infection, nasal polyps, anatomical deformities, such as a deviated septum, that block the sinus ducts. | Treat with antibiotics, decongestants, surgical drainage if necessary. | None |

**Source:** National Headache Foundation, "The Complete Headache Chart," 2010, www.headaches.org/education/Headache_Topic_Sheets/The_Complete_Headache_Chart.

# Maladies Specific to Women

Because of their different anatomies and lifestyles, men and women frequently experience different rates of chronic conditions. In addition, there are some conditions that are specific to one gender or the other because they affect body structures and organs associated with reproductive functions.

## FIBROCYSTIC BREAST CONDITION

A common, noncancerous problem among women in the United States is *fibrocystic breast condition.* Symptoms range in severity from one small, palpable lump to large masses of irregular tissue found in both breasts. Although most cyst formations consist of fibrous tissue, some are filled with fluid. Treatment often involves removing fluid from the affected area or surgically removing the cyst. The underlying causes of the condition are unknown; some experts believe it relates to an imbalance between estrogen and progesterone. Others relate it to hormonal changes that occur during the normal menstrual cycle. Likewise, caffeine has been discussed as a cause of fibrocystic breast condition. It's pretty clear that caffeine doesn't cause cysts, but it may increase hormone levels, which can increase susceptibility to fibrous tissue buildup. In most cases, the condition appears to run in families and to become progressively worse with age, irrespective of pregnancy or other hormonal disruptions. Today about 90 percent of all women have some degree of this condition, prompting experts to take it out of the disease category and begin referring to it as *benign breast changes*.

Experts believe that the risks for breast cancer among women with certain types of fibrocystic disease may be slightly higher than among the general populace, but this may be because fibrous tissue makes it more unlikely for a woman to notice an abnormal lump. As a result, women with fibrocystic tendencies may delay seeking medical advice.

## ENDOMETRIOSIS

*Endometriosis* is characterized by abnormal growth and development of endometrial tissue (the tissue lining the uterus) in regions of the body other than the uterus. It is most likely to appear between the ages of 20 and 40.

Symptoms of endometriosis include severe cramping during and between menstrual cycles, irregular periods, unusually

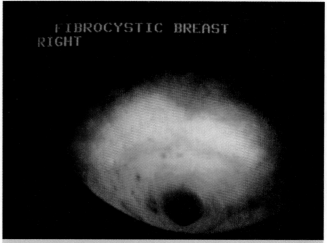

This image, created by computerized analysis of the light absorption of tissues, shows a fibrocystic breast.

heavy or light menstrual flow, abdominal bloating, fatigue, painful bowel movements with periods, painful intercourse, constipation, diarrhea, infertility, and low back pain. Among the most widely accepted theories concerning the causes of endometriosis are the transmission of endometrial tissue to other regions of the body during surgery or through the birthing process, the movement of menstrual fluid backward through the fallopian tubes during menstruation, and abnormal cell migration through body-fluid movement. Women with cycles shorter than 27 days or flows lasting over a week are at increased risk. The more aerobic exercise a woman engages in and the earlier she starts it, the less likely she is to develop endometriosis.

Treatment for endometriosis ranges from bed rest and stress reduction to *hysterectomy* (the removal of the uterus) or the removal of one or both ovaries and the fallopian tubes. More conservative treatments involve dilation and curettage, surgically scraping endometrial tissue off the fallopian tubes and other reproductive organs. Combinations of hormone therapy have also become more acceptable.

**Sources:** The Endometriosis Association, "Treatment Options," Accessed September 2010, www.endometriosisassn.org/treatment.html; American Congress of Obstetricians and Gynecologists, *Patient Education Pamphlet: Endometriosis* (Washington, DC: American Congress of Obstetricians and Gynecologists, 2008), Available at www.acog.org/publications/patient _education/bp013.cfm; National Institutes of Health, Medline Plus, "Endometriosis," Updated September 2010, www.nlm.nih.gov/medlineplus/ endometriosis.html; National Women's Health Information Center, "Endometriosis," Updated November 2009, www.womenshealth.gov/faq/ endometriosis.cfm.

vomiting, and sensitivity to light and sound.[18] In fact, 1 out of 4 households has a migraine sufferer. Usually migraine incidence peaks in young adulthood (between ages 20 and 45).[19]

Migraine appears to run in families: If both your parents experience migraines, you have a 75 percent chance of experiencing them too; if only one parent has them, you have a 50 percent chance. If any of your relatives have them, you have a

20 percent risk.[20] Although 4 out of 5 migraine sufferers report a family history, researchers do not know if this is a genetic or familial predisposition. Migraine is also an example of a condition that is more common among members of one gender than the other; three times as many women as men suffer from migraine (see the **Gender & Health** box for discussion of two other conditions that are unique to women).[21]

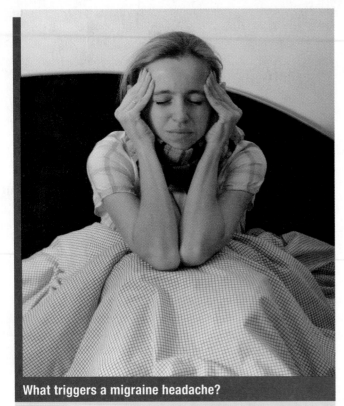

**What triggers a migraine headache?**

Patients report that migraines can be triggered by emotional stress, fatigue, too much or not enough sleep, fasting, caffeine, chocolate, alcohol, menses, hormone changes, altitude, weather, certain foods, and a litany of other causes. There is tremendous variability in these. What triggers a migraine in one person may relieve it in another.

Whereas all headaches can be painful, migraines can be disabling. Symptoms vary greatly by individual, and attacks can last anywhere from 4 to 72 hours, with distinct phases of symptoms. In about 25 percent of cases, migraines are preceded by a sensory warning sign called an *aura*, such as flashes of light, flickering vision, blind spots, tingling in arms or legs, or a sensation of odor or taste.[22] The triggers of a migraine vary widely from one person to the next. Although vascular abnormalities in the brain have long been thought to be underlying causes, experts are beginning to believe that migraines may be triggered within the brain itself as a result of a complex biochemical and inflammatory process.[23]

**epilepsy** A neurological disorder caused by abnormal electrical brain activity; can be accompanied by altered consciousness or convulsions.

When true migraines occur, relaxation is only minimally effective as a treatment. Often, strong pain-relieving prescription drugs are necessary. See your doctor for more information or go to the National Headache Foundation website (www.headaches.org) for the latest information on treatments.

**what do you think?**

Have you ever experienced a migraine or tension-type headache? How did you alleviate the pain? ● What actions can you take to reduce your risks of severe headaches in the future?

**70%** of people with epilepsy who take medication enter remission, defined as remaining seizure-free for 5 years or more.

## Seizure Disorders

Approximately 3 million people in the United States suffer from **epilepsy** or some other form of seizure-related disorder (the word *epilepsy* derives from the Greek *epilepsia*, meaning "seizure"). Each year, some 300,000 people in the United States will have a seizure for the first time, and an estimated 5 to 10 percent of the population will experience at least one seizure in their lives. Over a third of all new seizures this year will occur in people under the age of 18, with males having a slightly greater risk than females.[24]

Seizure disorders are generally caused by abnormal electrical activity in the brain and are characterized by loss of control of muscular activity and unconsciousness. People who take certain drugs, are withdrawing from drugs, have a high fever and abnormal levels of sodium or glucose in the blood, or experience physical, chemical, or temperature trauma may be at higher risk for seizures. Symptoms vary widely from person to person and can range from temporary confusion to major seizure activity.

About half of all cases of seizure disorder are of unknown origin. In addition to the above, possible causes include stroke, head injury, congenital abnormalities, injury or illness resulting in inflammation of the brain or spinal column, tumors, nutritional deficiency, and heredity. See the appendix for information on providing first aid to someone experiencing a seizure.

In most cases, people afflicted with seizure disorders can lead normal, seizure-free lives when under medical supervision. Public ignorance and stigma associated with having these disorders can have a significant impact on sufferers and their families as they cope with the challenges of treatment and daily living. Improvements in medication and surgical interventions to reduce some causes of seizures are among the most promising treatments today.

## Coping with Digestion-Related Disorders

Digestive disorders are on the increase in the United States, with more than 95 million people suffering from one or more of these ailments.[25] Unfortunately, the causes of digestive disorders are often complex, symptoms are often subtle, and there is great variability in type of treatment and effectiveness. For reasons that are not totally understood, rates are on the increase among younger adults. Two of the most common disorders, lactose intolerance and celiac disease (gluten intolerance), are discussed in Chapter 7; disorders that are not related to a specific nutrient are described below. See Table 17.2

| Disease | Who's Affected? | Causes and Risk Factors | Symptoms | Treatment | Prevention |
|---|---|---|---|---|---|
| **Fibromyalgia** Extreme fatigue, painful, aching joints and muscles. | Affects 3%–7% of population. Rates increase with age. | Unknown. Affects primarily women in their 30s and 40s. | Numbness, tingling, pain, headache, dizziness. | Pain medications, anti-inflammatories, rest, stress management. | Rest, dietary adjustments. Avoid extreme temperatures. |
| **Gallbladder diseases** Several types; most common are cholecystitis (inflammation) and cholelithiasis (gallstones). Often asymptomatic. | More than 25 million have gallstones (25% of women by age 60, 50% by age 75, 80% of men by age 75). Highest in Mexican Americans and Native Americans. | Repeated exposure to certain chemicals, infections, traumatic injury, obesity, cirrhosis of liver, rapid weight loss and yo-yo diets, diabetes, cholesterol-lowering drugs, excess weight gain during pregnancy. | Acute pain in the upper right quadrant of abdomen, particularly after eating fatty food; nausea, vomiting. | Medications to relieve inflammation or cause of inflammation; removal of gallstones through lithotripsy or surgery. | Reduce dietary fat; avoid alcohol, fried foods, whole grains. |
| **Multiple sclerosis** Degenerative neurological disease caused by breakdown of myelin, (protective sheath around nerves). Scarring occurs, resulting in faulty nerve transmissions. Form of autoimmune disease. | Over 400,000 cases, most between ages of 20 and 40. Most common disabling neurological disease to affect young adults today. Affects women 2 to 3 times more frequently than men. Overall risk for general population is 1 in 800. | Several causes suspected (none proven), including genetics, viruses, allergies, and environmental toxins. Caucasians are at greatest risk. | Vary by type, from minor numbness, blurred vision, fatigue, balance issues to severely disabling. Intermittent course for some, with flare-ups. | No cure, but drug therapy, climate change, and lifestyle choices can reduce symptoms and increase healthy years. | Prevention of flare-ups is possible with healthy lifestyle, adequate sleep, healthy diet, stress management, and avoidance of temperature extremes. |
| **Parkinson's disease** Chronic, progressive, neurological disease that affects motor function. | 50,000–60,000 new cases/year. Nearly 2 million total, mostly over age 50. | Cause unknown. Genetic and familial factors may play a part, but not yet proved. Environmental toxins, trauma, history of past illness, and low vitamin D level have all been implicated. | Tremor (shaking hands, arms, legs, jaw, head/face); rigidity, postural instability, slowness, lack of spontaneous movement; balance issues, shuffling gait; speech difficulties. | No cure, but prescription medications can relieve symptoms. Ibuprofen and NSAIDs may help. Deep brain stimulation (DBS) and gamma knife surgery have proved useful in some cases. | None obvious. Healthy lifestyle may help slow progression. |
| **Raynaud's syndrome** Exaggerated constriction of small arteries in the extremities. | 5%–10% of adults, primarily women. | Unknown. | Fingers and toes become numb, turn white or purple; throbbing pain. | Topical medications to reduce symptoms. | More common in those exposed to extreme weather repeatedly, so control temperatures, wear gloves or boots, avoid frostbite or medications that affect blood flow. |

*Continued on next page*

TABLE

17.2 **Other Modern Maladies (continued)**

| Disease | Who's Affected? | Cause/Risk Factors | Symptoms | Treatment | Prevention |
|---------|-----------------|--------------------|-----------|-----------|------------|
| **Rosacea** Inflammatory skin condition causing redness and small red bumps or pustules on the face. | Affects over 14 million Americans; underdiagnosed. Common in adults 30–60, more common in women and people with fair skin/sensitive skin. Menopausal women are at higher risk. | Still unknown, many suspects, ranging from genetic predisposition to blushing, skin mites, bacteria. None conclusive. | Can progress in stages: from frequent flushing to spider veins on face, to lumps and bumps, to red, angry skin. Skin thickening, primarily on the nose and face, red itchy eyes, bulbous nose in later stages. | No cure, but strategies for control include prescription medications and facial lotions, changes to soaps that are less irritating, antibiotics, surgery, new laser treatments, freezing. | Unknown. |
| **Systemic lupus erythematosus** Autoimmune disease in which antibodies destroy or injure organs such as kidneys, brain, and heart. | 1 in 700 Caucasians, 1 in 250 African Americans. 90% of patients are women between ages 18 and 45. Ratio of females to males is 10:1. | Cause unknown. Possible genetic predisposition combined with environment and hormones. | Different types/ severity present various symptoms: sensitivity to light, arthritis, swelling, tendency toward increased infections, butterfly-shaped rash across nose and cheeks. | Medications such as steroids to reduce symptoms and complications. | Healthy lifestyle; other possible preventive measures unknown. |

**Sources:** Data are from National Fibromyalgia Association, "About Fibromyalgia," Accessed September 2010, www.fmaware.org/site/PageServer?pagename =fibromyalgia; A. Assumpção et al., "Prevalence of Fibromyalgia in a Low Socioeconomic Status Population," BMC Musculoskeletal Disorders 10 (2009): 64–67; K. Maurer, M. Carey, and J. Fox, "Roles of Infection, Inflammation, and Immune System in Cholesterol Gallstone Formation," Gastroenterology 136, no. 2 (2009): 425–40; eMedicineHealth, "Gallstones," Accessed September 2010, www.emedicinehealth.com/gallstones/article_em.htm; WebMD, "Cholecystitis: Overview," Updated July 2009, www.webmd.com/digestive-disorders/tc/cholecystitis-overview; National Multiple Sclerosis Society, "Who Gets MS?" Accessed September 2010, www.nationalmssociety.org/about-multiple-sclerosis/what-we-know-about-ms/who-gets-ms/index.aspx; P. Sweeney, Cleveland Clinic, Center for Continuing Education, "Parkinson's Disease," Accessed September 2010, www.clevelandclinicmeded.com/medicalpubs/diseasemanagement/neurology/parkinsons-disease; The National Rosacea Society, "The Many Faces of Rosacea," Accessed September 2010, http://rosacea.org/patients/faces.php; What Health?, "Rosacea Statistics," Accessed September 2010, www.whathealth.com/rosacea/incidence.html; P. Schur and B. Hahn, "Epidemiology and Pathogenesis of Systemic Lupus Erythematosus," Updated June 2010, www.uptodate.com/patients/content/topic.do?topicKey=~/3ljrinen9.

for discussion of gallbladder disease, another common digestive disorder, as well as several other modern maladies.

# Inflammatory Bowel Disease

**Inflammatory bowel disease (IBD)** is an umbrella term for a group of disorders in which the intestines become inflamed. The cause is not known but the symptoms are typically severe stomach cramping, bloating, pain, and bloody bouts of diarrhea. For unknown reasons, adults between the ages of 15 and 35 are the most common victims, and numbers seem to be increasing on college campuses. More than 1 million people in the United States have been diagnosed, with the majority of cases being whites, particularly persons of Jewish descent. Numbers of cases in African Americans and Latinos are increasing without clear patterns by geographical region.[26] The most common types of IBD are **ulcerative colitis (UC),** which affects the colon and large intestine, and **Crohn's disease,** which can affect any part of the intestine from the mouth to the anus.

Ulcerative colitis often has symptoms that come and go. Typically, severe stomach cramping, diarrhea, and bloody stools are the key symptoms. People with severe cases may have as many as 20 bouts of bloody diarrhea a day. About 25 percent of those with those with UC develop it before the age of 20, especially those who have a family history of the disease. White and black Americans tend to have similar rates, but Asian Americans have lower rates. Among white Americans, rates are higher among those of Jewish descent.[27]

Although some experts believe that colitis occurs more frequently in people with high stress levels, this theory is controversial. Smokers have a higher risk of UC, as do those who have had measles and certain bacterial infections. Hypersensitive reactions to certain foods have also been considered a possible cause. Determining the cause of colitis is difficult because the disease can go into remission and then recur without apparent reason. This pattern often continues over periods of years and may be related to the later development of colorectal cancer.

**inflammatory bowel disease (IBD)** A group of disorders in which the intestines become inflamed.

**ulcerative colitis (UC)** An inflammatory disorder that affects the mucous membranes of the large intestine, producing bloody diarrhea.

**Crohn's disease** An autoimmune inflammatory disease of the gastrointestinal tract characterized by cramping and diarrhea.

Because the cause is unknown, treatment of symptoms and avoidance of substances that may trigger attacks are important. Treatment focuses on relieving the symptoms by decreasing foods that are hard to digest (raw vegetables, seeds, nuts, and high-fiber foods); taking probiotics; and taking anti-inflammatory drugs, steroids, and other medications to reduce inflammation and soothe irritated intestinal walls.

Crohn's disease is usually diagnosed in men and women in their twenties and thirties and is characterized by intense stomach pain, often in the lower right area, and diarrhea. Bleeding may also occur, and can be serious enough to cause anemia, fatigue, and immune system dysfunction. Those diagnosed with this disease must carefully monitor diet to ensure adequate nutrition and must take medications to reduce inflammation and infection.[28]

Students with IBD face a difficult and unique set of challenges: Studies show that victims have increased difficulty in adjusting to the demands of campus life.[29] More aggressive medical therapy and increased emotional support are suggested to increase positive college experiences and improve retention and graduation rates.

## Irritable Bowel Syndrome

Inflammatory bowel disease and **irritable bowel syndrome (IBS)** are not the same condition, although they may sound as if they were. Irritable bowel syndrome is a functional bowel disorder rather than an inflammatory process. The exact cause is unknown, but in individuals with IBS, the normal muscular contractions in the intestines don't work properly and food isn't processed or eliminated as it should be.[30]

Irritable bowel syndrome may begin after an infection, a stressful life event, or onset of maturity without any other medical indicators. Characterized by nausea, pain, gas, diarrhea, or cramps after eating certain foods or during unusual stress, IBS commonly begins in early adulthood. Symptoms may vary from week to week and can fade for long periods of time, only to return. Researchers suspect that people with IBS have digestive systems that are overly sensitive to what they eat and drink, to stress, and to certain hormonal changes. Often, because symptoms are so similar to other gastrointestinal tract diseases, IBS is only diagnosed after all the other gastrointestinal diseases have been ruled out. As many as 55 million Americans suffer from IBS.

Although there is no cure for IBS, treatments to attempt to relieve symptoms, stress management, relaxation techniques, regular activity, and diet changes can control it in the vast major-

ity of cases. Problems with diarrhea can be reduced by cutting down on fat and avoiding caffeine and sorbitol, a sweetener found in diet foods and chewing gum. Constipation can be relieved by a gradual increase in fiber and increased fluid consumption. Some sufferers benefit from drugs that relax the intestinal muscle, or from antidepressant drugs and counseling to reduce stress.

## Gastroesophageal Reflux Disease

**Gastroesophageal reflux disease (GERD),** commonly referred to as *heartburn* or *acid reflux,* affects millions of people throughout the world. Risk factors include age, diet, alcohol use, obesity, pregnancy, and smoking. At any given time, people of all ages and stages of life suffer from a sensation of heartburn, or backflow of stomach acid into the esophagus, characterized by discomfort or a burning sensation behind the breastbone. Symptoms usually occur after a meal and can include coughing, choking, heartburn, or vomiting. When these symptoms are severe and occur more than 2 to 3 times per week, GERD is often the diagnosis.

**irritable bowel syndrome (IBS)** Nausea, pain, gas, or diarrhea caused by certain foods or stress.
**gastroesophageal reflux disease (GERD)** Chronic condition in which stomach acid backflows into the esophagus, causing heartburn and potential damage to the esophagus.

Prevention of GERD is often focused on determining which foods or beverages trigger symptoms (coffee, sodas, and alcohol are the big culprits), and avoiding spicy or fried

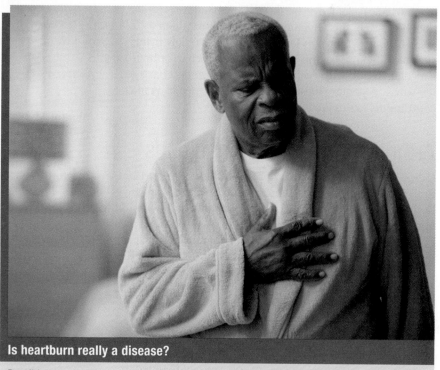

**Is heartburn really a disease?**

Possible complications of untreated heartburn (GERD) include bleeding of the stomach or esophagus, ulcers, and cancer of the esophagus. Regardless of the nature and extent of heartburn, it should not be ignored. If you have persistent heartburn, see your doctor.

foods. Dietary control is often a key in reducing heartburn symptoms. Also, it is important to find out whether there are mechanical causes of reflux, such as sleeping or sitting in positions that exacerbate symptoms. It may be helpful to elevate your upper body if acid rushes into the esophagus when you lie down. If repositioning doesn't work, taking medications to reduce stomach acids can help. If heartburn persists, see your doctor.

# Coping with Musculoskeletal Diseases

Musculoskeletal diseases, including back pain, arthritis, bodily injuries, and osteoporosis, are more common than any other health condition in the United States.[31] Based on the most recent statistics, over 108 million adults, or 1 in every 2 aged 18 or over, suffered from a musculoskeletal condition lasting 3 months or longer in the past year. The annual cost of such conditions is over $850 billion in treatment and lost wages. More than half of all days of work missed due to a major medical condition are a result of a musculoskeletal disease (Figure 17.4). In addition, because of this affliction, over 15 million adults are unable to perform at least one activity of daily living, such as self-care, walking, or getting out of a chair or bed, on a regular basis.[32] With each decade, these numbers have gotten worse. Sedentary lifestyle and obesity are listed as major contributors to this growing epidemic.[33]

## Arthritis and Related Conditions

Called "the nation's primary crippler," **arthritis** strikes 1 in 5 Americans, or over 47 million people.[34] Symptoms range from the occasional tendinitis of the weekend athlete to the horrific pain of rheumatoid arthritis. There are over 100 types of arthritis diagnosed today, the most common of which are osteoarthritis and rheumatoid arthritis. Arthritis accounts for over 30 million lost workdays annually and the cost to the U.S. economy was over $282 billion in 2005 for treatment alone.[35] Add in the cost of lost wages and productivity, prescriptions, and OTC pain relief medications and the numbers skyrocket. Unfortunately, as epidemic rates of obesity and sedentary lifestyle contribute to the development of arthritis, by 2030 over 67

**arthritis** Painful inflammatory disease of the joints.
**osteoarthritis (OA)** Progressive deterioration of bones and joints that has been associated with the wear-and-tear theory of aging.

## 437 million

**days of work are missed annually due to musculoskeletal conditions.**

million Americans aged 18 and over will be diagnosed with the disease, a number that will have staggering consequences for our health care system.[36]

**Osteoarthritis** Also called *degenerative joint disease*, **osteoarthritis (OA)** is the most common form of arthritis. If you notice that your parents or grandparents are slow to get out of their chairs or walk with a little "gimpy" stiffness after getting out of bed, they may be showing the early signs of OA. Over 27 million adults in the United States have this disease, most of whom are women.[37] This progressive deterioration of cartilage, bones and joints has been associated with the "wear-and-tear" theory of aging.

Although age and injury are undoubtedly factors in osteoarthritis, heredity, abnormal joint use, diet, abnormalities in joint structure, and impaired blood supply to

### "Why Should I Care?"

You may think arthritis and back pain are problems only your grandparents have to worry about, but they also affect young adults. Some of your habits today may increase your chances of experiencing musculoskeletal problems in the near—and distant—future. Managing your weight, wearing protective gear when engaging in recreational activities or sports, and avoiding repetitive joint usage are all things you can do now to lessen your chances of developing osteoarthritis and other musculoskeletal problems.

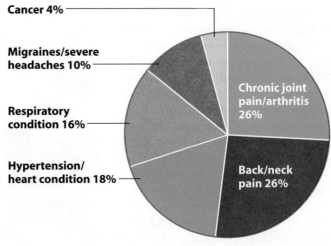

Cancer 4%
Migraines/severe headaches 10%
Respiratory condition 16%
Hypertension/heart condition 18%
Chronic joint pain/arthritis 26%
Back/neck pain 26%

FIGURE 17.4 **Proportion of Lost Work Days for Persons Aged 18 and Older by Major Medical Condition**

**Source:** United States Bone and Joint Decade, *The Burden of Musculoskeletal Diseases in the United States: Prevalence, Societal and Economic Costs* (Rosemont, IL: American Academy of Orthopaedic Surgeons, 2008), Available at www.boneandjointburden.org.

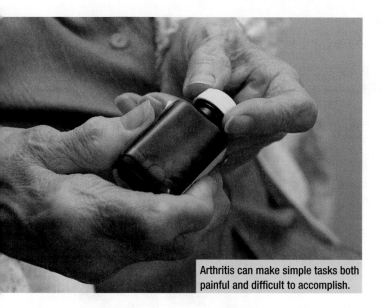
Arthritis can make simple tasks both painful and difficult to accomplish.

edy for this condition is typically bone fusion, which leaves the joint immobile. In some instances, joint replacement may be a viable alternative.

## Low Back Pain

If you're like 85 percent of the population, at some point you will injure your back. The resulting pain may be mild, involving short-lived muscle spasms, or it may be more severe, involving damage to discs, dislocation, a fracture, or another form of spinal trauma. Treatment may involve surgery, rehabilitation, and medications.

**Low back pain (LBP)**, in particular, is increasingly common, especially among young adults (see the **Student Health Today** box on page 572 for one of the possible

rheumatoid arthritis An autoimmune inflammatory joint disease.
low back pain (LBP) Pain or discomfort in the lumbosacral region of the back.

the joint may also contribute. For most people, anti-inflammatory drugs and pain relievers such as aspirin and cortisone-related agents ease discomfort. In some sufferers, applications of heat, mild exercise, and massage may also relieve the pain. When joints become so distorted that they impair activity, surgical intervention is often necessary. Joint replacement and bone fusion are increasingly common.

**Rheumatoid Arthritis** The most crippling form of arthritis, **rheumatoid arthritis** is an autoimmune disease involving chronic inflammation. It is most common in young adults, particularly those between the ages of 20 and 45, and affects more than 2.1 million Americans.[38] Symptoms include stiffness, pain, redness, and swelling of multiple joints, particularly those of the hands and wrists, and can be gradually progressive or sporadic, with occasional unexplained remissions. Although the cause of rheumatoid arthritis is unknown, some theorists believe that invading microorganisms take over the joint and cause the immune system to begin attacking the body's own tissues. Exposure to toxic chemicals and stress are also possible triggers. Genetic markers that seem to increase risk have also been identified. Regardless of the cause, treatment of rheumatoid arthritis is similar to that for osteoarthritis, emphasizing pain relief and improved functional mobility. In some instances, immunosuppressant drugs can reduce the inflammatory response and in advanced cases, surgery may be necessary. Advanced rheumatoid arthritis often involves destruction of the bony ends of joints. The rem-

## what do you think?

Do you know anyone who currently has problems with arthritis? ● Which joints seem to be most affected? ● What factors do you think might have contributed to their problems? ● What could they have done to reduce their risks?

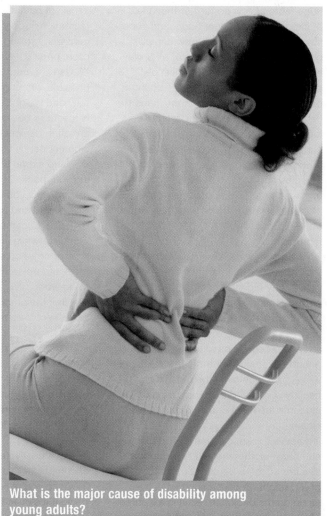

**What is the major cause of disability among young adults?**

Low back pain is the major cause of disability for people aged 20 to 45 in the United States, who suffer more frequently and severely from this problem than older people do. It is one of the most common chronic ailments among college students.

# STUDENT HEALTH Today

## COLLEGE STUDENTS AND LOW BACK PAIN: OH, MY ACHING BACKPACK?

**D**id you know that more than half of your college peers suffer from back problems? Many of them suffer in silence and simply ease up a bit in their activities or pop over-the-counter (OTC) pain relievers and keep going. Nearly 14 percent see a doctor for their pain or a physical therapist for treatment. Why are there so many issues with the back? Although athletics, exercise regimens, sitting for hours while studying, and a host of other normal activities can cause problems, modern conveniences may also be a huge factor. Look no further than the backpacks, messenger bags, and super-sized purses in vogue today. Laptops, books, bottled water, wallets, MP3 players, smartphones, headphones, cell phones, snacks, and a change of shoes or a T-shirt are but a few of the items that can be found in the typical "portable locker" students tote on their backs. Not surprisingly, lugging such an assortment around each day can cause flare-ups of muscles and other soft tissues. According to one study, 85 percent of college students report neck or back pain attributable to carrying heavy backpacks or laptops.

Whereas hikers have long recognized the importance of internal frames and heavy-duty hip straps to displace the weight of heavy packs, most college students carry less supportive (and cheaper) daypacks with only a shoulder strap that contain as much as 30 to 40 pounds of stuff. Over time, this weight can wreak havoc on even the most fit and healthy backs and shoulders. And college students are not alone; studies show that elementary schoolchildren are also carrying heavy backpacks in ever-increasing numbers—sometimes carrying amounts that are 10 to 15 percent of their total body weight. Because such repetitive strain on the back can result in a lifetime of pain and disability, prevention is imper-

ative. If you must carry a pack all day, protect your back health by following this advice:

✱ Opt for the lightest pack available and make sure that it has a heavy-duty hip strap so that you are not carrying the bulk of the weight around your back and shoulders. Adjust the strap so that the weight is primarily on the hips.

✱ If you can afford a small internal-frame pack, buy one. There are many excellent packs available from outdoor recreation supply companies, or consider a rolling version of a computer case, particularly in good weather.

✱ Use and carry the lightest computer possible. Although big screens are nice, they add weight. Remember that a laptop is meant to be portable. Larger devices are often designed for business travelers who frequently use packs with wheels.

✱ Keep extras to a minimum when loading your pack. Don't bring your books to class unless your instructor asks you to. Plan ahead and bring only those study materials to campus that you can complete while you're there; carry a smaller notepad; store files on a jump drive and upload to a campus computer to do work.

✱ Limit the amount of personal nonessential items you carry each day. Wallets, makeup, hair products, and so on should be kept to a minimum.

✱ When lifting your pack to put it on your back, make sure to stand with both feet on the ground, knees slightly flexed, and your back straight. Twisting the back while swinging up the load can cause back injuries.

✱ Pack heavy items as close to the back and the bottom as possible.

✱ Once you're ready to go, weigh the pack. If it's over 15 pounds, reassess what is necessary and ditch the rest.

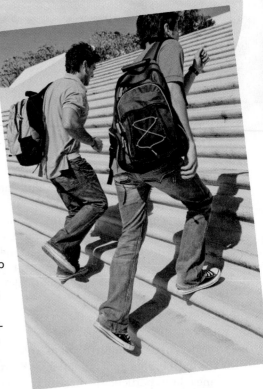

Overstuffed backpacks can lead to a lifetime of back pain.

**Sources:** L. Hestbaek et al., "The Course of Low Back Pain from Adolescence to Adulthood: Eight-Year Follow-Up of 9,600 Twins," *Spine* 31, no. 4 (2006): 468–72; American Occupational Therapy Association, "Study: Most University Students Self-Report Discomfort, Pain Due to Backpack Usage," Press release, September 3, 2008, www.prlog.org/10113114-study-most-university-students-self-report-discomfort-pain-due-to-backpack-usage.html; D. Gilkey et al., "Risk Factors Associated with Back Pain: A Cross Sectional Study of College Students," *Journal of Manipulative and Physiological Therapeutics* 33, no. 2 (2010): 88–95; American College Health Association, *American College Health Association—National College Health Assessment II (ACHA-NCHA II): Reference Group Executive Summary Fall 2009* (Baltimore: American College Health Association, 2010), Available at www.achancha.org/reports_ACHA-NCHAII.html.

causes).[39] Back injuries are the most frequently mentioned complaints in injury-related lawsuits and result in high medical and rehabilitation bills; in the United States direct and indirect costs (such as lost wages) relating to spinal injuries cost over $200 billion annually.[40] As a result, employers throughout the country have become increasingly interested in preventing these injuries.

Health experts believe that the following factors contribute to LBP:

- **Age.** People between the ages of 20 and 45 run the greatest risk of LBP. At age 50, the condition becomes less common. After age 65, the incidence again rises, apparently because of bone and joint deterioration.
- **Body type.** Many studies have indicated that people who are very tall, have a high body mass index (BMI), or have a lanky body type run an increased risk of LBP. However, much of this research is controversial.
- **Posture.** Poor posture may be one of the greatest

High-heeled shoes tilt the pelvis forward and stress the back. To avoid potential injury and back pain, wear flats whenever possible and save the heels for special occasions.

contributors to LBP. If you routinely slouch, particularly during daily tasks, you run an increased risk.
- **Strength and fitness.** People with LBP tend to have less overall trunk strength (core strength) than other people. In addition, one's total level of fitness and conditioning is a factor. The more fit you are, the better. Sedentary people who suddenly decide to "get fit" often are among those most at risk for LBP. They engage in strenuous activity without first strengthening supporting muscles. LBP is often the result.
- **Psychological factors.** Numerous psychological factors appear to increase risk for LBP. Depression, apathy, inattentiveness, boredom, emotional upsets, drug abuse, and family and financial problems all heighten risk.
- **Occupational risk.** The type of work you do and the conditions you do it in greatly affect risk. For example, truck drivers, who must endure the bumps and jolts of the road while in a sitting position, frequently suffer from back pain.

# Are You at Risk for Chronic Illness?

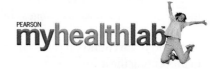

Certain characteristics place people at greater risk for chronic illness. Nevertheless, many people remain unaware of or ignore the symptoms of chronic illness until after the disease has progressed. Take the following quiz to help determine your risk for the chronic illnesses discussed in this chapter.

Fill out this assessment online at www.pearsonhighered.com/myhealthlab or www.pearsonhighered.com/donatelle.

## 1 Chronic Lung Disease

|  | Yes | No |
|---|---|---|
| 1. As part of your daily routine, are you exposed to environmental toxins, such as tobacco smoke, air pollution, asbestos, or silica dust? | ○ | ○ |
| 2. Do you smoke? | ○ | ○ |
| 3. Have you had cancer, infections, or degenerative changes that might impede lung function? | ○ | ○ |
| 4. Does your family have a history of lung disease? | ○ | ○ |

## 2 Musculoskeletal Diseases

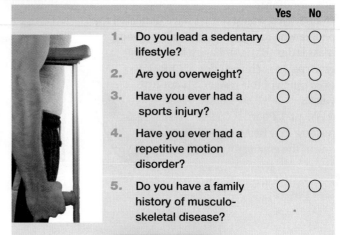

|  | Yes | No |
|---|---|---|
| 1. Do you lead a sedentary lifestyle? | ○ | ○ |
| 2. Are you overweight? | ○ | ○ |
| 3. Have you ever had a sports injury? | ○ | ○ |
| 4. Have you ever had a repetitive motion disorder? | ○ | ○ |
| 5. Do you have a family history of musculo-skeletal disease? | ○ | ○ |

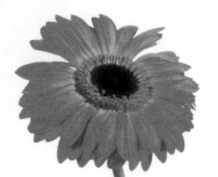

## 3 Headaches

|  | Yes | No |
|---|---|---|
| 1. Do you stress out about your "to do" list? | ○ | ○ |
| 2. Do you sometimes drink too much alcohol? | ○ | ○ |
| 3. Are you sleep-deprived? | ○ | ○ |
| 4. Do you lead a sedentary lifestyle? | ○ | ○ |
| 5. Do you ever fast? | ○ | ○ |
| 6. Does your family have a history of headaches? | ○ | ○ |

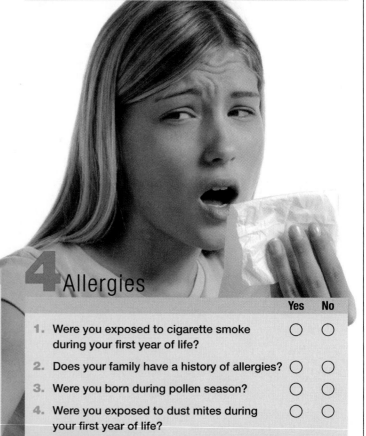

## 4 Allergies

|  | Yes | No |
|---|---|---|
| 1. Were you exposed to cigarette smoke during your first year of life? | ○ | ○ |
| 2. Does your family have a history of allergies? | ○ | ○ |
| 3. Were you born during pollen season? | ○ | ○ |
| 4. Were you exposed to dust mites during your first year of life? | ○ | ○ |

## 5 Digestion-Related Disorders

|  | Yes | No |
|---|---|---|
| 1. Do you smoke? | ○ | ○ |
| 2. Have you had measles or any other bacterial infection? | ○ | ○ |
| 3. Does your family have a history of digestion-related disorders? | ○ | ○ |

If you answered yes to any of these questions, you may be at risk for one or more of the chronic diseases discussed in this chapter. You probably should visit your health care provider to discuss ways you might avoid illness.

# YOUR PLAN FOR CHANGE

The **Assess yourself** activity asked you to evaluate whether you are at risk for a variety of chronic illnesses. Now that you have considered your results, you may need to take further steps to understand and address your risks.

### Today, you can:

○ Make an appointment with your doctor to find out more about any symptoms you've been having or to discuss your potential risk factors.

○ Call your parents and find out if they have ever had similar problems, or if they know of anyone in your family who has had these problems.

○ Weigh your full backpack and, if it's more than 10 percent of your body weight, unpack it and decide what you can leave at home.

### Within the next 2 weeks, you can:

○ Find out more about your family history of chronic illness, and what you can do to cut down your risk. Ask your parents what sorts of illnesses your family members have had, and use that information for your health. For example, if your parent has lung disease, find out ways to cut down on environmental exposure to smoke and other toxins yourself.

○ If you suffer from migraines, pay attention to what triggers them for you, and then work on creating a routine that keeps you out of harm's way.

○ If you suffer from heartburn, identify the foods or situations (such as sleeping postures) that bring it on. Make an effort to eliminate the problematic foods or positions.

### By the end of the semester, you can:

○ Make changes in your routine to avoid environmental toxins. Avoid going to parties where people smoke, for example.

○ Keep track of allergy-related symptoms to see if you can identify any likely triggers.

○ Replace all of your cleaning products for your house, apartment, or dorm room with less toxic ones made from vinegar, lemon juice, and other natural ingredients (see the Be Healthy, Be Green box on page 558 for tips on how to make these yourself). Find out how to safely dispose of the chemical-intensive products that you previously used.

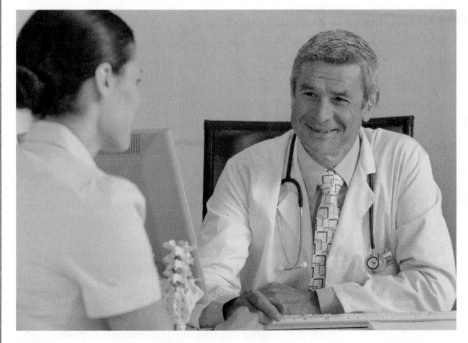

# Summary

* Chronic lung diseases include chronic bronchitis, emphysema, and asthma. Chronic obstructive pulmonary diseases (COPDs) are the fourth leading cause of death in the United States.
* Allergies occur as the immune system responds to allergens. They can be triggered by pollens, foods, or other substances.
* Neurological conditions include headaches and seizure disorders, such as epilepsy. The most common types of headache are tension and migraine.
* Inflammatory bowel disease includes ulcerative colitis and Crohn's disease. Irritable bowel syndrome, GERD, and other digestive problems affect increasing numbers of adults.
* Musculoskeletal diseases such as arthritis cause significant pain and disability in millions of people. Low back pain is common but usually preventable.

# Pop Quiz

1. Diseases and health conditions that appear to have no explanation or are of unknown cause are referred to as
   a. homeopathic.
   b. iatrogenic.
   c. idiopathic.
   d. psychotic.

2. Which of the following is NOT correct?
   a. Women have more migraine headaches; men have more cluster headaches.
   b. Inflammatory bowel diseases and irritable bowel syndrome are the same thing.
   c. An asthma attack can be fatal.
   d. Rheumatoid arthritis is also referred to as "wear and tear arthritis."

3. The gradual destruction of the alveoli in a smoker's lung usually causes

   which COPD characterized by difficulty in exhaling?
   a. Dyspnea
   b. Bronchitis
   c. Emphysema
   d. Asthma

4. School-aged children miss school for this condition more than any other illness.
   a. Bronchitis
   b. Common cold
   c. Attention-deficit disorder
   d. Asthma

5. Julie has found that she cannot eat nuts without suffering from itching and nausea. What condition is she likely to be suffering from?
   a. Irritable bowel syndrome
   b. Ulcerative colitis
   c. Food allergy
   d. Diabetes mellitus

6. Which of the following conditions is the leading cause of employee sick time and lost productivity in the United States?
   a. Low back pain
   b. Upper respiratory infections
   c. Asthma
   d. On-the-job injuries

7. If you experience an aura, a sensory warning sign that may include flickering vision or blind spots, you are likely to
   a. have an asthma attack.
   b. have a migraine headache.
   c. be suffering from an allergic reaction.
   d. be showing symptoms of glaucoma.

8. Margaret experiences attacks of wheezing, difficulty in breathing, shortness of breath, and coughing spasms on occasion. What chronic respiratory disorder is she likely suffering from?
   a. Sleep apnea
   b. Bronchitis
   c. Asthma
   d. COPD

9. Food allergies are
   a. immune responses to food.
   b. the same thing as food intolerance.
   c. sometimes confused with food-borne illnesses.
   d. not really allergies at all.

10. Which of the following is NOT correct?
    a. Asthma is an inflammatory disease in which airflow in and out of the lungs is compromised.
    b. Extrinsic asthma is usually triggered by emotional upset or anxiety.
    c. Acute bronchitis is often triggered by an infectious disease of the upper airways.
    d. Symptoms of chronic bronchitis last for at least 3 months of the year for 2 consecutive years.

*Answers to these questions can be found on page A-1.*

# Think about It!

1. What are some of the major non-infectious chronic diseases affecting Americans today? Do you think there is a pattern in the types of diseases that we get? What are the common risk factors?
2. List common respiratory diseases affecting Americans. Which of these has a genetic basis? An environmental basis? An individual basis?
3. Compare and contrast the different types of headaches.
4. Compare the symptoms of ulcerative colitis, gastroesophageal reflux disease, and Crohn's disease. How can you tell whether your stomach is reacting to final exams or telling you that you have a serious medical condition?
5. What is the difference between a food allergy and food intolerance?
6. What are the major disorders of the musculoskeletal system? Describe the difference between osteoarthritis and rheumatoid arthritis.

## Accessing Your Health on the Internet

The following websites explore further topics and issues related to personal health. For links to the websites below, visit the Companion Website for *Access to Health*, 12th Edition, at www.pearsonhighered.com/donatelle.

1. *American Academy of Allergy, Asthma, and Immunology.* This site provides an overview of asthma information, particularly as it applies to children with allergies. It also offers interactive quizzes to test your knowledge and an ask-the-expert section. www.aaaai.org

2. *American Lung Association.* This organization's site includes the latest news on asthma and lung disease. www.lungusa.org

3. *National Center for Chronic Disease Prevention and Health Promotion.* This site provides access to a wide range of information from this CDC-linked organization dedicated to chronic diseases and health promotion. www.cdc.gov/chronicdisease

4. *National Institute of Neurological Disorders and Stroke.* Many of the modern maladies result in chronic pain. This site provides up-to-date information to help individuals cope with pain-related difficulties. www.ninds.nih.gov

## References

1. American Lung Association, "Lung Disease," 2010, www.lungusa.org/lung-disease.
2. American Lung Association, "Chronic Obstructive Pulmonary Disease (COPD) Fact Sheet," 2010, www.lungusa.org/lung-disease/copd/resources/facts-figures/COPD-Fact-Sheet.html.
3. American Lung Association, "Chronic Obstructive Pulmonary Disease (COPD) Fact Sheet," 2010; S. J. Nolan, American Lung Association, *Statement of the American Lung Association on Fiscal Year 2010 Appropriations for the Veterans Affairs Medical Research Program, presented April 23, 2009 before the House Appropriations Subcommittee on Military Construction, Veterans Affairs, and Related Agencies,* 2009, Available at www.lungusa.org/get-involved/advocate/testimony.html.
4. National Center for Health Statistics, "FASTSTATS Chronic Obstructive Pulmonary Disease (COPD) Includes: Chronic Bronchitis and Emphysema," Updated January 2010, www.cdc.gov/nchs/fastats/copd.htm.
5. National Center for Health Statistics, "FASTSTATS Asthma," Updated May 2009, www.cdc.gov/nchs/fastats/asthma.htm; American Lung Association, "About Asthma," 2010, www.lungusa.org/lung-disease/asthma/about-asthma.
6. American Lung Association, "About Asthma," 2010.
7. Ibid.
8. Ibid.
9. Ibid.
10. Asthma and Allergy Foundation of America, "Allergy Overview," Accessed July 2010, www.aafa.org/display.cfm?id=9.
11. American Academy of Allergy, Asthma, and Immunology, "Allergy Statistics," 2010. www.aaaai.org/media/statistics/allergy-statistics.asp.
12. Ibid.
13. Ibid.
14. U.S. Food and Drug Administration, "Food Allergies; Reducing the Risks," January 2009, www.fda.gov/ForConsumers/ConsumerUpdates/ucm089307.htm.
15. National Institute of Neurological Disorders and Stroke "NINDS Overview," Updated February 2009, www.ninds.nih.gov/about_ninds/ninds_overview.htm.
16. National Headache Foundation, "Press Kits: Categories of Headache," 2010. www.headaches.org/press/NHF_Press_Kits/Press_Kits_-_Categories_of_Headache.
17. Mayo Clinic, "Tension Headache: Symptoms," February 2009, www.mayoclinic.com/health/tension-headache/ds00304/dsection=symptoms.
18. Mayo Clinic, "Migraine: Symptoms," June 2009, www.mayoclinic.com/health/migraine-headache/DS00120/DSECTION=symptoms.
19. National Headache Foundation, "The Complete Guide to Headache: Migraine," 2010, www.headaches.org/educational_modules/completeguide/migrindex.html.
20. Ibid.
21. Mayo Clinic, "Migraine: Risk Factors," June 2009, www.mayoclinic.com/health/migraine-headache/DS00120/DSECTION=risk%2Dfactors.
22. National Headache Foundation, "The Complete Guide to Headache: Migraine," 2010.
23. Ibid.
24. Epilepsy Foundation, "Epilepsy and Seizure Statistics," Accessed July 2010, www.epilepsyfoundation.org/about/statistics.cfm.
25. American College of Gastroenterology, "Common GI Problems, Volume 1," 2010, www.acg.gi.org/patients/cgp/cgpvol1.asp.
26. S. Kane, "Inflammatory Bowel Disease Defined," IBD Support Foundation, Accessed July 2010, www.ibdsf.com.
27. J. Markowitz et al., "Ulcerative Colitis," Updated September 2009, http://emedicine.medscape.com/article/930146-overview.
28. National Digestive Diseases Information Clearinghouse, "Crohn's Disease," NIH Publication no. 06–3410, February 2006, Available at www.digestive.niddk.nih.gov/ddiseases/pubs/crohns/index.htm.
29. J. Adler et al., "College Adjustment in University of Michigan Students with Crohn's and Colitis," *Inflammatory Bowel Diseases* 14, no. 9 (2008): 1281–86.
30. E. Roberts, "IBD and IBS Are Not the Same Thing." April 2009, www.healthcentral.com/ibd/c/2623/66985/ibd-ibs-thing.
31. U.S. Bone and Joint Decade, *The Burden of Musculoskeletal Diseases in the United States: Prevalence, Societal and Economic Costs* (Rosemont, IL: American Academy of Orthopaedic Surgeons, 2008), Available at www.boneandjointburden.org.
32. Ibid.
33. R. Shiri et al., "The Association between Obesity and Low Back Pain: A Meta-Analysis," *American Journal of Epidemiology,* 171, no. 2 (2010): 135–54.
34. Brigham and Women's Hospital, "Arthritis and Other Rheumatic Diseases Statistics," Modified March 2009, http://healthlibrary.brighamandwomens.org/RelatedItems/85,P00068; U.S. Bone and Joint Decade, *The Burden of Musculoskeletal Diseases in the United States,* 2008.
35. U.S. Bone and Joint Decade, *The Burden of Musculoskeletal Diseases in the United States,* 2008.
36. J. M. Hootman and C. G. Helmick, "Projections of U.S. Prevalence of Arthritis and Associated Activity Limitations," *Arthritis & Rheumatism* 54, no. 1 (2006): 226–29.
37. Arthritis Foundation, "Disease Center: Osteoarthritis: What Is It?" 2010, www.arthritis.org/disease-center.php?disease_id=32.
38. Ibid.
39. National Institute of Neurological Disorders and Stroke, "Low Back Pain Fact Sheet," NIH Publication no. 03-5161, Updated June 2010, www.ninds.nih.gov/disorders/backpain/detail_backpain.htm.
40. U.S. Bone and Joint Decade, *The Burden of Musculoskeletal Diseases in the United States,* 2008.

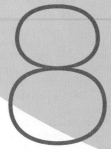

8

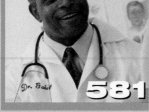

**581**

What questions should I ask my health care provider about proposed tests, treatments, or medications?

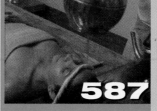

**587**

Why are so many people using alternative medicine?

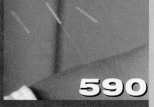

**590**

How does acupuncture work?

# Choosing Conventional and Complementary Health Care

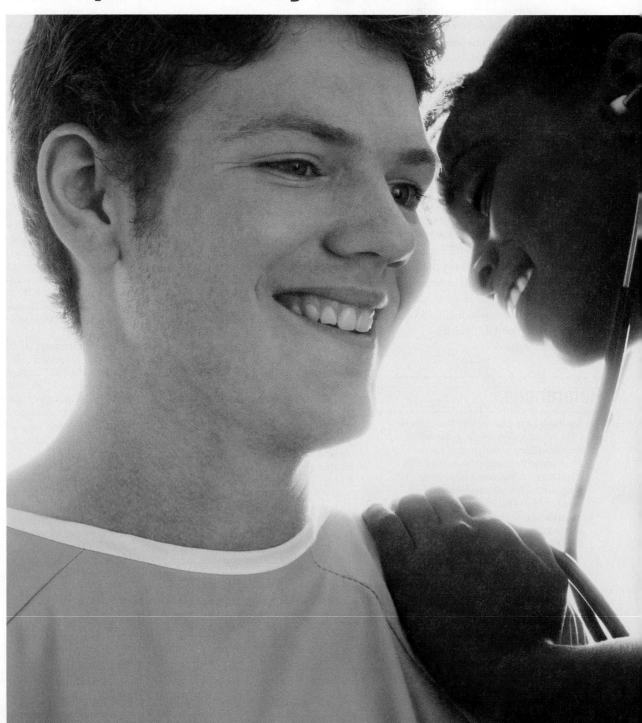

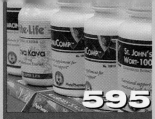

**Do herbal remedies have any risks or side effects?**

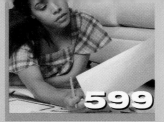

**What should I consider when choosing health insurance?**

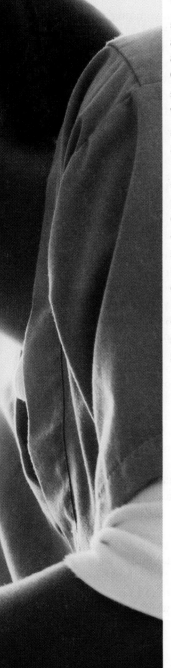

## Objectives

✳ Explain why it is important to be a responsible health care consumer and how to encourage health care consumers to take action.

✳ Understand what factors to consider when making health care decisions.

✳ Describe and discuss conventional and complementary and alternative health care.

✳ Discuss types of health care products and treatments available in conventional and complementary care, and their potential benefits and risks.

✳ Describe the U.S. health care system in terms of types of insurance; the changing structure of the system; and issues concerning cost, quality, and access to services.

✳ Discuss issues facing our health care system today.

Have there been times when you wondered whether you were sick enough to go to your campus health clinic? Have you left visits with your health care provider feeling that the doctor didn't give you a thorough exam or that you had more questions than you did when you arrived? Do you engage in risky behaviors, such as riding your bike without a helmet, and don't know where or how you would be treated if you were injured? Are you one of the 20 percent of college students without health insurance? Have you ever had to help a family member or loved one make health care decisions? If the answer to any of these questions is yes, then you will find the information in this chapter valuable in helping you become a better health care consumer.

There are many reasons for you to learn to make better decisions about your health and health care. Most important, you have only one body—if you don't treat it with care, you will pay a major price in terms of monetary costs and consequences to your health. Doing everything you can to stay healthy and to recover rapidly when you do get sick will enhance every other part of your life. Throughout this book we have emphasized the importance of healthy preventive behaviors. Learning how to navigate the health care system is an important part of taking charge of your health.

# Taking Responsibility for Your Health Care

As the health care industry has become more sophisticated in seeking your business, so must you become more sophisticated in purchasing its products and services. Acting responsibly in times of illness can be difficult, but the person best able to act on your behalf is you.

If you are not feeling well, you must first decide whether you really need to seek medical advice. Not seeking treatment, whether because of high costs or limited coverage, or trying to medicate yourself when more rigorous methods of treatment are needed, is potentially dangerous. Being knowledgeable about the benefits and limits of self-care is critical for responsible consumerism.

## Self-Care

Individuals can practice behaviors that promote health, prevent disease, and minimize reliance on the formal medical system. We can also treat minor afflictions without seeking professional help. Self-care consists of knowing your body, paying attention to its signals, and taking appropriate action to stop the progression of illness or injury. Common forms of self-care include the following:

● Diagnosing symptoms or conditions that occur frequently but may not require physician visits (e.g., the common cold, minor abrasions)
● Using over-the-counter remedies to treat minor, infrequent pains, scrapes, or cold or allergy symptoms

- Performing monthly breast or testicular self-examinations
- Learning first aid for common, uncomplicated injuries and conditions
- Checking blood pressure, pulse, and temperature
- Using home pregnancy tests and ovulation kits
- Using home HIV test kits
- Doing periodic checks for blood cholesterol level
- Learning from reliable self-help books, websites, and DVDs
- Benefiting from meditation and other relaxation techniques and nutrition, rest, and exercise

Be aware that there are many times that people use self-care methods inappropriately. Taking prescription drugs used for a previous illness to treat your current illness, using unproven self-treatment, or using other people's medications are examples of inappropriate self-care. Using self-care methods appropriately takes education and effort.

## When to Seek Help

With the vast array of home diagnostic devices available, it seems relatively easy for most people to take care of themselves. But some caution is in order here: Although many of these devices are valuable for making an initial diagnosis, home health tests are not substitutes for regular, complete examinations by a trained practitioner. Effective self-care also means paying attention to your own body's warning signs and understanding when to seek medical attention rather than treating a condition yourself. Deciding which conditions warrant professional advice is not always easy. Generally, you should consult a physician if you experience *any* of the following:

- A serious accident or injury
- Sudden or severe chest pains, especially if they cause breathing difficulties

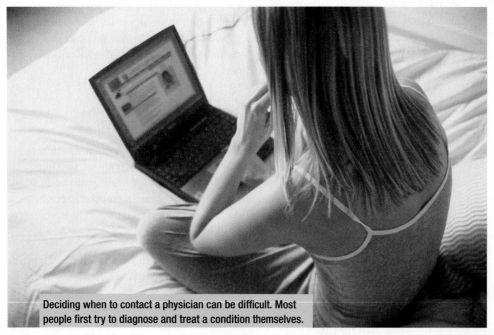

Deciding when to contact a physician can be difficult. Most people first try to diagnose and treat a condition themselves.

# 35 million

**Americans are admitted to the hospital each year.**

- Trauma to the head or spine accompanied by persistent headache, blurred vision, loss of consciousness, vomiting, convulsions, or paralysis
- Sudden high fever or recurring high temperature (over 102°F for children and 103°F for adults) and/or sweats
- Tingling sensation in the arm accompanied by slurred speech or impaired thought processes
- Adverse reactions to a drug or insect bite (shortness of breath, severe swelling, dizziness)
- Unexplained bleeding or loss of body fluid from any body opening
- Unexplained sudden weight loss
- Persistent or recurrent diarrhea or vomiting
- Blue-colored lips, eyelids, or nail beds
- Any lump, swelling, thickness, or sore that does not subside or that grows for over a month
- Any marked change or pain in bowel or bladder habits
- Yellowing of the skin or the whites of the eyes
- Any symptom that is unusual and recurs over time
- Pregnancy

See the **Skills for Behavior Change** box on the next page for information on taking an active role in your own health care.

## Assessing Health Professionals

Suppose you decide that you do need medical help. You must then identify what type of help you need and where to obtain it. Selecting a professional may seem simple, yet many people have no idea how to assess the qualifications of a health care provider.[1]

Numerous studies document the importance of good communication skills: The most satisfied patients are those who feel their health care provider explains diagnosis and treatment options thoroughly and involves them in decisions regarding their own care.

When evaluating a health care provider, consider the following questions:

- Do they listen to you, respect you as an individual, and give you time to ask questions? Do they return your calls, and are they available to answer questions between visits?

## Be Proactive in Your Health Care

Here are some tips for getting the most out of doctor visits and being proactive in your health care.

✳ Keep records of your own and your family's medical histories.

✳ Research your condition—causes, physiological effects, possible treatments, and prognosis. Don't rely on the health care provider for this information.

✳ If you use a CAM therapy such as acupuncture, choose the practitioner with care. Check with your insurer to see if the services will be covered.

✳ Bring a friend or relative along for medical visits to help you review what the doctor says. If you go alone, take notes. Write down what happened and what was said.

✳ Ask the practitioner to explain the problem and possible treatments, tests, and drugs in a clear and understandable way. If you don't understand something, ask for clarification.

✳ If the health care provider prescribes any medications, ask whether you can take generic equivalents that cost less.

✳ Ask for a written summary of the results of your visit and any lab tests.

✳ Find out what studies have been done on the safety and effectiveness of any treatment in which you are interested. Consult only reliable sources—texts, journals, and government resources. Start with the websites listed at the end of this and every chapter.

✳ If you have any doubt about the health care provider's recommended treatment, get a second opinion.

✳ Decisions regarding treatment should be made in consultation with your health care provider and based on your condition and needs. If you use any CAM therapy, inform your primary health care provider. It is particularly important to talk with your provider if you are thinking about replacing your prescribed treatment with one or more supplements, are currently taking a prescription drug, have a chronic medical condition, are planning to have surgery, are pregnant or nursing, or are thinking about giving supplements to children.

✳ When filling prescriptions, ask the pharmacist to show you the package inserts that list medical considerations. Request detailed information about potential drug and food interactions.

✳ Remember that *natural* and *safe* are not necessarily the same. You can become seriously ill from seemingly harmless "natural" products. Be cautious about combining herbal medications, just as you should be cautious about combining other drugs. Seek help if you notice any unusual side effects.

● What professional education and training have they had? What license or board certification(s) do they hold? Note that there is a difference between "board certified" and "board eligible" physicians. *Board certified* indicates that the physician has passed the national board examination for his or her specialty (e.g., pediatrics) and has been certified as competent in that specialty. In contrast, *board eligible* merely means that the physician is eligible to take the specialty board's exam, but not necessarily that he or she has passed it.

● Are they affiliated with an accredited medical facility or institution? The Joint Commission is an independent non-profit organization that evaluates and accredits more than 15,000 health care organizations and programs in the United States. Accreditation requires that these institutions verify all education, licensing, and training claims of their affiliated practitioners.

● Are they open to complementary or alternative strategies? Would they refer you for different treatments if appropriate?

● Do they indicate clearly how long a given treatment may last, what side effects you might expect, and what problems you should watch for?

● Who will be responsible for your care when your physician is on vacation or off call?

● Are there professional reviews and information on any lawsuits against them available online?

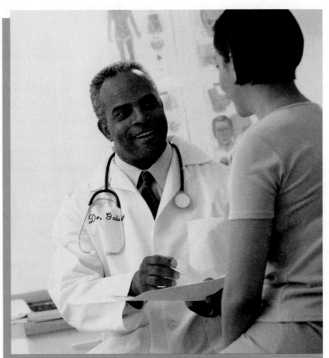

**What questions should I ask my health care provider about proposed tests, treatments, or medications?**

It's important to understand recommendations that your health care provider makes. Questions to ask include how often the practitioner has performed a procedure, the proportion of successful outcomes for the treatment or procedure, any side effects and whether they can be treated or reduced, whether a hospital stay will be required, and why a test has been ordered.

# 91%

of U.S. physicians admitted that they sometimes order unnecessary medical tests because they are concerned about being sued for malpractice.

Questions to ask yourself about the quality of care you are receiving include the following:

- Did your health care provider take a thorough health history and ask for any recent updates to your health history? Was your examination thorough?
- Did your health care provider listen to you?
- Did you feel comfortable asking questions? Did your health care provider answer thoroughly, in a way that was easy to understand? Did he or she admit to not knowing an answer to your question when appropriate?
- Would you feel comfortable seeing the health care provider again?

Asking the right questions at the right time may save you personal suffering and expense. Many patients find that writing their questions down before an appointment helps them get all the answers they need. You don't need to accept a defensive or hostile response; asking questions is your right as a patient.

Active participation in your treatment is the only sensible course in a health care environment that encourages **defensive medicine,** or the use of medical practices designed to avert the possibility of malpractice suits in the future.[2] It is estimated that between $250 and $325 billion per year are spent on medical tests and procedures that do not improve health outcomes. Unwarranted treatment such as the overuse of antibiotics and use of diagnostic laboratory tests to protect against malpractice exposure are two significant factors driving up the cost of medicine.[3] Unnecessary drugs and procedures are unlikely to improve health outcomes and may create new health problems.

In addition to asking the suggested questions above, being proactive in your health care also means that you should be aware of your rights as a patient, as follows:[4]

**1.** The right of informed consent means that before receiving any care, you should be fully informed of what is being planned; the risks and potential benefits; and possible alternative forms of treatment, including the option to refuse treatment. Your consent must be voluntary and without any form of coercion. It is critical that you read any consent forms carefully and amend them as necessary before signing.

**defensive medicine** The use of medical practices designed to avert the possibility of malpractice suits in the future.

**allopathic medicine** Conventional, Western medical practice; in theory, based on scientifically validated methods and procedures.

**evidence-based practice** Decisions regarding patient care based on clinical expertise, patient values, and current best scientific evidence.

**2.** You are entitled to know whether the treatment you are receiving is standard or experimental. In experimental conditions, you have the legal and ethical right to know if any drug is being used in the research project for a purpose not approved by the Food and Drug Administration (FDA), and whether the study is one in which some people receive treatment while others receive a placebo. (See the **Student Health Today** box for more on placebos and the placebo effect.)

**3.** You have the right to privacy, which includes the source of payment for treatment and care. It also includes protecting your right to make personal decisions concerning all reproductive matters.

**4.** You have the right to receive care. You also have the legal right to refuse treatment at any time and to cease treatment at any time.

**5.** You are entitled to have access to all of your medical records and to have those records remain confidential.

**6.** You have the right to seek the opinions of other health care professionals regarding your condition.

# Conventional Health Care

Conventional health care, also called **allopathic medicine,** mainstream medicine, or traditional Western medical practice, is the dominant type of health care delivered in the United States, Canada, Europe, and much of the developed world. Among U.S. health care providers, the majority currently receives conventional medical training and treats patients using conventional medicine. Allopathic medicine is based on the premise that illness is a result of exposure to pathogens, such as bacteria and viruses, or organic changes in the body. The prevention of disease and the restoration of health involve vaccines, drugs, surgery, and other treatments.

Be aware, however, that not all allopathic treatments have had the benefit of the extensive clinical trials and long-term studies of outcomes that would be necessary to conclusively prove effectiveness in different populations. Even when studies appear to support the health benefits of a particular treatment or product, other studies with equal or better scientific validity often refute these claims. Also, today's recommended treatment may change dramatically in the future as new technologies and medical advances replace older practices. Like other professionals, medical doctors are only as good as their training, continued acquisition of knowledge, and resources.

Health care providers strive to ensure the quality of care they provide to their patients, and one of the ways they do this is by using **evidence-based medicine.** Decisions

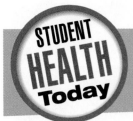

# THE PLACEBO EFFECT: MIND OVER MATTER?

The *placebo effect* is an apparent cure or improved state of health brought about by a substance, product, or procedure that has no generally recognized therapeutic value. Patients often report improvements in a condition based on what they expect, desire, or were told would happen after receiving a treatment, even though the treatment was, for example, simple sugar pills instead of powerful drugs.

Researchers are investigating how and why placebos work on some people. One theory is that expecting a positive outcome activates the same natural pathways in the brain as some medications do. One study involved patients with Parkinson's disease. The patients who thought that they were receiving the real treatment but actually received a placebo had the same changes in their brains on positron-emission tomography (PET) scans as those who received the medication. Similar chemical changes on brain imaging tests were seen with placebos in studies of pain and depression.

In a recent trial, a sample of alcohol-dependent patients received either the drugs naltrexone or acamprosate, or a placebo for a period of 12 weeks. They were also asked whether they thought they were receiving an active medication or a placebo. Those who believed they had been taking medication consumed fewer alcoholic drinks and reported less alcohol dependence and cravings, regardless of whether they really were receiving the drug.

Placebos are also used in clinical research studies. Patients with a particular condition are given either the treatment that is being tested or a placebo. If the patients receiving the treatment have a more beneficial outcome than the patients receiving the placebo, then the treatment can be considered effective. The patients and the doctors running the study are not told until the study ends who had the real treatment and who had the placebo.

People who mistakenly use placebos when medical treatment is needed increase their risk for health problems.

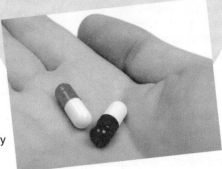

Is it a real medicine or a placebo? In some cases, it may not make a difference.

However, what we learn from the ways in which placebos work may someday help us harness the mind's power to treat certain diseases and conditions.

**Sources:** J. Friedman and R. Dubinsky, "The Placebo Effect," *Neurology* 71, no. 9 (2008): e25–e26; R. de la Fuente-Fernandez et al., "Expectation and Dopamine Release: Mechanism of the Placebo Effect in Parkinson's Disease," *Science* 293 (2001): 1164–66; N. Diedrich and C. Goetz, "The Placebo Treatments in Neurosciences: New Insights from Clinical and Neuroimaging Studies," *Neurology* 71 (2008): 677–84.

---

regarding patient care are based on clinical expertise, patient values, and current best scientific evidence. Clinical expertise refers to the clinician's cumulative experience, education, and clinical skills. The patient brings his or her own personal and unique concerns, expectations, and values. The best evidence is usually found in clinically relevant research that has been conducted using sound methodology.

## Conventional Health Care Practitioners

Selecting a **primary care practitioner (PCP)**—a medical practitioner whom you can visit for routine ailments, preventive care, general medical advice, and appropriate referrals—is not an easy task. The PCP for most people is a family practitioner, an internist, a pediatrician, or an obstetrician-gynecologist (ob-gyn). Many people routinely see nurse practitioners or physician assistants who work for an individual doctor or a medical group, and others use nontraditional providers as their primary source of care. As a college student, you may opt to visit a PCP at your campus health cen-

ter. The reputation of health care providers on college campuses is excellent. In national surveys, students have indicated that the health center medical staff is their most trusted source of health information.[5]

Doctors undergo rigorous training before they can begin practicing. After 4 years of undergraduate work, students typically spend 4 years studying for their medical degree (MD). After this general training, some students choose a specialty, such as pediatrics, cardiology, cancer, radiology, or surgery, and spend 1 year in an internship and several years doing a residency. Some doctors receive additional training in order to specialize in certain elective surgeries (see the **Consumer Health** box on page 584). Some specialties also require a fellowship; in all, the time spent in additional training after receiving an MD can be up to 8 years.

Specialists include **osteopaths,** general practitioners who receive training similar to that of a medical doctor but

**primary care practitioner (PCP)** A medical practitioner who treats routine ailments, advises on preventive care, gives general medical advice, and makes appropriate referrals when necessary.

**osteopath** General practitioner who receives training similar to a medical doctor's but with an emphasis on the skeletal and muscular systems; often uses spinal manipulation as part of treatment.

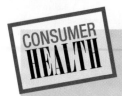
# Choosing Surgery: Elective Procedures

The National Center for Health Statistics states that over 40 million elective medical procedures—surgeries and treatments that are planned, nonemergency procedures—are performed every year, and that number seems to be growing. Although not considered medically necessary, many types of elective procedures enhance people's lives and benefit them in terms of raising their self-esteem. Some procedures, such as gastric bypass (discussed in Chapter 8), can improve the functional quality of life and reduce risks for chronic diseases, even though they are technically an "optional" or elective procedure and carry their own set of risks for patients.

If a procedure is considered not medically necessary, it may not be covered by insurance. In some cases, insurance companies may require a second opinion before approving payment on elective surgical procedures. If you are considering elective surgery, review your coverage requirements with your health insurance carrier before scheduling the procedure.

An elective surgical procedure is typically performed by a surgeon or qualified physician in either an inpatient, hospital environment or an outpatient, ambulatory center. Some simple, minimally invasive procedures may be performed in a doctor's office. The type of surgery will mandate the qualifications and background of the surgeon or physician who performs it. The following are some of the elective surgeries that some people opt to have performed.

## LASIK

Surgery to correct vision has been performed on millions of Americans to reduce their dependence on contact lenses or glasses. The most commonly used technique is called Lasik (laser-assisted in situ keratomileusis); a surgeon uses a razorlike instrument or laser to cut a flap in the cornea, the clear covering on the front of the eye, and then reshapes the exposed area using a laser. The surgery alters the way the eye focuses light, correcting nearsightedness, farsightedness, and some astigmatism. However, Lasik is not effective at treating close-up vision problems in middle-aged adults.

The procedure is an ambulatory procedure, meaning that you walk into the surgery center and walk out again. The actual surgery usually takes less than 5 minutes and you are awake the entire time. Numbing eye drops make the treatment painless, although there can be some burning and itchiness for up to a couple of hours after surgery. Postoperative complications can include infection or night glare—starbursts or halos that appear when you are viewing lights at night.

Lasik surgery costs about $2,150. Prices for Lasik have decreased over the years, but consumers should be cautious of "bargain" prices, as some surgery centers have cut corners to cut prices. By hiring inexperienced surgeons or using optometrists or technicians rather than MDs for postoperative checkups, surgery centers are able to reduce cost, but compromise patient care. Ideally the surgeon should be the one doing your pre- and post-op checkups.

## COSMETIC SURGERY

Approximately 1.5 million cosmetic surgeries are performed every year. Cosmetic surgery is performed to reshape normal structures of the body in order to improve the patient's appearance and thus their self-esteem.

The most common cosmetic surgery is breast augmentation, the surgical placement of an implant behind each breast to increase breast volume and enhance shape. Currently, all women undergoing breast augmentation receive implants that consist of a silicone shell filled with sterile saltwater. Considerations include changes in breast or nipple sensation and scarring, and difficulty in performing and reading mammograms.

Liposuction—the removal of fatty tissue with a vacuum-like device—is another common cosmetic surgery. This procedure can slim hips and thighs, flatten the abdomen, shape calves and ankles, or eliminate double chins. Liposuction works well on people of relatively normal weight who have pockets of fat. Although liposuction can be performed on people of almost any age, it works best on those whose skin is still elastic enough to achieve a smooth contour following removal of fat. Fat is removed by inserting a small, hollow *cannula,* or tube, through one or more tiny incisions near the area to be suctioned. The cannula is attached to a vacuum, which essentially sucks out the unwanted fat.

Risks and complications include infection, numbness, bleeding, and poor healing. Healing is gradual and may include fluid retention and swelling following surgery, so the desired appearance may be delayed. Liposuction is not a substitute for overall weight loss.

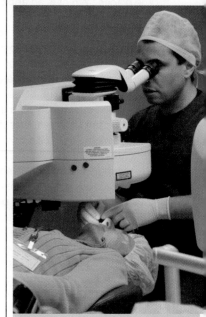

If you have imperfect vision and want to ditch your glasses or contact lenses for good, you may want to consider Lasik laser eye surgery.

**Sources:** U.S. Food and Drug Administration, "LASIK," 2009, www.fda.gov/MedicalDevices/ProductsandMedicalProcedures/SurgeryandLifeSupport/LASIK/default.htm; American Society for Aesthetic Plastic Surgery, "Quick Facts," 2010, www.surgery.org/media/statistics; American Society of Plastic Surgeons, "Plastic Surgery Information for Patients and Consumers," 2010, www.plasticsurgery.org/Patients_and_Consumers.html.

who place special emphasis on the skeletal and muscular systems. Their treatments may involve manipulation of the muscles and joints. Osteopaths receive the degree of doctor of osteopathy (DO) rather than MD.

Eye care specialists can be either ophthalmologists or optometrists. An **ophthalmologist** holds a medical degree and can perform surgery and prescribe medications. An **optometrist** typically evaluates visual problems and fits glasses but is not a trained physician. If you have an eye infection, glaucoma, or other eye condition needing diagnosis and treatment, you need to see an ophthalmologist.

**Dentists** are specialists who diagnose and treat diseases of the teeth, gums, and oral cavity. They attend dental school for 4 years and receive the title of doctor of dental surgery (DDS) or doctor of medical dentistry (DMD). They must also pass both state and national board examinations before receiving their licenses to practice. The field of dentistry includes many specialties. For example, *orthodontists* specialize in the alignment of teeth. *Oral surgeons* perform surgical procedures to correct problems of the mouth, face, and jaw.

**Nurses** are highly trained and strictly regulated health professionals who provide a wide range of services for patients and their families, including patient education, counseling, community health and disease prevention information, and administration of medications. They may choose from several training options. Registered nurses (RNs) in the United States complete either a 4-year program leading to a bachelor of science in nursing (BSN) degree or a 2-year associate degree program. Lower-level licensed practical or vocational nurses (LPN or LVN) complete a 1- to 2-year training program, which may be based in either a community college or a hospital.

**Nurse practitioners (NPs)** are nurses with advanced training obtained through either a master's degree program or a specialized nurse practitioner program. Nurse practitioners have the training and authority to conduct diagnostic tests and prescribe medications (in some states). They work in a variety of settings, particularly in HMOs (health maintenance organizations), clinics, and student health centers. Nurses and nurse practitioners may also earn the clinical doctor of nursing degree (ND), doctor of nursing science (DNS and DNSc degrees), or a research-based PhD in nursing.

**Physician assistants (PAs)** are licensed to examine and diagnose patients, offer treatment, and write prescriptions under a physician's supervision. An important difference between a PA and an NP is that the PA must practice under a physician's supervision. Like other health care providers, PAs are licensed by state boards of medicine.

# Complementary and Alternative Medicine (CAM)

Although the terms *complementary* and *alternative* are often used interchangeably when referring to therapies, there is a distinction between them. **Complementary medicine** is used *together with* conventional medicine, as part of the modern integrative-medicine approach.[6] An example of complementary medicine is to use massage therapy along with prescription medicine to treat anxiety. **Alternative medicine** has traditionally been used *in place of* conventional medicine, such as following a special diet or herbal remedy to treat cancer instead of using radiation, surgery, or other conventional treatments. A survey conducted by the National Center for Complementary and Alternative Medicine (NCCAM; part of the National Institutes of Health) and the National Center of Health Statistics (NCHS; part of the Centers for Disease Control and Prevention) revealed that 38 percent of adults use some form of CAM.[7] **Figure 18.1** on page 586 shows more results from this study.

The list of practices that are considered CAM changes continually as therapies become accepted as mainstream. In general, CAM therapies serve as alternatives to the conventional Western system of medicine, which some people regard as too invasive, too high-tech, and too toxic in terms of laboratory-produced medications. Complementary and alternative medical therapies incorporate a **holistic** approach to medicine that focuses on treating the mind and the whole body, rather than just an isolated part of the body. Often CAM users seek what they perceive as a more natural, gentle approach to healing. Other CAM patients distrust the traditional medical approach and believe that alternative practices will give them greater control over their own health care. CAM therapies can vary based on whether they have been scientifically studied and whether those studies have shown them to be beneficial. Research has shown that many types of CAM, including acupuncture and massage therapy, are beneficial in treating conditions such as chronic back pain and cancer.[8]

As the NCCAM/NCHS survey indicates, more than one-third of adults in the United States have used CAM. Why do so many people seek alternative therapy? Distinct patterns of CAM use emerge from this survey.[9] The following groups are likely to use or have used CAM:

- More women than men
- People with higher educational levels

## 36%
of 18- to 29-year-olds report having used some form of CAM.

**ophthalmologist** Physician who specializes in the medical and surgical care of the eyes, including prescriptions for glasses.

**optometrist** Eye specialist whose practice is limited to prescribing and fitting lenses.

**dentist** Specialist who diagnoses and treats diseases of the teeth, gums, and oral cavity.

**nurse** Health professional who provides many services for patients and who may work in a variety of settings.

**nurse practitioner (NP)** Professional nurse with advanced training obtained through either a master's degree program or a specialized nurse practitioner program.

**physician assistant (PA)** A midlevel practitioner trained to handle most standard cases of care under the supervision of a physician.

**complementary medicine** Treatment used in conjunction with conventional medicine.

**alternative medicine** Treatment used in place of conventional medicine.

**holistic** Relating to or concerned with the whole body and the interactions of systems, rather than treatment of individual parts.

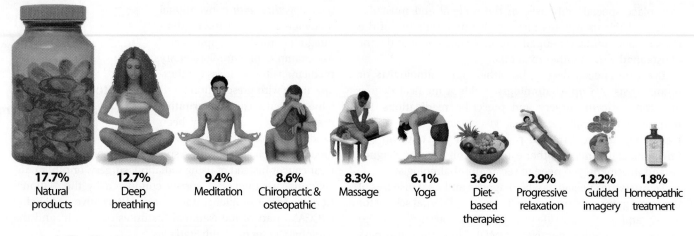

| 17.7% | 12.7% | 9.4% | 8.6% | 8.3% | 6.1% | 3.6% | 2.9% | 2.2% | 1.8% |
|---|---|---|---|---|---|---|---|---|---|
| Natural products | Deep breathing | Meditation | Chiropractic & osteopathic | Massage | Yoga | Diet-based therapies | Progressive relaxation | Guided imagery | Homeopathic treatment |

**FIGURE** 18.1 **The 10 Most Common CAM Therapies Among U.S. Adults**

**Source:** Data are from P. M. Barnes, B. Bloom, and R. Nahin, "Complementary and Alternative Medicine Use among Adults and Children: United States, 2007," *CDC National Health Statistics Report*, no. 12 (December 2008).

- People who have been hospitalized in the past year
- Former smokers (compared with current smokers or those who have never smoked)
- People with back, neck, head, or joint aches or other painful conditions
- People with gastrointestinal disorders or sleeping problems

Figure 18.2 summarizes the conditions for which respondents to the NCCAM/NCHS survey used CAM.

As with traditional Western medicine, practitioners of most complementary and alternative therapies spend years learning their practice. Various forms of CAM are increasingly being taught in U.S. medical schools and are available to patients in some clinics and hospitals. Some, such as acupuncture, are even covered under many health insurance policies. However, it is important to note that complementary and alternative therapies vary widely in terms of the nature of treatment, extent of therapy, and types of problems for which they offer help. There is no national training or licensure standard, and states differ in their practices (this is also true for conventional medicine). Whereas practitioners of conventional medicine have graduated from U.S.-sanctioned schools of medicine or are licensed medical practitioners recognized by the American Medical Association (AMA)—the governing body for all physicians—each CAM domain has a different set of training standards, guidelines for practice, and licensure procedures.

## Alternative Medical Systems

**Alternative (whole) medical systems** are built on specific systems of theory and practice. There are many alternative systems of medicine that have been practiced by various cultures throughout the world. Some have evolved from centuries-old prac-

**alternative (whole) medical systems** Complete systems of theory and practice that involve several CAM domains.

tices, such as traditional Chinese medicine and Ayurveda, which are at the root of much of our CAM thinking today. Other alternative medical systems include homeopathy and naturopathy.

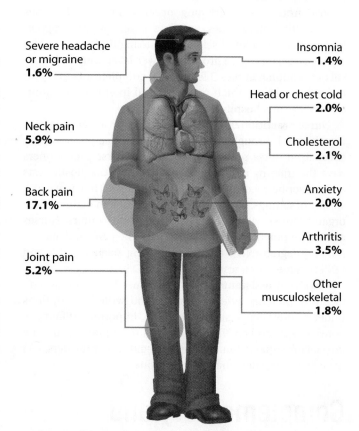

Severe headache or migraine **1.6%**

Insomnia **1.4%**

Head or chest cold **2.0%**

Neck pain **5.9%**

Cholesterol **2.1%**

Back pain **17.1%**

Anxiety **2.0%**

Arthritis **3.5%**

Joint pain **5.2%**

Other musculoskeletal **1.8%**

**FIGURE** 18.2 **Diseases and Conditions for Which CAM is Most Frequently Used Among Adults, 2007**

**Source:** Data are from P. M. Barnes, B. Bloom, and R. Nahin, "Complementary and Alternative Medicine Use among Adults and Children: United States, 2007," *CDC National Health Statistics Report*, no. 12 (December 2008).

**Traditional Chinese Medicine** Traditional Chinese medicine (TCM) emphasizes the proper balance or disturbances of *qi* (pronounced "chee"), or vital energy, in health and disease, respectively. Diagnosis is based on personal history, observation of the body (especially the tongue), palpation, and pulse diagnosis, an elaborate procedure requiring considerable skill and experience by the practitioner. Techniques such as acupuncture, herbal medicine, massage, and *qigong* (a form of energy therapy) are among the TCM approaches to health and healing.

Traditional Chinese medicine practitioners within the United States must complete a graduate program at a college or university approved by the Accreditation Commission for Acupuncture and Oriental Medicine (ACAOM). Graduate programs vary based on the specific area of concentration within TCM but usually involve an extensive 3- or 4-year clinical internship. In addition, an examination by the National Commission for the Certification of Acupuncture and Oriental Medicine, a standard for licensing in the United States, must be completed. Specific practices incorporated in TCM are discussed later in the chapter under the different CAM domains.

**Ayurveda** Ayurveda (Ayurvedic medicine) relates to the "science of life," an alternative medical system that began and evolved over thousands of years in India. Ayurveda seeks to integrate and balance the body, mind, and spirit and to restore harmony in the individual.[10] Ayurvedic practitioners use various techniques, including questioning, observing, touching patients, and classifying patients into one of three body types, or *doshas*, before establishing a treatment plan. The goals of Ayurvedic treatment are to eliminate impurities in the body and reduce symptoms. Dietary modification and herbal remedies drawn from the botanical wealth of the Indian subcontinent are common. Treatments may also include animal and mineral ingredients, powdered gemstones, yoga, stretching, meditation, massage, steam baths, exposure to the sun, and controlled breathing.

Training of Ayurvedic practitioners varies. There is no national standard for certifying or training Ayurvedic practitioners, although professional groups are working toward creating licensing guidelines.

**Homeopathy** Homeopathic medicine is an unconventional Western system based on the principle that "like cures like." In other words, the same substance that in large doses produces the symptoms of an illness will in very small doses cure the illness. It was developed in the late 1700s by Samuel Hahnemann, a German physician, as an approach to medicine that was not as harsh as other treatments of the time, such as bloodletting and blistering.[11] Homeopathic physicians use herbal medicine, minerals, and chemicals in extremely diluted forms to kill infectious agents or ward off illnesses that are caused by more potent forms or doses of those substances.

Homeopathic training varies considerably and is offered through diploma programs, certificate programs, short courses, and correspondence courses. Laws that detail requirements to practice vary from state to state.

**Naturopathy** Naturopathic medicine views disease as a manifestation of an alteration in the processes by which the body naturally heals itself. Disease results from the body's effort to ward off impurities and harmful substances from the environment. Naturopathic physicians emphasize restoring health rather than curing disease. They employ an array of

---

**traditional Chinese medicine (TCM)** Ancient comprehensive system of healing that uses herbs, acupuncture, and massage to bring the body into balance and to remove blockages of vital energy flow that lead to disease.

***qi*** Element of traditional Chinese medicine that refers to the vital energy force that courses through the body; when *qi* is in balance, health is restored.

**Ayurveda (Ayurvedic medicine)** A comprehensive system of medicine, derived largely from ancient India, that places equal emphasis on the body, mind, and spirit, and strives to restore the body's innate harmony through diet, exercise, meditation, herbs, massage, exposure to sunlight, and controlled breathing.

**homeopathic medicine** Unconventional Western system of medicine based on the principle that "like cures like."

**naturopathic medicine** System of medicine originating from Europe that views disease as a manifestation of alterations in the body's natural self-healing processes, and that emphasizes health restoration as well as disease treatment.

---

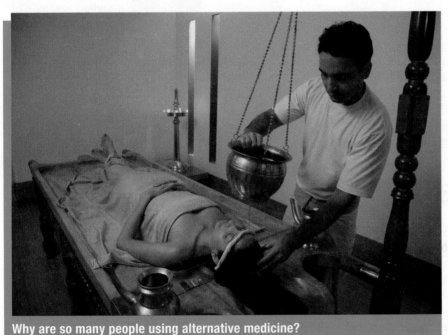

**Why are so many people using alternative medicine?**

People use alternative medicine for multiple reasons, and many treatments can benefit a variety of physical and mental ailments. For example, *shirodhara*—a traditional Ayurvedic treatment in which warm herbalized oil is poured over the forehead in guided rhythmic patterns—is said to relieve stress and anxiety, treat insomnia and chronic headaches, and improve memory.

healing practices, including diet and clinical nutrition; home-opathy; acupuncture; herbal medicine; hydrotherapy (the use of water in a range of temperatures and methods of application); spinal and soft-tissue manipulation; physical therapies involving electric currents, ultrasound, and light therapy; therapeutic counseling; and pharmacology.

Several major naturopathic schools in the United States and Canada provide training, conferring the *naturopathic doctor* (*ND*) degree on students who have completed a 4-year graduate program that emphasizes humanistically oriented family medicine.

**Other Alternative Medical Systems** Native American, Aboriginal, African, Middle Eastern, and South American cultures also have their own unique alternative systems. As the number of alternative therapists grows and systems become intertwined, so do the number of options available to consumers. Before considering any treatments, wise consumers will consult the most reliable resources to thoroughly evaluate risks, the scientific basis of claimed benefits, and any contraindications to using the CAM product or service. Avoid practitioners who promote their treatments as a cure-all for every health problem or who seem to promise remedies for ailments that have thus far defied the best scientific efforts of mainstream medicine. In short, apply the same strategies to researching CAM as you would to choosing allopathic care.

# Major Domains of Complementary and Alternative Medicine

The U.S. government has created the National Center for Complementary and Alternative Medicine (NCCAM) within the National Institutes of Health (NIH) to provide a mechanism for reliable information about CAM practices. The NCCAM serves as a clearinghouse for CAM information and a focal point for research initiatives, policy development, and general recommendations. It has grouped the many varieties of CAM into four domains of practice (Figure 18.3), recognizing that the domains may overlap and aspects of them may be part of larger alternative medical systems.

# Manipulative and Body-Based Practices

The CAM domain of **manipulative and body-based practices** includes methods that are based on manipulation or movement of the body. For example, chiropractors focus on the relationship between the body's structures (primarily the spine) and function and on how that relationship affects the preservation and restoration of health. Massage therapists use various hand techniques to move muscles and soft tissues to increase the flow of blood and oxygen to these areas or to release muscle tension.

**manipulative and body-based practices** Treatments involving manipulation or movement of one or more body parts.

**chiropractic medicine** Manipulation of the spine to allow proper energy flow.

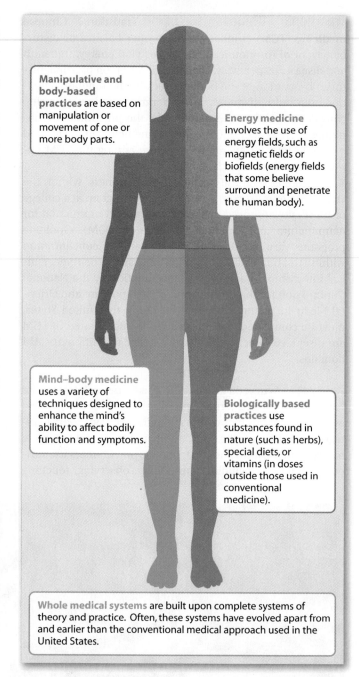

**FIGURE 18.3 The Domains of Complementary and Alternative Medicine (CAM)**
NCCAM groups CAM practices into four domains, recognizing that there can be some overlap. In addition, NCCAM studies CAM whole medical systems, which cut across all domains.

**Source:** National Center for Complementary and Alternative Medicine, "The Use of Complementary and Alternative Medicine in the United States," NCCAM Publication no. D434, 2009.

**Chiropractic Medicine** **Chiropractic medicine** has been practiced for more than 100 years and focuses on manipulation as a key therapy.[12] A century ago, allopathic medicine and chiropractic medicine were in direct competition. Today, however, many health care organizations work closely with chiropractors, and many insurance companies will pay for chiropractic treatment, particularly if it is recommended by a medical doctor.

Chiropractic medicine is based on the idea that a life-giving energy flows through the spine by way of the nervous system. If the spine is partly misaligned or dislocated, that force is disrupted. Chiropractors use a variety of techniques to manipulate the spine back into proper alignment so the energy can flow unimpeded. It has been established that their treatment can be effective for back pain, neck pain, and headaches.

The average chiropractic training program requires 4 years of intensive courses in biochemistry, anatomy, physiology, diagnostics, pathology, nutrition, and related topics, combined with hands-on clinical training. Many chiropractors continue their training to obtain specialized certification, for instance, in neurology, geriatrics, or pediatrics. Most state licensing boards require a 4-year course of study after completing at least a 2-year undergraduate program. Although states vary, increasing numbers require a 4-year undergraduate degree prior to entrance into chiropractic colleges. After completion of these requirements, applicants must pass an extensive examination given by the National Board of Chiropractic Examiners to obtain a license. The practice of chiropractic is licensed and regulated in all 50 states.[13]

### Massage Therapy

*Massage therapy* is defined as soft tissue manipulation by trained therapists for healing purposes.[14] References to massage have been found in ancient writings from many cultures, including those of ancient Greece, ancient Rome, Japan, China, Egypt, and the Indian subcontinent.[15] Today, massage therapy is used as a means of treating painful conditions, including low back pain, relaxing tired and overworked muscles, reducing stress and anxiety, rehabilitating sports injuries, and promoting general health.[16] This is accomplished by manipulating soft tissues to improve the body's circulation and to remove waste products from the muscles. There are many different types of massage therapy; the following are some of the more popular:

● *Swedish massage* uses long strokes, kneading, and friction on the muscles and moves the joints to aid flexibility.
● *Deep tissue massage* uses patterns of strokes and deep finger pressure on parts of the body where muscles are tight or knotted, focusing on layers of muscle deep under the skin.
● *Trigger point massage* (also called *pressure point massage*) uses a variety of strokes but applies deeper, more focused pressure on myofascial trigger points—"knots" that can form in the muscles, are painful when pressed, and cause symptoms elsewhere in the body as well.
● *Shiatsu massage* uses varying, rhythmic pressure from the fingers on parts of the body that are believed to be important for the flow of vital energy.

Other varieties include massage of specific body parts, such as the feet or fingers, application of hot rocks, water

massage, or other techniques. Massage techniques are important aspects of both traditional Chinese medicine and Ayurvedic medicine.

There are about 1,500 massage therapy schools, college programs, and training programs in the United States.[17] The course of study typically covers subjects such as anatomy and physiology; kinesiology; therapeutic evaluation; massage techniques; first aid; business, ethical, and legal issues; and hands-on practice. These educational programs vary in respect to length, quality, and whether they are accredited. Many require 500 hours of training, which is the same number of hours that many states require for certification. Some therapists also pursue specialty or advanced training. Massage therapists work in an array of settings both private and public: private offices, studios, hospitals, nursing homes, fitness centers, and sports medicine facilities, for example.[18]

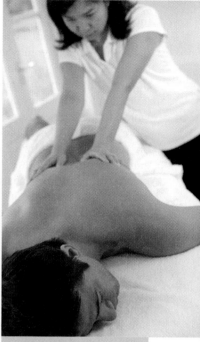

Oh, my aching back? Try massage!

### Bodywork

Bodywork actually consists of several forms of exercise. The *Feldenkrais method* is a system of movements, floor exercises, and bodywork designed to retrain the central nervous system to find new pathways around areas of blockage or damage. It is gentle and effective in rehabilitating trauma victims. *Rolfing,* a more invasive form of bodywork, aims to restructure the musculoskeletal system by working on patterns of tension held in deep tissue. The therapist applies firm—sometimes painful—pressure to different areas of the body. Rolfing can release repressed emotions as well as dissipate muscle tension. *Shiatsu* (also known as finger massage), is a traditional healing art from Japan that applies firm finger pressure to specified points on the body and is intended to increase the circulation of vital energy. *Trager bodywork* employs gentle, shaking motions of the patient's limbs in a rhythmic fashion to induce states of deep, pleasant relaxation.[19]

## Energy Medicine

**Energy medicine** therapies focus either on energy fields thought to originate within the body (biofields) or on fields from other sources (electromagnetic fields). The existence of these fields has not been experimentally proven. Some forms of energy therapy manipulate biofields by applying pressure and/or manipulating the body by placing the hands in, or through, these fields.[20]

**energy medicine** Therapies using energy fields, such as magnetic fields or biofields.

Popular examples of biofield therapy include qigong, Reiki, and therapeutic touch. *Qigong,* a component of traditional Chinese medicine, combines movement, meditation, and regulation of breathing to enhance the flow of vital energy (*qi*), improve blood circulation, and enhance immune function. *Reiki,* whose name derives from the Japanese word representing "universal life energy," is based on the belief that by channeling spiritual energy through the practitioner, the spirit is healed, and it in turn heals the physical body. *Therapeutic touch* derives from the ancient technique of "laying on" of hands and is based on the premise that the healing force of the therapist brings about the patient's recovery and that healing is promoted when the body's energies are in balance. By passing the hands over the body, the healers identify bodily imbalances.

Bioelectromagnetic-based therapies involve the unconventional use of electromagnetic fields—such as pulsed fields, magnetic fields, or alternating current or direct current fields—to treat asthma, cancer, pain, migraines, and other conditions. There is little scientific documentation to support claims for energy field techniques at this point. However, two derivatives of energy medicine have gained much wider acceptance in recent years: acupuncture and acupressure.

**Acupuncture** Acupuncture, one of the oldest forms of traditional Chinese medicine (and one of the most popular among Americans), is sought for a wide variety of health conditions, including musculoskeletal dysfunction, mood enhancement, and wellness pro-

**361**

points along 14 meridians exist on the human body, according to classic acupuncture theory.

**acupuncture** Branch of traditional Chinese medicine that uses the insertion of long, thin needles to affect flow of energy (*qi*) along pathways (meridians) within the body.
**acupressure** Branch of traditional Chinese medicine related to acupuncture. Uses application of pressure to selected body points to balance energy.
**mind–body medicine** Techniques designed to enhance the mind's ability to affect bodily functions and symptoms.

motion. It describes a family of procedures that involve stimulating anatomical points of the body with a series of precisely placed needles. The placement and manipulation of acupuncture needles is based on traditional Chinese theories of life-force energy (*qi*) flow through *meridians,* or energy pathways, in the body. Following acupuncture, most respondents and participants in clinical studies report high levels of satisfaction with the treatment, improved quality of life, improvement in or cure of the condition, and reduced reliance on prescription drugs and surgery. In particular, results have been promising in the treatment of nausea associated with chemotherapy, dental pain, and knee pain.[21] Some Western researchers believe that acupuncture may work through stimulating or repressing the autonomic nervous system.[22]

Acupuncturists in the United States are state licensed, and each state has specific requirements regarding training programs. Most acupuncturists either have completed a 2- to 3-year postgraduate program to obtain a master of traditional Oriental medicine (MTOM) degree or have attended a shorter certification program in North America or Asia.

**Acupressure** Acupressure is similar to acupuncture but does not use needles. Instead, the practitioner applies pressure to points critical to balancing *yin* and *yang,* the two Chinese principles that interact to influence overall harmony (health) of the body. Practitioners must have the same basic training and understanding of energy pathways as do acupuncturists.

## Mind–Body Medicine

**Mind–body medicine** employs a variety of techniques designed to facilitate the mind's capacity to affect bodily functions and symptoms. Many therapies fall under this category, but some areas, such as biofeedback and cognitive-behavioral techniques, have been so well investigated that they are no longer considered alternative. However, meditation, yoga, tai chi, certain uses of hypnosis, dance, music and art therapies, prayer and mental healing, and several others are still categorized as complementary and alternative. (See Chapter 9 for more on yoga and tai chi, and Chapters 2 and 3 and Focus On: Cultivating Your Spiritual Health beginning on page 60 for more on the mind–body connection.)

**Psychoneuroimmunology** As discussed in Chapter 3, *psychoneuroimmunology* (*PNI*) is a relatively new field of study. It is defined as the "interaction of consciousness (*psycho*), the brain and central nervous system (*neuro*), and the body's defense against external infection and internal aberrant cell division (*immunology*)."[23] Many researchers have postulated over the years that excessive stress and maladaptive coping can lead to immune system dysfunction and can increase the risk of disease. Scientists are exploring ways in which relaxation, biofeedback, meditation, yoga, laughter,

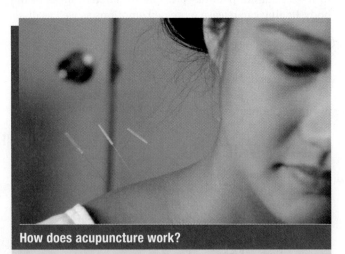

**How does acupuncture work?**

In acupuncture, long, thin needles are inserted into specific points along the body. This is thought to increase the flow of life-force energy, providing many physical and mental benefits.

exercise, and activities that involve either conscious or unconscious mind "quieting" may counteract negative stressors.

A classic study of PNI and mind–body health attempted to assess the effects of relaxation and coping techniques on the immune system by studying nursing home patients. Participants were divided into three groups: those who were taught relaxation techniques, those who were provided with abundant social contact, and those who received no special techniques or contact. After 1 month, immune system function greatly improved in participants who received stress management therapy as compared to the other groups. Several studies have shown promising positive effects of mind–body techniques that encourage relaxation and other stress-reduction strategies for people with cancer or other health problems.[24]

## what do you think?

Why do you think more and more people are opting for complementary and alternative treatments? ● What are the potential benefits of these treatments? ● What are the potential risks?

## Biologically Based Practices

**Biologically based practices** are perhaps the most controversial domain of CAM therapies because of the sheer number of options available and the many claims that are made about their effects. Many of these claims have not been thoroughly investigated, and the FDA's regulation of this aspect of CAM has been slow in coming. Biologically based practices include natural treatments, interventions, and products, many of which overlap with conventional medicine's use of dietary supplements. The FDA defines a dietary supplement as a "product (other than tobacco) that is intended to supplement or add to the diet; contains one or more dietary ingredients (including vitamins, minerals, herbs or other botanicals, amino acids, and other substances) or their constituents; is intended to be taken by mouth as a pill, capsule, tablet, or liquid; and is labeled on the front panel as being a dietary supplement."[25] Included among biologically based practices are herbal remedies, special dietary supplements, individual biological therapies, and functional foods. Typically, people take these supplements and remedies—often without guidance from any CAM practitioner—to improve health, prevent disease, or enhance mood. These products are discussed further in the section Choosing Health Products later in this chapter.

### The Role of Functional Foods in CAM Therapies

Changes to the diet are often part of CAM therapies, and such changes commonly involve increased intake of certain *functional foods*—foods or supplements designed to improve some specific aspect of physical or mental functioning. Sometimes referred to as **nutraceuticals** for their combined nutritional and pharmaceutical benefit, several are believed to work in much the same way as pharmaceutical drugs in making a person well or bolstering the immune system.

In recent years, the most commonly advertised functional foods have been those containing *antioxidants*. Antioxidants are chemicals that combat free radicals and oxidative damage in cells. They are present in many plant foods (including green tea). Although covered in depth in Chapter 7, it should be noted here that antioxidants are among the most sought-after functional foods on the market. Primary antioxidants include beta-carotene, selenium, vitamin C, and vitamin E.

Other common functional foods and their purported benefits include the following:

- **Plant stanols/sterols.** Can lower "bad" (low-density lipoprotein [LDL]) cholesterol.
- **Oat fiber.** Can lower LDL cholesterol; serves as a natural soother of nerves; stabilizes blood sugar levels.
- **Sunflower seeds and oil.** Can lower risk of heart disease; may prevent angina.
- **Soy protein.** May lower heart disease risk by reducing LDL cholesterol and triglycerides.
- **Garlic.** Lowers cholesterol and reduces clotting tendency of blood; lowers blood pressure; may serve as form of antibiotic.
- **Ginger.** May prevent motion sickness, stomach pain, and stomach upset; discourages blood clots; may relieve rheumatism.
- **Yogurt.** Yogurt that is labeled "Live Active Culture" contains active, friendly bacteria that can fight off infections.

**"Why Should I Care?"**

The ultimate choice about health care remains with you. In order to make sound decisions about what is best for your health, you need to understand as much as you can about your options.

**biologically based practices** Treatments using substances found in nature, such as herbs, special diets, or vitamin megadoses.
**nutraceuticals** Term often used interchangeably with *functional foods*; refers to the combined nutritional and pharmaceutical benefit derived through use of foods or food supplements.

# Choosing Health Products

Recall from Chapter 13 that prescription drugs can be obtained only with a written prescription from a physician, whereas over-the-counter drugs can be purchased without a prescription. Just as making wise decisions about providers is an important aspect of responsible health care, so is making wise decisions about medications.

## Prescription Drugs

In about two-thirds of doctor visits, the physician administers or prescribes at least one medication. In fact, prescription drug use has risen by 25 percent over the past decade.

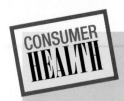

# MEDICATIONS ONLINE: BUYER BEWARE

The U.S. Food and Drug Administration (FDA) cannot warn people enough about the possible dangers of buying medications online. Buying prescription and over-the-counter drugs online from a company you don't recognize means that you may not know exactly what you're getting.

Consumers may choose to have prescriptions filled online for convenience and to save money. Although many websites are operating legally and observe the safeguards of traditional procedures for dispensing drugs, consumers must be wary of rogue websites that often sell unapproved drugs, or sidestep required practices meant to protect consumers.

Some websites sell counterfeit drugs. Counterfeit drugs are of unknown quality and safety and may be contami-

nated, contain the wrong active ingredient, or be made with the wrong amounts of ingredients. Sometimes they contain no active ingredients at all or contain too much of an active ingredient. As a result of these inconsistencies, they may not help the condition or disease that the medicine is intended to treat, and may even cause dangerous side effects.

The Verified Internet Pharmacy Practice Sites seal, also known as the VIPPS seal, is given by the National Association of Boards of Pharmacy (NABP) to Internet pharmacy sites that apply and meet state licensure requirements and other VIPPS criteria.

Follow these tips to protect yourself from fraudulent sites:

✱ Buy only from state-licensed pharmacy sites based

in the United States (preferably from VIPPS-certified sites, when possible).

✱ Don't buy from sites that sell prescription drugs without a prescription or that offer to prescribe a medication for the first time without a physical exam by your doctor.

✱ Check with your state board of pharmacy or the NABP to see if an online pharmacy has a valid pharmacy license and meets state quality standards.

✱ Use legitimate websites that have a licensed pharmacist to answer your questions.

✱ Look for privacy and security policies that are easy to find and easy to understand.

✱ Don't provide any personal information, such as a Social Security number, credit card information, or medical or

**Be very cautious if you consider ordering from an online pharmacy.**

health history, unless you are sure the website will keep your information safe and private.

**Source:** U.S. Food and Drug Administration, "The Possible Dangers of Buying Medicine over the Internet," 2010, www.fda.gov/ForConsumers/ConsumerUpdates/ucm048396.htm.

---

Even though these drugs are administered under medical supervision, the wise consumer still takes precautions. Hazards and complications arising from the use of prescription drugs are common. There are also potential risks to ordering prescription drugs from online sources; see the **Consumer Health** box above.

Consumers have a variety of resources available to determine the risks of various prescription medicines and to make educated decisions about whether to take a certain drug. One of the best resources is the FDA's Center for Drug Evaluation and Research website (www.fda.gov/drugs). This consumer-specific section of the FDA website provides current information on risks and benefits of prescription drugs. Being knowledgeable about what you are taking or thinking about taking is a sound strategy to ensure safety. Common types of prescription drugs discussed in

## 45%

**of Americans report taking at least one prescription drug in the past month; 18% report taking three or more such drugs.**

this text include antidepressants and antianxiety drugs (Chapter 2), hormonal contraceptives (Chapter 6), weight-loss aids (Chapter 8), smoking-cessation aids (Chapter 12), stimulants and sedatives (Chapter 13), antibiotics (Chapter 14), and statins and other cholesterol-lowering drugs (Chapter 15).

**Generic drugs,** medications sold under a chemical name rather than a brand name, contain the same active ingredients as brand-name drugs but are less expensive. Not all drugs are available as generics. If your doctor prescribes a drug, always ask if a generic equivalent exists and if it would be safe and effective for you to try.

Be aware, though, that there is some controversy about the effectiveness of generic drugs, because substitutions sometimes are made in minor ingredients that can affect the way the drug is absorbed, potentially causing discomfort or even allergic reactions in some patients. Always note any reactions you have to medications and tell your doctor about them.

**generic drugs** Medications marketed by chemical names rather than brand names.

# 18.1  Common Over-the-Counter Drugs, Their Uses, and Potential Side Effects

| Type/Name of Drug | Use | Examples | Potential Hazards/Common Side Effects |
|---|---|---|---|
| Acetaminophen | Pain reliever, fever reducer | Tylenol | Bloody urine, painful urination; skin rash; bleeding and bruising; yellowing of the eyes or skin; difficulty in diagnosing overdose because reaction may be delayed up to a week; liver damage from chronic low-level use |
| Antacids | Relieve "heartburn" | Tums Maalox | Reduced mineral absorption from food; possible concealment of ulcer; reduced effectiveness of anticlotting medications; interference with the function of certain antibiotics (for antacids that contain aluminum); worsened high blood pressure (for antacids that contain sodium); aggravated kidney problems |
| Anticholinergics | Often added to cold preparations to reduce nasal secretions and tears | atropine scopolamine | None of the preparations tested by the FDA have been found to be Generally Recognized as Effective (GRAE) or Generally Recognized as Safe (GRAS). Some cold compounds contain alcohol in concentrations greater than 40%. |
| Antihistamines | Central nervous system depressants that dry runny noses, clear postnasal drip and sinus congestion, and reduce tears | Claritin Benadryl Xyzal | Drowsiness, sedation, dizziness, disturbed coordination |
| Aspirin | Pain reliever; reduces fever and inflammation | Bayer Bufferin | Stomach upset and vomiting; stomach bleeding; worsening of ulcers; enhancement of the action of anticlotting medications; hearing damage from loud noise; severe allergic reaction; association with Reye's syndrome in children and teenagers; prolonged bleeding when combined with alcohol |
| Decongestants | Reduce nasal stuffiness due to colds | Sudafed DayQuil Allermed | Nervousness; restlessness; excitability; dizziness; drowsiness; headache; nausea; weakness; sleep problems |
| Diet pills, caffeine | Aid to weight loss | Dexatrim | Organ damage or death from cerebral hemorrhage; nervousness; irritability; dehydration |
| Expectorants | Loosen phlegm, which allows the user to cough it up and clear congested respiratory passages | Mucinex | Safety issues may arise when combined with other medications, particularly in frail or very ill individuals. Effectiveness is sometimes in question. |
| Ibuprofen | Pain reliever; reduces fever and inflammation | Advil Motrin | Allergic reaction in some people with aspirin allergy; fluid retention or swelling (edema); liver damage similar to that from acetaminophen; enhancement of anticlotting medications; digestive disturbances |
| Laxatives | Relieve constipation | ex-lax Citrucel | Reduced absorption of minerals from food; dehydration; dependency |
| Naproxen sodium | Pain reliever; reduces fever and inflammation | Aleve Naprosyn | Potential bleeding in the digestive tract; possible stomach cramps or ulcers |
| Sleep aids and relaxants | Help relieve occasional sleeplessness | Nytol Sleep-Eze Sominex | Drowsiness the next day; dizziness; lack of coordination; reduced mental alertness; constipation; dry mouth and throat; dependency |

# Over-the-Counter (OTC) Drugs

Over-the-counter (OTC) drugs are nonprescription substances used in the course of self-diagnosis and self-medication. More than one-third of the time, people treat their routine health problems with OTC medications. In fact, American consumers spend billions of dollars yearly on OTC preparations for relief of everything from runny noses to ingrown toenails. Those most commonly used are analgesics; cold, cough, allergy, and asthma relievers; stimulants; sleeping aids and relaxants; and dieting aids (Table 18.1).

Despite a common belief that OTC products are safe and effective, indiscriminate use and abuse can occur with these drugs as with all others. For example, people who

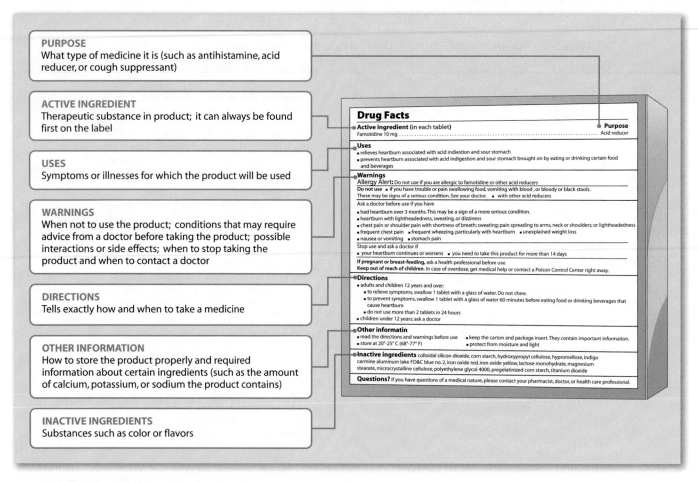

**PURPOSE**
What type of medicine it is (such as antihistamine, acid reducer, or cough suppressant)

**ACTIVE INGREDIENT**
Therapeutic substance in product; it can always be found first on the label

**USES**
Symptoms or illnesses for which the product will be used

**WARNINGS**
When not to use the product; conditions that may require advice from a doctor before taking the product; possible interactions or side effects; when to stop taking the product and when to contact a doctor

**DIRECTIONS**
Tells exactly how and when to take a medicine

**OTHER INFORMATION**
How to store the product properly and required information about certain ingredients (such as the amount of calcium, potassium, or sodium the product contains)

**INACTIVE INGREDIENTS**
Substances such as color or flavors

**Drug Facts**

**Active ingredient** (in each tablet)      **Purpose**
Famotidine 10 mg . . . . . . . . . . . . . . . . . . . . . . . . . . . . . . . . . . . . . . . . . . . . . . . . . . Acid reducer

**Uses**
- relieves heartburn associated with acid indigestion and sour stomach
- prevents heartburn associated with acid indigestion and sour stomach brought on by eating or drinking certain food and beverages

**Warnings**
**Allergy Alert:** Do not use if you are allergic to famotidine or other acid reducers
**Do not use** • if you have trouble or pain swallowing food, vomiting with blood , or bloody or black stools. These may be signs of a serious condition. See your doctor. • with other acid reducers
Ask a doctor before use if you have
- had heartburn over 3 months. This may be a sign of a more serious condition.
- heartburn with lightheadedness, sweating, or dizziness
- chest pain or shoulder pain with shortness of breath; sweating; pain spreading to arms, neck or shoulders; or lightheadedness
- frequent chest pain • frequent wheezing, particularly with heartburn • unexplained weight loss
- nausea or vomiting • stomach pain
Stop use and ask a doctor if
- your heartburn continues or worsens • you need to take this product for more than 14 days
**If pregnant or breast-feeding,** ask a health professional before use.
**Keep out of reach of children.** In case of overdose, get medical help or contact a Poison Control Center right away.

**Directions**
- adults and children 12 years and over:
  - to relieve symptoms, swallow 1 tablet with a glass of water. Do not chew.
  - to prevent symptoms, swallow 1 tablet with a glass of water 60 minutes before eating food or drinking beverages that cause heartburn
  - do not use more than 2 tablets in 24 hours
- children under 12 years: ask a doctor

**Other informatin**
- read the directions and warnings before use • keep the carton and package insert. They contain important informaiton.
- store at 20°-25° C (68°-77° F) • protect from moisture and light

**Inactive ingredients** colloidal silicon dioxide, corn starch, hydroxypropyl cellulose, hypromellose, indigo carmine aluminum lake FD&C blue no. 2, iron oxide red, iron oxide yellow, lactose monohydrate, magnesium stearate, microcrystalline cellulose, polyethylene glycol 4000, pregelatinized corn starch, titanium dioxide

**Questions?** If you have questions of a medical nature, please contact your pharmacist, doctor, or health care professional.

FIGURE 18.4 **The Over-the-Counter Medicine Label**
**Source:** Consumer Healthcare Products Association, OTC Label, www.otcsafety.org. Used with permission.

frequently drop medication into their eyes to "get the red out" or pop antacids after every meal are likely to become dependent. Many people also experience adverse side effects because they ignore the warnings on the labels or simply do not read them.

The FDA has developed a standard label that appears on most OTC products (Figure 18.4). It provides directions for use, warnings, and other useful information. Diet supplements, which are regulated as food products, have their own type of label that includes a Supplement Facts panel.

## Herbal Remedies and Special Supplements

People have been using herbal remedies for thousands of years. Herbs were the original sources for compounds found in approximately 25 percent of the pharmaceutical drugs we use today, including aspirin (white willow bark), the heart medication digitalis (foxglove), and the cancer treatment Taxol (Pacific yew tree plant). In addition, scientists continue to make pharmacological advances by studying the herbal remedies used in cultures throughout the world. With conventional scientists now recognizing the benefits of herbs, it is no wonder that more and more consumers are turning to herbal products.

However, herbal remedies are not to be taken lightly. Just because something is natural does not necessarily mean that it is safe. For example, in recent years, the FDA has warned that certain herbal products containing kava may be associated with severe liver damage.[26] Even rigorously tested products can be risky. Many plants are poisonous, and some can be toxic if ingested in high doses. Others may be dangerous when combined with prescription or over-the-counter drugs, could disrupt the normal action of the drugs, or could cause unusual side effects.[27] Properly trained herbalists and homeopaths receive graduate-level training in special programs such as herbal nutrition or traditional Chinese medicine. These practitioners are trained in diagnosis; in mixing herbs, titrations, and dosages; and in the follow-up care of patients.

Herbal remedies come in several different forms. **Tinctures** (extracts of fresh or dried plants) usually contain a high percentage of grain alcohol to prevent spoilage and

**tinctures** Herbal extracts usually combined with grain alcohol to prevent spoilage.

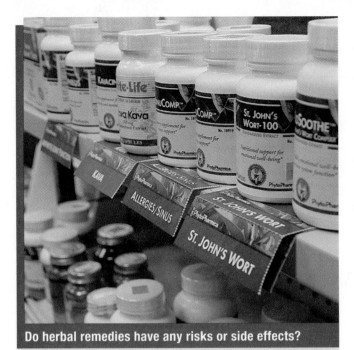

**Do herbal remedies have any risks or side effects?**

Herbs do have the potential to cause negative side effects. St. John's wort, for example, has potentially dangerous interactions with some prescription antidepressants and should never be taken with them. Other herbs, such as kava, can have negative effects even when taken alone.

lists popular nonherbal supplements and their risks and benefits.

## Strategies to Protect Supplement Consumers' Health

The burgeoning popularity of nutraceuticals and functional foods concerns many scientists. Although some alternative therapies, such as acupuncture, have been widely studied, there is little quality research to support the many claims in the area of nutraceuticals and supplements. It is important to gather whatever information you can on both the safety and efficacy of any CAM treatment you are considering (see Figure 18.5). In the case of herbal supplements or functional foods, start your own research with NCCAM (www.nccam.nih .gov) and the Cochrane Collaboration's review on complementary and alternative medicine (www.cochrane.org).

Herbal supplements and functional foods can currently be sold without FDA approval. This raises issues of consumer safety to new levels. Even when products are dispensed by CAM practitioners, the situation can be risky. Some homeopaths and herbalists who mix their own tonics may not use standardized measures. Lack of standard regulation means that some unskilled and untrained people may be treating patients without fully understanding the potential chemical interactions of their preparations.

Pressure has mounted to establish consistent standards for herbal supplements and functional foods similar to those used in Germany and other countries. Many scientists have advocated a more stringent FDA approval process for

are among the best herbal options. Freeze-dried extracts are very stable and offer good value for your money. Standardized extracts, often available in pill or capsule form, are also among the more reliable forms of herbal preparations.

In general, herbal medicines tend to be milder than chemical drugs and produce their effects more slowly; they also are much less likely to cause toxicity because they are diluted rather than concentrated forms of drugs. But diluted or not, and no matter how natural they are, herbs still contain many of the same chemicals as synthetic prescription drugs. Too much of any herb, particularly one from nonstandardized extracts, can cause problems. Table 18.2 gives an overview of some of the most common herbal supplements on the market.

Not all the supplements on the market today are directly derived from plant sources. In recent years, there have been increasing reports in the media on the health benefits of various vitamins, minerals, amino acids, and other specific biological compounds. Table 18.3

**May be safe; efficacy unclear**
**Treatment examples:** Acupuncture for chronic pain; homeopathy for seasonal allergies; low-fat diet for some cancers; massage therapy for low back pain; mind–body techniques for cancer
**Advice:** Physician monitoring recommended

**Likely safe and effective**
**Treatment examples:** Chiropractic care for acute low back pain; acupuncture for nausea from chemotherapy; acupuncture for dental pain; mind–body techniques for chronic pain and insomnia
**Advice:** Treatment is reasonable; physician monitoring advised

MORE SAFE

LESS EFFECTIVE ──────────────▶ MORE EFFECTIVE

LESS SAFE

**Dangerous or ineffective**
**Treatment examples:** Injections of unapproved substances; use of toxic herbs; delaying essential medical treatments; taking herbs known to interact dangerously with conventional medications (e.g., St. John's wort and indinavir)
**Advice:** Avoid treatment

**May work, but safety uncertain**
**Treatment examples:** St. John's wort for depression; saw palmetto for an enlarged prostate; chondroitin sulfate for osteoarthritis; ginkgo biloba for improving cognitive function in dementia
**Advice:** Physician monitoring is important

FIGURE 18.5 **Assessing the Risks and Benefits of CAM Treatments**
Medical experts devised this chart to gauge the potential liability of recommending alternative treatments, but by categorizing treatments according to their relative safety and effectiveness, it can also help patients and consumers make appropriate choices.

**Source:** M. H. Cohen and D. M. Eisenberg, "Potential Physician Malpractice Liability Associated with Complementary and Integrative Medical Therapies," *Annals of Internal Medicine* 136, no. 8 (2002): 596–603. Copyright © 2002 American College of Physicians. Used with permission.

**Common Herbs and Herbal Supplements: Benefits, Research, and Risks**

| | Herb | Claims of Benefits | Research Findings | Potential Risks |
|---|---|---|---|---|
| | Echinacea (purple coneflower, *Echinacea purpurea*, *E. angustifolia*, *E. pallida*) | Stimulates the immune system and increases the effectiveness of white blood cells that attack bacteria and viruses. Useful in preventing and treating colds or the flu. | Many studies in Europe have provided preliminary evidence of its effectiveness, but a recent controlled study in the United States indicated that it is no more effective than a placebo in preventing or treating a cold. | Allergic reactions, including rashes, increased asthma, gastrointestinal problems, and anaphylaxis (a life-threatening allergic reaction). Pregnant women and those with diabetes, autoimmune disorders, or multiple sclerosis should avoid it. |
| | Ephedra (ma huang, Chinese ephedra, *Ephedra sinica*) | Useful for weight loss and athletic performance. | Comprehensive research has found that ephedra has only limited positive effects on weight loss and athletic performance but has numerous adverse effects. | Heart attack, stroke, heart palpitations, psychiatric problems, upper gastrointestinal effects, tremor, insomnia, and death. The FDA has banned the sale of supplements containing ephedra. |
| | Flaxseed (*Linum usitatissimum*) | Useful as a laxative and for hot flashes and breast pain; the oil is used for arthritis; both flaxseed and flaxseed oil have been used for cholesterol level reduction and cancer prevention. | Study results are mixed on whether flaxseed decreases hot flashes or lowers cholesterol levels. | Delays absorption of medicines, but otherwise has few side effects. Should be taken with plenty of water. |
| | Ginkgo (*Ginkgo biloba*) | Useful for depression, impotence, premenstrual syndrome, dementia and Alzheimer's disease, diseases of the eye, and general vascular disease. | Some promising results have been seen for Alzheimer's disease and dementia, and research continues on its ability to enhance memory and reduce the incidence of cardiovascular disease. | Gastric irritation, headache, nausea, dizziness, difficulty thinking, memory loss, and allergic reactions. |
| | Ginseng (*Panax ginseng*) | Affects the pituitary gland, increasing resistance to stress, affecting metabolism, aiding skin, muscle tone, and sex drive; improves concentration and muscle strength. | Studies have raised questions about appropriate dosages. Because the potency of plants varies considerably, dosage is difficult to control and side effects are fairly common. | Nervousness, insomnia, high blood pressure, headaches, chest pain, depression, and abnormal vaginal bleeding. |
| | Green tea (*Camellia sinensis*) | Useful for lowering cholesterol and risk of some cancers, protecting the skin from sun damage, bolstering mental alertness, and boosting heart health. | Although some studies have shown promising links between green and white tea consumption and cancer prevention, recent research questions the ability of tea to significantly reduce the risk of breast, lung, or prostate cancer. | Insomnia, liver problems, anxiety, irritability, upset stomach, nausea, diarrhea, or frequent urination. |
| | Kava (*Piper methysticum*) | Useful for relaxation; relief of anxiety, insomnia, and menopausal symptoms; sometimes used topically as a numbing agent. | Scientific studies provide some evidence that kava may be beneficial for the management of anxiety. | Increases the effect of alcohol and other drugs; causes drowsiness; the FDA has issued a warning that using kava supplements has been linked to a risk of severe liver damage. |
| | St. John's wort (SJW, Klamath weed, *Hypericum perforatum*) | Useful for depression, anxiety, and sleep disorders. | There is evidence that SJW is useful for treating mild to moderate depression, but two large studies showed that it was no more effective than a placebo in treating major depression of moderate severity. | Gastrointestinal upset, fatigue, dry mouth, anxiety, sexual dysfunction, dizziness, skin rashes, itching, and extreme sensitivity to sunlight. |
| | Valerian (*Valeriana officinalis*) | Useful for relaxation, sleep disorders, anxiety, headaches, depression, irregular heartbeat, and trembling. | Research suggests it may be helpful for insomnia, but there is not enough evidence to determine whether it works for anxiety, depression, or headaches. | Mild side effects, such as headaches, dizziness, upset stomach, and tiredness, occur the morning after use. |

**Sources:** National Center for Complementary and Alternative Medicine, "Herbs at a Glance," 2009, http://nccam.nih.gov/health/herbsataglance.htm; Office of Dietary Supplements, National Institutes of Health, "Dietary Supplement Fact Sheets," 2009, http://ods.od.nih.gov/Health_Information/Information_About_Individual_Dietary_Supplements.aspx; U.S. Food and Drug Administration, "Final Rule Declaring Dietary Supplements Containing Ephedrine Alkaloids Adulterated Because They Present an Unreasonable Risk," 2008, www.fda.gov/Food/GuidanceComplianceRegulatoryInformation/GuidanceDocuments/DietarySupplements/ucm072997.htm; American Cancer Society, "Green Tea," 2008, www.cancer.org/docroot/ETO/content/ETO_5_3x_Green_Tea.asp.

TABLE
18.3 Common Nonherbal Supplements: Benefits, Research, and Risks

| Supplement | Claims of Benefits | Research Findings | Potential Risks |
|---|---|---|---|
| Dehydroepiandrosterone (DHEA) (hormone) | Fights aging, boosts immunity, strengthens bones, and improves brain functioning. | No proven antiaging benefits. | Could increase cancer risk and lead to liver damage, even when taken briefly. |
| Vitamin E | Reduces risk of heart disease; better chance of survival after heart attack. | Research results on prevention of heart disease are mixed. Some researchers are curious to see if it is most protective for young, healthy people against eventual heart disease. | High doses cause bleeding when taken with blood thinners. |
| Glucosamine (biological substance that helps the body grow cartilage) | Useful for arthritis and related degenerative joint diseases; relieves swelling and decreases pain. | When it is taken with chondroitin sulfate, preliminary research shows that it helps reduce pain in people with moderate to severe joint pain. | Few side effects noted. |
| L-Carnitine (amino acid derivative) | Improves athletic performance, increases fat-burning enzymes, used to combat fatigue and aging. | No consistent evidence that it improves performance in healthy athletes. Some evidence that it enhances mental function in older adults with mild cognitive impairment. | Nausea, vomiting, abdominal cramps, diarrhea, "fishy" body odor; more rarely, muscle weakness, seizures in patients with seizure disorders; interacts with some medications. |
| Melatonin (hormone) | Useful in regulating circadian rhythms and sleep patterns and treating insomnia; claims of antiaging benefits. | Some evidence supports its usefulness in regulating sleep patterns. No scientific support for antiaging claims. | Nausea, headaches, dizziness, blood vessel constriction; possibly a danger for people with high blood pressure or other cardiovascular problems. |
| SAMe (pronounced "sammy") (biological compound that aids over 40 functions in the body) | Useful in treatment of mild to moderate depression and in treatment of arthritis pain. | Studies have supported its usefulness in treating depression and arthritis pain. | Fewer side effects than prescription antidepressants have. Questions remain over how much a person should take, in what form, and whether there are long-term side effects. |
| Zinc (mineral) | Supports immune system; used to lessen duration and severity of cold symptoms; aids wound healing. | Research results are mixed, possibly due to the wide variety of cold viruses and differences of formulations and dosages in zinc lozenges. | Excessive intake associated with reduced immune function, reduced levels of high-density lipoproteins ("good" cholesterol). |

**Source:** Office of Dietary Supplements, National Institutes of Health, "Dietary Supplement Fact Sheets," Modified August 2010, http://ods.od.nih.gov/Health _Information/Information_About_Individual_Dietary_Supplements.aspx.

supplements sold in the United States. As a result, the FDA has instituted new regulations to oversee the manufacture of dietary supplements, including herbal supplements. These new regulations require manufacturers to evaluate the identity, purity, strength, and composition of the supplements to ensure they contain what the label claims.

The official public standards-setting authority for all medicines, supplements, and other health care products manufactured and sold in the United States is the U.S. Pharmacopeia, which tests select products, including herbal supplements, to ensure that they comply with safety and purity standards. Products that meet these standards display a "USP Dietary Supplement Verified" seal (Figure 18.6). In addition, dietary supplements are required to include specific information on their labels, as regulated by the Dietary Supplement Health and Education Act.

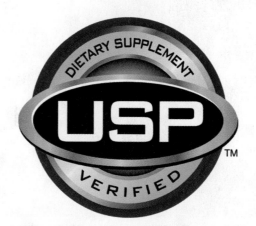

FIGURE 18.6 **The U.S. Pharmacopeia Verified Mark**
**Source:** Used with permission of The United States Pharmacopeial Convention.

# Health Insurance

Whether you're visiting your regular doctor, consulting a specialist, or preparing for a hospital stay, chances are that you'll be using some form of health insurance to pay for your care. Insurance typically allows you, the consumer, to pay into a pool of funds and then bill the insurance carrier for health care charges you incur. The fundamental principle of insurance underwriting is that the cost of health care can be predicted for large populations. This is how health care premiums (payments) are determined. Policyholders pay premiums into a pool, which is held in reserve until needed. When you are sick or injured, the insurance company pays out of the pool, regardless of your total amount of contribution. Depending on circumstances, you may never pay for what your medical care costs, or you may pay much more for insurance than your medical bills ever total. The idea is that you pay affordable premiums so that you never have to face catastrophic bills. In today's profit-oriented system, insurers prefer to have healthy people in their plans who pour money into risk pools without taking money out.

Unfortunately, not everyone has health insurance. Over 46 million Americans are uninsured—that is, they have no private health insurance and are not eligible for Medicare, Medicaid, or other government health programs.[28] Lack of health insurance has been associated with delayed health care and increased mortality. *Underinsurance* (i.e., the inability to pay out-of-pocket expenses despite having insurance) also may result in adverse health consequences.

Another 25 million Americans between the ages of 19 and 64 are estimated to be underinsured (at risk for spending more than 10% of their income on medical care because their insurance is inadequate).[29]

Contrary to the common belief that the uninsured are unemployed, 75 percent of them are either workers or the dependents of workers. Almost 15 percent of all the uninsured are children under age 18. Among young adults aged 18 to 24, more than 29 percent reported being uninsured at some point in time. This age group is almost twice as likely to be uninsured as are people aged 45 to 64.[30]

However, for young adults who are college students, the statistics are different. According to a recent study, approximately 20 percent of college students report not having health insurance.[31] Those who are covered only under their school's health care plan may not realize that such plans are usually short term and have low upper limits of benefits, which is problematic in the event of an emergency illness or accident. Few students buy the higher level catastrophic plans, however.

Racial and ethnic minorities are overly represented in the number of uninsured Americans. Close to 40 percent of the American Indian or Alaskan Natives population and more than a third of the Latino population are uninsured compared to 16 percent of whites.[32] The number of uninsured African Americans is also higher than that of whites. Issues such as citizenship and language barriers contribute to some of the disparities in access to health insurance for many in our country.

For the uninsured and many of the underinsured, health care from any source may be too expensive to be obtainable. People without health care coverage are less likely than other Americans to have their children immunized, seek early prenatal care, obtain annual blood pressure checks, and seek attention for serious symptoms. Experts believe that this ultimately leads to higher system costs, because their conditions deteriorate to a more debilitating and costly stage before they are forced to seek help.

## Private Health Insurance

Originally, health insurance consisted solely of coverage for hospital costs (it was called *major medical*), but gradually it was extended to cover routine physicians' treatment and other areas, such as dental services and pharmaceuticals. These payment mechanisms laid the groundwork for today's steadily rising health care costs. Hospitals were reimbursed for the costs of providing care plus an amount for profit. This system provided no incentive to contain costs, limit the number of procedures, or curtail capital investment in redundant equipment and facilities. Physicians were reimbursed on a fee-for-service (indemnity) basis determined by

People without insurance can't gain access to preventive care, so they seek care only in an emergency or crisis. Because emergency care is extraordinarily expensive, they often are unable to pay, and the cost is absorbed by those who can pay—the insured or taxpayers.

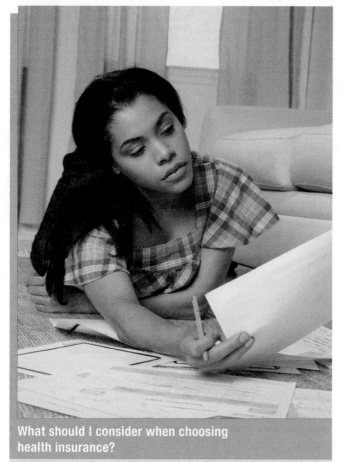

**What should I consider when choosing health insurance?**

Choosing a health insurance plan can be confusing. Some things to think about include how comprehensive your coverage needs to be, how convenient your care must be, how much you are willing to spend on premiums and co-payments, what the overall cost will be, and whether the services of the plan meet your needs.

throughout the course of treatment (e.g., 20% of the total bill). *Preexisting condition clauses* limit the insurance company's liability for medical conditions that a consumer had before obtaining coverage (i.e., if a woman takes out coverage while she is pregnant, the insurance company may cover pregnancy complications and infant care but may not cover charges related to "normal pregnancy"). Because many insurance companies use a combination of these mechanisms, keeping track of the costs that you are responsible for can become very difficult.

Group plans of large employers (e.g., government agencies, school districts, and corporations) generally do not have preexisting condition clauses in their plans, but smaller group plans (a group may be as small as two people) often do. Some plans never cover preexisting conditions, whereas others specify a *waiting period* (e.g., 6 months) before they will provide coverage. All insurers set some limits on the types of services they cover (e.g., most exclude cosmetic surgery, private rooms, and experimental procedures). Some insurance plans may also include an *upper* or *lifetime limit,* after which coverage will end. Although $250,000 may seem like an enormous sum, medical bills for a sick child or chronic disease can easily run this high within a few years.

> **what do you think?**
> Why is it important that private insurance cover preventive or lower-level care as well as hospitalization and high-technology interventions?
> ● What kinds of incentives would cause you to seek care early rather than delay care?

"usual, customary, and reasonable" fees. This system encouraged physicians to charge high fees, raise them often, and perform as many procedures as possible. At the same time, because most insurance did not cover routine or preventive services, consumers were encouraged to use hospitals whenever possible (the coverage was better) and to wait until illness developed to seek care instead of seeking preventive care. Consumers were also free to choose any provider or service they wished, including even inappropriate—and often very expensive—levels of care.

Private insurance companies have increasingly employed several mechanisms to limit potential losses: cost sharing (in the form of deductibles, co-payments, and coinsurance), exclusions, "preexisting condition" clauses, waiting periods, and upper limits on payments. *Deductibles* are front-end payments (commonly $250 to $1,000) that you must make to your provider before your insurance company will start paying for any services you use. *Co-payments* are set amounts that you pay per service received, regardless of the cost of the service (e.g., $20 per doctor visit or per prescription). *Coinsurance* is the percentage of the bill that you must pay

## Managed Care

**Managed care** describes a health care delivery system consisting of the following elements:

**1.** A network of physicians, hospitals, and other providers and facilities linked contractually to deliver comprehensive health benefits within a predetermined budget, sharing economic risk for any budget deficit or surplus

**2.** A budget based on an estimate of the annual cost of delivering health care for a given population

**3.** An established set of administrative rules requiring patients to follow the advice of participating health care providers in order to have their health care paid for under the terms of the health plan

> **managed care** Cost-control procedures used by health insurers to coordinate treatment.
> **capitation** Prepayment of a fixed monthly amount for each patient without regard to the type or number of services provided.

Types of managed care plans include health maintenance organizations (HMOs), preferred provider organizations (PPOs), and point of service (POS). Approximately 64 million Americans are enrolled in HMOs, the most common type.[33]

Many managed care plans pay their contracted health care providers through **capitation,** that is, prepayment of a fixed monthly amount for each patient without regard for the type or number of health services provided. Some plans pay health care providers a salary, and some are still fee-for-service plans.

As with other insurance plans, enrollees are members of a risk pool, and it is expected that some persons will use no services, some will use a modest amount, and others will have high-cost usage over a given year. Doctors have the incentive to keep their patient pool healthy and avoid catastrophic ailments that are preventable; usually such incentives come back in terms of increased salaries, bonuses, and other benefits. As such, prevention and health education to reduce risk and intervene early to avoid major problems are often capstone components of such plans.

Managed care plans have grown steadily over the past decade with a proportionate decline of enrollment in traditional indemnity insurance plans. The reason for this shift is that indemnity insurance, which pays providers and hospitals on a fee-for-service basis with no built-in incentives to control costs, has become unaffordable or unavailable for most Americans.

### Health Maintenance Organizations

Health maintenance organizations (HMOs) provide a wide range of covered health benefits (e.g., checkups, surgery, doctor visits, lab tests) for a fixed amount prepaid by the patient, the employer, Medicaid, or Medicare (discussed later). Usually, HMO premiums are the least expensive form of managed care (saving between 10% and 40% more than other plans) but also are the most restrictive (offering little or no choice in doctors and certain services). These premiums are 8 to 10 percent lower than for traditional plans, there are low or no deductibles or coinsurance payments, and co-payments are approximately $20 per office visit.

**diagnosis-related groups (DRGs)** Diagnostic categories established by the federal government to determine in advance how much hospitals will be reimbursed for the care of a particular Medicare patient.

The downside of HMOs is that patients are typically required to use the plan's doctors and hospitals and to get approval from a "gatekeeper" or PCP for treatment and referrals. As more and more people enroll in HMOs, criticisms about them are mounting. Concerns about HMOs include questions about care allocation, profit-motivated medical decision making, and the degree of focus on prevention and intervention.

### Preferred Provider Organizations

Preferred provider organizations (PPOs) are networks of independent doctors and hospitals that contract to provide care at discounted rates. Although they offer greater choices in doctors than HMOs do, they are less likely to coordinate a patient's care. Members do have a choice of seeing doctors who are not on the preferred list, but this choice may come at considerable cost (e.g., having to pay 30% of the charges out of pocket, rather than 10% to 20% for PPO doctors and services).

### Point of Service

Point of service (POS) plans—offered by many HMOs—provide a more acceptable form of managed care for people used to the traditional indemnity plan of insurance, which probably explains why it is among the fastest growing of the managed care plans. Under POS plans, the patient selects a primary care physician from a list of participating providers, and this physician becomes the patient's "point of service." If referrals are made outside of the network, then the patient is still partially covered.

## Medicare and Medicaid

The government, through programs such as Medicare and Medicaid, currently funds 35 percent of the total U.S. health spending. Under Medicare, the federal government pays 80 percent of most medical bills, after a deductible fee, for people over 65. Medicare also offers options for coverage of prescription medications.[34]

Medicare is a federal insurance program that covers a broad range of services except long-term care. Medicare covers 99 percent of individuals over age 65, all totally and permanently disabled people (after a waiting period), and all people with end-stage kidney failure—currently over 45 million people, or 1 in 7 Americans, in all.[35] By 2030, it is estimated that 1 in 5—or 77 million—Americans will be insured by Medicare. As the costs of medical care have continued to increase, Medicare has placed limits on the amount of reimbursement to providers. As a result, some physicians and managed care programs have stopped accepting Medicare patients.

To control hospital costs, in 1983 the federal government set up a prospective payment system based on **diagnosis-related groups (DRGs)** for Medicare. Using a complicated formula, nearly 500 groupings of diagnoses were created to establish how much a hospital would be reimbursed for a particular patient. If a hospital can treat the patient for less than that amount, it can keep the difference. However, if a patient's care costs more than the set amount, the hospital must absorb the difference (with a few exceptions that must be reviewed by a panel). This system gives hospitals the incentive to discharge patients quickly after doing as little as possible for them, to provide more ambulatory care, and to admit only patients in favorable (profitable) DRGs. Many private health insurance companies have followed the federal government in adopting this type of reimbursement. In 1998, the federal Health Care Financing Administration (HCFA) expanded the prospective payment system to include payments for outpatient surgery and skilled nursing care.

In its continuing effort to control rising costs, the HCFA has encouraged the growth of prepaid HMO senior plans for Medicare-eligible persons. Under this system, commercial managed care insurance plans receive a fixed per capita premium from the HCFA and then offer more preventive services with lower out-of-pocket co-payments. These managed care plans encourage providers and patients to utilize health care resources under administrative rules similar to commercial HMO plans.

In contrast to Medicare, Medicaid is a federal/state welfare program for people who are defined as poor, including many who are blind, disabled, elderly, or receiving Aid to Families with Dependent Children monies. Medicaid covers about 36 million people and it relies on matching funds provided by federal and state sources.[36] Because each state determines income eligibility and payments to providers, there are vast differences in the way Medicaid operates from state to state.

# Issues Facing Today's Health Care System

Many Americans believe that our health care system needs fundamental reform. In recent years, the number of individuals who are underinsured has risen dramatically, and, without reform, the rise will likely continue. Individuals with preexisting conditions and those who are self-employed are just two groups whose members often find themselves unable to find or afford health care. The significant costs of a major procedure, course of treatment, or hospital stay mean many families are one catastrophic illness or accident away from financial ruin. In addition to cost and access, malpractice, restricted choices in providers and treatments, unnecessary procedures, complicated insurance rules, and dramatic ranges in quality are also issues of concern. See the **Be Healthy, Be Green** box on page 602 for a discussion of another concern about the health care system: the amount of waste it produces and its impact on the environment.

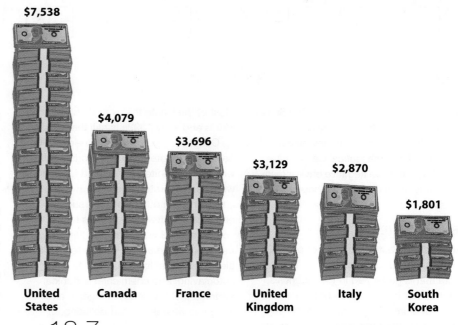

$7,538 United States
$4,079 Canada
$3,696 France
$3,129 United Kingdom
$2,870 Italy
$1,801 South Korea

FIGURE 18.7 **Health Care Spending per Person, 2008 (in thousands of U.S. dollars)**

Source: Data are from Organisation for Economic Co-Operation and Development, *OECD Health Data 2010*, 2010, www.oecd.org/health.

## Cost

Both per capita and as a percentage of gross domestic product (GDP), we spend more on health care than any other nation. Yet, unlike the rest of the industrialized world, we do not provide access for our entire population. We spend over $2 trillion annually on health care, over $7,500 for every man, woman, and child (Figure 18.7). This translates into 18.3 percent of our GDP. Does this sound like a lot? Consider that health care expenditures are projected to grow by 6.1 percent each year, reaching over $4 trillion annually by 2019—nearly 20 percent of our projected GDP.[37]

Why do health care costs continue to skyrocket? Many factors are involved: excess administrative costs; duplication of services; an aging population; growing rates of obesity, inactivity, and related health problems; demand for new diagnostic and treatment technologies; an emphasis on crisis-oriented care instead of prevention; and inappropriate use of services by consumers.

Our system has more than 2,000 health insurance companies, each with different coverage structures and administrative requirements. This lack of uniformity prevents our system from achieving the *economies of scale* (bulk purchasing at a reduced cost) and administrative efficiency realized in countries where there is a single-payer delivery system. According to the Health Insurance Association of America, commercial insurance companies commonly experience administrative costs greater than 10 percent of the total health care insurance premium, whereas the administrative cost of the government's Medicare program is less than 4 percent. These administrative expenses contribute to the high cost of health care and force companies to require employees to share more of the costs, cut back on benefits, and drop some benefits altogether. These costs are largely passed on to consumers in the form of higher prices for goods and services. See Figure 18.8 on page 603 for a breakdown of how health care dollars are spent.

## Access

Over 133 million people in the United States suffer from at least one chronic health condition.[38] Their access to care is largely determined by whether they have health insurance. Catastrophic or chronic illness among only 10 percent of the population accounts for 75 percent of all health expenditures.[39] Because we cannot perfectly predict who will fall into that 10 percent, every American is potentially vulnerable to the high cost and devastating effects of such illnesses.

Access to health care is determined by numerous factors, including the supply of providers and facilities, proximity to care, ability to maneuver in the system, health status, and insurance coverage. Although there are almost 700,000 physicians in the United States, many Americans lack adequate access to health services because of insurance barriers or maldistribution of providers.[40] There is an oversupply of higher-paid specialists and a shortage of lower-paid primary care physicians (family practitioners, pediatricians, internists, ob-gyns, geriatricians). Inner cities and some rural areas face constant shortages of physicians.

Until recently, many employees lost their insurance benefits when they changed jobs; this led the federal government to pass legislation mandating the "portability" of health insurance

## The Perils of Medical Waste

The health care system in the United States is massive, and it affects many aspects of our daily lives, including our environment. Medical and pharmaceutical wastes have been shown to have negative environmental impacts on air and water resources, as well as on human and animal health.

### MEDICAL WASTE

The Medical Waste Tracking Act of 1988 defines medical waste as "any solid waste that is generated in the diagnosis, treatment, or immunization of human beings or animals, in research pertaining thereto, or in the production or testing of biologicals." This definition includes, but is not limited to, blood-soaked bandages; culture dishes and other glassware; discarded surgical gloves; discarded surgical instruments; discarded needles used to give shots or draw blood (e.g., medical sharps); cultures, stocks, or swabs used to inoculate cultures; removed body parts (e.g., tonsils, appendices, limbs); and discarded lancets.

Due to concern about the spread of infectious diseases, especially in hospital and clinic settings, there is a vital need for sterility. This leads to excessive one-time-use items such as latex gloves, needles, bandages, and much more. All these items contribute substantially to the amount of medical waste.

Some estimate that the volume of hospital-generated medical waste is as much as 2 million tons each year. Approximately 15 percent of potentially infectious medical waste is combined with medical waste that is not deemed infectious and then disposed of in landfills. As water percolates through solid-waste disposal sites such as landfills, it collects contaminants and forms a substance called *leachate*. This can contaminate groundwater and surface water. Pollution in the ocean is also a major problem, as it directly affects all sea life and indirectly affects human health. In 1988, the Environmental Protection Agency banned dumping waste into the ocean, but the ban wasn't enforced until January 1992.

Most of the waste that was dumped in the 1980s and early 1990s is still there today.

Currently, the vast majority—over 90 percent—of potentially infectious medical waste in the United States and around the world is incinerated, resulting in carbon emissions and other pollution such as particulate matter. Alternatives to incineration of medical waste include thermal treatment, such as microwave technologies; steam sterilization, such as autoclaving; and chemical mechanical systems that break down organic and inorganic wastes without polluting.

### PHARMACEUTICAL WASTE

In addition to medical waste, hospitals generate a substantial amount of pharmaceutical waste—both hazardous and nonhazardous—that requires proper disposal. Generally, this waste comprises drugs that have been dispensed but not completely used. There is also a large amount of individual-generated pharmaceutical waste. Studies have shown that nearly 54 percent of consumers put unwanted medications in the trash, and 35 percent flush them down the toilet.

Prescription drug waste can contaminate our water supply through a number of avenues. First, medicines disposed of down the toilet or drain can easily be incorporated into groundwater, lakes, rivers, and streams. This may harm fish and wildlife that live in lakes, rivers, and the ocean. In addition, these drugs can end up back in our drinking water supply. This leads to elevated levels of chemicals that many water treatment facilities are not equipped to filter. Pharmaceutical drugs have been detected in the drinking water supplies of major metropolitan areas all across the United States. To date, the federal government has not set limits on the amount of pharmaceutical drugs that can be present in drinking water and does not require any testing for their presence.

Prescription drugs that are thrown away rather than flushed add to our growing landfills and can contribute to the toxicity of leachate. However, many

**Extra precautions must be taken when disposing of medical waste.**

sources still encourage throwing away unused prescription drugs, as it is a better method of disposal than flushing or dumping down the drain. Alternatively, here are some more green ways to manage unused medications:

✱ Send your medicine to those in need. Some organizations collect unused, unexpired medicine to send to other countries where prescription drugs are harder to get. Many states have passed legislation for recycling unused medications in nursing homes or other locations, but implementation has proven difficult. Nonprofits, such as the Iowa Prescription Drug Corporation (www.iowapdc.org), have developed and administered statewide drug-donation programs.

✱ Take your drugs back to the pharmacy. Many community pharmacies are starting take-back programs for unused or unneeded prescriptions. The pharmacy then disposes of these drugs safely. In some cases, pharmacies return unused pharmaceuticals to manufacturers for processing; in other cases, unused prescription medications are destroyed safely. It is still recommended to throw away (instead of flush) nonprescription drugs such as aspirin or ibuprofen.

**Sources:** Environmental Protection Agency, "Medical Waste Frequent Questions," 2010, www.epa.gov/wastes/nonhaz/industrial/medical/mwfaqs.htm; National Conference of State Legislatures, "State Prescription Drug Return, Reuse, and Recycling Laws," 2010, www.ncsl.org/default.aspx?tabid=14425; U.S. Food and Drug Administration, "How to Dispose of Unused Medicines," 2009, www.fda.gov/ForConsumers/ConsumerUpdates/ucm101653.htm.

**Total expenditures = $2.2 trillion**

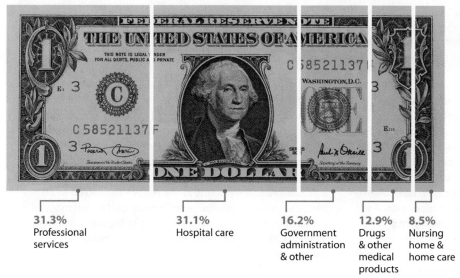

31.3%
Professional
services

31.1%
Hospital care

16.2%
Government
administration
& other

12.9%
Drugs
& other
medical
products

8.5%
Nursing
home &
home care

FIGURE 18.8 **Where Do We Spend Our Health Care Dollars?**

**Source:** Data are from National Center for Health Statistics, *Health, United States, 2009, with Special Feature on Medical Technology* (Hyattsville, MD: National Center for Health Statistics, 2010).

benefits from one job to the next, thereby guaranteeing coverage during the transition. Today, individuals who leave their jobs can continue their group health insurance benefits under the Consolidated Omnibus Budget Reconciliation Act (COBRA). COBRA allows former employees, retirees, spouses, and dependents to continue their insurance at group rates. COBRA beneficiaries pay a higher amount than they did when they were employed, as they're covering both the personal premium and the amount previously covered by the employer. As a result, COBRA benefits are more expensive than benefits through an employer, but usually less expensive than purchasing individual insurance. COBRA coverage is only temporary—it usually lasts for up to 18 months.

Managed care health plans determine access on the basis of participating providers, health plan benefits, and administrative rules. Often this means that consumers do not have the freedom to choose specialists, facilities, or treatment options beyond those contracted with the health plan and recommended by their PCP.

See the **Points of View** box on page 604 for a discussion of the pros and cons of national health insurance that would address concerns over access to health care.

**Increasing Support for CAM from Insurers and Providers** In the United States, consumer demand has led to an expansion of benefits to include nonallopathic therapies such as chiropractic and acupuncture. More and more insurers are covering alternative care, at least to some degree. This is especially true as criticisms of managed care increase and government agencies get involved.

Today, nearly all health insurance providers cover at least one form of CAM, with acupuncture and massage therapy being the most common. In spite of this progress, many patients will continue to pay out of pocket for alternative ther-

apies until the scientific evidence supporting these alternative medical care choices is impossible to ignore. What is known is that the numbers are increasing despite a reimbursement system that favors traditional treatments.

Support from professional organizations, such as the AMA, is also increasing as more physician training programs require or offer electives in alternative treatment modes. In many cases, medical schools are educating doctors to be better prepared to advise patients about the pros and cons of alternative treatments and how to follow integrative practices. Although alternative medicine is becoming increasingly integrated into today's health care programs and plans, there is still a long way to go.

## Quality and Malpractice

The U.S. health care system has several mechanisms for ensuring quality services: education, licensure, certification/registration, accreditation, peer review, and the legal system of malpractice litigation. Some of these mechanisms are mandatory before a professional or an organization may provide care, whereas others are purely voluntary. (Be aware that licensure, although mandated by the state for some practitioners and facilities, is only a minimum guarantee of quality.) Insurance companies and government payers may also require a higher level of quality by linking payment to whether a practitioner is board certified or a facility is

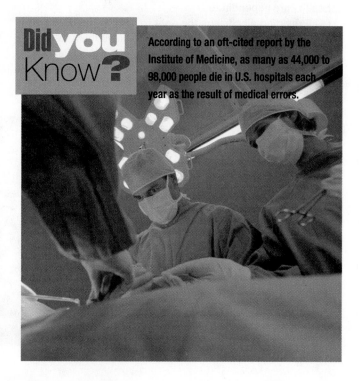

**Did you Know?**

According to an oft-cited report by the Institute of Medicine, as many as 44,000 to 98,000 people die in U.S. hospitals each year as the result of medical errors.

# National Health Care:
## IS IT A GOVERNMENT RESPONSIBILITY?

Whether universal health care coverage will—or should—be achieved in the United States and through what mechanism remain hotly debated topics. Proponents of reform argue that health care should be available and affordable for everyone. They point to other Western countries, such as Canada and France, that currently have successful universal coverage. Opponents of health care reform feel that the high cost of changing the system is more than the United States can afford, and state that the government should not interfere in what has been largely a free-market industry.

However, analysts believe that health care reform has failed in the past due to a combination of factors that have little to do with the quality of the nation's health. Lobbying efforts by the insurance industry and the medical community, overcomplicated proposed plans, and special interest groups that contended that the plans either went "too far" or "not far enough" have all played a role in thwarting reform.

In 2010, Congress passed the Patient Protection and Affordable Care Act. The reforms in this Act are scheduled to be implemented over several years, through 2014, and many of their actual effects are uncertain. It remains to be seen what the next steps will be in the ongoing discussion over health insurance for those who remain uninsured.

## Arguments for National Health Insurance

◯ Health care is a human right. The United Nations Universal Declaration of Human Rights states that "everyone has the right to a standard of living adequate for the health and well-being of oneself and one's family, including . . . medical care."

◯ Americans would be more likely to engage in preventive health behaviors and clinicians would be encouraged to practice preventive medicine; people without insurance often avoid preventive care checkups and inquiring early about suspected symptoms due to cost concerns.

◯ Medical professionals could concentrate on the care of patients rather than on insurance procedures, malpractice liability, and other administrative distractions.

◯ Taxes already pay for a substantial amount of our health care expenditures.

◯ Providing all citizens the right to health care is good for economic productivity because it allows them to live longer and healthier lives, thus contributing to society for a longer time.

## Arguments against National Health Insurance

◯ Health care is not a right, because it is not in the Bill of Rights in the U.S. Constitution, which lists rights that the government cannot infringe upon, not services or goods that the government must ensure for the people.

◯ It is the individual's responsibility, not the government's, to ensure personal health. Diseases and health problems can often be prevented by individuals choosing to live healthier lifestyles.

◯ Expenses for health care would have to be paid for with higher taxes or spending cuts in other areas such as defense and education.

◯ Profit motives, competition, and individual ingenuity have always led to greater cost control and effectiveness. These concepts should be brought to health care reform.

◯ Providing a right to health care is socialistic and is bad for economic productivity.

## Where Do You Stand?

◯ Do you think that all Americans should have the right to health care?

◯ Is health insurance a personal responsibility?

◯ Do you currently have health insurance? If you don't, what are the barriers that prevent you from having health insurance?

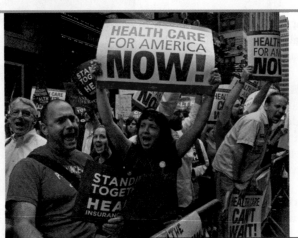

◯ If you do have health insurance, are you currently paying for it? If you are not paying for it, who is?

**Sources:** Right to Health Care ProCon.org, "Should All Americans Have the Right (Be Entitled) to Health Care?" Updated October 2010, http://healthcare.procon.org; The White House, "Health Care Reform: The Affordable Care Act," 2010, www .whitehouse.gov/healthreform/healthcare -overview.

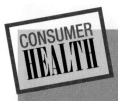

# PERSONAL ADVOCACY DURING A HEALTH CARE CRISIS

If you or a loved one faces a health care crisis, such as a heart attack, stroke, or unexpected surgery, it is important to act with knowledge, strength, and assertiveness. The following suggestions will help you deal with hospitals and health care providers.

**1. Know your rights as a patient.** Ask about the risks and costs of various diagnostic tests. Some procedures may pose significant risks for people who are older and can be replaced or supplemented by less invasive tests. When you get the results, ask for an explanation of any abnormalities. If you still don't understand them, ask for further clarification.

**2. Find out about informed consent procedures, living wills, durable power of attorney, organ donation, and other legal issues before you become sick.** Having someone shove a clipboard in your face and ask if life support can be terminated in case of a problem is one of the great horrors of many people's hospital experiences. Be prepared by taking care of these issues well in advance. If your parents or loved ones have not done so, encourage them to think about these

issues (see Chapter 21 for more on these topics).

**3. Remain with your loved one as a personal advocate.** If your loved one is weak and unable to ask questions, ask the questions for them. Inquire about new medications, tests, and other potentially risky procedures that may be undertaken during the course of treatment or recovery. If you feel that your loved one is being removed from intensive care or other closely monitored areas prematurely, ask if the hospital is taking this action to comply with diagnosis-related groups (DRGs) and if this action is warranted.

**4. Check the credentials of the health care providers.** Find out if the persons staffing the surgery unit, giving anaesthesia, and so on, are all part of your preferred provider insurance group. Many people are shocked to find that part-time staff members from unaffiliated hospitals are treating them, even in a preferred provider facility. When this happens, you may have to pay a much larger co-payment for out-of-group practitioners. Ask about the patient-to-staff ratio, and make sure that people monitoring you or your loved ones have appropriate credentials.

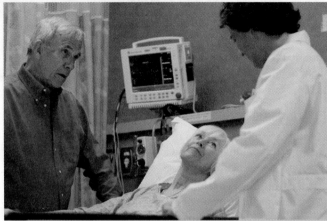

Facing a medical procedure is often frightening, but having a loved one present can help.

**5. Be considerate of the care providers.** One of the most stressful jobs is caring for a critically ill person. Although questions are appropriate and your emotions are running high, be as considerate and tactful as possible. Nurses often carry a disproportionately large responsibility for patient care and have a higher-than-optimal patient load. Try to remain out of their way, ask questions as necessary, and report any problems to the supervisor.

**6. Be patient with the patient.** The pain, suffering, and fears associated with surgery or other major medical events can cause otherwise nice

people to act in not-so-nice ways. Be patient and helpful, and allow time for the person to rest. Talk with the patient about his or her feelings, concerns, and fears. Do not ignore these concerns to ease your own anxieties. A wide range of psychological and physical problems, including severe depression, can occur in the aftermath of illness, as people struggle to deal with physical limitations, rehabilitation, lifestyle changes, and the recognition of their own vulnerability and mortality. Guilt and frustration can be challenges for survivors and their families.

accredited by the appropriate agency. In addition, most insurance plans now require prior authorization and/or second opinions, not only to reduce costs but also to improve quality of care.

Consumer, provider, and advocacy groups focus on the great variation in quality as a major problem. A new form of quality measurement uses "outcome" as the primary indicator for measuring health care quality at the individual level. With outcome measurements, we don't look just at what is done to the patient, but at what subsequently happens to the patient's health status. Thus, mortality rates and complication rates (e.g.,

infections) become important in assessing individual practitioners and facilities. On a personal level, perhaps the most important measurement is how you and your loved ones experience the health care provided. The **Consumer Health** box above offers some guidelines for ensuring that you receive the best care possible.

## what do you think?

Do you believe prospective patients should have access to information about practitioners' and facilities' malpractice records? ● How about their success and failure rates or outcomes of various procedures?

## Are You a Smart Health Care Consumer?

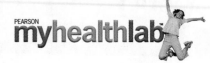

Fill out this assessment online at www.pearsonhighered.com/myhealthlab or www.pearsonhighered.com/donatelle.

Answer the following questions to determine what you might do to become a better health care consumer.

| | Yes | No |
|---|---|---|
| 1. Do you have health insurance? | ○ | ○ |
| 2. If you answered yes to question 1, do you understand the coverage available to you under your plan? | ○ | ○ |
| 3. Do you know which health care services are available for free or at a reduced cost at your student health center or local clinic? | ○ | ○ |
| 4. When you receive a prescription, do you ask the doctor or pharmacist if a generic brand could be substituted? | ○ | ○ |
| 5. When you receive a prescription, do you ask the doctor or pharmacist about potential side effects and interactions? | ○ | ○ |
| 6. Do you report any unusual drug side effects to your health care provider? | ○ | ○ |
| 7. Do you read labels carefully before buying over-the-counter (OTC) medications? | ○ | ○ |

| | Yes | No |
|---|---|---|
| 8. Do you take medication as directed? | ○ | ○ |
| 9. When you receive a diagnosis, do you seek more information about the diagnosis and treatment? | ○ | ○ |
| 10. When considering a CAM technique, do you research and identify scientific findings about the specific CAM therapy? | ○ | ○ |
| 11. Do you research the credentials of your practitioner before receiving treatment? | ○ | ○ |
| 12. Do you inform new practitioners of all the treatments you are currently receiving, including all CAM and traditional therapies? | ○ | ○ |
| 13. Do you choose only supplements with the USP (United States Pharmacopeia) seal on their labels? | ○ | ○ |
| 14. Do you consult a physician before taking a supplement? | ○ | ○ |

# YOUR PLAN FOR CHANGE

Once you have considered your responses to the **Assess yourself** questions, you may want to change or improve certain behaviors in order to get the best treatment from your health care provider and the heath care system.

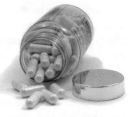

### Today, you can:

○ Research your insurance plan. Find out which health care providers and hospitals you can visit, the amounts of co-payments and premiums you are responsible for, and the drug coverage of your plan.

○ Update your medicine cabinet. Dispose properly of any expired prescriptions or OTC medications. Keep on hand a supply of basic items, such as pain relievers, antiseptic cream, bandages, cough suppressants, and throat lozenges.

### Within the next 2 weeks, you can:

○ Find a regular health care provider if you do not already have one and make an appointment for a general checkup.

○ Check with your insurance provider and see what CAM practitioners and therapies are covered.

○ Find out what alternative therapies your college's health clinic offers.

### By the end of the semester, you can:

○ Become an advocate for others' health. Write to your congressperson or state legislature to express your interest in health care reform.

○ Make relaxation and mind–body stress-reducing techniques a part of your everyday life. This can simply mean practicing meditation, deep breathing, or even taking long walks in nature. You don't need to visit a CAM practitioner or follow a specific therapeutic practice to benefit from methods of relaxation, meditation, and spiritual awakening.

# Summary

* Self-care and individual responsibility are key factors in reducing rising health care costs and improving health status. Advance planning can help you navigate health care treatment in unfamiliar situations or emergencies. Assess health professionals by considering their qualifications, their record of treating similar problems, and their ability to work with you.

* In theory, conventional Western (allopathic) medicine is based on scientifically validated methods and procedures. Medical doctors, specialists of various kinds, nurses, physician assistants, and other health care professionals practice allopathic medicine.

* Throughout the world people are using complementary and alternative medicine (CAM) in increasing numbers. Alternative medical systems include traditional Chinese medicine (TCM), Ayurveda, homeopathy, and naturopathy. CAM also includes manipulative and body-based practices, use of energy medicine, mind–body medicine, and biologically based practices.

* Consumers need to understand the risks and benefits of prescription drugs, over-the-counter (OTC) medications, and herbal products and supplements. Regulations governing drug labels help ensure that information about these products is available.

* Health insurance is based on the concept of spreading risk. Insurance is provided by private insurance companies (which charge premiums) and the government Medicare and Medicaid programs (which are funded by taxes). Managed care (in the form of HMOs, POS plans, and PPOs) attempts to control costs by streamlining administrative procedures and stressing preventive care, among other initiatives.

* Concerns about the U.S. health care system include cost, access, choice of treatment modality, quality and malpractice.

# Pop Quiz

1. Which of the following is not a condition that would indicate a visit to a physician is needed?
   a. Recurring high temperature (over 103°F in adults)
   b. Persistent or recurrent diarrhea
   c. The common cold
   d. Yellowing of the skin or the whites of the eyes

2. What medical practice is based on procedures whose objective is to heal by countering the patient's symptoms?
   a. Allopathic medicine
   b. Nonallopathic medicine
   c. Osteopathic medicine
   d. Chiropractic medicine

3. What mechanism used by private insurance companies requires that the subscriber pay a certain amount directly to the provider before the insurance company will begin paying for services?
   a. Coinsurance
   b. Cost sharing
   c. Co-payments
   d. Deductibles

4. Deborah, 28, is a single parent on welfare. Her medical bills are paid by a federal health insurance program for the poor. This agency is
   a. an HMO.
   b. Social Security.
   c. Medicaid.
   d. Medicare

5. CAM therapies focus on treating both the mind and the whole body, which makes them part of a
   a. natural approach.
   b. psychological approach.
   c. holistic approach.
   d. gentle approach.

6. What type of medicine addresses imbalances of *qi*?
   a. Chiropractic medicine
   b. Naturopathic medicine
   c. Traditional Chinese medicine
   d. Homeopathic medicine

7. The alternative system of medicine based on the principle that "like cures like" is
   a. naturopathic medicine.
   b. homeopathic medicine.
   c. Ayurvedic medicine.
   d. chiropractic medicine.

8. The use of techniques to improve the psychoneuroimmunology of the human body is called
   a. acupressure.
   b. mind–body medicine.
   c. Reiki.
   d. bodywork.

9. What system places equal emphasis on body, mind, and spirit and strives to restore the innate harmony of the individual?
   a. Ayurvedic medicine
   b. Homeopathic medicine
   c. Naturopathic medicine
   d. Traditional Chinese medicine

10. The "USP Dietary Supplement Verified" seal indicates that a supplement is
    a. safe and pure.
    b. effective.
    c. low cost.
    d. child safe.

*Answers for these questions can be found on page A-1.*

# Think about It!

1. List several conditions (resulting from illness or accident) for which you wouldn't need to seek medical help. When would you consider each condition to be bad enough to require medical attention? How would you decide where to go for treatment?

2. Describe your rights as a patient. Have you ever received treatment that violated these rights? If so, what action, if any, did you take?
3. Discuss how medical and pharmaceutical waste has a negative impact on the environment. What are two ways in which you personally can reduce such waste?
4. What are some of the potential benefits and risks of CAM? Why do you think these practices and products are becoming so popular?
5. What can you do to ensure that you are receiving accurate information regarding CAM treatments or medicines? Which federal agency oversees CAM in the United States?

# Accessing Your Health on the Internet

The following websites explore further topics and issues related to personal health. For links to the websites below, visit the Companion Website for *Access to Health*, 12th Edition, at www.pearsonhighered.com/donatelle.

1. *Agency for Healthcare Research and Quality (AHRQ)*. AHRQ's website is a gateway to consumer health information. It provides links to sites that can address health care concerns and provide information on what questions to ask, what to look for, and what you should know when making critical decisions about personal care. www.ahrq.gov
2. *Food and Drug Administration (FDA)*. The FDA provides news on the latest government-approved home health tests and other health-related products. www.fda.gov
3. *The Leapfrog Group*. A nationwide coalition of more than 150 public and private organizations, the Leapfrog Group focuses on identifying and devising solutions for problems in the U.S. hospital system that can lead to medical errors. www.leapfroggroup.org
4. *National Committee for Quality Assurance (NCQA)*. The NCQA

assesses and reports on the quality of managed care plans, including HMOs. www.ncqa.org
5. *HealthCare.Gov*. This site provides up-to-date information regarding the 2010 Patient Protection and Affordable Care Act, which mandates health insurance for previously uninsured Americans. www.healthcare.gov
6. *National Center for Complementary and Alternative Medicine (NCCAM)*. A division of the National Institutes of Health, NCCAM is dedicated to providing the latest information and research on complementary and alternative practices. http://nccam.nih.gov
7. *National Institutes of Health, Office of Dietary Supplements*. This excellent resource includes access to a database of federally funded research projects pertaining to dietary supplements. http://ods.od.nih.gov

# References

1. American Academy of Orthopaedic Surgeons, "Information Statement: The Importance of Good Communication in the Physician-Patient Relationship," September 2005, www.aaos.org/about/papers/advistmt/1017.asp.
2. MedicineNet, "Definition of Defensive Medicine," Reviewed June 2004, www.medterms.com/script/main/art.asp?articlekey=33262.
3. D. Merenstein et al., "Use and Costs of Nonrecommended Tests during Routine Preventive Health Exams," *American Journal of Preventive Medicine* 30, no. 6 (2006): 521–27; Thomson Reuters, "Waste in the U.S. Healthcare System Pegged at $700 Billion in Report from Thomson Reuters," October 26, 2009, http://thomsonreuters.com/content/press_room/tsh/waste_US_healthcare_system.
4. N. Kwon, "Patient Rights," 2006, www.emedicinehealth.com/patient_rights/article_em.htm.
5. American College Health Association, *American College Health Association–National College Health Assessment (ACHA-NCHA) Reference Group Data Report Spring 2008* (Baltimore: American College Health Association, 2008), Available at www.achancha.org/reports_ACHA-NCHAoriginal.html.
6. Mayo Clinic Staff, "Complementary and Alternative Medicine: What Is It?" Mayo Clinic, October 2009, www.mayoclinic.com/health/alternative-medicine/PN00001.
7. National Center for Complementary and Alternative Medicine, "The Use of Complementary and Alternative Medicine in the United States," Updated December 2008, http://nccam.nih.gov/news/camstats/2007/camsurvey_fs1.htm.
8. J. Tsao, "Effectiveness of Massage Therapy for Chronic, Non-Malignant Pain: A Review," *Evidence-Based Complementary and Alternative Medicine* 4, no. 2 (2007): 165–79; National Cancer Institute, "Acupuncture: Human/ Clinical Studies," 2008, www.cancer.gov/cancertopics/pdq/cam/acupuncture/HealthProfessional/page6.
9. National Center for Complementary and Alternative Medicine, "The Use of Complementary and Alternative Medicine in the United States," 2008.
10. National Center for Complementary and Alternative Medicine, "Ayurvedic Medicine: An Introduction," NCCAM Publication no. D287, Updated July 2009, http://nccam.nih.gov/health/ayurveda/introduction.htm.
11. American Institute of Homeopathy, "Homeopathy: Efficacy and Evidence Base," 2007, http://homeopathyusa.org/homeopathy-now.html; Health Alternatives Online, "Homeopathy," 2008, www.healthalternativesonline.com/homeopathy.html.
12. National Center for Complementary and Alternative Medicine, "Chiropractic: An Introduction," NCCAM Publication no. D403, Modified November 2009, http://nccam.nih.gov/health/chiropractic/#intro.
13. Bureau of Labor Statistics, U.S. Department of Labor, "Chiropractors," *Occupational Outlook Handbook, 2010–11 Edition*, December 2009, www.bls.gov/oco/ocos071.htm.
14. J. Tsao, "Effectiveness of Massage Therapy for Chronic, Non-Malignant Pain," 2007.
15. National Center for Complementary and Alternative Medicine, "Massage Therapy: An Introduction," NCCAM Publication no. D327, Updated June 2009, http://nccam.nih.gov/health/massage.
16. Mayo Clinic Staff, "Massage: Get in Touch with Its Many Health Benefits," January 2010, www.mayoclinic.com/health/massage/SA00082; National Center for Complementary and Alternative Medicine, "Massage Therapy," 2009.
17. National Center for Complementary and Alternative Medicine, "Massage Therapy," 2009.

18. Bureau of Labor Statistics, U.S. Department of Labor, "Massage Therapists," *Occupational Outlook Handbook, 2010–11 Edition,* Modified December 2009, www.bls.gov/oco/ocos295.htm.

19. National Center for Complementary and Alternative Medicine, "What Is CAM?" Updated April 2010, http://nccam.nih.gov/health/whatiscam; U.S. Trager Association, "The Trager Approach," 2010, www.trager-us.org/trager-approach.html.

20. National Center for Complementary and Alternative Medicine, "What Is CAM?" 2010.

21. American Cancer Society, "Acupuncture," 2010, www.cancer.org/docroot/ETO/content/ETO_5_3X_Acupuncture.asp.

22. National Center for Complementary and Alternative Medicine, "Acupuncture: An Introduction," NCCAM Publication no. D404, Modified October 2009, http://nccam.nih.gov/health/acupuncture/introduction.htm.

23. B. Seaward, *Managing Stress,* 6th ed. (Sudbury, MA: Jones and Bartlett, 2009); D. Tosevski and M. Milovancevic, "Stressful Life Events and Physical Health," *Current Opinion in Psychiatry* 19, no. 2 (2006): 184–89.

24. J. Robins et al., "Research in Psychoneuroimmunology: Tai Chi as a Stress Management Approach for Individuals with HIV Disease," *Applied Nursing Research* 19, no. 1 (February 2006): 2–9; M. Opp et al., "Sleep and Psychoneuroimmunology," *Immunology and Allergy Clinics of North America* 29, no. 2 (May 2009): 295–307; A. Starkweather et al., "Immune Function, Pain, and Psychological Stress in Patients Undergoing Spinal Surgery," *Spine* 31, no. 18 (August 2006): E641–E647.

25. Office of Dietary Supplements, National Institutes of Health, "Dietary Supplements: Background Information," Updated July 2009, http://ods.od.nih.gov/factsheets/dietarysupplements.asp.

26. National Center for Complementary and Alternative Medicine, "Kava," June 2008, http://nccam.nih.gov/health/kava/ataglance.htm.

27. Mayo Clinic Staff, "Herbal Supplements: What to Know before You Buy," November 2009, www.mayoclinic.com/health/herbal-supplements/SA00044.

28. R. A. Cohen et al., "Health Insurance Coverage: Early Release of Estimates from the *National Health Interview Survey,* 2009," 2010, www.cdc.gov/nchs/data/nhis/earlyrelease/insur201006.htm.

29. C. Schoen et al., "How Many Are Underinsured? Trends among U.S. Adults, 2003 and 2007," *Health Affairs* Web Exclusive (June 10, 2008): w298–w309.

30. R. A. Cohen et al., "Health Insurance Coverage," 2010.

31. Lookout Mountain Group, "Analysis and Policy Recommendations for Providing Health Insurance and Health Care for the College Student Population," June 2, 2009, www.hbc-slba.com/LMG/LMG_abstract_3.5.pdf.

32. National Center for Health Statistics, *Health, United States, 2009, with Special Feature on Medical Technology* (Hyattsville, MD: National Center for Health Statistics, 2010), Available at www.cdc.gov/nchs/hus.htm.

33. Kaiser Family Foundation, "Total HMO Enrollment, July 2008," 2009, www.statehealthfacts.org/comparemaptable.jsp?ind=348&cat=7.

34. Centers for Medicare and Medicaid Services, "NHE Fact Sheet," Modified June 29, 2010, https://www.cms.gov/NationalHealthExpendData/25_NHE_Fact_Sheet.asp.

35. Centers for Medicare and Medicaid Services, "Medicare Enrollment: National Trends 1966–2008," Modified October 2009, https://www.cms.gov/MedicareEnRpts/01_Overview.asp.

36. Centers for Medicare and Medicaid Services, "Medicaid Data Sources—General Information," Modified December 2005, www.cms.gov/MedicaidDataSourcesGenInfo.

37. National Center for Health Statistics, *Health, United States, 2009, with Special Feature on Medical Technology,* 2010; Centers for Medicare and Medicaid Services, "National Health Care Expenditures Projections: 2009–2019," 2009, Available at www.cms.gov/NationalHealthExpendData/03_NationalHealthAccountsProjected.asp.

38. National Center for Chronic Disease Prevention and Health Promotion, "Chronic Diseases and Health Promotion," Updated July 2010, www.cdc.gov/chronicdisease/overview/index.htm.

39. Ibid.

40. Bureau of Labor Statistics, U.S. Department of Labor, "Physicians and Surgeons," *Occupational Outlook Handbook, 2010–11,* Modified December 2009, www.bls.gov/oco/ocos074.htm.

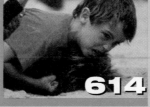
**614**
What makes some people act out their anger with violence?

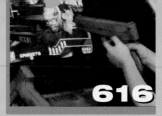
**616**
Does violence in the media cause violence in real life?

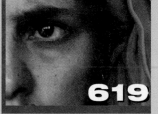
**619**
Why do people stay in abusive relationships?

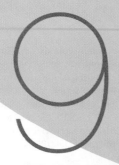

# 19
# Preventing Violence and Abuse

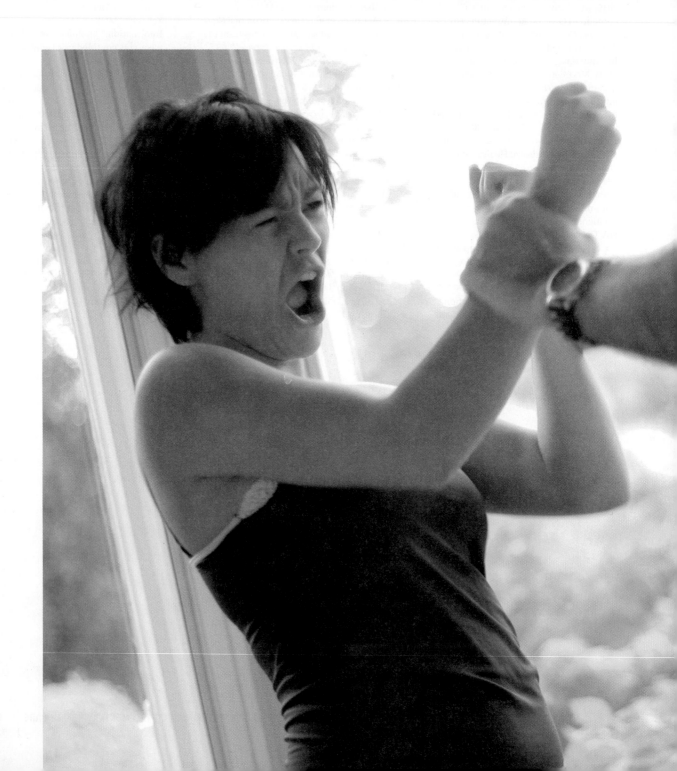

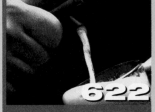
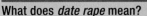

**622**

What does *date rape* mean?

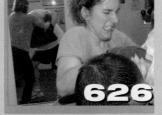

**626**

How can I protect myself from becoming a victim of violence?

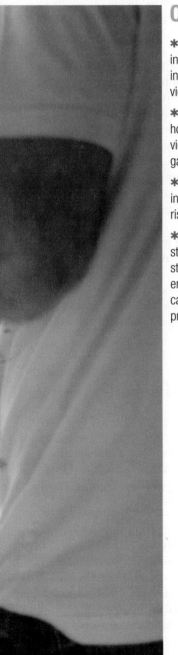

## Objectives

✳ Discuss the various types of intentional injuries, and societal and individual factors that contribute to violence in American society.

✳ Discuss factors that contribute to homicide, domestic violence, sexual victimization, child and elder abuse, gang violence, and terrorism.

✳ Discuss strategies to prevent intentional injuries and reduce their risk of occurrence.

✳ Explain potential risks of violence to students on campus and potential strategies that campus leaders, law enforcement officials, and individuals can develop to protect themselves and prevent others from becoming victims.

*Fear follows crime, and is its punishment.*
*—Voltaire, 1694–1778*

Acts of hatred and brutality have always played a major role in human history as humans struggle to dominate one another. Today, violence is pervasive and takes all forms, whether it be in the news report of a murdered child; the images of the terrorist attacks of September 11, 2001; or the Internet predator who hacks into online accounts to stalk a former girlfriend. In the wake of such violence, many people live in fear, even though they may not have experienced the violence personally. Are our fears justified? Is violence in the United States worse than ever? And what about college campuses—are they safe?

Before we can discuss the extent and nature of violence, it's important that we understand what the word *violence* means. The World Health Organization (WHO) defines **violence** as "the intentional use of physical force or power, threatened or actual, against oneself, another person, or against a group or community, that either results in or has a high likelihood of resulting in injury, death, pyschological harm, maldevelopment or deprivation."[1] Today, most experts realize that emotional and psychological forms of violence can be as devastating as physical blows to the body.

The U.S. Public Health Service categorizes violence resulting in injuries into either intentional injuries or unintentional injuries. **Intentional injuries**—those committed with intent to harm—typically include assaults, homicides, and self-directed injuries. **Unintentional injuries** are those committed without intent to harm.[2] Unintentional injuries are discussed in detail in Focus On: Reducing Your Risk of Unintentional Injury beginning on page 636.

Why do we focus attention on violence in an introductory health text for college and university students? The answer is simple: Violent and abusive interactions are common problems for young adults. In fact, homicides and suicides are the second and third leading causes of death in Americans aged 15 to 24.[3] Intimate partner violence, assaults, harassment, and psychological abuse are possible threats to student health. These forms of intentional injuries can hurt emotional health, leading to maladaptive behavior, suicide, drug abuse, poor grades, and high drop-out rates, among other problems.

**violence** A set of behaviors that produces injuries, as well as the outcomes of these behaviors (the injuries themselves).

**intentional injuries** Injury, death, psychological harm, maldevelopment, or deprivation that involves the intentional use of physical force or power, threatened or actual, against oneself, another person, or against a group or community.

**unintentional injuries** Injury, death, or harm that involves accidents committed without intent to harm, often as a result of circumstances, or without premeditation.

# Violence in the United States

Violence has been a part of the American landscape since colonial times; however, it wasn't until the 1980s that the U.S. Public Health Service identified violence as a leading cause of

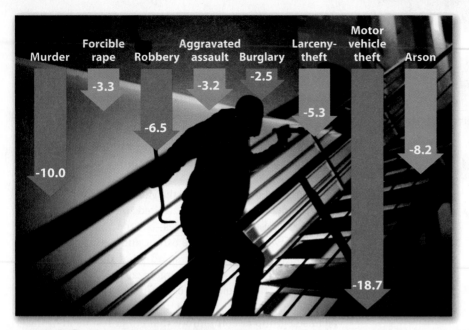

Murder  Forcible rape  Robbery  Aggravated assault  Burglary  Motor vehicle theft  Larceny-theft  Arson

-3.3  -6.5  -3.2  -2.5  -5.3  -8.2  -10.0  -18.7

**93%** of crimes against college students occur at off-campus locations.

**FIGURE 19.1 Declining Crime Rates**

According to the FBI's *Preliminary Semiannual Uniform Crime Report,* violent crime in the nation dropped 4.4 percent and property crime declined 6.1 percent during the first 6 months of 2009, compared to the same period in 2008.

**Source:** Adapted from U.S. Department of Justice, Federal Bureau of Investigation, *Crime in the United States, Preliminary Semiannual Uniform Crime Report 2009,* 2009.

death and disability and gave it chronic disease status, indicating that it was a pervasive threat to society. Statistics from the Federal Bureau of Investigation (FBI) have shown that, after steadily increasing from 1973 to 2006, the rates of overall crime and certain types of violent crime have been decreasing over the past few years. Violent crimes involve force or threat of force, and include four offenses: *murder and nonnegligent manslaughter, forcible rape, robbery,* and *aggravated assault.* During the first 6 months of 2009, violent crime in the United States decreased 4.4 percent compared to the same time period in 2008 and property crime also showed significant decreases **(Figure 19.1).**[4]

Why be so concerned about violence if the major forms of violent crime are on a downward trend? The answer is that *any* violence affects us all. Even if we have never been victimized personally, we all are victimized by violent acts that cause us to be fearful; impinge on our liberty; and damage the reputation of our campus or city, or our nation in the international community.

## Violence on U.S. Campuses

On April 16, 2007, the most deadly mass shooting in U.S. history took place at Virginia Tech. The tragedy sparked dialogue and action on campuses across the nation and throughout the world. A year later, when the February 14, 2008, shootings at Northern Illinois University sent another shock wave across college campuses, increased priorities were put on campus security and student and faculty safety. Today, it would be hard to find a campus without a safety

plan in place to prevent and respond to this type of violent crime.

Relationship violence is one of the most prevalent problems on college campuses. In the most recent American College Health Association's survey, 11 percent of women and 7 percent of men reported being emotionally abused in the past 12 months by a significant other. Two percent of men and 2 percent of women reported being involved in a physically abusive relationship. Another 1 percent of men and 2 percent of women reported being in a sexually abusive relationship.[5]

The statistics on reported violence on campus represent only a glimpse of the big picture. It is believed that fewer than 25 percent of campus crimes in general are reported to *any* authority. Even though as many as 20 to 25 percent of college women will be raped or sexually assaulted before they graduate, 95 percent of these women never report these crimes.[6] Why would students fail to report crimes? Typical reasons include concerns over privacy, fear of retaliation, embarrassment or shame, lack of support, perception that the crime was too minor, or uncertainty that it was a crime. This is particularly true in the case of crimes such as acquaintance rape, stalking, and hazing. See the **Student Health Today** boxes on pages 613 and 614 for further exploration of these issues.

## Factors Contributing to Violence

Several social, community, relationship, and individual factors increase the likelihood of violent acts, as discussed in the following list:[7]

- **Poverty.** Low socioeconomic status can create an environment of hopelessness in which some people view violence as the only way of obtaining what they want.
- **Unemployment.** Financial strain, losing or fear of losing a job, economic downturns, and living in economically depressed areas can increase rates and severity of violence.[8]
- **Parental influence.** Children raised in environments in which shouting, hitting, emotional abuse, antisocial

# SEXUAL ASSAULT: A CULTURE OF SILENCE?

How many students do you think are sexually assaulted during a typical year on campus? Would it surprise you to know that the majority of colleges and universities indicate that there were zero rapes or sexual assaults on their campuses during the past year? A sexual assault prevention program at one major university had over 46 sexual assault clients in a recent academic year, yet none of these reports showed up in the university's annual security report. Likewise, a counseling and victim advocacy program at a large midwestern university served 62 students, faculty, and staff who reported being raped or almost raped in the past fiscal year. Those assaults didn't show up on university reports either. In fact, in 2006, out of 3,068 four-year colleges and universities 77 percent reported zero sexual offenses! Another 501 reported just one or two sexual offenses. How can this be?

A federal law known as the Clery Act requires colleges and universities to solicit information about crime from women's centers, student health centers, residence hall directors, coaches, and the like and to report this information. But Clery statistics are "official statistics," meaning that a victim must report an assault to campus security for the assault to be listed. If victims talk only with campus counselors and not to security officers as well, confidentiality issues prevent counselors from reporting these cases. Thus, for a variety of reasons, the Clery Act isn't working as it was intended.

Why are victims so unwilling to report crimes? The answers are complex. According to the Center for Public Integrity, which has been conducting an ongoing investigation into the problem, they typically include the following:

✴ Victims often blame themselves for getting into a dangerous situation.

✴ Drinking too much is often cited as a contributor and many feel if they hadn't had so much to drink, their assault might not have happened.

✴ Often there are no witnesses and the difficulty in proving that sexual assault occurred in a "he said, she said" situation is more than victims can manage.

✴ Conflicting lines of authority among local police, campus police, and university officials can block swift action. Rape is a felony, so some question whether hearings and other disciplinary actions should be conducted on campus or whether police should handle such matters exclusively.

✴ Lengthy university hearings and investigations can pose a heavy burden on victims and their families, leading many to drop charges.

✴ Victims fear retaliation or ostracism or being labeled as promiscuous or a troublemaker.

Although efforts are underway to change campus culture by educating students about their options, informing counselors and support staff of their responsibilities

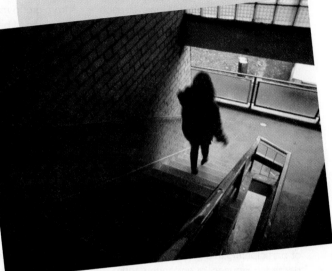

The reluctance to report sexual assault on campus, and the difficulty of pursuing criminal proceedings in the campus environment can create turmoil in victims' lives while too rarely leading to punishment of offenders.

and legal ramifications of their acts, including men in the dialogue about appropriate and inappropriate intimate partner behaviors, and improving reporting protocols, the process is slow. Campuses fear negative public relations when reports of rape and sexual assault appear in the newspaper. Should such reports be used for comparative data as parents help their children pick schools, campus images could be tarnished, having direct effects on enrollments.

**Sources:** Center for Public Integrity, "Sexual Assault on Campus: A Frustrating Search for Justice," Updated February 2010, www.publicintegrity.org/investigations/campus_assault; Center for Public Integrity, "Barriers Curb Reporting on Campus Sexual Assault," 2009, www.publicintegrity.org/investigations/campus_assault/articles/entry/1822.

behavior, and other forms of violence are commonplace are more apt to act out these behaviors as adults.[9]

● **Cultural beliefs.** Cultures that objectify women and empower men to be tough and aggressive show higher rates of violence in the home.[10]

● **Discrimination or oppression.** Whenever one group is oppressed or perceives that its members are oppressed by those of another group, violence against others is more likely.

● **Religious beliefs and differences.** Strong religious beliefs can lead people to think that violence against others is justified.

● **Political differences.** Civil unrest and differences in political party affiliations and beliefs have historically been triggers for violent acts.

● **Breakdowns in the criminal justice system.** Overcrowded prisons, lenient sentences, early releases from prison, and trial errors subtly encourage violence in many ways.

# HAZING: OVER THE TOP AND DANGEROUS FOR MANY

We've all seen instances of hazing—those silly, humiliating things sorority or fraternity initiates, rookie team members, or new club recruits are asked to do to show their willingness to belong. However, each year on U.S. campuses, students are asked to do things for "initiation" that may actually put them in harm's way. In fact, each year there are reports of deaths and injuries, as well as lawsuits brought against various campus organizations for real or perceived harm caused by hazing. Currently, hazing is considered a crime in 44 states. Most institutions have policies against hazing, but few students ever report it, and only when high-profile cases make it to the mainstream media do most of us pay attention to what goes on in these selective organizations.

Just what is hazing? Essentially it is "any activity expected of someone joining or participating in a group that humiliates, degrades, abuses, or endangers them regardless of a person's willingness to participate." Typically, it involves forcing students to consume excessive alcohol; dress in humiliating garb; undergo forced sleep deprivation; endure verbal abuse from group members; or physical abuse in the form of beatings, heat or cold exposure, or forced sexual acts. These activities can range from practical jokes to situations where life and limb are endangered. For those who are victimized and don't find their forced hazing humorous, psychological and physical damage can be serious.

But how much of a problem is hazing on today's campuses? According to a recent national study, 55 percent of college students involved in clubs, teams, and organizations experience hazing and 47 percent of students come to college already having experienced hazing. Yet many students are unaware of the dangers or legal implications of hazing, and, in fact, 9 out of 10 students who experience hazing in college do not think they've been hazed.

In 95 percent of the cases in which students identified their experience as hazing, they did not report the events to campus officials. There may be several reasons for this underreporting, but one reason seems to be that more students perceive positive rather than negative outcomes of hazing, for example, feeling a sense of accomplishment or belonging. Students also report their schools' administrations do little to prevent hazing beyond maintaining a "hazing is not tolerated" stance. If schools are to have an impact on the prevalence of hazing on their campuses, they will need to design broader intervention and prevention efforts, and work to educate their campus community on the physical and legal perils of hazing.

**Source:** Adapted from E. Allan and M. Madden, *Hazing in View: College Students at Risk* (Orono, ME: National Collaborative for Hazing Research and Prevention, 2008), www.hazingstudy.org. Used with permission.

- **Stress.** People who are in crisis or under stress are more apt to be highly reactive, striking out at others or acting irrationally.
- **Heavy use of alcohol and other substances.** Alcohol and drug abuse are often catalysts for violence and are risk factors for domestic violence and other crimes.[11]

## What Makes Some People Prone to Violence?

In addition to the broad, societally based factors that contribute to crime, personal factors also can increase risks for violence. Why might two children from the same neighborhood, or even from the same family, be affected differently by violence? There are several predictors of future aggressive behavior.[12]

**Anger** *Anger* is a spontaneous, usually temporary, biological feeling or emotional

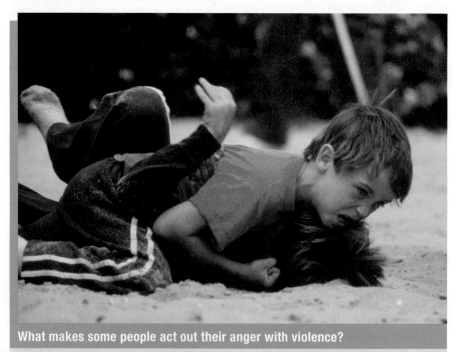

**What makes some people act out their anger with violence?**

If you are like most people, you probably acted out your anger more as a child than you do today. With age and maturity, most people learn to control outbursts of anger in a socially acceptable and rational manner. However, some people go through life acting out their aggressive tendencies in much the same way they did as children—with anger and violence that are a form of self-assertion or a response to frustration.

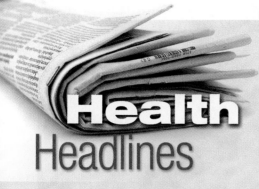

# Health Headlines

## ROAD RAGE: SEETHING BEHIND THE WHEEL

Has someone ever scared you with a bout of road rage while you were in a car? If so, you are not alone. According to a study conducted by the National Institute of Mental Health, intermittent explosive disorder (IED) affects over 7.3 percent of all adults—up to 16 million Americans—in their lifetime. One common form of IED is *road rage,* an episode that occurs while a person is driving and that is believed to be a leading cause of highway deaths.

Although you cannot control or predict the behavior of others, there are several steps you can take to avoid becoming a victim of road rage:

* **Avoid eye contact and engagement.** If you are driving or out in public and someone tries getting a reaction from you, avoid confrontation, and remove yourself from the situation.
* **Don't antagonize.** Slowing down in traffic to bug someone in an obvious hurry, honking your horn, flashing your high beams at someone, or other passive-aggressive gestures can upset even the most mild-mannered people.
* **If someone follows you after a nasty interaction, either in a car or on foot, do not immediately drive home or walk into your workplace.** If you are driving, head for the nearest police station or area where there are lots of cars and traffic. Never isolate yourself.
* **Take names.** If you don't know the person, try keeping a mental description or get a license plate number if driving. Report offenders, even if you are afraid of getting involved.

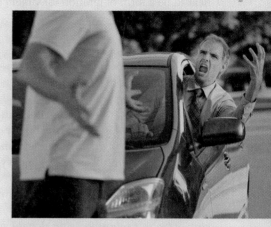

For people prone to road rage, even minor inconveniences occurring while they are driving can prompt a violent reaction.

* **Stay calm.** Think before opening your mouth, and practice stress management whenever possible.

**Source:** Data point from R. Kessler, "The Prevalence and Correlates of *DSM-IV* Intermittent Explosive Disorder in the National Comorbidity Survey Replication,"*Archives of General Psychiatry* 63, no. 6 (2006): 669–78. Copyright © 2006 American Medical Association. All rights reserved.

---

state of displeasure that occurs most frequently during times of personal frustration. If life is stressful, anger can become a daily experience. Anger can range from slight irritation to *rage,* a violent and extreme form of anger.

People who anger quickly often have a low tolerance for frustration. The cause may be genetic or physiological; there is evidence that some people are born with strong tendencies toward being angry. Family background may be the most important factor. Typically, anger-prone people come from families that are disruptive, chaotic, and unskilled in emotional expression.[13] Another root of explosive anger is a sociocultural one. People who are taught not to express anger in public do not know how to handle it when it reaches a level they can no longer hide.

Aggressive behavior is often a key aspect of violent interactions. **Primary aggression** is goal-directed, hostile self-

### "Why Should I Care?"

The amount you drink tonight can directly affect your chances of becoming a victim of injury or assault. College students are particularly at risk for crimes committed under the influence of alcohol, including assault, rape, and intimate partner violence, but understanding the impact of alcohol in escalating potentially violent situations can help you stay out of harm's way.

assertion that is destructive in nature. **Reactive aggression** is more often part of an emotional reaction brought about by frustrating life experiences. Whether aggression is reactive or primary, it is most likely to flare up in times of acute stress.

For some people, sudden episodes of rage are related to a psychological disorder known as **intermittent explosive disorder (IED).** This disorder is characterized by repeated episodes of aggressive, violent behavior that are grossly out of proportion to the situation. When a person acts out his or her rage at home or on the road, the consequences can be deadly; see the **Health Headlines** box above on IED and road rage.

**Substance Abuse** Substance abuse and violence are closely linked, even though research has yet to show that substance abuse actually causes violence. In some

**primary aggression** Goal-directed, hostile self-assertion that is destructive in character.
**reactive aggression** Hostile emotional reaction brought about by frustrating life experiences.
**intermittent explosive disorder (IED)** A behavioral disorder characterized by repeated episodes of aggression and violent behavior that are disproportionate to the situation.

situations, psychoactive substances appear to be a form of ignition for violence. Consider the following:[14]

- Consumption of alcohol—by perpetrators of the crime, the victim, or both—immediately precedes over half of all violent crimes, including murder.
- Criminals using illegal drugs commit robberies and assaults more frequently than criminals who do not use them, and do so especially during periods of heavy drug use.
- In domestic assault cases, more than 86 percent of the assailants and 42 percent of victims reported using alcohol at the time of the attack. Nearly 15 percent of victims and assailants reported using cocaine at the time of the attack.
- Alcohol abuse, particularly binge drinking, is associated with physical victimization among males and sexual victimization (particularly rape) among females on college and university campuses.

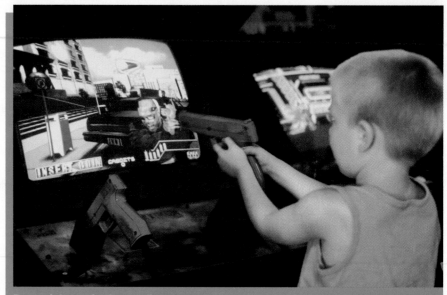

**Does violence in the media cause violence in real life?**

Evidence of the real-world effects of violence in the media is inconclusive. Arguably, Americans today—especially children—are exposed to more depictions of violence in the news, movies, music, and games than ever before, but research has not shown a clear link between a person's exposure to violent media and his or her propensity to engage in violent acts. Regardless, many people are concerned that children today are being exposed to more violence than they have the emotional or cognitive maturity to handle.

## How Much Impact Do the Media Have?

Does watching TV or playing video games make people violent? Although the media are blamed for having a major role in the escalation of violence, this association is not as clear as you might suspect. Several early studies in which people were surveyed about self-reported media use and involvement in various forms of violence seemed to support a link between excessive exposure to violent media and subsequent violent behavior. A recent study of the self-reported perceived behavior of nearly 1,600 young people, aged 10 to 15, indicated that there was a perception of significantly higher levels of shootings, stabbings, assault, robbery, and sexual assault among those who had watched higher amounts of violence in the media.[15]

Critics of such studies point out that today's young people are exposed to more media violence—on the Internet and TV, and in movies and video games—than any previous generation has been without any measurable impact on crime rates. Yet, just as media violence has exploded into our homes and lives, rates of violent crime and victimization among teens aged 10 to 17 have fallen to the lowest rates ever recorded.[16] According to the National Crime Victimization Survey, the violent crime rate declined by 41 percent and the property crime rate fell by 32 percent over the 10-year period from 1999 to 2008.[17] A meta-analysis of 26 studies examining the relationship between exposure to media violence and violent aggression did not support the idea that media violence and criminal aggression are positively associated.[18] In a rather unusual twist, some critics argue that playing violent video games or watching violent movies is actually cathartic for some and that people who engage in these activities report relieved stress and even feelings of exhaustion afterward.[19]

Concern has been raised that people who spend too much time in front of their big screen TV or online may miss the important communication lessons that come from talking with people in person, and learning to get along with others. In addition, debate continues over whether a person who sees so much violence enacted in the media becomes *desensitized* to violence. Most experts believe that multiple factors in a person's background and environment converge to precipitate violent deeds. Media exposure to violence may be only one piece of a very complex series of events in a person's history.

## Interpersonal Violence

Intentional injury can be categorized into three major types: *interpersonal violence, collective violence,* and *self-directed violence,* although there is some degree of overlap among these groups.[20] Interpersonal violence and collective violence

## TABLE 19.1 Per Capita Homicide Rates in Selected Nations

| Rank | Country | Homicide Rate |
|------|---------|---------------|
| 1 | Colombia | 0.617847 per 1,000 people |
| 2 | South Africa | 0.496008 per 1,000 people |
| 5 | Russia | 0.201534 per 1,000 people |
| 6 | Mexico | 0.130213 per 1,000 people |
| 16 | Zimbabwe | 0.0749938 per 1,000 people |
| 24 | United States | 0.042802 per 1,000 people |
| 26 | India | 0.0344083 per 1,000 people |
| 40 | France | 0.0173272 per 1,000 people |
| 43 | Australia | 0.0150324 per 1,000 people |
| 44 | Canada | 0.0149063 per 1,000 people |
| 55 | Ireland | 0.00946215 per 1,000 people |
| 60 | Japan | 0.00499933 per 1,000 people |
| 61 | Saudi Arabia | 0.00397456 per 1,000 people |

**Source:** Nationmaster, "Crime Statistics: Murders (per capita) (most recent) by Country," www.nationmaster.com/graph/cri_mur_percap-crime-murders-per -capita, Accessed March 2010. Used with permission.

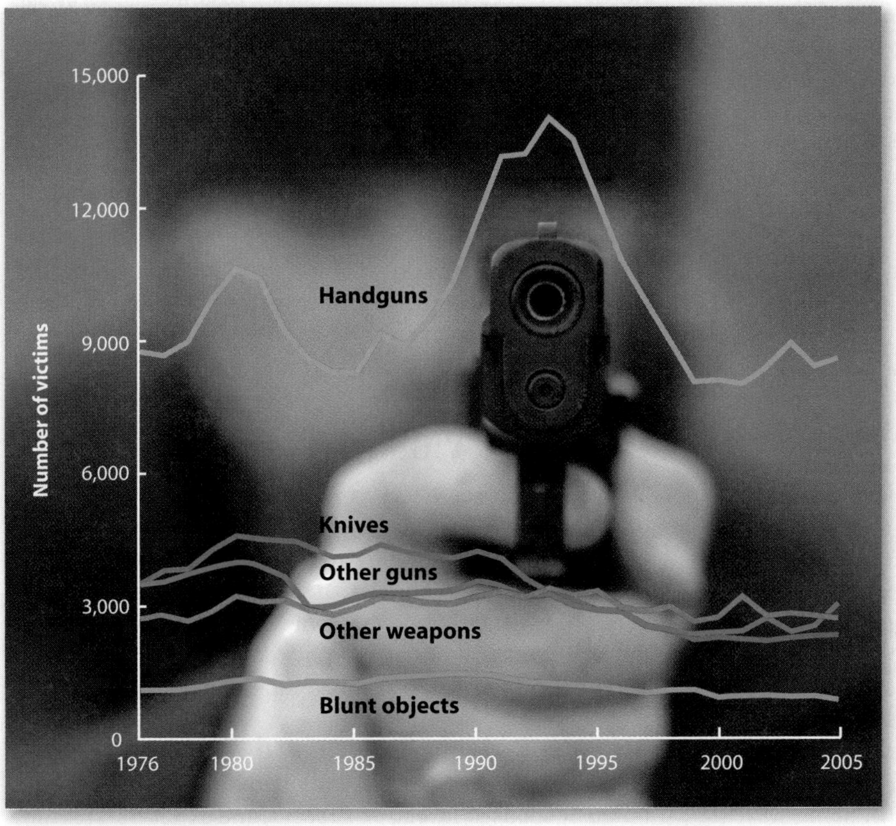

FIGURE 19.2 **Homicide in the United States by Weapon Type, 1976–2005**
Like the homicide rate generally, gun-involved incidents increased sharply in the late 1980s and early 1990s before falling to a low in 1999. The number of gun-involved homicides increased thereafter to levels experienced in the mid-1980s.

**Source:** Adapted from J. Fox and M. Zawitz, *Homicide Trends in the United States,* U.S. Department of Justice, Office of Justice Programs, Bureau of Justice Statistics, Revised 2007, http://bjs.ojp.usdoj.gov/ content/homicide/weapons.cfm.

are discussed below. Self-directed violence, including suicide and self-mutilation, is discussed in Chapter 2. **Interpersonal violence** includes violence inflicted against one individual by another, or a small group of others; homicide, hate crimes, domestic violence, child abuse, elder abuse, and sexual victimization all fit into this category.

**interpersonal violence** Violence inflicted against one individual by another, or a small group of others.
**homicide** Death that results from intent to injure or kill.

## Homicide

**Homicide,** defined as murder or non-negligent manslaughter, is the fifteenth leading cause of death in the United States, but the second leading cause of death for persons aged 15 to 24. It accounts for more than 17,000 premature deaths in the United States annually.[21] Most homicides are not random acts of violence: Over half of all homicides occur among people who know one another. In two-thirds of these cases, the perpetrator and the victim are friends or acquaintances; in one-third, they belong to the same family.[22]

**what do you think?**
Do you think the general populace should be allowed to carry guns? ● Should students be allowed to carry guns? ● If you think guns should be controlled, what is the best way for government agencies to regulate their use?

Homicide rates reveal clear differences across races and ages. Whereas overall homicide rates in the United States have fluctuated minimally and have even decreased in some populations, those involving young victims and perpetrators, particularly young black males, have surged. From 2002 to 2007, the number of homicides involving black male victims, aged 15 to 24, rose by 31 percent, and those involving them as perpetrators increased by 41 percent.[23] How do homicide rates compare by race in general? Overall, in 2008 in the United States, population-based rates of homicide were 3.3 per 100,000 for whites, 20.6 per 100,000 for blacks, and 2.5 per 100,000 for all other races combined.[24]

The rates of homicide in the United States are higher than in many other developed nations (Table 19.1). As Figure 19.2 shows, the number of gun-related homicides in the United States is particularly high; handguns are consistently responsible for more murders than any other single type of weapon.[25] Today, 35 percent of American homes have a gun on the premises, with more than 283 million privately owned guns registered—40 percent of which are handguns.[26] However, the number of guns available doesn't entirely account for the high rates of gun-related homicide in the United States. Countries such as Canada with similar household possessions of guns have much different gun-related crime rates than does the United States: In 2006, there were 12,791 murders by firearms in the United States, compared to only 190 in Canada.[27]

## Hate and Bias-Motivated Crimes

A **hate crime** is a crime committed against a person, property, or group of people that is motivated by the offender's bias against a race, religion, disability, sexual orientation, or ethnicity. In spite of national efforts to promote understanding and appreciation of diversity in workplaces, schools, and communities, intolerance of differences continues to smolder in many parts of U.S. society. According to the FBI's most recent *Hate Crime Statistics* report, there were 9,691 reported victims of hate crimes in 2008 (Figure 19.3).[28] Over 61 percent of the persons who committed these crimes were white, 20 percent were black, and the remaining offenders' race was unknown.[29]

*Bias-related crime*, both on campus and in the community, is sometimes referred to as **ethnoviolence,** a word that describes violence among ethnic groups in the larger society that is based on prejudice and discrimination. **Prejudice** is an irrational attitude of hostility directed against an individual; a group; a race; or the supposed characteristics of an individual, group, or race. **Discrimination** constitutes actions that deny equal treatment or opportunities to a group of people, often based on prejudice. Often prejudice and discrimination stem from a fear of change and a desire to blame others when forces such as the economy and crime seem to be out of control.

**hate crime** A crime targeted against a particular societal group and motivated by bias against that group.
**ethnoviolence** Violence directed at persons affiliated with a particular, usually ethnic, group.
**prejudice** A negative evaluation of an entire group of people that is typically based on unfavorable and often wrong ideas about the group.
**discrimination** Actions that deny equal treatment or opportunities to a group, often based on prejudice.
**domestic violence** The use of force to control and maintain power over another person in the home environment, including both actual harm and the threat of harm.

# 70%
**of all hate crimes are committed against a person or persons; the rest are crimes against property.**

Common reasons given to explain bias-related and hate crimes include (1) *thrill seeking* by multiple offenders through a group attack; (2) *feeling threatened* that others will take their jobs or property or best them in some way; (3) *retaliating* for some real or perceived insult or slight; and (4) *fearing the unknown or differences.* For other people, hate crimes are a part of their mission in life, either due to religious zeal or distorted moral beliefs.

Nearly 12 percent of all bias-related and hate crimes occur on campuses, and schools and colleges have the fastest growing risks for such crimes.[30] Campuses have responded to

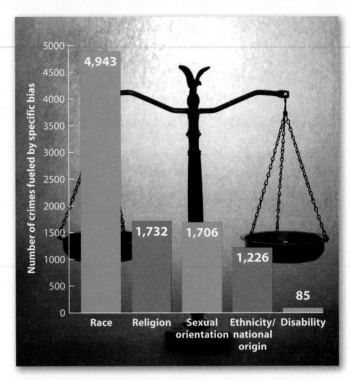

FIGURE 19.3 **Bias-Motivated Crimes, 2008, Breakdown by Bias**
There were 9,691 reported victims (including individuals, businesses, and institutions) of bias-motivated hate crimes in the United States in 2008.

**Source:** Adapted from Federal Bureau of Investigation, "Hate Crime: New Stats and a New Law," Press release, November 23, 2009, www.fbi.gov/page2/nov09/hatecrimes_112309.html.

reports of hate crimes by offering courses that emphasize diversity, training faculty appropriately, and developing policies that strictly enforce punishment for hate crimes.[31] Sadly, many minor assaults do go unreported, because the victims fear retaliation or continued stigmatization.

## Domestic Violence

**Domestic violence** refers to the use of force to control and maintain power over another person in the home environment. It can occur between parent and child, between spouses or intimate partners, or between siblings or other family members. The violence may involve emotional abuse; verbal abuse; threats of physical harm; and physical violence ranging from slapping and shoving to beatings, rape, and homicide.

**Intimate Partner Violence and Women** Women are more likely than men to become victims of violent acts perpetrated by spouses, lovers, ex-spouses, and ex-lovers. This form of domestic violence is known as **intimate partner violence (IPV).** The aggression often includes pushing, slapping, and shoving, but it can take more severe forms.

In 2008, about 552,000 nonfatal violent victimizations from an intimate partner were experienced by U.S. females aged 12 and older and about 101,000 were experienced by U.S. men.[32] Every year IPV results in more than 1,500 deaths, about 78 percent of which are women.[33] Homicide committed by a current or former intimate partner is the leading cause of death of pregnant women in the United States.[34] In addition, 74 percent of all murder-suicides in the United States involve an intimate partner.[35] Women are not the only victims of intimate partner violence; the **Gender & Health** box on page 620 explores some of the issues surrounding male victimization.

**The Cycle of Violence** Have you ever heard of a woman who is repeatedly beaten by her partner and wondered, "Why doesn't she just leave him?" There are many reasons some women find it difficult to break their ties with their abusers. Some women, particularly those with small children, are financially dependent on their partners. Others fear retaliation against themselves or their children. Some hope the situation will change with time, and others stay because cultural or religious beliefs forbid divorce. Finally, some women still love the abusive partner and are concerned about what will happen to him if they leave.

In the 1970s, psychologist Lenore Walker developed a theory called the *cycle of violence* that explained predictable, repetitive patterns of psychological and/or physical abuse that seemed to occur in abusive relationships.[36] Over the years, Walker's initial work has been criticized for its lack of scientific rigor, anecdotal approach, and seeming overstatement of selected patterns as universal truths. In her most recent book, *The Battered Woman Syndrome,* Walker responds to many of her early critics with improved quantitative analysis, reviews of recent research, and an extensive list of experts in the field of violence.[37]

Today, the cycle of violence continues to be important to understanding why people stay in otherwise unhealthy relationships. The cycle consists of three major phases:

**1. Tension building.** This phase typically occurs prior to the overtly abusive act and includes breakdowns in communication, anger, psychological aggression and violent language, growing tension, and fear.

**2. Incident of acute battering.** At this stage, the batterer usually is trying to "teach her a lesson," and when he feels he has inflicted enough pain, he'll stop. When the acute attack is over, he may respond with shock and denial about his own behavior or blame her for making him do it.

**3. Remorse/reconciliation.** During this "honeymoon" period, the batterer may be kind, loving, and apologetic, swearing that he will never act violently again and will work to change his behavior. However, when the same things that triggered past abuse begin to resurface, the cycle starts over again.

For a woman who gets caught in this cycle, it is often very hard to summon the resolution to extricate herself. Most need effective outside intervention.

**Causes of Domestic Violence** There is no single reason to explain why people tend to be abusive in relationships. Alcohol abuse is often associated with such violence, and marital dissatisfaction is also a predictor. Numerous studies also point to differences in the communication patterns between abusive and nonabusive relationships. Many experts believe

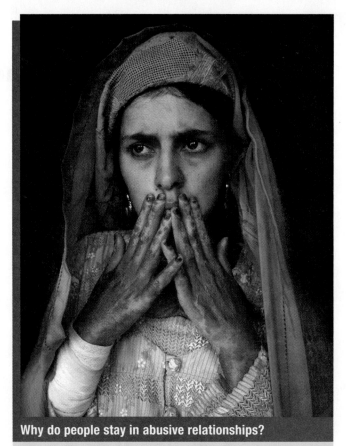

**Why do people stay in abusive relationships?**

People who stay with their abusers may do so because they are dependent on the abuser, because they fear the abuser, or even because they love the abuser. In some cultures, women may not be free to leave an abusive relationship because of restrictive laws, religious beliefs, or social mores. Such women sometimes turn to drastic measures in order to escape; this young Afghani woman bears burn scars from the time that she set herself on fire in an attempt to end her life with an abusive husband.

that men who engage in severe violence are more likely than other men to suffer from personality disorders.[38]

# Child Abuse and Neglect

Children living in families in which domestic violence or sexual abuse occurs are at great risk for damage to personal health and well-being. **Child abuse** refers to the harm of a child by a caregiver, generally a parent. The abuse may be sexual, psychological, physical, or any combination of these. **Neglect** includes failure to provide for a child's basic needs for food, shelter, clothing, medical care, education, or proper supervision.

How serious are the problems of child abuse and neglect? Although exact figures are difficult to obtain, a new report to Congress includes results of several

**intimate partner violence (IPV)** Violent behavior, including physical violence, sexual violence, threats, and emotional abuse, occurring between current or former spouses or dating partners.

**child abuse** The systematic harming of a child by a caregiver, typically a parent.

**neglect** Failure to provide for a child's basic needs such as food, shelter, medical care, and clothing.

# Intimate Partner Violence: Men as Victims

We may think that intimate partner violence happens only to women, but every year in the United States men experience about 2.9 million physical assaults by an intimate partner, male or female. In fact, gay men appear to be just as susceptible to male-perpetrated violence as are women in heterosexual populations, and abuse of heterosexual men by their female partners is likely more common than statistics show. We may never know the exact nature and extent of intimate partner violence against men. However, several studies indicate that between 20 and 24 percent of men have experienced physical, sexual, or psychological intimate partner violence during their lifetime. Why don't men report this? In part, they don't because of the stigma associated with a man reporting that he has been brutalized. And, when women assault men, the injuries are usually emotional or psychological in nature and hard to identify. Physical injuries tend to be minor in nature and consist of scratches, bruises, or property damage. Other possible reasons include the following:

* Fear that no one will believe them
* Belief that "taking it" and never hitting back is a badge of honor, strength, and masculinity
* Humiliation and fear of being found out; machismo attitude
* Belief that they deserve bad treatment because they are so emotionally abused

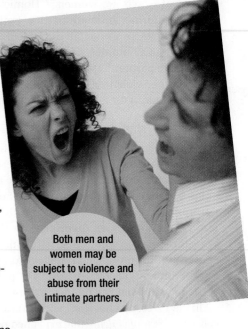

Both men and women may be subject to violence and abuse from their intimate partners.

* Lack of awareness and support services for men in abusive relationships

Recognizing that a real problem exists, communities across the nation are responding with education and awareness about various forms of violence, support groups, resources, and options that potential victims can take to protect themselves.

**Sources:** CDC, National Center for Injury Prevention and Control, "Understanding Intimate Partner Violence Fact Sheet," 2009, www.cdc.gov/violenceprevention/pdf/IPV_factsheet-a.pdf; National Domestic Violence Hotline, "Abuse in America," www.ndvh.org/get-educated/abuse-in-america, Accessed June 2009; Medical Review Board, "Men as Victims of Abusive Relationships," http://menshealth.about.com/od/relationships/a/Battered_Men.htm, Updated January 2007; Oregon Counseling Center, "About Domestic Violence against Men," www.oregoncounseling.org/Handouts/DomesticViolenceMen.htm, Revised May 2007.

studies based largely on information obtained from nearly 11,000 sentinels—people who deal with probable cases on a daily basis and report their findings. These studies indicate that an estimated 1.25 million children (1 out of every 58) experienced maltreatment in one form or another between 2005 and 2006. Of those children, an estimated 553,000 (44%) were abused. Most of the abused children (58%) experienced physical abuse, slightly more than 27 percent were emotionally abused, and slightly more than 24 percent experienced sexual abuse.[39] **Figure 19.4** shows the rates of abuse among children of different ages.

There is no single profile of a child abuser. The most common perpetrators in child maltreatment cases are biological parents. Frequently, the perpetrator is a young adult in his or her mid-twenties without a high school diploma, living at or below the poverty level, depressed, socially isolated, with a poor self-image, and having difficulty coping

## "Why Should I Care?"

You may be too young to be at risk for elder abuse, but your parents and grandparents could become victims—of domestic violence; of caregiver abuse; of financial abuse; and of sexual, physical, and emotional abuse. If you're aware of this possibility, you may be able to help identify a problem and take steps to fix it.

with stressful situations. In many instances, the perpetrator has experienced violence and is frustrated by life.

Not all violence against children is physical. Health can be severely affected by psychological violence—assaults on personality, character, competence, independence, or general dignity as a human being. The negative consequences of this kind of victimization can include depression, low self-esteem, and a pervasive fear of offending the abuser.

## Elder Abuse

By 2030, the number of people in the United States over the age of 65 will exceed 71 million—nearly double their number in 2000. This growing population will need increasing levels of care in the coming decades, and there will be fewer and fewer people who are willing and able to provide it.

Elder abuse is a problem for many of today's seniors; best estimates indicate that between 700,000 and 3.5 million older Americans are abused, neglected, or exploited each year, with fewer than 1 in 6 cases

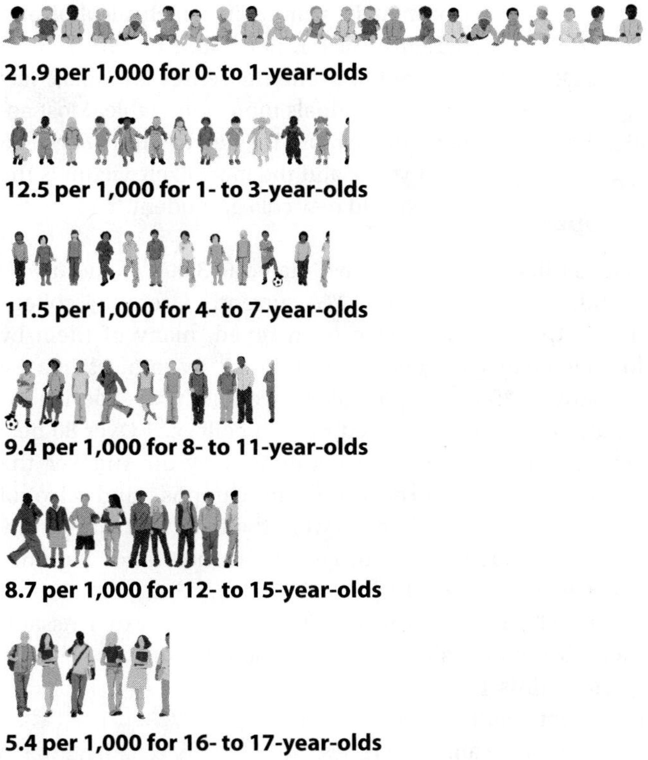

**21.9 per 1,000 for 0- to 1-year-olds**

**12.5 per 1,000 for 1- to 3-year-olds**

**11.5 per 1,000 for 4- to 7-year-olds**

**9.4 per 1,000 for 8- to 11-year-olds**

**8.7 per 1,000 for 12- to 15-year-olds**

**5.4 per 1,000 for 16- to 17-year-olds**

FIGURE 19.4 **Child Maltreatment Rates by Age, 2007**
In 2007, U.S., state, and local child protective services reported that approximately 794,000 children were nonfatal victims of maltreatment, and an estimated 1,760 children died of abuse or neglect. Younger children are victimized at much higher rates than are older children.

**Source:** Data are from U.S. Department of Health and Human Services, Administration on Children, Youth and Families, *Child Maltreatment 2007* (Washington, DC: U.S. Government Printing Office, 2009), Available at www.acf.hhs.gov/programs/cb/pubs/cm07/index.htm.

ever identified.[40] Many victims fail to report because they are embarrassed that a family member is an abuser; they don't want the abuser to get in trouble or retaliate by putting them in a nursing home; they feel guilty because someone has to take care of them; or they fear that after a report, things will get worse. Others suffer from dementia and therefore aren't even aware that the abuse is happening. Today, a variety of social service and public health groups are exploring options for protecting our elderly citizens in much the same way that we endeavor to protect children in our society.

## Sexual Victimization

The term *sexual victimization* refers to any situation in which an individual is coerced or forced to comply with or endure another's sexual acts or overtures. It can run the gamut from harassment to stalking to assault and rape. As with all forms of violence, both men and women are susceptible to sexual victimization. Young people are especially vulnerable; 60 percent of female victims of sexual violence and 69 percent of male victims were first raped before the age of 18.[41] Sexual victimization and violence can have devastating and far-reaching effects on people of any age. Depression, suicide risks, drug and alcohol abuse, traumatic stress disorders, self-harm, and a host of interpersonal problems often increase among women and men who have been victimized sexually.[42]

**Sexual Assault and Rape** **Sexual assault** is any act in which one person is sexually intimate with another person without that person's consent. This may range from simple touching to forceful penetration and may include, for example, ignoring indications that intimacy is not wanted, threatening force or other negative consequences, and actually using force.

Considered to be the most extreme form of sexual assault, **rape** is defined as "penetration without the victim's consent."[43] Incidents of rape generally fall into one of two types—aggravated or simple. An **aggravated rape** is any rape involving one or multiple attackers, strangers, weapons, or physical beatings. A **simple rape** is a rape perpetrated by one person, whom the victim knows, and does not involve a physical beating or use of a weapon. Most rapes are classified as simple rape, but that terminology should not be taken to mean that a simple rape is any less violent or criminal. The FBI ranks rape as the second most violent crime, trailing only murder.[44]

According to the National Center for Injury Prevention and Control, 1 in 6 women and 1 in 33 men reported experiencing an attempted or completed rape at some time in their lives.[45] An estimated 63 percent of all sexual assaults reported by women victims in 2008 were committed by someone the victim knew: 42 percent of perpetrators were the victim's friend or acquaintance; 18 percent were intimates; and 3 percent were relatives.[46] Men can also be victims of rape and sexual assault, and a growing number have come forward to report their abusers. Over 41 percent of male victims were first raped before the age of 12, and 28 percent were first raped between the ages of 12 and 17. These first rapes were committed by acquaintances (32.3%), family members (17.7%), friends (17.6%), or intimate partners (15.9%).[47]

By most indicators, reported cases of rape appear to have declined in the United States since the early 1990s, even as reports of other forms of sexual assault have increased. This decline is thought to be due to shifts in public awareness and attitudes about rape, combined with tougher crime policies, major educational campaigns, and media attention. These changes enforce the idea that rape is a violent crime and should be treated as such.

Although these declines in reported cases may be encouraging, studies indicate that only 16 percent of all rapes are actually reported to law enforcement![48] Why do so many victims never report the crimes committed against them? Typically major barriers include not wanting others to know

**sexual assault** Any act in which one person is sexually intimate with another without that person's consent.
**rape** Sexual penetration without the victim's consent.
**aggravated rape** Rape that involves one or multiple attackers, strangers, weapons, or physical beating.
**simple rape** Rape by one person, usually known to the victim, that does not involve physical beating or use of a weapon.

about the rape, fear of retaliation, perception of insufficient evidence, uncertainty about how to report, and uncertainty whether a crime was committed or harm was intended.

**Acquaintance Rape** The terms *date rape* and *acquaintance rape* have been used interchangeably in the past. However, most experts now believe that the term *date rape* is inappropriate because it implies a consensual interaction in an arranged setting and may, in fact, minimize the crime of rape when it occurs. Today, *acquaintance rape* refers to any rape in which the rapist is known to the victim. It may be a dating situation, but it may also be a situation in which two strangers happen to meet at a bar or social setting. Acquaintance rape is more

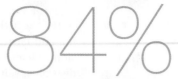

**84%**

**of sexual assaults that occur on college campuses are acquaintance rapes.**

common in venues in which alcohol and partying are the norm and in which drugs are used to numb the senses and make targeted individuals more vulnerable. Most acquaintance rapes happen to women aged 15 to 24 years, and the most likely victim is the 18-year-old new college student.[49]

**Rape on U.S. Campuses** An estimated 673,000 of the nearly 6 million women (about 12%) currently attending college in the United States have been raped, many of them by forcible means that resulted in injury.[50] By some estimates, as many as 25 percent of college women have experienced an attempted or completed rape in college.[51] Over 80 percent of these rapes were committed by an attacker the victim knew, most occurred on campus, and alcohol was commonly involved, as were the two most commonly used rape-facilitating drugs, Rohypnol and gamma-hydroxybutyrate (GHB).[52]

In 1992, Congress passed the Campus Sexual Assault Victim's Bill of Rights, known as the *Ramstad Act.* The act gives victims the right to call in off-campus authorities to investigate serious campus crimes. In addition, it requires universities to set up educational programs and to notify students of available counseling. More recent provisions of the act specify notification procedures and options for victims, rights of victims and the accused perpetrators, and consequences if schools do not comply. It also requires the Department of Education to publish campus crime statistics annually.

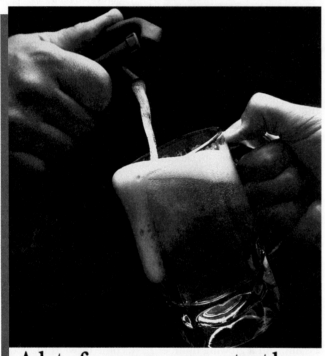

# A lot of campus rapes start here.

Whenever there's drinking or drugs, things can get out of hand. So it's no surprise that many campus rapes involve alcohol. But you should know that under any circumstances, sex without the other person's consent is considered rape. A felony, punishable by prison. And drinking is no excuse.

That's why, when you party, it's good to know what your limits are. You see, a little sobering thought now can save you from a big problem later.

**What does *date rape* mean?**

The term *date rape* was formerly applied to a sexual assault occurring in the context of a dating relationship. The term has fallen out of favor because the word *date* implies something reciprocal or arranged, thus minimizing the crime. The term *acquaintance rape* is now more commonly used, referring to any rape in which the rapist is known to the victim, even if only minimally. Acquaintance rape is particularly common on college campuses, where alcohol and drug use can impair young people's judgment and self-control.

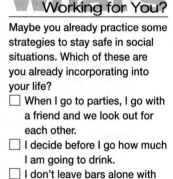

**What's Working for You?**

Maybe you already practice some strategies to stay safe in social situations. Which of these are you already incorporating into your life?

☐ When I go to parties, I go with a friend and we look out for each other.

☐ I decide before I go how much I am going to drink.

☐ I don't leave bars alone with people I've just met.

**Marital Rape** Although its legal definition varies within the United States, *marital rape* can be any unwanted intercourse or penetration (vaginal, anal, or oral) obtained by force, threat of force, or when the spouse is unable to consent.[53] Some researchers estimate that marital rape may account for 25 percent of all rapes. This problem has undoubtedly existed since the origin of marriage as a social institution, and it is noteworthy that marital rape did not become a crime in all 50 states until 1993. Even more noteworthy is the fact that 33 states still allow exemptions from marital rape prosecution, meaning that the judicial system may treat it as a lesser crime.

In general, women under the age of 25 and those from lower socioeconomic groups are at highest risk of marital rape. Women from homes where other forms of domestic violence are common and where there is a high rate of alcoholism or substance abuse also tend to be victimized at greater rates. Women who are subjected to marital rape often report multiple offenses over a period of time; these events are likely to be forced anal and oral experiences.[54]

## Child Sexual Abuse

**Sexual abuse of children** by adults or older children includes sexually suggestive conversations; inappropriate kissing; touching; petting; oral, anal, or vaginal intercourse; and other kinds of sexual interaction. Between 20 and 30 percent of all adult women report having had an unwanted childhood sexual encounter with an adult male, usually a father, uncle, brother, or grandfather.[55] Girls are more commonly abused than boys, although young boys are also frequent victims, usually by male family members.

The most frequent abusers are a child's parent or a parent's companion or spouse. The next most frequent abusers are grandfathers and siblings. About 87 percent of cases of sexual abuse of children are perpetrated by males.[56] Unfortunately, the "stranger danger" programs taught in schools today may give children the false impression that they are more likely to be assaulted by some seedy-looking stranger lurking in the bushes. They may not recognize that they are being victimized by the very people whom they trust and love.

People who were abused as children bear spiritual, psychological, or physical scars. Studies have shown that child sexual abuse has an impact on later life; children who experience maltreatment and abuse are at increased risk for smoking, alcoholism, drug abuse, eating disorders, mental health problems, and suicide.[57] In some cases, people who are victimized at a young age later become perpetrators themselves.

## Sexual Harassment

**Sexual harassment** is defined as unwelcome sexual conduct that is related to any condition of employment or evaluation of student performance. Typically, it has one or more of the following components: (1) Submission to such conduct is a condition of employment, academic progress, or participation in a university program; (2) submission to or rejection of such conduct influences employment, academic or university program decisions, or grades; and (3) the conduct interferes with an employee's work or a student's academic career, or creates an intimidating, hostile, or offensive work, learning, or program environment.[58] Commonly, people think of harassment as involving only faculty members or persons in power, where sex is used to exhibit control of a situation. However, peers can harass one another too.

## 80%
**of college students who have experienced sexual harassment report being harassed by another student or former student.**

Sexual harassment may include unwanted touching; unwarranted sex-related comments or subtle pressure for sexual favors; deliberate or repeated humiliation or intimidation based on sex; and gratuitous comments, jokes, questions, or remarks about clothing or bodies, sexuality, or past sexual relationships. Making derogatory jokes based on sex or appearance, speaking in crude or offensive language, spreading rumors about a person's sexuality, posting compromising photos on the Web, or ogling are all forms of sexual harassment as well.

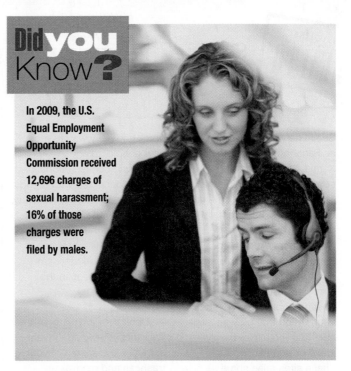

Most schools and companies have sexual harassment policies in place, as well as procedures for dealing with harassment problems. If you feel you are being harassed, the most important thing you can do is to be assertive:

**sexual abuse of children** Sexual interaction between a child and an adult or older child.

**sexual harassment** Any form of unwanted sexual attention related to any condition of employment or performance evaluation.

- **Tell the harasser to stop.** Be clear and direct about what is bothering you and why you are upset. Tell the person if it continues that you will report it to the proper legal authorities. If harassing is via phone or Internet, block the person from your listings.
- **Document the harassment.** Make a record of the incident. If the harassment becomes intolerable, a record of exactly what occurred (and when and where) will help make your case. Save copies of all communication that the harasser sends you.
- **Try to make sure you aren't alone in the harasser's presence.** Witnesses to harassment can ensure appropriate validation of the event.
- **Complain to a higher authority.** Talk to your instructor, adviser, or counseling center psychologist about

### what do you think?

What policies does your school have regarding consensual relationships between faculty members and students? ● Should consenting adults have the right to become intimate or interact socially, regardless of their positions within a school system or workplace? ● What are the potential dangers of such interactions? Are there ever situations in which such interactions are okay?

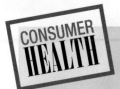
# Social Networking Safety

Social networking sites such as Facebook, MySpace, Bebo, Xanga, and Twitter; dating services; personal blogs; and other such virtual arenas have become almost universally accepted as the norm in recent years. At any given time, millions of people are chatting away with friends, family, and strangers, and posting photos and personal information that may be available to people they barely know or don't know at all. These sites raise some concerns about potential risks—from stalking and identity theft, to gossip and slander, to embarrassment and defamation.

Although real threats to health, reputation, financial security, and future employment lie in wait for those who post indiscriminately and unwisely to the Web, social networking sites can have many benefits, particularly for college students. Social networking sites provide a quick and easy way to meet new people, to engage in interesting conversations, and to stay connected with friends and relatives who are far away.

To enjoy the benefits safely and to avoid the risks of social networking sites, practice a little caution and use some common sense, as in the following tips:

✱ Don't post anything on the Web that you wouldn't want someone to pick out of your trashcan and read. Your address, phone numbers, banking information, calendar, family secrets, and other information should be kept off the sites. Assume that there will be at least one unscrupulous person viewing your information,

✱ Don't post compromising pictures, videos, or other things that you wouldn't want your mother or coworkers to see.

✱ Never meet a stranger in person whom you've met only online without bringing a trusted friend along, or at the very least, notifying a close friend of where you will be and when you will return. Arrange a ride home with a friend in advance and choose a well-established, public place to meet during daylight hours. Don't give your address or traceable phone numbers to the person you are meeting.

*To stay safe online, think before you tweet.*

---

what happened. If he or she doesn't take you seriously, investigate your school's internal grievance procedures.

● **Remember that you have not done anything wrong.** You will likely feel awful after being harassed (especially if you have to complain to superiors). However, feel proud that you are not keeping silent.

### Stalking

The crime of **stalking** can be defined as a course of conduct directed at a specific person that would cause a reasonable person to feel fear. This may include repeated visual or physical proximity, nonconsensual written or verbal communication, and implied or explicit threats.[59] Stalking can even occur online (see the **Consumer Health** box above about staying safe when using social networking sites). Over 1 in 4 victims report being stalked through the use of some form of technology, such as cell phones, e-mail, instant messaging, Internet sites,

**stalking** The willful, repeated, and malicious following, harassing, or threatening of another person.

Global Positioning Systems (GPS), listening devices, and video cameras.[60]

Millions of women and men are stalked annually in the United States, and the vast majority of stalkers are persons involved in relationship breakups or other dating acquaintances. Adults between the ages of 18 and 24 experience the highest rates of stalking, making college campuses a high-risk setting for stalking incidents. However, like harassment, stalking is an underreported crime, both on campuses and in the nation at large. Often students do not think a stalking incident is serious enough to report, or they worry that the police will not take it seriously.

Researchers suggest several reasons for stalking: (1) Stalkers may have deficits in social skills; (2) they are young and have not yet learned how to deal with complex social relationships and situations; (3) they may not realize that their behavior constitutes stalking; (4) they have a flexible schedule and free time; and (5) they are not accountable to authority figures for their daily activities.[61] Stalkers may call a person constantly to monitor his or her actions, follow the victim to bars or parties to see whom he or she is with, or go on clandestine drive-bys to see what a former intimate is doing. Student stalkers may not view such behaviors as criminal in nature, or they may be surprised to find out that their showing interest and persistence in the other party is causing that person to be anxious and fearful.

### Emotional and Psychological Abuse

A common and insidious form of violence between intimate partners is emotional or psychological abuse. Emotional abuse can occur in any intimate relationship but is particularly prevalent in romantic and sexual relationships. This abuse can take the form of constant criticisms, personal verbal attacks, displays of explosive anger meant to intimidate, and controlling behavior. Psychological abusers seek to intimidate, denigrate, and debase their partners, thereby gaining control over the partner and the relationship. Often this form of abuse can lead to or accompany physical abuse and sexual coercion. If you note that your friend's or a family member's intimate partner is verbally or emotionally abusive or controlling, encourage them to seek counseling before the situation escalates further.

### Social Contributors to Sexual Violence

Sexual violence and intimate partner violence share common factors that increase the likelihood of their occurrence. Even as we do our best to engage in more progressive thinking and actions, certain societal assumptions and traditions in our society continue to be present, including the following:[62]

- **Minimization.** Many people assume that sexual assault is rare because official crime statistics, including the uniform crime statistics reports of the FBI, show few rapes per thousand population. However, rape is the most underreported of all serious crimes; 1 out of every 6 women in the United States has been a victim of sexual assault.
- **Trivialization.** Because rape is underreported, many are not aware that they know rape victims. In addition, many consider rape by a husband or intimate partner not to count or not to be serious.
- **Blaming the victim.** In spite of efforts to combat this type of thinking, there is still the belief that a scantily clad woman "asks" for sexual advances.
- **Pressure to be macho.** Males are taught from a young age that "big boys don't cry," that showing emotions is a sign of weakness. This portrayal often depicts men as aggressive and predatory and females as passive targets.
- **Male socialization.** Many still believe that "sowing wild oats" and "boys will be boys" are merely normal parts of development to adulthood in males. Women are often *objectified,* or treated as sexual objects, in the media, which contributes to the idea that it's only natural for men to be predatory.
- **Male misperceptions.** With media implying that sex is the focus of life, it's not surprising that some men believe that when a woman says no, she is really asking to be seduced.

Later, these same men may be surprised when the woman says she was raped.

- **Situational factors.** Dates in which the male makes all the decisions, pays for everything, and generally controls the entire situation are more likely to end in an aggressive sexual scenario. Alcohol and other drugs increase the risk and severity of assaults. If two people have been seeing each other for a long time, the chances of aggression escalate, particularly if there has already been a sexual incident that didn't turn out as the male expected.

# Collective Violence

**Collective violence** is violence perpetrated by groups and includes political party, militia, and governmental violence; religious or cultural clashes; national or international violence; mobs; riots after sporting events; and other group-against-group forms of violence. Gang violence and terrorist threats are two forms of collective violence that have surfaced as major threats in recent years.

**collective violence** Violence perpetrated by groups against other groups.

## Gang Violence

The growing influence of street gangs has had a harmful impact on our country. Gang violence, including drug trafficking, sex trafficking, shootings, beatings, thefts, carjackings, and bystanders literally being caught in the crossfire of gang shootouts, have caused entire neighborhoods to live in fear. Once thought to occur only in urban areas, gang violence now is a growing threat in rural and suburban communities as well, particularly in the West, Pacific Northwest, Southwest, and Midwest regions of the country.[63]

Why do young people join gangs? Although the reasons are complex, gangs seem to meet many of the personal needs of young people. Often, gangs give members a sense of self-worth, companionship, security, and excitement. In other cases, gangs provide economic security through criminal activity, drug sales, or prostitution. Once young people become involved in gang subculture, it is difficult for them to leave. Threats of violence or fear of not making it on their own discourage even those who are seriously trying to get out.

Who is at risk for joining a gang? The age range of gang members is typically 12 to 22. Risk factors include low self-esteem, academic problems, low socioeconomic status, alienation from family and society, a history of family violence, and living in gang-controlled neighborhoods.[64]

## Terrorism

On September 11, 2001, terrorist attacks on the World Trade Center and the Pentagon revealed the vulnerability of our nation to domestic and international threats. Today, threats against our airlines, mass transportation systems, cities, national monuments, and our population fuel our fears of

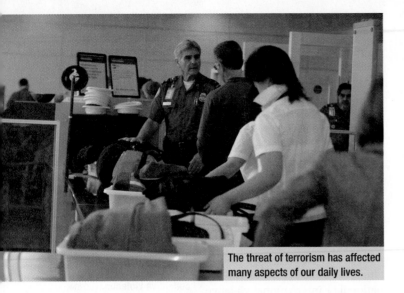

The threat of terrorism has affected many aspects of our daily lives.

looming terrorist attacks. Effects on our economy, travel restrictions, additional security measures, and military buildups are but a few of the examples of how terrorist threats have affected our lives. As defined in the Code of Federal Regulations, **terrorism** is the "unlawful use of force or violence against persons or property to intimidate or coerce a government, the civilian population, or any segment thereof in furtherance of political or social objectives."[65]

**terrorism** The unlawful use of force or violence against persons or property to intimidate or coerce a government, the civilian population, or any segment thereof in furtherance of political or social objectives.

Over the past decade the Centers for Disease Control and Prevention (CDC) consolidated many resources into its Emergency Preparedness and Response division. The division is set up to monitor potential problems, develop a plan for mobilizing communities in the case of attack, and provide resources and information to help Americans respond to terrorist threats and prepare for possible attacks. The Department of Homeland Security has been established to prevent future attacks, and the FBI and other government agencies have also prepared a set of procedures and guidelines to ensure citizens' health and safety.

## What's Working for You?

Maybe you already use street smarts to stay safe. Do you practice any of these safety tips?

☐ I keep to lighted paths instead of dark alleys.

☐ I pay attention to my surroundings.

☐ I don't let strangers into my home.

☐ I arrange rides home beforehand with trusted friends who will remain sober.

# How to Avoid Becoming a Victim of Violence

After a violent act is committed against someone we know, we acknowledge the horror of the event, express sympathy, and go on with our lives—but it may take the brutalized person months or years to recover both physically and emotionally. For this reason, preventing a violent act is far better than recovering from it. Both individuals and communities can play important roles in the prevention of violence and intentional injuries.

## Self-Defense against Rape and Personal Assault

Assault can occur no matter what preventive actions you take, but commonsense self-defense tactics can lower the risk. Self-defense is a process that includes increasing your awareness, developing self-protective skills, taking reasonable precautions, and having the judgment necessary to respond quickly to changing situations. Because rape on campus often occurs in social or dating settings, it is important to know ways to avoid and extract yourself from potentially dangerous situations. The Skills for Behavior Change box on the next page identifies practical tips for preventing dating violence.

Most attacks by unknown assailants are planned in advance. Many rapists use certain ploys to initiate their attacks. Examples include asking for help, offering help, staging a deliberate "accident" such as bumping into you, or posing as a police officer or other authority figure. Sexual assault frequently begins with a casual, friendly conversation.

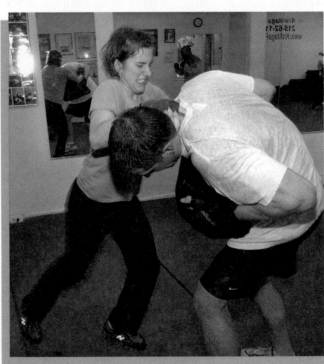

How can I protect myself from becoming a victim of violence?

One of the best ways to protect yourself from violence is to avoid situations or circumstances that could lead to it. Another way to protect yourself is to learn self-defense techniques. College campuses often offer safety workshops and self-defense classes to arm students with the physical and mental skills that may help them to repel or deter an assailant.

## Reducing Your Risk of Dating Violence

* Prior to your date, think about your values and set personal boundaries before you walk out the door.

* If the situation feels like it is getting out of control, stop and talk, speak directly, and don't worry about hurting feelings. Be firm.

* Watch your alcohol consumption. Drinking might get you into situations you'd otherwise avoid.

* Do not accept beverages or open-container drinks from anyone you do not know well and trust. At a bar or a club, accept drinks only from the bartender or waitstaff.

* Never leave a drink or food unattended. If you get up to dance, have someone you trust watch your drink or take it with you.

* Go out with several couples or in groups when dating someone new.

* Stick with your friends. Agree to keep an eye out for one another at parties, and have a plan for leaving together and checking in with one another. Never leave a bar or party alone with a stranger.

* Pay attention to your date's actions. If there is too much teasing and all the decisions are made for you, it may mean trouble. Trust your intuition.

* Practice what you will say to your date if things go in an uncomfortable direction. You have the right to express your feelings, and it is OK to be assertive. Do not be swayed by arguments such as "What about my feelings?" "You were leading me on," and "If you really cared about me, you would."

Listen to your feelings and trust your intuition. Be assertive and direct to someone who is getting out of line or becoming threatening. Stifle your tendency to be nice, and don't fear making a scene. Use the following tips to let a potential assailant know that you mean what you say and are prepared to defend yourself:

- **Speak in a strong voice.** Use commands such as, "Leave me alone!" rather than questions such as, "Will you please leave me alone?" Avoid apologies and excuses. Sound like you mean it.
- **Maintain eye contact with the would-be attacker.** Eye contact keeps you aware of the person's movements and conveys an aura of strength and confidence.
- **Stand up straight, act confident, and remain alert.** Walk as if you own the sidewalk.

If you are attacked, act immediately. Draw attention to yourself and your assailant. Scream, "Fire!" Research has shown that passersby are much more likely to help if they hear the word *fire* rather than just a scream.

## What to Do If a Rape Occurs

If you are a rape victim, report the attack. This gives you a sense of control. Follow these steps:

- Call 9-1-1 (if a phone is available).
- Do not bathe, shower, douche, clean up, or touch anything that the attacker may have touched.
- Save the clothes you were wearing, and do not launder them. They will be needed as evidence. Bring a clean change of clothes to the clinic or hospital.
- Contact the rape assistance hotline in your area, and ask for advice on therapists or counseling if you need additional help or advice.

If a friend is raped, here's how you can help:

- Believe her. Don't ask questions that may appear to implicate her in the assault.
- Recognize that rape is a violent act and the victim was not looking for this to happen.
- Encourage your friend to see a doctor immediately, because she may have medical needs but feel too embarrassed to seek help on her own. Offer to go with her.
- Encourage her to report the crime.
- Be understanding, and let her know you will be there for her.
- Recognize that this is an emotional recovery, and it may take months or years for her to bounce back.
- Encourage your friend to seek counseling.

# Campuswide Responses to Violence

Increasingly, campuses have become microcosms of the greater society, complete with the risks, hazards, and dangers that people face in the world. They also are uniquely different, in that they are open to the public and offer an opportunity for predators of all types to exploit young men and women in environments where they feel safe. Many college administrators have been proactive in establishing violence-prevention policies, programs, and services. They have also begun to examine the aspects of campus culture that promote and tolerate violent acts.[66]

## Prevention and Early Response Efforts

The Virginia Tech and Northern Illinois tragedies of 2007 and 2008 prompted vast restructuring of existing policies and strategies for prevention, as well as implementation of methods for notifying students and faculty of immediate risk. Historically, prevention efforts have focused on rape-awareness programs, safety workshops, antitheft programs, and grounds

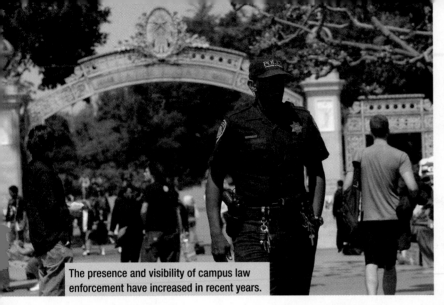
The presence and visibility of campus law enforcement have increased in recent years.

safety measures such as good lighting, escort services, and well-placed emergency call boxes. Newer programs being developed include emergency response drills that enable campus police, campus administration, community law enforcement, and emergency medical teams to practice how they would respond in the event of a major threat, such as a shooter on campus.

Campuses are reviewing the effectiveness of emergency messaging systems. E-mail alerts can reach only those campus community members who are either at their computers or who receive e-mail updates on mobile devices, so campuses are also working to implement cell phone alert systems. The REVERSE 9-1-1 system uses database and geographic information system (GIS) mapping technologies to notify campus police and community members in the event of problems, whereas systems developed by companies such as Rave Wireless allow campus administrators to send out alerts in text, voice, e-mail, or instant message format. Some schools program the phone numbers, photographs, and basic student information for all incoming first-year students into a university security system, so that, in the event of a threat, students need only hit a button on their phones, whereupon campus police will be notified and tracking devices will pinpoint their location.

## Changes in the Campus Environment

Recognizing that they may be liable for not protecting their students, and out of a genuine concern for faculty, staff, and student health, administrators are asking key questions about the safety of the campus environment. Campus lighting, parking lot security, call boxes for emergencies, removal of overgrown shrubbery along bike paths and walking trails, and stepped-up security are increasingly on the radar of campus safety personnel. Buildings themselves are designed with better lighting and more security provisions, and in some cases security cameras have been installed in hallways, classrooms,

and in public places throughout campus. Safe rides are provided for students who have consumed too much alcohol; campus leaders have become more involved in campus safety issues; and health promotion programs have stepped up their violence prevention efforts through seminars on acquaintance rape, sexual assault, harassment, and other topics.

## Campus Law Enforcement

Campus law enforcement has changed over the years by increasing both numbers of its members and its authority to prosecute student offenders. Campus police are responsible for emergency responses to situations that threaten safety, human resources, the general campus environment, traffic and bicycle riders, and other dangers. They have the power to enforce laws with students in the same way they are handled in the general community. In fact, many campuses now hire state troopers or local law enforcement officers to deal with campus issues rather than maintain a separate police staff.

Many of these law enforcement groups follow a community policing model in which officers have specific responsibilities for certain areas of campus, departments, or events. By narrowing the scope of each officer's territory, officers get to know people in the area and are better able to anticipate risky situations and prevent problems from erupting. Schools around the country are also enhancing the ability of campus law enforcement to respond in case of an emergency. Many officers receive special training in handling crisis and hostage situations, as well as being issued stun guns and other equipment meant to disable potential offenders.

# Community Strategies for Preventing Violence

There are many steps you can take to ensure your personal safety (see the Skills for Behavior Change box on the next page); however, it is also necessary to address the issues of violence and safety at a community level. Because the factors that contribute to violence are complex and interrelated, community strategies for prevention must also be multidimensional, focusing on individuals, schools, families, communities, policies, programs, and services designed to reduce risk. As part of the CDC's Injury Response initiatives, recommended strategies include a variety of interventions designed to prevent violence before it begins:

● Develop policies, intervention programs, and laws that prevent violence, such as counseling services, education programs focused on parenting skills or dating behavior, and assistance in giving individuals the confidence to protect themselves against physical and emotional assaults.
● Work with individuals in skills-based educational programs that teach the basics of interpersonal communication,

## Stay Safe on All Fronts

There are many steps you can take to protect yourself from assault. Follow these tips to increase your awareness and reduce your risk of a violent attack.

### OUTSIDE ALONE

✳ Carry a cell phone; keep it turned on, but don't use it. Be aware of what is happening around you.

✳ If you are being followed, don't go home. Head for a location where there are other people. If you decide to run, run fast and scream loudly to attract attention.

✳ Vary your routes; walk or jog with others. Stay close to others.

✳ Park near lights; avoid dark areas where people could hide.

✳ Carry pepper spray or other deterrents. Consider using your campus escort service.

✳ Tell others where you are going and when you expect to be back.

### IN YOUR CAR

✳ Lock your doors. Do not open your doors or windows to strangers.

✳ If someone hits your car while you are driving, drive to the nearest gas station or other public place. Call the police or road service for help, and stay in your car until help arrives.

✳ If a car appears to be following you, do not drive home. Drive to the nearest police station.

### IN YOUR HOME

✳ Install dead bolts on all doors and locks on all windows. Make sure the locks work, and don't leave a spare key outside. Consider installing a home alarm system.

✳ Lock doors when at home, even during the day. Close blinds and drapes whenever you are away and in the evening when you are home.

✳ Rent apartments that require a security code or clearance to gain entry, and avoid easily accessible apartments, such as first-floor units. When you move into a new residence, pay a locksmith to change the keys and locks.

✳ Don't let repair people in without asking for their identification, and have someone else with you when repairs are being made in your home or apartment.

✳ Keep a phone near your bed and program it to dial 9-1-1.

✳ If you return home to find your residence has been broken into, don't enter. Call the police. If you encounter an intruder, it is better to give up your money than to fight back.

anger management, conflict resolution, appropriate assertiveness, stress management, and other health-based behaviors.

● Beginning at an early age, involve families, schools, community programs, athletics, music, faith-based groups, and so on, in providing experiences that help young people to develop self-esteem and self-efficacy.

● Promote tolerance and acceptance, and establish and enforce policies that forbid discrimination on the basis of religion, gender, race, sexual orientation, age, marital status, income, or other differences.

● Improve community services focused on family planning, mental health services, day care and respite care, and alcohol and substance abuse prevention.

● Improve the built environment in communities by making sure walking trails, parking lots, and other public areas are well lit, unobstructed, and patrolled regularly to reduce threats to users.

● Improve community-based support and treatment for victims, and ensure that individuals have choices available when trying to stop the violence in their lives.

## Are You at Risk for Violence?

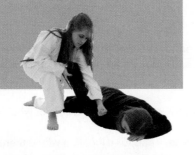

PEARSON
**myhealthlab**

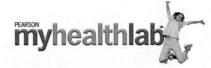

Fill out this assessment online at www.pearsonhighered.com/myhealthlab or www.pearsonhighered.com/donatelle.

How often are you at risk of being a victim of violence? Answer the questions below to find out.

### 1 Relationship Risk

How often does your partner:

| | Never | Sometimes | Often |
|---|---|---|---|
| 1. Criticize you for your appearance? | ○ | ○ | ○ |
| 2. Embarrass you in front of others by putting you down? | ○ | ○ | ○ |
| 3. Blame you or others for his or her mistakes? | ○ | ○ | ○ |
| 4. Curse at you, shout at you, say mean things, insult, or mock you? | ○ | ○ | ○ |
| 5. Demonstrate uncontrollable anger? | ○ | ○ | ○ |
| 6. Criticize your friends, family, or others who are close to you? | ○ | ○ | ○ |
| 7. Threaten to leave you if you don't behave in a certain way? | ○ | ○ | ○ |
| 8. Express jealousy, distrust, and anger when you spend time with other people? | ○ | ○ | ○ |
| 9. Intimidate or threaten you, or make threats to harm others you care about? | ○ | ○ | ○ |
| 10. Control your telephone calls, listen in on your messages, or read your e-mail? | ○ | ○ | ○ |
| 11. Punch, hit, slap, or kick you? | ○ | ○ | ○ |
| 12. Use money or possessions to control you? | ○ | ○ | ○ |
| 13. Force you to have sex or perform sexual acts that make you uncomfortable? | ○ | ○ | ○ |
| 14. Threaten to kill himself or herself if you leave? | ○ | ○ | ○ |
| 15. Follow you, call to check on you, or demonstrate a constant obsession with what you are doing? | ○ | ○ | ○ |

### 2 Online Safety

How often do you:

| | Never | Sometimes | Often |
|---|---|---|---|
| 1. Put personal identifying information on your blog, Web page, or networking sites? | ○ | ○ | ○ |
| 2. Post personal pictures and other private material on networking sites such as Facebook or MySpace? | ○ | ○ | ○ |
| 3. Date people you meet online? | ○ | ○ | ○ |
| 4. Use a shared or public computer to check e-mail without clearing the browser cache afterward? | ○ | ○ | ○ |
| 5. Make financial transactions online without confirming security measures? | ○ | ○ | ○ |

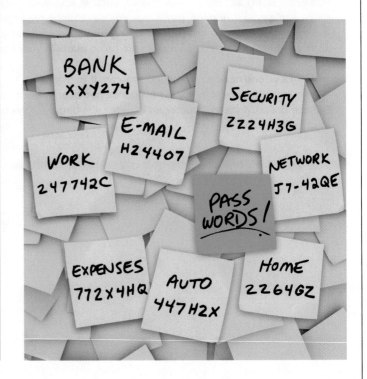

# 3 Risk for Assault or Rape

How often do you:

| | Never | Sometimes | Often |
|---|---|---|---|
| 1. Drink more than one or two drinks while out with friends or at a party? | ○ | ○ | ○ |
| 2. Accept drinks from strangers while out at a bar or party? | ○ | ○ | ○ |
| 3. Leave parties with people you barely know or just met? | ○ | ○ | ○ |
| 4. Walk alone in poorly lit or unfamiliar places? | ○ | ○ | ○ |
| 5. Leave your car or home door unlocked? | ○ | ○ | ○ |

## Analyzing Your Responses

Now look at your responses to the list of questions in each of these sections. Part 1 focused on relationships—if you answered "sometimes" to one or more of these questions, you may be at risk for emotional or physical abuse. Typically, such potentially abusive patterns only get worse over time. If you are anxious about talking to your partner, seek counseling through your campus counseling center, student health center, or community services. In each of the other sections, if you answered "often" to any question, you may need to adjust your behavior and educate yourself about steps you can take to remain safe.

# YOUR PLAN FOR CHANGE

The **Assessyourself** activity gave you the chance to consider symptoms of abuse in your relationships and signs of unsafe behavior in other realms of your life. Now that you are aware of these signs and symptoms, you can work on changing behaviors to reduce your risk.

### Today, you can:

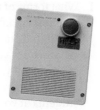

○ Pay attention as you walk your normal route around campus, and think about whether you are taking the safest route. Is it well lit? Are there any emergency phone boxes along your route? Does campus security patrol the area? If part of your route seems unsafe, look around for alternate routes.

○ Look at your residence's safety features. Is there a secure lock, dead bolt, or keycard entry system on all outer doors? Can windows be shut and locked? Are the outside areas well lit? If you notice any potential safety hazards, report them to your landlord or campus residential life administrator right away.

### Within the next 2 weeks, you can:

○ Visit the campus counseling center and ask about resources on campus or in your community to help you deal with potential relationship abuse if you are worried about such abuse. Consider talking to a counselor about your concerns or sitting in on a support group.

○ Set limits for yourself the next time you attend a party in order to remain in control of your behavior and to avoid putting yourself in a dangerous or compromising position. Decide ahead of time on the number of drinks you will have, arrange with a friend to monitor each other's behavior during the party, and be sure you have a reliable, safe way of getting home.

### By the end of the semester, you can:

○ Learn ways to protect yourself by signing up for a self-defense workshop on campus or in the community.

○ Get involved in an on-campus or community group dedicated to promoting safety. You might want to attend a meeting of an antiviolence group, join in a Take Back the Night rally, or volunteer at a local rape crisis center or battered women's shelter.

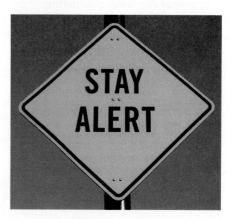

## Summary

* Violence affects everyone in society—from the direct victims, to children and families who witness it, and those who modify their behaviors because they are fearful.
* Factors that lead people to be violent include economic difficulties, parental influence, cultural beliefs, discrimination, political differences, stress, alcohol and substance abuse, stress, excessive fear, anger, and a history of violence.
* Interpersonal violence includes homicide, domestic violence, child abuse, elder abuse, and sexual victimization. Each of these causes significant emotional, social, and physical risks to health.
* Forms of collective violence, including gang violence and terrorism, continue to result in fear, anxiety, and issues of discrimination.
* Recognizing how to protect yourself and your friends; knowing where to turn for help; and having honest, straightforward dialogue about sexual matters in dating situations are sound strategies to reduce risk of becoming a victim of violence. Alcohol moderation is another key factor in reducing your risks.
* Shootings and extreme acts of violence on campuses have resulted in a groundswell of activities designed to protect students and ensure their safety. Preventing violence is a public health priority. It means community activism; prioritizing mental and emotional health; and providing skills training in anger management, coping, parenting, and other key areas.

## Pop Quiz

1. _____ is an example of an *intentional injury.*
   a. A car accident
   b. Murder
   c. Accidental drowning
   d. Road rage

2. Emotional reaction brought about by frustrating life experience is called
   a. reactive aggression.
   b. primary aggression.
   c. secondary aggression.
   d. tertiary aggression.

3. When Jane began her new job with all male coworkers, her supervisor told her that he enjoyed having an attractive woman in the workplace, and he winked at her. His comment constitutes
   a. acquaintance rape.
   b. sexual assault.
   c. sexual harassment.
   d. sexual battering.

4. Psychologist Lenore Walker developed a theory known as the
   a. aggression cycle.
   b. sexual harassment cycle.
   c. cycle of child abuse.
   d. cycle of violence.

5. What is the single greatest cause of injury to women?
   a. Rape
   b. Mugging
   c. Auto accidents
   d. Domestic violence

6. In a sociology class, some students were discussing sexual assault. One student commented that some women dress too provocatively. The social assumption this student made is
   a. minimization.
   b. trivialization.
   c. blaming the victim.
   d. "boys will be boys."

7. Rape by a person the victim knows and that does not involve a physical beating or use of a weapon is called
   a. simple rape.
   b. sexual assault.
   c. simple assault.
   d. aggravated rape.

8. Which of the following is *not* a contributor to violence?
   a. Cultural beliefs
   b. Poverty
   c. Physical appearance
   d. Unemployment

9. Which of the following is an example of stalking?
   a. Making intimate and sexually implied comments to another person
   b. Repeated visual, physical, or virtual seeking out of another person
   c. Unwelcome sexual conduct by the perpetrator
   d. Sexual abuse of a child

10. Jack beats his wife Melissa "to teach her a lesson." Afterward, he denies attacking her. This illustrates which phase of the cycle of violence?
    a. Acute battering
    b. Fear/depression
    c. Remorse/reconciliation
    d. Tension building

*Answers to these questions can be found on page A-1.*

## Think about It!

1. What forms of violence do you think are most significant or prevalent in the United States today? Why?
2. What type of violence is most common on your campus? How do you think campus violence affects students at your school? Are there differences in how men and women respond to news that there has been a rape or violent assault on campus? If so, why?
3. Have you known anyone personally who has been sexually assaulted on campus? What actions were taken to help him or her cope with the assault? What campus services, if any, were used?
4. Should students be able to obtain licenses to carry weapons on your campus? Why or why not?

5. Why do some people develop into violent or abusive adults and others become pacifists or peaceful adults? What key factors influence violent offenders to be violent?

6. What actions need to be taken to stem the tide of violence in America at the individual level? At the community level? In schools? On college campuses? Nationally?

## Accessing Your Health on the Internet

The following websites explore further topics and issues related to personal health. For links to the websites below, visit the Companion Website for *Access to Health,* 12th Edition, at www.pearsonhighered.com/donatelle.

1. *Communities against Violence Network.* This is an extensive, searchable database for information about violence against women, with articles about everything from domestic violence to legal information and statistics. www.cavnet2.org

2. *Men Can Stop Rape.* Practical suggestions for men interested in helping to protect women from sexual predators and assault. www.mencanstoprape.org

3. *National Center for Injury Prevention and Control.* The Web-based Injury Statistics Query and Reporting System (WISQARS) database of this CDC section provides statistics and information on fatal and nonfatal injuries, both intentional and unintentional. www.cdc.gov/injury

4. *National Center for Victims of Crime.* Provides information and resources for victims of crimes ranging from hate crimes to sexual assault. www.ncvc.org

5. *National Sexual Violence Resources Center.* An excellent resource for victims of sexual violence. www.nsvrc.org

6. *CyberAngels.* This site provides information on online safety, as well as help and advice for victims of cyber- stalking, identity theft, and related personal invasions via technology. www.cyberangels.org

## References

1. World Health Organization, *World Report on Violence and Health* (Geneva: World Health Organization, 2002), Available at www.who.int/violence_injury_prevention/ violence/world_report/en.
2. Ibid.
3. J. Xu, K. Kochanek, and B. Tejada-Vera, "Deaths: Preliminary Data for 2007," *National Vital Statistics Reports* 58, no. 1 (2009): 1–52.
4. U.S. Department of Justice, Federal Bureau of Investigation, "Crime Rates Fall in the First Half of 2009," December 2009, www.fbi.gov/news/stories/2009/ december/crimestats_122109.
5. American College Health Association, *American College Health Association— National College Health Assessment II: Reference Group Data Report Fall 2009* (Baltimore: American College Health Association, 2010), Available at www .acha-ncha.org/reports_ACHA-NCHAII .html.
6. Center for Public Integrity, "Sexual Assault on Campus: A Frustrating Search for Justice," Updated February 2010, www .publicintegrity.org/investigations/ campus_assault.
7. World Health Organization Violence Prevention Alliance, "The Ecological Framework," 2010, www.who.int/ violenceprevention/approach/ecology/ en/index.html; Centers for Disease Control and Prevention, National Center for Injury Prevention and Control, "Understanding Youth Violence," 2009, Available at www.cdc.gov/violenceprevention/ youthviolence.
8. U.S. Department of Justice, National Institute of Justice, "Economic Distress and Intimate Partner Violence," 2009, www.ojp.usdoj.gov/nij/topics/crime/ intimate-partner-violence/economic -distress.htm.
9. C. Ferguson, C. San Miguel, and R. Hartley, "A Multivariate Analysis of Youth Violence and Aggression: The Influences of Family, Peers, Depression, and Media Violence," *Journal of Pediatrics* 155, no. 6 (2009): 904–08; A. Gover, C. Kaukinen, and K. Fox, "The Relationship between Violence in the Family of Origin and Dating Violence among College Students," *Journal of Interpersonal Violence* 23, no. 12 (2008): 1667–93.
10. M. Flood and B. Pease, "Factors Influencing Attitudes to Violence against Women," *Trauma, Violence and Abuse* 10, no. 2 (2009): 125–42.
11. G. Stuart et al., "Examining the Interface between Substance Misuse and Intimate Partner Violence," *Substance Abuse Research and Treatment* 3 (2009): 25–29.
12. M. Teicher et al., "Sticks, Stones and Hurtful Words: Relative Effects of Various Forms of Childhood Maltreatment," *American Journal of Psychiatry* 163 (2006): 993–1000; A. Gover, C. Kaukinen, and K. Fox, "The Relationship between Violence in the Family of Origin and Dating Violence among College Students," 2008.
13. M. Teicher et al., "Sticks, Stones and Hurtful Words: Relative Effects of Various Forms of Childhood Maltreatment," 2006.
14. M. Randolph, H. Torres, C. Gore-Felton, B. Lloyd, and E. McGarvey, "Alcohol Use and Sexual Risk Behavior among College Students: Understanding Gender and Ethnic Differences," *American Journal of Drug & Alcohol Abuse* 35, no. 2 (2009): 80–84; E. Reed, H. Amaro, A. Matsumoto, and D. Kaysen, "The Relation between Interpersonal Violence and Substance Use among a Sample of University Students: Examination of the Role of Victim and Perpetrator Substance Use," *Addictive Behaviors* 34, no. 3 (2009): 316–18; T. Messman-Moore, R. Ward, and A. Brown, "Substance Use and PTSD Symptoms Impact the Likelihood of Rape and Revictimization in College Women," *Journal of Interpersonal Violence* 24, no. 3 (2009): 499–521; P. Giancola et al., "Men and Women, Alcohol and Aggression," *Experimental and Clinical Psychopharmacology* 17, no. 3 (2009): 154–64; J. McCauley, K. Calhoun, and C. Gidycz, "Binge Drinking and Rape: A Prospective Examination of College Women with a History of Previous Sexual Victimization," *Journal of Interpersonal Violence* 25, no. 9 (2010): 1655–68.
15. M. Ybares, M. Diner-West, D. Markow, and P. Leaf, "Linkages between Internet and Other Media Violence with Serious Violent Behavior by Youth," *Pediatrics* 122, no. 5 (2008): 929–37; C. Anderson et al., "Longitudinal Effects of Violent Video Games on Aggression in Japan and the United States," *Pediatrics* 122 (2008): e1067– e1072; J. Savage, "The Effects of Media Violence Exposure on Criminal Aggression," *Criminal Justice and Behavior* 35, no. 6 (2008): 772–91.
16. M. Ferguson, "Weak Results: Misleading Conclusions—Response to Anderson Article," *Pediatrics,* "eLetters," http:// pediatrics.aappublications.org/cgi/ eletters/122/5/e1067, 2008; C. Ferguson et al., "Personality, Parental and Media

Influences on Aggressive Personality and Violent Crime in Youth," *Journal of Aggression, Maltreatment and Trauma* 17, no. 4 (2008): 395–414; B. Wilson, "Media and Children's Aggression, Fear, and Altruism," *The Future of Children* 18, no. 1 (2008): 1550–54; L. Price and V. Maholmes, "Understanding the Nature and Consequences of Children's Exposure to Violence: Research Perspectives," *Clinical Child and Family Psychology Review* 12, no. 2 (2009): 65–70.

17. U.S. Department of Justice, Office of Justice Programs, Bureau of Justice Statistics, *National Crime Victimization Survey: Criminal Victimization, 2008* (Washington, DC: Bureau of Justice Statistics, 2009) NCJ 227777, Available at http://bjs.ojp.usdoj .gov/index.cfm?ty=pbdetail&iid=1975.

18. J. Savage and C. Yancey, "The Effects of Media Violence Exposure on Criminal Aggression: A Meta-Analysis," *Criminal Justice and Behavior* 35, no. 6 (2008): 772–91.

19. C. Ferguson, *Violent Crime: Clinical and Social Implications* (Thousand Oaks, CA: Sage, 2010).

20. World Health Organization, *World Report on Violence and Health*, 2002.

21. J. Xu, K. Kochanek, and B. Tejada-Vera, "Deaths: Preliminary Data for 2007," *National Vital Statistics Reports* 58, no. 1 (2009): 1–52.

22. U.S. Department of Justice, Federal Bureau of Investigation, *Crime in the United States 2009*, 2010, http://www2.fbi.gov/ ucr/cius2009.

23. J. Fox and M. Swatt, *The Recent Surge in Homicides Involving Young Black Males and Guns: Time to Reinvest in Prevention and Crime Control* (Alexandria, VA: American Statistical Association, 2008), Available at www.ncjrs.gov/App/publications/ abstract.aspx?ID=248092.

24. Centers for Disease Control and Prevention, "FastStats: Assault or Homicide," 2009, www.cdc.gov/nchs/FASTATS/ homicide.htm.

25. J. Fox and M. Zawitz, *Homicide Trends in the United States*, U.S. Department of Justice, Office of Justice Programs, Bureau of Justice Statistics, Revised 2007, http://bjs .ojp.usdoj.gov/content/homicide/ weapons.cfm.

26. L. Hepburn, M. Miller, and D. Hemenway, "The U.S. Gun Stock: Results from the 2004 National Firearms Survey," *Injury Prevention* 13 (2007): 15–19.

27. National Center for Injury Prevention and Control, "WISQARS Fatal Injury Reports 1999–2007," Updated 2010, Available at www.cdc.gov/injury/wisqars/fatal.html; Statistics Canada, "CANSIM," Updated 2010, http://cansim2.statcan.gc.ca.

28. Federal Bureau of Investigation, "Hate Crime Statistics, 2008," November 2009, www.fbi.gov/about-us/cjis/ucr/ hate-crime/2008.

29. Ibid.

30. Ibid.

31. J. Carr, *American College Health Association Campus Violence White Paper*, (Baltimore: American College Health Association, 2005), Available at www.acha.org/ Publications/Guidelines_WhitePapers.cfm.

32. S. Catalano et al., *Female Victims of Violence* (Washington, DC: Bureau of Justice Statistics, 2009), DOJ (US) NCJ228356, Available at http://bjs.ojp.usdoj.gov/index .cfm?ty=pbdetail&iid=2020.

33. Centers for Disease Control and Prevention, National Center for Injury Prevention and Control, "Understanding Sexual Violence Fact Sheet," 2009, Available at www.cdc.gov/violenceprevention/ sexualviolence/index.html.

34. J. Chang, C. Berg, L. Saltzman, and J. Herndon, "Homicide: A Leading Cause of Injury Deaths among Pregnant and Postpartum Women in the United States, 1991–1999," *American Journal of Public Health* 96, no. 3 (2005): 471–77.

35. Violence Policy Center, *American Roulette: Murder-Suicide in the United States*. 3rd ed. (Washington, DC: Violence Policy Center, 2008), Available at www.vpc.org/ studyndx.htm.

36. L. Walker, *The Battered Woman* (New York: Harper and Row, 1979).

37. L. Walker, *The Battered Woman Syndrome*. 3rd ed. (New York: Springer, 2009).

38. L. Rosen and J. Fontaine, *Compendium of Research on Violence against Women, 1993–Present* (Washington, DC: National Institute of Justice, 2009). DOJ (US) NCJ223572, Available at www.ojp.usdoj .gov/nij/pubs-sum/vaw-compendium .htm.

39. A. J. Sedlak et al., *Fourth National Incidence Study of Child Abuse and Neglect (NIS-4): Report to Congress, Executive Summary* (Washington, DC: U.S. Department of Health and Human Services, Administration for Children and Families, 2010), Available at www.acf.hhs.gov/programs/ opre/abuse_neglect/natl_incid/index .html.

40. C. Cooper, A. Selwood, and G. Livingston, "The Prevalence of Elder Abuse and Neglect: A Systematic Review," *Age and Ageing* 37, no. 2 (2008): 151–60; National Center on Elder Abuse, "Fact Sheet: Elder Abuse Prevalence and Incidence," 2005, Available at www.ncea.aoa.gov/ncearoot/ main_site/library/statistics_research/ abuse_statistics/statistics_at_glance.aspx.

41. Centers for Disease Control and Prevention, National Center for Injury Prevention

and Control, "Sexual Violence: Facts at a Glance," 2008, Available at www.cdc.gov/ violenceprevention/sexualviolence/ index.html.

42. D. Kilpatrick et al., "Drug-Facilitated, Incapacitated, and Forcible Rape: A National Study," National Crime Victims Research and Treatment Center, February 1, 2007, www.ncjrs.gov/pdffiles1/nij/grants/ 219181.pdf.

43. Centers for Disease Control and Prevention, National Center for Injury Prevention and Control, "Sexual Violence: Facts at a Glance," 2008.

44. M. Rand, *National Crime Victimization Survey: Criminal Victimization, 2008* (Washington, DC: Bureau of Justice Statistics, 2009) NCJ 227777, Available at http://bjs.ojp.usdoj.gov/index.cfm?ty =pbdetail&iid=1975.

45. Centers for Disease Control and Prevention, National Center for Injury Prevention and Control, "Understanding Sexual Violence Fact Sheet," 2009.

46. M. Rand, *National Crime Victimization Survey*, 2009.

47. Centers for Disease Control and Prevention, "Sexual Violence: Facts at a Glance," 2008; L. Schneider, L. Mori, P. Lambert, and A. Wong, "The Role of Gender and Ethnicity in Perceptions of Rape and Its Aftereffects," *Sex Roles* 60, no. 5/6 (2009): 410–21.

48. D. Kilpatrick et al., "Drug-Facilitated, Incapacitated, and Forcible Rape," 2007.

49. J. Carr, *American College Health Association Campus Violence White Paper*, 2005.

50. D. Kilpatrick et al., "Drug-Facilitated, Incapacitated, and Forcible Rape," 2007.

51. Centers for Disease Control and Prevention, National Center for Injury Prevention and Control, "Understanding Sexual Violence Fact Sheet," 2009.

52. University of Illinois at Chicago, "Most Sexual Assaults Drug Facilitated, Study Claims," *ScienceDaily* (May 13, 2006), Retrieved May 18, 2008, www.sciencedaily .com/releases/2006/05/060513122928 .htm.

53. R. Bergen and E. Barnhill, "Marital Rape: New Research and Directions," National Online Resource Center on Violence against Women, 2006, http://new.vawnet.org/ category/Main_Doc.php?docid=248.

54. Ibid.

55. D. Rungan et al., "Child Abuse and Neglect by Parents and Caregivers," in *World Health Report on Violence and Health*, eds. E. Krug et al. (Geneva: World Health Organization, 2002), 59–86.

56. A. J. Sedlak et al., *Fourth National Incidence Study of Child Abuse and Neglect (NIS-4): Report to Congress, Executive Summary* (Washington, DC: U.S. Department

of Health and Human Services, Administration for Children and Families, 2010), Available at www.acf.hhs.gov/programs/opre/abuse_neglect/natl_incid/index.html.

57. D. Rungan et al., "Child Abuse and Neglect by Parents and Caregivers," 2002.

58. University of Wisconsin–Madison, "What Is Sexual Harassment?", Sexual Harassment Information and Resources, Updated February 2007, www.oed.wisc.edu/sexualharassment/what.html.

59. K. Baum et al., *National Crime Victimization Survey: Stalking Victimization in the United States* (Bureau of Justice Statistics:

Washington, DC, 2009) NCJ 224527, Available at http://bjs.ojp.usdoj.gov/index.cfm?ty=pbdetail&iid=1211.

60. Ibid.

61. Ibid.

62. CDC Injury Center, "Preventing Intimate Partner Violence, Sexual Violence and Child Maltreatment," 2006, www.cdc.gov/ncipc/pub-res/research_agenda/07_violence.htm; P. York, "Traditional Gender Role Attitudes and Violence against Women: A Test of Feminist Theory," Paper presented at the annual meeting of the American Society of Crimi-

nology, November 13, 2007, Accessed June 2008, www.allacademic.com/meta/p200649_index.html.

63. U.S. Department of Justice, National Drug Intelligence Center, *National Gang Threat Assessment 2009* (Washington, DC: National Drug Intelligence Center, 2009) 2009-M0335-001, Available at www.justice.gov/ndic/pubs32/32146/index.htm.

64. Ibid.

65. U.S. Code of Federal Regulations, Title 28CFR0.85.

66. J. Carr, *American College Health Association Campus Violence White Paper,* 2005.

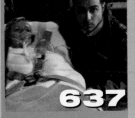

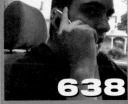

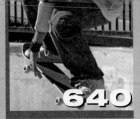

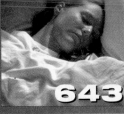

How many Americans die from unintentional injuries each year?

What's wrong with talking on a cell phone while driving?

Do I really have to wear a helmet while I'm skateboarding?

What's the top cause of fire-related deaths?

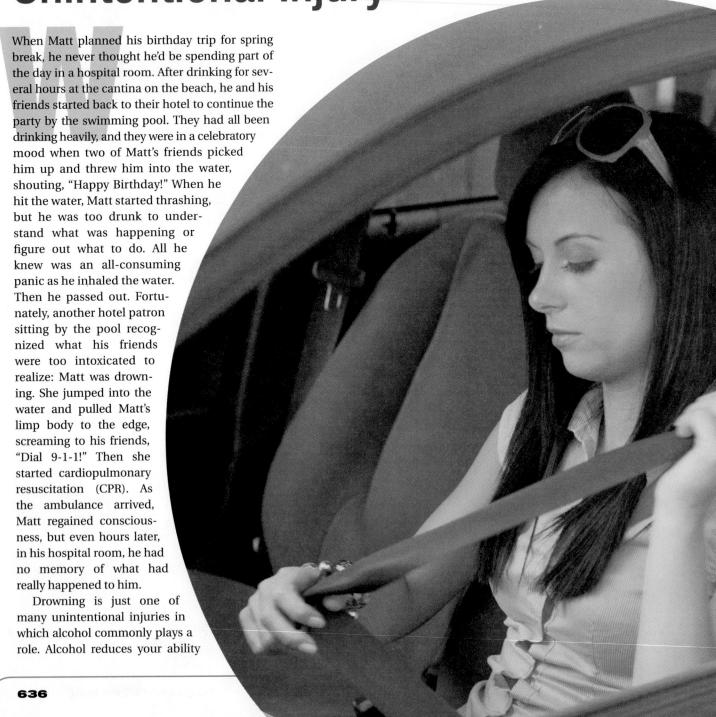

# FOCUS ON Reducing Your Risk of Unintentional Injury

When Matt planned his birthday trip for spring break, he never thought he'd be spending part of the day in a hospital room. After drinking for several hours at the cantina on the beach, he and his friends started back to their hotel to continue the party by the swimming pool. They had all been drinking heavily, and they were in a celebratory mood when two of Matt's friends picked him up and threw him into the water, shouting, "Happy Birthday!" When he hit the water, Matt started thrashing, but he was too drunk to understand what was happening or figure out what to do. All he knew was an all-consuming panic as he inhaled the water. Then he passed out. Fortunately, another hotel patron sitting by the pool recognized what his friends were too intoxicated to realize: Matt was drowning. She jumped into the water and pulled Matt's limp body to the edge, screaming to his friends, "Dial 9-1-1!" Then she started cardiopulmonary resuscitation (CPR). As the ambulance arrived, Matt regained consciousness, but even hours later, in his hospital room, he had no memory of what had really happened to him.

Drowning is just one of many unintentional injuries in which alcohol commonly plays a role. Alcohol reduces your ability to stay alert, to maintain an awareness of your surroundings, and to make good decisions. Other factors—such as drowsiness, distraction, and failing to take sensible precautions—increase your risk for injury for similar reasons. In fact, although the term **unintentional injury** might sound academic, most health professionals shy away from the more familiar term *accidental injury* because it implies that these injuries occur without individuals having any control over their situation. As we saw with Matt's near-drowning, "accidents" often occur as a consequence of people's poor choices. Car "accidents," for example, often occur because the driver was distracted by cell phone use or another activity, or impaired by sub-

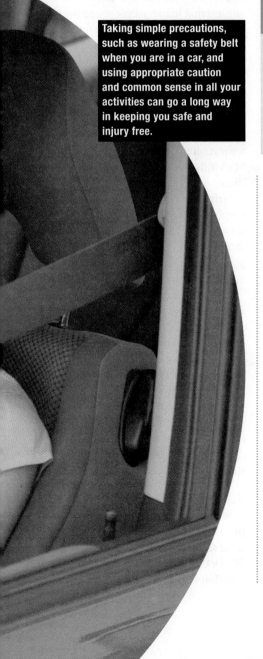

Taking simple precautions, such as wearing a safety belt when you are in a car, and using appropriate caution and common sense in all your activities can go a long way in keeping you safe and injury free.

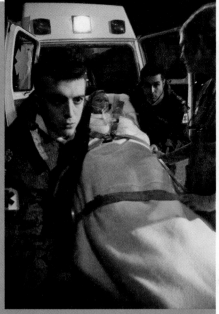

**How many Americans die from unintentional injuries each year?**

Unintentional injuries kill nearly 100,000 Americans each year. That's over 270 people per day. Most strategies for preventing unintentional injuries focus on changing something about the person, the environment, or the circumstances that put people in harm's way.

stance abuse, sleep deprivation, or other circumstances.

How big a problem is unintentional injury? For adults aged 18 to 44, unintentional injuries are the leading cause of death, killing approximately 45,000 young adults in the prime of life.[1] In fact, unintentional injuries are responsible for about 1 of every 4 deaths in this age group.[2] As you might expect, motor vehicle accidents are responsible for the greatest percentage of unintentional injury deaths. However, many other mechanisms are responsible for significant mortality each year, most notably poisonings, drownings, falls, and fires.[3]

In this chapter, we'll discuss the most common unintentional injuries, beginning with motor vehicle crashes, which are the leading cause of death of young adults.[4] For each injury type, we'll identify steps you can take to reduce your risk as well as strategies for managing an injury situation should one occur.

# Are You at Risk on the Road?

According to the National Highway Traffic Safety Administration, almost 34,000 people died in motor vehicle accidents (MVAs) in 2009.[5] That's nearly 100 Americans every day. What factors contribute to MVAs? And how can you reduce your risk?

## Five Factors Affect Motor Vehicle Safety

In the blink of an eye, your actions could transform your vehicle from a pleasant mode of transportation into a deadly weapon. Five factors—distracted driving, impaired driving, speeding, vehicle safety issues, and driver age—contribute to the majority of MVAs.[6] As you read about each of these, notice that most are within your personal control.

**Distracted Driving** In 2008, an estimated 11 percent of drivers were talking on a cell phone at any daylight moment. Not surprisingly, in the same year, 1.4 million crashes were attributed to cell phone use. Texting while driving is even more dangerous. Although only an estimated 1 percent of drivers were text-messaging in 2008, the behavior was responsible for an estimated 200,000 to 1 million crashes![7] Given these statistics, it's no wonder that laws regulating cell phone use while driving have been passed in several states, and 30 states now ban text-messaging for all drivers.[8]

Other common distractions for drivers include manipulating handheld music and Internet devices, adjusting CD players or the radio, looking in the mirror, calling out the window, and eating. Nearly 8 out of 10 MVAs happen within just 3 seconds of a driver becoming distracted.[9] The next time you're tempted to text, make a call, or even swat an insect while driving, don't do it. Pull over. Handle the distraction.

**unintentional injury** Any injury committed or sustained without intent of harm.

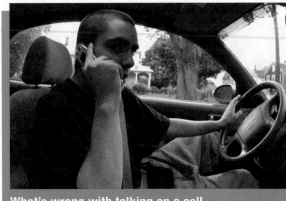

**What's wrong with talking on a cell phone while driving?**

Talking on a cell phone while driving puts you at a four times greater risk of being in a motor vehicle accident. It also increases the risk of injury and death to other drivers, passengers, and pedestrians and is illegal in many states.

Then rejoin the traffic when you're ready to give it your full attention.

**Impaired Driving** Every day, 32 people in the United States die in MVAs that involve an alcohol-impaired driver. This amounts to nearly 12,000 deaths, or 1 death every 45 minutes. If you think these deaths occur mainly among older adults, think again: 65 percent of alcohol-impaired drivers involved in fatal crashes are between the ages of 21 and 34.[10]

Although alcohol is the primary cause of impairment while driving, other substances and situations are also responsible. For example, use of drugs other than alcohol, including marijuana, cocaine, and prescription medications are increasing problems among young adult drivers and a significant cause of MVA injury and death.[11] Drowsiness can impair driving, too; many researchers contend that driving while sleep deprived is as dangerous as driving drunk.

Both public health and law enforcement agencies are cooperating on several measures to keep impaired drivers off the road. These include the following:

- Promotion of designated driver programs, including measures such as public funding of "safe rides" for people who have been drinking, and provision of nonalcoholic beverages free of charge to designated drivers.
- Strict enforcement of existing laws defining impaired driving and the legal drinking age

- Implementation of measures to prevent repeat offenses by anyone previously convicted of driving while impaired:
  - ✳ Mandatory alcohol or other drug abuse treatment
  - ✳ Installation of ignition interlock systems that prevent vehicle operation by anyone with a blood alcohol concentration above a specified safe level
  - ✳ Revoking the driver's license
- Stricter testing for and punishment of those who abuse prescription medicines and/or drive when sleep impaired.

**Speeding** Speeding is a factor in 1 out of every 3 fatal crashes. Driver surveys suggest that many people speed because they don't perceive it as dangerous—they believe that traffic laws are overly restrictive and don't apply to them! Unfortunately, such attitudes lead to more than 13,000 deaths each year.[12]

**Vehicle Safety Issues** Failure to wear a safety belt increases your risk of MVA injury and death, so buckle up and insist any passengers do the same. Wearing a safety belt cuts your risk of death or serious injury in a crash by about half.[13] If you're transporting an infant or child in your vehicle, follow state laws governing use and location of age-appropriate safety seats.

Vehicles can include many safety features, from air bags to stability control. Unfortunately, people who don't have the financial resources to drive vehicles with all of the state-of-the-art features—and that group often includes college students—are at increased risk during MVAs. Still, the next time you're planning to purchase a car, new or used, look for the following features recommended by the Insurance Institute for Highway Safety:

**1.** Does the car have front air bags? Side air bags? Remember, air bags do not eliminate the need for everyone to wear safety belts.
**2.** Does the car have antilock brakes? Traction and stability control? Each of

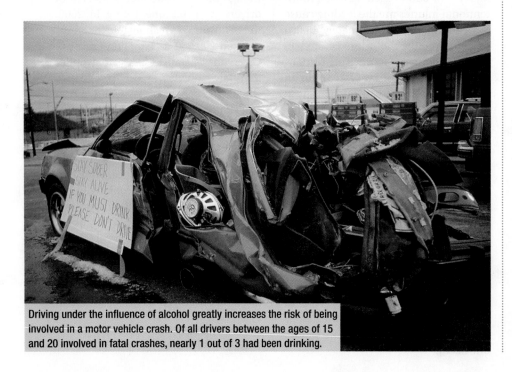

Driving under the influence of alcohol greatly increases the risk of being involved in a motor vehicle crash. Of all drivers between the ages of 15 and 20 involved in fatal crashes, nearly 1 out of 3 had been drinking.

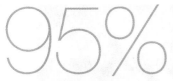

**95%** of college students surveyed reported that they mostly or always wear a safety belt when driving or riding in a car.

these features can mean the difference between life, injury, or death.

**3.** Does the car have impact-absorbing crumple zones?

**4.** Are there strengthened passenger compartment side walls?

**5.** Is there a strong roof support? (The center doorpost on four-door models gives you an extra roof pillar.)

Another factor in MVA safety is the size of the vehicles involved. All cars sold in the United States must meet U.S. Department of Transportation standards for crash worthiness, no matter their size. However, in crashes involving multiple vehicles, the death rate in 2007 for people in minicars was almost twice the rate for people in very large cars.[14] Many college students drive minicars because they are more affordable and use less gas, but the laws of physics make such cars more dangerous, especially in frontal collisions with larger cars.

What about motorcycles? Per vehicle mile traveled, motorcyclists are about 37 times more likely than passenger car occupants to die in an MVA, and 9 times more likely to be injured. In 2008, this translated into more than 5,000 motorcyclist deaths and 96,000 injuries.

Many motorcyclists involved in MVAs have avoided severe injuries because they were wearing a helmet. Although the benefits of helmets and protective clothing are well established, only 20 states have full helmet requirements for anyone riding a motorcycle. To find out what your state requirements are, go to www.iihs.org/laws/helmetusecurrent.aspx. An estimated 823 lives could have been saved in 2008—more than 16 percent—if all motorcyclists had worn helmets.[15]

**Driver Age** Many of us assume that seniors are the age group most often involved in MVAs. Sensory impairments and slowed reflexes can increase accident rates among people 65 and older,

but rates are at their peak among teen drivers, especially the first year that a teen has a license.[16] Graduated driver licensing (GDL) programs, which have been implemented in many states, have been shown to reduce MVA fatalities in crashes involving teens by nearly 20 percent.[17] They are also thought to reduce the risk of all MVAs involving teen drivers by 20 to 40 percent.[18] Typically, GDL programs involve several stages for teens to complete before becoming fully licensed.

## what do you think?

Should the use of handheld electronic devices while driving be outlawed throughout the United States? What about hands-free cell phone use? ● How does talking on a hands-free cell phone differ from gabbing with a friend in the passenger seat? ● Should graduated driver licensing be mandatory for all teen drivers in the United States?

## Practice Risk-Management Driving Techniques

Although you can't control what other drivers are doing, you can reduce your risk of injury in an MVA by practicing risk-management driving techniques. These include the following:

● Don't manipulate electronic devices while driving. Avoid talking on a cell phone while driving, even if the phone is hands free.
● Don't drink and drive. If you plan to party with friends, designate a sober driver or arrange in advance for a taxi or "safe ride," or plan to spend the night where you are.
● Don't drive when tired or when in a highly emotional or stressed state.
● Surround your car with a safety "bubble." The rear bumper of the car ahead of you should be at least 3 seconds away.
● Scan the road ahead of you and to both sides.

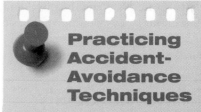

● Drive with your low-beam headlights on, *day and night,* to make your car more visible to other drivers.
● Anticipate the actions of other drivers as much as you can, and be on the alert for unsignaled lane changes, sudden braking, or other unexpected maneuvers.
● Obey all traffic laws.
● Whether you are the driver or a passenger, always wear a seat belt.

Even the most careful drivers may find themselves having to avoid an accident at some time in their lives. See the **Skills for Behavior Change** box above for tips on how to manage your risk.

## Can You Play It Safe and Still Have Fun?

Recreational activities among young people that commonly involve injury include biking, skateboarding, snow sports, swimming and boating, and using fireworks. By following some basic guidelines while doing these activities, you can have fun and be safe.

## Follow Bike Safety Rules

Currently, over 63 million Americans of all ages ride bicycles for transportation, recreation, and fitness. The National Highway Traffic Safety Administration (NHTSA) reports about 700 to 750 deaths per year from cycling accidents. The great majority of cycling deaths (87%) involve cyclists aged 16 and older.[19] Most fatal collisions are due to cyclists' errors, usually failure to yield at intersections. However, alcohol also plays a significant role in bicycle deaths and injuries: In 2008, nearly one-fourth (23%) of cyclists killed were legally drunk.[20]

All cyclists should wear a properly fitted bicycle helmet every time they ride (Figure 1). In spite of this, fewer than half of all college students report wearing a helmet while biking.[21] The NHTSA reports that a helmet is the single most effective way to prevent head injury resulting from a bicycle crash. Moreover, bear in mind that cyclists are considered vehicle operators; they are required to obey the same rules of the road as do drivers.

Cyclists should consider the following suggestions:

- Wear a helmet approved by the American National Standards Institute (ANSI) or the Snell Memorial Foundation.
- Watch the road and listen for traffic sounds! Never listen to an MP3 player or talk on a cell phone, even hands free, while cycling.
- Don't drink and ride.
- Follow all traffic laws, signs, and signals.
- Ride with the flow of traffic.
- Wear light or brightly colored, reflective clothing that is easily seen at dawn, dusk, and during full daylight.
- Avoid riding after dark. If you must ride at night, use a front light and a red reflector or flashing rear light, as well as reflective tape or other markings on your bike and clothing.
- Know and use proper hand signals.
- Keep your bicycle in good condition.
- Use bike paths whenever possible.
- Stop at stop signs and traffic lights.

## Stay Safe on Your Board

According to the U.S. Consumer Product Safety Commission (CPSC), approximately 26,000 people are treated in hospital emergency rooms each year with skateboard-related injuries. These

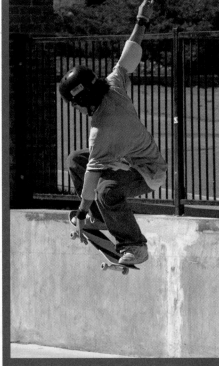

**Do I really have to wear a helmet while I'm skateboarding?**

The majority of skateboarding injuries occur among people who have been practicing the sport for more than a year, often when they attempt a stunt beyond their level of skill. Wearing a helmet, no matter how experienced a skateboarder you are, will help protect you in case of a fall.

injuries are most commonly due to falls or collisions, and some are fatal. Three factors commonly contribute to skateboard injury: lack of protective equipment, poor board maintenance, and irregular riding surfaces. Both inexperience and overconfidence also play a role: One-third of all injuries happen to people who have been skateboarding for less than a week, but the majority of injuries occur among people who have been skating for more than a year, typically when they are attempting difficult stunts.[22]

Skateboard safety tips from the CPSC include the following:

- Wear an approved helmet, padded clothes, special skateboarding gloves, and padding for your knees and other joints. Padding should be snug but loose enough to allow movement.

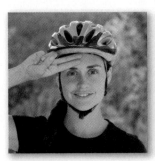 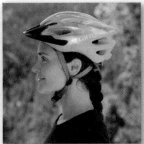 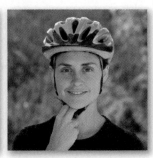

❶ The helmet should sit level on your head and low on your forehead—one or two finger-widths above your eyebrows.

❷ The sliders on the side straps should be adjusted to form a "V" shape under, and slightly in front of, your ears. Lock the sliders if possible.

❸ The chin strap buckle should be centered under your chin. Tighten the strap until it is snug, so that no more than two fingers fit under the strap.

**FIGURE 1** **Fitting a Bicycle Helmet**
When your helmet is fitted correctly, opening your mouth wide in a yawn should cause the helmet to pull down on your head. Also, you should not be able to rock the helmet back more than the width of two fingers above the eyebrows or forward into your eyes.

- Maintain your board. Between uses, check it for loose, broken, sharp, or cracked parts, and have it repaired if necessary.
- Examine the surface where you'll be riding for holes, bumps, and debris.
- Never skateboard in the street.
- Never hitch a ride from a car, bicycle, or other vehicle.
- Practice complicated stunts in specially designed areas, wearing lots of protective padding.
- Practice safe falling: If you start to lose your balance, crouch down; if you fall, try to "relax and roll."
- Don't drink and ride.

## Stay Safe in the Snow

The National Ski Areas Association (NSAA) reports that a skiing or snowboarding fatality occurs at the rate of 3.9 per 1 million participants per year.[23] Severe nonfatal injuries, such as head trauma and spinal cord injury, also occur, but at a similarly low rate. This makes snow sports much safer, overall, than bicycling, swimming, and many others. More good news is that the rate of injury has been declining for decades, largely because of the use of shorter skis, improved safety features on equipment, and increased safety efforts at resorts, such as having more monitors on the slopes, setting aside special family skiing areas, and encouraging helmet use.

These safety measures are critical, because when collisions and other accidents occur on the slopes, they can be fatal or leave the victim permanently paralyzed. One of the most important ways to protect yourself while skiing or snowboarding is to wear an approved helmet. The NSAA reports that helmet use reduces the risk of any head injury by 30 to 50 percent. It's also important to keep skis and snowboards in good condition, and to ski according to your ability. Pay attention to the locations of other skiers, and if you stop, move to the side of the trail. Finally, observe all posted signs and warnings.

## Stay Safe in the Water

Drowning is the fourth most common cause of accidental death among Americans of all ages, with 1 in 5 of those deaths occurring in children aged 14 and younger. Males are nearly four times more likely than females to die from unintentional drowning.[24] As we saw with Matt at the beginning of this chapter, alcohol plays a significant role in many drownings: About half of all fatal drownings involve alcohol.[25]

**Swimming** The American Red Cross reports that almost half of adults surveyed say they've had an experience in which they nearly drowned.[26] Most drownings occur during water recreation—swimming, diving, or just simply having fun—in unorganized or unsupervised areas, such as ponds or pools without lifeguards present. Many drowning victims were strong swimmers, so all swimmers should take the following precautions:

- Don't drink alcohol before or while swimming.
- Don't enter the water without a lifejacket unless you can swim at least 50 feet unassisted.
- Know your limitations; get out of the water when you start to feel even slightly fatigued.
- Never swim alone, even if you are a skilled swimmer. You never know what might happen.
- Never leave a child unattended, even in extremely shallow water.
- Before entering the water, check the depth. Most neck and back injuries result from diving into water that is too shallow.
- Never swim in a river with currents too swift for easy, relaxed swimming.
- Never swim in muddy or dirty water that obstructs your view of the bottom. Water that is discolored and choppy or foamy may indicate a rip current.
- If you are caught in a rip current, swim parallel to the shore. Once you are free of the current, swim toward the shore.
- Learn cardiopulmonary resuscitation (CPR). In the event of an emergency, in the time it might take for paramedics to arrive, your CPR skills could make a difference in someone's life. CPR performed by bystanders has been shown to improve outcomes in drowning victims.[27]

**Boating** In 2006, the U.S. Coast Guard received reports of 3,474 injured boaters and 710 deaths. About 70 percent of boating fatalities are drownings, and among those who drown, 9 out of 10 are not wearing a **personal flotation device**—that is, a lifejacket. Other boating fatalities are due to trauma, hypothermia, carbon monoxide poisoning, and other causes.[28]

Alcohol sharply raises the death risk for boaters: About one-third of all

---

**personal flotation device** A device worn to provide buoyancy and keep the wearer, conscious or unconscious, afloat with the nose and mouth out of the water; also known as a life jacket.

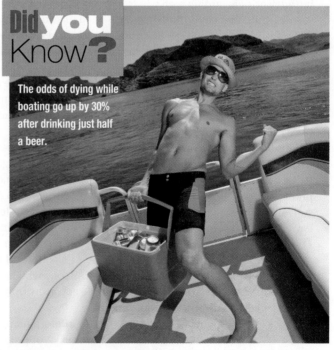

**Did you Know?**

The odds of dying while boating go up by 30% after drinking just half a beer.

**Source:** Data are from American Boating Association, "ABA Boating Safety Program," Accessed September 2010, www.americanboating.org/safety.asp.

boating fatalities involve alcohol. In fact, the effects of alcohol can be more pronounced during boating than they are during driving. This is due to boat and engine noise, vibration, wind, sun, glare, temperature, and wave action. When boat operators are drinking, both collisions with other boats and falls overboard are much more likely. If someone who has been drinking does fall overboard, he or she is more likely to drown or to die of hypothermia. Unfortunately, the "designated driver" concept does not apply to boating because intoxicated passengers often cause or directly contribute to boating accidents. The U.S. Coast Guard and every state have "Boating Under the Influence" (BUI) laws that carry stringent penalties for violation, including fines, license revocation, and even jail time.[29]

The following boating safety tips are from the American Boating Association:[30]

- Share your plans for your outing. Before leaving home, let others know where you are going, who will be with you, and when you expect to return.
- Check the weather. Listen to boating advisories regarding high winds, storms, and other environmental factors.
- Make sure your boat is seaworthy. Even if you are just going for a short trip, make sure the vessel doesn't leak, has enough fuel (if powered), and has the proper safety equipment.
- Make sure you have enough life jackets for all who are on board and that they are easily accessible.
- Carry an emergency radio and cell phone.
- Don't drink alcohol before you leave, and don't bring any aboard.

In addition, the U.S. Coast Guard recommends that before setting out, you put on your lifejacket. Most modern lifejackets are thin and flexible and

can be worn comfortably all day. Children must wear a lifejacket once the vessel is under way, unless they are below deck. If you decide not to put on your lifejacket initially, you must have one immediately available for every person aboard. Bear in mind that you need to wear a lifejacket not only when sailing or motorboating, but also when canoeing, kayaking, and rafting!

## Have Fun with Fireworks—Safely

It's the Fourth of July, and you're celebrating with friends and family. Your cousin has fished out of his basement a box of old fireworks and invites you to help him shoot them off. Should you do it? Each year, fireworks cause an estimated 7,000 injuries in the United States, often the loss of fingers or hands. And using improperly stored fireworks is a risk factor. Here are some safety tips for fireworks use from the National Council on Fireworks Safety:[31]

- Only use fireworks outdoors in an open area, at least 50 feet from spectators, buildings, dry grasses, and the like.
- Have plenty of water handy—either a hose or a bucket.
- When lighting fireworks, crouch down and reach out. Never bend over them. Don't hold onto them or throw them: Light the fuse and step away.
- Use only commercial fireworks, never homemade ones: They can kill you.
- Never tamper with fireworks, for example, trying to combine the powders. Use them only as intended.
- Never try to relight a "dud" firework. It could explode in your hand. Set it aside for 20 minutes, then soak it in a bucket of water.
- Alcohol and fireworks don't mix. Anyone who has been drinking should keep away from fireworks.

Before using any type of fireworks, check your state laws. You can find a state-by-state directory of fireworks-related laws at www.fireworksafety.com.

## How Can You Avoid Injuries at Home?

Injuries within the home typically occur in the form of poisonings, falls, or burns. Some populations, such as the elderly, are particularly vulnerable. However, older adults are not the only victims; each year, hundreds of young adults, teens, and children are brought to hospital emergency rooms for treatment of home-based injuries.

## Prevent Poisoning

A **poison** is any substance that is harmful to your body when ingested, inhaled, injected, or absorbed through the skin. Any substance can be poisonous if too much is taken. Every day in the United States, about 75 people die as a result of unintentional poisoning, and another 2,000 are treated in emergency departments.[32] This makes poisonings the second most common cause of unintentional injury deaths.

**Tips to Prevent Poisonings** The safety tips below were adapted from the American Association of Poison Control Centers:

- Read and follow all usage and warning labels before taking medications or working with chemicals, including household products.
- Never share or sell your prescription drugs.
- Never mix household products together, as combinations of products can give off toxic fumes.
- When working with chemicals, wear a protective mask and make sure the area in which you are working is well ventilated. Wear gloves and other protective clothing if there is any possibility of skin contact, and eyeglasses or an eye guard if splashing could occur.
- Be especially careful with medications, dietary supplements, and alcohol around children. Keep such items out of sight, preferably in a locked cabinet, and never refer to medication as "candy."

**poison** Any substance harmful to the body when ingested, inhaled, injected, or absorbed through the skin.

- Program the national poison control number, 1-800-222-1222, into your cell phone. The line is open 24 hours a day, 7 days a week.

### What to Do in Case of Poisoning

If you suspect you have ingested or inhaled a poison, or you are with someone who has collapsed, dial 9-1-1. If you are with someone who is not breathing and you are trained in CPR, provide CPR until paramedics arrive. If the victim is awake and alert, dial the poison control hot line (1-800-222-1222). Follow the instructions you are given: If you are told to take the person to a hospital emergency room, bring along the suspected poison, if possible.

## Avoid Falls

Falls are the third most common cause of death from unintentional injury, and a very common source of injury in the home. About 20 to 30 percent of people who fall suffer moderate to severe injury such as bruises, a fracture, a dislocation, or a head injury. In fact, falls are the most common cause of traumatic brain injury.[33] Although falls are most common among older adults, people of all ages experience them, and many are preventable.

Observe the following measures to reduce your risk of falls:

- Leave nothing lying around on the floor and nothing on the stairs.
- Avoid using small scatter rugs and mats, which can slide out from under your feet. Use rubberized liners or strips to secure large rugs to the floor.
- Train your pets to stay away from your feet.
- Install slip-proof mats, treads, or decals in showers and tubs and on the stairs.
- If you need to reach something in a high cupboard or closet, or to change a ceiling light, use an appropriate step stool or short ladder. Don't try to balance on a ledge or on any piece of furniture not designed to bear and balance body weight.
- When using a ladder, make sure it's stable before climbing.

- Wear supportive shoes. Flip flops and shoes without laces can trip you up.

## Reduce Your Risk of Fire

In the United States, a residential fire claims a life every 3 hours.[34] On an average day, nine college campuses in the United States will experience a fire in a residential structure. The three main causes of fires in campus housing are cooking, careless smoking, and arson. However, a variety of other factors typically contribute to injuries from dormitory fires:[35]

**1.** Alcohol is often a key factor. In more than 50 percent of fire fatalities, victims were intoxicated at the time of the fire.
**2.** Student apathy. Many students do not believe that fire is a risk to them, and ignore both fire drills and actual fire alarms.
**3.** Lack of preparation. Building evacuations are delayed because of inadequate fire drills, inability to recall exit routes, and so on.
**4.** Failure of early detection. Smoke alarms and fire alarm systems have not been maintained in working order, or have been vandalized and not repaired.
**5.** Delayed response. Students fail to properly notify the fire department using the 9-1-1 system.

**Fire Prevention** Tips to prevent fires include the following:

- Extinguish all cigarettes in ashtrays before bed, and never smoke in bed!
- Set lamps away from drapes, linens, and paper.
- In the kitchen, keep hot pads and kitchen cloths away from stove burners, avoid reaching over hot pans. Use caution when lighting barbecue grills.
- Keep candles under control and away from combustibles. Never leave candles unattended or burning while you sleep.
- Avoid overloading electrical circuits with appliances and cords. Older

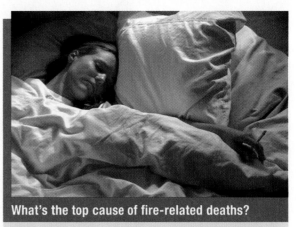

**What's the top cause of fire-related deaths?**

Smoking is the number one cause of fire-related deaths. If you fall asleep with a lit cigarette, bedding and clothing can quickly ignite. If you can't quit, take it outside.

buildings are at particular risk for fire from such overloads.
- Have the proper fire extinguishers ready in case of fire, and replace batteries in smoke alarms and test them periodically.

**What to Do in a Fire** If a fire breaks out in your dorm or apartment, your priority is to get out. Don't take time to phone before leaving. Don't gather up your stuff. First, feel the door handle: If it's hot, don't open the door! Go to a window, open it as fully as possible, and call for help. Hang a sheet from the window to let rescuers know where you are. If no one is outside, call 9-1-1. If smoke is entering your room, seal the cracks in the door with blankets or towels. Then stay low until you're rescued—there is less smoke close to the floor.

If the door handle is not hot, open the door cautiously. If the hallway is clear to the exit, get out, yelling, "Fire!" and knocking on doors as you leave. If you encounter smoke, stay low to the floor—crawl if necessary—to make your way out. If you pass a fire alarm on your way out, pull it. Always use the stairs, never an elevator. Once you're outside, dial 9-1-1.

The same tips apply when you're staying in a hotel or motel. Always bring a flashlight with you when traveling, and study the evacuation plan posted in your room. Before going to bed, locate the two exits nearest your room and the fire alarms on your floor.

## Learn First Aid and CPR

**25%** of all emergency room hospital visits could be avoided if people knew basic first aid and CPR.

If you were to encounter someone who is injured, would you offer assistance? Many bystanders don't, because they lack training and are afraid their efforts will do more harm than good. However, one simple action can help any injury victim: Dial 9-1-1. As soon as your call is answered, describe the situation, then follow the advice you're given. First aid measures are provided in Appendix B.

If you witness someone who has collapsed and you cannot detect a pulse, the American Heart Association advises that you call 9-1-1 and then begin chest compressions.[36] This technique simply requires you to push down in the middle of the victim's chest hard and fast (about 100 compressions per minute). Traditional **cardiopulmonary resuscitation (CPR)**, which includes mouth-to-mouth resuscitation as well as chest compression, is preferable for victims of near-drowning and other forms of respiratory collapse. Everyone is encouraged to get training in CPR, and the course is offered on most college campuses.

### "Why Should I Care?"

If you know first aid and CPR, someday you may be able to save someone's life. Less than one-third of people who suffer cardiac arrest outside of a hospital receive CPR from a bystander. When a person's heart stops beating, his or her chance of survival decreases by 7% to 10% each minute, and bystander CPR doubles or triples a victim's chances of surviving.

**cardiopulmonary resuscitation (CPR)** Emergency technique to provide lifesaving chest compression and mouth-to-mouth resuscitation when an individual has stopped breathing and has no pulse.

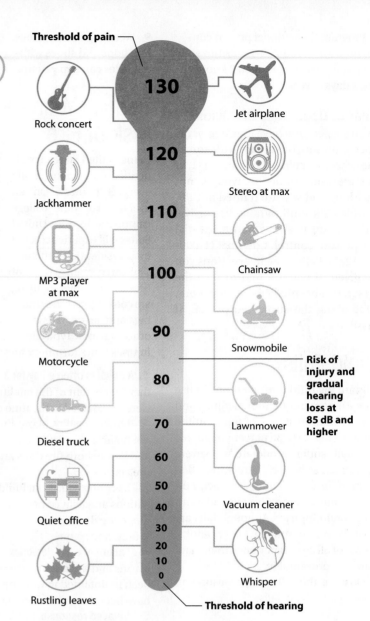

Threshold of pain — 130

Rock concert

Jet airplane

120

Jackhammer

Stereo at max

110

MP3 player at max

Chainsaw

100

Motorcycle

90

Snowmobile

80

Diesel truck

70

Lawnmower

60

50

40

Quiet office

30

Vacuum cleaner

20

10

0

Rustling leaves

Whisper

— Threshold of hearing

Risk of injury and gradual hearing loss at 85 dB and higher

**FIGURE 2 Noise Levels of Various Sounds (dB)**
Decibels increase logarithmically, so each increase of 10 db represents a tenfold increase in loudness.

**Source:** Adapted from National Institute on Deafness and Other Communication Disorders, "How Loud Is Too Loud? Bookmark," Updated June 2010, www.nidcd.nih.gov/health/hearing/ruler.asp.

## Limit Your Exposure to Loud Noise

Our modern society is too often filled with excess noise. Take a look at **Figure 2**, which shows the decibel (dB) levels of various common sounds. In general, noise levels above 85 dB (about as loud as a diesel truck) increase risks for hearing loss. When you consider the many such noises people are exposed to every day, it should be no surprise that hearing loss is becoming increasingly common. In fact, more than 36 million U.S. adults have hearing loss. Although you might think hearing loss is only a problem for the very old, 26 million Americans between the ages of 20 and 69 have hearing loss due to exposure to loud sounds either at work or in leisure activities.[37] In fact, according to the Bureau of Labor Statistics, occupational hearing loss is the most commonly recorded occupational illness in manufacturing, accounting for 1 in 9

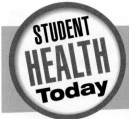

# STUDENT HEALTH Today | TURNING DOWN THE TUNES

Increasingly, children and young adults are experiencing hearing loss due to use of portable music devices such as MP3 players. Three factors make these devices more likely to damage hearing than simply listening to music from an external speaker: frequency of use, duration of use, and volume. The high level of sound quality, small size, and portability of the new MP3 players mean that people are listening to music more often, and for longer periods of time. Moreover, playing a tune at high volume on modern MP3 players doesn't distort its sound, so people may not be as likely to turn down the volume as they would have with older music devices. Any sound above 90 decibels (dB) can cause hearing loss if the exposure is prolonged and many people listen to music at volumes higher than this throughout the day, every day.

What can you do to avoid hearing loss while still enjoying your music?

The most important step is to keep the volume at or below 80 dB—or at a level at which you can still comfortably carry on a conversation. If you do that, you won't need to limit the amount of time you spend listening to music. Another way to tell if your volume is set too loud is to ask someone nearby if they can hear your music. If they can, it's definitely too loud. Finally, debate continues over the relative safety of over-the-ear earphones versus in-the-ear ear buds; however, experts agree that earphones are probably safer.

**Sources:** Mayo Clinic, "Hearing Loss: MP3 Players Can Pose Risk," 2006, www .riversideonline.com/health_reference/Ear -Nose-Throat/GA00046.cfm; H. Keppler et al., "Short-Term Auditory Effects of Listening to an MP3 Player," *Archives of Otolaryngology— Head & Neck Surgery* 136, no. 6 (2010): 538–48.

Hearing loss is becoming more frequent as music lovers increase the frequency, duration, and volume of their listening time.

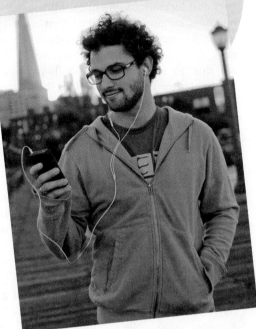

---

reportable illnesses.[38] These numbers may be just the tip of the iceberg, as a person's hearing loss must be determined to be work-related and severe enough to cause hearing impairment in order to be recordable by the Occupational Safety and Health Administration (OSHA). Many more workers are likely to have measurable occupational hearing loss, though they have not yet become hearing impaired.

Noise-induced hearing loss results when exposure to high-decibel (dB) noise, usually over extended periods of time, damages sensory receptors in the cochlea, or inner ear. Hearing loss can be temporary or permanent, and in general worsens with age. One of the highest rates of sudden noise-induced hearing loss is among adults aged 20 to 29. Ironically, many students (more than 75%) in a recent study reported being aware of the danger, yet more than 50 percent continued to expose themselves.[39] More than 66 percent of

these students reported having experienced tinnitus (ringing in the ears), but most said they weren't worried about it. However, tinnitus can be a precursor to hearing loss, and students who experience it or find themselves frequently in noisy settings should take steps to avoid prolonged exposure. Most rock musicians use earplugs when performing or rehearsing, and their audiences would be wise to do the same. Hearing loss may result from one evening in front of huge speakers at a rock concert. If you can't hear the person standing next to you at a concert, then you should put in earplugs or look for a quieter spot. In addition, you should rest your ears in between nights out partying, or attending concerts or loud sporting events.

Another source of hearing impairment is the use of portable listening devices such as MP3 players. Although they may deliver a lower level of deci-

bels than rock concerts, the frequent and prolonged exposure increases the potential for damage. Check out the **Student Health Today** box for more details and tips for protecting your hearing while enjoying your tunes.

## How Can You Avoid Injury While Working?

American adults spend most of their waking hours on the job. Although most job situations are pleasant and productive, others pose hazards. Transportation incidents make up the largest number of fatal work injuries (41%). An additional 23 percent of fatal work injuries occur on highways, mostly involving truck drivers. Overall, workers in the transportation and material moving, construction and extraction, and service industries are at the highest risk of fatal injuries, and those who fish for a living and related fishing workers, farmers, and loggers are also at high risk.[40]

Although on-the-job deaths capture media attention, workers may also be seriously injured or disabled at their jobs. Common work injuries include cuts and lacerations, chemical burns, fractures, sprains, and strains (often of the back), and repetitive motion disorders. Because so many work injuries are due to overexertion, poor body mechanics, or repetitive motion, they are largely preventable. We discuss these problems and share some prevention strategies here.

## Protect Your Back

Low back pain (LBP), usually as a result of injury, is epidemic throughout the world and is the major cause of disability for people aged 20 to 45 in the United States, who suffer more frequently and severely from this problem than older people do.[41] It is one of the most commonly experienced chronic ailments among college students.

Because most injuries to the back are in the lumbar spine area (lower back), strengthening core muscle groups and stretching muscles to avoid cramping and spasms are key strategies to reduce risks. Frequently, sports injuries, stress on spinal bones and tissues, the sudden jolt of a car accident, or other obvious causes are the culprits. Other times, sitting too long in the same position or hunching over your computer while you're pulling an all-nighter can leave you with pain so severe that you can't stand up or walk comfortably. Carrying heavy backpacks between classes is another frequent source of LBP.

You can avoid typical risks by using common sense and thinking "safety" when engaging in activities that could injure your back. Getting up and stretching after long hours in a static position is another great strategy to avoid problems. Maintaining good posture can also reduce back problems.

Other measures you can take to reduce the risk of back pain include the following:

- Invest in a high-quality, supportive mattress.
- Avoid high-heeled shoes, which tilt the pelvis forward.
- Control your weight. Extra weight puts increased strain on your knees, hips, and back.
- Warm up and stretch before exercising or lifting heavy objects.
- When lifting something heavy, use your leg muscles and use proper form (Figure 3). Do not bend from the waist or take the weight load on your back.
- Buy a desk chair with good lumbar support.

- Move your car seat forward so your knees are elevated slightly.
- Engage in exercise regularly, particularly in core exercises that strengthen the abdominal muscles and stretch the back muscles.
- Downsize your backpack.

## Maintain Alignment while Sitting

Think back over your day: How many hours have you sat glued to a workstation, laptop, netbook, tablet computer, pocket computer, mobile device, or an ordinary book? And while you were at it, were you slouching, hunched over, or sitting up straight? Your answers are probably reflected in the degree of aching and stiffness you may be feeling right now. So how can you maintain a healthy alignment while you sit and work? Try these strategies:

**1.** Sit comfortably with your feet flat on the floor or on a footrest, and your knees level with your hips. Raise or lower your chair, or move to a different chair, to achieve this position.
**2.** Your middle back should be firmly against the back of the chair. The small of your back should be supported, too. If you can't feel the chair back supporting your lumbar region, try placing a small cushion or even a rolled towel behind the curve of your lower back.
**3.** Keep your shoulders relaxed and straight, not rolled or hunched forward.
**4.** The angle of your elbows should be 90 degrees to your upper arms. Change your position or the position of your device to achieve this angle.
**5.** Ideally, you should be looking straight ahead, not peering down at the device's screen.

## Avoid Repetitive Motion Disorders

It's the end of the term, and you have finished the last of several papers. After hours of nonstop typing, your hands are numb and you feel an

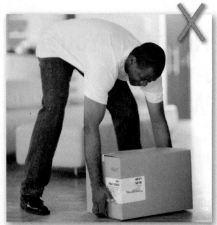

ⓐ Attempting to lift a heavy object by bending at your waist is a common cause of back injury.

FIGURE 3 **Lifting a Heavy Object**

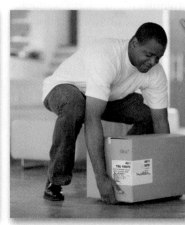

ⓑ Start as close to the object as possible, with it positioned between your knees as you squat down. Keep your feet parallel, or stagger one foot in front of the other. Keep the object close to your body as you stand, using your legs, not your back, to lift.

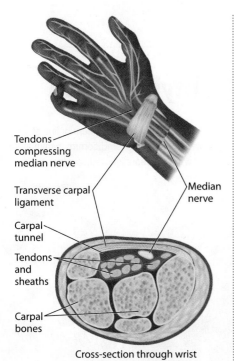

Tendons
compressing
median nerve

Transverse carpal
ligament

Median
nerve

Carpal
tunnel

Tendons
and
sheaths

Carpal
bones

Cross-section through wrist

FIGURE 4 **Carpal Tunnel Syndrome**
The carpal tunnel is a space beneath the transverse carpal ligament and above the carpal bones of the wrist. The median nerve and the tendons that allow you to flex your fingers run through this tunnel. Carpal tunnel syndrome occurs when repetitive use prompts inflammation of the tissues and fluids of the tunnel. This in turn compresses the median nerve.

intense, burning pain that makes the thought of typing one more word almost unbearable. If this happens, you may be suffering from one of several **repetitive motion disorders (RMDs)**, sometimes called *overuse syndrome, cumulative trauma disorders,* or *repetitive stress injuries.* These refer to a family of painful soft tissue injuries that begin with inflammation and gradually become disabling.

Repetitive motion disorders include carpal tunnel syndrome, bursitis, tendonitis, and ganglion cysts, among others.[42] Twisting of the arm or wrist, overexertion, and incorrect posture or position are usually contributors. The areas most likely to be affected are the hands, wrists, elbows, and shoulders, but the neck, back, hips, knees, feet, ankles, and legs can be affected, too. Over time, RMDs can

cause permanent damage to nerves, soft tissue, and joints. Usually, RMDs are associated with repeating the same task in an occupational setting and gradually irritating the area in question. However, certain sports (tennis, golf, and others), gripping the wheel while driving, keyboarding or texting, and a number of newer technology-driven activities can also result in RMDs.

Because many of these injuries occur in everyday work, play, and athletics, they are often not reported to national agencies that keep track of injury statistics. Many people just pop over-the-counter pain remedies and continue working until the pain becomes unbearable. Nevertheless, reports of increasing numbers of cases of disorders like "BlackBerry thumb," carpal tunnel syndrome, and other maladies are widespread.

One of the most common RMDs is **carpal tunnel syndrome (CTS)**, an inflammation of the soft tissues and fluids within the "tunnel" through the carpal bones of the wrist (Figure 4). This puts pressure on the median nerve, which runs down the forearm through the tunnel to innervate the hand. Symptoms include numbness, tingling, and pain in the fingers and hands. Carpal tunnel syndrome typically results from spending hours typing at the computer keyboard, flipping groceries through computerized scanners, or manipulating other objects in jobs "made simpler" by technology. The risk for CTS can be reduced by proper design of workstations, protective wrist pads, and worker training. Physical and occupational therapy is an important part of treatment and recovery.

# Are You Prepared for Environmental Events?

A **natural disaster** is any extreme environmental event that causes widespread destruction of land and/or property, injuries, and sometimes

deaths. Some, such as hurricanes and volcanic eruptions, may be predictable, whereas others, like earthquakes and many tornadoes, can occur without warning. If a natural disaster were to strike without warning in your region, would you be prepared?

The first step in preparedness is to learn what types of natural disasters typically affect the area where you live. If you've relocated from New England to the Midwest to attend school, for example, you may want to learn about tornado preparedness. If you attend school in the Southeast, hurricanes would be a key concern. To learn more about specific types of disasters, log on to the Centers for Disease Control and Prevention (CDC) website at www.cdc.gov and search the event name. For instance, the CDC's hurricane page provides key facts; basic steps to prepare yourself, your residence, and even your pets; a list of emergency supplies you'd need; information on how to evacuate safely; and steps to take to get through the storm safely if you're ordered *not* to evacuate. You can always find advisories and other information about weather-related events in your area—from blizzards to gales to flash floods—by visiting the National Weather Service website at www.weather.gov.

# Assess Yourself

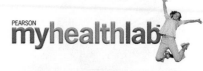

## Are You at Risk for a Motor Vehicle Accident?

Fill out this assessment online at
www.pearsonhighered.com/myhealthlab or
www.pearsonhighered.com/donatelle.

How often are you at risk for becoming involved in a motor vehicle accident? Answer the questions below to find out.

**How often do you:**

| | Never | Sometimes | Often |
|---|---|---|---|
| 1. Drive after you have had one or two drinks? | ○ | ○ | ○ |
| 2. Drive after you have had three or more drinks? | ○ | ○ | ○ |
| 3. Drive when you are tired? | ○ | ○ | ○ |
| 4. Drive while you are extremely upset? | ○ | ○ | ○ |
| 5. Drive while texting or talking on your cell phone? | ○ | ○ | ○ |
| 6. Drive or ride in a car while not wearing a seat belt? | ○ | ○ | ○ |
| 7. Drive faster than the speed limit? | ○ | ○ | ○ |
| 8. Accept rides from friends who have been drinking? | ○ | ○ | ○ |

If you answered "often" or "sometimes" to any question, you may need to adjust your behavior and educate yourself about the steps you can take to be safer on the road.

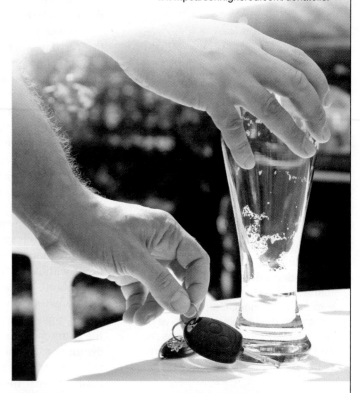

# YOUR PLAN FOR CHANGE

The **Assess Yourself** activity should help you identify the ways you take risks on the road. Depending on your responses, you might choose to make some of the following changes.

**Today, you can:**

○ Fasten your seat belt before you turn the ignition key, and ask everyone in your vehicle to do the same.

○ Commit to turning off your cell phone and other handheld devices before you drive.

○ Drive within the posted speed limit.

**Within the next 2 weeks, you can:**

○ Offer to be the designated driver the next time you go out with friends.

○ Get 7 to 8 hours of sleep before setting out on a long drive.

**By the end of the semester, you can:**

○ Bring your car in for a tune-up, and have the mechanic check that the seat belts and air bags are functioning properly.

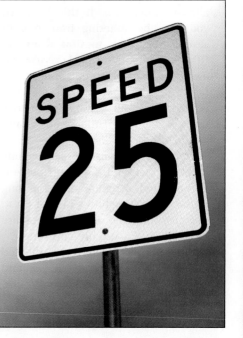

# References

1. Centers for Disease Control and Prevention, "Leading Causes of Death, United States, 2007—All Races, Both Sexes," 2007, Available at www.cdc.gov/injury/wisqars/index.html.
2. M. Heron, Centers for Disease Control and Prevention, "Deaths: Leading Causes for 2006," *National Vital Statistics Reports*, 58, no. 14 (March 2010), Available at www.cdc.gov/nchs/products/nvsr.htm.
3. Centers for Disease Control and Prevention, "Injury Mortality: Unintentional Injury: U.S. 2001–2006," 2009, http://205.207.175.93/HDI/TableViewer/tableView.aspx?ReportId=71.
4. National Safety Council, "Defensive Driving," 2010, www.nsc.org/safety _road/DefensiveDriving/Pages/defensive_driving.aspx.
5. National Highway Traffic Safety Administration, "Traffic Safety Facts: Early Estimate of Motor Vehicle Traffic Fatalities in 2009," DOT HS 811 291, 2010, www-nrd.nhtsa.dot.gov/Pubs/811291.PDF.
6. National Safety Council, "Driver Safety," 2010, www.nsc.org/safety_road/DriverSafety/Pages/driver_safety.aspx.
7. National Safety Council, "Summary of Estimate Model," 2010, www.nsc.org/news_resources/Resources/Documents/NSC%20Estimate%20Summary.pdf.
8. Governors Highway Safety Association, "Cell Phone and Texting Laws," Updated October 2010, www.ghsa.org/html/stateinfo/laws/cellphone_laws.html.
9. Centers for Disease Control and Prevention, "Parents Are the Key: Eight Danger Zones," Updated October 2009, www.cdc.gov/parentsarethekey/danger/index.html.
10. National Highway Traffic Safety Administration, *Traffic Safety Facts 2008 Data: Alcohol-Impaired Driving* (Washington, DC: NHTSA's National Center for Statistics and Analysis, 2009), DOT HS 811 155, Available at www-nrd.nhtsa.dot.gov/cats/listpublications.aspx?Id=A&ShowBy=DocType.
11. National Institute on Drug Abuse, "NIDA InfoFacts: Drugged Driving," Revised September 2009, http://drugabuse.gov/infofacts/driving.html.
12. National Safety Council, "Speeding," 2010, Available at www.nsc.org/safety_road/DriverSafety/Pages/speeding.aspx.
13. Centers for Disease Control and Prevention, "Eight Danger Zones," 2009, www.cdc.gov/parentsarethekey/danger/index.html.
14. Insurance Institute for Highway Safety, "New Crash Tests Demonstrate the Influence of Vehicle Size and Weight on Safety in Crashes; Results Are Relevant to Fuel Economy Policies," April 2009, www.iihs.org/news/rss/pr041409.html.
15. National Highway Traffic Safety Administration, *Traffic Safety Facts 2008 Data: Motorcycles* (Washington, DC: NHTSA's National Center for Statistics and Analysis, 2009), DOT HS 811 159, Available at www-nrd.nhtsa.dot.gov/cats/listpublications.aspx?Id=A&ShowBy=DocType.
16. Centers for Disease Control and Prevention, "Eight Danger Zones," 2009.
17. A. Williams and R. Shults, "Graduated Driver Licensing Research, 2007–Present: A Review and Commentary," *Journal of Safety Research* 41, no. 2 (2010): 77–84.
18. National Safety Council, "Graduated Driver Licensing," 2010, www.nsc.org/safety_road/TeenDriving/GDL/Pages/GraduatedDriverLicensing.aspx.
19. National Highway Traffic Safety Administration, *Traffic Safety Facts 2008 Data: Bicyclists and Other Cyclists* (Washington, DC: NHTSA's National Center for Statistics and Analysis, 2009), DOT HS 811 156, Available at www-nrd.nhtsa.dot.gov/cats/listpublications.aspx?Id=A&ShowBy=DocType.
20. Ibid.
21. American College Health Association, *ACHA-NCHA Reference Group Executive Summary Fall 2009*, 2009, Available at www.achancha.org/docs/ACHA-NCHA_Reference_Group_ExecutiveSummary_Fall2009.pdf.
22. Consumer Product Safety Commission, "Fact Sheet: Skateboards," 2009, Available at www.cpsc.gov/cpscpub/pubs/rec_sfy.html.
23. National Ski Areas Association, "Facts about Skiing/Snowboarding Safety," 2009, www.nsaa.org/nsaa/press/facts-ski-snbd-safety.asp.
24. Centers for Disease Control and Prevention, "Unintentional Drowning: Fact Sheet," June 2010, www.cdc.gov/HomeandRecreationalSafety/Water-Safety/waterinjuries-factsheet.html.
25. Ibid.
26. American Red Cross, "Summer Water Safety Guide," March 2009, http://american.redcross.org/site/DocServer/watersafety0609.pdf?docID=735.
27. Centers for Disease Control and Prevention, "Unintentional Drowning," 2010.
28. Ibid.
29. U. S. Coast Guard, "Boating Safety Resource Center: Boating Under the Influence Initiatives," 2009, www.uscgboating.org/safety/boating_under_the_influence_initiatives.aspx.
30. American Boating Association, "Boating Safety—It Could Mean Your Life," 2010, www.americanboating.org/safety.asp.
31. National Council on Fireworks Safety, "Key Fireworks Safety Information," 2010, www.fireworksafety.com.
32. Centers for Disease Control and Prevention, "Poisoning in the United States: Fact Sheet," 2010, www.cdc.gov/HomeandRecreationalSafety/Poisoning/poisoning-factsheet.htm.
33. Centers for Disease Control and Prevention, "Falls among Older Adults: An Overview," 2009, www.cdc.gov/HomeandRecreationalSafety/Falls/adultfalls.html.
34. Fire Safety Council, "Home Fires: The Big Picture," 2007, www.firesafety.gov/media/overview/index.shtm.
35. Fire Safety Council, "Campus Fire Safety," 2008, www.firesafety.gov/citizens/firesafety/college.shtm.
36. M. R. Sayre et al., "Hands-Only (Compression-Only) Cardiopulmonary Resuscitation: A Call to Action for Bystander Response," *Circulation* 177, no. 16 (2008): 2162–67.
37. National Institute on Deafness and Other Communication Disorders, "Quick Statistics," 2010, www.nidcd.nih.gov/health/statistics/quick.htm.
38. National Institute for Occupational Safety and Health, "Occupationally Induced Hearing Loss," 2010, www.cdc.gov/niosh/docs/2010-136.
39. V. Rawool and L. Colligon-Wayne, "Auditory Lifestyles and Beliefs Related to Hearing Loss among College Students in the USA," *Noise and Health* 10, no. 38 (January–March 2008): 1–10.
40. U.S. Bureau of Labor Statistics, "Census of Fatal Occupational Injuries (CFOI)-Current and Revised Data," 2010, www.bls.gov/iif/oshcfoi1.htm.
41. National Institute of Neurological Disorders and Stroke, "Low Back Pain Fact Sheet," June 2010, www.ninds.nih.gov/disorders/backpain/detail_backpain.htm.
42. National Institute of Neurological Disorders and Stroke, "NINDS Repetitive Motion Disorders Information Page," 2007, www.ninds.nih.gov/disorders/repetitive_motion/repetitive_motion.htm.

## 20

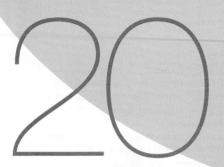

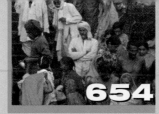

**654**

Why is population growth an environmental issue?

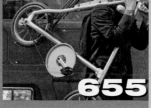

**655**

What's a carbon footprint and why should I worry about it?

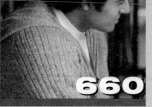

**660**

How can air pollution be a problem indoors?

# Preserving and Protecting Your Environment

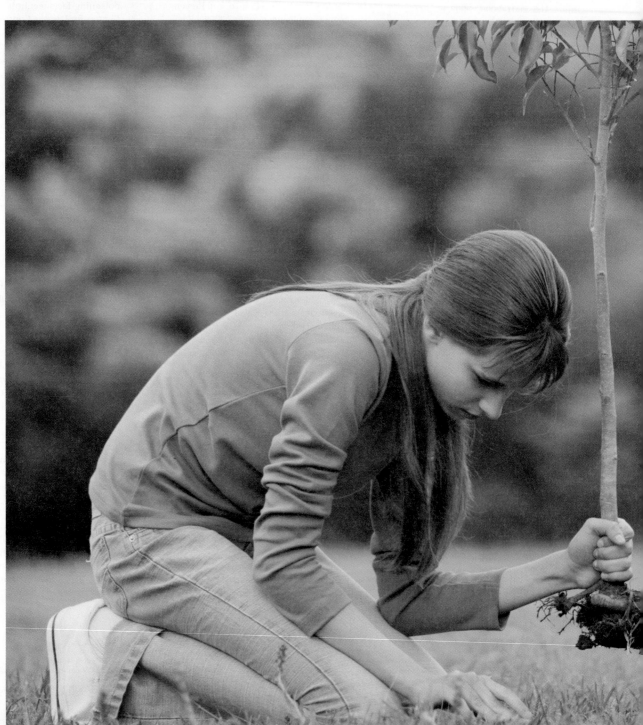

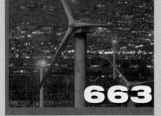

**663**

How can I help prevent global warming?

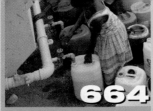

**664**

Is there such a thing as water scarcity?

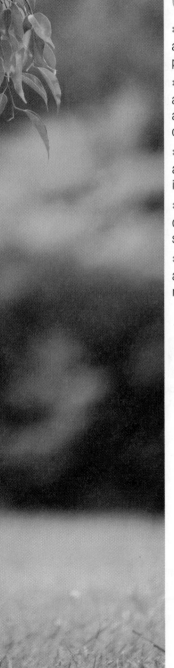

## Objectives

✳ Explain the environmental impact associated with the current global population and its projected growth.

✳ Discuss major causes of air pollution and the global consequences of the accumulation of greenhouse gases and ozone depletion.

✳ Identify sources of water pollution and chemical contaminants often found in water.

✳ Explain how municipal solid waste is different from hazardous waste, and list strategies for reducing land pollution.

✳ Discuss the health concerns associated with ionizing and nonionizing radiation.

*We have arrived at a moment of decision. Our home—Earth—is in grave danger. What is at risk of being destroyed is not the planet itself, of course, but the conditions that have made it hospitable for human beings.*
*—Al Gore, opening statement before the Senate Foreign Relations Committee, January 28, 2009*

We live in an especially dangerous time—dangerous for us, dangerous for future generations, and dangerous to our very existence. Our global population has grown more in the past 50 years than at any other time in human history. Population growth poses a potentially devastating threat to the water we drink, the air we breathe, the food we eat, and our capacity to survive. Our polar ice caps and glaciers are melting at rates that defy even the most dire predictions of just a decade ago, and threats of rising sea levels loom large. One in four existing mammals in the world is now threatened with extinction as humans destroy habitat, exacerbate drought and flooding through climate change, and pollute the environment. Clean water is becoming increasingly scarce, fossil fuels are being depleted at unprecedented rates, and our solid and hazardous wastes are growing in direct proportion to our global population.

Have we already crossed the "tipping-point"—the point at which we will be unable to restore the balance between humans and nature—or are there actions we can take to slowly improve our environmental situation? To bring the environmental health of Earth back into balance, individuals, communities, and political powers must take action now to make positive change. Americans must reduce consumption, waste less, discover new "green energy," be less selfish when it comes to personal comfort and perceived needs, and force governments to enact and enforce environmentally responsible legislation. This chapter provides an overview of the factors contributing to our global environmental crisis. Staying informed and becoming involved in the process are key things you can do to help.

## Overpopulation

Anthropologist Margaret Mead wrote, "Every human society is faced with not one population problem but two: how to beget and rear enough children and how not to beget and rear too many."[1] As noted environmental scientist Robert H. Friis described it, "Every day we share Earth and its resources with 250,000 more people than the day before. Although rates are slowing, every year, there are more than 80 million new mouths to feed. This is the equivalent to adding a city the size of Philadelphia to the world population every week, a Los Angeles every 2 weeks, a Mexico or Germany every year, and a United States and Canada every 3 years."[2] Although the United Nations projected that the world population would grow from 7 billion in 2011 to 9.4 billion by 2050 and to 11.5 billion by 2150, 2009 population growth already surpasses 6.8 billion (see **Figure 20.1** on page 652).[3]

Although our population continues to expand, and people live longer, Earth's resources are not expanding. Fertile land, clean water, rain forests, and all natural resources are disappearing at a phenomenal rate. According to a recent United Nations Global Environmental Outlook report (GEO-4), the human population is living far beyond its means and is inflicting damage on the environment that may already be irreparable.[4] Population experts believe that the most critical environmental challenge today is to slow the world's population growth.

## Bursting with People: Measuring the Impact

While many people question *when* we will reach the tipping point, others argue that it is too late now. Evidence of the effects of unchecked population growth, excessive consumption, and toxic by-products of human use and waste is everywhere:

**ecosystem** The collection of physical (nonliving) and biological (living) components of an environment and the relationships between them.

**fossil fuels** Carbon-based material used for energy; includes oil, coal, and natural gas.

● **Impact on other species.** Based on current reporting, changes in the **ecosystem** are resulting in destruction of whole species. Twelve percent of birds are threatened with extinction, and 23 percent of mammals and more than 30 percent of amphibians are already gone or nearly gone. Many that survive have chemically induced ailments or genetic disfigurement.[5]

● **Impact on our food supply.** We are currently fishing our oceans at rates that are 250 percent more than they can regenerate. At current rates, scientists project a global collapse of all fish species by 2050. Food shortages and famine are occurring in many regions of the world with increasing frequency. Faced with decreasing supplies of food products, fish, and the capacity to feed livestock, we may be forced to change the way we think about food. Many experts say we should "eat lower on the food chain" by eating more plants.

● **Land degradation and contamination of drinking water.** The per capita availability of freshwater is declining rapidly, and contaminated water remains the greatest single environmental cause of human disease. Unsustainable land use and climate change are increasing land degradation, including erosion, nutrient depletion, and deforestation that will inevitably affect human life.

● **Impact on energy consumption.** "Use it *and* lose it" is an apt saying for the use of nonrenewable energy sources in the form of **fossil fuels** (oil, coal, natural gas).

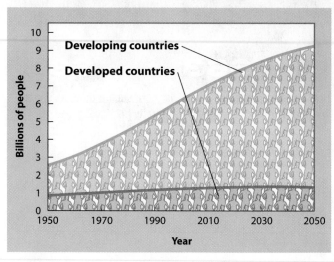

FIGURE 20.1 **World Population Growth, 1950–2050 (Projected)**

**Source:** Data are from Population Division of the Department of Economic and Social Affairs of the United Nations Secretariat, *World Population Prospects: The 2008 Revision*, 2009, http://esa.un.org/unpp.

Although we are seeing a shift toward renewable energy sources, such as hydropower, solar and wind power, and biomass power, most of us still use fossil fuels. In many developing regions of the world, demand for limited fossil fuels is growing at unprecedented rates (see Figure 20.2).

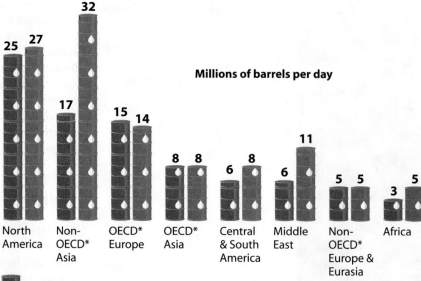

**Millions of barrels per day**

**2007 actual; each barrel = 5 million**

**2035 projected; each barrel = 5 million**

FIGURE 20.2 **World Liquid Fuels Consumption by Region and Country Group, 2007 and 2035 (Projected)**

*OECD is the Organization for Economic Cooperation and Development.

**Source:** Data are from U.S. Energy Information Administration, *International Energy Outlook 2010*, DOE/EIA-0484 (Washington, DC: U.S. Energy Information Administration, 2010), Available at www.eia.gov/oiaf/ieo/index.html.

## Factors That Affect Population Growth

Changes in fertility and mortality rates are key factors in population increase. The **total fertility rate** is a measure of the hypothetical average number of children born to women during their lifetime (typically assessed between the ages of 15 and 44), given prevailing fertility and mortality rates. In the United States today, the fertility rate is just over 2 births per woman, as compared to nearly 3.5 births per woman during the baby boom years after World War II.[6] In other regions of the world, particularly in certain African countries and the Middle East, fertility rates range from over 5 to nearly 8 (see Table 20.1).[7]

High fertility rates lead to rapid increases in overall population in these poorer countries and create a significant impact on environmental resources. Even in higher income countries slight changes in fertility rates affect energy use.

Mortality rates from both chronic and infectious diseases have declined in both developed and developing regions of the world as a result of improved public health infrastructure, increased availability of drugs and vaccines, better disaster preparedness, and other factors. Consequently, people are living longer. This, too, contributes to pressure on the environment.

TABLE 20.1 | **Selected Total Fertility Rates Worldwide, 2010**

| Country | Number of Children Born per Woman* | Rank |
|---|---|---|
| Niger | 7.68 | 1 |
| Uganda | 6.73 | 2 |
| Afghanistan | 5.50 | 12 |
| Saudi Arabia | 3.77 | 44 |
| India | 2.65 | 82 |
| Mexico | 2.31 | 104 |
| United States | 2.06 | 124 |
| Australia | 1.78 | 156 |
| Canada | 1.58 | 178 |
| China | 1.54 | 182 |
| Russia | 1.41 | 196 |
| Japan | 1.20 | 219 |

*Indicates the average number of children that would be born per woman if all women lived to the end of their childbearing years and bore children according to a given fertility rate at each age.

**Source:** Data are from Central Intelligence Agency, "The World Factbook: Country Comparison: Total Fertility Rate," 2010, https://www.cia.gov/library/publications/the-world-factbook/rankorder/2127rank.html.

## Different Nations, Different Growth Rates

The country projected to have the largest increase in population in coming decades is India, which is expected to add another 600 million people by the year 2050, surpassing China as the most populous country in the world.[8] The preference for large families in many developing nations has historically been related to several factors: high infant mortality rates; the traditional view of children as "social security" (working from a young age to assist families in daily survival and supporting parents when they grow too old to work); the low educational and economic status of women, which often leaves women with few reproductive choices; and the traditional desire for sons, which keeps parents of daughters reproducing until they have male offspring.

In contrast to developing nations, the population sizes in wealthier nations are static or declin-

**"Why Should I Care?"**

Imagine waking up in the morning and finding that you have no water for a shower; that your lights can be used only a few hours each day or not at all; and that you have to choose between using electricity for your laptop, flat-screen TV, or your refrigerator. Imagine having very little gas for your car, and going to the grocery store to find half-empty shelves of items you can't afford. Such scenarios are not the imaginings of science fiction. Major difficulties loom unless we take action to change our current rate of population growth and our consumption of natural resources, and unless the global community acts together to enforce policies and programs to check rampant population growth.

ing, with one notable exception—the United States. With a population of over 310 million, the United States continues to lead most other industrialized nations in population growth with a growth rate of nearly 1 percent in 2010.[9] Currently, we are 123 out of 233 nations of the world in population growth, exceeding industrialized nations such as Australia, New Zealand, France, Canada, and England. Each year, the United States adds nearly 3 million more people, or 8,000 per day.[10]

**total fertility rate** The hypothetical average number of children born to women during their lifetime, given prevailing fertility and mortality rates.

Although the United States makes up only 5 percent of the world's population, it is responsible for nearly 25 percent of total global resource consumption.[11] According to the Worldwatch Institute, "between 1950 and 2000, the United States was responsible for 212 gigatons of carbon dioxide, whereas India was responsible for less than 10 percent as much. So it is clear that the richest people on the planet are appropriating more than their fair share of 'environmental space.'"[12] In fact, industrial countries with less than 20 percent of the world's population contributed roughly 40 percent of global carbon emissions and are responsible for more than 60 percent of the total

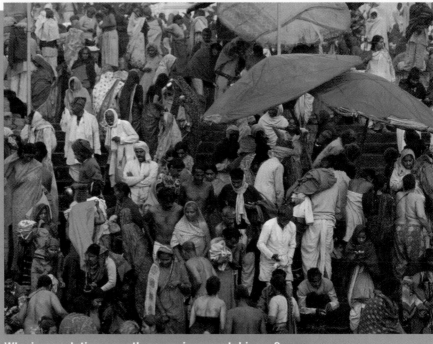

# 4 million

barrels of oil, the amount spilled into the Gulf of Mexico in 2010, is as much oil as Americans use every 5 hours.

carbon dioxide that fossil fuels have added to the atmosphere.[13]

These numbers are significant, and another alarming trend is occurring. China and other regions of the world are becoming major consumers of fossil fuels as they emulate Western lifestyles. Based on current estimates, emissions in China are now rising at a rate of 10 percent a year—ten times the rate of increase in industrialized nations.[14]

## Zero Population Growth

Recognizing that population control will be essential in the decades ahead, many countries have already enacted strict population control measures or have encouraged their citizens to limit the size of their families. Proponents of *total zero population growth* think that each couple should produce only two offspring. When the parents die, these two children are their replacements, allowing the population to stabilize or even decrease. Currently, there are over 20 countries in the world with zero or negative population growth, meaning that deaths surpass births or there are an equal number of births and deaths (this does not include the effects of immigration or emigration). Based on current rates, Ukraine is expected to lose 28 percent of its population between the present and 2050, with Russia losing 22 percent and Japan losing 21 percent.[15] Although environmentalists praise these population declines, economists and cultures worry that such declines may have significant social and cultural implications.

Education may be the single biggest contributor to zero population growth. As education levels of women increase and women achieve equality in pay, job status, and social status with men, fertility rates decline. Also, as women gain choices in birth control, access to health care, and informa-

**pollutant** A substance that contaminates some aspect of the environment and causes potential harm to living organisms.

**what do you think?**

Should individuals get tax breaks for having fewer children, living in smaller homes, or producing less garbage? ● How would such policies compare to our current policies? ● Can you think of other policies that might be effective in encouraging population control and resource conservation in the United States?

**Why is population growth an environmental issue?**

Every year the global population grows by 90 million, but Earth's resources are not expanding. Population increases are believed to be responsible for most of the current environmental stress.

tion about family planning, they tend to marry later and have fewer children.[16] Policies that encourage low birth rates in society and that educate citizens about the consequences of unchecked population growth may be effective. In countries such as the United States, policies that encourage zero population growth or provide incentives to young parents through tax breaks for reduced family size may be a viable option.

## Air Pollution

The term *air pollution* refers to the presence, in varying degrees, of those substances (suspended particles and vapors) not found in perfectly clean air.[17] Natural events, living creatures, and toxic by-products have always polluted the environment. What is new is the vast array of **pollutants,** their concentrations, and the potential interactive effects of many of these substances.

Generally, air pollutants are either *naturally occurring* or *anthropogenic* (human caused). Naturally occurring air pollutants include particulate matter, such as ash from volcanic eruptions. Anthropogenic sources include those caused by *stationary sources* (e.g., the BP oil spill in the Gulf of Mexico in 2010) and *mobile sources* such as vehicles. Mobile sources are *on-road* vehicles (e.g., passenger cars) or *off-road* sources (e.g., construction equipment) and *non-road* vehicles such as airplanes.[18] According to Environmental Protection Agency estimates, mobile sources are the major contributors of key air pollutants, such as carbon monoxide (CO), sulfur oxides ($SO_x$), and nitrogen oxides ($NO_x$). In fact, motor vehicles alone contribute about 60 percent of all CO emissions nationwide, whereas non-road sources contribute another 22 percent. Some say that "clean coal" offers a good alternative to oil, but critics argue that coal-burning plants contribute the major portion of sulfur oxide pollution, and that petroleum refineries and some older diesel engines continue to be large sources of pollution. Primary sources of $NO_x$ pollution also include motor vehicles, electric utilities, and other fuel-burning sources.[19]

## Components of Air Pollution

Concern about air quality prompted Congress to pass the Clean Air Act in 1970 and to amend it in 1977 and again in 1990. Since then, several minor amendments have been made to the Act. The goal was to develop standards for six of the most widespread air pollutants that seriously affect health: sulfur dioxide, particulates, carbon monoxide, nitrogen dioxide, ground-level ozone, and lead. Other common air pollutants include carbon dioxide and hydrocarbons. Today, ozone and particle air pollution are the most widespread and most dangerous of the air pollutants.[20] Table 20.2 on page 656, lists the major sources of the most common air pollutants, and their effects on health and welfare. Some of the components of air pollution, most notably carbon dioxide, are also greenhouse gases that play a role in global warming and climate change (discussed later in this chapter).

## Photochemical Smog

**Photochemical smog** is a mix of particulates and gases that forms when oxygen-containing compounds of nitrogen and hydrocarbons react in the presence of sunlight. It is sometimes called *ozone pollution,* because ozone is one of the products of this reaction. In most cases, smog forms in areas that experience a **temperature inversion,** a weather condition in which a cool layer of air is trapped under a layer of warmer air, which prevents the air from circulating. When gases such as hydrocarbons and nitrogen oxides are released into the cool air layer, they remain suspended until winds remove the warmer air layer. Smog is more likely to occur in valley regions blocked by hills or mountains—for example, Los Angeles.

The most noticeable adverse effects of smog are difficulty breathing, burning eyes, headaches, and nausea. Long-term exposure poses serious health risks, particularly for children,

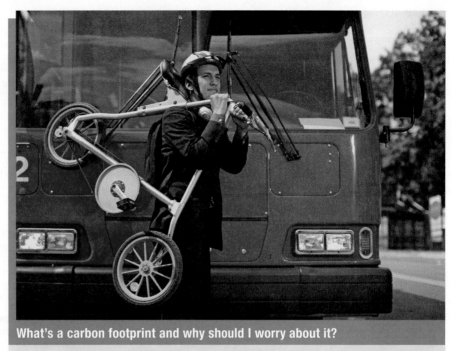

**What's a carbon footprint and why should I worry about it?**

Much of the rise in air pollution is directly related to excess carbon dioxide ($CO_2$) released from burning carbon-containing fossil fuels. As one of the largest $CO_2$ emitters in the world, the United States has the largest *carbon footprint*—the measure of impact that human activities have on the environment in terms of greenhouse gases produced, measured in units of $CO_2$. When you drive your car or heat your house with oil, gas, or coal, the burning of these fossil fuels emits $CO_2$ into the atmosphere. Each time you turn up your thermostat or leave lights on in your house, the fuel burned adds to your individual carbon footprint. Reducing our individual carbon footprint is a key goal in the struggle to combat air pollution, global warming, and climate change. Making small changes such as driving less, riding your bike more, taking public transportation or carpooling, turning off lights when you leave a room, and recycling and composting can all help reduce your carbon footprint.

older adults, pregnant women, and people with chronic respiratory disorders such as asthma and emphysema.

**Air Quality Index** Like the weather, air quality can change from day to day or even hour to hour. The U.S. Environmental Protection Agency (EPA) and other groups make information about outdoor air quality readily available. A key tool in this effort is the Air Quality Index (AQI).

A measure of daily air quality, the AQI tells you how clean or polluted your air is and what associated health concerns you should be aware of. The AQI focuses on health effects that can happen within a few hours or days after breathing polluted air. It reflects national air quality standards for five of the major air pollutants regulated by the Clean Air Act.

The AQI runs from 0 to 500. The higher the AQI value is, the greater the level of air pollution and associated health risks will be. Air Quality Index values below 100 are generally considered satisfactory. When AQI values rise above 100, air quality is considered unhealthy—at first for certain groups of people, then for everyone. The EPA has divided the AQI scale

**photochemical smog** The brownish yellow haze resulting from the combination of hydrocarbons and nitrogen oxides.

**temperature inversion** A weather condition occurring when a layer of cool air is trapped under a layer of warmer air.

# 20.2 Sources, Health Effects, and Welfare Effects for Criteria Pollutants

| Pollutant | Description | Sources | Health Effects | Welfare Effects |
|---|---|---|---|---|
| Carbon monoxide (CO) | Colorless, odorless gas | Motor vehicle exhaust; indoor sources include kerosene or wood-burning stoves | Headaches, reduced mental alertness, heart attack, cardiovascular diseases, impaired fetal development, death | Contribute to the formation of smog |
| Sulfur dioxide (SO$_2$) | Colorless gas that dissolves in water vapor to form acid, and interact with other gases and particles in the air | Coal-fired power plants, petroleum refineries, manufacture of sulfuric acid, and smelting of ores containing sulfur | Eye irritation, wheezing, chest tightness, shortness of breath, lung damage | Contribute to the formation of acid rain, visibility impairment, plant and water damage, aesthetic damage |
| Nitrogen dioxide (NO$_2$) | Reddish brown, highly reactive gas | Motor vehicles, electric utilities, and other industrial, commercial, and residential sources that burn fuels | Susceptibility to respiratory infections, irritation of the lungs and respiratory symptoms (e.g., cough, chest pain, difficulty breathing) | Contribute to the formation of smog, acid rain, water quality deterioration, global warming, and visibility impairment |
| Ozone (O$_3$) | Gaseous pollutant when it is formed in the troposphere | Vehicle exhaust and certain other fumes; formed from other air pollutants in the presence of sunlight | Eye and throat irritation, coughing, respiratory tract problems, asthma, lung damage | Plant and ecosystem damage |
| Lead (Pb) | Metallic element | Metal refineries, lead smelters, battery manufacturers, iron and steel producers | Anemia, high blood pressure, brain and kidney damage, neurological disorders, cancer, lowered IQ | Affects animals, plants, and the aquatic ecosystem |
| Particulate matter (PM) | Very small particles of soot, dust, or other matter, including tiny droplets of liquids | Diesel engines, power plants, industries, windblown dust, wood stoves | Eye irritation, asthma, bronchitis, lung damage, cancer, heavy metal poisoning, cardiovascular effects | Visibility impairment, atmospheric deposition, aesthetic damage |

**Source:** U.S. Environmental Protection Agency, "Air and Radiation: Air Pollutants," 2009, www.epa.gov/air/airpollutants.html.

**acid deposition** The acidification process that occurs when pollutants are deposited by precipitation, directly on the land, or by clouds.

into six categories and color codes (Figure 20.3). This makes it easy for the general public to assess the daily quality of the air we breathe.

| When the AQI is in this range: | ...air quality conditions are | ...as symbolized by this color: |
|---|---|---|
| 0 to 50 | Good | Green |
| 51 to 100 | Moderate | Yellow |
| 101 to 150 | Unhealthy for sensitive groups | Orange |
| 151 to 200 | Unhealthy | Red |
| 201 to 300 | Very unhealthy | Purple |
| 301 to 500 | Hazardous | Maroon |

FIGURE 20.3 **Air Quality Index (AQI)**
The EPA provides individual AQIs for ground-level ozone, particle pollution, carbon monoxide, sulfur dioxide, and nitrogen dioxide. All of the AQIs are presented using the general values, categories, and colors of this figure.
**Source:** U.S. Environmental Protection Agency, "Air Quality Index: A Guide to Air Quality and Your Health," Updated July 2010, www.airnow.gov/index.cfm?action=aqibasics.aqi.

# Acid Deposition and Acid Rain

**Acid deposition** is replacing the term *acid rain* in scientific circles and is used to refer to precipitation that has fallen through acidic air pollutants, particularly those containing sulfur dioxides and nitrogen dioxides.

In the United States, roughly two-thirds of all sulfur dioxide and one-fourth of all nitrogen oxides come from electric power generation that relies on burning fossil fuels, such as coal.[21] When coal-powered plants, ore smelters, oil refineries, and steel mills burn fuels, the sulfur and nitrogen in the emissions combine with oxygen and sunlight in the air to become sulfur dioxide and nitrogen oxides (precursors of sulfuric acid and nitric acids, respectively). Small acid particles are then carried by the wind and combine with moisture to produce acidic rain or snow. Acidic pollutants can be deposited in two ways. *Wet deposition* refers to acidic rain, fog, and snow. In *dry deposition*, chemicals may become incorporated into dust or smoke before falling to the ground.[22]

When it falls into lakes and ponds, acid deposition gradually acidifies the water. Once the acid content of the water reaches a certain level, plant and animal life cannot survive.[23] Ironically, acidified lakes and ponds become a crystal-clear deep blue, giving the illusion of beauty and health. Every year, acid deposition destroys millions of trees in

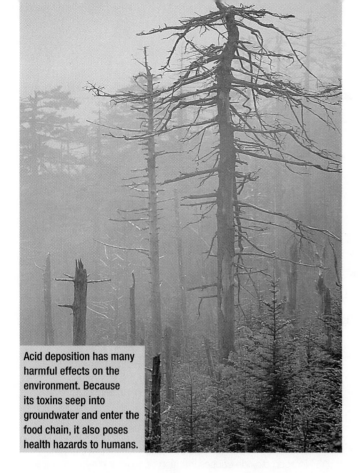

Acid deposition has many harmful effects on the environment. Because its toxins seep into groundwater and enter the food chain, it also poses health hazards to humans.

Europe and North America. Scientists have concluded that much of the world's forestlands are now experiencing damaging levels of acid deposition.[24]

Doctors believe that acid deposition aggravates and may even cause bronchitis, asthma, and other respiratory problems, and people with emphysema or heart disease may suffer from exposure.[25] It may also be hazardous to a pregnant woman's unborn child. Acid deposition can cause metals such as aluminum, cadmium, lead, and mercury to **leach** out of the soil. If these metals make their way into water or food supplies, they can cause cancer in humans.

## Indoor Air Pollution

Do you ever think about what's in the air you breathe in your home? In the past several years, a growing body of scientific evidence has indicated that the air inside buildings can be much more hazardous than outdoor air even in the most industrialized cities. There are 20 to 100 potentially dangerous chemical compounds in the average American home. The higher the dose of these pollutants there is in the air, and the more airtight the house is, the greater the risk becomes for individuals' health.

Factors including age; preexisting medical conditions; individual sensitivity; room temperature and humidity; and functioning of the liver, immune, and respiratory systems can influence immediate reactions to indoor air pollution and affect your level of risk for being affected by indoor air pollution.[26] Those with allergies may be particularly vulnerable. However, the relative dose of any given chemical and the degree of its toxicity are key variables in determining risk. Health effects may develop over years of exposure or may occur in response to toxic levels of pollutants. Table 20.3 on page 658 describes major sources of indoor air pollution and possible health effects from these pollutants.

There are strategies to limit your exposure to indoor air pollution. Today, more and more manufacturers are offering green building products and furnishings, such as natural fiber fabrics, untreated wood for furniture and floors, and low-volatile organic compound paints in an attempt to reduce pollutants. The Skills for Behavior Change box above offers ideas for being an environmentally conscious consumer.

**leach** To dissolve and filter through soil.

TABLE
20.3 | Health Effects of Indoor Air Pollution

| Pollutant | Sources | Health Effects |
|---|---|---|
| Asbestos | Deteriorating, damaged, or disturbed insulation; fireproofing; acoustical materials; and floor tiles | Long-term risk of chest and abdominal cancers and lung diseases. Smokers are at higher risk of developing asbestos-induced lung cancer. |
| Lead | Lead-based paint, contaminated soil, dust, and drinking water | Lead affects practically all systems within the body. Lead at high levels (at or above 80 ug/dL) of blood) can cause convulsions, coma, and even death. Lower levels of lead can cause adverse health effects on central nervous system, kidneys, and blood cells. Blood lead levels as low as 10 ug/dL can impair mental and physical development. |
| Radon | Uranium in the soil or rock on which homes are built; well water also can be a source | Major cause of lung cancer from exposure in air; other health risks from drinking contaminated water; a synergistic effect with smoking exposure |
| Environmental tobacco smoke | Smoke that comes from burning end of cigarettes, pipes, or cigars; consists of a complex mixture of more than 4,000 compounds | Over 40 compounds linked to increased risk of lung cancer; increased risk of asthma and lower respiratory infections; increased risk of sudden infant death syndrome (SIDS) and heart disease. |
| Biological contaminants (molds, mildew, viruses, animal dander and cat saliva, dust mites, cockroaches, and pollen) | Improper ventilation and moisture buildup, lack of cleanliness/sanitation, contaminated heating systems, faulty construction, household pets, rodents, insects, damp carpets | Allergic reactions, including hypersensitivity, rhinitis, asthma, infectious illnesses, sneezing, watering eyes, coughing, shortness of breath, dizziness, lethargy, fever, digestive problems |
| Combustion products | Unvented kerosene heaters, woodstoves, fireplaces, gas stoves | Carbon monoxide causes headaches, dizziness, weakness, nausea, confusion and disorientation, chest pain, death. Nitrogen dioxide causes irritation of nose and eyes, respiratory distress. Particles cause lung damage and irritation. |
| Benzene | Paint, new carpet, new drapes, upholstery, fast-drying glues, caulks | Headaches, eye/skin irritation, fatigue, cancer |
| Formaldehyde | Tobacco smoke, plywood, cabinets, furniture, particleboard, new carpet and drapes, wallpaper, ceiling tile, paneling | Headaches, eye/skin irritation, drowsiness, fatigue, respiratory problems, memory loss, depression, gynecological problems, cancer |
| Chloroform | Paint, new drapes, new carpet, upholstery | Headaches, asthma attacks, dizziness, eye/skin irritations |
| Toluene | All paper products, most finished wood products | Headaches, eye/skin irritation, sinus problems, dizziness, cancer |
| Hydrocarbons | Tobacco smoke, gas burners and furnaces | Headaches, fatigue, nausea, dizziness, breathing difficulty |
| Ammonia | Tobacco smoke, cleaning supplies, animal urine | Eye/skin irritation, headaches, nosebleeds, sinus problems |
| Trichloroethylene | Paints, glues, caulking, vinyl coatings, wallpaper | Headaches, eye/skin irritation, upper respiratory irritation |

**Source:** U.S. Environmental Protection Agency, "The Inside Story: A Guide to Indoor Air Quality," Updated April 2010, www.epa.gov/iaq/pubs/insidest.html.

Prevention of indoor air pollution should focus on three main areas: *source control* (eliminating or reducing individual contaminants), *ventilation improvements* (increasing the amount of outdoor air coming indoors), and *air cleaners* (removing particulates from the air).[27]

**Environmental Tobacco Smoke** Perhaps the greatest source of indoor air pollution is *environmental tobacco smoke* (*ETS*)—the smoke that comes from cigarette, cigar, and pipe smoking. The only truly effective way to eliminate ETS in public places is to enact strict no-smoking policies; ventilation and separate smoking areas are not sufficient. Today, many major U.S. cities ban smoking in public places, in worksites, and in automobiles where children are present.

**Home Heating** If you rely on wood for heating or oil- or gas-fired furnaces, make sure that the appliance you use is properly installed, vented, and maintained. In wood stoves, burning properly seasoned wood reduces particulates. Thorough cleaning and maintenance can prevent carbon monoxide buildup in the home. Inexpensive home monitors are available to detect high carbon monoxide levels.

# 20–100

**potentially dangerous chemical compounds can be found in the air of the average American home.**

**Asbestos** **Asbestos** is a mineral compound used in insulating materials, vinyl flooring, shingles/roofing materials, heating pipe coverings, and many other products in buildings constructed before 1970. When bonded to other materials, asbestos is relatively harmless, but if its tiny fibers become loosened and airborne, they can embed themselves in the lungs. If asbestos is detected in the home, it must be removed or sealed off by a professional.

**Formaldehyde** **Formaldehyde** is a colorless, strong-smelling gas. It may be released into the air from building materials or new carpet, among other things, in a process called *offgassing*. Offgassing is highest in new products, but the process can continue for many years.

How can you limit the amount of formaldehyde in your home? Ask about the formaldehyde content of products you purchase, and avoid those that contain it. Some houseplants, such as philodendrons and spider plants, help clean formaldehyde from the air.

**Radon** **Radon,** an odorless, colorless gas, penetrates homes through openings in the basement or foundation, such as cracks, pipes, or sump pits. The U.S. Surgeon General warns that radon is the second leading cause of lung cancer, after smoking, each year.[28]

The EPA estimates that as many as 8.1 million homes (1 out of every 15) throughout the country have elevated levels of radon.[29] Short-term testing, taking from 2 to 90 days to complete, is the quickest way to determine whether a potential problem exists. Low-cost radon test kits are available by mail order, in hardware stores, and through other retail outlets. If these short-term tests show levels of radon at 4 pCi/L (pico Curies per liter) or higher, a follow-up test is recommended. Since 1988, the EPA and the Office of the Surgeon General have recommended that homes below the third floor be tested for radon and that Americans test their homes every 2 years or when they move into a new home. Typically, radon sources in the home come primarily from the soil; however, the water supply can also be a source.

**Lead** **Lead** is a metal pollutant sometimes found in paint, batteries, drinking water, pipes, dishes with lead-based glazes, dirt, soldered cans, and some candies made in Mexico. Recently, toys produced in China and other regions of the world have been recalled due to unsafe levels of lead in their paint.

By some estimates, as many as 25 percent of U.S. homes still have lead-based paint hazards, and an estimated 250,000 American children aged 1 to 5 have unsafe blood lead levels.[30]

To reduce unsafe exposure, keep areas where children play as dust free and clean as possible, leave lead-based paint undisturbed if it is in good condition, and do not remove lead paint yourself.

**Mold** **Molds** are fungi that live both indoors and outdoors in most regions of the country. They produce tiny reproductive spores that continually waft through the indoor and outdoor air. Cleaning with bleach, controlling moisture, and improving ventilation are all methods of addressing mold in homes. For more ways to reduce your exposure to mold, see the **Skills for Behavior Change** box above.

**Sick Building Syndrome** **Sick building syndrome (SBS)** is said to exist when 80 percent of a building's

**asbestos** A mineral compound that separates into stringy fibers and lodges in the lungs, where it can cause various diseases.
**formaldehyde** A colorless, strong-smelling gas released through offgassing; causes respiratory and other health problems.
**radon** A naturally occurring radioactive gas resulting from the decay of certain radioactive elements.
**lead** A highly toxic metal found in emissions from lead smelters and processing plants; also sometimes found in pipes or paint in older houses.
**sick building syndrome (SBS)** Problem that exists when 80 percent of a building's occupants report maladies that tend to lessen or vanish when they leave the building.

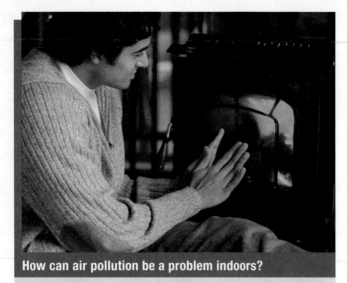

**How can air pollution be a problem indoors?**

The air within homes can be 10 to 40 times more hazardous than outside air. Indoor air pollution comes from woodstoves, furnaces, cigarette smoke, asbestos, formaldehyde, radon, lead, mold, and household chemicals.

**chlorofluorocarbons (CFCs)** Chemicals that contribute to the depletion of the atmospheric ozone layer.

**greenhouse gases** Gases that accumulate in the atmosphere, where they contribute to global warming by trapping heat near Earth's surface.

**carbon dioxide (CO$_2$)** Gas created by the combustion of fossil fuels, exhaled by animals, and used by plants for photosynthesis; the primary greenhouse gas in Earth's atmosphere.

**enhanced greenhouse effect** The warming of Earth's surface as a direct result of human activities that release greenhouse gases into the atmosphere, trapping more of the sun's radiation than is normal.

---

**what do you think?**

Many of us would rather use strong cleaning products than good old-fashioned elbow grease to clean showers, appliances, and other home devices. Think of the products you use each day. How many of these could you do without? ● What other options do you have for cleaning products that won't pollute the water supply or contaminate the air in your home?

---

occupants report air pollution-related problems. Poor ventilation is a primary cause of SBS. Other causes include faulty furnaces that emit carbon monoxide, nitrogen dioxide, and sulfur dioxide; biological air pollutants such as dander (dried skin and hair from pets), molds, and dust; volatile organic compounds from products such as hairspray, cleaners, and adhesives; and heavy metals such as lead, particularly in older buildings. Symptoms include eye irritation, sore throat, queasiness, and worsened asthma.

Indoor air pollution and SBS are increasing concerns in the classroom and workplace. Many people who work indoors complain of maladies that lessen or vanish when they leave the building. Studies show that significant numbers of U.S. schools have unsatisfactory indoor air quality, often due to poor ventilation, tighter construction techniques that block outside air, and the use of increasing numbers of synthetic materials in construction.[31] Poor air quality can trigger allergies, asthma, and other health problems among students.[32]

## Ozone Layer Depletion

The ozone layer forms a protective stratum in Earth's stratosphere—the highest level of our atmosphere, located 12 to 30 miles above Earth's surface. The ozone layer in the stratosphere protects our planet and its inhabitants from ultraviolet B (UVB) radiation, a primary cause of skin cancer. Such radiation damages DNA and weakens immune systems in both humans and animals (radiation in general is discussed later in the chapter).

In the 1970s, scientists began to warn of a breakdown in the ozone layer. Instruments developed to test atmospheric contents indicated that chemicals used on Earth, especially **chlorofluorocarbons (CFCs),** were contributing to the ozone layer's rapid depletion. Chlorofluorocarbons were used in many common products like refrigerants and hair sprays. When released into the air through spraying or offgassing, CFCs migrate into the ozone layer, where they decompose and release chlorine atoms. These atoms cause ozone molecules to break apart and levels to be depleted.

The U.S. government banned the use of aerosol sprays containing CFCs in the 1970s. The discovery of an ozone "hole" over Antarctica led to the 1987 Montreal Protocol treaty, whereby the United States and other nations agreed to further reduce the use of CFCs and other ozone-depleting chemicals. The treaty was amended in 1995 to ban CFC production in developed countries. Today, over 190 countries have signed the treaty as the international community strives to preserve the ozone layer.[33]

## Global Warming

More than 100 years ago, scientists theorized that carbon dioxide emissions from the burning of fossil fuels would create a buildup of greenhouse gases in Earth's atmosphere that could have a warming effect on Earth's surface.[34] In recent years, these predictions have been supported by reports from leading international scientists in the field and accounts in the popular media, such as the 2006 documentary film, *An Inconvenient Truth,* all detailing startling indicators of a planet in trouble.

The *greenhouse effect* is a natural phenomenon in which **greenhouse gases,** such as **carbon dioxide (CO$_2$),** warm the planet (see **Figure 20.4**). Human activities such as burning fossil fuels and land clearing have increased greenhouse gases in the atmosphere, resulting in the **enhanced greenhouse effect,** in which excess solar heat is trapped, raising the planet's temperature. According to data from the National Oceanic and Atmospheric Administration (NOAA) and the National Aeronautics and Space Administration (NASA), Earth's surface temperature has risen about 1.2 to 1.4 degrees Fahrenheit since 1900, with accelerated warming occurring in the past two decades.[35] Furthermore, the consensus is that temperatures will continue to rise, perhaps by as much as 5 to 10 degrees in the next 100 years, unless immediate steps are taken to reverse the trend. Results of such a temperature increase—which might

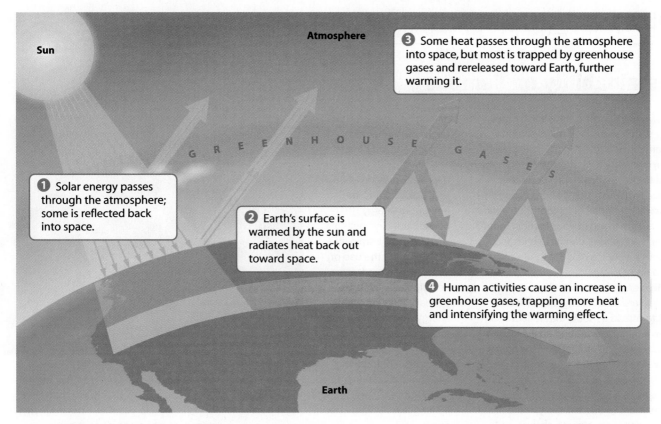

FIGURE 20.4 **The Enhanced Greenhouse Effect**
The natural greenhouse effect is responsible for making Earth habitable; it keeps the planet 33° Celsius (60° Fahrenheit) warmer than it would otherwise be. An increase in greenhouse gases resulting from human activities is creating the enhanced greenhouse effect, trapping more heat and causing dangerous global climate change.

include rising sea levels (potentially flooding entire countries), glacier retreat, arctic shrinkage at the poles, altered patterns of agriculture (including changes in growing seasons and alterations of climatic zones), deforestation, drought, extreme weather events, increases in tropical diseases, changes in disease trends and patterns, loss of biological species, and economic devastation—would be catastrophic.

The greenhouse gases include carbon dioxide, nitrous oxide, methane, CFCs, and hydrocarbons. The most predominant is carbon dioxide, which accounts for 49 percent of all greenhouse gases. The United States is the greatest producer of greenhouse gases, responsible for over 22 percent of all output, and this output is expected to increase by 43 percent by 2025.[36] Rapid deforestation of the tropical rain forests of Central and South America, Africa, and southeast Asia also contributes to the rapid rise in greenhouse gases. Trees take in carbon dioxide, transform it, store the carbon for food, and release oxygen into the air. As we lose forests, at the rate of hundreds of acres per hour, we lose the capacity to dissipate carbon dioxide.

A United Nations treaty signed in Kyoto in 1997 outlined an international plan to reduce the manmade emissions responsible for climate change. The Kyoto Protocol, which went into effect in 2005, required participating countries to reduce their emissions between 2008 and 2012 by at least 5 percent below 1990 levels.[37] More than 160 countries signed on to the Kyoto Protocol, including more than 30 industrialized countries.[38] The treaty would require the United States to reduce emissions by 33 percent, but the United States opted out of this proposal, ostensibly because of concerns that major developing nations, including India and China, are not required to reduce emissions under the treaty. A follow-up summit in Copenhagen in 2009 sought to restrict global temperatures to a rise of 2 degrees Celsius by 2050. To date, talks are stalled with disagreement between the West and developing countries; the next climate change summit, scheduled to take place in Cancun, Mexico, in late 2010, seems unlikely to result in a definite agreement.[39]

# Reducing Air Pollution and the Threat of Global Warming

Air pollution and climate change problems are rooted in our energy, transportation, and industrial practices. Clearly, we must develop comprehensive national strategies that encourage the use of renewable resources such as solar, wind, and water power. Because industrial production is a

# BE HEALTHY, BE GREEN

## Sustainability on Campus

You are moving into a new dorm room, along with hundreds of other students, and are excited to decorate, meet your new roommate, and make your room the place to be. As a student, this is also your chance to make a positive difference and minimize your ecological footprint. Your actions, and those of your friends, roommates, and school, can have a lasting impact on your life and the future of the environment.

More and more universities and colleges are recognizing that students want to attend schools that reflect their values and beliefs around sustainable movements. The annual College Sustainability Report Card (www.greenreportcard.org) grades colleges and universities on their reponses to a survey assessing their commitment to sustainability in the areas of administration, climate change and energy, food and recycling, green building, student involvement, transportation, endowment transparency, investment priorities, and shareholder engagement.

The green sustainability movement is picking up steam and turning ideas into realities. You do not need to be an environmental science major or a self-proclaimed "hippie" to make a difference. Going green on campus can be part of the goal for your apartment, your sorority or fraternity, or your residence hall.

Start making a positive impact by turning off lights when you leave a room or bathroom. See if your residence has a way of minimizing the amount of lights used on a floor. Sometimes lights might be connected through several outlets, and turning off a strand might still provide enough light but minimize the amount of energy consumed. Find out whether your administration supports the use of CFLs—compact fluorescent lights—which are typically longer-lasting, energy-conserving bulbs that give off the same amount of light as an incandescent bulb at a fraction of the energy used. Next time you go to the store, buy a couple for your new lighting fixtures and start making a positive impact.

When buying a new appliance, look for the Energy Star logo, indicating that the appliance meets energy-efficiency standards set by the Environmental Protection Agency (EPA) and U.S. Department of Energy. Adjust the controls on your new appliances so that they do not run at full power all the time. This will help curb unnecessary energy usage and lower the cost of your monthly energy bills. Better yet, consider unplugging items such as iPods, TVs, laptops, desktop computers, hair dryers, coffee pots, and cell phones, all of which still consume energy when not in use.

What about your computer? While in school, you will probably use it for every-

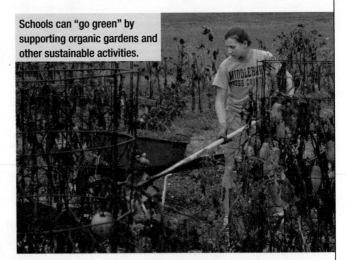

Schools can "go green" by supporting organic gardens and other sustainable activities.

thing from checking your e-mail to writing your papers. Fortunately, you have many options to help you make better energy-conserving choices when it comes to your computer use. When buying your computer, always look for the Energy Star logo. (Go to www.energystar.gov/index.cfm?c=higher_ed.bus_dormroom for more information about creating an Energy Star dorm room.)

Consider buying a laptop rather than a desktop computer, as laptops use less energy. You can also set your computer to sleep or hibernate mode when not in use. When you look for a printer, choose one that prints double-sided, which will help reduce the amount of paper you use. Do not print unnecessary documents, and make sure you recycle used paper—don't just throw it away.

---

key contributor to fossil fuel emission, clean energy, green factories, improved technology, and governmental regulation are necessary for preventing climate change.

Most experts agree that reducing consumption of fossil fuels in cars and shifting to alternative fuels, improving gas mileage, and using mass transportation are crucial to air pollution reduction. Many cities have taken steps in this direction by setting high parking fees and road-usage tolls in congested areas and by imposing bans on city driving. Local governments should be encouraged to provide convenient and inexpensive public transportation and to motivate people to use it regularly.

Meanwhile, many U.S. communities are creating bicycle lanes and holding "bike to work" days. Scooters and other low-energy modes of transportation are becoming increasingly popular. Some college campuses have enacted new policies allowing increased skateboard and in-line skate use on campus. Other campuses provide scooter and bike garages to protect students from theft and vandalism and to encourage students to bring energy-efficient vehicles to

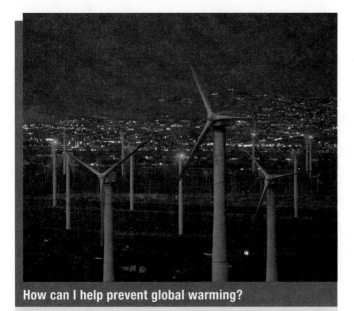

**How can I help prevent global warming?**

Global warming, sometimes referred to as *climate change,* is a global problem. We need to work with other nations to ensure that everyone does their part. By reducing your use of fossil fuels; using high-efficiency vehicles; and supporting increased use of renewable resources such as solar, wind, and water power, you can help combat global warming. For example, the National Renewable Energy Laboratory predicts that, with proper development, wind power could provide 20% of U.S. energy needs.

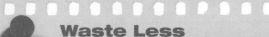
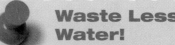

## Waste Less Water!

### IN THE KITCHEN

✳ Turn off the tap while washing dishes.
✳ Check faucets and pipes for leaks. Leaky faucets can waste more than 3,000 gallons of water each year.
✳ Equip faucets with aerators to reduce water use by 4 percent.
✳ Run dishwashers only when they are full, and use the energy-saving mode.

### IN THE LAUNDRY ROOM

✳ Wash only full laundry loads.
✳ Upgrade to a high-efficiency washing machine to use 30 percent less water per load.

### IN THE BATHROOM

✳ Detect and fix leaks. A leaky toilet can waste about 200 gallons of water every day.
✳ Replace your old toilet with a high-efficiency model that uses 60 percent less water per flush.
✳ Take showers instead of baths and limit showers to the time it takes to lather up and rinse off.
✳ Replace old showerheads with new, more efficient models that use 60 percent less water per minute.
✳ Turn off the tap while brushing your teeth to save up to 8 gallons of water per day.

campus. You can participate in this effort by finding ways to reduce your own **carbon footprint,** or the amount of $CO_2$ emissions you contribute to the atmosphere in your daily life. See the **Be Healthy, Be Green** box at left for more ideas about reducing energy use on campus.

# Water Pollution and Shortages

Seventy-five percent of Earth is covered with water in the form of oceans, seas, lakes, rivers, streams, and wetlands. Beneath the landmass are reservoirs of groundwater. We draw our drinking water from either this underground source or from surface freshwater. However, just 1 percent of the entire water supply is available for human use—the rest is too salty, too polluted, or locked away in polar ice caps.[40]

Over half the global population faces a shortage of clean water. More than 2.6 billion people, about 40 percent of the planet's population, have no access to basic sanitation or adequate toilet facilities. More than 1 billion have no access to clean water, and more than 4,500 children die every day from illnesses caused by lack of safe water and sanitation.[41] Two regions of the world that have the most severe water shortages also have some of the highest population growth rates—Africa and the Near East, which encompass 20 countries. Estimates suggest that by the year 2025, approximately

2.8 billion people will live in countries with severe shortages of clean water. By 2050, these numbers will increase to 4 billion people in 54 countries.[42]

**carbon footprint** The amount of greenhouse gases produced by an individual, nation, or other entity, usually expressed in equivalent tons of carbon dioxide emissions.

Considering how little water is available to meet the world's agricultural, manufacturing, community, personal, and sanitation needs, it is no wonder that clean water is a precious commodity that must not be wasted. Each U.S. resident uses an average of 1,500 gallons of water daily for all purposes—domestic consumption, recreation, energy (primarily from cooling at power plants), food production, and industry—about three times the world average.[43] The **Skills for Behavior Change** box presents simple conservation measures that you can adopt to save water in your home. In addition to conserving clean water, we must make efforts to prevent and reverse contamination and pollution of our water supplies.

## Water Contamination

Any substance that gets into the soil can enter the water supply. Industrial pollutants and pesticides eventually work their way into the soil, then into groundwater. Underground storage tanks containing gasoline may leak. Drugs we use, from

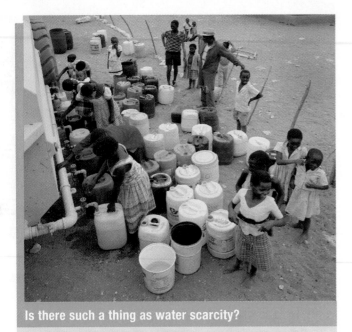

**Is there such a thing as water scarcity?**

The lack of clean water and sanitation is a major global problem. Another issue is the lack of water available relative to demand. "Closed basins" are defined as regions where existing water cannot meet the agricultural, industrial, municipal, and environmental needs of all, and the Stockholm International Water Institute estimates that 1.4 billion people live in a closed basin. The problem is expected to worsen rapidly. The Food and Agriculture Organization estimates that those suffering from water scarcity will increase to 1.8 billion by 2025.

# 2 million

**kilograms of water pollutants are released daily in the United States.**

states, localities, and water suppliers who implement those standards. Cities and municipalities have strict policies and procedures governing water treatment, filtration, and disinfection to screen out pathogens and microorganisms. However, their ability to filter out an ever-growing list of chemical by-products and other substances is increasingly questioned. According to a recent Associated Press (AP) inquiry, a "vast array of pharmaceuticals—including antibiotics, anti-convulsants, mood stabilizers and sex hormones—have been found in the drinking water supplies of at least 41 million Americans."[46]

In addition to prescription and over-the-counter medications and personal care products, a wide array of other toxic substances flow into our waterways and streams. Congress has coined two terms, *point source* and *nonpoint source,* to describe the general sources of water pollution. **Point source pollutants** enter a waterway at a specific location such as a ditch or pipe. The two major sources of point source pollution are sewage treatment plants and industrial facilities. **Nonpoint source pollutants**—commonly known as *runoff* and *sedimentation*—drain or seep into waterways from broad areas of land. Nonpoint source pollution results from our faulty land use practices. Forms of pollution include soil erosion and sedimentation, construction wastes, pesticide and fertilizer runoff, urban street runoff, acid mine drainage, wastes from engineering projects, leakage from septic tanks, and sewage sludge (see Figure 20.5).

**point source pollutants** Pollutants that enter waterways at a specific location.

**nonpoint source pollutants** Pollutants that run off or seep into waterways from broad areas of land.

pain killers to deodorants, eventually wind up in the sewer, making their way into waste treatment plants. A comprehensive survey by a group of U.S. Geological Survey researchers discovered the presence of low levels of many chemical compounds in a network of 139 targeted streams across the United States. Both surface water and some of our deepest underground aquifers appear to be affected.[44] Although some studies appear to indicate that concentrations of these contaminants are not yet high enough to result in high risks of reproductive disruptions, developmental toxicity or cancer development, others question the potential risk of long-term, continued low-dose exposure and/or cumulative effects of exposure.[45]

Tap water in the United States is among the safest in the world. The Safe Drinking Water Act (SDWA) is the main federal law that ensures the quality of Americans' drinking water. Under SDWA, the EPA sets standards for drinking water quality and oversees the

**Point-source** contamination can be traced to specific points of discharge from wastewater treatment plants and factories or from combined sewers.

**Air pollution** spreads across the landscape and is often overlooked as a major nonpoint souce of pollution. Airborne nutrients and pesticides can be transported far from their area of origin.

**Eroded soil and sediment** can transport considerable amounts of some nutrients, such as organic nitrogen and phosphorus, and some pesticides, such as DDT, to rivers and streams.

Wastewater

Runoff

Runoff

Seepage

Groundwater discharge to streams

Seepage

FIGURE 20.5 **Potential Sources of Groundwater Contamination**

**Source:** Adapted from U.S. Geological Survey, Wisconsin Water Science Center, "Learn More about Groundwater," 2008, http://wi.water.usgs.gov/gwcomp/learn.

The pollutants causing the most concern and the greatest potential harm are the following:

● **Gasoline and petroleum products.** In the mid-1980s, Congress authorized a leaking underground storage tank cleanup as part of the Solid Waste Disposal Act. Since then, the frequency and severity of leaks has declined markedly in the United States. Through 2009, cleanup or containment has occurred at over 80 percent of the nearly 500,000 remaining confirmed release sites. Funding challenges remain for the remaining sites, posing potential threats to the underground water sources that could easily be contaminated. Programs to replace tanks, secure tanks, and remove threats are ongoing.[47]

● **Chemical contaminants.** *Organic solvents* are chemicals designed to dissolve grease and oil. These extremely toxic substances are used to clean clothing, painting equipment, plastics, and metal parts. Many household products (e.g., stain and spot removers, degreasers, drain cleaners, septic system cleaners, and paint removers) also contain these toxic chemicals. Organic solvents work their way into the water supply in different ways. Consumers often dump leftover products into the toilet or into street drains. Industries pour leftovers into large barrels, which are then buried. After a while, the chemicals eat through the barrels and leach into groundwater.

● **Polychlorinated biphenyls.** Fire resistant and stable at high temperatures, **polychlorinated biphenyls (PCBs)** were used for many years as insulating materials in high-voltage electrical equipment, such as transformers and older fluorescent lights. The human body does not excrete ingested PCBs but rather stores them in fatty tissues and the liver (i.e., they *bioaccumulate*). Exposure to PCBs is associated with birth defects, cancer, and various skin problems. The manufacture of PCBs was discontinued in the United States in 1977, but approximately 500 million pounds of them have been dumped into landfills and waterways, where they continue to pose an environmental threat.[48]

● **Dioxins.** **Dioxins** are chlorinated hydrocarbons found in herbicides (chemicals that are used to kill vegetation) and are produced during certain industrial processes. Dioxins also bioaccumulate and are much more toxic than PCBs. Long-term effects include possible damage to the immune system and increased risk of infections and cancer. Exposure to high concentrations of PCBs or dioxins for a short period of time can also have severe consequences, including nausea; vomiting; diarrhea; painful rashes and sores; and chloracne, an ailment in which the skin develops hard, black, painful pimples that may never go away.

● **Pesticides.** **Pesticides** are chemicals designed to kill insects, rodents, plants, and fungi. There are over 1,055 active ingredients sold as pesticides throughout the world.[49] Americans use millions of pounds of pesticides each year, but only small amounts reach targeted organisms. The rest settles on the land, floats in the air, or runs off into our waterways. Pesticides evaporate readily, often being dispersed by winds over a large area or carried to the sea.

This is particularly true in tropical regions, where many farmers use pesticides heavily and the climate promotes their rapid release into the atmosphere. Pesticide residues cling to fresh fruits and vegetables and can accumulate in the body when people eat these items. Several groups have published consumer guides to the fruits and vegetables likely to be the best and worst when it comes to pesticide contaminants; see www.foodnews.org for one example. Potential hazards associated with exposure to pesticides include birth defects, liver and kidney damage, and nervous system disorders.

● **Lead.** Lead can leach into tap water from lead pipes or water lines, usually in older homes. The EPA has issued new standards to dramatically reduce the levels of lead in drinking water. The new rules stipulate that tap water lead values must not exceed 15 parts per billion (ppb). (The previous standard allowed an average lead level of 50 ppb.) If lead is present in your home's water, you can reduce your risk by running tap water for several minutes before taking a drink or cooking with it. This flushes out water that has been standing overnight in lead-contaminated lines.

**polychlorinated biphenyls (PCBs)** Toxic chemicals that were once used as insulating materials in high-voltage electrical equipment.
**dioxins** Highly toxic chlorinated hydrocarbons contained in herbicides and produced during certain industrial processes.
**pesticides** Chemicals that kill pests such as insects, weeds, and rodents.
**municipal solid waste (MSW)** Solid wastes such as durable goods; nondurable goods; containers and packaging; food waste; yard waste; and miscellaneous wastes from residential, commercial, institutional, and industrial sources.

# Land Pollution

Much of the waste that ends up polluting the water starts out polluting the land. For generations humans have gathered their garbage together in designated areas, creating uninhabitable dumps and landfills. The more people on the planet, the more waste they create, and the more pressure is put on the land to accommodate increasing amounts of refuse, much of which is nonbiodegradable, and some of which is directly harmful to living organisms including ourselves.

## Solid Waste

Each day, every person in the United States generates more than 4.5 pounds of **municipal solid waste (MSW),** more commonly known as trash or garbage—containers and packaging; discarded food; yard debris; and refuse from residential, commercial, institutional, and industrial sources (see **Figure 20.6** on page 666).[50] The total comes to about 250 million tons of MSW each year.[51] Although experts believe that up to 90 percent of our trash is recyclable, we still fall far short of this goal

**52%** of all waste produced in Switzerland is recycled, whereas only 31.5% of all waste produced in the U.S. is recycled.

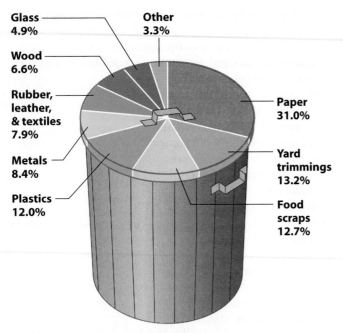

Glass
4.9%

Other
3.3%

Wood
6.6%

Rubber,
leather,
& textiles
7.9%

Metals
8.4%

Plastics
12.0%

Paper
31.0%

Yard
trimmings
13.2%

Food
scraps
12.7%

FIGURE 20.6 **What's in Our Trash?**

**Source:** Data are from U.S. Environmental Protection Agency, *Municipal Solid Waste Generation, Recycling, and Disposal in the United States: Facts and Figures for 2008* (Washington, DC: U.S. Environmental Protection Agency, 2009), Available at www.epa.gov/epawaste/nonhaz/municipal/msw99.htm.

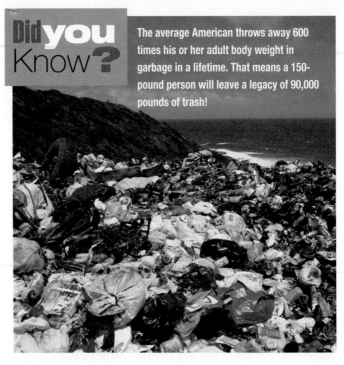

with respect to most types of trash (Figure 20.7). Currently in the United States, 33.2 percent of all MSW is recovered and recycled or composted, over 13 percent is burned at combustion facilities, and the remaining 54 percent is disposed of in landfills.[52]

The number of landfills in the United States has actually decreased in the past decade, but their sheer mass has increased. Many people worry that we are rapidly losing our ability to dispose of all of the waste we create. As communities run out of landfill space, it is becoming more common to haul garbage out to sea to dump, where it contaminates ocean ecosystems, or to ship it to landfills in other states or to developing countries, where it becomes someone else's problem. In today's throwaway society, we need to become aware of the amount of waste we generate every day and to look for ways to recycle, reuse, and—most desirable of all—reduce what we consume.

Communities, businesses, and individuals can adopt several strategies to control waste:

● *Source reduction* (*waste prevention*) involves altering the design, manufac-

ture, or use of products and materials to reduce the amount and toxicity of what gets thrown away. The most effective MSW-reducing strategy is to prevent waste from ever being generated in the first place.

● *Recycling* involves sorting, collecting, and processing materials to be reused in the manufacture of new products. This process diverts items such as paper, glass, plastics, and metals from the waste stream.

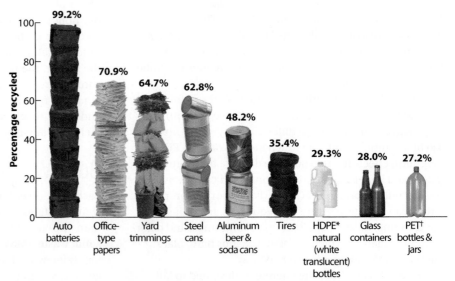

99.2%

70.9%

64.7%

62.8%

48.2%

35.4%

29.3%

28.0%

27.2%

Percentage recycled

Auto
batteries

Office-
type
papers

Yard
trimmings

Steel
cans

Aluminum
beer &
soda cans

Tires

HDPE*
natural
(white
translucent)
bottles

Glass
containers

PET†
bottles &
jars

†High-density polyethylene
*Polyethylene terephthalate

FIGURE 20.7 **How Much Do We Recycle?**

**Source:** Data are from U.S. Environmental Protection Agency, *Municipal Solid Waste Generation, Recycling, and Disposal in the United States: Facts and Figures for 2008* (Washington, DC: U.S. Environmental Protection Agency, 2009), Available at www.epa.gov/epawaste/nonhaz/municipal/msw99.htm.

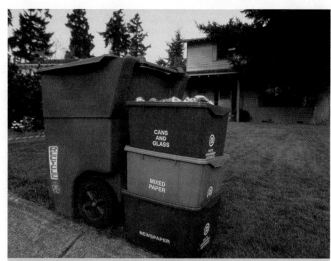

Curbside recycling programs offer convenient recycling of a variety of materials, including paper, glass, aluminum, and yard waste. Participation in these programs ranges widely. In San Francisco, 70% of waste is recycled and in Portland, Oregon, 63% of waste is recycled. In comparison, the recycling rate in Detroit is 10.5%, and 13% in Denver.

- *Composting* involves collecting organic waste, such as food scraps and yard trimmings, and allowing it to decompose with the help of microorganisms (mainly bacteria and fungi). Individuals and communities have increased composting processes in recent years and composted waste is increasingly used for a variety of products. Most commonly, organic waste is combined to produce a humus-like substance that is suitable for use in gardens and for soil enhancement.

- *Combustion with energy recovery* typically involves the use of boilers and industrial furnaces to generate energy and material recovery or incinerators, which primarily destroy waste but can also recover waste for material use. Energy recovery has become an increasing source of energy for many communities.

## Hazardous Waste

**Hazardous waste** is defined as waste with properties that make it capable of harming human health or the environment. In 1980, the Comprehensive Environmental Response, Compensation, and Liability Act, known as the **Superfund,** was enacted to provide funds for cleaning up hazardous waste dump sites that endanger public health and land. This fund is financed through taxes on the chemical and petroleum industries (87%) and through general federal tax revenues (13%). To date, 32,500 potentially hazardous waste sites have been identified across the nation, and 90 percent of these have been cleared or "recovered."[53] Currently there are 50 priority sites being actively cleared, with thousands more sites, costing billions of dollars, possible for future clean up. Newer technologies for cleanup are being investigated, including nanotechnologies that could reduce these costs by as much as 75 percent.

The large number of hazardous waste dump sites in the United States indicates the severity of our toxic chemical problem. Many wastes are now banned from land disposal or are being treated to reduce their toxicity before they become part of land disposal sites. The EPA has developed protective requirements for land disposal facilities, such as double liners, detection systems for substances that may leach into groundwater, and groundwater monitoring systems.

## Radiation

Radiation is energy that travels in waves or particles. There are many different types of radiation, ranging from radio waves to gamma rays, all making up the electromagnetic spectrum. Exposure to radiation is an inescapable part of life on this planet, and only some of it poses a threat to human health.

### Nonionizing Radiation

**Nonionizing radiation** is radiation at the lower end of the electromagnetic spectrum. This radiation moves in relatively long wavelengths and has enough energy to move atoms around, or cause them to vibrate, but not enough to remove electrons or alter molecular structure. Examples of nonionizing radiation are radio waves, TV signals, microwaves, infrared waves, and visible light.

If you believe what you hear on TV, *electromagnetic fields* (*EMFs*) generated by electric power delivery systems place you at risk for cancer, reproductive dysfunction, birth defects, neurological disorders, Alzheimer's disease, and other ailments. Does research support these claims about EMFs? Although many believe that the threat is legitimate, others point to major discrepancies and inconsistencies in the research. The **Consumer Health** box on page 668 discusses some of the findings regarding the radio frequency waves generated by cell phones. In spite of many questions, fears have increased,

**hazardous waste** Waste that, due to its toxic properties, poses a hazard to humans or to the environment.
**Superfund** Fund established under the Comprehensive Environmental Response, Compensation, and Liability Act to be used for cleaning up toxic waste dumps.
**nonionizing radiation** Electromagnetic waves having relatively long wavelengths and enough energy to move atoms around or cause them to vibrate.

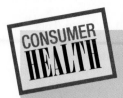
# ARE CELL PHONES HAZARDOUS TO YOUR HEALTH?

Cell phone usage has increased worldwide at over 21 percent annually each year over the past 5 years. By the end of 2010, subscriptions are projected to reach 5 billion. Although everyone today seems to have a cell phone, most users are unaware that their phone may pose a health risk. Much of the concern to date has centered on the radio-frequency (RF) energy that cell phones emit. Depending on how close the cell phone antenna is to the head, as much as 60 percent of the microwave radiation emitted by the phone may actually penetrate the area around the head, some of it reaching an inch to an inch-and-a-half into the brain. In infants and children, whose skull and bone tissues are thinner, the potential penetration may be even greater.

The theory behind this concern is that at high-power levels, radio-frequency energy can rapidly heat biological tissue and cause damage. However, cell phones operate at power levels well below the level at which such heating occurs. Many countries, including the United States and most European nations, use standards set by the Federal Communications Commission (FCC) for radio-frequency energy based on research by several scientific groups. These groups identified a whole-body *specific absorption rate* (*SAR*) value for exposure to radio-frequency

energy. Four watts per kilogram was identified as a threshold level of exposure at which harmful biological effects may occur. The FCC requires wireless phones to comply with a safety limit of 1.6 watts per kg. (To find out the SAR level for your phone, go to www.fcc.gov/cgb/sar.) This amount is much lower than the level shown to cause changes in laboratory animals.

Although there is controversy about potential negative effects of radio-frequency energy on the body, research to date has by and large not shown radio-frequency energy emitted from cell phones to be harmful. Still, these groups point to the need for more research, because cell phones have only been in widespread use for less than two decades, and no long-term studies have been done to determine that cell phones are risk free. As well, studies haven't assessed effects on small children and youth. Three large studies have compared cell phone use among brain cancer patients and individuals free of brain cancer, finding no correlation between cell phone use and brain tumors. However, preliminary results from smaller, well-designed studies have continued to raise questions and a recent large scale study by the International Agency for Research on Cancer found the risk of developing gliomas (a type of tumor) seemed to be higher among those who used their cell phones the most.

To lower any potential risk of problems related to cell phone use there are several things you can do:

* If your "talk time" is long, switch to a land-line phone on which RF levels are lower. If you talk a lot, buy a hands-free device and keep the calls short.
* Children under 14 should be limited in their talk time. Text messages (within limits) or using headsets and hands-free devices or speaker phones are the best option.
* When your signal level is low, stay off the phone. Phones that have to work harder to pull in a signal may increase RF levels.
* Don't wander through your day with a wireless earpiece in your ear. Put it in when you're using it and take it out otherwise. The earpiece is always searching for a signal and emitting RFs, even when you are fully engaged elsewhere
* Men shouldn't keep a cell phone in their pocket or hooked on their belt. Studies have shown that cell phone radiation can reduce sperm counts.

**Sources:** World Health Organization, "Electromagnetic Fields and Public Health: Mobile Phones," Fact Sheet no. 193, May 2010, www.who.int/

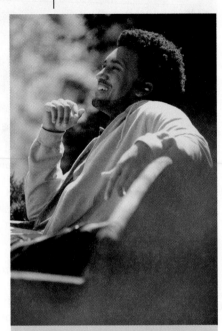
A hands-free device lets you keep your phone—and any radio-frequency energy it may emit—away from your head.

mediacentre/factsheets/fs193/en/; U.S. Food and Drug Administration, "Radiation-Emitting Products: Health Issues: Do Cell Phones Pose a Health Hazard?" Updated May 2010, www.fda.gov/Radiation-Emitting Products/RadiationEmitting ProductsandProcedures/Home BusinessandEntertainment/Cell Phones/ucm116282.htm; D. Hoch, MedlinePlus, "Cell Phones—Do They Cause Cancer?" Updated September 2008, www.nlm.nih.gov/ medlineplus/ency/article/007151 .htm; R. Snowden, American Cancer Society, "Major Study Complicates Debate over Cell Phone Use and Cancer Risks," May 2010, www .cancer.org/Cancer/news/News/ major-study-complicates-debate -over-cell-phone-use-and-cancer -risk; E. Assadourian and V. Damelio, Worldwatch Institute, "Mobile Phone and Internet Use Grows Robustly," July 2010, http://vitalsigns.world watch.org/vs-trend/mobile-phone -and-internet-use-grows-robustly.

and the potential from exploiting consumers is probably greater than the real hazard to health.

## Ionizing Radiation

**Ionizing radiation** is caused by the release of particles and electromagnetic rays from atomic nuclei during the normal process of disintegration. This type of radiation has enough energy to remove electrons from the atoms it passes through. Some naturally occurring elements, such as uranium, emit radiation. The sun is another source of ionizing radiation, in the form of high-frequency ultraviolet rays—those against which the ozone layer protects us.

There are three major types of ionizing radiation: alpha particles, beta particles, and gamma rays. *Alpha particles* are relatively massive and are not capable of penetrating human skin. They pose health hazards only when inhaled or ingested. *Beta particles* can penetrate the skin slightly and are harmful if ingested or inhaled. *Gamma rays* and *X rays* are the most dangerous, because they can pass straight through the skin, wreaking havoc on human cells and leading to mutations, cancer, miscarriages, and other problems. Radon, nuclear weapons, nuclear energy plants, and medical X-ray machines are all sources of this type of radiation.

Reactions to radiation differ from person to person. Exposure is measured in **radiation absorbed doses (rads)**, also called *roentgens*. Radiation can cause damage with dosages as low as 100 to 200 rads. At this level, signs of radiation sickness include nausea, diarrhea, fatigue, anemia, sore throat, and hair loss. At 350 to 500 rads, these symptoms become more severe, and death may result because the radiation hinders bone marrow production of the white blood cells we need to protect us from disease. Dosages above 600 to 700 rads are invariably fatal.

Recommended maximum "safe" dosages range from 0.5 to 5 rads per year. Approximately 50 percent of the radiation to which we are exposed comes from natural sources, including radon and cosmic radiation. Another 48 percent comes from medical exposure (e.g., CAT scans and X rays). The remaining 2 percent is nonionizing radiation that comes from such sources as computer monitors, microwave ovens, television sets, and radar screens.[54] Most of us are exposed to far less radiation than the safe maximum dosage per year. The effects of long-term exposure to relatively low levels of radiation are unknown.

## Nuclear Power Plants

Nuclear power plants account for less than 1 percent of the total radiation to which we are exposed, but are symbols to many of the dangers of radiation and a controversial source of energy. The debate over nuclear energy has gone on for many years. The lure of nuclear energy, some think, is that it's relatively cheap to make. Initial costs of building nuclear power plants are high, but actual power generation is relatively inexpensive. A 1,000-megawatt reactor produces enough energy for 650,000 homes and saves 420 million gallons of fossil fuels each year. In some areas where nuclear power plants were decommissioned, electricity bills tripled when power companies turned to hydroelectric or fossil fuel sources to generate electricity. Nuclear reactors discharge fewer carbon oxides into the air than fossil fuel–powered generators.

However, there are many difficulties with nuclear power. Currently, disposal of nuclear wastes is extremely problematic. Another major concern is the possibility of a **nuclear meltdown,** which occurs when the temperature in a nuclear reactor's core increases enough to melt both the nuclear fuel and the containment vessel that holds it. Most modern facilities seal their reactors and containment vessels in concrete buildings with pools of cold water on the bottom. If a meltdown occurs, the building and the pool are supposed to prevent the escape of radioactivity.

One serious nuclear accident in particular contributed to a steep decline in public support for nuclear energy: the 1986 reactor core fire and explosion at the Chernobyl nuclear power plant in Russia. Radioactive fallout from the Chernobyl disaster spread over most of the Northern Hemisphere. Milk, meat, and vegetables in Scandinavian countries were contaminated with radioactive elements and were declared unfit for human consumption. Thousands of reindeer in Lapland and sheep in Great Britain were contaminated and had to be destroyed.

See the **Points of View** box on page 670 for further discussion of the pros and cons of nuclear power.

**ionizing radiation** Electromagnetic waves and particles having short wavelengths and energy high enough to ionize atoms.

**radiation absorbed doses (rads)** Units that measure exposure to radiation.

**nuclear meltdown** An accident that results when the temperature in the core of a nuclear reactor increases enough to melt the nuclear fuel and the containment vessel housing it.

# Nuclear Power:
## IS IT WORTH THE RISKS?

The issues raised by our ongoing dependence on declining oil reserves have increased public interest in the potential benefits of nuclear power. Federal support for building more nuclear plants, and for relying more heavily on them in a power-hungry future, has increased under the Obama administration. These initiatives may increase further after the recent Gulf of Mexico oil spill involving BP provided a wake-up call about the hazards of many current energy production efforts. However, nuclear accidents continue to pose risks to human health, even in well-controlled settings. For some, the BP oil spill is a reminder of the dangers of accidents such as the incident in Chernobyl in 1986.

### Arguments for Nuclear Power

◯ Nuclear power is more efficient and cheaper than fossil fuels.

◯ Nuclear power generation emits relatively low amounts of $CO_2$. Greenhouse gas emissions and the contribution of nuclear power plants to global warming are relatively minor.

◯ The technology is readily available—it does not have to be developed, unlike solar power, for example.

◯ The construction and staffing of new nuclear power plants create jobs.

### Arguments against Nuclear Power

◯ Nuclear power may appear cheap, but the building of nuclear reactors is heavily dependent on taxpayer subsidies.

◯ We still have no foolproof way of disposing of nuclear waste.

◯ The risks of having another major nuclear accident are not worth any savings in cost of generating electricity.

◯ Uranium is a scarce resource—as with fossil fuels, it will run out one day.

### Where Do You Stand?

◯ Do you think America should build more nuclear power plants?

◯ If so, where do you think they should be built?

◯ If not, how should Americans meet their growing energy needs?

◯ What are the dangers associated with other forms of power generation? How do you think these compare to those associated with nuclear power?

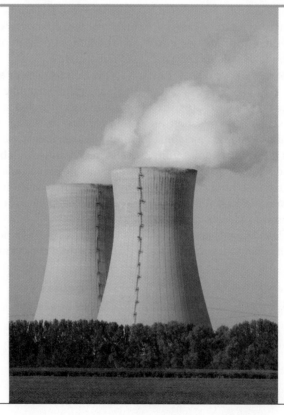

**Sources:** J. Deutch et al., *Update of the MIT 2003 Future of Nuclear Power: An Interdisciplinary MIT Study* (Cambridge, MA: Massachusetts Institute of Technology, 2009), Available at http://web.mit.edu/nuclearpower; Nuclear Energy Institute, "Key Issues," 2010, www.nei.org/keyissues; Public Citizen, "Just the Facts: A Look at the Five Fatal Flaws of Nuclear Power," 2010, www.citizen.org/cmep/article_redirect.cfm?ID=13447; Friends of the Earth, "Nuclear Reactors," 2010, www.foe.org/energy/nuclear-reactors.

## Are You Doing All You Can to Preserve the Environment?

**PEARSON**
**myhealthlab**

Fill out this assessment online at
www.pearsonhighered.com/myhealthlab
or www.pearsonhighered.com/donatelle.

Environmental problems often seem too big for one person to make a difference. Each day, though, there are things you can do that contribute to the planet's health. For each statement below, indicate how often you follow the described behavior.

| | Always | Usually | Sometimes | Never |
|---|---|---|---|---|
| 1. Whenever possible, I walk or ride my bicycle rather than drive a car. | 1 | 2 | 3 | 4 |
| 2. I carpool with others to school or work. | 1 | 2 | 3 | 4 |
| 3. I have my car tuned up and inspected every year. | 1 | 2 | 3 | 4 |
| 4. When I change the oil in my car, I make sure the oil is properly recycled, rather than dumped on the ground or into a floor drain. | 1 | 2 | 3 | 4 |
| 5. I avoid using the air conditioner except during extreme conditions. | 1 | 2 | 3 | 4 |
| 6. I turn off the lights when a room is not being used. | 1 | 2 | 3 | 4 |
| 7. I take a shower rather than a bath most of the time. | 1 | 2 | 3 | 4 |
| 8. I have water-saving devices installed on my shower, toilet, and sinks. | 1 | 2 | 3 | 4 |
| 9. I make sure faucets and toilets in my home do not leak. | 1 | 2 | 3 | 4 |
| 10. I use my bath towels more than once before putting them in the wash. | 1 | 2 | 3 | 4 |
| 11. I wear my clothes more than once between washings when possible. | 1 | 2 | 3 | 4 |
| 12. I make sure that the washing machine is full before I wash a load of clothes. | 1 | 2 | 3 | 4 |
| 13. I purchase biodegradable soaps and detergents. | 1 | 2 | 3 | 4 |
| 14. I use biodegradable trash bags. | 1 | 2 | 3 | 4 |
| 15. At home, I use dishes and silverware rather than disposable products. | 1 | 2 | 3 | 4 |
| 16. When I buy prepackaged foods, I choose the ones with the least packaging. | 1 | 2 | 3 | 4 |
| 17. I do not subscribe to newspapers and magazines that I can view online. | 1 | 2 | 3 | 4 |
| 18. I do not use a hair dryer. | 1 | 2 | 3 | 4 |
| 19. I recycle plastic bags that I get when I bring something home from the store. | 1 | 2 | 3 | 4 |
| 20. I don't run water continuously when washing the dishes, shaving, or brushing my teeth. | 1 | 2 | 3 | 4 |
| 21. I use unbleached or recycled paper. | 1 | 2 | 3 | 4 |
| 22. I use both sides of printer paper and other paper when possible. | 1 | 2 | 3 | 4 |
| 23. If I have items I do not want to use anymore, I donate them to charity so someone else can use them. | 1 | 2 | 3 | 4 |
| 24. I carry a reusable mug for my coffee or tea and have it filled rather than using a new paper cup each time I buy a hot beverage. | 1 | 2 | 3 | 4 |
| 25. I carry and use a refillable water bottle rather than frequently buying bottled water. | 1 | 2 | 3 | 4 |
| 26. I clean up after myself while enjoying the outdoors (picnicking, camping, etc.). | 1 | 2 | 3 | 4 |
| 27. I volunteer for cleanup days in the community in which I live. | 1 | 2 | 3 | 4 |
| 28. I consider candidates' positions on environmental issues before casting my vote. | 1 | 2 | 3 | 4 |

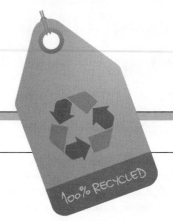

## For Further Thought

Review your scores. Are your responses mostly 1s and 2s? If not, what actions can you take to become more environmentally responsible? Are there ways to help the environment on this list that you had not thought of before? Are there behaviors not on the list that you are already doing?

# YOUR PLAN FOR **CHANGE**

The **Assess**yourself activity gave you the chance to look at your behavior and consider ways to conserve energy, save water, reduce waste, and otherwise help protect the planet. Now that you have considered these results, you can take steps to become more environmentally responsible.

### Today, you can:

◯ Find out how much energy you are using. Visit www.carbonfund.org, www.carbonoffsets.org, or www.greatest planet.org to find out what your carbon footprint is and to learn about projects you can support to offset your own emissions and energy usage. New carbon offset programs and organizations are popping up all the time, so watch for other opportunities to counter your carbon usage.

◯ Reduce the amount of paper waste in your mailbox. You can stop junk mail, such as credit card offers and unwanted catalogs, by visiting the Direct Marketing Association's Mail Preference Service site at www.dmachoice.org. You can also call 1-888-5-OPT-OUT to put an end to unwanted mail. In addition, the website www.catalogchoice.org is a free service that lets you decline paper catalogs you no longer want to receive.

### Within the next 2 weeks, you can:

◯ Look into joining an on-campus environmental group, attending an environmental campus event, or taking an environmental science course.

◯ Take part in a local cleanup day or recycling drive. These can be fun opportunities to meet like-minded people while benefiting the planet.

### By the end of the semester, you can:

◯ Start a compost pile for all your organic waste. You don't need a yard to do this; the EPA provides information on setting up an indoor compost bin at www.epa.gov/epawaste/conserve/rrr/composting/by_compost.htm.

◯ Make a habit of recycling everything you can rather than adding things to the trash. Find out what items can be recycled in your neighborhood and designate a box or trash can in your apartment or dorm to hold recyclable materials—cans, bottles, newspapers, junk mail, and so on—until you can carry them out to the curbside bins or a drop-off center.

◯ Work to influence the environment on a larger scale. Take part in an environmental activism group on campus or in your community. Listen carefully to what political candidates say about the environment. Let your legislators know how you feel about environmental issues and that you will vote according to their record on the issues.

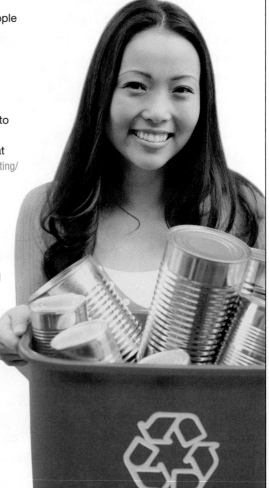

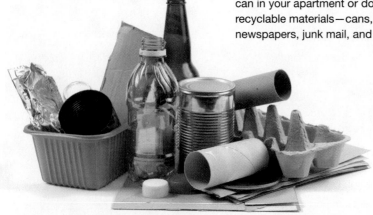

## Summary

* Population growth is the single largest factor affecting the environment. Demand for more food, water, and energy—as well as places to dispose of waste—places great strain on Earth's resources. The United States is among the greatest consumers of natural resources per person of any nation in the world. We can do more to reduce, reuse, and recycle.

* The primary constituents of air pollution are sulfur dioxide, particulate matter, carbon monoxide, nitrogen dioxide, ground-level ozone, lead, carbon dioxide, and hydrocarbons. Indoor air pollution is caused primarily by tobacco smoke, woodstove smoke, furnace emissions, asbestos, formaldehyde, radon, lead, and mold. Pollution is depleting Earth's protective ozone layer and contributing to global warming by enhancing the greenhouse effect.

* Water pollution can be caused by either point sources (direct entry) or nonpoint sources (runoff or seepage). Major contributors to water pollution include petroleum products, organic solvents, polychlorinated biphenyls (PCBs), dioxins, pesticides, and lead. Solid waste pollution includes household trash, plastics, glass, metal products, and paper. Limited landfill space creates problems. Hazardous waste is toxic; improper disposal creates health hazards for people in surrounding communities.

* Nonionizing radiation comes from electromagnetic fields, such as those around power lines. Ionizing radiation results from the natural erosion of atomic nuclei. The disposal and storage of radioactive waste from nuclear power plants pose potential problems for public health.

## Pop Quiz

1. The United States is responsible for what percentage of total global resource consumption?
   a. 10 percent
   b. 25 percent
   c. 50 percent
   d. 70 percent

2. Which of the following statements about population growth is NOT correct?
   a. Higher fertility rates and decreases in mortality rates are key factors in population growth.
   b. Populations of wealthier nations are static or declining overall.
   c. As education levels of women increase and women achieve equality in pay, job, and social status with men, fertility rates go down.
   d. Zero population growth has proved to be impossible and no countries of the world have been able to achieve it.

3. One possible source of indoor air pollution is a gas present in some carpets called
   a. lead.
   b. asbestos.
   c. radon.
   d. formaldehyde.

4. What substance separates into stringy fibers that can become embedded in the lungs?
   a. Asbestos
   b. Particulate matter
   c. Radon
   d. Formaldehyde

5. The terms *point source* and *nonpoint source* are used to describe the two general sources of
   a. water pollution.
   b. air pollution.
   c. noise pollution.
   d. ozone depletion.

6. The air pollutant that originates primarily from motor vehicle emissions is
   a. particulates.
   b. nitrogen dioxide.
   c. sulfur dioxide.
   d. carbon monoxide.

7. Which gas is considered radioactive and could become cancer causing when it seeps into a home?
   a. Carbon monoxide
   b. Radon
   c. Hydrogen sulfide
   d. Natural gas

8. The phenomenon that creates a barrier to protect us from the sun's harmful ultraviolet radiation rays is
   a. photochemical smog.
   b. ozone layer.
   c. gray air smog.
   d. greenhouse effect.

9. Your most recent DVD purchase came with less packaging than it previously had. This is an example of controlling municipal solid waste via
   a. source reduction.
   b. recycling.
   c. composting.
   d. incineration.

10. Some herbicides contain toxic substances called
   a. THMs.
   b. PCPs.
   c. dioxins.
   d. PCBs.

*Answers for these questions can be found on page A-1.*

## Think about It!

1. How are the rapid increases in global population and consumption of resources related? Is population control the best solution? Why or why not?
2. What are the primary sources of air pollution? What can be done to reduce air pollution?
3. What are the causes and consequences of global warming? What can individuals do to reduce the threat of global warming?
4. What are point and nonpoint sources of water pollution? What can be done to reduce or prevent water pollution?

5. How do you think communities and governments could encourage recycling efforts in the United States?

## Accessing Your Health on the Internet

The following websites explore further topics and issues related to personal health. For links to the websites below, visit the Companion Website for *Access to Health*, 12th Edition, at www.pearsonhighered.com/donatelle.

1. *Environmental Literacy Council.* This website is an excellent source of information about environmental issues in general. Topics range from how the ozone layer works to why the rain forests are important ecosystems. www.enviroliteracy.org
2. *Environmental Protection Agency (EPA).* The EPA is the government agency responsible for overseeing environmental regulation and protection issues in the United States. www.epa.gov
3. *National Center for Environmental Health (NCEH).* This site provides information on a wide variety of environmental health issues and includes a series of helpful fact sheets. www.cdc.gov/nceh
4. *National Environmental Health Association (NEHA).* This organization provides educational resources and opportunities for environmental health professionals. www.neha.org

## References

1. R. Caplan, *Our Earth, Ourselves* (New York: Bantam, 1990), 247.
2. R. H. Friis, *Essentials of Environmental Health* (Boston: Jones and Bartlett, 2007), 7; R. Engelman, "Population Growth Steady in Recent Years," 2009, http://vitalsigns.worldwatch.org/vs-trend/population-growth-steady-recent-years.
3. Population Reference Bureau, *2010 World Population Data Sheet* (Washington, DC: Population Reference Bureau, 2010), Available at www.prb.org/Publications/Datasheets/2010/2010wpds.aspx.
4. United Nations Environment Programme, *Global Environment Outlook: Environment for Development (GEO-4)* (Valletta, Malta: United Nations Environment Programme, 2007), Available at www.unep.org/geo/geo4.asp.
5. Ibid.
6. N. Eberstadt, "Born in the USA," American Enterprise Institute for Public Policy Research, 2007, www.aei.org/article/25988.
7. Central Intelligence Agency, "The World Factbook: Country Comparison: Total Fertility Rate," Updated August 2010, https://www.cia.gov/library/publications/the-world-factbook/rankorder/2127rank.html.
8. U.S. Census Bureau, Population Division, "International Data Base Country Rankings," 2010, http://sasweb.ssd.census.gov/idb/ranks.html.
9. U.S. Census Bureau, U.S. and World Population Clocks, "U.S. POPClock Projection," 2010, www.census.gov/population/www/popclockus.html.
10. Central Intelligence Agency, "The World Factbook: United States," Updated August 2010, https://www.cia.gov/library/publications/the-world-factbook/geos/us.html.
11. V. Markham, *U.S. National Report on Population and the Environment* (New Canaan, CT: Center for Environment and Population, 2006), Available at www.cepnet.org.
12. C. Flavin et al., *State of the World 2008: Innovations for a Sustainable Economy* (Washington, DC: Worldwatch Institute, 2008), Available at www.worldwatch.org/node/5560.
13. Ibid.
14. Ibid.
15. Population Reference Bureau, "World Population Growth, 1950–2050," 2010, www.prb.org/educators/teachersguides/humanpopulation/populationgrowth.aspx?p=1; M. Rosenberg, "Negative Population Growth," 2010, http://geography.about.com/od/populationgeography/a/zero.htm.
16. U.S. Department of Health and Human Services, *Healthy People 2010*, 2nd ed., vol. 1, *Objectives for Improving Health: Focus Area 9 Family Planning* (Washington, DC: U.S. Government Printing Office, 2000), Available at www.healthypeople.gov/document/HTML/volume1/09Family.htm; Women Deliver, "Women Deliver 2010: Ministers' Forum Statement," 2010, www.womendeliver.org/updates/entry/women-deliver-2010-ministers-forum-statement/.
17. R. H. Friis, *Essentials of Environmental Health*, 2007, 232.
18. U.S. Environmental Protection Agency, "Air Pollution Control Orientation Course: Criteria Pollutants," Updated January 2010, www.epa.gov/apti/course422/ap5.html.
19. Ibid.
20. American Lung Association, "Health Effects of Ozone and Particle Pollution," in *State of the Air 2010* (Washington, DC: American Lung Association, 2010), Available at www.stateoftheair.org/2010/health-risks.
21. Ibid.
22. U.S. Environmental Protection Agency, "Acid Rain: What Is Acid Rain?" Updated June 2007, www.epa.gov/acidrain/what/index.html.
23. U.S. Environmental Protection Agency, "Acid Rain: Effects of Acid Rain—Surface Waters and Aquatic Animals," Updated December 2008, www.epa.gov/acidrain/effects/surface_water.html.
24. U.S. Environmental Protection Agency, "Acid Rain: Effects of Acid Rain—Forests," Updated June 2007, www.epa.gov/acidrain/effects/forests.html.
25. U.S. Environmental Protection Agency, "Acid Rain: Effects of Acid Rain—Human Health," Updated May 2009, www.epa.gov/acidrain/effects/health.html.
26. U.S. Environmental Protection Agency, "An Introduction to Indoor Air Quality," Updated April 2010, www.epa.gov/iaq/ia-intro.html.
27. Ibid.
28. U.S. Environmental Protection Agency, "Indoor Air Quality: Radon: Health Risks," Updated March 2010, www.epa.gov/radon/healthrisks.html.
29. U.S. Environmental Protection Agency, "U.S. Homes above EPA's Radon Action Level," Updated June 2010, http://cfpub.epa.gov/eroe/index.cfm?fuseaction=detail.viewInd&lv=list.listByAlpha&r=201747.
30. Centers for Disease Control and Prevention, "Lead," Updated July 2010, www.cdc.gov/nceh/lead.
31. North Carolina Department of Health and Human Services, Epidemiology, "Indoor Air Quality: Schools," Updated July 2010, http://www.epi.state.nc.us/epi/air/schools.html.
32. U.S. Environmental Protection Agency, "IAQ Tools for Schools: Improved Academic Performance: Evidence from Scientific Literature," Updated May 2010, www.epa.gov/iaq/schools/student_performance/evidence.html.
33. U.S. Environmental Protection Agency, "Ozone Layer Depletion: Ozone Science: Brief Questions and Answers on Ozone Depletion," Updated February 2010, www.epa.gov/ozone/science/q_a.html.
34. S. Arrhenius, "On the Influence of Carbonic Acid in the Air upon the Temperature of the Ground," *Philosophical*

*Magazine and Journal of Science* (fifth series) 41 (1896): 237–75.

35. U.S. Environmental Protection Agency, "Climate Change: Basic Information," Updated May 2010, www.epa.gov/climatechange/basicinfo.html.

36. U.S. Government Accountability Office, "Climate Change: Trends in Greenhouse Gas Emissions and Emissions Intensity in the United States and Other High-Emitting Nations," GAO-04-146R, October 2003, www.gao.gov/products/GAO-04-146R.

37. United Nations Framework Convention on Climate Change, "Kyoto Protocol," 2010, http://unfccc.int/kyoto_protocol/items/2830.php.

38. D. Malakoff and E. M. Williams, "Q & A: An Examination of the Kyoto Protocol," June 2007, www.npr.org/templates/story/story.php?storyId=5042766.

39. J. Vidal, "Climate Change Talks Yield Small Chance of Global Treaty," 2010, www.guardian.co.uk/environment/2010/apr/11/climate-change-talks-deal-treaty.

40. U.S. Geological Survey, "Water Science for Schools: Where Is Earth's Water Located?" Modified July 2010, http://ga.water.usgs.gov/edu/earthwherewater.html.

41. World Health Organization, "World in Danger of Missing Sanitation Target; Drinking-Water Target Also at Risk, New Report Shows," September 2006, www.who.int/mediacentre/news/releases/2006/pr47/en; UNICEF, "Water, Sanitation, and Hygiene: Children and Water: Global Statistics," Updated March 2006, www.unicef.org/wash/index_31600.html; United Nations General Assembly, "Sustainable Management of Water Resources Vital to Achieving Anti-Poverty Goals," March 2010, www.un.org/News/Press/docs/2010/ga10925.doc.htm.

42. R. H. Friis, *Environmental Health*, 2007, 204.

43. V. Markham, *U.S. National Report on Population and the Environment*, 2006.

44. D. W. Kolpin et al., "Pharmaceuticals, Hormones, and Other Organic Wastewater Contaminants in U.S. Streams, 1999–2000: A National Reconnaissance," *Environmental Science & Technology* 36, no. 6 (2002): 1202–11.

45. G. Bruce et al., "Toxicological Relevance of Pharmaceuticals in Drinking Water," *Environmental Science & Technology* 44, no.14 (2010): 5619–26; J. Donn et al., "AP Probe Finds Drugs in Drinking Water," March 2010, www.breitbart.com/article.php?id=D8VADOP80.

46. J. Donn et al., "AP Probe Finds Drugs in Drinking Water," 2010.

47. M. Tiemann, "Environmental Legislation: Leaking Underground Storage Tanks (USTs): Prevention and Cleanup," May 2010, http://environmental-legislation.blogspot.com/2010/05/leaking-underground-storage-tanks-usts.html.

48. Agency for Toxic Substances and Disease Registry (ATSDR), "Toxic Substances Portal: Polychlorinated Biphenyls (PCBs)," Updated April 2010, www.atsdr.cdc.gov/substances/toxsubstance.asp?toxid=26.

49. U.S. Environmental Protection Agency, "Pesticides: Topical and Chemical Fact Sheets: Assessing Health Risks from Pesticides," Updated September 2009, www.epa.gov/pesticides/factsheets/riskassess.htm.

50. U.S. Environmental Protection Agency, *Municipal Solid Waste Generation, Recycling, and Disposal in the United States: Facts and Figures for 2008* (Washington, DC: U.S. Environmental Protection Agency, 2009), Available at www.epa.gov/epawaste/nonhaz/municipal/msw99.htm.

51. Ibid.

52. Ibid.

53. U.S. Environmental Protection Agency, "Superfund: Superfund National Accomplishments Summary, Fiscal Year 2009," Updated May 2010, www.epa.gov/superfund/accomp/numbers09.html.

54. National Council on Radiation Protection and Measurements, "NCRP Report No. 160 Section 1 Pie Chart," Accessed September 2010, Available at www.ncrponline.org/Publications/160_Pie_charts.html.

# 21

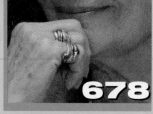

**678**

Is it really possible to "age gracefully"?

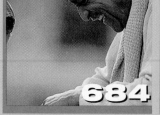

**684**

Is memory loss an inevitable part of aging?

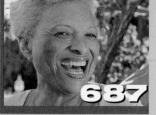

**687**

Is there any way to slow down the aging process?

# Preparing for Aging, Death, and Dying

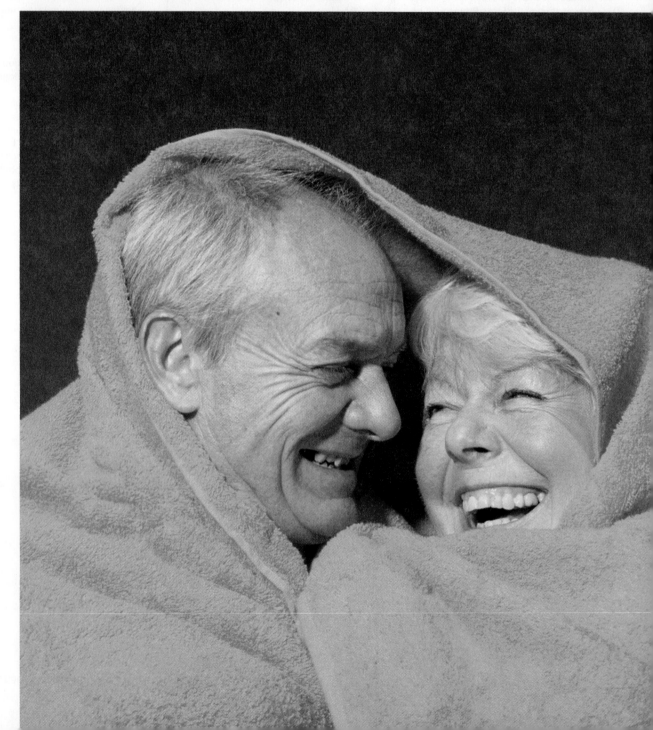

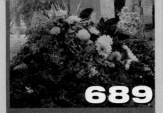

**689**

How can I help a friend who has just experienced a loss?

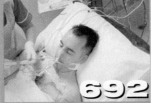

**692**

Why should I create a living will?

## Objectives

✳ Define *aging* and explain the related concepts of biological, psychological, social, legal, and functional age.

✳ Explain how the growing population of older adults will affect society, including considerations of economics, health care, living arrangements, and ethical and moral issues.

✳ Discuss the biological and psychosocial theories of aging, and summarize major physiological changes that occur as a result of the normal aging process.

✳ Discuss unique health challenges faced by older adults, and describe strategies for successful and healthy aging that can begin during young adulthood.

✳ Discuss death, the stages of the grieving process, and strategies for coping with death.

✳ Explain the ethical concerns that arise from the concepts of the right to die and rational suicide.

✳ Review the decisions that need to be made when someone is dying or has died, including hospice care, funeral arrangements, wills, and organ donation.

In a society that seems to worship youth, researchers have begun to offer good—even revolutionary—news about the aging process. Growing older doesn't have to mean a slow slide into declining physical and mental health. Health promotion, disease prevention, and wellness-oriented activities can prolong vigor and productivity, even among those who haven't always led model lifestyles or made healthful habits a priority. Numerous research studies show that people who make even modest lifestyle changes can reap significant health benefits. In fact, getting older can mean getting better in many ways—particularly socially, psychologically, spiritually, and intellectually.

**Aging** has traditionally been described as the patterns of life changes that occur in members of all species as they grow older. Some believe that aging begins at the moment of conception. Others contend that it starts at birth. Still others believe that true aging does not begin until we reach our forties.

Typically, experts and laypersons alike have used chronological age to assign people to particular life cycle stages. However, people of different chronological ages view age very differently. To the 4-year-old, a first-year college student seems quite old. To the 20-year-old, parents in their forties are over the hill. A 75-year-old may still think of himself as that 30-year-old he once was. Views of aging are also colored by occupation. For example, most professional athletes are considering other careers by the time they reach 40, whereas writers, musicians, and even college professors may work well into their seventies and eighties. Clearly, definitions of aging that consider only years lived rather than quality of life warrant reexamination.

> **aging** The patterns of life changes that occur in members of all species as they grow older.
> **gerontology** The study of individual and collective aging processes.

## Redefining Aging

The study of individual and collective aging processes, known as **gerontology,** explores the reasons for aging and the ways in which people cope with and adapt to this process. Gerontologists have identified several age-related characteristics that define where a person is in terms of biological, psychological, social, legal, and functional life-stage development:[1]

● *Biological age* refers to the relative age or condition of the person's organs and body systems. There are 70-year-old runners who have the cardiovascular system of a 40-year-old and 40-year-olds with the cardiovascular system of someone in their late sixties or seventies. Research shows that healthy lifestyle behaviors such as being active, eating a healthy diet, and not smoking are the most influential factors on how your body ages.[2]

● *Psychological age* refers to a person's adaptive capacities, such as coping abilities and intelligence, and to the person's awareness of his or her individual capabilities, self-efficacy, and general ability to adapt to new situations.

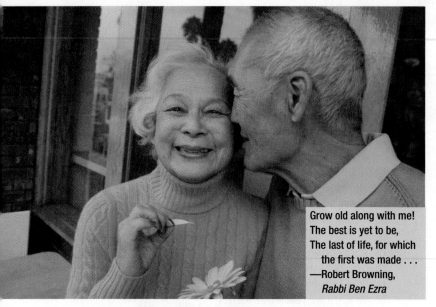

Grow old along with me!
The best is yet to be,
The last of life, for which
the first was made . . .
—Robert Browning,
*Rabbi Ben Ezra*

Typically, people who have aged successfully have the following characteristics:

- In general, they have managed to avoid serious debilitating diseases and disability.
- They function well physically, live independently, and engage in most normal activities of daily living.
- They have maintained cognitive function and are actively engaged in mentally challenging and stimulating activities and in social and productive pursuits.
- They are resilient and able to cope reasonably well with physical, social, and emotional changes.
- They feel a sense of control over circumstances in their lives.[6]

The question is not how many years someone has lived, but how much life the person has packed into those years. This quality-of-life index, combined with the chronological process, appears to be the best indicator of the phenomenon of "aging gracefully." Most experts agree that the best way to experience a productive, full, and satisfying old age is to lead a productive, full, and satisfying life prior to old age.

Research documents that many older adults maintain a positive attitude and do successfully cope with the physical and cognitive changes associated with aging.[3]

- *Social age* refers to a person's habits and roles relative to society's expectations. People in a particular life stage often share similar tastes in music and television shows, for example.
- *Legal age* is probably the most common definition of age in the United States. Based on chronological years, legal age is used as a factor in determining voting rights, driving privileges, drinking rights, eligibility for Social Security payments, and other rights and obligations.
- *Functional age* refers to the ways—heart rate, hearing, and so on—in which people compare to others of a similar age. It can be difficult to separate functional aging from many of the other types of aging, particularly chronological and biological aging.

## What Is Successful Aging?

Many of today's "elderly" individuals lead active, productive lives. For instance, nearly 20.5 percent of Americans aged 65 or over have completed bachelor's through doctoral or professional degrees.[4] The majority of adults over 65 continue to work, volunteer, serve in public office, travel, and remain otherwise active.[5]

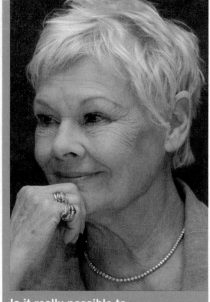

**Is it really possible to "age gracefully"?**

Growing old will happen to anyone who hangs around long enough, but aging gracefully requires embracing the progress of your years. The people we often think of as aging gracefully—such as actress Dame Judi Dench—are those who continue to be active and productive; who are not frightened or ashamed of growing older; who adapt to the changing circumstances of their lives; and who strive to be healthy, vibrant, and alive at any age.

## Older Adults: A Growing Population

The United States and much of the developed world are on the brink of a *longevity revolution*, one that will affect society in ways that we have not yet begun to understand. According to the latest statistics, life expectancy for a child born in 2007 is 77.9 years, about 30 years longer than for a child born in 1900.[7] Today there are nearly 39 million people aged 65 or older in the United States, making up over 12 percent of the total population.[8] By 2030, the older population is expected to be twice as large as in 2007, growing to 72.1 million and representing 19.3 percent of the population. In comparison, a mere 3 million people were aged 65 and older in 1900 (see Figure 21.1).[9] Other nations report a similar trend. The World Health Organization (WHO) predicts that by 2050, the percentage of adults over 60 years old will double to 22 percent.[10]

Within the United States, the population of those over 65 will increase substantially over the next two decades, due to the aging "baby boomer" generation. The baby boomers, born between 1946 and 1964, start turning 65 in 2011. The needs of this generation of Americans—who are better educated and more racially diverse than past generations—will have a major

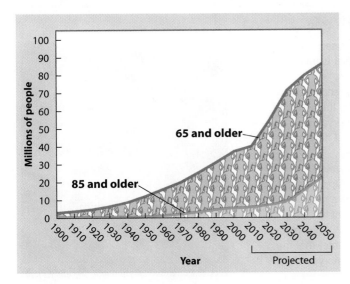

FIGURE 21.1 **Number of Americans 65 and Older (in millions), Years 1900–2008, and Projected 2010–2050**

Note: Data for 2010–2050 are projections of the population.

**Source:** Data are from U.S. Census Bureau, Decennial Census, Population Estimates and Projections.

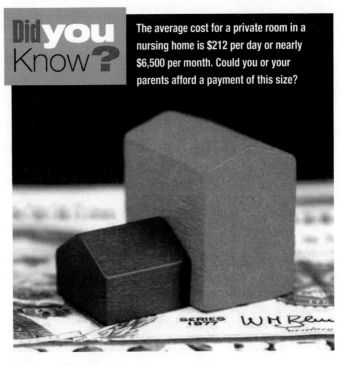

Did**you** Know**?** The average cost for a private room in a nursing home is $212 per day or nearly $6,500 per month. Could you or your parents afford a payment of this size?

impact on the economy, housing market, health care system, and Social Security.

## Health Issues for an Aging Society

Meeting an older population's financial and medical needs, providing health care and adequate housing, and addressing end-of-life ethical considerations are all of concern in an aging society. You may have heard discussions on the potential bankruptcy of the Social Security system and the large increases in out-of-pocket costs for people on Medicare. Many fear the combination of fewer younger workers paying into the system and more older people drawing for more years than ever before will result in tremendous shortfalls in the future. This is particularly true as the federal government borrows against the existing Social Security revenues and as federal debt continues to soar.

**Health Care Costs** Older Americans averaged $4,605 in out-of-pocket medical expenses in 2008, an increase of 57 percent since 1998.[11] These costs included $2,844 (62%) for insurance, $793 (17%) for drugs, $821 (18%) for medical services, and $145 (3%) for medical supplies.[12] As people live longer, the chances of developing a costly chronic disease increase, and as technology improves, chronic illnesses that once were quickly fatal may now be treated successfully for years. Most older adults have at least one chronic condition and many have multiple conditions. It is estimated that 41 percent of older adults have hyper-

tension, 49 percent have been diagnosed with arthritis, 39 percent with heart disease, and 22 percent with cancer.[13] Among people turning 65 today, nearly 69 percent will need some form of long-term care, whether in the community or in a residential care facility.[14]

**Housing and Living Arrangements** Most older people (over 95%) never live in a true nursing home. Many live with a spouse, while others live alone or with relatives or friends (Figure 21.2). Increasing numbers of people live their later years in communities that offer various levels of assistance for their clients. Some of these communities allow individuals to purchase their own homes and live fairly independently, sometimes with electronically monitored devices that allow some

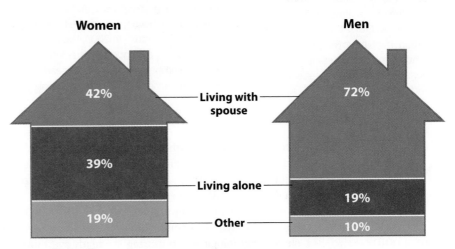

FIGURE 21.2 **Living Arrangements of Americans Aged 65 and Older**

Percentages may not total 100% due to rounding.

**Source:** Administration on Aging, U.S. Dept. of Health and Human Services, "A Profile of Older Americans: Living Arrangements, 2009," 2010, www.aoa.gov/AoAroot/Aging_Statistics/Profile/2009/6.aspx.

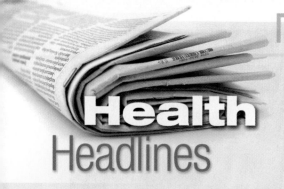

# Health Headlines

## THE DEBATE OVER STEM CELLS

Stem cells are unique and controversial. Stem cells have two important characteristics: (1) They are capable of renewing themselves by dividing repeatedly; and (2) they are unspecialized, and so can be induced to become specialized cells that perform specific functions, such as muscle cells that make the heart beat or nerve cells that enable the brain to function.

Many scientists believe that stem cells have the potential to cure debilitating health conditions that involve the destruction of crucial cells—in the case of type 1 diabetes, for example, the pancreatic cells that secrete insulin. In the laboratory, researchers are working to coax stem cells to develop into these pancreatic cells. The plan is to transplant the new cells into diabetic patients, where they could replace the patients' damaged cells and produce insulin. If successful, this approach could prevent the destructive complications of the disease and free diabetics from the painful burden of injecting insulin for the rest of their lives. Other therapies under investigation involve growing new cells to replace those ravaged by spinal injuries, Alzheimer's disease, heart disease, and vision and hearing loss.

Generally, stem cells used in research are derived from eggs that were fertilized in vitro. Typically these are "extra" embryos created during fertility treatments at clinics but not used for implantation. Only 4 to 5 days old, embryonic stem cells are *pluripotent* (capable of developing into many different cell types).

Embryonic stem cell research has provoked fierce debate. Opponents believe that an embryo is a human being and that no one has a right to create life and then destroy it, even for humanitarian purposes. Advocates counter that the eggs from which these embryos developed were given freely by donors and would otherwise be discarded.

Are adult stem cells a solution? An adult stem cell is an undifferentiated cell that is found in some body tissues and can specialize to replace certain types of cells. For example, human bone marrow contains at least two kinds of adult stem cells. One kind gives rise to the various types of blood cells, whereas the other can differentiate into bone, cartilage, fat, or fibrous connective tissue. Although research indicates that adult stem cells may be more versatile than previously thought, many scientists think that embryonic stem cells are more medically promising.

In the United States, embryonic stem cell research has been limited by law. In recent years federal funding—a major source of support for universities and labs—has been restricted to experiments on only a small number of stem cell lines (a stem cell line refers to a set of pluripotent, embryonic stem cells that have grown in the laboratory for at least 6 months). In 2009, President Barack Obama expanded federal funding for human embryonic stem cell research, rescinding previous policy. The new policy

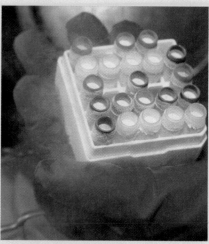

Using stored embryos to derive stem cells for research is a highly controversial matter.

allows researchers to utilize the many hundreds of lines created since 2001, and relieves them from the challenges of duplicating equipment and other resources in order to separate privately or state-funded stem cell research from federally funded efforts. However, challenges to the federal funding continue, and uncertainties remain regarding federal support of research.

**Sources:** National Institutes of Health, Stem Cell Information, "Stem Cell Basics," http://stemcells .nih.gov/info/basics/defaultpage, Revised April 2009; Presidential Documents, "Executive Order 13505 of March 9, 2009: Removing Barriers to Responsible Scientific Research Involving Human Stem Cells," *Federal Register* 74, no. 46 (2009), http://edocket.access.gpo.gov/2009/pdf/E9-5441 .pdf; International Society for Stem Cell Research (ISSCR), "ISSCR Scientists Elated for Future of Human Embryonic Stem Cell Research after Obama Lifts Funding Ban," Press release, March 9, 2009, www.isscr.org/press_releases/obama _repeals.html; International Society for Stem Cell Research (ISSCR), "ISSCR Decries Negative Impact of Stem Cell Injunction on Science and Medicine," Press release, September 2, 2010, www.isscr.org/ press_releases/injunction.html.

## 95%
**of older adults never live in a nursing home.**

form of supervision. Other communities and facilities can also include 24/7 monitoring of unique needs, such as Alzheimer's cases or other disabilities. Newer, technologically advanced housing includes physiological monitoring that actually records heart rate and other life indicators to ensure prompt emergency services in case of problems.

Essentially, if you have the money, the sky's the limit in terms of superb care for your later years. However, tremendous income-based disparities exist in caring for the elderly. Those without means are more likely to be homeless or shut out of all but the most meager care situations.

**Ethical and Moral Considerations** Difficult ethical questions arise when we consider the implications of an already overburdened health care system. Given the shortage of donor organs, will we be forced to decide whether a 50-year-old should receive a heart transplant instead of a 75-year-old? Questions have already surfaced regarding the efficacy of hooking up a terminally ill older person to costly machines that prolong life for a few weeks or months but overtax health care resources, or performing costly surgeries such as hip replacements on people in their eighties and nineties. Is the prolongation of life at all costs a moral imperative, or will future generations devise a set of criteria for deciding who will be helped and who will not? The debate over stem cell research asks us to balance scientific achievements with questions of morality (see the **Health Headlines** box at left).

## Theories of Aging

Social gerontologists, behaviorists, biologists, geneticists, and physiologists continue to explore various potential explanations for why the body breaks down over time. One explanation for the biological cause of aging is the *wear-and-tear theory*, which states that, like everything else in the world, the human body wears out. Inherent in this theory is the idea that the more you abuse your body, the faster it will wear out. Another theory, the *cellular theory*, proposes that at birth we have only a certain number of usable cells, which are genetically programmed to reproduce a limited number of times. Once cells reach the end of their reproductive cycle, they die, and the organs they make up begin to deteriorate.

According to the *genetic mutation theory*, the number of body cells exhibiting unusual or different characteristics increases with age. Proponents of this theory believe that aging is related to the amount of mutational damage within the genes. The more mutation there is, the greater the chance becomes that cells will not function properly.

Finally, the *autoimmune theory* attributes aging to the decline of the body's immunological system. Studies indicate that as we age, the ability to produce necessary antibodies declines, and our immune systems become less effective in fighting disease. At the same time, the white blood cells active in the immune response become less able to recognize foreign invaders and more likely to mistakenly attack the body's own proteins.

## Physical and Mental Changes of Aging

Although the physiological consequences of aging can differ in severity and timing, certain standard changes occur as a result of the aging process. Many of these changes are physical (see **Figure 21.3**), whereas others are mental or psychosocial.

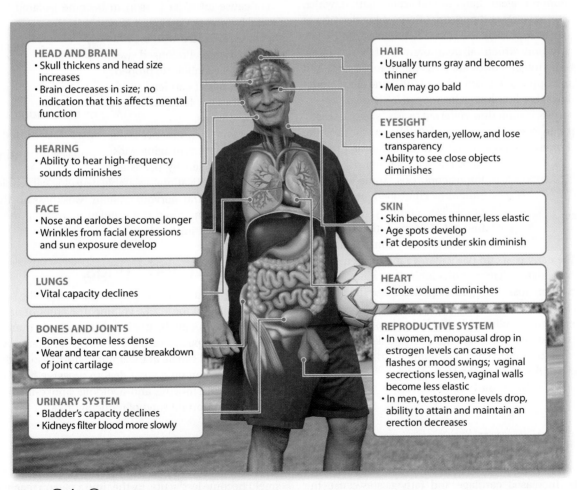

**HEAD AND BRAIN**
• Skull thickens and head size increases
• Brain decreases in size; no indication that this affects mental function

**HEARING**
• Ability to hear high-frequency sounds diminishes

**FACE**
• Nose and earlobes become longer
• Wrinkles from facial expressions and sun exposure develop

**LUNGS**
• Vital capacity declines

**BONES AND JOINTS**
• Bones become less dense
• Wear and tear can cause breakdown of joint cartilage

**URINARY SYSTEM**
• Bladder's capacity declines
• Kidneys filter blood more slowly

**HAIR**
• Usually turns gray and becomes thinner
• Men may go bald

**EYESIGHT**
• Lenses harden, yellow, and lose transparency
• Ability to see close objects diminishes

**SKIN**
• Skin becomes thinner, less elastic
• Age spots develop
• Fat deposits under skin diminish

**HEART**
• Stroke volume diminishes

**REPRODUCTIVE SYSTEM**
• In women, menopausal drop in estrogen levels can cause hot flashes or mood swings; vaginal secretions lessen, vaginal walls become less elastic
• In men, testosterone levels drop, ability to attain and maintain an erection decreases

FIGURE 21.3 **Normal Effects of Aging on the Body**

## The Skin

As a normal part of aging, the skin becomes thinner and loses elasticity, particularly in the outer surfaces. Fat deposits, which add to the soft lines and shape of the skin, diminish. Starting at about age 30, lines develop on the forehead as a result of smiling, squinting, and other facial expressions. During the forties, these lines become more pronounced, with added "crow's feet" around the eyes. In a person's fifties and sixties, the skin begins to sag and lose color, which leads to pallor in the seventies. Body fat in underlying layers of skin continues to be redistributed away from the limbs and extremities into the body's trunk region. Age spots become more numerous because of excessive pigment accumulation under the skin, particularly in areas of the skin exposed to heavy sun.

## Bones and Joints

Throughout the life span, bones are continually changing because of the accumulation and loss of minerals. By the third or fourth decade of life, mineral loss from bones becomes more prevalent than mineral accumulation, which results in a weakening and porosity (diminishing density) of bony tissue. **Osteoporosis** is a disease characterized by low bone density and structural deterioration of bone tissue. These porous, fragile bones are susceptible to fracture and may lead to crippling malformation of the spine characteristic of the dowager's hump seen in stooped individuals.

Osteoporosis is sometimes referred to as a "silent disease," because it can occur at any age, develops slowly over the years, and often has no symptoms until late in its progression. There are several risk factors for osteoporosis, some of which cannot be controlled (gender, age, body size, ethnicity, and family history). However, there are factors that can be controlled, starting from the early years. In particular, young women should consume adequate calcium and vitamin D to reduce risk of accelerated bone loss during menopause.[15] See the **Gender & Health** box for more information on preventing osteoporosis.

Another bone condition that afflicts almost 27 million Americans is *osteoarthritis*, a progressive breakdown of joint cartilage that becomes more common with age and is a major cause of disability in the United States.[16] For information on osteoarthritis and other forms of arthritis, see Chapter 17.

**osteoporosis** A degenerative bone disorder characterized by increasingly porous bones.

**urinary incontinence** Inability to control urination.

## The Head and Face

With age, features of the head enlarge and become more noticeable. Increased cartilage and fatty tissue cause the nose to grow a half inch wider and another half inch longer.

Earlobes get fatter and grow longer. As the skull becomes thicker with age, the overall head circumference increases one-quarter of an inch per decade, even though the brain itself shrinks.

**"Why Should I Care?"**

Aging isn't a distant process somewhere in the future—it's something that is happening to every one of us every day of our lives. The way you live your life now has a direct impact on how you will live it in the future. Learning to cope with challenges and changes early in life develops attitudes and skills that contribute to a full and satisfying old age.

## The Urinary Tract

At age 70, the kidneys can filter waste from the blood only half as fast as they could at age 30. The need to urinate more frequently occurs because the bladder's capacity declines from 2 cups of urine at age 30 to 1 cup at age 70.

One problem sometimes associated with aging is **urinary incontinence**, which ranges from passing a few drops of urine while laughing or sneezing to having no control over urination. Urinary incontinence affects 30 percent of the general geriatric population and affects more than half of all persons in long-term facilities.[17]

Incontinence can pose major social, physical, and emotional problems. Embarrassment and fear of wetting oneself may cause an older person to become isolated and avoid social functions. Caregivers may become frustrated with incontinent patients. Prolonged wetness and the inability to properly care for oneself can lead to tissue irritation, infections, and other problems.

However, incontinence is not an inevitable part of aging. Most cases are caused by persistent infections, medications, treatable neurological problems that affect the central nervous system, weakness in the pelvic wall, and so on. When the problem is treated, the incontinence usually vanishes.[18]

**50%** of older adults in long-term care facilities experience urinary incontinence.

## The Heart and Lungs

Resting heart rate stays about the same over the course of a person's life, but the stroke volume (the amount of blood the heart pushes out per beat) diminishes as heart muscle deteriorates. Vital capacity, or the amount of air that moves when you inhale and exhale at maximum effort, also declines with age. Exercise can do a great deal to preserve heart and lung function. Not smoking and avoiding smoke-filled environments are important ways of reducing risks.

## The Senses

With aging, the senses (vision, hearing, touch, taste, and smell) become less acute. By the time a person reaches age 30, the lens of the eye begins to harden, which causes problems

# Osteoporosis: Preventing an Age-Old Problem

Many people think osteoporosis is a disease only of older women; however, it can occur at any age, and it can pose a problem for men, too. In the United States, osteoporosis affects more than 44 million Americans, almost a third of whom (32%) are men. Each year, osteoporosis causes 1.5 million fractures: 300,000 at the hip, 700,000 in the vertebrae, 250,000 in the wrists, and more than 300,000 at other sites. Bone density scans using dual-energy X-ray absorptiometry can screen for osteoporosis. With early detection, steps can be taken to reverse the bone loss and prevent fractures.

Some of the factors that predispose a person to developing osteoporosis are intrinsic and cannot be controlled, including the following:

\* **Gender.** Women have a higher risk of developing osteoporosis. They have less bone tissue and lose bone more rapidly than men do because of the hormonal changes resulting from menopause.

\* **Age.** Bones become less dense and weaker with age, so the older you are, the greater your risk of osteoporosis.

\* **Body size.** Small, thin-boned women are at greatest risk.

\* **Ethnicity.** Caucasian and Asian women are at highest risk; African American and Latina women have a lower but still significant risk.

\* **Family history.** Susceptibility to fracture may be, in part, hereditary. People whose parents have a history of fractures also seem to have reduced bone mass.

Regular weight-bearing exercise such as walking will help keep your bones healthy and strong.

You cannot modify your age, gender, or ethnicity to prevent osteoporosis, but there *are* things you can do to prevent the disease, starting when you are still young. During your lifetime, bone is constantly being added (formation) and being broken down and removed (reabsorption). Through childhood and the young adult years, formation outpaces reabsorption, and bone grows heavier, stronger, and denser. At around 30 years of age, a person reaches *peak bone mass*. After this peak mass is reached, a slow and steady decline occurs. Individuals who accrue strong, dense, healthy bones through proper diet and exercise begun in young adulthood and continued into middle age and beyond can minimize this decline and reduce their risk for osteoporosis later in life.

In order to create strong, healthy bones you need to consume sufficient calcium. Adequate vitamin D, which helps the body absorb and use calcium more efficiently, is also important for creating strong bones. In addition, bone is a living tissue that grows stronger with exercise and weight-bearing activity; therefore, bone loss can be slowed or prevented with regular weight-bearing exercise, such as walking, jogging, dancing, and weight training. To further protect yourself from developing osteoporosis, avoid unhealthy behaviors that contribute to bone loss, including cigarette smoking, excessive alcohol consumption, and anorexia nervosa.

**Sources:** Osteoporosis and Related Bone Diseases—National Resource Center, "Fast Facts about Osteoporosis," May 2009, www .niams.nih.gov/bone/hi/ff_osteoporosis.htm; National Institute of Arthritis and Musculoskeletal Diseases, "Osteoporosis," Reviewed May 2009, www.niams.nih.gov/Health_Info/Bone/ Osteoporosis/default.asp.

---

by the early forties. The lens begins to yellow and loses transparency, and the pupil shrinks, allowing less light to penetrate. By age 60, depth perception declines, and far-sightedness often develops. **Cataracts** (clouding of the lens) and **glaucoma** (elevated pressure within the eyeball) become more likely. Eventually, a tendency toward color blindness may develop, especially for shades of blue and green. **Macular degeneration** is the breakdown of the light-sensitive area of the retina responsible for the sharp, direct vision needed to read or drive. Its effects can be devastating to independent older adults; the causes are still being investigated.

With age, the ear structure also experiences changes and often deteriorates. The eardrum thickens and the inner ear bones are affected. The inner ear is the portion that controls balance (equilibrium). As a result, it often becomes difficult for a person to maintain balance. The ability to hear high-frequency consonants (e.g., *s, t,* and *z*) also diminishes with age. Much of the actual hearing loss lies in the inability to distinguish extreme ranges of sound rather than in the inability to distinguish normal conversational tones.

Many studies have indicated that with age, there is a reduced or changed sensation of pain, vibration, cold, heat, pressure, and touch. It may be that some of these changes are caused by decreased blood flow to the touch receptors or to the brain and spinal cord.[19] It may become difficult, for example, to tell the difference between cool and cold.

**cataracts** Clouding of the lens that interrupts the focusing of light on the retina, resulting in blurred vision or eventual blindness.
**glaucoma** Elevation of pressure within the eyeball, leading to hardening of the eyeball, impaired vision, and possible blindness.
**macular degeneration** Breakdown of the macula, the light-sensitive part of the retina responsible for sharp, direct vision.

Decreased temperature sensitivity increases the risk of injuries such as hypothermia and frostbite.

The senses of taste and smell are closely connected. The number of taste buds decreases starting at about age 40 in women and age 50 in men. Each remaining taste bud also begins to atrophy (lose mass). The sense of smell may diminish, especially after age 70. This may be related to loss of nerve endings in the nose. Studies about the cause of decreased sense of taste and smell have conflicting results. Some studies have indicated that normal aging by itself produces very little change in taste and smell.[20] Therefore, changes may be related to chronic diseases, smoking, and environmental exposures over a lifetime.

For some people, the need for reading glasses is one of the earliest signs of aging.

## Changes in Sexual Function

As men age, they experience noticeable alterations in sexual function. Although the degree and rate of change vary greatly from man to man, several changes generally occur, including a slowed ability to obtain an erection, diminished ability to maintain an erection, and a decline in angle of the erection. Men may also experience a longer refractory period between orgasms and shortened duration of orgasm.

Women also experience several changes in sexual function as they age. Menopause usually occurs between the ages of 45 and 55. Women may experience hot flashes, mood swings, weight gain, development of facial hair, or other hormone-related symptoms. The walls of the vagina become less elastic, and the epithelium thins, possibly making intercourse painful. Vaginal secretions, particularly during sexual activity, diminish. The breasts become less firm, and loss of fat in various areas leads to fewer curves, with a decrease in the soft lines of body contours.

Although these physiological changes may sound discouraging, sex is still an essential component in the lives of those in their middle fifties and older, and many people remain sexually active throughout their entire adult lives. Indeed, in a study by the University of Chicago's National Social Life, Health and Aging Project, sex was identified as an important part of overall health for those in their fifties to middle eighties.[21] Results of this survey and others conducted by the AARP indicated that the proportion of sexually active couples who engaged in sexual activity was approximately 50 percent for those under the age of 75.[22] The study reported that among those who were sexually active, nearly half reported at least one sexual problem, such as lack of desire (43% of women), vaginal dryness (39% of women), or erectile dysfunction (37% of men). With the advent of drugs and medical interventions designed to treat sexual dysfunction, such as Viagra, many older adults are able to be sexually active.

## Body Temperature Regulation

Because of the loss of body fat, thinning of the epithelium, and diminished glandular activity, older adults experience greater difficulty regulating body temperature. This limits their ability to withstand extreme cold or heat, which increases the risks of hypothermia, heatstroke, and heat exhaustion.

## Intelligence and Memory

Given an appropriate length of time, older people learn and develop skills in a similar manner to younger people. Researchers have also determined that what many older adults lack in speed of learning they make up for in practical knowledge—that is, the "wisdom of age." Nor is memory loss necessarily a normal part of aging; however, as a person ages, drug interactions, vascular deficiencies, hormonal or biochemical imbalances, and other physiological changes can make memory lapses occur more frequently. Although short-term memory may fluctuate on a daily basis, the ability to remember events from past decades seems to remain largely unchanged in the absence of disease.

What can you do to help improve memory and overall mental functioning as you age? Here the research is less clear, but several common themes have emerged. Generally those who maintain their memory in old age have exercised and kept their cardiovascular system and other body systems healthy over the years. Another key to maintaining memory is keeping your mind active as well. Those people who foster

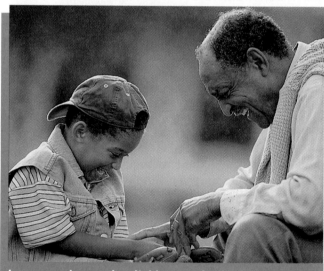

**Is memory loss an inevitable part of aging?**

No. In fact, all of us have periods in our lives when remembering things seems more difficult than other times, due to stress, illness, grief, task overload, injury or trauma, relationship problems, or other life challenges. Certain physiological conditions or diseases may cause older people to experience memory loss, but in general, the knowledge and memories gained through a lifetime of experience remain intact.

their creative side and engage their minds with reading books, solving mental puzzles (crossword, Sudoku), learning to play musical instruments, becoming involved in volunteer activities, and, in general, sharpening their brains seem to fare much better in the memory department. As with the physical aspects of the body, "use it or lose it" applies to your brain acuity.

## Depression

Most older adults continue to lead healthy, fulfilling lives. However, some older people do suffer from mental and emotional disturbances. Some research indicates that depression may be the most common psychological problem facing older adults. However, the rate of major depression is actually lower among older people than it is among younger adults. Regardless of age, people who have a poor perception of their health, have multiple chronic illnesses, take a lot of medications, abuse alcohol and other drugs, lack social support, and do not exercise face more challenges that may require emotional strength.

## Dementias and Alzheimer's Disease

Memory failure, errors in judgment, disorientation, or erratic behavior can occur at any age and for various reasons, including nutrient deficiency (such as vitamin B deficiency), alcohol abuse, medication interactions, vascular problems, tumors, hormonal or metabolic imbalances, or any number of problems. Often, when the underlying issues are corrected, the memory loss and disorientation also improve. The terms *dementing diseases,* or **dementias,** are used to describe either reversible symptoms or progressive forms of brain malfunctioning.

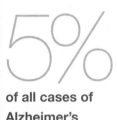

**of all cases of Alzheimer's disease occur before age 65.**

Although there are many types of dementia, one of the most common forms is **Alzheimer's disease (AD).** Affecting an estimated 5.3 million Americans, this disease is one of the most painful and devastating conditions that families can endure.[23] It kills its victims twice: first through a slow loss of personhood (memory loss, disorientation, personality changes, and eventual loss of independent functioning), and then through the deterioration of body systems as they gradually succumb to the powerful impact of neurological problems.

The number of individuals with AD has significantly increased in the United States, and by 2050, a projected 11 to 16 million individuals could suffer from the disease. An estimated 10.9 million family members and friends cared for a person with Alzheimer's disease or another dementia in 2009.[24] Patients with AD live for an average of 4 to 6 years after diagnosis, although the disease can last for up to 20 years.[25] Caring for a person with AD can be a heavy financial burden; the average cost of nursing care is between $72,000

and almost $80,000 each year.[26] Most people associate the disease with the aged, but AD has been diagnosed in people in their late forties.

Alzheimer's disease is a degenerative illness in which areas of the brain develop "tangles" that impair the way nerve cells communicate with one another, eventually causing them to die. This degeneration occurs in the sections of the brain that affect memory, speech, and personality, leaving the parts that control other bodily functions, such as heartbeat and breathing, functioning at near-normal levels. Thus, the mind begins to go while the body lives on.

This disease characteristically progresses in stages, each of which is marked by increasingly impaired memory and judgment. In later stages of the disease these symptoms can be accompanied by agitation and restlessness (especially at night), loss of sensory perceptions, muscle twitching, and repetitive actions. Many patients become depressed, combative, and aggressive. In the final stage of AD, disorientation is often complete. The person becomes dependent on others for eating, dressing, and other activities. Identity loss and speech problems are common. Eventually, control of bodily functions may be lost.

Researchers are investigating several possible causes of the disease, including genetic predisposition, immune system malfunction, a slow-acting virus, chromosomal or genetic defects, chronic inflammation, uncontrolled hypertension, and neurotransmitter imbalance. There is no treatment that can stop the progression of AD, but there are medications that can prevent some symptoms from progressing for a short period of time or relieve symptoms such as sleeplessness, anxiety, and depression. Some researchers are looking at anti-inflammatory drugs, theorizing that AD may develop in response to an inflammatory ailment. Others are focusing on stimulating the brains of AD-prone individuals, believing that as people learn, more connections among cells are formed that may offset those that are lost.[27]

> **dementias** Progressive brain impairments that interfere with memory and normal intellectual functioning.
> **Alzheimer's disease (AD)** A chronic condition involving changes in nerve fibers of the brain that results in mental deterioration.

## Alcohol and Drug Use and Abuse

A person who is prone to alcoholism during the younger and middle years is more likely to continue during later years. Men tend to have a higher risk for alcoholism at all ages. Alcohol abuse is more common among older men than it is among older women. Yet, those aged 65 and older have the lowest rates of drinking among any age group. Those who do drink do so less than younger persons, consuming only five to six drinks weekly.[28]

If the recent studies are accurate, the reason there aren't many heavy drinkers among older adults may be that very heavy drinkers tend to either die of alcoholic complications before they live long enough to grow old, because they find they cannot process alcohol as readily as they did when they were younger, or because they are afraid of combining it with their prescription drugs. Most older adults who consume alcohol are neither alcoholics nor using alcohol to cope with their losses but rather are those who drink socially.

Older people rarely use illicit drugs, but some do overuse or misuse prescription drugs. *Polypharmacy,* or the use of multiple medications, is common in older adults. It is estimated that 89 percent of adults aged 65 years and older reported taking at least one prescription drug compared to 38 percent of adults aged 18 to 44 years and 65 percent of adults aged 45 to 64. Furthermore, 65 percent of adults aged 65 years and over reported taking three or more prescribed drugs compared to 11 percent of adults aged 18 to 44 years and 35 percent of adults aged 45 to 64 years old. Anyone who combines different drugs runs the risk of dangerous drug interactions.[29] The risks of adverse effects are even greater for people with impaired circulation and declining kidney and liver function.

Currently there is no one system that tracks all of a patient's prescriptions. Pharmacists may not know about other drugs, vitamins, or herbal supplements that a patient is taking and thus may not warn them of possible drug interactions. To avoid drug interactions and other problems, older adults should use the same pharmacy consistently; ask questions about medicines, dosages, and possible drug interactions; and read the directions carefully.

A substantial segment of the over-60 population avoids orthodox medical treatment and views it only as a last resort. This is becoming increasingly true as Medicare coverage becomes less adequate and older adults are forced to pay larger medical bills out of their own resources. The poor are particularly prone to using folk medicine and over-the-counter (OTC) drugs as cheaper, less intimidating alternatives.

# Strategies for Healthy Aging

As you know from reading this book, you can do many things to prolong and improve the quality of your life. To provide for healthy older years, make each of the following part of your younger years.

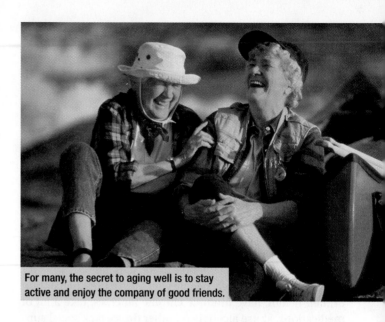

For many, the secret to aging well is to stay active and enjoy the company of good friends.

you. By experiencing diverse people and interacting with different points of view, we gain a new perspective on life.

## Enrich the Spiritual Side of Life

Although we often take the spiritual side of life for granted, cultivating a relationship with nature, the environment, a higher being, and yourself is a key factor in personal growth and development. Take time for thought and quiet contemplation, and enjoy the sunsets, sounds, and energy of life. These moments spent in time you have set aside for yourself will leave you invigorated and refreshed—better able to cope with the ups and downs of life. See Focus On: Cultivating Your Spiritual Health beginning on page 60 for more on ways to enhance this aspect of your life.

## Improve Fitness

If you're basically sedentary, just about any moderate-intensity exercise that gets your heart beating faster and increases strength and/or flexibility will maximize your physical health and functional years. One of the physical changes that the body undergoes is *sarcopenia,* age-associated loss of muscle mass. The less muscle you have, the less energy you will burn even while resting. The lower your metabolic rate, the more likely you will gain weight. With regular strength training, you can increase your muscle mass, boost your metabolism, strengthen your bones, prevent osteoporosis, and, in general, feel better and function more efficiently.

Both aerobic and muscle-strengthening activities are critical for healthy aging. Table 21.1 lists the basic recommendations for aerobic and strength-training exercises in older adults. In addition to these, the American College of Sports Medicine (ACSM) and the American Heart Association (AHA) recommend that people who are at risk of falling perform regular balance exercises.[30] It is also recommended that older adults or adults with chronic conditions develop an activity plan with a health professional to manage risks and

### What's Working for You?

Maybe you're already on the path to aging well. Which of these are you already incorporating into your life?

☐ I like to try new things and meet new people.

☐ I keep busy with several different things that interest me.

☐ I stay in touch with old friends, and get out socially on a regular basis.

☐ I exercise on a regular basis.

## Develop and Maintain Healthy Relationships

Social bonds lend vigor and energy to life. Be willing to give to others, and seek variety in your relationships rather than befriending only people who agree with

take therapeutic needs into account.[31] This will maximize the benefits of physical activity and ensure your safety.

## Eat for Health

Although other chapters in this text provide detailed information about nutrition and weight control, certain nutrients are especially essential to healthy aging:

- **Calcium.** Bone loss tends to increase in women, particularly in the hip region, shortly before menopause. During perimenopause and menopause, this bone loss accelerates rapidly, with an average of about 3 percent skeletal mass lost per year over a 5-year period. The result is an increased risk for fracture and disability. Adequate consumption of calcium throughout one's life can help prevent this bone loss.
- **Vitamin D.** Vitamin D is necessary for adequate calcium absorption, yet as people age, particularly in their fifties and sixties, they do not absorb vitamin D from foods as readily as they did in their younger years. If vitamin D is unavailable, calcium levels are also likely to be lower.
- **Protein.** As older adults become more concerned about cholesterol and fatty foods, and as their budgets shrink, one nutrient that they often cut back on is protein. It costs more, takes longer to cook, and has that "fat" stigma associated with animal products. Because protein is necessary for muscle mass, protein insufficiencies can spell trouble.

Other nutrients, including vitamin E, folic acid (folate), iron, potassium, and vitamin $B_{12}$ (cobalamin), are important

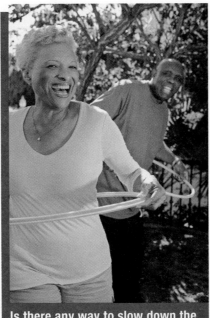

**Is there any way to slow down the aging process?**

Aging is inevitable, but if you take good care of your body, mind, and spirit, you can prevent disease and delay the deterioration of abilities that can lead to disability or a poor quality of life in old age. Participating in regular physical activity and following a healthy diet are two of the most important things you can do to stay active and thriving throughout all the years of your life.

to the aging process, and most of these are readily available in any diet that follows the U.S. Department of Agriculture's (USDA) MyPyramid recommendations (www.mypyramid.gov).

# Understanding the Final Transitions: Dying and Death

Throughout history, humans have attempted to determine the nature and meaning of death. Individuals' feelings about death vary widely, depending on many factors, including age, religious beliefs, family orientation, health, personal experience with death, and the circumstances of the death itself. To cope effectively with dying, we must address the individual needs of those involved. See the **Assess Yourself** box on page 698 to evaluate your personal level of anxiety about death.

Large-scale and impersonal death seems to surround us. Often sensationalized by the news media, it is regularly woven into our entertainment. In the context of this routine exposure, it seems paradoxical that modern Western society has been characterized as "death denying." Why do we wish to deny, or even postpone, death? Let's begin by investigating what death means, at least in medical terms.

## Defining Death

According to the *Shorter Oxford English Dictionary*, **death** can be defined as the "final cessation of the vital functions" and also refers to a state in which these functions are "incapable of being restored."[32] This definition has become more significant as medical advances make it increasingly possible to postpone death. Legal and ethical issues led to the Uniform Determination of Death Act in 1981. This act, which several states have adopted, reads as follows: "An individual who has sustained either (1) irreversible cessation of circulatory and respiratory functions, or (2) irreversible cessation of all functions of the entire brain, including the brainstem, is dead. A determination of death must be made in accordance with accepted medical standards."[33]

**death** The permanent ending of all vital functions.
**brain death** The irreversible cessation of all functions of the entire brainstem.

The concept of **brain death,** defined as the irreversible cessation of all functions of the entire brainstem, has gained increasing credence. As defined by the Ad Hoc Committee

**Source:** M. Nelson et al., "Physical Activity and Public Health in Older Adults: Recommendations from the American College of Sports Medicine and the American Heart Association," *Medicine and Science in Sports and Exercise* 39, no. 8 (2007): 1435–45. Reprinted by permission of Wolters/Kluwer. http://lww.com.

**TABLE 21.1** **Exercise Recommendations for Adults over Age 65**

| Activity | Duration | Frequency |
|---|---|---|
| Moderately intense aerobic exercise | 30 minutes | 5 days a week |
| *or* | | |
| Vigorously intense aerobic exercise | 20 minutes | 3 days a week |
| Strength-training exercises for all major muscle groups | 8 to 12 repetitions for each exercise | 2 to 3 times per week |

of the Harvard Medical School, brain death occurs when the following criteria are met:[34]

- Unreceptivity and unresponsiveness—that is, no response even to painful stimuli
- No movement for a continuous hour after observation by a physician, and no breathing after 3 minutes off a respirator
- No reflexes, including brainstem reflexes (the brainstem is a relay site for sensory and motor pathways and mediates such critical body functions as respiration and heart rate); fixed and dilated pupils
- A "flat" electroencephalogram (EEG, which monitors electrical activity of the brain) for at least 10 minutes
- All of these tests repeated at least 24 hours later with no change
- Certainty that hypothermia (extreme loss of body heat) or depression of the central nervous system caused by use of drugs such as barbiturates are not responsible for these conditions

The Harvard report provides useful guidelines; however, the definition of *death* and all its ramifications continues to concern us.

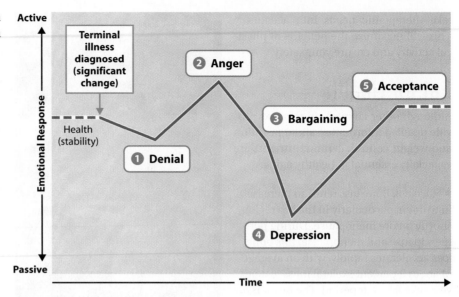

FIGURE 21.4 Kübler-Ross's Stages of Dying
Kübler-Ross developed this model while working with terminally ill patients. She later expanded the model to apply to people experiencing grief or significant loss of any kind.

## what do you think?

Why is there so much concern over the definition of *death*?
● How does modern technology complicate the understanding of when death occurs?

# The Process of Dying

**Dying** is the process of decline in body functions that results in the death of an organism. It is a complex process that includes physical, intellectual, social, spiritual, and emotional dimensions. Now that we have examined the physical indicators of death, we must consider the emotional aspects of dying and "social death."

**dying** The process of decline in body functions, resulting in the death of an organism.
**thanatology** The study of death and dying.

## Coping Emotionally with Death

Science and medicine have enabled us to understand many changes throughout the life span, but they have not fully explained the nature of death. This may explain why the transition from life to death evokes so much mystery and emotion. Although emotional reactions to dying vary, many people share similar experiences during this process. Terms such as *tasks, stages,* and *phases* have been used in models that have been developed to understand the process of dying.

**Kübler-Ross and the Stages of Dying** Much of our knowledge about reactions to dying stems from the work of Elisabeth Kübler-Ross, a pioneer in **thanatology,** the study of death and dying. In 1969, Kübler-Ross published *On Death and Dying,* a sensitive analysis of the reactions of terminally ill patients. This pioneering work encouraged the development of death education as a discipline and prompted efforts to improve the care of dying patients. Kübler-Ross identified five psychological stages (Figure 21.4) that people coping with death often experience:[35]

**1.** **Denial.** ("Not me, there must be a mistake.") A person intellectually accepts the impending death but rejects it emotionally and feels a sense of shock and disbelief. The patient is too confused and stunned to comprehend "not being" and thus rejects the idea.
**2.** **Anger.** ("Why me?") The person becomes angry at having to face death when others, including loved ones, are healthy and not threatened. The dying person perceives the situation as unfair or senseless and may be hostile to friends, family, physicians, or the world in general.
**3.** **Bargaining.** ("If I'm allowed to live, I promise . . .") The dying person may resolve to be a better person in return for an extension of life or may secretly pray for a short postponement of death in order to experience a special event, such as a family wedding or birth.
**4.** **Depression.** ("It's really going to happen to me, and I can't do anything about it.") Depression eventually sets in as vitality diminishes and the person begins to experience symptoms with increasing frequency. The person's deteriorating condition becomes impossible for him or her to deny. Common feelings experienced during this stage include doom, loss, worthlessness, and guilt over the emotional

suffering of loved ones and arduous but seemingly futile efforts of caregivers.

**5. Acceptance.** ("I'm ready.") This is often the final stage. The patient stops battling with emotions and becomes tired and weak. With acceptance, the person does not "give up" and become sullen or resentfully resigned to death, but rather becomes passive.

Some of Kübler-Ross's contemporaries consider her stage theory too neat and orderly. Subsequent research has indicated that the experiences of dying people do not fit easily into specific stages, and patterns vary from person to person. Some people never go through this process and instead remain emotionally calm; others may pass back and forth between the stages. Even if it is not accurate in all its particulars, however, Kübler-Ross's theory offers valuable insights for those seeking to understand or deal with the process of dying.

**Corr's Coping Approach** Others have developed alternative models for understanding the ways in which we cope with death and other significant losses. Charles Corr believes that there are unique challenges and responses for the dying person and those who love them.[36] He suggests four dimensions of coping with loss: *physical*—doing everything possible to make ourselves comfortable and minimize pain; *psychological*—living to the fullest, focusing on life accomplishments, and seeking satisfaction in daily activities; *social*—nurturing relationships, keeping loved ones involved, and sharing emotions; and *spiritual*—identifying what matters in life and reaffirming meaningful experiences.

## Social Death

The need for recognition and appreciation within a social group is nearly universal. Loss of being valued or appreciated by others can lead to **social death,** a situation in which a person is not treated like an active member of society. Dramatic examples of social death include the exile of nonconformists from their native countries or the excommunication of dissident members of religious groups. More often, however, social death is inflicted by denying a person normal social interaction. Numerous studies indicate that people are treated differently when they are dying, leading them to feel more isolated and unable to talk about their feelings: The dying person may be excluded from conversations or referred to as if he or she were already dead.[37] Dying patients are often moved to terminal wards and may be given minimal care; medical personnel may make degrading or impersonal comments about dying patients in their presence. In addition, inadequate pain control may contribute to patient suffering and anger or hostility, making caregiver assistance more difficult.

A decrease in meaningful social interaction often strips dying and bereaved people of their identity as valued members of society at a time when being able to talk, share, and make important decisions or say important things is critical. Some dying people choose not to speak of their inevitable fate in an attempt to make others feel more comfortable and thus preserve vital relationships.

**social death** A seemingly irreversible situation in which a person is not treated like an active member of society.

**bereavement** The loss or deprivation experienced by a survivor when a loved one dies.

# Coping with Loss

Coping with the loss of a loved one is extremely difficult. The dying person, as well as close family and friends, frequently suffers emotionally and physically from the loss of critical relationships and roles. Words used to describe feelings and behaviors related to losses resulting from death include *bereavement, grief, grief work,* and *mourning.* The meanings of these terms are related but not identical. Understanding them will help you comprehend the emotional processes associated with a terminal person's accepting his or her fate and the cultural constraints that often inhibit normal coping behavior.

**Bereavement** is generally defined as the loss or deprivation that a survivor experiences when a loved one dies. Because relationships vary in type and intensity, reactions to losses also vary. The death of a parent, spouse, sibling, child,

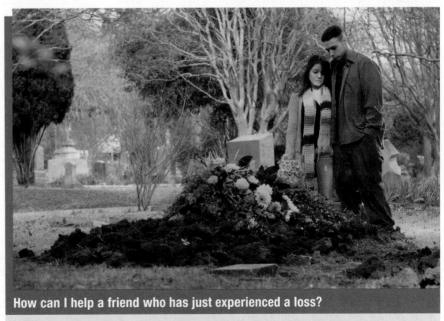

**How can I help a friend who has just experienced a loss?**

The most important thing you can do for a grieving friend is offer emotional support and a caring presence. Knowing what to say is less important than knowing how to listen. Acknowledge the loss, let your friend know you care, and be there when he or she needs to talk or express grief.

friend, or pet will result in different kinds of feelings for different people. We should not make assumptions about the value a person places on his or her relationship with the deceased or the nature of his or her feelings about the loss. For example, often people fail to recognize the importance a pet can have, especially in single people's lives; for some, the loss of a pet may be as significant as the loss of a child. In the lives of the bereaved or of close survivors, the loss of loved ones leaves "holes" and inevitable changes. Loneliness and despair may envelop the survivors. Understanding of these normal reactions, time, patience, and support from loved ones can do much to help the bereaved heal and move on, even though they will not forget.

**Grief** occurs in reaction to significant loss, including one's own impending death, the death of a loved one, or a *quasi-death* experience (a loss, such as the end of a relationship or job, that resembles death because it involves separation or change in personal identity). Grief may be experienced as a mental, physical, social, or emotional reaction, and often includes changes in patterns of eating, sleeping, working, and even thinking.

When a person experiences a loss that cannot be openly acknowledged, publicly mourned, or socially supported, coping may be much more difficult. This type of grief is referred to as *disenfranchised grief.* It may occur among people who experience a miscarriage, who are developmentally disabled, or who are close friends rather than blood relatives of the deceased. It may be even more challenging for those in relationships that are hidden, such as extramarital affairs, or that lack approval in some social groups, such as homosexual relationships.

Symptoms of grief vary in severity and duration, depending on the situation and the individual. However, the bereaved person can benefit from emotional and social support from family, friends, clergy, employers, and traditional support organizations, including the medical community and the funeral industry. The larger and stronger the support system, the easier readjustment is likely to be. See the **Skills for Behavior Change** box at right to learn about how you can best help a grieving friend.

The term *mourning* is often incorrectly equated with the term *grief.* As we have noted, *grief* refers to a wide variety of feelings and actions that occur in response to bereavement. **Mourning,** in contrast, refers to culturally prescribed and accepted time periods and behavior patterns for the expression of grief. In Judaism, for example, *sitting shivah* is a designated mourning period of 7 days that involves prescribed rituals and prayers. Depending on a person's relationship with the deceased, various other rituals may continue for up to a year.

Religion provides comfort to many dying and grieving people. Although some people question the existence of an afterlife, others take comfort from religious beliefs that provide a purpose and meaning to life. By accepting dying as a

**grief** An individual's reaction to significant loss, including one's own impending death, the death of a loved one, or a quasi-death experience; grief can involve mental, physical, social, or emotional responses.
**mourning** The culturally prescribed behavior patterns for the expression of grief.

## Talking to Friends When Someone Dies

It's always hard to know just what to say and how to say it when talking with grieving friends or relatives. Here are some dos and don'ts.

### DO . . .
* Let your genuine concern and caring show; say you are sorry about their loss and pain.
* Be available to listen, run errands, help with the children, or whatever else seems needed at the time.
* Allow them to express as much grief as they are feeling at the moment and are willing to share.
* Encourage them to be patient with themselves and not worry about things they should be doing.
* Allow them to talk about the person who has died as much and as often as they want to.
* Reassure them that they did everything they could, that the medical care given was the best, or whatever else you know to be true and positive about the care given.

### DON'T . . .
* Let your own sense of helplessness keep you from reaching out to those who are bereaved.
* Avoid them because you are uncomfortable (this adds pain to an already unbearably painful experience).
* Say you know how they feel (unless you've suffered a similar loss, you probably don't).
* Say, "You ought to be feeling better by now" or anything else that implies judgment about their feelings or what they should be doing.
* Change the subject when they mention the person who has died.

part of the continuum of life, many people are able to make necessary readjustments after the death of a loved one. This holistic concept is shared by both believers and nonbelievers.

## What Is "Typical" Grief?

Grief responses vary widely from person to person but frequently include such symptoms as periodic waves of prolonged physical distress, a feeling of tightness in the throat, choking and shortness of breath, a frequent need to sigh, feelings of emptiness and muscular weakness, or intense anxiety that is described as actually painful.

Other common symptoms of grief include insomnia, memory lapses, loss of appetite, difficulty concentrating, a tendency to engage in repetitive or purposeless behavior, an "observer" sensation or feeling of unreality, difficulty in

## Living with Grief

The reality of death and loss touches everyone. Coping with death is vital to your mental health. The National Mental Health Association offers these suggestions for living with grief and coping effectively with pain:

❋ Seek out caring people. Find relatives and friends who can understand your feelings of loss. Join support groups with others who are experiencing similar losses.
❋ Express your feelings. Tell others how you feel; it will help you to work through the grieving process.
❋ Take care of your health. Maintain regular contact with your family physician and be sure to eat well and get plenty of rest. Be aware of the danger of developing a dependence on medication or alcohol to deal with your grief.
❋ Accept that life is for the living. It takes effort to begin living again in the present and not dwell on the past.
❋ Postpone major life decisions. Try to put off making any significant changes, such as moving, remarrying, changing jobs, or having another child. You need time to adjust to your loss.
❋ Be patient. It can take months or even years to absorb a major loss and accept your changed life.

**3.** Adjust to an environment in which the deceased is missing. The bereaved may feel lonely and uncertain about a new identity without the person who has died. This loss confronts them with the challenge of adjusting their own sense of self.

**4.** Emotionally relocate the deceased and move on with life. Individuals never lose memories of a significant relationship. They may need help in letting go of the emotional energy that used to be invested in the person who has died, and they may need help in finding an appropriate place for the deceased in their emotional lives.

Models of the grief process can be viewed as "generalized maps"—each theory is an attempt by an investigator to understand and guide grieving people through their pain. However, each individual will travel through grief at his or her own speed using an appropriate route. See the **Skills for Behavior Change** box at left for more suggestions on living with grief.

### what do you think?

If you have experienced a death among your family or friends, how did you grieve? ● Did you accomplish Worden's tasks? ● Did any of the models above match your experience?

## Children and Death

At the beginning of the twentieth century, children under the age of 15 made up 34 percent of the U.S. population but accounted for

**grief work** The process of accepting the reality of a person's death and coping with memories of the deceased.

making decisions, lack of organization, excessive speech, social withdrawal or hostility, guilty feelings, and preoccupation with the image of the deceased. Susceptibility to disease increases with grief and may even be life threatening in severe and enduring cases.

A bereaved person may suffer emotional pain and exhibit a variety of grief responses for many months after the death. The rate of the healing process depends on the amount and quality of grief work that a person does. **Grief work** is the process of integrating the reality of the loss into everyday life and learning to feel better. Often, the bereaved person must deliberately and systematically work at reducing denial and coping with the pain that comes from remembering the deceased.

## Worden's Model of Grieving Tasks

William Worden, a researcher into the death process, developed an active grieving model that suggests four developmental tasks that a grieving person must complete in the grief work process:[38]

**1.** Accept the reality of the loss. This task requires acknowledging and realizing that the person is dead. Traditional rituals, such as the funeral, help many bereaved people move toward acceptance.
**2.** Work through the pain of grief. It is necessary to acknowledge and work through the pain associated with loss, or it will manifest itself through other symptoms or behaviors.

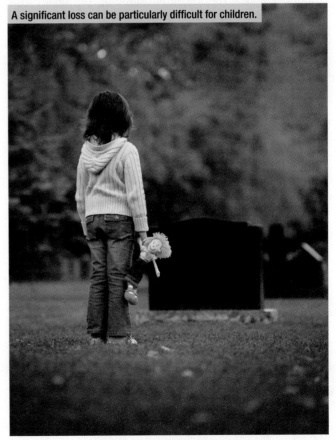

A significant loss can be particularly difficult for children.

53 percent of total deaths. Today, children continue to benefit from advances in medicine and social policy that have reduced mortality rates by more than 90 percent since 1900.[39] Children are highly valued in our society, and their deaths are considered major tragedies. No matter what the cause of death—miscarriage, fatal birth defects, childhood illness, accident, suicide, homicide, natural disaster, neglect, or war injuries—the grief experienced when a child dies may be overwhelming.

Siblings of a deceased child may have a particularly hard time with grief work. Because so much attention and energy are devoted to the deceased child, the surviving children may feel emotionally abandoned by their parents. They may feel uncomfortable talking about death, and they may also receive less social support and sympathy than their parents do.

In the past, children were thought to be miniature adults and were expected to behave as such. We now understand that children and adults react to death quite differently. Bereaved children usually have limited experience with death and therefore have not yet learned how to deal with major loss. Often, when children suffer a loss, they will continue to behave "normally" to the adult observer. When it comes to complex emotional issues, like those surrounding the death of a loved one, children do not always show their feelings as openly as adults do.

Children tend to experience more prolonged grieving periods. They often worry about whether they caused the death and whether they will die or will lose someone else they love, and they worry about what will happen to them and to the person who died. When family members and others involve the children in the dying process and talk with them about the death while reassuring them of their safety, things may go easier for all concerned.

# Life-and-Death Decision Making

When a loved one is dying, many complex and emotional—and often expensive—life-and-death decisions must be made during a highly distressing period in people's lives. We will not attempt to present definitive answers to moral and philosophical questions about death; instead, we offer these topics for your consideration.

**advance directive** A document that stipulates an individual's wishes about medical care; used to make treatment decisions when and if the individual becomes physically unable to voice their preferences.
**living will** A type of advance directive.

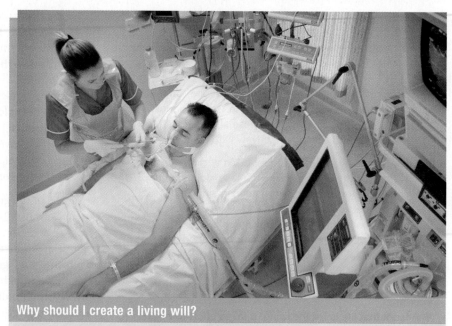

**Why should I create a living will?**

Unexpected end-of-life situations can happen at any age. Today's sophisticated life-support technology can prolong a patient's life even in cases of terminal illness or mortal injury, yet not everyone would choose to have their life extended by such means. Unfortunately, by the time the situation arises, you may no longer be conscious and able to speak for yourself. Living wills, advance directives, and health care proxies are all legal documents that can protect your wishes and aid your loved ones should you become incapacitated.

# The Right to Die

Few people would object to the right to a dignified death. Going beyond that concept, however, many people today believe that they should be allowed to die if their condition is terminal and their existence depends on mechanical life-support devices or artificial feeding or hydration systems. Artificial life-support techniques that may be legally refused by competent patients include electrical or mechanical heart resuscitation, mechanical respiration by machine, nasogastric tube feedings, intravenous nutrition, gastrostomy (tube feeding directly into the stomach), and medications to treat life-threatening infections.

As long as a person is conscious and competent, he or she has the legal right to refuse treatment, even if this decision will hasten death. However, when a person is in a coma or otherwise incapable of speaking on his or her own behalf, medical personnel, family members, and administrative policy will dictate treatment. This issue has evolved into a battle involving personal freedom, legal rulings, health care administration policy, and physician responsibility. The living will and other **advance directives** were developed to assist in solving these conflicts.

Even young, apparently healthy people need a **living will.** Consider Terri Schiavo, who collapsed at age 26 from heart failure that led to irreversible brain damage. Schiavo, unable to survive without life support, never left any written guidelines about her wishes should she become incapacitated. After a 15-year legal battle between her parents, who wanted her to be kept alive, and her husband, who felt she should be allowed to die, the courts sided with her husband, and she was removed from life support.

Many legal experts suggest that you take the following steps to ensure that your wishes are carried out:[40]

● **Be specific.** Complete an advance directive that permits you to make very specific choices about a variety of procedures, including cardiopulmonary resuscitation (CPR); being placed on a ventilator; being given food, water, or medication through tubes; being given pain medication; and organ donation.
● **Get an agent.** You may want to also appoint a family member or friend to act as your agent, or *proxy,* by completing a form known as either a *durable power of attorney for health care* or a *health care proxy.*
● **Discuss your wishes.** Discuss your preferences in detail with your proxy and your doctor. Going over the situations described in the form will give them a clear idea of just how much you are willing to endure to preserve your life.
● **Deliver the directive.** Distribute several copies, not only to your doctor and your agent, but also to your lawyer and to immediate family members or a close friend. Make sure *someone* knows to bring a copy to the hospital in the event you are hospitalized.

One alternative to the traditional advance directive or living will is a document called *Five Wishes* that meets the legal requirements for advance directive statutes in most states. This document differs from most other living wills because it addresses personal, emotional, and spiritual needs, as well as medical needs.[41] It is available at low cost online at www.agingwithdignity.org. Written in uncomplicated language, *Five Wishes* allows you to outline the following:

**1.** Which person you want to make health care decisions for you when you can't make them
**2.** The kind of medical treatment you want or don't want
**3.** How comfortable you want to be
**4.** How you want people to treat you
**5.** What you want your loved ones to know

Although every state has different guidelines and laws for living wills and advance directives, the above questions are important things to think about now. How would you answer each of the above?

## Rational Suicide and Euthanasia

Although exact numbers are not known, medical ethicists and specialists in forensic medicine (the study of legal issues in medicine) estimate that thousands of terminally ill people every year decide to kill themselves rather than endure constant pain and slow decay. This alternative to the extended dying process is known as **rational suicide.** To these people, the prospect of an undignified death is unacceptable. This issue has been complicated by advances in death prevention techniques that allow terminally ill patients to exist in an irreversible disease state for extended periods of time.

According to public opinion polls, most Americans believe that suicide is morally wrong but are divided on whether physician-assisted suicide is morally acceptable. Roughly 70 percent of Americans believe doctors should be allowed to help end an incurably ill patient's life painlessly at the patient's request.[42]

Physician-assisted suicide is not a new phenomenon. It has been practiced in many societies throughout history and currently is legal in some European countries, such as Belgium and the Netherlands. Legalization of assisted suicide has been debated in many states across the United States. Currently, more than 30 states have statutes explicitly prohibiting assisted suicide and only three states—Oregon, Washington, and Montana—have laws allowing for physician-assisted suicide under certain circumstances.[43] See the **Points of View** box on page 694 for a discussion of this topic.

Euthanasia is often referred to as "mercy killing." The term **active euthanasia** refers to ending the life of a person (or animal) who is suffering greatly and has no chance of recovery. An example might be a physician-prescribed lethal injection, as in physician-assisted suicide. **Passive euthanasia** refers to the intentional withholding of treatment that would prolong life. Deciding not to place a person with massive brain trauma on life support is an example of passive euthanasia. Advance directives, such as "do not resuscitate" orders, can provide legal justification for various forms of passive euthanasia.

# Making Final Arrangements

Caring for dying people and dealing with the practical and legal questions surrounding death can be difficult and painful. The problems of the dying person and his or her bereaved loved ones involve a wide variety of psychological, legal, social, spiritual, economic, and interpersonal issues.

## Hospice Care: Positive Alternatives

Since the mid-1970s, **hospice** programs in the United States have grown from a mere handful to more than 4,800 and are available in nearly every community.[44] These programs are a form of **palliative care** that focus on reducing pain and suffering while attending to the emotional and spiritual needs of dying individuals and their caregivers. Hospice

**rational suicide** The decision to kill oneself rather than endure constant pain and slow decay.
**active euthanasia** "Mercy killing" in which a person or organization knowingly acts to end the life of a terminally ill person.
**passive euthanasia** The intentional withholding of treatment that would prolong life.
**hospice** A concept of end-of-life care designed to maximize quality of life and help dying people have peace, comfort, and dignity.
**palliative care** Any form of medical care focused on relieving the pain, symptoms, and stress of serious illness in order to improve the quality of life for patients and their families.

# Physician-Assisted Suicide:
## SHOULD IT BE LEGALIZED?

*Physician-assisted suicide* (also known as *physician aid-in-dying*) refers to a practice in which the physician provides, after a terminally ill patient's request, a lethal dose of medication that the patient intends to use to end his or her own life. Currently, more than 30 states have statutes explicitly prohibiting assisted suicide. Only Oregon, Montana, and Washington allow physician-assisted suicide under certain circumstances. Oregon's Death with Dignity Act states that a person must be 18 years or older, a resident of Oregon, competent to make health decisions, and diagnosed with a terminal illness that will lead to death within 6 months. The physician must determine that all of these factors have been met. The arguments for and against the legalization of physician-assisted suicide within individual states continue to be debated. Below are some of the major points from both sides of the issue.

### Arguments in Favor of Legalization of Physician-Assisted Suicide

○ Decisions about time and circumstances regarding death are personal and a competent person with a terminal illness should have the right to choose death.

○ For some patients, treatment refusal does not lead quickly enough to death; therefore, their only option is to commit suicide. Justice requires that patients should be allowed to choose death.

○ Many terminal conditions are accompanied by tremendous suffering and pain. Physician-assisted suicide is a compassionate response to unbearable suffering.

○ Physician-assisted suicide already occurs, but behind closed doors and in secret. Legalization of physician-assisted suicide would promote open discussion of existing practices.

### Arguments against Legalization of Physician-Assisted Suicide

○ It is unethical to take a human life and historical, ethical traditions of medicine strongly oppose taking life. The Hippocratic Oath states, "I will not administer poison to anyone where asked," and "Be of benefit, or at least do no harm."

○ There is an important difference between passively letting someone die and actively killing. Treatment refusal or withholding treatment equates to letting a patient die (passive) and is justifiable, whereas physician-assisted suicide equates to killing (active) and is not morally justifiable.

○ Certain groups of terminally ill people, lacking access to care and support, may be pushed into assisted suicide. Physician-assisted suicide may become a cost-containment strategy. Burdened family members and health care providers may encourage the option of assisted suicide.

○ There may be uncertainty in the diagnosis and prognosis of the terminal illness. There may be errors in diagnosis and treatment of depression, or inadequate treatment of pain.

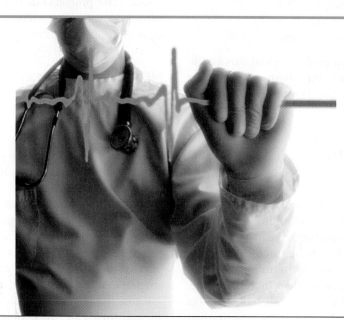

### Where Do You Stand?

○ Do you think physician-assisted suicide should be legalized in your state?

○ What criteria do you think should be used to monitor physician-assisted suicide if it were widely legalized?

○ What are your feelings on physician-assisted suicide in general? Is it an appropriate option for patients diagnosed with devastating, terminal illnesses?

**Sources:** C. H. Braddock III and M. R. Tonelli, University of Washington, School of Medicine, "Physician Aid-in-Dying," Revised April 2009, http://depts.washington.edu/bioethx/topics/pad.html; Oregon Department of Human Services, "FAQ's about the Death with Dignity Act," Updated May 2010, www.oregon.gov/DHS/ph/pas/faqs.shtml; International Task Force on Euthanasia and Assisted Suicide, "Assisted Suicide Laws," Updated January 2009, www.internationaltaskforce.org/assisted_suicide_laws.htm.

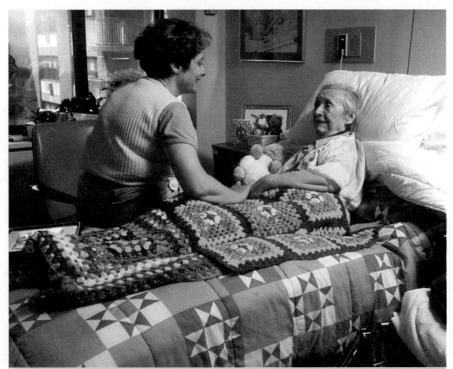

A hospice program provides support services to family members, ensures that the dying loved one is comfortable, and allows family and friends to be involved in their loved one's care.

Despite the growing number of people considering hospice, many people prefer to die in a hospital. Others choose to die at home, without the intervention of medical staff or life-prolonging equipment. Each dying person and his or her family should decide as early as possible what type of terminal care is most desirable and feasible. This will allow time for necessary emotional, physical, and financial preparations.

## Making Funeral Arrangements

Anthropological evidence indicates that all cultures throughout human history have developed some sort of funeral ritual. For this reason, social scientists agree that funerals assist survivors of the deceased in coping with their loss. In the United States, with its diversity of religious, regional, and ethnic customs, funeral patterns vary. (See the **Be Healthy, Be Green** box on page 696 for information on how concern about environmental responsibility is influencing modern funeral, burial, and memorial practices.) In some faiths, the deceased may be displayed to formalize last respects and increase social support of the bereaved. This part of the funeral ritual is referred to as a *wake* or *viewing*. The deceased's body is usually embalmed prior to viewing to retard decomposition and minimize odors. The funeral service may be held in a church, in a funeral chapel, or at the burial site. Some people choose to replace the funeral service with a simple memorial service held within a few days of the burial. Social interaction associated with funeral and memorial services is valuable in helping survivors cope with their losses.

Common methods of body disposal include burial in the ground, entombment above ground in a mausoleum, cremation, and anatomical donation. Expenses vary according to the method chosen and the available options. If burial is selected, an additional charge may be assessed for a burial vault. Burial vaults—concrete or metal containers that hold the casket—are required by most cemeteries to limit settling of the gravesite as the casket disintegrates and collapses.

Choosing the actual container for the remains is only one of many tasks that must be dealt with when a person dies. In addition to the method and details of body disposal, the type of memorial service, display of the body, and the site of burial or body disposition, loved ones must also consider the cost of funeral options, organ donation, and floral displays. Then, they usually have to contact friends and relatives, plan for the arrival of guests, choose markers, gather and submit obituary information to newspapers, and print memorial folders, in addition to many other details. Even though funeral directors

care may help the survivors cope better with the death experience. Hospice volunteers provide much needed "respite" care for caregivers who often face emotional and physical challenges in caring for dying loved ones.

The primary goals of hospice programs are to relieve the dying person's pain; offer emotional support to the dying person and loved ones; and restore a sense of control to the dying person, family, and friends. Hospice programs usually include the following characteristics:

- Both the patient and family constitute the unit of care, because the physical, psychological, social, and spiritual problems of dying confront the family as well as the patient.
- Emphasis is placed on symptom control, primarily the alleviation of pain. Curative treatments are curtailed as requested by the patient, but sound judgment must be applied to avoid a feeling of abandonment.
- There is overall medical direction of the program, with all health care provided under the direction of a qualified physician.
- Services are provided by an interdisciplinary team, because no one person can provide all the needed care.
- Coverage is provided 24 hours a day, 7 days a week, with emphasis on the availability of medical and nursing skills.
- Carefully selected and extensively trained volunteers who augment but do not replace staff service are an integral part of the health care team.
- Care of the family extends through the bereavement period.
- Patients are accepted on the basis of their health needs, not their ability to pay.

# BE HEALTHY, BE GREEN

## Green Goodbyes

Worldwide, more than 56 million people die each year. Nearly all of those people are given some form of burial, funeral, or cremation, and yet traditional burial, funeral, and cremation practices can have significant and negative environmental impacts. With growing awareness of these impacts has come an increased interest in ways to "go green" in funeral, burial, and cremation practices.

Each year, more than 20,000 cemeteries in the United States bury millions of feet of hardwood; tens of thousands of tons of steel, copper, and bronze; and more than a million tons of reinforced concrete. In addition, it is estimated that more than 1 million gallons of embalming fluid are buried in the United States every year. These chemicals (including formaldehyde, glutaraldehyde, phenol, methanol, antibiotics, dyes, and more) eventually make their way into the soil and can potentially contaminate water supplies.

Instead of traditional cemetery and burial sites, you can opt for a green burial site that prohibits the use of formaldehyde-based embalming fluids, metal caskets, and concrete burial vaults. Typically, these sites are located in nature preserves that eschew the manicured expanses of lawn present in modern cemeteries. They have restrictions on the density of burials allowed, as well as strict guidelines aimed at conservation and preservation of the ecosystem. To find global locations of natural cemeteries, start by checking out www.naturalburial.coop or www.greenburialcouncil.org.

Many green cemeteries and other burial sites choose to plant living markers instead of erecting tombstones. Traditional grave markers are made of stone, a nonrenewable resource, and most leave a carbon footprint, as both the mining and

shipping of them produce excess carbon. In contrast, a living marker is a tree, bush, plant, or flowers planted in memory of the deceased loved one. This not only reduces waste and negative environmental impact, but also contributes to the development of green landscape.

Green coffins are also available as an alternative to traditional coffins made of metal, plastic, endangered hardwood, or particleboard with formaldehyde glues. Greener options include coffins made of oak, pine, cardboard, willow, seagrass, wicker, fair-trade bamboo, and other natural materials that are more sustainable, biodegradeable, and renewable. In addition, some burial sites allow one to forgo the coffin altogether and bury loved ones in natural-cloth shrouds.

Cremation has historically been viewed as a more ecofriendly option, because the environmental footprint is much less than that of traditional burials. Although cremation does not involve the land use that burial does, it takes a lot of energy, approximately the same amount required to power an average car for a distance of 4,800 miles, and the burning process releases carbon and particulate emissions into the air. However, these emissions are relatively low in comparison to others in our society. Some fast-food restaurants release 0.46 pound of carbon an hour, whereas the human cremation process emits only 0.08 pound an hour. Environmental monitoring agencies have imposed emission standards on crematoriums that help to keep the levels down. Furthermore, some crematoriums are installing

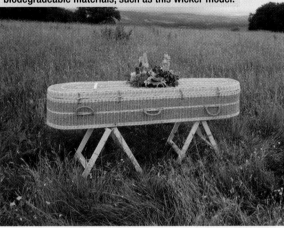

Ecofriendly burial options include coffins made of biodegradeable materials, such as this wicker model.

additional filters to catch smaller particulate matter.

Another alternative to traditional burial is the controversial and relatively new process of "promession," or freeze-drying. This technique, developed by Swedish biologist Susanne Wiigh-Mäsak, was patented in 1999 and first introduced to the public in May 2001. Currently, there are a few facilities in Europe that perform promession. The first step in promession involves freezing the body in a vat of liquid nitrogen, a process that makes the body very brittle. Next, the body is gently broken apart with ultrasonic vibration. This creates a damp powder that is then dried and packaged in a small biodegradable coffin that can be buried alongside a living memorial plant. As the "promains" become wet from rain and watering, they naturally decompose, composting the soil and providing nourishment to the living memorial.

**Sources:** S. Grover, "How to Go Green: Funerals," Planet Green, 2009, http://planetgreen.discovery.com/go-green/funerals/funerals-basics.html; Green Burial Council, "Frequently Asked Questions," 2010, www.greenburialcouncil.org/faqs-fiction/.

are available to facilitate decision making, the bereaved may experience undue stress, especially if the death is sudden and unexpected. People who make their own funeral arrangements ahead of time can save their loved ones from having to deal with unnecessary problems.

## Wills

The issue of inheritance is controversial in some families and should be resolved before the person dies to reduce both conflict and needless expense. Unfortunately, many people are so intimidated by the thought of making a will that they never do so and die **intestate** (without a will). This is tragic, especially because the procedure for establishing a legal will is relatively simple and inexpensive. In addition, if you don't make a will before you die, the courts (as directed by state laws) will make a will for you. Legal issues, rather than your wishes, will preside. Furthermore, settling an estate takes longer when a person dies without a will.

In some cases, other types of wills may substitute for the traditional legal will. One alternative is the **holographic will,** which is written in the handwriting of the **testator** (person who leaves a will) and is unwitnessed. However, be very cautious if considering alternatives to legally written and witnessed wills, because they are not honored in all states. Holographic wills are contestable in court.

## Organ Donation

In recent years, organ transplant techniques have become so refined, and the demand for transplant tissues and organs has become so great, that many people are encouraged to donate these gifts of life upon death. Uniform donor cards are available through the U.S. Department of Health and Human Services and through many health care foundations and nonprofit organizations (Figure 21.5); donor information is printed on drivers' licenses; and many hospitals include the opportunity for organ donor registration in their admission procedures. Although some people are opposed to organ transplants and tissue donation, others experience personal fulfillment from knowing that their organs may extend and improve someone else's life after their own death.

**intestate** Dying without a will.
**holographic will** A will written in the testator's own handwriting and unwitnessed.
**testator** A person who leaves a will or testament at death.

**UNIFORM DONOR CARD**

I, ______________________, have spoken to my family about organ and tissue donation. The following people have witnessed my commitment to be a donor. I wish to donate the following:

☐ any needed organs and tissues

☐ only the following organs and tissues: ______________

______________________________

Donor Signature ______________ Date ____________

Witness ______________________

Witness ______________________

FIGURE 21.5 **Organ Donor Card**
Each organ and tissue donor can save or improve the lives of as many as 50 people.

# Assess yourself

## Are You Afraid of Death?

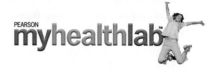

How anxious or accepting are you about the prospect of your death? Indicate how well each statement describes your attitude.

Not True at All = **0**  Mainly Not True = **1**  Not Sure = **2**
Somewhat True = **3**  Very True = **4**

1. I tend not to be very brave in times of crisis situations. 0 1 2 3 4

2. I am something of a hypochondriac. 0 1 2 3 4

3. I tend to be unusually frightened in airplanes at takeoff and landing. 0 1 2 3 4

4. I would give a lot to be immortal in this body. 0 1 2 3 4

5. I am superstitious that preparing for dying might hasten my death. 0 1 2 3 4

6. My experience of friends and family dying has been wholly negative. 0 1 2 3 4

7. I would feel easier being with a dying relative if he or she had not been told he or she was dying. 0 1 2 3 4

8. I have fears of dying alone without friends around me. 0 1 2 3 4

9. I have fears of dying slowly. 0 1 2 3 4

10. I have fears of dying suddenly. 0 1 2 3 4

11. I have fears of dying before my time or while my children are still young. 0 1 2 3 4

12. I have fears of what could happen to my family after my death. 0 1 2 3 4

13. I have fears of dying in a hospital or an institution. 0 1 2 3 4

14. I have fears of not getting help with euthanasia. 0 1 2 3 4

15. I have fears of dying without adequately having expressed my love to those I am close to. 0 1 2 3 4

16. I have fears of being given unofficial and unwanted euthanasia. 0 1 2 3 4

17. I have fears of getting insufficient pain control while dying. 0 1 2 3 4

18. I have fears of being overmedicated and unconscious while dying. 0 1 2 3 4

19. I have fears of being declared dead when not really dead or being buried alive. 0 1 2 3 4

20. I have fears of what may happen to my body after death. 0 1 2 3 4

Total points: _____

### Interpreting Your Score

If you are extremely anxious (scoring 38 or more), you might consider counseling or therapy; if you are unusually anxious (scoring between 24 and 37), you might want to find a method of meditation, philosophy, or spiritual practice to help experience, explore, and accept your feelings about death. Average anxiety is a score under 24.

---

# YOUR PLAN FOR CHANGE

The **Assess yourself** activity encouraged you to explore your death-related anxiety. Now that you have considered your results, you may want to take steps to lessen your fears about death and dying.

### Today, you can:

○ Learn about advance directives. Visit a low-cost legal clinic for information and a sample. You can also locate samples online, including the *Five Wishes* document, which is available at www.agingwithdignity.org.

○ Fill out an organ donation card. Knowing that you may be able to prolong another person's life after your death can help you feel more at peace with your mortality.

### Within the next 2 weeks, you can:

○ Write down a list of goals you want to attain by ages 30, 40, and 50. Think about the steps you need to take to attain these goals.

○ Talk to family members about their life goals. What have they achieved, and what do they wish they had done differently? What can you learn from their experiences?

### By the end of the semester, you can:

○ Consider how you feel about various medical techniques that might be used in the event you become incapacitated. Do you feel comfortable being kept alive by a machine? Make your wishes on these matters known to family members and friends, and put them in writing.

○ Talk to your parents or grandparents about the arrangements they prefer in the event of their death. Do they want a burial or cremation? A full funeral or a small service? Making these decisions now will save you and your loved ones stress later.

# Summary

* Aging can be defined in terms of biological age, psychological age, social age, legal age, or functional age. The growing number of older adults (people aged 65 and older) has an increasing impact on society in terms of the economy, health care, housing, and ethical considerations.
* Biological explanations of aging include the wear-and-tear theory, the cellular theory, the genetic mutation theory, and the autoimmune theory. Psychosocial theories center on adaptation and adjustments related to self-development.
* Aging changes the body and mind in many ways. Physical changes occur in the skin, bones and joints, head, urinary tract, heart and lungs, senses, sexual function, and temperature regulation. Major physical concerns are osteoporosis, urinary incontinence, and changes in eyesight and hearing. Most older people maintain a high level of intelligence and memory. Potential mental problems include depression and Alzheimer's disease.
* Lifestyle choices we make today will affect health status later in life. Choosing to exercise, eat a healthy diet, foster lasting relationships, and avoid tobacco will contribute to healthy aging. Special challenges for older adults include alcohol abuse, and prescription drug and OTC interactions.
* *Death* can be defined biologically in terms of brain death or the cessation of vital functions. Denial of death results in limited communication about death, which can lead to further denial. Death is a multifaceted emotional process, and individuals may experience emotional stages of dying such as denial, anger, bargaining, depression, and acceptance. Social death results when a person is no longer treated as living.
* Grief is the state of distress felt after loss. People differ in their responses to grief. Children need to be helped through the process of grieving.
* The right to die by rational suicide involves ethical, moral, and legal issues. Choices of care for the terminally ill include hospice care. After death, funeral arrangements must be made almost immediately, which adds to pressures on survivors. Decisions should be made in advance of death through wills and organ donation cards.

# Pop Quiz

1. Which biological theory of aging supports the concept that body cells are able to reproduce only so many times throughout life?
   a. Wear-and-tear theory
   b. Cellular theory
   c. Autoimmune theory
   d. Genetic mutation theory

2. The progressive breakdown of joint cartilage is known as
   a. osteoporosis.
   b. osteoarthritis.
   c. calcium loss.
   d. vitamin D deficiency.

3. Martha's ophthalmologist tells her that she has a condition that involves the breakdown of the light-sensitive area of the retina that is affecting her sharp, direct vision needed to read or drive. What is this condition?
   a. Cataracts
   b. Glaucoma
   c. Macular degeneration
   d. Nearsightedness

4. What is the most common form of dementia in older adults?
   a. Alzheimer's disease
   b. Incontinence
   c. Depression
   d. Psychosis

5. The keys to successful aging include
   a. being physically active.
   b. eating a healthy diet.
   c. not smoking.
   d. All of the above

6. The study of death and dying is called
   a. thanatology.
   b. gerontology.
   c. biology.
   d. a living will.

7. Grief work is
   a. the process of integrating the reality of the loss with everyday life and learning to feel better.
   b. the total acceptance that a loved one has died.
   c. assigning feelings to the loss of a loved one.
   d. completing the cultural rituals required to express one's grief.

8. Kerri's elderly grandmother is terminally ill and wants to die without medical intervention. Her family has agreed to withhold treatment that may prolong her life. This is called
   a. rational suicide.
   b. health care proxy.
   c. passive euthanasia.
   d. active euthanasia.

9. The Kübler-Ross stage of dying in which the individual rejects death emotionally and feels a sense of shock and disbelief is known as
   a. acceptance.
   b. bargaining.
   c. denial.
   d. anger.

10. A culturally prescribed and accepted period of grief for someone who has died is known as
   a. bereavement.
   b. grief work.
   c. coping with loss.
   d. mourning.

*Answers for these questions can be found on page A-1.*

## Think about It!

1. Discuss when you think people should start deciding whether to have an advance directive. What are some important considerations when preparing an advance directive?
2. As the percentage of the population that is older continues to grow larger, how will it affect your life? Would you be willing to pay higher taxes to support government social programs for older adults? Why or why not?
3. List the major physical and mental changes that occur with aging. Which of these, if any, can you change? Discuss actions you can start taking now to ensure a healthier aging process.
4. Discuss why so many of us deny death. How could death become a more acceptable topic to discuss?
5. Explain the importance of recognizing mental conditions such as depression in the older population. Do you think loneliness and isolation are common in the older population as a result of life transitions? How could this be addressed?

## Accessing Your Health on the Internet

The following websites explore further topics and issues related to personal health. For links to the websites below, visit the Companion Website for *Access to Health*, 12th Edition, at www.pearsonhighered.com/donatelle.

1. *Administration on Aging.* This is a link to the U.S. Department of Health and Human Services, dedicated to addressing the health needs of older adults. www.aoa.gov
2. *Alzheimer's Association.* This site includes media releases, position statements, fact sheets, and research on Alzheimer's disease. www.alz.org

3. *Beyond Indigo.* This site addresses all aspects of grief and loss, including terminal illness, legal issues, and funeral planning. www.beyondindigo.com
4. *National Hospice and Palliative Care Organization.* This site offers information on hospice care, including resources for finding a hospice, end-of-life issues, and advance directives. www.nhpco.org
5. *AARP.* This site includes comprehensive information on issues related to aging that include longevity and caregiving. www.aarp.org/

## References

1. J. C. Cavanaugh and F. Blanchard-Fields, *Adult Development and Aging,* 6th ed. (Belmont, CA: Wadsworth, Cengage Learning, 2011); S. Hillier and G. Barrow, *Aging, the Individual, and Society,* 9th ed. (Belmont, CA: Wadsworth, Cengage Learning, 2011).
2. Centers for Disease Control and Prevention and the Merck Company Foundation, *The State of Aging and Health in America 2007* (Whitehouse Station, NJ: The Merck Company Foundation, 2007), Available at www.cdc.gov/aging/data/stateofaging .htm.
3. Ibid.
4. Administration on Aging, U.S. Dept. of Health and Human Services, "A Profile of Older Americans: Education," Modified April 2010, www.aoa.gov/AoAroot/ Aging_Statistics/Profile/2009/13.aspx.
5. Centers for Disease Control and Prevention and the Merck Company Foundation, *The State of Aging and Health in America 2007,* 2007.
6. M. Lachman, "Aging under Control?" *Psychological Science Agenda* 19, no. 1 (2005): 1–3.
7. J. Xu et al., "Deaths: Final Data for 2007," *National Vital Statistics Reports* 58, no. 19 (May 2010): 1–73; National Center for Health Statistics, *Health, United States, 2009, with Special Feature on Medical Technology* (Hyattsville, MD: National Center for Health Statistics, 2010), table 26, Available at www.cdc.gov/nchs/hus.htm.
8. Administration on Aging, U.S. Department of Health and Human Services, "A Profile of Older Americans: The Older Population," Modified January 2010, www.aoa .gov/AoAroot/Aging_Statistics/Profile/ 2009/3.aspx.
9. Federal Interagency Forum on Aging-Related Statistics, *Older Americans 2010:*

*Key Indicators of Well-Being* (Washington, DC: U.S. Government Printing Office, 2010), Available at www.agingstats.gov/ agingstatsdotnet/main_site/default.aspx; Administration on Aging, "A Profile of Older Americans 2009," Modified January 2010, www.aoa.gov/AoAroot/Aging _Statistics/Profile/index.aspx.
10. United Nations, Department of Economic and Social Affairs, Population Division, "World Population Prospects: The 2008 Revision, Population Database," Updated March 2009, http://esa.un.org/unpp/ index.asp; "Networks of Cities Tackle Age-Old Problem," *Bulletin of the World Health Organization* 88 (2010): 406–07.
11. Administration on Aging, "A Profile of Older Americans 2009: Health and Health Care," Modified April 2010, www.aoa.gov/ AoARoot/Aging_Statistics/Profile/2009/14 .aspx.
12. Ibid.
13. Ibid.
14. American Association of Homes and Services for the Aging, "Aging Services: The Facts," 2010, www.aahsa.org/facts.
15. National Institute of Arthritis and Musculoskeletal Diseases, "Osteoporosis Overview," Reviewed June 2010, www .niams.nih.gov/Health_Info/Bone/ Osteoporosis/overview.asp.
16. Arthritis Foundation, "Osteoarthritis Fact Sheet," 2008, Available at www.arthritis .org/osteoarthritis-educate.php.
17. National Association for Continence, "Statistics," Updated March 2009, www.nafc .org/media/statistics.
18. Ibid.
19. U.S. National Library of Medicine and National Institutes of Health, Medline Plus, "Aging Changes in the Senses," Updated February 2009, www.nlm.nih .gov/medlineplus/ency/article/004013 .htm.
20. D. Kemmet and S. Brotherson, "Making Sense of Sensory Losses as We Age—Childhood, Adulthood, Elderhood?" September 2008, North Dakota State University, www .ag.ndsu.edu/pubs/yf/famsci/fs1378.html.
21. S. T. Lindau et al., "A National Study of Sexuality and Health among Older Adults in the U.S.," *New England Journal of Medicine* 357, no. 8 (2007): 762–74.
22. S. T. Lindau et al., "A National Study of Sexuality and Health among Older Adults in the U.S.," 2007; L. Fisher, *Sex, Romance, and Relationships: AARP Survey of Midlife and Older Adults* (Washington, DC: AARP, 2010), Available at www.aarp.org/ relationships/love-sex/info-05-2010/ srr_09.html.
23. Alzheimer's Association, *2010 Alzheimer's Disease Facts and Figures* (Chicago: Alzheimer's Association, 2010), Available at

www.alz.org/alzheimers_disease_facts _figures.asp.

24. Ibid.

25. B. Kantrowitz and K. Springen, "Confronting Alzheimer's," *Newsweek,* June 15, 2007, www.newsweek.com/2007/06/17/ confronting-alzheimer-s.html.

26. Alzheimer's Association, *2010 Alzheimer's Disease Facts and Figures,* 2010.

27. Ibid.

28. National Center for Health Statistics, *Health, United States, 2009, with Special Feature on Medical Technology* (Hyattsville, MD: National Center for Health Statistics, 2010), table 66, Available at www.cdc.gov/nchs/hus.htm; National Institute on Aging, "AgePage: Alcohol Use in Older People," Updated February 2010, www.nia.nih.gov/HealthInformation/Publications/alcohol.htm.

29. Centers for Disease Control and Prevention, "Information Sheets: NCHS Data on Prescription Drugs," Updated October 2009, www.cdc.gov/nchs/data/infosheets/ infosheet_prescription_drugs.htm.

30. M. Nelson et al., "Physical Activity and Public Health in Older Adults: Recommendations from the American College of Sports Medicine and the American Heart Association," *Medicine and Science in Sports and Exercise* 39, no. 8 (2007): 1435–45.

31. M. Nelson et al., "Physical Activity and Public Health in Older Adults," 2007; National Institute on Aging, *Exercise &*

*Physical Activity: Your Everyday Guide from the National Institute on Aging* (Bethesda, MD: National Institutes of Health, 2009) NIH Publication no. 09-4258, Available at www.nia.nih.gov/HealthInformation/ Publications/ExerciseGuide.

32. SHORTER OXFORD ENGLISH DICTIONARY 6E edited by Stevenson (2007) definition of "death." By permission of Oxford University Press.

33. President's Commission on the Uniform Determination of Death, *Defining Death: Medical, Ethical and Legal Issues in the Determination of Death* (Washington, DC: U.S. Government Printing Office, 1981).

34. Ad Hoc Committee of the Harvard Medical School to Examine the Definition of Brain Death, "A Definition of Irreversible Coma," *Journal of the American Medical Association* 205 (1968): 377.

35. E. Kübler-Ross, and D. Kessler, *On Grief and Grieving: Finding the Meaning of Grief through the Five Stages of Loss* (New York: Scribner, 2005).

36. C. Corr, C. Nabe, and D. Corr, *Death and Dying, Life and Living,* 6th ed. (Belmont, CA: Wadsworth, 2009).

37. Ibid.

38. J. W. Worden, *Grief Counseling and Grief Therapy: A Handbook for the Mental Health Practitioner,* 4th ed. (New York: Springer, 2004).

39. Federal Interagency Forum on Child and Family Statistics, *America's Children in Brief: Key National Indicators of Well-Being 2010* (Washington, DC: U.S. Government Printing Office, 2010), Available at www .childstats.gov/americaschildren/index .asp.

40. American Bar Association, Commission on Law and Aging, *Consumer's Tool Kit for Health Care Advance Planning,* 2d ed., (Washington, DC: American Bar Association, 2005), Available at www.abanet.org/ aging/toolkit/home.html.

41. Aging with Dignity, "Five Wishes," 2010, www.agingwithdignity.org/five-wishes.php.

42. Public Agenda, "Right to Die," 2010, www .publicagenda.org/articles/right-die.

43. Oregon Department of Human Services, "FAQ's about the Death with Dignity Act," Updated May 2010, www.oregon.gov/DHS/ ph/pas/faqs.shtml; International Task Force on Euthanasia and Assisted Suicide, "Assisted Suicide Laws," Updated January 2009, www.internationaltaskforce.org/ assisted_suicide_laws.htm.

44. National Hospice and Palliative Care Organization, *NHPCO Facts and Figures: Hospice Care in America, 2009 Edition* (Alexandria, VA: National Hospice and Palliative Care Organization, 2009), Available at www.nhpco.org/i4a/pages/ index.cfm?pageid=3296.

# Answers to Chapter Review Questions

**Chapter 1**
1. d; 2. b; 3. b; 4. d; 5. a;
6. a; 7. a; 8. a; 9. c; 10. c

**Chapter 2**
1. a; 2. b; 3. a; 4. b; 5. c;
6. a; 7. b; 8. b; 9. c; 10. b

**Chapter 3**
1. c; 2. c; 3. d; 4. d; 5. c;
6. d; 7. c; 8. c; 9. c; 10. b

**Chapter 4**
1. b; 2. b; 3. c; 4. c; 5. a;
6. c; 7. a; 8. d; 9. a; 10. d

**Chapter 5**
1. a; 2. d; 3. c; 4. a; 5. a;
6. b; 7. b; 8. b; 9. b; 10. a

**Chapter 6**
1. b; 2. b; 3. a; 4. c; 5. b;
6. a; 7. c; 8. d; 9. c; 10. a

**Chapter 7**
1. d; 2. a; 3. a; 4. b; 5. b;
6. a; 7. b; 8. b; 9. b; 10. c

**Chapter 8**
1. c; 2. c; 3. b; 4. b; 5. c;
6. b; 7. a; 8. a; 9. d; 10. a

**Chapter 9**
1. c; 2. d; 3. c; 4. b; 5. a;
6. a; 7. d; 8. c; 9. b; 10. a

**Chapter 10**
1. d; 2. d; 3. b; 4. c; 5. d;
6. b; 7. d; 8. b; 9. b; 10. a

**Chapter 11**
1. c; 2. d; 3. d; 4. d; 5. b;
6. b; 7. c; 8. d; 9. c; 10. a

**Chapter 12**
1. b; 2. b; 3. c; 4. b; 5. d;
6. c; 7. d; 8. d; 9. b; 10. c

**Chapter 13**
1. c; 2. c; 3. a; 4. b; 5. c;
6. c; 7. a; 8. d; 9. c; 10. b

**Chapter 14**
1. a; 2. c; 3. c; 4. d; 5. a;
6. d; 7. c; 8. b; 9. c; 10. a

**Chapter 15**
1. c; 2. b; 3. a; 4. d; 5. c;
6. d; 7. b; 8. d; 9. a; 10. c

**Chapter 16**
1. b; 2. d; 3. d; 4. a; 5. c;
6. d; 7. a; 8. d; 9. a; 10. c

**Chapter 17**
1. c; 2. b; 3. c; 4. d; 5. c;
6. a; 7. b; 8. c; 9. a; 10. b

**Chapter 18**
1. c; 2. a; 3. d; 4. c; 5. c;
6. c; 7. b; 8. b; 9. a; 10. a

**Chapter 19**
1. b; 2. a; 3. c; 4. d; 5. d;
6. c; 7. a; 8. c; 9. b; 10. a

**Chapter 20**
1. b; 2. d; 3. d; 4. a; 5. a;
6. d; 7. b; 8. b; 9. a; 10. c

**Chapter 21**
1. b; 2. b; 3. c; 4. a; 5. d;
6. a; 7. a; 8. c; 9. c; 10. d

# Providing Emergency Care

Ideally, first-aid procedures should be performed only by someone who has received formal training from the American Red Cross or another reputable institution. (There are numerous classes and opportunities in most communities for updating your skills in these areas. Check for such classes at your university, or local community colleges.) If you do not have such training, contact a physician or call your local emergency medical service (EMS) by dialing 9-1-1 or your local emergency number. In life-threatening situations, however, you may need to begin first aid immediately and continue until help arrives. This section contains basic information for various emergency situations. Simply reading these directions, however, may not prepare you fully to handle these situations. For this reason, you may want to enroll in a first-aid course.

## Calling for Emergency Assistance

When calling for emergency assistance, be prepared to give exact details. Be clear and thorough, and do not panic. Never hang up until the dispatcher has informed you that he or she has all the information needed. Be ready to answer the following questions:

● Where are you and the victim located? (This is the most important information that the EMS will need.)
● What is your phone number and name?
● What has happened? Was there an accident, or is the victim ill?
● How many people need help?
● What is the nature of the emergency? What is the victim's apparent condition?
● Are there any life-threatening situations that the EMS should know about (for example, fires, explosions, or fallen electrical lines)?
● Is the victim wearing a medic-alert tag (a tag indicating a specific medical condition such as diabetes)?

## Administering First Aid

According to the laws in most states, you are not required to administer first aid unless you have a special obligation to the victim. For example, parents must provide first aid for their children, and a lifeguard must provide aid to a swimmer.

Before administering first aid, you should obtain the victim's consent. If the victim refuses aid, you must respect that person's rights. However, you should make every reasonable effort to persuade the victim to accept your help. In emergency situations, consent is *implied* if the victim is unconscious. Once you begin to administer first aid, you are required by law to continue. You must remain with the victim until someone of equal or greater competence takes over.

Can you be held liable if you fail to provide adequate care or if the victim is further injured? To protect people who render first aid, most states have Good Samaritan laws, which grant immunity (protection from civil liability) if you act in good faith to provide care to the best of your ability, according to your level of training. Because these laws vary, you should become familiar with the Good Samaritan laws in your state.

## First-Aid Supplies

Every home, car, and boat should be supplied with a basic first-aid kit, which should be stored in a convenient place but kept out of the reach of children. Following is a list of supplies that should be included:

● Bandages, including triangular bandages (36 inches by 6 inches), butterfly bandages, a roller bandage, rolled white gauze bandages (2- and 3-inch widths), adhesive bandages
● Sterile gauze pads and absorbent pads
● Adhesive tape (2- and 3-inch widths)
● Cotton-tip applicators
● Scissors
● Thermometer
● Antibiotic ointment
● Aspirin
● Calamine lotion
● Antiseptic cream or petroleum jelly
● Safety pins
● Tweezers
● Latex gloves
● Flashlight
● Paper cups
● Blanket

You cannot be prepared for every medical emergency, but these essential tools and a knowledge of basic first aid will help you cope with many emergency situations, including the ones discussed below.

## Cessation of Breathing

If someone has stopped breathing, you should perform mouth-to-mouth resuscitation. This involves the following steps:

1. Check for responsiveness by gently tapping or shaking the victim. Ask loudly, "Are you okay?"
2. Call the local EMS for help (usually 9-1-1).
3. Gently roll the victim onto his or her back.
4. Open the airway by tilting the victim's head back—place your hand nearest the victim's head on the victim's forehead, and apply backward pressure to tilt the head back and lift the chin.
5. Check for breathing (3 to 5 seconds): look, listen, and feel for breathing.
6. Give two slow breaths.
   - Keep the victim's head tilted back.
   - Pinch the victim's nose shut.
   - Seal your lips tightly around the victim's mouth.
   - Give two slow breaths, each lasting 1.5 to 2 seconds.
   - Watch for the chest to rise and fall.
7. Check for pulse at side of neck; feel for pulse for 5 to 10 seconds.
8. Begin rescue breathing.
   - Keep the victim's head tilted back.
   - Pinch the victim's nose shut.
   - Give one breath about every 5 seconds (12 breaths per minute).
   - Look, listen, and feel for breathing between breaths.
9. Recheck pulse every minute.
   - Keep the victim's head tilted back.
   - Feel for pulse for 5 to 10 seconds.
   - If the victim has a pulse but is not breathing, continue rescue breathing. If there is no pulse, begin CPR (see below).

There are some variations when performing this procedure on infants and children. For infants, at step 8, you should give one slow breath every 3 seconds. You should not pinch the nose. Instead, seal your lips tightly around the infant's nose and mouth. For children aged 1 to 8, at step 8, give one slow breath every 4 seconds.

## Sudden Collapse

If an adult has a sudden cardiac arrest, his or her survival depends largely on being given immediate cardiopulmonary resuscitation (CPR). People are often afraid to offer aid for fear of doing something wrong or making matters worse. In addition, some people are squeamish about performing the artificial respiration that is part of traditional CPR. However, studies have shown that simply providing hands-only CPR to an adult who has collapsed can double that person's chance of survival. The American Heart Association now recommends that anyone, trained or untrained, who witnesses an adult's sudden collapse should call 9-1-1 and then immediately begin hands-only CPR. That means uninterrupted chest compressions—pushing hard in the center of the victim's chest—at a rate of about 100 per minute until the EMS arrives.

Conventional CPR, a technique that involves a combination of artificial respiration and chest compressions, is still recommended for infants or children, drowning victims, drug overdose, or other respiratory problems, and on adult victims who are found already unconscious and not breathing normally. The American Red Cross, the American Heart Association, and other organizations offer courses in mouth-to-mouth resuscitation and CPR as well as general first aid. If you have taken a CPR course in the past, you should be aware that certain changes have been made in the procedure. Consider taking a refresher course.

## Choking

Choking occurs when an object obstructs the trachea (windpipe), thus preventing normal breathing. Failure to expel the object and restore breathing can lead to death within 6 minutes. The universal signal of distress related to choking is the clasping of the throat with one or both hands. Other signs of choking include not being able to talk and/or noisy and difficult breathing. If a victim can cough or speak, do not interfere. The most effective method for assisting choking victims is the Heimlich maneuver (Figure 1), which involves the application of pressure to the victim's abdominal area to expel the foreign object, as described below.

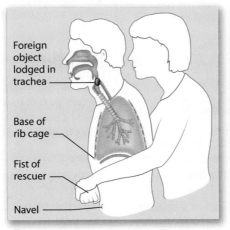

Foreign object lodged in trachea

Base of rib cage

Fist of rescuer

Navel

(a) Standing behind the victim, place a fist thumb-side in just above the victim's navel and cover it with your other hand.

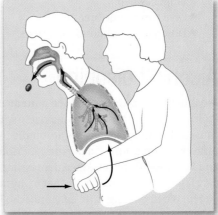

(b) Press sharply upward and inward, using enough force to push the diaphragm and lungs up and create air pressure that will expel the object.

FIGURE 1 **Heimlich Maneuver**
The Heimlich maneuver can be used to dislodge an object that is blocking a person's airway, causing him or her to choke. The technique shown here is appropriate for use on a person who is either sitting or standing.

**Source:** Adapted from JOHNSON, MICHAEL D., HUMAN BIOLOGY: CONCEPTS AND CURRENT ISSUES, 5th, © 2010. Printed and Electronically reproduced by permission of Pearson Education, Inc., Upper Saddle River, New Jersey.

### If the Choking Victim Is Standing or Seated

**1.** Recognize that the victim is choking. Without startling him or her, approach from behind.
**2.** Wrap your arms around the victim's waist, making a fist with one hand.
**3.** Place the thumb side of the fist on the middle of the victim's abdomen, just above the navel and well below the tip of the sternum.
**4.** Cover your fist with your other hand.
**5.** Press fist into victim's abdomen, with up to five quick upward thrusts.
**6.** After every five abdominal thrusts, check the victim and your technique.
**7.** If the victim becomes unconscious, gently lower him or her to the ground.
**8.** Try to clear the airway by using your finger to sweep the object from the victim's mouth or throat.
**9.** Give two rescue breaths. If the passage is still blocked and air will not go in, repeat the Heimlich maneuver.

### If the Choking Victim Is Lying Down

**1.** Facing the person, kneel with your legs astride the victim's hips. Place the heel of one hand against the abdomen, slightly above the navel and well below the tip of the sternum. Put the other hand on top of the first hand.
**2.** Press inward and upward using both hands with up to five quick abdominal thrusts.
**3.** Repeat the following steps in this sequence until the airway becomes clear or the EMS arrives:
  - Finger sweep.
  - Give two rescue breaths.
  - Do up to five abdominal thrusts.

## Alcohol Poisoning

Alcohol overdose is considered a medical emergency when an irregular heartbeat or coma occurs. The two immediate causes of death in such cases are cardiac arrhythmia and respiratory depression. If a person is seriously uncoordinated and has possibly also taken a depressant, the risk of respiratory failure is serious enough that a physician should be contacted. When dealing with someone who is drunk, remember these points:

**1.** Stay calm. Assess the situation.
**2.** Keep your distance. Before approaching or touching the person, explain what you intend to do.
**3.** Speak in a clear, firm, reassuring manner.
**4.** Keep the person still and comfortable.
**5.** Stay with the person if she or he is vomiting. When helping him or her to lie down, turn the head to the side to prevent it from falling back. This helps to keep the person from choking on vomit.
**6.** Monitor the person's breathing.

## Seizures

If you are with someone experiencing a seizure, there are several steps you can take to help ensure his or her safety during and after the episode:

**1.** Note the length of the attack. Seizures in which a person remains unconscious for long periods of time should be monitored closely. If medical help arrives, be sure to tell them how long the person has been unconscious.
**2.** Remove obstacles that could harm the victim. Because seizure victims may lose motor control during a convulsion, they inadvertently thrash around. To reduce the chances of serious injury, clear away any objects that could pose a threat.
**3.** Loosen clothing, and turn the victim's head to the side. This will help ensure that the person can breathe freely and will allow fluids or vomit to drain from the mouth.
**4.** Do not force objects into the victim's mouth. Although seizure victims may bite their tongues, causing possible damage, they will not swallow them. If the victim's mouth is clamped shut, forcing objects into the mouth may break teeth or cause more harm than doing nothing.
**5.** Get help. After you have completed steps 1 through 4, get help or send someone for help. This is particularly important if the victim does not regain consciousness within a few minutes.
**6.** Reassure the victim. Too often, the seizure victim regains consciousness only to face a crowd of staring people. When administering first aid, try to dissuade curious bystanders from hanging around. Calmly reassure the victim that everything is okay.
**7.** Allow the person to rest. After a seizure, many people will be exhausted. Allow them to sleep if possible.

## Bleeding

**External Bleeding**  Control of external bleeding is an important part of emergency care. Survival is threatened by the loss of 1 quart of blood or more. There are three major procedures for the control of external bleeding:

- **Direct pressure.** The best method is to apply firm pressure by covering the wound with a sterile dressing, bandage, or clean cloth. Wearing disposable latex gloves or an equally protective barrier, apply pressure for 5 to 10 minutes to stop bleeding.
- **Elevation.** Elevate the wounded section of the body to slow the bleeding. For example, a wounded arm or leg should be raised above the level of the victim's heart.
- **Pressure points.** Pressure points are sites where an artery that is close to the body's surface lies directly over a bone (Figure 2). Pressing the artery against the bone can limit the flow of blood to the injury. This technique should be used only as a last resort when direct pressure and elevation have failed to stop bleeding.

For serious wounds, seek medical attention immediately.

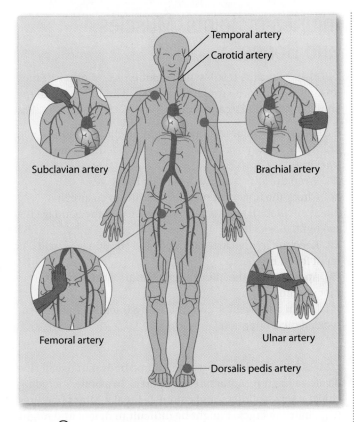

FIGURE 2 **Pressure Points**
Pressure can be applied to these points to stop bleeding. However, unless absolutely necessary, avoid applying pressure to the carotid arteries, which supply blood to the brain. Never apply pressure to both carotid arteries at the same time.

**Internal Bleeding**  Although internal bleeding may not be immediately obvious, you should be aware of the following signs and symptoms:

- Symptoms of shock (discussed below)
- Coughing up or vomiting blood
- Bruises or contusions of the skin
- Bruises on chest or fractured ribs
- Black, tarlike stools
- Abdominal discomfort or pain (rigidity or spasms)

In some cases, a person who has suffered an injury (such as a blow to the head, chest, or abdomen) that does not cause external bleeding may bleed internally. If you suspect internal bleeding, follow these steps:

**1.** Have the person lie on his or her back on a flat surface with knees bent.
**2.** Treat for shock. Keep the victim warm. Cover the person with a blanket, if possible.
**3.** Expect vomiting. If this occurs, keep the victim on his or her side for drainage, to prevent inhalation of vomit, and to prevent expulsion of vomit from the stomach.
**4.** Do *not* give the victim any medications or fluids.
**5.** Send someone to call for emergency medical help immediately.

### Nosebleeds

**1.** Have the victim sit down and lean slightly forward to prevent blood from running into the throat. If you do not suspect a fracture, pinch the person's nose firmly closed using the thumb and forefinger. Keep the nose pinched for at least 5 minutes.
**2.** While the nose is pinched, apply a cold compress to the surrounding area.
**3.** If pinching does not work, gently pack the nostril with gauze or a clean strip of cloth. Do not use absorbent cotton, which will stick. Be sure that the ends of the gauze or cloth hang out so that it can be easily removed later. Once the nose is packed with gauze, pinch it closed again for another 5 minutes.
**4.** If the bleeding persists, seek medical attention.

## Shock

Shock is a condition in which the cardiovascular system fails to provide sufficient blood circulation to all parts of the body. Victims of shock display some or all of the following symptoms:

- Dilated pupils
- Cool, moist skin
- Weak, rapid pulse
- Vomiting
- Delayed or unrelated responses to questions

All injuries result in some degree of shock. Therefore, treatment for shock should be given after every major injury. The following are basic steps for treating shock:

**1.** Have the victim lie flat with his or her feet elevated approximately 8 to 12 inches. (In the case of chest injuries, difficulty breathing, or severe pain, the victim's head should be slightly elevated if there is no sign of spinal injury.)
**2.** Keep the victim warm. If possible, wrap him or her in blankets or other material. Keep the victim calm and reassured.
**3.** Seek medical help.

## Treatment for Burns

**Minor Burns**  For minor burns caused by fire or scalding water, apply running cold water or cold compresses for 20 to 30 minutes. Never put butter, grease, salt water, aloe vera, or topical burn ointments or sprays on burned skin. If the burned area is dirty, gently wash it with soap and water, and blot it dry with a sterile dressing.

**Major Burns**  For major burn injuries, call for help immediately. Wrap the victim in a clean, dry sheet. Do not clean the burns or try to remove any clothing attached to burned skin. Remove jewelry near the burned skin immediately, if possible. Keep the victim lying down and calm.

**Chemical Burns**  Remove clothing surrounding the burn. Wash skin that has been burned by chemicals by flushing with water for at least 20 minutes. Seek medical assistance as soon as possible.

# Electrical Shock

Do not touch a victim of electrical shock until the power source has been turned off. Approach the scene carefully, avoiding any live wires or electrical power lines. Pay attention to the following:

**1.** If the victim is holding on to the live electrical wire, do not remove it unless the power has been shut off at the plug, circuit breaker, or fuse box.

**2.** Check the victim's breathing and pulse. Electrical current can paralyze the nerves and muscles that control breathing and heartbeat. If necessary, give mouth-to-mouth resuscitation. If there is no pulse, CPR might be necessary. (Remember that only trained people should perform CPR.)

**3.** Keep the victim warm and treat for shock. Once the person is breathing and stable, seek medical help or send someone else for help.

# Poisoning

Among adults, almost all poisonings are caused by an overdose of a prescription drug, most commonly an opioid pain medication, or an illegal drug, such as cocaine or heroin. Among children, the majority of poisonings are caused by household products.

You should keep emergency telephone numbers for the poison control center and the local EMS close at hand. Many people keep these numbers on labels on their telephones. Check the front of your telephone book for these numbers. Be prepared to answer the following questions and to give the following information when calling for help:

● What was ingested? Have the container of the product and the remaining contents ready so you can describe it. Bring the container with you to the emergency room.
● When was the substance taken?
● How much was taken?
● Has vomiting occurred? If the person has vomited, save a sample to take to the hospital.
● Are there any other symptoms?
● How long will it take to get to the nearest emergency room?

When caring for a person who has ingested poison, keep these basic principles in mind:

**1.** Maintain an open airway. Make sure the person is breathing.

**2.** Call the local poison control center. Follow their advice for neutralizing the poison.

**3.** If the poison control center or another medical authority advises you to induce vomiting, then do so.

**4.** If a corrosive or caustic (that is, acid or alkali) substance was swallowed, immediately dilute it by having the victim drink at least one or two 8-ounce glasses of cold water or milk.

**5.** Place the victim on his or her left side. This position will delay advancement of the poison into the small intestine, where absorption into the victim's circulatory system is faster.

# Injuries of Joints, Muscles, and Bones

**Sprains** Sprains result when ligaments and other tissues around a joint are stretched or torn. The following steps should be taken to treat sprains:

**1.** Elevate the injured joint to a comfortable position.
**2.** Apply an ice pack or cold compress to reduce pain and swelling.
**3.** Wrap the joint firmly with a roller bandage.
**4.** Check the fingers or toes periodically to ensure that blood circulation has not been obstructed. If the bandage is too tight, loosen it.
**5.** Keep the injured area elevated, and continue ice treatment for 24 hours.
**6.** Apply heat to the injury after 48 hours if there is no further swelling.
**7.** If pain and swelling continue or if a fracture is suspected, seek medical attention.

**Fractures** Any deformity of an injured body part usually indicates a fracture. A fracture is any break in a bone, including chips, cracks, splinters, and complete breaks. Minor fractures (e.g., hairline cracks) might be difficult to detect and might be confused with sprains. If there is doubt, treat the injury as a fracture until X rays have been taken.

Do not move the victim if a fracture of the neck or back is suspected, because this could result in a spinal cord injury. If the victim must be moved, splints should be applied to immobilize the fracture in order to prevent further damage and to decrease pain. Following are some basic steps for treating fractures and applying splints to broken limbs:

**1.** If the person is bleeding, apply direct pressure above the site of the wound.
**2.** If a broken bone is exposed, do not try to move it back into the wound. This can cause contamination and further injury.
**3.** Do not try to straighten out a broken limb. Splint the limb as it lies.
**4.** The following materials are needed for splinting:
   ● *Splint:* wooden board, pillow, or rolled up magazines and newspapers
   ● *Padding:* towels, blankets, socks, or cloth
   ● *Ties:* cloth, rope, or tape
**5.** Place splints and padding above and below the joint. Never put padding directly over the break. Padding should protect bony areas and the soft tissue of the limb.
**6.** Tie splints and padding into place.
**7.** Check the tightness of the splints periodically. Pay attention to the skin color, temperature, and pulse below the fracture to make sure the blood flow is adequate.
**8.** Elevate the fracture and apply ice packs to prevent swelling and reduce pain.

# Head Injuries

All head injuries can potentially lead to brain damage, which may result in a cessation of breathing and pulse.

## Minor Head Injuries

**1.** For a minor bump on the head resulting in a bruise without bleeding, apply ice to decrease the swelling.

**2.** If there is bleeding, apply even, moderate pressure. Do not use excessive pressure because the skull may be fractured.

**3.** Observe the victim for a change in consciousness. Observe the size of pupils, including whether both pupils are dilated to the same degree, and note signs of inability to think clearly. Check for any signs of numbness or paralysis. Allow the victim to sleep, but wake him or her periodically to check for awareness.

## Severe Head Injuries

**1.** If the victim is unconscious, check the airway for breathing. If necessary, perform mouth-to-mouth resuscitation.

**2.** If the victim is breathing, check the pulse. If it is less than 55 or more than 125 beats per minute, the victim may be in danger.

**3.** Check for bleeding. If fluid is flowing from the ears or nose, do not stop it.

**4.** Do not remove any objects embedded in the victim's skull.

**5.** Cover the victim with blankets to maintain body temperature, but guard against overheating.

**6.** Seek medical help as soon as possible.

# Temperature-Related Emergencies

**Frostbite** Frostbite is damage to body tissues caused by intense cold, generally occurring at temperatures below 32°F. When skin is exposed to the cold, ice crystals form beneath the skin. Avoid rubbing frostbitten tissue, because the ice crystals can scrape and break blood vessels. The body parts most likely to suffer frostbite are the toes, ears, fingers, nose, and cheeks. To treat frostbite, follow these steps:

**1.** Bring the victim to a medical facility as soon as possible.

**2.** Cover and protect the frostbitten area. If possible, apply a steady source of external warmth, such as a warm compress. Avoid walking if the feet are frostbitten.

**3.** If the victim cannot be transported, warm the body part by immersing it in warm water (100°F to 105°F). Continue to warm until the frostbitten area is warm to the touch when removed from the bath. Do not allow the body part to touch the sides or bottom of the water container. After warming, dry gently and wrap the body part in bandages to protect from refreezing.

**Hypothermia** Hypothermia is a condition of generalized cooling of the body, resulting from exposure to cold temperatures or immersion in cold water. It can occur at any temperature below 65°F and can be made more severe by wind chill and moisture. The following are key symptoms of hypothermia:

- Shivering
- Vague, slow, slurred speech
- Poor judgment
- A cool abdomen
- Lethargy, or extreme exhaustion
- Slowed breathing and heartbeat
- Numbness and loss of feeling in extremities

After contacting the EMS, take the following steps:

**1.** Get the victim out of the cold.

**2.** Keep the victim in a flat position. Do not raise the legs.

**3.** Squeeze as much water as possible from wet clothing, and layer dry clothing over wet clothing. Removal of clothing may jostle the victim and lead to other problems.

**4.** Give the victim warm drinks only if he or she is able to swallow. Do not give the victim alcohol or caffeinated beverages, and do not allow the victim to smoke.

**5.** Do not allow the victim to exercise.

**Heatstroke** Heatstroke, the most serious heat-related disorder, results from the failure of the brain's heat-regulating mechanism (the hypothalamus) to cool the body. The following are signs and symptoms of heatstroke:

- Rapid pulse
- Hot, dry, flushed skin (absence of sweating)
- Disorientation leading to unconsciousness
- High body temperature

Body temperature should be reduced as quickly as possible. Immerse the victim in a cool bath, lake, or stream. If there is no water nearby, loosen clothing and use a fan to help lower the victim's body temperature.

**Heat Exhaustion** Heat exhaustion results from excessive loss of salt and water. The onset is gradual, with the following symptoms:

- Fatigue and weakness
- Anxiety
- Nausea
- Profuse sweating and clammy skin
- Normal body temperature

Move the victim to a cool place and have him or her lie down flat, with feet elevated 8 to 12 inches. Replace lost fluids slowly and steadily. Sponge or fan the victim.

**Heat Cramps** Heat cramps result from excessive sweating, resulting in an excessive loss of salt and water. Although heat cramps are the least serious heat-related emergency, they are the most painful. The symptoms include muscle cramps, usually starting in the arms and legs. To relieve symptoms, the victim should drink electrolyte-rich beverages or a light saltwater solution or eat salty foods.

# Nutritive Value of Selected Foods and Fast Foods

This section presents nutritional information about a wide array of foods, including many fast foods. Values are given for calories, protein, carbohydrates, fiber, fat, saturated fat, and cholesterol for common foods and serving sizes. Use this information to assess your diet and make improvements. This is only a sampling of the most common foods. See the MyDietAnalysis database for a more extensive list of foods.

| MDA Code | Food Name | Amt | Wt (g) | Ener (kcal) | Prot (g) | Carb (g) | Fiber (g) | Fat (g) | Sat (g) | Chol (g) |
|---|---|---|---|---|---|---|---|---|---|---|
| **Beverages** | | | | | | | | | | |
| *Alcoholic Beverages* | | | | | | | | | | |
| 22831 | Beer | 12 fl. oz | 360 | 157 | 1 | 13 | | 0 | 0 | 0 |
| 34053 | Beer, light | 12 fl. oz | 353 | 105 | 1 | 5 | 0 | 0 | 0 | 0 |
| 22606 | Beer, nonalcoholic | 12 fl. oz | 353 | 73 | 1 | 14 | 0 | 0 | 0 | 0 |
| 22884 | Wine, red | 1 fl. oz | 29 | 24 | 0 | 1 | | 0 | 0 | |
| 22861 | Wine, white | 1 fl. oz | 29 | 24 | 0 | 1 | | 0 | 0 | |
| 22514 | Gin, 80 proof | 1 fl. oz | 28 | 64 | 0 | 0 | 0 | 0 | 0 | 0 |
| 22593 | Rum, 80 proof | 1 fl. oz | 28 | 64 | 0 | 0 | 0 | 0 | 0 | 0 |
| 22515 | Tequila, 80 proof | 1 fl. oz | 28 | 64 | 0 | 0 | 0 | 0 | 0 | 0 |
| 22594 | Vodka, 80 proof | 1 fl. oz | 28 | 64 | 0 | 0 | 0 | 0 | 0 | 0 |
| 22670 | Whiskey, 80 proof | 1 fl. oz | 28 | 64 | 0 | 0 | 0 | 0 | 0 | 0 |
| *Coffee, Tea, and Dairy Drink Mixes* | | | | | | | | | | |
| 20012 | Coffee, brewed | 1 cup | 237 | 2 | 0 | 0 | 0 | 0 | 0 | 0 |
| 20686 | Coffee, decaffeinated, brewed | 1 cup | 237 | 0 | 0 | 0 | 0 | 0 | 0 | 0 |
| 20439 | Coffee, espresso | 1 cup | 237 | 5 | 0 | 0 | 0 | 0 | 0.2 | 0 |
| 20402 | Coffee, from mix, French vanilla, sugar & fat free | 1 ea | 7 | 25 | 0 | 5 | 0 | 0 | 0.1 | 0 |
| 85 | Chocolate milk, prepared w/ syrup | 1 cup | 282 | 254 | 9 | 36 | 1 | 8 | 4.7 | 25 |
| 46 | Hot cocoa, w/ aspartame, sodium, vitamin A, prepared w/ water | 1 cup | 256 | 74 | 3 | 14 | 2 | 1 | 0.4 | 0 |
| 48 | Hot cocoa, prep from dry mix w/ water | 1 cup | 275 | 151 | 3 | 32 | 1 | 2 | 0.9 | 0 |
| 166 | Hot cocoa, w/ marshmallows, from dry packet | 1 ea | 28 | 112 | 1 | 21 | 1 | 4 | 4.2 | 0 |
| 39 | Chocolate flavor, dry mix, prepared w/ milk | 1 cup | 266 | 226 | 9 | 32 | 1 | 9 | 4.9 | 24 |
| 41 | Strawberry flavor, dry mix, prepared w/ milk | 1 cup | 266 | 234 | 8 | 33 | 0 | 8 | 5.1 | 32 |
| 20014 | Tea, brewed | 1 cup | 237 | 2 | 0 | 1 | 0 | 0 | 0 | 0 |
| 20036 | Tea, herbal (not chamomile) brewed | 1 cup | 237 | 2 | 0 | 0 | 0 | 0 | 0 | 0 |
| *Fruit and Vegetable Beverages and Juices* | | | | | | | | | | |
| 71080 | Apple juice, canned or bottled, unsweetened | 1 ea | 262 | 121 | 0 | 30 | 1 | 0 | 0.1 | 0 |
| 20277 | Capri Sun All Natural Juice Drink, Fruit Punch | 1 ea | 210 | 99 | 0 | 26 | 0 | 0 | 0 | 0 |
| 5226 | Carrot juice, canned | 1 cup | 236 | 94 | 2 | 22 | 2 | 0 | 0.1 | 0 |
| 3042 | Cranberry juice cocktail | 1 cup | 253 | 137 | 0 | 34 | 0 | 0 | 0 | 0 |
| 20024 | Fruit punch, canned | 1 cup | 248 | 117 | 0 | 30 | 0 | 0 | 0 | 0 |
| 20035 | Fruit punch, from frozen concentrate | 1 cup | 247 | 114 | 0 | 29 | 0 | 0 | 0 | 0 |
| 20101 | Grape drink, canned | 1 cup | 250 | 152 | 0 | 39 | 0 | 0 | 0 | 0 |
| 3053 | Grapefruit juice, from frozen concentrate, unsweetened | 1 cup | 247 | 101 | 1 | 24 | 0 | 0 | 0 | 0 |
| 20045 | Lemonade flavor drink, from dry mix | 1 cup | 266 | 72 | 0 | 18 | 0 | 0 | 0 | 0 |
| 20047 | Lemonade w/ aspartame, low kcal, from dry mix | 1 cup | 237 | 7 | 0 | 2 | 0 | 0 | 0 | 0 |
| 20070 | Orange drink, canned | 1 cup | 248 | 122 | 0 | 31 | 0 | 0 | 0 | 0 |
| 20004 | Orange flavor drink, from dry mix | 1 cup | 248 | 122 | 0 | 31 | 0 | 0 | 0 | 0 |
| 71108 | Orange juice, canned, unsweetened | 1 ea | 263 | 124 | 2 | 29 | 1 | 0 | 0 | 0 |
| 3090 | Orange juice, fresh | 1 cup | 248 | 112 | 2 | 26 | 0 | 0 | 0.1 | 0 |
| 3091 | Orange juice, from frozen concentrate, unsweetened | 1 cup | 249 | 112 | 2 | 27 | 0 | 0 | 0 | 0 |
| 5397 | Tomato juice, canned w/o salt | 1 cup | 243 | 41 | 2 | 10 | 1 | 0 | 0 | 0 |
| 20849 | Vegetable and fruit, mixed juice drink | 4 oz | 113 | 33 | 0 | 8 | 0 | 0 | 0 | 0 |
| 20080 | Vegetable juice cocktail, canned | 1 cup | 242 | 46 | 2 | 11 | 2 | 0 | 0 | 0 |

**Ener** = energy (kilocalories); **Prot** = protein; **Carb** = carbohydrate; **Fiber** = dietary fiber; **Fat** = total fat; **Sat** = saturated fat; **Chol** = cholesterol.

| MDA Code | Food Name | Amt | Wt (g) | Ener (kcal) | Prot (g) | Carb (g) | Fiber (g) | Fat (g) | Sat (g) | Chol (g) |
|---|---|---|---|---|---|---|---|---|---|---|
| *Soft Drinks* | | | | | | | | | | |
| 20006 | Club soda | 1 cup | 237 | 0 | 0 | 0 | 0 | 0 | 0 | 0 |
| 20685 | Low-calorie cola, w/ aspartame, caffeine free | 12 fl. oz | 355 | 4 | 0 | 1 | 0 | 0 | 0 | 0 |
| 20843 | Cola, w/ higher caffeine | 12 fl. oz | 370 | 152 | 0 | 39 | 0 | 0 | 0 | 0 |
| 20008 | Ginger ale | 1 cup | 244 | 83 | 0 | 21 | 0 | 0 | 0 | 0 |
| 20032 | Lemon-lime soft drink | 1 cup | 246 | 98 | 0 | 25 | 0 | 0 | 0 | 0 |
| 20027 | Pepper-type soft drink | 1 cup | 246 | 101 | 0 | 26 | 0 | 0 | 0.2 | 0 |
| 20009 | Root beer | 1 cup | 246 | 101 | 0 | 26 | 0 | 0 | 0 | 0 |
| *Other* | | | | | | | | | | |
| 20033 | Soy milk | 1 cup | 245 | 132 | 8 | 15 | 1 | 4 | 0.5 | 0 |
| 20041 | Water, tap | 1 cup | 237 | 0 | 0 | 0 | 0 | 0 | 0 | 0 |
| **Breakfast Cereals** | | | | | | | | | | |
| 40095 | All-Bran/Kellogg | 0.5 cup | 30 | 78 | 4 | 22 | 9 | 1 | 0.2 | 0 |
| 40032 | Cap'n Crunch/Quaker | 0.75 cup | 27 | 109 | 1 | 23 | 1 | 2 | 1.1 | 0 |
| 40297 | Cheerios/Gen Mills | 1 cup | 30 | 110 | 3 | 22 | 3 | 2 | 0.3 | 0 |
| 40126 | Cinnamon Toast Crunch/Gen Mills | 0.75 cup | 30 | 130 | 2 | 24 | 1 | 3 | 0.4 | 0 |
| 40195 | Corn Flakes/Kellogg | 1 cup | 28 | 101 | 2 | 24 | 1 | 0 | 0 | 0 |
| 40089 | Corn Grits, instant, plain, prepared/Quaker | 1 pkg | 137 | 104 | 2 | 22 | 2 | 1 | 0.1 | |
| 40206 | Corn Pops/Kellogg | 1 cup | 31 | 117 | 1 | 28 | 0 | 0 | 0.1 | 0 |
| 40179 | Cream of Rice, prepared w/ salt | 1 cup | 244 | 127 | 2 | 28 | 0 | 0 | 0 | 0 |
| 40182 | Cream of Wheat, instant, prepared w/ salt | 1 cup | 241 | 149 | 4 | 32 | 1 | 1 | 0.1 | 0 |
| 40104 | Crispix/Kellogg | 1 cup | 29 | 109 | 2 | 25 | 0 | 0 | 0.1 | 0 |
| 40218 | Froot Loops/Kellogg | 1 cup | 30 | 112 | 2 | 26 | 3 | 1 | 0.6 | 0 |
| 40217 | Frosted Flakes/Kellogg | 0.75 cup | 31 | 114 | 1 | 28 | 1 | 0 | 0 | 0 |
| 11916 | Frosted Mini-Wheats, bite size/Kellogg | 1 cup | 55 | 189 | 6 | 45 | 6 | 1 | 0.2 | 0 |
| 40209 | Raisin Bran/Kellogg | 1 cup | 61 | 196 | 5 | 47 | 7 | 1 | 0.2 | 0 |
| 40210 | Rice Krispies/Kellogg | 1.25 cup | 33 | 128 | 2 | 28 | 0 | 0 | 0.1 | 0 |
| 60887 | Shredded wheat, large biscuit | 2 ea | 38 | 127 | 4 | 30 | 5 | 1 | 0.2 | 0 |
| 40211 | Special K/Kellogg | 1 cup | 31 | 117 | 7 | 22 | 1 | 0 | 0.1 | 0 |
| **Dairy and Cheese** | | | | | | | | | | |
| 500 | Cream, half & half | 2 Tbs | 30 | 39 | 1 | 1 | 0 | 3 | 2.1 | 11 |
| 11 | Milk, condensed, sweetened, canned | 2 Tbs | 38 | 123 | 3 | 21 | 0 | 3 | 2.1 | 13 |
| 19 | Milk, lowfat, 1% fat, chocolate | 1 cup | 250 | 158 | 8 | 26 | 1 | 2 | 1.5 | 8 |
| 218 | Milk, 2%, w/ added vitamins A & D | 1 cup | 245 | 130 | 8 | 13 | 0 | 5 | 3 | 20 |
| 6 | Milk, nonfat/skim, w/ added vitamin A | 1 cup | 245 | 83 | 8 | 12 | 0 | 0 | 0.1 | 5 |
| 1 | Milk, whole, 3.25% | 1 cup | 244 | 149 | 8 | 12 | 0 | 8 | 4.6 | 24 |
| 20 | Milk, whole, chocolate | 1 cup | 250 | 208 | 8 | 26 | 2 | 8 | 5.3 | 30 |
| 72088 | Yogurt, fruit variety, nonfat | 1 cup | 245 | 233 | 11 | 47 | 0 | 0 | 0.3 | 5 |
| 1287 | American cheese, nonfat slices | 1 pce | 21 | 32 | 5 | 2 | 0 | 0 | 0.1 | 3 |
| 13349 | Cheez Whiz cheese sauce/Kraft | 2 Tbs | 33 | 91 | 4 | 3 | 0 | 7 | 4.3 | 25 |
| 1014 | Cottage cheese, 2% fat | 0.5 cup | 113 | 97 | 13 | 4 | 0 | 3 | 1.1 | 11 |
| 1015 | Cream cheese | 2 Tbs | 29 | 99 | 2 | 1 | 0 | 10 | 5.6 | 32 |
| 1452 | Cream cheese, fat free | 2 Tbs | 29 | 30 | 5 | 2 | 0 | 0 | 0.2 | 3 |
| 1016 | Feta, crumbled | 0.25 cup | 38 | 99 | 5 | 2 | 0 | 8 | 5.6 | 33 |
| 47887 | Mozzarella, whole milk, slice | 1 ea | 34 | 102 | 8 | 1 | 0 | 8 | 4.5 | 27 |
| 1075 | Parmesan, grated | 1 Tbs | 5 | 22 | 2 | 0 | 0 | 1 | 0.9 | 4 |
| 1024 | Ricotta, part skim | 0.25 cup | 62 | 86 | 7 | 3 | 0 | 5 | 3.1 | 19 |
| 1064 | Ricotta, whole milk | 0.25 cup | 62 | 108 | 7 | 2 | 0 | 8 | 5.1 | 32 |
| **Eggs and Egg Substitutes** | | | | | | | | | | |
| 19525 | Egg substitute, liquid | 0.25 cup | 63 | 53 | 8 | 0 | 0 | 2 | 0.4 | 1 |
| 19506 | Egg, white, raw | 1 ea | 33 | 16 | 4 | 0 | 0 | 0 | 0 | 0 |
| 19509 | Egg, whole, fried | 1 ea | 46 | 90 | 6 | 0 | 0 | 7 | 2 | 210 |
| 19515 | Egg, whole, hard boiled | 1 ea | 37 | 57 | 5 | 0 | 0 | 4 | 1.2 | 157 |
| 19521 | Egg, whole, poached | 1 ea | 37 | 53 | 5 | 0 | 0 | 4 | 1.1 | 156 |
| 19516 | Egg, whole, scrambled | 1 ea | 61 | 102 | 7 | 1 | 0 | 7 | 2.2 | 215 |
| 19508 | Egg, yolk, raw, fresh | 1 ea | 17 | 53 | 3 | 1 | 0 | 4 | 1.6 | 205 |

| MDA Code | Food Name | Amt | Wt (g) | Ener (kcal) | Prot (g) | Carb (g) | Fiber (g) | Fat (g) | Sat (g) | Chol (g) |
|---|---|---|---|---|---|---|---|---|---|---|
| **Fruit** | | | | | | | | | | |
| 72101 | Apricots, canned, heavy syrup, drained | 1 cup | 182 | 151 | 1 | 39 | 5 | 0 | 0 | 0 |
| 3164 | Fruit cocktail canned in juice | 1 cup | 237 | 109 | 1 | 28 | 2 | 0 | 0 | 0 |
| 71079 | Apple w/ skin, raw | 1 cup | 125 | 65 | 0 | 17 | 3 | 0 | 0 | 0 |
| 3331 | Applesauce w/ added vitamin C | 0.5 cup | 128 | 97 | 0 | 25 | 2 | 0 | 0 | 0 |
| 3657 | Apricot, raw | 1 cup | 165 | 79 | 2 | 18 | 3 | 1 | 0 | 0 |
| 3210 | Avocado, California, peeled, raw | 1 ea | 173 | 289 | 3 | 15 | 12 | 27 | 3.7 | 0 |
| 71082 | Banana, peeled, raw | 1 ea | 81 | 72 | 1 | 19 | 2 | 0 | 0.1 | 0 |
| 71976 | Grapefruit, fresh | 0.5 ea | 154 | 60 | 1 | 16 | 6 | 0 | 0 | 0 |
| 3055 | Grapes, Thompson seedless, fresh | 0.5 cup | 80 | 55 | 1 | 14 | 1 | 0 | 0 | 0 |
| 3642 | Melon, fresh, wedge | 1 pce | 69 | 23 | 1 | 6 | 1 | 0 | 0 | 0 |
| 3168 | Mixed fruit (prune, apricot, & pear) dried | 1 oz | 28 | 69 | 1 | 18 | 2 | 0 | 0 | 0 |
| 3216 | Nectarine, raw | 1 cup | 138 | 61 | 1 | 15 | 2 | 0 | 0 | 0 |
| 3726 | Peach, peeled, raw | 1 ea | 79 | 31 | 1 | 8 | 1 | 0 | 0 | 0 |
| 3106 | Pear, raw | 1 ea | 209 | 121 | 1 | 32 | 6 | 0 | 0 | 0 |
| 3766 | Raisins, seedless | 50 ea | 26 | 78 | 1 | 21 | 1 | 0 | 0 | 0 |
| 72113 | Pineapple, fresh, slice | 1 pce | 84 | 38 | 0 | 10 | | 0 | | |
| 3085 | Orange, fresh | 1 ea | 184 | 86 | 2 | 22 | 4 | 0 | 0 | 0 |
| 3135 | Strawberries, halves/slices, raw | 1 cup | 166 | 53 | 1 | 13 | 3 | 0 | 0 | 0 |
| **Grain Products** | | | | | | | | | | |
| *Breads, Rolls, and Bread Crumbs* | | | | | | | | | | |
| 71170 | Bagel, cinnamon-raisin | 1 ea | 26 | 71 | 3 | 14 | 1 | 0 | 0.1 | 0 |
| 71167 | Bagel, egg | 1 ea | 26 | 72 | 3 | 14 | 1 | 1 | 0.1 | 6 |
| 71152 | Bagel, plain/onion/poppy/sesame, enriched | 1 ea | 26 | 67 | 3 | 13 | 1 | 0 | 0.1 | 0 |
| 42433 | Biscuit, w/ butter | 1 ea | 82 | 273 | 5 | 28 | 1 | 16 | 3.9 | 1 |
| 71192 | Biscuit, plain or buttermilk, refrig dough, baked, reduced fat | 1 ea | 21 | 63 | 2 | 12 | 0 | 1 | 0.3 | 0 |
| 42004 | Bread crumbs, dry, plain, grated | 1 Tbs | 7 | 27 | 1 | 5 | 0 | 0 | 0.1 | 0 |
| 49144 | Bread, crusty Italian w/ garlic | 1 pce | 50 | 186 | 4 | 21 | | 10 | 2.4 | 6 |
| 70964 | Bread, garlic, frozen/Campione | 1 pce | 28 | 101 | 2 | 12 | 1 | 5 | 0.8 | |
| 42069 | Bread, oat bran | 1 pce | 30 | 71 | 3 | 12 | 1 | 1 | 0.2 | 0 |
| 42095 | Bread, wheat, reduced kcal | 1 pce | 23 | 46 | 2 | 10 | 3 | 1 | 0.1 | 0 |
| 71247 | Bread, white, commercially prepared, crumbs/cubes/slices | 1 pce | 9 | 24 | 1 | 5 | 0 | 0 | 0.1 | 0 |
| 42084 | Bread, white, reduced kcal | 1 pce | 23 | 48 | 2 | 10 | 2 | 1 | 0.1 | 0 |
| 26561 | Buns, hamburger, Wonder | 1 ea | 43 | 117 | 3 | 22 | 1 | 2 | 0.4 | |
| 42021 | Hamburger/hot dog bun, plain | 1 ea | 43 | 120 | 4 | 21 | 1 | 2 | 0.5 | 0 |
| 42115 | Cornbread, prepared from dry mix | 1 pce | 60 | 188 | 4 | 29 | 1 | 6 | 1.6 | 37 |
| 71227 | Pita bread, white, enriched | 1 ea | 28 | 77 | 3 | 16 | 1 | 0 | 0 | 0 |
| 71228 | Pita bread, whole wheat | 1 ea | 28 | 74 | 3 | 15 | 2 | 1 | 0.1 | 0 |
| 71368 | Roll, dinner, plain, homemade w/ reduced fat (2%) milk | 1 ea | 43 | 136 | 4 | 23 | 1 | 3 | 0.8 | 15 |
| 42161 | Roll, French | 1 ea | 38 | 105 | 3 | 19 | 1 | 2 | 0.4 | 0 |
| 71056 | Roll, hard/kaiser | 1 ea | 57 | 167 | 6 | 30 | 1 | 2 | 0.3 | 0 |
| 42297 | Tortilla, corn, w/o salt, ready to cook | 1 ea | 26 | 58 | 1 | 12 | 1 | 1 | 0.1 | 0 |
| 90645 | Taco shell, baked | 1 ea | 5 | 23 | 0 | 3 | 0 | 1 | 0.3 | 0 |
| *Crackers* | | | | | | | | | | |
| 71451 | Cheez-its/Goldfish crackers, low sodium | 55 pce | 33 | 166 | 3 | 19 | 1 | 8 | 3.2 | 4 |
| 43507 | Oyster/soda/soup crackers | 1 cup | 45 | 189 | 4 | 33 | 1 | 4 | 0.9 | 0 |
| 70963 | Ritz crackers/Nabisco | 5 ea | 16 | 79 | 1 | 10 | 0 | 4 | 0.9 | |
| 43587 | Saltine crackers, original premium/Nabisco | 5 ea | 14 | 56 | 1 | 10 | 0 | 1 | 0 | 0 |
| 43545 | Sandwich crackers, cheese filled | 4 ea | 28 | 134 | 3 | 17 | 1 | 6 | 1.7 | 1 |
| 43546 | Sandwich crackers, peanut butter filled | 4 ea | 28 | 138 | 3 | 16 | 1 | 7 | 1.4 | 0 |
| 44677 | Snackwell Wheat Cracker/Nabisco | 1 ea | 15 | 62 | 1 | 12 | 1 | 2 | | |
| 43581 | Wheat Thins, baked/Nabisco | 16 ea | 29 | 140 | 3 | 20 | 1 | 6 | 0.9 | 0 |
| 43508 | Whole wheat cracker | 4 ea | 32 | 137 | 3 | 22 | 3 | 5 | 0.7 | 0 |

| MDA Code | Food Name | Amt | Wt (g) | Ener (kcal) | Prot (g) | Carb (g) | Fiber (g) | Fat (g) | Sat (g) | Chol (g) |
|---|---|---|---|---|---|---|---|---|---|---|
| *Muffins and Baked Goods* | | | | | | | | | | |
| 42723 | English muffin, plain | 1 ea | 57 | 132 | 5 | 26 | | 1 | 0.2 | |
| 62916 | Muffin, blueberry, commercially prepared | 1 ea | 11 | 43 | 1 | 5 | 0 | 2 | 0.4 | 4 |
| 44521 | Muffin, corn, commercially prepared | 1 ea | 57 | 174 | 3 | 29 | 2 | 5 | 0.8 | 15 |
| 44514 | Muffin, oatbran | 1 ea | 57 | 154 | 4 | 28 | 3 | 4 | 0.6 | 0 |
| 44518 | Toaster muffin, blueberry | 1 ea | 33 | 103 | 2 | 18 | 1 | 3 | 0.5 | 2 |
| *Noodles and Pasta* | | | | | | | | | | |
| 38048 | Chow mein noodles, dry | 1 cup | 45 | 237 | 4 | 26 | 2 | 14 | 2 | 0 |
| 38047 | Egg noodles, enriched, cooked | 0.5 cup | 80 | 110 | 4 | 20 | 1 | 2 | 0.3 | 23 |
| 38060 | Spaghetti, whole wheat, cooked | 1 cup | 140 | 174 | 7 | 37 | 6 | 1 | 0.1 | 0 |
| 38251 | Egg noodles, enriched, cooked w/ salt | 0.5 cup | 80 | 110 | 4 | 20 | 1 | 2 | | 23 |
| 38102 | Macaroni noodles, enriched, cooked | 1 cup | 140 | 221 | 8 | 43 | 3 | 1 | 0.2 | 0 |
| 38118 | Spaghetti noodles, enriched, cooked | 0.5 cup | 70 | 111 | 4 | 22 | 1 | 1 | 0.1 | 0 |
| *Grains* | | | | | | | | | | |
| 38076 | Couscous, cooked | 0.5 cup | 78 | 88 | 3 | 18 | 1 | 0 | 0 | 0 |
| 38080 | Oats | 0.25 cup | 39 | 152 | 7 | 26 | 4 | 3 | 0.5 | 0 |
| 38010 | Rice, brown, long grain, cooked | 1 cup | 195 | 216 | 5 | 45 | 4 | 2 | 0.4 | 0 |
| 38256 | Rice, white, long grain, enriched, cooked w/ salt | 1 cup | 158 | 205 | 4 | 45 | 1 | 0 | 0.1 | 0 |
| 38019 | Rice, white, long grain, instant, enriched, cooked | 1 cup | 165 | 193 | 4 | 41 | 1 | 1 | 0 | 0 |
| *Pancakes, French Toast, and Waffles* | | | | | | | | | | |
| 42156 | French toast, homemade, w/reduced fat (2%) milk | 1 pce | 65 | 149 | 5 | 16 | | 7 | 1.8 | 75 |
| 45192 | Pancake/waffle, buttermilk/Eggo/Kellogg | 1 ea | 42 | 99 | 3 | 16 | 0 | 3 | 0.6 | 5 |
| 45117 | Pancakes, plain, homemade | 1 ea | 77 | 175 | 5 | 22 | 1 | 7 | 1.6 | 45 |
| 45193 | Waffle, lowfat, homestyle, frozen | 1 ea | 35 | 83 | 2 | 15 | 0 | 1 | 0.3 | 9 |
| **Meat and Meat Substitutes** | | | | | | | | | | |
| *Beef* | | | | | | | | | | |
| 10093 | Beef, average of all cuts, lean & fat (1/4" trim), cooked | 3 oz | 85 | 260 | 22 | 0 | 0 | 18 | 7.3 | 75 |
| 10705 | Beef, average of all cuts, lean (1/4" trim), cooked | 3 oz | 85 | 184 | 25 | 0 | 0 | 8 | 3.2 | 73 |
| 10133 | Beef, whole rib, roasted, 1/4" trim | 3 oz | 85 | 305 | 19 | 0 | 0 | 25 | 10 | 71 |
| 58129 | Ground beef (hamburger), 25% fat, cooked, pan-browned | 3 oz | 85 | 236 | 22 | 0 | 0 | 15 | 6 | 76 |
| 58119 | Ground beef (hamburger), 15% fat, cooked, pan-browned | 3 oz | 85 | 218 | 24 | 0 | 0 | 13 | 5 | 77 |
| 58109 | Ground beef (hamburger), 5% fat, cooked, pan-browned | 3 oz | 85 | 164 | 25 | 0 | 0 | 6 | 2.9 | 76 |
| 10791 | Porterhouse steak, lean & fat (1/4" trim), broiled | 3 oz | 85 | 280 | 19 | 0 | 0 | 22 | 8.7 | 61 |
| 58257 | Rib eye steak, small end (ribs 10–12), 0" trim, broiled | 3 oz | 85 | 210 | 23 | 0 | 0 | 13 | 4.9 | 94 |
| 58094 | Skirt steak, trimmed to 0" fat, broiled | 3 oz | 85 | 187 | 22 | 0 | 0 | 10 | 4 | 51 |
| 58328 | Strip steak, top loin, 1/8" trim, broiled | 3 oz | 85 | 171 | 25 | 0 | 0 | 7 | 2.7 | 67 |
| 10805 | T-Bone steak, lean & fat (1/4" trim), broiled | 3 oz | 85 | 260 | 20 | 0 | 0 | 19 | 7.6 | 55 |
| 11531 | Veal, average of all cuts, cooked | 3 oz | 85 | 197 | 26 | 0 | 0 | 10 | 3.6 | 97 |
| *Chicken* | | | | | | | | | | |
| 15057 | Chicken breast, w/o skin, fried | 3 oz | 85 | 159 | 28 | 0 | 0 | 4 | 1.1 | 77 |
| 15080 | Chicken, dark meat, w/ skin, roasted | 3 oz | 85 | 215 | 22 | 0 | 0 | 13 | 3.7 | 77 |
| 15026 | Chicken, dark meat, w/o skin, fried | 3 oz | 85 | 203 | 25 | 2 | 0 | 10 | 2.7 | 82 |
| 15042 | Chicken drumstick, w/o skin, fried | 3 oz | 85 | 166 | 24 | 0 | 0 | 7 | 1.8 | 80 |
| 15048 | Chicken, wing, w/o skin, fried | 3 oz | 85 | 180 | 26 | 0 | 0 | 8 | 2.1 | 71 |
| 15059 | Chicken, wing, w/o skin, roasted | 3 oz | 85 | 173 | 26 | 0 | 0 | 7 | 1.9 | 72 |
| *Turkey* | | | | | | | | | | |
| 51151 | Turkey bacon, cooked | 1 oz | 28 | 108 | 8 | 1 | 0 | 8 | 2.4 | 28 |
| 51098 | Turkey patty, breaded, fried | 1 ea | 42 | 119 | 6 | 7 | 0 | 8 | 2 | 32 |
| 16110 | Turkey breast w/ skin, roasted | 3 oz | 85 | 130 | 25 | 0 | 0 | 3 | 0.7 | 77 |
| 16038 | Turkey breast, no skin, roasted | 3 oz | 85 | 115 | 26 | 0 | 0 | 1 | 0.2 | 71 |
| 16101 | Turkey, dark meat w/ skin, roasted | 3 oz | 85 | 155 | 24 | 0 | 0 | 6 | 1.8 | 100 |
| 16003 | Turkey, ground, cooked | 1 ea | 82 | 193 | 22 | 0 | 0 | 11 | 2.8 | 84 |
| *Lamb* | | | | | | | | | | |
| 13604 | Lamb, average of all cuts (1/4" trim), cooked | 3 oz | 85 | 250 | 21 | 0 | 0 | 18 | 7.5 | 83 |
| 13616 | Lamb, average of all cuts, lean (1/4" trim), cooked | 3 oz | 85 | 175 | 24 | 0 | 0 | 8 | 2.9 | 78 |

| MDA Code | Food Name | Amt | Wt (g) | Ener (kcal) | Prot (g) | Carb (g) | Fiber (g) | Fat (g) | Sat (g) | Chol (g) |
|---|---|---|---|---|---|---|---|---|---|---|
| *Pork* | | | | | | | | | | |
| 12000 | Bacon, broiled, pan-fried, or roasted | 3 pcs | 19 | 103 | 7 | 0 | 0 | 8 | 2.6 | 21 |
| 28143 | Canadian bacon | 1 pce | 56 | 68 | 9 | 1 | | 3 | 1 | 27 |
| 12211 | Ham, cured, boneless, regular fat (11% fat), roasted | 1 cup | 140 | 249 | 32 | 0 | 0 | 13 | 4.4 | 83 |
| 12309 | Pork, average of retail cuts, cooked | 3 oz | 85 | 203 | 22 | 0 | 0 | 12 | 4.2 | 75 |
| 12097 | Pork, ribs, backribs, roasted | 3 oz | 85 | 315 | 21 | 0 | 0 | 25 | 9.4 | 100 |
| 12099 | Pork, ground, cooked | 3 oz | 85 | 253 | 22 | 0 | 0 | 18 | 6.6 | 80 |
| *Lunchmeats* | | | | | | | | | | |
| 13000 | Beef, thin slices | 1 oz | 28 | 33 | 5 | 1 | 0 | 1 | 0.3 | 14 |
| 58275 | Bologna, beef and pork, low fat | 1 ea | 14 | 32 | 2 | 0 | 0 | 3 | 1 | 5 |
| 13157 | Chicken breast, oven roasted deluxe | 1 oz | 28 | 29 | 5 | 1 | 0 | 1 | 0.2 | 14 |
| 13306 | Corned beef, cooked, chopped, pressed | 1 ea | 71 | 101 | 14 | 1 | 0 | 5 | 2 | 46 |
| 13264 | Ham, slices, regular (11% fat) | 1 cup | 135 | 220 | 22 | 5 | 2 | 12 | 4 | 77 |
| 13101 | Pastrami, beef, cured | 1 oz | 28 | 42 | 6 | 0 | 0 | 2 | 0.8 | 19 |
| 13215 | Salami, beef, cotto | 1 oz | 28 | 59 | 4 | 1 | 0 | 4 | 1.9 | 24 |
| 16160 | Turkey breast slice | 1 pce | 21 | 22 | 4 | 1 | 0 | 0 | 0.1 | 9 |
| 58279 | Turkey ham, sliced, extra lean, prepackaged or deli-sliced | 1 cup | 138 | 171 | 27 | 4 | 0 | 5 | 1.5 | 92 |
| *Sausage* | | | | | | | | | | |
| 13070 | Chorizo, pork & beef | 1 ea | 60 | 273 | 14 | 1 | 0 | 23 | 8.6 | 53 |
| 57877 | Frankfurter, beef | 1 ea | 45 | 148 | 5 | 2 | 0 | 13 | 5.3 | 24 |
| 13012 | Frankfurter, turkey | 1 ea | 45 | 100 | 6 | 2 | 0 | 8 | 1.8 | 35 |
| 57890 | Italian sausage, pork, cooked | 1 ea | 83 | 286 | 16 | 4 | 0 | 23 | 8 | 47 |
| 13021 | Pepperoni sausage | 1 pce | 6 | 27 | 1 | 0 | 0 | 2 | 0.8 | 6 |
| 13185 | Pork sausage links, cooked | 2 ea | 48 | 165 | 8 | 0 | 0 | 15 | 5.1 | 37 |
| 58227 | Sausage, pork, precooked | 3 oz | 85 | 321 | 12 | 0 | 0 | 30 | 9.9 | 63 |
| 58007 | Turkey sausage, breakfast links, mild | 2 ea | 56 | 132 | 9 | 1 | 0 | 10 | 2.1 | 90 |
| *Meat Substitutes* | | | | | | | | | | |
| 7509 | Bacon substitute, vegetarian, strips | 3 ea | 15 | 46 | 2 | 1 | 0 | 4 | 0.7 | 0 |
| 7722 | Garden patties, frozen/Worthington, Morningstar | 1 ea | 67 | 118 | 12 | 9 | 3 | 4 | 0.5 | 1 |
| 7674 | Harvest burger, original flavor, vegetable protein patty | 1 ea | 90 | 138 | 18 | 7 | 6 | 4 | 1 | 0 |
| 90626 | Sausage, vegetarian, meatless | 1 ea | 28 | 72 | 5 | 3 | 1 | 5 | 0.8 | 0 |
| 7726 | Spicy Black Bean Burger/Worthington, Morningstar | 1 ea | 78 | 133 | 13 | 15 | 5 | 4 | 0.6 | 1 |
| **Nuts** | | | | | | | | | | |
| 4519 | Cashews, dry roasted w/ salt | 0.25 cup | 34 | 196 | 5 | 11 | 1 | 16 | 3.1 | 0 |
| 4728 | Macadamia nuts, dry roasted, unsalted | 1 cup | 134 | 962 | 10 | 18 | 11 | 102 | 16 | 0 |
| 4592 | Mixed nuts, w/ peanuts, dry roasted, salted | 0.25 cup | 34 | 203 | 6 | 9 | 3 | 18 | 2.4 | 0 |
| 4626 | Peanut butter, chunky w/ salt | 2 Tbs | 32 | 188 | 8 | 7 | 3 | 16 | 2.6 | 0 |
| 4756 | Peanuts, dry roasted w/o salt | 30 ea | 30 | 176 | 7 | 6 | 2 | 15 | 2.1 | 0 |
| 4696 | Peanuts, raw | 0.25 cup | 36 | 207 | 9 | 6 | 3 | 18 | 2.5 | 0 |
| 4540 | Pistachio nuts, dry roasted, salted | 0.25 cup | 32 | 182 | 7 | 9 | 3 | 15 | 1.8 | 0 |
| **Seafood** | | | | | | | | | | |
| 17029 | Bass, freshwater, cooked w/ dry heat | 3 oz | 85 | 124 | 21 | 0 | 0 | 4 | 0.9 | 74 |
| 17037 | Cod, Atlantic, baked/broiled (dry heat) | 3 oz | 85 | 89 | 19 | 0 | 0 | 1 | 0.1 | 47 |
| 19036 | Crab, Alaskan King, boiled/steamed | 3 oz | 85 | 83 | 16 | 0 | 0 | 1 | 0.1 | 45 |
| 17090 | Haddock, baked or broiled (dry heat) | 3 oz | 85 | 95 | 21 | 0 | 0 | 1 | 0.1 | 63 |
| 17291 | Halibut, Atlantic & Pacific, baked or broiled (dry heat) | 3 oz | 85 | 119 | 23 | 0 | 0 | 3 | 0.4 | 35 |
| 17181 | Salmon, Atlantic, farmed, cooked w/ dry heat | 3 oz | 85 | 175 | 19 | 0 | 0 | 11 | 2.1 | 54 |
| 17099 | Salmon, Sockeye, baked or broiled (dry heat) | 3 oz | 85 | 184 | 23 | 0 | 0 | 9 | 1.6 | 74 |
| 71707 | Squid, fried | 3 oz | 85 | 149 | 15 | 7 | 0 | 6 | 1.6 | 221 |
| 17066 | Swordfish, baked or broiled (dry heat) | 3 oz | 85 | 132 | 22 | 0 | 0 | 4 | 1.2 | 43 |
| 56007 | Tuna salad, lunchmeat spread | 2 Tbs | 26 | 48 | 4 | 2 | 0 | 2 | 0.4 | 3 |
| 17151 | White tuna, canned in water, drained | 3 oz | 85 | 109 | 20 | 0 | 0 | 3 | 0.7 | 36 |
| 17083 | White tuna, canned in oil, drained | 3 oz | 85 | 158 | 23 | 0 | 0 | 7 | 1.1 | 26 |

| MDA Code | Food Name | Amt | Wt (g) | Ener (kcal) | Prot (g) | Carb (g) | Fiber (g) | Fat (g) | Sat (g) | Chol (g) |
|---|---|---|---|---|---|---|---|---|---|---|
| **Vegetables and Legumes** | | | | | | | | | | |
| *Beans* | | | | | | | | | | |
| 7038 | Baked beans, plain or vegetarian, canned | 1 cup | 254 | 239 | 12 | 54 | 10 | 1 | 0.2 | 0 |
| 5197 | Bean sprouts, mung, canned, drained | 1 cup | 125 | 15 | 2 | 3 | 1 | 0 | 0 | 0 |
| 7012 | Black beans, boiled w/o salt | 1 cup | 172 | 227 | 15 | 41 | 15 | 1 | 0.2 | 0 |
| 5862 | Beets, boiled w/ salt, drained | 0.5 cup | 85 | 37 | 1 | 8 | 2 | 0 | 0 | 0 |
| 90018 | Cowpeas, cooked w/ salt | 1 cup | 171 | 198 | 13 | 35 | 11 | 1 | 0.2 | 0 |
| 7081 | Hummus, garbanzo or chickpea spread, homemade | 1 Tbs | 15 | 27 | 1 | 3 | 1 | 1 | 0.2 | 0 |
| 7087 | Kidney beans, canned | 1 cup | 256 | 215 | 13 | 37 | 14 | 2 | 0.3 | 0 |
| 7006 | Lentils, boiled w/o salt | 1 cup | 198 | 230 | 18 | 40 | 16 | 1 | 0.1 | 0 |
| 7051 | Pinto beans, canned | 1 cup | 240 | 206 | 12 | 37 | 11 | 2 | 0.4 | 0 |
| 6748 | Snap green beans, raw | 10 ea | 55 | 17 | 1 | 4 | 1 | 0 | 0 | 0 |
| 5320 | Snap yellow beans, raw | 0.5 cup | 55 | 17 | 1 | 4 | 2 | 0 | 0 | 0 |
| 90026 | Split peas, boiled w/ salt | 0.5 cup | 98 | 114 | 8 | 20 | 8 | 0 | 0.1 | 0 |
| 7054 | White beans, canned | 1 cup | 262 | 299 | 19 | 56 | 13 | 1 | 0.2 | 0 |
| *Fresh Vegetables* | | | | | | | | | | |
| 9577 | Artichokes (globe or French) boiled w/ salt, drained | 1 ea | 20 | 11 | 1 | 2 | 2 | 0 | 0 | 0 |
| 6033 | Arugula/roquette, raw | 1 cup | 20 | 5 | 1 | 1 | 0 | 0 | 0 | 0 |
| 90406 | Asparagus, raw | 10 ea | 35 | 7 | 1 | 1 | 1 | 0 | 0 | 0 |
| 5558 | Broccoli stalks, raw | 1 ea | 114 | 32 | 3 | 6 | 3 | 0 | 0.1 | 0 |
| 5036 | Cabbage, raw | 1 cup | 70 | 18 | 1 | 4 | 2 | 0 | 0 | 0 |
| 90605 | Carrots, baby, raw | 1 ea | 15 | 5 | 0 | 1 | 0 | 0 | 0 | 0 |
| 5049 | Cauliflower, raw | 0.5 cup | 50 | 12 | 1 | 2 | 1 | 0 | 0 | 0 |
| 90436 | Celery, raw | 1 ea | 17 | 3 | 0 | 1 | 0 | 0 | 0 | 0 |
| 7202 | Corn, white, sweet, ears, raw | 1 ea | 73 | 63 | 2 | 14 | 2 | 1 | 0.1 | 0 |
| 5900 | Corn, yellow, sweet, boiled w/ salt, drained | 0.5 cup | 82 | 79 | 3 | 17 | 2 | 1 | 0.2 | 0 |
| 5908 | Eggplant (brinjal) boiled w/ salt, drained | 1 cup | 99 | 33 | 1 | 8 | 2 | 0 | 0 | 0 |
| 5087 | Lettuce, looseleaf, raw | 2 pcs | 20 | 3 | 0 | 1 | 0 | 0 | 0 | 0 |
| 51069 | Mushrooms, brown, Italian, or crimini, raw | 2 ea | 28 | 6 | 1 | 1 | 0 | 0 | 0 | 0 |
| 90472 | Onions, chopped, raw | 1 ea | 70 | 28 | 1 | 7 | 1 | 0 | 0 | 0 |
| 5116 | Peas, green, raw | 1 cup | 145 | 117 | 8 | 21 | 7 | 1 | 0.1 | 0 |
| 7932 | Peppers, jalapeno, raw | 1 cup | 90 | 27 | 1 | 5 | 2 | 1 | 0.1 | 0 |
| 90493 | Peppers, sweet green, chopped/sliced, raw | 10 pcs | 27 | 5 | 0 | 1 | 0 | 0 | 0 | 0 |
| 6990 | Pepper, sweet red, raw | 1 ea | 10 | 3 | 0 | 1 | 0 | 0 | 0 | 0 |
| 9251 | Potatoes, red, flesh and skin, baked | 1 ea | 138 | 123 | 3 | 27 | 2 | 0 | 0 | 0 |
| 9245 | Potatoes, russet, flesh and skin, baked | 1 ea | 138 | 134 | 4 | 30 | 3 | 0 | 0 | 0 |
| 5146 | Spinach, raw | 1 cup | 30 | 7 | 1 | 1 | 1 | 0 | 0 | 0 |
| 90525 | Squash, zucchini w/ skin, slices, raw | 1 ea | 118 | 20 | 1 | 4 | 1 | 0 | 0.1 | 0 |
| 6924 | Sweet potato, baked in skin w/ salt | 0.5 cup | 100 | 92 | 2 | 21 | 3 | 0 | 0.1 | 0 |
| 5180 | Tomato sauce, canned | 0.5 cup | 123 | 30 | 2 | 7 | 2 | 0 | 0 | 0 |
| 90532 | Tomato, red, ripe, whole, raw | 1 pce | 15 | 3 | 0 | 1 | 0 | 0 | 0 | 0 |
| 5306 | Yam, peeled, raw | 0.5 cup | 75 | 88 | 1 | 21 | 3 | 0 | 0 | 0 |
| *Soy and Soy Products* | | | | | | | | | | |
| 7564 | Tempeh | 0.5 cup | 83 | 160 | 15 | 8 | | 9 | 1.8 | 0 |
| 7015 | Soybeans, cooked | 1 cup | 172 | 298 | 29 | 17 | 10 | 15 | 2.2 | 0 |
| 7542 | Tofu, firm, silken, 1" slice | 3 oz | 85 | 53 | 6 | 2 | 0 | 2 | 0.3 | 0 |
| **Meals and Dishes** | | | | | | | | | | |
| 92216 | Tortellini with cheese filling | 1 cup | 108 | 332 | 15 | 51 | 2 | 8 | 3.9 | 45 |
| 57658 | Chili con carne w/ beans, canned entree | 1 cup | 222 | 269 | 16 | 25 | 9 | 12 | 3.9 | 29 |
| 57703 | Chili, vegetarian chili w/ beans, canned entree/Hormel | 1 cup | 247 | 205 | 12 | 38 | 10 | 1 | 0.1 | 0 |
| 57068 | Macaroni and cheese, unprepared/Kraft | 1 ea | 70 | 260 | 9 | 48 | 1 | 4 | 2 | 15 |
| 70958 | Stir fry, rice & vegetables, w/ soy sauce/Hanover | 1 cup | 137 | 130 | 5 | 27 | 2 | 0 | | |
| 70943 | Beef & bean burrito/Las Campanas | 1 ea | 114 | 296 | 9 | 38 | 1 | 12 | 4.2 | 13 |
| 16195 | Chicken & vegetables/Lean Cuisine | 1 ea | 297 | 232 | 20 | 26 | 4 | 5 | 1.9 | 30 |
| 70917 | Hot Pockets, beef & cheddar, frozen | 1 ea | 142 | 403 | 16 | 39 | | 20 | 8.8 | 53 |
| 70918 | Hot Pockets, croissant pocket w/ chicken, broccoli, & cheddar, frozen | 1 ea | 128 | 301 | 11 | 39 | 1 | 11 | 3.4 | 37 |

| MDA Code | Food Name | Amt | Wt (g) | Ener (kcal) | Prot (g) | Carb (g) | Fiber (g) | Fat (g) | Sat (g) | Chol (g) |
|---|---|---|---|---|---|---|---|---|---|---|
| 56757 | Lasagna w/ meat sauce/Stouffer's | 1 ea | 215 | 249 | 17 | 27 | 2 | 8 | 4.1 | 28 |
| 11029 | Macaroni & beef in tomato sauce/Lean Cuisine | 1 ea | 283 | 326 | 21 | 40 | 3 | 9 | 3.7 | 32 |
| 5587 | Mashed potatoes, from granules w/ milk, prep w/ water & margarine | 0.5 cup | 105 | 122 | 2 | 17 | 1 | 5 | 1.2 | 2 |
| 70898 | Pizza, pepperoni, frozen | 1 ea | 146 | 432 | 16 | 42 | 3 | 22 | 7 | 22 |
| 56703 | Spaghetti w/ meat sauce/Lean Cuisine | 1 ea | 326 | 284 | 14 | 49 | 5 | 4 | 1.1 | 13 |

**Snack Foods**

| MDA Code | Food Name | Amt | Wt (g) | Ener (kcal) | Prot (g) | Carb (g) | Fiber (g) | Fat (g) | Sat (g) | Chol (g) |
|---|---|---|---|---|---|---|---|---|---|---|
| 10051 | Beef jerky | 1 pce | 20 | 81 | 7 | 2 | 0 | 5 | 2.1 | 10 |
| 63331 | Breakfast bars, oats, sugar, raisins, coconut | 1 ea | 43 | 200 | 4 | 29 | 1 | 8 | 5.5 | 0 |
| 61251 | Cheese puffs and twists, corn based, low fat | 1 oz | 28 | 123 | 2 | 21 | 3 | 3 | 0.6 | 0 |
| 44032 | Chex snack mix | 1 cup | 42 | 180 | 4 | 32 | 2 | 4 | 0.6 | |
| 23059 | Granola bar, hard, plain | 1 ea | 24 | 115 | 2 | 16 | 1 | 5 | 0.6 | 0 |
| 23104 | Granola bar, soft, plain | 1 ea | 28 | 126 | 2 | 19 | 1 | 5 | 2.1 | 0 |
| 44012 | Popcorn, air-popped | 1 cup | 8 | 31 | 1 | 6 | 1 | 0 | 0 | 0 |
| 44076 | Potato chips, plain, no salt | 1 oz | 28 | 152 | 2 | 15 | 1 | 10 | 3.1 | 0 |
| 5437 | Potato chips, sour cream & onion | 1 oz | 28 | 151 | 2 | 15 | 1 | 10 | 2.5 | 2 |
| 44015 | Pretzels, hard | 5 pcs | 30 | 114 | 3 | 24 | 1 | 1 | 0.1 | 0 |
| 44021 | Rice cake, brown rice, plain, salted | 1 ea | 9 | 35 | 1 | 7 | 0 | 0 | 0.1 | 0 |
| 44058 | Trail mix, regular | 0.25 cup | 38 | 173 | 5 | 17 | | 11 | 2.1 | 0 |

**Soups**

| MDA Code | Food Name | Amt | Wt (g) | Ener (kcal) | Prot (g) | Carb (g) | Fiber (g) | Fat (g) | Sat (g) | Chol (g) |
|---|---|---|---|---|---|---|---|---|---|---|
| 50398 | Beef barley, canned/Progresso Healthy Classics | 1 cup | 241 | 142 | 11 | 20 | 3 | 2 | 0.7 | 19 |
| 50081 | Chicken noodle, chunky, canned | 1 cup | 240 | 89 | 8 | 10 | 1 | 2 | 1 | 12 |
| 50085 | Chicken rice, chunky, ready to eat, canned | 1 cup | 240 | 127 | 12 | 13 | 1 | 3 | 1 | 12 |
| 50088 | Chicken vegetable, chunky, canned | 1 cup | 240 | 166 | 12 | 19 | | 5 | 1.4 | 17 |
| 90238 | Chicken, chunky, canned | 1 cup | 240 | 170 | 12 | 17 | 1 | 6 | 1.9 | 29 |
| 50697 | Cup of Noodles, ramen, chicken flavor, dry/Nissin | 1 ea | 64 | 296 | 6 | 37 | | 14 | 6.3 | |
| 50009 | Minestrone, canned, made w/ water | 1 cup | 241 | 82 | 4 | 11 | 1 | 3 | 0.6 | 2 |
| 92163 | Ramen noodle, any flavor, dehydrated, dry | 0.5 cup | 38 | 166 | 4 | 24 | 1 | 6 | 2.9 | 0 |
| 50043 | Tomato vegetable, from dry mix, made w/ water | 1 cup | 253 | 56 | 2 | 10 | 1 | 1 | 0.4 | 0 |
| 50028 | Tomato, canned, made w/ water | 1 cup | 244 | 73 | 2 | 16 | 1 | 1 | 0.2 | 0 |
| 50014 | Vegetable beef, canned, made w/ water | 1 cup | 244 | 76 | 5 | 10 | 2 | 2 | 0.8 | 5 |
| 50013 | Vegetarian vegetable, canned, made w/ water | 1 cup | 241 | 67 | 2 | 12 | 1 | 2 | 0.3 | 0 |

**Desserts**

| MDA Code | Food Name | Amt | Wt (g) | Ener (kcal) | Prot (g) | Carb (g) | Fiber (g) | Fat (g) | Sat (g) | Chol (g) |
|---|---|---|---|---|---|---|---|---|---|---|
| 62904 | Brownie, commercially prepared, square, lrg, 2-3/4" × 7/8" | 1 ea | 56 | 227 | 3 | 36 | 1 | 9 | 2.4 | 10 |
| 46062 | Cake, chocolate, homemade, w/o icing | 1 pce | 95 | 352 | 5 | 51 | 2 | 14 | 5.2 | 55 |
| 46091 | Cake, yellow, homemade, w/o icing | 1 pce | 68 | 245 | 4 | 36 | 0 | 10 | 2.7 | 37 |
| 71337 | Doughnut, cake, w/ chocolate icing, lrg, 3 1/2" | 1 ea | 57 | 258 | 3 | 29 | 1 | 14 | 7.7 | 11 |
| 45525 | Doughnut, cake, glazed/sugared, med, 3" | 1 ea | 45 | 192 | 2 | 23 | 1 | 10 | 2.7 | 14 |
| 47026 | Animal crackers/Arrowroot/Tea Biscuits | 10 ea | 12 | 56 | 1 | 9 | 0 | 2 | 0.4 | 0 |
| 90636 | Chocolate chip cookie, commercially prepared 3.5" to 4" | 1 ea | 40 | 190 | 2 | 26 | 1 | 9 | 4 | 0 |
| 47006 | Chocolate sandwich cookie, creme filled | 3 ea | 30 | 141 | 2 | 21 | 1 | 6 | 1.9 | 0 |
| 62905 | Fig bar, 2 oz | 1 ea | 57 | 197 | 2 | 40 | 3 | 4 | 0.6 | 0 |
| 90640 | Oatmeal cookie, commercially prepared, 3-1/2" to 4" | 1 ea | 25 | 112 | 2 | 17 | 1 | 5 | 1.1 | 0 |
| 47010 | Peanut butter cookie, homemade, 3" | 1 ea | 20 | 95 | 2 | 12 | | 5 | 0.9 | 6 |
| 62907 | Sugar cookie, refrigerated dough, baked | 1 ea | 23 | 111 | 1 | 15 | 0 | 5 | 1.4 | 7 |
| 57894 | Pudding, chocolate, ready to eat | 1 ea | 113 | 160 | 2 | 26 | 0 | 5 | 1.4 | 1 |
| 2612 | Pudding, vanilla, ready to eat | 1 ea | 113 | 147 | 2 | 26 | 0 | 4 | 1.1 | 1 |
| 2651 | Rice pudding, ready to eat | 1 ea | 142 | 168 | 5 | 28 | 1 | 4 | 2.5 | 26 |
| 57902 | Tapioca pudding, ready to eat | 1 ea | 113 | 147 | 2 | 25 | 0 | 4 | 1.1 | 1 |
| 71819 | Frozen yogurts, chocolate, nonfat | 1 cup | 186 | 199 | 8 | 37 | 4 | 1 | 0.9 | 7 |
| 72124 | Frozen yogurts, flavors other than chocolate | 1 cup | 174 | 221 | 5 | 38 | 0 | 6 | 4 | 23 |
| 2010 | Ice cream, light, vanilla, soft serve | 0.5 cup | 88 | 111 | 4 | 19 | 0 | 2 | 1.4 | 11 |
| 90723 | Ice popsicle | 1 ea | 59 | 47 | 0 | 11 | 0 | 0 | 0 | 0 |
| 42264 | Cinnamon rolls w/ icing, refrigerated dough/Pillsbury | 1 ea | 44 | 145 | 2 | 23 | 0 | 5 | 1.5 | 0 |
| 71299 | Croissant, butter | 1 ea | 67 | 272 | 5 | 31 | 2 | 14 | 7.8 | 45 |
| 45572 | Danish, cheese | 1 ea | 71 | 266 | 6 | 26 | 1 | 16 | 4.8 | 16 |
| 45593 | Toaster pastry, Pop Tart, apple-cinnamon/Kellogg | 1 ea | 52 | 205 | 2 | 37 | 1 | 5 | 0.9 | 0 |

| MDA Code | Food Name | Amt | Wt (g) | Ener (kcal) | Prot (g) | Carb (g) | Fiber (g) | Fat (g) | Sat (g) | Chol (g) |
|---|---|---|---|---|---|---|---|---|---|---|
| 23014 | Chocolate syrup, fudge-type | 2 Tbs | 38 | 133 | 2 | 24 | 1 | 3 | 1.5 | 0 |
| 510 | Whipped cream topping, pressurized | 2 Tbs | 8 | 19 | 0 | 1 | 0 | 2 | 1 | 6 |
| 54387 | Whipped topping, frozen, low fat | 2 Tbs | 9 | 21 | 0 | 2 | 0 | 1 | 1.1 | 0 |

**Fats, Oils, and Condiments**

| MDA Code | Food Name | Amt | Wt (g) | Ener (kcal) | Prot (g) | Carb (g) | Fiber (g) | Fat (g) | Sat (g) | Chol (g) |
|---|---|---|---|---|---|---|---|---|---|---|
| 90210 | Butter, unsalted | 1 Tbs | 14 | 100 | 0 | 0 | 0 | 11 | 7.2 | 30 |
| 8084 | Oil, vegetable, canola | 1 Tbs | 14 | 124 | 0 | 0 | 0 | 14 | 1 | 0 |
| 8008 | Oil, olive, salad or cooking | 1 Tbs | 14 | 119 | 0 | 0 | 0 | 14 | 1.9 | 0 |
| 8111 | Oil, safflower, salad or cooking, greater than 70% oleic | 1 Tbs | 14 | 120 | 0 | 0 | 0 | 14 | 0.8 | 0 |
| 44483 | Shortening, household | 1 Tbs | 13 | 113 | 0 | 0 | 0 | 13 | 3.2 | 0 |
| 1708 | Barbecue sauce, original | 2 Tbs | 36 | 63 | 0 | 15 | | 0 | | |
| 27001 | Ketchup | 1 ea | 6 | 6 | 0 | 2 | 0 | 0 | 0 | 0 |
| 53523 | Cheese sauce, ready to eat | 0.25 cup | 63 | 110 | 4 | 4 | 0 | 8 | 3.8 | 18 |
| 54388 | Cream substitute, powdered, light | 1 Tbs | 6 | 25 | 0 | 4 | 0 | 1 | 0.2 | 0 |
| 50939 | Gravy, brown, homestyle, canned | 0.25 cup | 60 | 25 | 1 | 3 | 0 | 1 | 0.3 | 2 |
| 23003 | Jelly | 1 Tbs | 19 | 51 | 0 | 13 | 0 | 0 | 0 | 0 |
| 25002 | Maple syrup | 1 Tbs | 20 | 52 | 0 | 13 | 0 | 0 | 0 | 0 |
| 44476 | Margarine, regular, 80% fat, with salt | 1 Tbs | 14 | 101 | 0 | 0 | 0 | 11 | 2 | 0 |
| 8145 | Mayonnaise, safflower/soybean oil | 1 Tbs | 14 | 99 | 0 | 0 | 0 | 11 | 1.2 | 8 |
| 8502 | Miracle Whip, light/Kraft | 1 Tbs | 16 | 37 | 0 | 2 | 0 | 3 | 0.5 | 4 |
| 435 | Mustard, yellow | 1 tsp | 5 | 3 | 0 | 0 | 0 | 0 | 0 | 0 |
| 23042 | Pancake syrup | 1 Tbs | 20 | 47 | 0 | 12 | 0 | 0 | 0 | 0 |
| 23172 | Pancake syrup, reduced kcal | 1 Tbs | 15 | 25 | 0 | 7 | 0 | 0 | 0 | 0 |
| 53524 | Pasta sauce, spaghetti/marinara | 0.5 cup | 125 | 109 | 2 | 17 | 3 | 3 | 0.9 | 2 |
| 53646 | Salsa picante, mild | 2 Tbs | 30 | 8 | 0 | 1 | 0 | 0 | | 0 |
| 504 | Sour cream, cultured | 2 Tbs | 29 | 56 | 1 | 1 | 0 | 6 | 3.3 | 15 |
| 53063 | Soy sauce | 1 Tbs | 18 | 11 | 2 | 1 | 0 | 0 | 0 | 0 |
| 53652 | Taco sauce, red, mild | 1 Tbs | 16 | 7 | 0 | 1 | 0 | 0 | | 0 |
| 53004 | Teriyaki sauce | 1 Tbs | 18 | 16 | 1 | 3 | 0 | 0 | 0 | 0 |
| 8024 | Thousand Island, regular | 1 Tbs | 16 | 58 | 0 | 2 | 0 | 5 | 0.8 | 4 |
| 8013 | Blue/Roquefort cheese, regular | 2 Tbs | 31 | 146 | 0 | 1 | 0 | 16 | 2.5 | 9 |
| 90232 | French, regular | 1 Tbs | 12 | 56 | 0 | 2 | 0 | 6 | 0.7 | 0 |
| 44498 | Italian, fat-free | 1 Tbs | 14 | 7 | 0 | 1 | 0 | 0 | 0 | 0 |
| 44696 | Ranch, reduced fat | 1 Tbs | 15 | 29 | 0 | 3 | 0 | 2 | 0.2 | 2 |
| 8035 | Vinegar & oil, homemade | 2 Tbs | 31 | 140 | 0 | 1 | 0 | 16 | 2.8 | 0 |

**Fast Food**

| MDA Code | Food Name | Amt | Wt (g) | Ener (kcal) | Prot (g) | Carb (g) | Fiber (g) | Fat (g) | Sat (g) | Chol (g) |
|---|---|---|---|---|---|---|---|---|---|---|
| 6177 | Baked potato, topped w/ cheese sauce | 1 ea | 296 | 474 | 15 | 47 | | 29 | 10.6 | 18 |
| 56629 | Burrito w/ beans & cheese | 1 ea | 93 | 189 | 8 | 27 | | 6 | 3.4 | 14 |
| 66023 | Burrito w/ beans, cheese, & beef | 1 ea | 102 | 166 | 7 | 20 | | 7 | 3.6 | 62 |
| 66024 | Burrito w/ beef | 1 ea | 110 | 262 | 13 | 29 | | 10 | 5.2 | 32 |
| 56600 | Biscuit w/ egg sandwich | 1 ea | 136 | 373 | 12 | 32 | 1 | 22 | 4.7 | 245 |
| 66029 | Biscuit w/ egg, cheese, & bacon sandwich | 1 ea | 144 | 433 | 17 | 35 | 0 | 25 | 8.5 | 239 |
| 66013 | Cheeseburger, double, condiments & vegetables | 1 ea | 166 | 417 | 21 | 35 | | 21 | 8.7 | 60 |
| 56649 | Cheeseburger, large, one meat patty w/ condiments & vegetables | 1 ea | 219 | 451 | 25 | 37 | 3 | 23 | 8.5 | 74 |
| 15063 | Chicken, breaded, fried, dark meat (drumstick or thigh) | 3 oz | 85 | 248 | 17 | 9 | | 15 | 4.1 | 95 |
| 15064 | Chicken, breaded, fried, light meat (breast or wing) | 3 oz | 85 | 258 | 19 | 10 | | 15 | 4.1 | 77 |
| 56000 | Chicken filet, plain | 1 ea | 182 | 515 | 24 | 39 | | 29 | 8.5 | 60 |
| 56635 | Chimichanga w/ beef & cheese | 1 ea | 183 | 443 | 20 | 39 | | 23 | 11.2 | 51 |
| 5461 | Cole slaw | 0.75 cup | 99 | 151 | 1 | 15 | 2 | 10 | 1.6 | 4 |
| 56606 | Croissant w/ egg & cheese sandwich | 1 ea | 127 | 368 | 13 | 24 | | 25 | 14.1 | 216 |
| 56607 | Croissant w/ egg, cheese, & bacon sandwich | 1 ea | 129 | 413 | 16 | 24 | | 28 | 15.4 | 215 |
| 66021 | Enchilada w/ cheese | 1 ea | 163 | 319 | 10 | 29 | | 19 | 10.6 | 44 |
| 66020 | Enchirito w/ cheese, beef, & beans | 1 ea | 193 | 344 | 18 | 34 | | 16 | 7.9 | 50 |
| 66031 | English muffin w/ cheese & sausage sandwich | 1 ea | 115 | 389 | 15 | 29 | 1 | 24 | 9.4 | 49 |
| 66010 | Fish sandwich w/ tartar sauce | 1 ea | 158 | 431 | 17 | 41 | | 23 | 5.2 | 55 |
| 90736 | French fries fried in vegetable oil, medium | 1 ea | 134 | 427 | 5 | 50 | 5 | 23 | 5.3 | 0 |
| 56638 | Frijoles (beans) w/ cheese | 0.5 cup | 84 | 113 | 6 | 14 | | 4 | 2 | 18 |

| MDA Code | Food Name | Amt | Wt (g) | Ener (kcal) | Prot (g) | Carb (g) | Fiber (g) | Fat (g) | Sat (g) | Chol (g) |
|---|---|---|---|---|---|---|---|---|---|---|
| 56664 | Ham & cheese sandwich | 1 ea | 146 | 352 | 21 | 33 | | 15 | 6.4 | 58 |
| 56662 | Hamburger, large, double, w/ condiments & vegetables | 1 ea | 226 | 540 | 34 | 40 | | 27 | 10.5 | 122 |
| 56659 | Hamburger, one patty w/ condiments & vegetables | 1 ea | 110 | 279 | 13 | 27 | | 13 | 4.1 | 26 |
| 66007 | Hamburger, plain | 1 ea | 90 | 266 | 13 | 30 | 1 | 10 | 3.2 | 30 |
| 5463 | Hash browns | 0.5 cup | 72 | 235 | 2 | 23 | 2 | 16 | 3.6 | 0 |
| 66004 | Hot dog, plain | 1 ea | 98 | 242 | 10 | 18 | | 15 | 5.1 | 44 |
| 2032 | Ice cream sundae, hot fudge | 1 ea | 158 | 284 | 6 | 48 | 0 | 9 | 5 | 21 |
| 6185 | Mashed potatoes | 0.5 cup | 121 | 100 | 3 | 20 | | 1 | 0.6 | 2 |
| 56639 | Nachos w/ cheese | 7 pcs | 113 | 346 | 9 | 36 | | 19 | 7.8 | 18 |
| 6176 | Onion rings, breaded, fried | 8 pcs | 78 | 259 | 3 | 29 | | 15 | 6.5 | 13 |
| 6173 | Potato salad | 0.33 cup | 95 | 108 | 1 | 13 | | 6 | 1 | 57 |
| 56619 | Pizza w/ pepperoni 12" or 1/8 | 1 pce | 108 | 275 | 15 | 30 | | 11 | 3.4 | 22 |
| 66003 | Roast beef sandwich, plain | 1 ea | 139 | 346 | 22 | 33 | | 14 | 3.6 | 51 |
| 56671 | Submarine sandwich, cold cuts | 1 ea | 228 | 456 | 22 | 51 | | 19 | 6.8 | 36 |
| 57531 | Taco | 1 ea | 171 | 371 | 21 | 27 | | 21 | 11.4 | 56 |
| 71129 | Shake, chocolate, 12 fl. oz | 1 ea | 250 | 318 | 8 | 51 | 5 | 9 | 5.8 | 32 |
| 71132 | Shake, vanilla, 12 fl. oz | 1 ea | 250 | 370 | 8 | 49 | 2 | 16 | 9.9 | 58 |

**Source:** This food composition table has been prepared for Pearson Education, Inc., and is copyrighted by ESHA Research in Salem, Oregon, the developer of the MyDietAnalysis software program.

# Glossary

**1 RM** *See* one repetition maximum.

**5-year survival rates** The percentage of people in a study or treatment group who are alive 5 years after they were diagnosed with or treated for a disease such as cancer.

**AA** *See* Alcoholics Anonymous.

**abortion** The termination of a pregnancy by expulsion or removal of an embryo or fetus from the uterus.

**abstinence** Refraining from a behavior.

**accountability** Accepting responsibility for personal decisions, choices, and actions.

**acid deposition** The acidification process that occurs when pollutants are deposited by precipitation, directly on the land, or by clouds.

**acquired immunodeficiency syndrome (AIDS)** A disease caused by a retrovirus, the human immunodeficiency virus (HIV), that attacks the immune system, reducing the number of helper T cells and leaving the victim vulnerable to infections, malignancies, and neurological disorders.

**active euthanasia** "Mercy killing" in which a person or organization knowingly acts to end the life of a terminally ill person.

**acupressure** Branch of traditional Chinese medicine related to acupuncture. Uses application of pressure to selected body points to balance energy.

**acupuncture** Branch of traditional Chinese medicine that uses the insertion of long, thin needles to affect flow of energy (*qi*) along pathways (meridians) within the body.

**acute stress** The short-term physiological response to an immediate perceived threat.

**AD** *See* Alzheimer's disease.

**adaptive response** Form of adjustment in which the body attempts to restore homeostasis.

**adaptive thermogenesis** Theoretical mechanism by which the brain regulates metabolic activity according to caloric intake.

**addiction** Persistent, compulsive dependence on a behavior or substance, including mood-altering behaviors or activities, despite ongoing negative consequences.

**adrenaline** *See* epinephrine.

**advance directive** A document that stipulates an individual's wishes about medical care; used to make treatment decisions when and if the individual becomes physically unable to voice their preferences.

**aerobic capacity** (or **power**) The functional status of the cardiorespiratory system; refers specifically to the volume of oxygen the muscles consume during exercise.

**aerobic exercise** Any type of exercise that increases heart rate.

**aggravated rape** Rape that involves one or multiple attackers, strangers, weapons, or physical beating.

**aging** The patterns of life changes that occur in members of all species as they grow older.

**AIDS** *See* acquired immunodeficiency syndrome.

**alcohol abuse** Use of alcohol that interferes with work, school, or personal relationships or that entails violations of the law.

**alcohol dependency** *See* alcoholism.

**alcohol poisoning** A potentially lethal blood alcohol concentration that inhibits the brain's ability to control consciousness, respiration, and heart rate; usually occurs as a result of drinking a large amount of alcohol in a short period of time. Also known as *acute alcohol intoxication*.

**alcoholic hepatitis** A condition resulting from prolonged use of alcohol in which the liver is inflamed; can be fatal.

**Alcoholics Anonymous (AA)** An organization whose goal is to help alcoholics stop drinking; includes auxiliary branches such as Al-Anon and Alateen.

**alcoholism (alcohol dependency)** Condition in which personal and health problems related to alcohol use are severe and stopping alcohol use results in withdrawal symptoms.

**allele** One of potentially several variants of the same gene.

**allergy** Hypersensitive reaction in which the body produces antibodies to a normally harmless substance in the environment.

**allopathic medicine** Conventional, Western medical practice; in theory, based on scientifically validated methods and procedures.

**allostatic load** Wear and tear on the body caused by prolonged or excessive stress responses.

**alternative insemination** Fertilization accomplished by depositing a partner's or a donor's semen into a woman's vagina via a thin tube; almost always done in a doctor's office.

**alternative (whole) medical systems** Complete systems of theory and practice that involve several CAM domains.

**alternative medicine** Treatment used in place of conventional medicine.

**altruism** The giving of oneself out of genuine concern for others.

**alveoli** Tiny air sacs of the lungs where gas exchange occurs (oxygen enters the blood and carbon dioxide is removed).

**Alzheimer's disease (AD)** A chronic condition involving changes in nerve fibers of the brain that results in mental deterioration.

**amino acids** The nitrogen-containing building blocks of protein.

**amniocentesis** A medical test in which a small amount of fluid is drawn from the amniotic sac to test for Down syndrome and other genetic diseases.

**amniotic sac** The protective pouch surrounding the fetus.

**amphetamines** A large and varied group of synthetic agents that stimulate the central nervous system.

**anabolic steroids** Artificial forms of the hormone testosterone that promote muscle growth and strength.

**anal intercourse** The insertion of the penis into the anus.

**androgyny** High levels of traditional masculine and feminine traits in a single person.

**anemia** Condition that results from the body's inability to produce hemoglobin.

**aneurysm** A weakened blood vessel that may bulge under pressure and, in severe cases, burst.

**angina pectoris** Chest pain occurring as a result of reduced oxygen flow to the heart.

**angiography** A technique for examining blockages in heart arteries.

**angioplasty** A technique in which a catheter with a balloon at the tip is inserted into a clogged artery; the balloon is inflated to flatten fatty deposits against artery walls and a stent is typically inserted to keep the artery open.

**anorexia nervosa** Eating disorder characterized by excessive preoccupation with food, self-starvation, or extreme exercising to achieve weight loss.

**ANS** *See* autonomic nervous system.

**antagonism** A drug interaction in which two drugs compete for the same available receptors, potentially blocking each other's actions.

**antibiotic resistance** The ability of bacteria or other microbes to withstand the effects of an antibiotic.

**antibiotics** Medicines used to kill microorganisms, such as bacteria.

**antibodies** Substances produced by the body that are individually matched to specific antigens.

**antigen** Substance capable of triggering an immune response.

**antioxidants** Substances believed to protect against oxidative stress and resultant tissue damage at the cellular level.

**anxiety disorders** Mental illnesses characterized by persistent feelings of threat and worry in coping with everyday problems.

**appetite** The desire to eat; normally accompanies hunger but is more psychological than physiological.

**appraisal** The interpretation and evaluation of information provided to the brain by the senses.

**arrhythmia** An irregularity in heartbeat.

**arteries** Vessels that carry blood away from the heart to other regions of the body.

**arterioles** Branches of the arteries.

**arthritis** Painful inflammatory disease of the joints.

**asbestos** A mineral compound that separates into stringy fibers and lodges in the lungs, where it can cause various diseases.

**asthma** A chronic respiratory disease characterized by attacks of wheezing, shortness of breath, and coughing spasms.

**atherosclerosis** Condition characterized by deposits of fatty substances (plaque) on the inner lining of an artery.

**atria** (singular: *atrium*) The heart's two upper chambers, which receive blood.

**autoerotic behaviors** Sexual self-stimulation.

**autoimmune disease** Disease caused by an overactive immune response against the body's own cells.

**autoinoculate** Transmit a pathogen from one part of your body to another part.

**autonomic nervous system (ANS)** The portion of the central nervous system regulating body functions that a person does not normally consciously control.

**autosomal dominant disorder** Single-gene disorder that occurs in individuals who have inherited at least one copy of an autosome with the affected dominant allele.

**autosomal recessive disorder** Single-gene disorder that occurs in individuals who have inherited two copies of an autosome with the affected recessive allele.

**Ayurveda (Ayurvedic medicine)** A comprehensive system of medicine, derived largely from ancient India, that places equal emphasis on the body, mind, and spirit, and strives to restore the body's innate harmony through diet, exercise, meditation, herbs, massage, exposure to sunlight, and controlled breathing.

**BAC** *See* blood alcohol concentration.

**background distressors** Environmental stressors of which people are often unaware.

**bacteria** (singular: *bacterium*) Simple, single-celled microscopic organisms; about 100 known species of bacteria cause disease in humans.

**barbiturates** Drugs that depress the central nervous system and have sedating, hypnotic, and anesthetic effects.

**barrier methods** Contraceptive methods that block the meeting of egg and sperm by means of a physical barrier (such as condom, diaphragm, or cervical cap), a chemical barrier (such as spermicide), or both.

**basal metabolic rate (BMR)** The rate of energy expenditure by a body at complete rest in a neutral environment.

**BDD** *See* body dysmorphic disorder.

**behavioral genetics** The science that studies the role of inheritance in human behavior.

**belief** Appraisal of the relationship between some object, action, or idea and some attribute of that object, action, or idea.

**benign** Harmless; refers to a noncancerous tumor.

**benzodiazepines** A class of central nervous system depressant drugs with sedative, hypnotic, and muscle relaxant effects.

**bereavement** The loss or deprivation experienced by a survivor when a loved one dies.

**bidis** Hand-rolled flavored cigarettes.

**binge drinking** *See* heavy episodic drinking.

**binge-eating disorder** A type of eating disorder characterized by binge eating once a week or more, but not typically followed by a compensatory behavior.

**biofeedback** A technique using a machine to self-monitor physical responses to stress.

**biologically based practices** Treatments using substances found in nature, such as herbs, special diets, or vitamin megadoses.

**biopsy** Microscopic examination of tissue to determine if a cancer is present.

**biopsychosocial model of addiction** Theory of the relationship between an addict's biological (genetic) nature and psychological and environmental influences.

**bipolar disorder** A form of mood disorder characterized by alternating mania and depression; also called manic depression.

**birth control** *See* contraception.

**bisexual** Experiencing attraction to and preference for sexual activity with people of both sexes.

**blood alcohol concentration (BAC)** The ratio of alcohol to total blood volume; the factor used to measure the physiological and behavioral effects of alcohol.

**BMI** *See* body mass index.

**BMR** *See* basal metabolic rate.

**body composition** Describes the relative proportions of fat and lean (muscle, bone, water, organs) tissues in the body.

**body dysmorphic disorder (BDD)** Psychological disorder characterized by an obsession with a minor or imagined flaw in appearance.

**body image** Most fundamentally, how you see yourself when you look in a mirror or picture yourself in your mind and how you feel about your body.

**body mass index (BMI)** A number calculated from a person's weight and height that is used to assess risk for possible present or future health problems.

**brain death** The irreversible cessation of all functions of the entire brainstem.

**bronchitis** Inflammation of the lining of the bronchial tubes.

**bulimia nervosa** Eating disorder characterized by binge eating followed by inappropriate measures, such as vomiting, to prevent weight gain.

**CAD** *See* coronary artery disease.

**calorie** A unit of measure that indicates the amount of energy obtained from a particular food.

**cancer** A large group of diseases characterized by the uncontrolled growth and spread of abnormal cells.

**candidiasis** Yeastlike fungal infection often transmitted sexually; also called *moniliasis* or *yeast infection.*

**capillaries** Minute blood vessels that branch out from the arterioles and venules; their thin walls permit exchange of oxygen, carbon dioxide, nutrients, and waste products among body cells.

**capitation** Prepayment of a fixed monthly amount for each patient without regard to the type or number of services provided.

**carbohydrates** Basic nutrients that supply the body with glucose, the energy form most commonly used to sustain normal activity.

**carbon dioxide ($CO_2$)** Gas created by the combustion of fossil fuels, exhaled by animals, and used by plants for photosynthesis; the primary greenhouse gas in Earth's atmosphere.

**carbon footprint** The amount of greenhouse gases produced by an individual, nation, or other entity, usually expressed in equivalent tons of carbon dioxide emissions.

**carbon monoxide** A gas found in cigarette smoke that binds at oxygen receptor sites in the blood.

**carcinogens** Cancer-causing agents.

**cardiometabolic risks** Physical and biochemical changes that are risk factors for the development of cardiovascular disease and type 2 diabetes.

**cardiopulmonary resuscitation (CPR)** Emergency technique to provide lifesaving chest compression and mouth-to-mouth resuscitation when an individual has stopped breathing and has no pulse.

**cardiorespiratory fitness** The ability of the heart, lungs, and blood vessels to supply oxygen to skeletal muscles during sustained physical activity.

**cardiovascular disease (CVD)** Diseases of the heart and blood vessels.

**cardiovascular system** Organ system, consisting of the heart and blood vessels, that transports nutrients, oxygen, hormones, metabolic wastes, and enzymes throughout the body.

**carotenoids** Fat-soluble plant pigments with antioxidant properties.

**carpal tunnel syndrome** A common occupational injury in which the median nerve in the wrist becomes irritated, causing numbness, tingling, and pain in the fingers and hands.

**carrier** Individual who has one copy of an autosome with a recessive allele for a particular trait, but is unaffected by it.

**cataracts** Clouding of the lens that interrupts the focusing of light on the retina, resulting in blurred vision or eventual blindness.

**CAT scan** *See* computerized axial tomography scan.

**celiac disease** An inherited autoimmune disorder affecting the digestive process of the small intestine and triggered by the consumption of gluten.

**celibacy** State of abstaining from sexual activity.

**cell-mediated immunity** Aspect of immunity that is mediated by specialized white blood cells that attack pathogens and antigens directly.

**cerebrospinal fluid** Fluid within and surrounding the brain and spinal cord tissues.

**cervical cap** A small cup made of latex or silicone that is designed to fit snugly over the entire cervix.

**cervix** Lower end of the uterus that opens into the vagina.

**cesarean section (C-section)** A surgical birthing procedure in which a baby is removed through an incision made in the mother's abdominal and uterine walls.

**CFCs** *See* chlorofluorocarbons.

**chancre** Sore often found at the site of syphilis infection.

**CHD** *See* coronary heart disease.

**chemotherapy** The use of drugs to kill cancerous cells.

**chewing tobacco** A stringy type of tobacco that is placed in the mouth and then sucked or chewed.

**CHF** *See* congestive heart failure.

**chickenpox** A highly infectious disease caused by the herpes varicella zoster virus.

**child abuse** The systematic harming of a child by a caregiver, typically a parent.

**chiropractic medicine** Manipulation of the spine to allow proper energy flow.

**chlamydia** Bacterially caused sexually transmitted infection of the urogenital tract.

**chlorofluorocarbons (CFCs)** Chemicals that contribute to the depletion of the atmospheric ozone layer.

**cholesterol** A form of fat circulating in the blood that can accumulate on the inner walls of arteries, causing a narrowing of the channel through which blood flows.

**chorionic villus sampling (CVS)** A prenatal test that involves snipping tissue from the fetal sac to be analyzed for genetic defects.

**chromosome** Discrete bundle of DNA, 46 of which are present in the nucleus of almost all cells of the human body.

**chromosome disorder** A disorder arising from a missing or extra chromosome, or damage to part of a chromosome.

**chronic disease** A disease that typically begins slowly, progresses, and persists, with a variety of signs and symptoms that can be treated but not cured by medication.

**chronic mood disorder** Experience of persistent emotional states, such as sadness, despair, and hopelessness.

**chronic obstructive pulmonary diseases (COPDs)** The chronic lung diseases of emphysema and chronic bronchitis.

**chronic stress** An ongoing state of physiological arousal in response to ongoing or numerous perceived threats.

**circadian rhythm** The 24-hour cycle by which you are accustomed to going to sleep, waking up, and performing habitual behaviors.

**cirrhosis** The last stage of liver disease associated with chronic heavy alcohol use, during which liver cells die and damage becomes permanent.

**clinical depression** *See* major depression.

**clitoris** A pea-sized nodule of tissue located at the top of the labia minora; central to sexual arousal in women.

**club drugs** Synthetic analogs (drugs that produce similar effects) of existing illicit drugs.

**$CO_2$** *See* carbon dioxide.

**codependence** A self-defeating relationship pattern in which a person is "addicted to the addict."

**cognitive restructuring** The modification of thoughts, ideas, and beliefs that contribute to stress.

**cohabitation** Living together without being married.

**coitus interruptus** *See* withdrawal (1).

**collateral circulation** Adaptation of the heart to partial damage accomplished by rerouting needed blood through unused or underused blood vessels while the damaged heart muscle heals.

**collective violence** Violence perpetrated by groups against other groups.

**colonization** The process of bacteria or some other infectious organisms establishing themselves in a host without causing infection.

**common-law marriage** Cohabitation lasting a designated period of time (usually 7 years) that is considered legally binding in some states.

**comorbidities** The presence of one or more diseases at the same time.

**complementary medicine** Treatment used in conjunction with conventional medicine.

**complete (high-quality) proteins** Proteins that contain all nine of the essential amino acids.

**complex carbohydrates** A major type of carbohydrate, which provides sustained energy.

**compulsion** Preoccupation with a behavior and an overwhelming need to perform it.

**compulsive exercise** Disorder characterized by a compulsion to engage in excessive amounts of exercise, and feelings of guilt and anxiety if the level of exercise is perceived as inadequate.

**compulsive shoppers** People who are preoccupied with shopping and spending.

**computerized axial tomography (CAT) scan** A scan by a machine that uses radiation to view internal organs not normally visible in X rays.

**conception** The fertilization of an ovum by a sperm.

**conflict** An emotional state that arises when the behavior of one person interferes with the behavior of another.

**conflict resolution** A concerted effort by all parties to constructively resolve points of contention.

**congeners** Forms of alcohol that are metabolized more slowly than ethanol and produce toxic by-products.

**congenital cardiovascular defect** Cardiovascular problem that is present at birth.

**congestive heart failure (CHF)** An abnormal cardiovascular condition that reflects impaired cardiac pumping and blood flow; pooling blood leads to congestion in body tissues.

**contemplation** A practice of concentrating the mind on a spiritual or ethical question or subject, a view of the natural world, or an icon or other image representative of divinity.

**contraception (birth control)** Methods of preventing conception.

**COPDs** *See* chronic obstructive pulmonary diseases.

**coping** Managing events or conditions to lessen the physical or psychological effects of excess stress.

**coronary artery disease (CAD)** A narrowing or blockage of coronary arteries, usually caused by atherosclerotic plaque build up.

**coronary bypass surgery** A surgical technique whereby a blood vessel taken from another part of the body is implanted to bypass a clogged coronary artery.

**coronary heart disease (CHD)** A narrowing of the small blood vessels that supply blood to the heart.

**coronary thrombosis** A blood clot occurring in a coronary artery.

**corpus luteum** A body of cells that forms from the remains of the graafian follicle following ovulation; it secretes estrogen and progesterone during the second half of the menstrual cycle.

**cortisol** Hormone released by the adrenal glands that makes stored nutrients more readily available to meet energy demands.

**countering** Substituting a desired behavior for an undesirable one.

**Cowper's glands** Glands that secrete a fluid that lubricates the urethra and neutralizes any acid remaining in the urethra after urination.

**CPR** *See* cardiopulmonary resuscitation.

**Crohn's disease** An autoimmune inflammatory disease of the gastrointestinal tract characterized by cramping and diarrhea.

**cross-tolerance** Development of a physiological tolerance to one drug that reduces the effects of another, similar drug.

**C-section** *See* cesarean section.

**cunnilingus** Oral stimulation of a woman's genitals.

**CVD** *See* cardiovascular disease.

**CVS** *See* chorionic villus sampling.

**Daily Values (DVs)** Percentages listed as "% DV" on food and supplement labels; made up of the RDIs and DRVs together.

**D&E** *See* dilation and evacuation.

**death** The permanent ending of all vital functions.

**defensive medicine** The use of medical practices designed to avert the possibility of malpractice suits in the future.

**dehydration** Abnormal depletion of body fluids; a result of lack of water.

**delirium tremens (DTs)** A state of confusion brought on by withdrawal from alcohol; symptoms include hallucinations, anxiety, and trembling.

**dementias** Progressive brain impairments that interfere with memory and normal intellectual functioning.

**denial** Inability to perceive or accurately interpret the self-destructive effects of the addictive behavior.

**dentist** Specialist who diagnoses and treats diseases of the teeth, gums, and oral cavity.

**deoxyribonucleic acid** *See* DNA.

**Depo-Provera** An injectable method of birth control that lasts for 3 months.

**depressants** Drugs that slow down the activity of the central nervous system.

**depression** *See* major depression.

**determinants of health** The array of critical influences that determine the health of individuals and communities.

**detoxification** The early abstinence period during which an addict adjusts physically and cognitively to being free from the influences of the addiction.

**diabetes mellitus** A group of diseases characterized by elevated blood glucose levels.

**diagnosis-related groups (DRGs)** Diagnostic categories established by the federal government to determine in advance how much hospitals will be reimbursed for the care of a particular Medicare patient.

**diaphragm** A latex, cup-shaped device designed to cover the cervix and block access to the uterus; should always be used with spermicide.

**diastolic pressure** The lower number in the fraction that measures blood pressure, indicating pressure on arterial walls during the relaxation phase of heart activity.

**dietary supplements** Vitamins and minerals taken by mouth that are intended to supplement existing diets.

**digestive process** The process by which the body breaks down foods and either absorbs or excretes them.

**dilation and evacuation (D&E)** An abortion technique that uses a combination of instruments and vacuum aspiration; fetal tissue is both sucked and scraped out of the uterus.

**dioxins** Highly toxic chlorinated hydrocarbons contained in herbicides and produced during certain industrial processes.

**dipping** Placing a small amount of chewing tobacco between the front lip and teeth for rapid nicotine absorption.

**disaccharides** Combinations of two monosaccharides.

**discrimination** Actions that deny equal treatment or opportunities to a group, often based on prejudice.

**disease prevention** Actions or behaviors designed to keep people from getting sick.

**disordered eating** A pattern of atypical eating behaviors that is used to achieve or maintain a lower body weight.

**disordered gambling** Compulsive gambling that cannot be controlled.

**disorders of sexual development (DSDs)** *See* intersex.

**distillation** The process whereby mash is subjected to high temperatures to release alcohol vapors, which are then condensed and mixed with water to make the final product.

**distress** Stress that can have a detrimental effect on health; negative stress.

**DNA (deoxyribonucleic acid)** Acid molecule that resides in the nucleus of a cell and stores in its sequence of chemical subunits the instructions for assembling body proteins.

**domestic violence** The use of force to control and maintain power over another person in the home environment, including both actual harm and the threat of harm.

**dominant** Term describing an allele that is expressed even if there is only one copy in the pair.

**Down syndrome** A genetic disorder characterized by mental retardation and a variety of physical abnormalities.

**DRGs** *See* diagnosis-related groups.

**drug abuse** Excessive use of a drug.

**drug misuse** Use of a drug for a purpose for which it was not intended.

**DSDs** *See* intersex.

**DTs** *See* delirium tremens.

**D&X** *See* intact dilation and extraction.

**DVs** *See* Daily Values.

**dying** The process of decline in body functions, resulting in the death of an organism.

**dysfunctional families** Families in which there is violence; physical, emotional, or sexual abuse; parental discord; or other negative family interactions.

**dysmenorrhea** Condition of pain or discomfort in the lower abdomen just before or after menstruation.

**dyspareunia** Pain experienced by women during intercourse.

**dyspnea** Shortness of breath, usually associated with disease of the heart or lungs.

**dysthymic disorder (dysthymia)** A type of depression that is milder and harder to recognize than major depression; chronic; and often characterized by fatigue, pessimism, or a short temper.

**eating disorder** A psychiatric disorder characterized by severe disturbances in body image and eating behaviors.

**eating disorders not otherwise specified (EDNOS)** Eating disorders that are a true psychiatric illness but do not fit the strict diagnostic criteria for anorexia nervosa, bulimia nervosa, or binge-eating disorder.

**ECG** *See* electrocardiogram.

**ecological** or **public health model** A view of health in which diseases and other negative health events are seen as a result of an individual's interaction with his or her social and physical environment.

**ECPs** *See* emergency contraceptive pills.

**ectopic pregnancy** Implantation of a fertilized egg outside the uterus, usually in a fallopian tube; a medical emergency that can end in death from hemorrhage or peritonitis.

**ED** *See* erectile dysfunction.

**EDNOS** *See* eating disorders not otherwise specified.

**ejaculation** The propulsion of semen from the penis.

**ejaculatory duct** Tube formed by the junction of the seminal vesicle and the vas deferens that carries semen to the urethra.

**electrocardiogram (ECG)** A record of the electrical activity of the heart; may be measured during a stress test.

**embolus** A blood clot that becomes dislodged from a blood vessel wall and moves through the circulatory system.

**embryo** The fertilized egg from conception until the end of 2 months' development.

**emergency contraceptive pills (ECPs)** Drugs taken within 3 days after unprotected intercourse to prevent fertilization or implantation.

**emotional health** The feeling part of psychosocial health; includes your emotional reactions to life.

**emotions** Intensified feelings or complex patterns of feelings we constantly experience.

**emphysema** A chronic lung disease in which the tiny air sacs in the lungs are destroyed, making breathing difficult.

**EMR** *See* exercise metabolic rate.

**enablers** People who knowingly or unknowingly protect addicts from the natural consequences of their behavior.

**endemic** Describing a disease that is always present to some degree.

**endometriosis** A disorder in which uterine lining tissue establishes itself outside the uterus; the leading cause of infertility in women in the United States.

**endometrium** Soft, spongy matter that makes up the uterine lining.

**endorphins** Opioid-like hormones that are manufactured in the human body and contribute to natural feelings of well-being.

**energy medicine** Therapies using energy fields, such as magnetic fields or biofields.

**enhanced greenhouse effect** The warming of Earth's surface as a direct result of human activities that release greenhouse gases into the atmosphere, trapping more of the sun's radiation than is normal.

**environmental stewardship** A responsibility for environmental quality shared by all those whose actions affect the environment.

**environmental tobacco smoke (ETS)** Smoke from tobacco products, including sidestream and mainstream smoke; commonly called secondhand smoke.

**epidemic** Disease outbreak that affects many people in a community or region at the same time.

**epididymis** The duct system atop the testis where sperm mature.

**epilepsy** A neurological disorder caused by abnormal electrical brain activity; can be accompanied by altered consciousness or convulsions.

**epinephrine** Also called adrenaline, a hormone that stimulates body systems in response to stress.

**erectile dysfunction (ED)** Difficulty in achieving or maintaining a penile erection sufficient for intercourse.

**ergogenic drug** Substance believed to enhance athletic performance.

**erogenous zones** Areas of the body that, when touched, lead to sexual arousal.

**essential amino acids** Nine of the basic nitrogen-containing building blocks of protein, which must be obtained from foods to ensure health.

**estrogens** Hormones secreted by the ovaries that control the menstrual cycle.

**ethanol** *See* ethyl alcohol.

**ethnoviolence** Violence directed at persons affiliated with a particular, usually ethnic, group.

**ethyl alcohol (ethanol)** An addictive drug produced by fermentation and found in many beverages.

**ETS** *See* environmental tobacco smoke.

**eustress** Stress that presents opportunities for personal growth; positive stress.

**evidence-based practice** Decisions regarding patient care based on clinical expertise, patient values, and current best scientific evidence.

**exercise** Planned, structured, and repetitive bodily movement done to improve or maintain one or more components of physical fitness.

**exercise addicts** People who exercise compulsively to try to meet needs of nurturance, intimacy, self-esteem, and self-competency.

**exercise metabolic rate (EMR)** The energy expenditure that occurs during exercise.

**extensively drug resistant TB (XDR-TB)** Form of tuberculosis that is resistant to nearly all existing antibiotics.

**fallopian tubes (oviducts)** Tubes that extend from near the ovaries to the uterus; site of fertilization and passageway for fertilized eggs.

**family of origin** People present in the household during a child's first years of life—usually parents and siblings.

**FAMs** *See* fertility awareness methods.

**FAS** *See* fetal alcohol syndrome.

**fats** Basic nutrients composed of carbon and hydrogen atoms; needed for the proper

functioning of cells, insulation of body organs against shock, maintenance of body temperature, and healthy skin and hair.

**fellatio** Oral stimulation of a man's genitals.

**female athlete triad** A syndrome of three interrelated health problems seen in some female athletes: disordered eating, amenorrhea, and poor bone density.

**female condom** A single-use polyurethane sheath for internal use during vaginal or anal intercourse to catch semen on ejaculation.

**female orgasmic disorder** A woman's inability to achieve orgasm.

**fermentation** The process whereby yeast organisms break down plant sugars to yield ethanol.

**fertility** A person's ability to reproduce.

**fertility awareness methods (FAMs)** Several types of birth control that require alteration of sexual behavior rather than chemical or physical intervention in the reproductive process.

**fetal alcohol syndrome (FAS)** A disorder involving physical and mental impairment that may affect the fetus when the mother consumes alcohol during pregnancy.

**fetus** The word for a developing baby from the third month of pregnancy until birth.

**fiber** The indigestible portion of plant foods that helps move food through the digestive system and softens stools by absorbing water.

**fibrillation** A sporadic, quivering pattern of heartbeat that results in extreme inefficiency in moving blood through the cardiovascular system.

**fight-or-flight response** Physiological arousal response in which the body prepares to combat or escape a real or perceived threat.

**FITT** Acronym for Frequency, Intensity, Time, and Type; the terms that describe the essential components of a program or plan to improve a parameter of physical fitness.

**flexibility** The range of motion, or the amount of movement possible, at a particular joint or series of joints.

**food allergy** Overreaction by the body to normally harmless proteins, which are perceived as allergens. In response, the body produces antibodies, triggering allergic symptoms.

**food intolerance** Adverse effects resulting when people who lack the digestive chemicals needed to break down certain substances eat those substances.

**food irradiation** Treating foods with gamma radiation from radioactive cobalt, cesium, or other sources of X rays to kill microorganisms.

**formaldehyde** A colorless, strong-smelling gas released through offgassing; causes respiratory and other health problems.

**frequency** As part of the FITT prescription, refers to how many days per week a person should exercise to improve a parameter of physical fitness.

**functional foods** Foods believed to have specific health benefits and/or to prevent disease.

**fungi** A group of multicellular and unicellular organisms that obtain their food by infiltrating the bodies of other organisms, both living and dead; several microscopic varieties are pathogenic.

**GAD** *See* general anxiety disorder.

**GAS** *See* general adaptation syndrome.

**gastroesophageal reflux disease (GERD)** Chronic condition in which stomach acid backflows into the esophagus, causing heartburn and potential damage to the esophagus.

**gay** Sexual orientation involving primary attraction to people of the same sex.

**gender** The psychological condition of being feminine or masculine as defined by the society in which one lives.

**gender identity** Personal sense or awareness of being masculine or feminine, a male or a female.

**gender-role stereotypes** Generalizations concerning how men and women should express themselves and the characteristics each possesses.

**gender roles** Expressions of maleness or femaleness in everyday life.

**gene** Discrete segment of DNA in a chromosome that stores the code for assembling a particular body protein.

**general adaptation syndrome (GAS)** The pattern followed in the physiological response to stress, consisting of the alarm, resistance, and exhaustion phases.

**generalized anxiety disorder (GAD)** A constant sense of worry that may cause restlessness, difficulty in concentrating, tension, and other symptoms.

**generic drugs** Medications marketed by chemical names rather than brand names.

**genetically modified (GM) foods** Foods derived from organisms whose DNA has been altered using genetic engineering techniques.

**genital herpes** Sexually transmitted infection caused by the herpes simplex virus.

**genital warts** Warts that appear in the genital area or the anus; caused by the human papillomavirus (HPV).

**genome** All of the genetic information an organism possesses.

**GERD** *See* gastroesophageal reflux disease.

**German measles** *See* rubella.

**gerontology** The study of individual and collective aging processes.

**gestational diabetes** Form of diabetes mellitus in which women who have never had diabetes before have high blood sugar (glucose) levels during pregnancy.

**glaucoma** Elevation of pressure within the eyeball, leading to hardening of the eyeball, impaired vision, and possible blindness.

**glycogen** The polysaccharide form in which glucose is stored in the liver and, to a lesser extent, in muscles.

**GM foods** *See* genetically modified foods.

**gonads** The reproductive organs in a male (testes) or female (ovaries) that produce sperm (male), eggs (female), and sex hormones.

**gonorrhea** Second most common bacterial sexually transmitted infection in the United States; if untreated, may cause sterility.

**graafian follicle** Mature ovarian follicle that contains a fully developed ovum, or egg.

**greenhouse gases** Gases that accumulate in the atmosphere, where they contribute to global warming by trapping heat near Earth's surface.

**grief** An individual's reaction to significant loss, including one's own impending death, the death of a loved one, or a quasi-death experience; grief can involve mental, physical, social, or emotional responses.

**grief work** The process of accepting the reality of a person's death and coping with memories of the deceased.

**habit** A repeated behavior in which the repetition may be unconscious.

**hallucinogens** Substances capable of creating auditory or visual distortions and heightened states.

**hangover** The physiological reaction to excessive drinking, including headache, upset stomach, anxiety, depression, diarrhea, and thirst.

**hate crime** A crime targeted against a particular societal group and motivated by bias against that group.

**hay fever** A chronic allergy-related respiratory disorder that is most prevalent when ragweed and flowers bloom.

**hazardous waste** Waste that, due to its toxic properties, poses a hazard to humans or to the environment.

**HBM** *See* health belief model.

**HCG** *See* human chorionic gonadotropin.

**HDLs** *See* high-density lipoproteins.

**health** The ever-changing process of achieving individual potential in the physical, social, emotional, mental, spiritual, and environmental dimensions.

**health belief model (HBM)** Model for explaining how beliefs may influence behaviors.

**health disparities** Differences in the incidence, prevalence, mortality, and burden of diseases and other health conditions among specific population groups.

**health promotion** The combined educational, organizational, procedural, environmental, social, and financial supports that help individuals and groups reduce negative health behaviors and promote positive change.

**healthy life expectancy** Expected number of years of full health remaining at a given age, such as at birth.

**heart attack** *See* myocardial infarction.

**heat cramps** Involuntary and forcible muscle contractions that occur during or following exercise in hot and/or humid weather.

**heat exhaustion** A heat stress illness caused by significant dehydration resulting from exercise in hot and/or humid conditions.

**heatstroke** A deadly heat stress illness resulting from dehydration and overexertion in hot and/or humid conditions.

**heavy episodic (binge) drinking** A binge is a pattern of drinking alcohol that brings blood alcohol concentration (BAC) to 0.08 grampercent or above; for a typical adult, this pattern corresponds to consuming five or more drinks (male) or four or more drinks (female) in about 2 hours.

**hepatitis** A viral disease in which the liver becomes inflamed, producing symptoms such as fever, headache, and possibly jaundice.

**herpes gladiatorum** A skin infection caused by the herpes simplex type 1 virus and seen among athletes participating in contact sports.

**heterosexual** Experiencing primary attraction to and preference for sexual activity with people of the opposite sex.

**high-density lipoproteins (HDLs)** Compounds that facilitate the transport of cholesterol in the blood to the liver for metabolism and elimination from the body.

**high-quality proteins** *See* complete proteins.

**histamine** Chemical substance that dilates blood vessels, increases mucous secretions, and triggers other allergy symptoms.

**HIV** *See* human immunodeficiency virus.

**holistic** Relating to or concerned with the whole body and the interactions of systems, rather than treatment of individual parts.

**holographic will** A will written in the testator's own handwriting and unwitnessed.

**homeopathic medicine** Unconventional Western system of medicine based on the principle that "like cures like."

**homeostasis** A balanced physiological state in which all the body's systems function smoothly.

**homicide** Death that results from intent to injure or kill.

**homosexual** Experiencing primary attraction to and preference for sexual activity with people of the same sex.

**hormonal methods** Contraceptive methods that introduce synthetic hormones into the woman's system to prevent ovulation, thicken cervical mucus, or prevent a fertilized egg from implanting.

**hormone** A "chemical messenger" that is released from one of body's endocrine glands and travels in the bloodstream to another site where it helps to regulate body functions.

**hormone replacement therapy** or **menopausal hormone therapy** Use of synthetic or animal estrogens and progesterone to compensate for decreases in estrogens in a woman's body during menopause.

**hospice** A concept of end-of-life care designed to maximize quality of life and help dying people have peace, comfort, and dignity.

**hostility** The cognitive, affective, and behavioral tendencies toward anger and cynicism.

**HPV** *See* human papillomavirus.

**human chorionic gonadotropin (HCG)** Hormone detectable in blood or urine samples of a mother within the first few weeks of pregnancy.

**human immunodeficiency virus (HIV)** The virus that causes AIDS by infecting helper T cells.

**human papillomavirus (HPV)** A group of viruses, many of which are transmitted sexually; some types of HPV can cause genital warts or cervical cancer.

**humoral immunity** Aspect of immunity that is mediated by antibodies secreted by white blood cells.

**hunger** The physiological impulse to seek food, prompted by the lack or shortage of basic foods needed to provide the energy and nutrients that support health.

**hymen** Thin tissue covering the vaginal opening in some women.

**hyperglycemia** Elevated blood glucose level.

**hyperplasia** A condition characterized by an excessive number of fat cells.

**hypertension** Sustained elevated blood pressure.

**hypertrophy** The act of swelling or increasing in size, as with cells.

**hypnosis** A trancelike state that allows people to become unusually responsive to suggestion.

**hyponatremia** or **water intoxication** The overconsumption of water, which leads to a dilution of sodium concentration in the blood with potentially fatal results.

**hypothalamus** A structure in the brain that acts as a control center for the many functions of the autonomic nervous system and coordinates activities of the endocrine system through its interactions with the pituitary gland; plays a role in the stress response and in control of reproductive functions.

**hypothermia** Potentially fatal condition caused by abnormally low body core temperature.

**hysterectomy** Surgical removal of the uterus.

**hysterotomy** The surgical removal of the fetus from the uterus.

**IBD** *See* inflammatory bowel disease.

**IBS** *See* irritable bowel syndrome.

**idiopathic** Of unknown cause.

**IED** *See* intermittent explosive disorder.

**imagined rehearsal** Practicing, through mental imagery, to become better able to perform an event in actuality.

**immunocompetence** The ability of the immune system to respond to attack.

**immunocompromised** Having an immune system that is impaired.

**immunotherapy** Treatment strategies based on the concept of regulating the immune system, as by administering antibodies or desensitization shots of allergens.

**incomplete proteins** Proteins that lack one or more of the essential amino acids.

**incubation period** The time between exposure to a disease and the appearance of symptoms.

**induction abortion** An abortion technique in which chemicals are injected into the uterus through the uterine wall; labor begins, and the woman delivers a dead fetus.

**infection** The state of pathogens being established in or on a host and causing disease.

**infertility** Inability to conceive after a year or more of trying.

**inflammatory bowel disease (IBD)** A group of disorders in which the intestines become inflamed.

**influenza** A common viral disease of the respiratory tract.

**inhalants** Products that are sniffed or inhaled in order to produce highs.

**inhalation** The introduction of drugs through breathing into the lungs.

**inheritance** Process by which physical and biological characteristics—called traits—are transmitted from parents to their offspring.

**inhibited sexual desire** Lack of sexual appetite or simply a lack of interest and pleasure in sexual activity.

**inhibition** A drug interaction in which the effects of one drug are eliminated or reduced by the presence of another drug at the same receptor site.

**injection** The introduction of drugs into the body via a hypodermic needle.

**insomnia** A disorder characterized by difficulty in falling asleep quickly, frequent arousals during sleep, or early morning awakening.

**insulin** Hormone secreted by the pancreas and required by body cells for the uptake and storage of glucose.

**insulin resistance** State in which body cells fail to respond to the effects of insulin; obesity increases the risk that cells will become insulin resistant.

**intact dilation and extraction (D&X)** A late-term abortion procedure in which the body of the fetus is extracted up to the head and then the contents of the cranium are aspirated.

**intensity** As part of the FITT prescription, refers to how hard or how much effort is needed when a person exercises to improve a parameter of physical fitness.

**intentional injuries** Injury, death, psychological harm, maldevelopment, or deprivation that involves the intentional use of physical force or power, threatened or actual, against oneself, another person, or against a group or community.

**intermittent explosive disorder (IED)** A behavioral disorder characterized by repeated episodes of aggression and violent behavior that are disproportionate to the situation.

**Internet addiction** Compulsive use of the computer, PDA, cell phone, or other forms of technology to access the Internet for activities such as e-mail, games, shopping, or blogging.

**interpersonal violence** Violence inflicted against one individual by another, or a small group of others.

**intersex** General term for a variety of conditions in which a person is born with reproductive or sexual anatomy that doesn't seem to fit the typical definitions of female or male. Also termed disorders of sexual development (DSDs).

**intervention** A planned process of confronting an addict; carried out by close family, friends, and significant others.

**intestate** Dying without a will.

**intimate partner violence (IPV)** Violent behavior, including physical violence, sexual violence, threats, and emotional abuse, occurring between current or former spouses or dating partners.

**intimate relationships** Relationships with family members, friends, and romantic partners, characterized by behavioral interdependence, need fulfillment, emotional attachment, and emotional availability.

**intolerance** A drug interaction in which the combination of two or more drugs in the body produces extremely uncomfortable symptoms.

**intrauterine device (IUD)** A device, often T-shaped, that is implanted in the uterus to prevent pregnancy.

**in vitro fertilization (IVF)** Fertilization of an egg in a nutrient medium and subsequent transfer back to the mother's body.

**ionizing radiation** Electromagnetic waves and particles having short wavelengths and energy high enough to ionize atoms.

**IPV** *See* intimate partner violence.

**irritable bowel syndrome (IBS)** Nausea, pain, gas, or diarrhea caused by certain foods or stress.

**ischemia** Reduced oxygen supply to a body part or organ.

**IUD** *See* intrauterine device.

**IVF** *See* in vitro fertilization.

**jealousy** An aversive reaction evoked by a real or imagined relationship involving a person's partner and a third person.

**labia majora** "Outer lips," or folds of tissue covering the female sexual organs.

**labia minora** "Inner lips," or folds of tissue just inside the labia majora.

**LBP** *See* low back pain.

**LDLs** *See* low-density lipoproteins.

**leach** To dissolve and filter through soil.

**lead** A highly toxic metal found in emissions from lead smelters and processing plants; also sometimes found in pipes or paint in older houses.

**learned behavioral tolerance** The ability of heavy drinkers to modify behavior so that they appear to be sober even when they have high BAC levels.

**learned helplessness** Pattern of responding to situations by giving up because of repeated failure in the past.

**learned optimism** Teaching oneself to think positively.

**lesbian** Sexual orientation involving attraction of women to other women.

**leukoplakia** A condition characterized by leathery white patches inside the mouth; produced by contact with irritants in tobacco juice.

**libido** Sexual drive or desire.

**life expectancy** Expected number of years of life remaining at a given age, such as at birth.

**life jacket** *See* personal flotation device.

**living will** A type of advance directive.

**locavore** A person who primarily eats food grown or produced locally.

**locus of control** The location, external (outside oneself) or internal (within oneself), that an individual perceives as the source and underlying cause of events in his or her life.

**loss of control** Inability to reliably predict whether a particular instance of involvement with the addictive substance or behavior will be healthy or damaging.

**low back pain (LBP)** Pain or discomfort in the lumbosacral region of the back.

**low-density lipoproteins (LDLs)** Compounds that facilitate the transport of cholesterol in the blood to the body's cells.

**low sperm count** A sperm count below 20 million sperm per milliliter of semen; the leading cause of infertility in men.

**lymphocyte** A type of white blood cell involved in the immune response.

**macrominerals** Minerals that the body needs in fairly large amounts.

**macrophage** A type of white blood cell that ingests foreign material.

**macular degeneration** Breakdown of the macula, the light-sensitive part of the retina responsible for sharp, direct vision.

**magnetic resonance imaging (MRI)** A device that uses magnetic fields, radio waves, and computers to generate an image of internal tissues of the body for diagnostic purposes without the use of radiation.

**mainstream smoke** Smoke that is drawn through tobacco while inhaling.

**major depression** Severe depressive disorder that entails chronic mood disorder, physical effects such as sleep disturbance and exhaustion, and mental effects such as the inability to concentrate; also called clinical depression.

**male condom** A single-use sheath of thin latex or other material designed to fit over an erect penis and to catch semen upon ejaculation.

**malignant** Very dangerous or harmful; refers to a cancerous tumor.

**malignant melanoma** A virulent cancer of the melanocytes (pigment-producing cells) of the skin.

**managed care** Cost-control procedures used by health insurers to coordinate treatment.

**manipulative and body-based practices** Treatments involving manipulation or movement of one or more body parts.

**marijuana** Chopped leaves and flowers of *Cannabis indica* or *Cannabis sativa* plants (hemp); a psychoactive stimulant.

**masturbation** Self-stimulation of genitals.

**MDR-TB** *See* multidrug resistant TB.

**measles** A viral disease that produces symptoms such as an itchy rash and a high fever.

**medical abortion** The termination of a pregnancy during its first 9 weeks using hormonal medications that cause the embryo to be expelled from the uterus.

**medical model** A view of health in which health status focuses primarily on the individual and a biological or diseased organ perspective.

**meditation** A practice of mental exercise, usually involving concentration and deep breathing, undertaken to realize some

benefit, such as relaxation or heightened spiritual awareness.

**menarche** The first menstrual period.

**meningitis** An infection of the meninges, the membranes that surround the brain and spinal cord.

**menopausal hormone therapy** *See* hormone replacement therapy.

**menopause** The permanent cessation of menstruation, generally between the ages of 40 and 60.

**mental health** The thinking part of psychosocial health; includes your values, attitudes, and beliefs.

**mental illnesses** Disorders that disrupt thinking, feeling, moods, and behaviors, and that impair daily functioning.

**metabolic syndrome (MetS)** A group of metabolic conditions occurring together that increase a person's risk of heart disease, stroke, and diabetes.

**metastasis** Process by which cancer spreads from one area to different areas of the body.

**MetS** *See* metabolic syndrome.

**methicillin-resistant *Staphylococcus aureus* (MRSA)** Highly resistant form of staph infection that is growing in international prevalence.

**MI** *See* myocardial infarction.

**migraine** A condition characterized by localized headaches that possibly result from alternating dilation and constriction of blood vessels.

**mind–body medicine** Techniques designed to enhance the mind's ability to affect bodily functions and symptoms.

**mindfulness** A practice of purposeful, nonjudgmental observation in which we are fully present in the moment.

**minerals** Inorganic, indestructible elements that aid physiological processes.

**miscarriage** Loss of the fetus before it is viable; also called spontaneous abortion.

**modeling** Learning specific behaviors by watching others perform them.

**moniliasis** *See* candidiasis.

**monogamy** Exclusive sexual involvement with one partner.

**mononucleosis** A viral disease that causes pervasive fatigue and other long-lasting symptoms.

**monosaccharides** Simple sugars that contain only one molecule of sugar.

**mons pubis** Fatty tissue covering the pubic bone in females; in physically mature women, the mons is covered with coarse hair.

**morbidly obese** Having a body weight 100 percent or more above healthy recommended levels; in an adult, having a BMI of 40 or more.

**mortality** The proportion of deaths to population.

**motivation** A social, cognitive, and emotional force that directs human behavior.

**mourning** The culturally prescribed behavior patterns for the expression of grief.

**MRI** *See* magnetic resonance imaging.

**MRSA** *See* methicillin-resistant *Staphylococcus aureus.*

**MSW** *See* municipal solid waste.

**multidrug resistant TB (MDR-TB)** Form of tuberculosis that is resistant to at least two of the best antibiotics available.

**multifactorial disease** Disease caused by interactions of several factors.

**multifactorial disorder** A disorder attributable to more than one of a variety of factors.

**municipal solid waste (MSW)** Solid wastes such as durable goods; nondurable goods; containers and packaging; food waste; yard waste; and miscellaneous wastes from residential, commercial, institutional, and industrial sources.

**muscle dysmorphia** Body image disorder in which men believe that their body is insufficiently lean or muscular.

**muscular endurance** A muscle's ability to exert force repeatedly without fatiguing or the ability to sustain a muscular contraction for a length of time.

**muscular strength** The amount of force that a muscle is capable of exerting in one contraction.

**mutant cells** Cells that differ in form, quality, or function from normal cells.

**myocardial infarction (MI) or heart attack** A blockage of normal blood supply to an area in the heart.

**narcolepsy** Excessive, intrusive sleepiness.

**natural disaster** Any extreme environmental event that causes widespread destruction of land and/or property, injuries, and sometimes deaths.

**naturopathic medicine** System of medicine originating from Europe that views disease as a manifestation of alterations in the body's natural self-healing processes, and that emphasizes health restoration as well as disease treatment.

**negative consequences** Severe problems associated with addiction, such as physical damage, legal trouble, financial problems, academic failure, or family dissolution.

**neglect** Failure to provide for a child's basic needs such as food, shelter, medical care, and clothing.

**neoplasm** A new growth of tissue that serves no physiological function and results from uncontrolled, abnormal cellular development.

**neurotransmitter** One of many chemical substances, such as acetylcholine or dopamine, that transmit nerve impulses between nerve fibers.

**nicotine poisoning** Symptoms often experienced by beginning smokers, including dizziness, diarrhea, lightheadedness, rapid and erratic pulse, clammy skin, nausea, and vomiting.

**nicotine** The primary stimulant chemical in tobacco products; nicotine is highly addictive.

**nicotine withdrawal** Symptoms, including nausea, headaches, irritability, and intense tobacco cravings, suffered by addicted smokers who stop using tobacco.

**nonionizing radiation** Electromagnetic waves having relatively long wavelengths and enough energy to move atoms around or cause them to vibrate.

**nonpoint source pollutants** Pollutants that run off or seep into waterways from broad areas of land.

**non-REM (NREM) sleep** A period of restful sleep dominated by slow brain waves; during non-REM sleep, rapid eye movement is rare.

**nonverbal communication** All unwritten and unspoken messages, both intentional and unintentional.

**NP** *See* nurse practitioner.

**NREM sleep** *See* non-REM sleep.

**nuclear meltdown** An accident that results when the temperature in the core of a nuclear reactor increases enough to melt the nuclear fuel and the containment vessel housing it.

**nurse** Health professional who provides many services for patients and who may work in a variety of settings.

**nurse practitioner (NP)** Professional nurse with advanced training obtained through either a master's degree program or a specialized nurse practitioner program.

**nutraceuticals** Term often used interchangeably with functional foods; refers to the combined nutritional and pharmaceutical benefit derived through use of foods or food supplements.

**nutrients** The constituents of food that sustain humans physiologically: proteins, carbohydrates, fats, vitamins, minerals, and water.

**nutrition** The science that investigates the relationship between physiological function and the essential elements of foods eaten.

**NuvaRing** A soft, flexible ring inserted into the vagina that releases hormones, preventing pregnancy.

**OA** *See* osteoarthritis.

**obesity** A body weight more than 20 percent above healthy recommended levels; in an adult, a BMI of 30 or more.

**obesogenic** Characterized by environments that promote increased food intake, non-healthful foods, and physical inactivity; refers to conditions that lead people to become excessively fat.

**obsession** Excessive preoccupation with an addictive object or behavior.

**obsessive-compulsive disorder (OCD)** A form of anxiety disorder characterized by recurrent, unwanted thoughts and repetitive behaviors.

**OCD** *See* obsessive-compulsive disorder.

**oncogenes** Suspected cancer-causing genes present on chromosomes.

**one repetition maximum (1 RM)** The amount of weight or resistance that can be lifted or moved only once.

**open relationship** A relationship in which partners agree that sexual involvement can occur outside the relationship.

**ophthalmologist** Physician who specializes in the medical and surgical care of the eyes, including prescriptions for glasses.

**opioids** Drugs that induce sleep and relieve pain; includes derivatives of opium and synthetics with similar chemical properties; also called narcotics.

**opium** The parent drug of the opioids; made from the seedpod resin of the opium poppy.

**opportunistic infections** Infections that occur when the immune system is weakened or compromised.

**optometrist** Eye specialist whose practice is limited to prescribing and fitting lenses.

**oral contraceptives** Pills containing synthetic hormones that prevent ovulation by regulating hormones.

**oral ingestion** Intake of drugs through the mouth.

**organic** Grown without use of pesticides, chemicals, or hormones.

**Ortho Evra** A patch that releases hormones similar to those in oral contraceptives; each patch is worn for 1 week.

**osteoarthritis (OA)** Progressive deterioration of bones and joints that has been associated with the wear-and-tear theory of aging.

**osteopath** General practitioner who receives training similar to a medical doctor's but with an emphasis on the skeletal and muscular systems; often uses spinal manipulation as part of treatment.

**osteoporosis** A degenerative bone disorder characterized by increasingly porous bones.

**ovarian follicles** Areas within the ovary in which individual eggs develop.

**ovaries** Almond-sized organs that house developing eggs and produce hormones.

**overload** A condition in which a person feels overly pressured by demands.

**overuse injuries** Injuries that result from the cumulative effects of day-after-day stresses placed on tendons, muscles, and joints.

**overweight** Having a body weight more than 10 percent above healthy recommended levels; in an adult, having a BMI of 25 to 29.

**oviducts** *See* fallopian tubes.

**ovulation** The point of the menstrual cycle at which a mature egg ruptures through the ovarian wall.

**ovum** A single mature egg cell.

**PA** *See* physician assistant.

**PAD** *See* peripheral artery disease.

**palliative care** Any form of medical care focused on relieving the pain, symptoms, and stress of serious illness in order to improve the quality of life for patients and their families.

**pancreas** Organ that secretes digestive enzymes into the small intestine, and hormones, including insulin, into the bloodstream.

**pandemic** Global epidemic of a disease.

**panic attack** Severe anxiety reaction in which a particular situation, often for unknown reasons, causes terror.

**Pap test** A procedure in which cells taken from the cervical region are examined for abnormal cellular activity.

**parasitic worms** The largest of the pathogens, most of which are more a nuisance than they are a threat.

**parasomnia** A disorder characterized by the occurrence of undesirable events while a person is sleeping.

**parasympathetic nervous system** Branch of the autonomic nervous system responsible for slowing systems stimulated by the stress response.

**passive euthanasia** The intentional withholding of treatment that would prolong life.

**pathogen** A disease-causing agent.

**PCBs** *See* polychlorinated biphenyls.

**PCP** *See* primary care practitioner.

**pelvic inflammatory disease (PID)** Inflammation of the female reproductive tract that occurs especially as a result of sexually transmitted infections and is a leading cause of infertility in women.

**penis** Male sexual organ that releases sperm into the vagina.

**peptic ulcer** Damage to the stomach or intestinal lining, usually caused by digestive juices; most ulcers result from infection by the bacterium *Helicobacter pylori*.

**perfect-use failure rate** The number of pregnancies (per 100 users) that are likely to occur in the first year of use of a particular birth control method if the method is used consistently and correctly.

**perineum** Tissue that forms the "floor" of the pelvic region in both men and women.

**peripheral artery disease (PAD)** Atherosclerosis occurring in the lower extremities, such as in the feet, calves, or legs, or in the arms.

**personal flotation device** A device worn to provide buoyancy and keep the wearer, conscious or unconscious, afloat with the nose and mouth out of the water; also known as a life jacket.

**personality disorders** A class of mental disorders that are characterized by inflexible patterns of thought and beliefs that lead to socially distressing behavior.

**pesticides** Chemicals that kill pests such as insects, weeds, and rodents.

**PET scan** *See* positron emission tomography scan.

**phobia** A deep and persistent fear of a specific object, activity, or situation that results in a compelling desire to avoid the source of the fear.

**photochemical smog** The brownish yellow haze resulting from the combination of hydrocarbons and nitrogen oxides.

**physical activity** Refers to all body movements produced by skeletal muscles resulting in substantial increases in energy expenditure.

**physical fitness** Refers to a set of attributes that allow you to perform moderate- to vigorous-intensity physical activities on a regular basis without getting too tired and with energy left over to handle physical or mental emergencies.

**physician assistant (PA)** A midlevel practitioner trained to handle most standard cases of care under the supervision of a physician.

**physiological dependence** The adaptive state that occurs with regular addictive behavior and results in withdrawal syndrome.

**PID** *See* pelvic inflammatory disease.

**pituitary gland** The endocrine gland controlling the release of hormones from the gonads.

**placenta** The network of blood vessels connected to the umbilical cord that carries nutrients, oxygen, and wastes between the developing infant and the mother.

**plant sterols** Essential components of plant membranes that, when consumed in the diet, appear to help lower cholesterol levels.

**plaque** Buildup of deposits in the arteries.

**platelet adhesiveness** Stickiness of red blood cells associated with blood clots.

**PMDD** *See* premenstrual dysphoric disorder.

**PMS** *See* premenstrual syndrome.

**pneumonia** Inflammatory disease of the lungs characterized by chronic cough, chest pain, chills, high fever, and fluid accumulation; may be caused by bacteria, viruses, fungi, chemicals, or other substances.

**PNI** *See* psychoneuroimmunology.

**point source pollutants** Pollutants that enter waterways at a specific location.

**poison** Any substance harmful to the body when ingested, inhaled, injected, or absorbed through the skin.

**pollutant** A substance that contaminates some aspect of the environment and causes potential harm to living organisms.

**polychlorinated biphenyls (PCBs)** Toxic chemicals that were once used as insulating materials in high-voltage electrical equipment.

**polydrug use** Taking several medications, vitamins, recreational drugs, or illegal drugs simultaneously.

**polysaccharides** Complex carbohydrates formed by the combination of long chains of monosaccharides.

**pornography** Visual or literary depictions of sexual activity intended to be sexually arousing.

**positive reinforcement** Presenting something positive following a behavior that is being reinforced.

**positron emission tomography (PET) scan** Method for measuring heart activity by injecting a patient with a radioactive tracer that is scanned electronically to produce a three-dimensional image of the heart and arteries.

**postpartum depression** Energy depletion, anxiety, mood swings, and depression that women may feel during the postpartum period.

**post-traumatic stress disorder (PTSD)** A collection of symptoms that may occur as a delayed response to a serious trauma.

**potentiation** *See* synergism.

**power** The ability to make and implement decisions.

**prayer** Communication with a transcendent Presence.

**preconception care** Medical care received prior to becoming pregnant that helps a woman assess and address potential maternal health issues.

**pre-diabetes** Condition in which blood glucose levels are higher than normal, but not high enough to be classified as diabetes.

**preeclampsia** A complication in pregnancy characterized by high blood pressure, protein in the urine, and edema.

**pre-gaming** A strategy of drinking heavily at home before going out to an event or other location.

**prejudice** A negative evaluation of an entire group of people that is typically based on unfavorable and often wrong ideas about the group.

**premature ejaculation** Ejaculation that occurs prior to or almost immediately following penile penetration of the vagina.

**premenstrual dysphoric disorder (PMDD)** Collective name for a group of negative symptoms similar to but more severe than PMS, including severe mood disturbances.

**premenstrual syndrome (PMS)** Comprises the mood changes and physical symptoms that occur in some women during the 1 or 2 weeks prior to menstruation.

**primary aggression** Goal-directed, hostile self-assertion that is destructive in character.

**primary care practitioner (PCP)** A medical practitioner who treats routine ailments, advises on preventive care, gives general medical advice, and makes appropriate referrals when necessary.

**prion** A recently identified self-replicating, protein-based pathogen.

**process addictions** Behaviors such as disordered gambling, compulsive buying, compulsive Internet or technology use, work addiction, compulsive exercise, and sexual addiction that are known to be addictive because they are mood altering.

**procrastinate** To intentionally put off doing something.

**progesterone** Hormone secreted by the ovaries; helps the endometrium develop and helps maintain pregnancy.

**proof** A measure of the percentage of alcohol in a beverage.

**prostate gland** Gland that secretes nutrients and neutralizing fluids into the semen.

**prostate-specific antigen (PSA)** An antigen found in prostate cancer patients.

**prostitution** The practice of engaging in sexual acts for money.

**proteins** The essential constituents of nearly all body cells; necessary for the development and repair of bone muscle, skin, and blood; the key elements of antibodies, enzymes, and hormones.

**protozoans** Microscopic single-celled organisms that can be pathogenic.

**PSA** *See* prostate-specific antigen.

**psychoactive drugs** Drugs that have the potential to alter mood or behavior.

**psychological hardiness** A personality trait characterized by control, commitment, and the embrace of challenge.

**psychological health** The mental, emotional, social, and spiritual dimensions of health.

**psychoneuroimmunology (PNI)** The science that examines the relationship between the brain and behavior and how this affects the body's immune system.

**PTSD** *See* post-traumatic distress disorder.

**puberty** The period of sexual maturation.

**pubic lice** Parasitic insects that can inhabit various body areas, especially the genitals.

**public health model** *See* ecological or public health model.

*qi* Element of traditional Chinese medicine that refers to the vital energy force that courses through the body; when *qi* is in balance, health is restored.

**rabies** A viral disease of the central nervous system; often transmitted through animal bites.

**radiation absorbed doses (rads)** Units that measure exposure to radiation.

**radiotherapy** The use of radiation to kill cancerous cells.

**radon** A naturally occurring radioactive gas resulting from the decay of certain radioactive elements.

**rads** *See* radiation absorbed doses.

**rape** Sexual penetration without the victim's consent.

**rational suicide** The decision to kill oneself rather than endure constant pain and slow decay.

**RDAs** *See* Recommended Dietary Allowances.

**reactive aggression** Hostile emotional reaction brought about by frustrating life experiences.

**receptor sites** Specialized areas of cells and organs where chemicals, enzymes, and other substances interact.

**recessive** Term describing an allele that is expressed only in the absence of a dominant allele, that is, if both alleles are recessive, or if the recessive gene is on the X chromosome of the twenty-third pair.

**Recommended Dietary Allowances (RDAs)** The average daily intakes of energy and nutrients considered adequate to meet the needs of most healthy people in the United States under usual conditions.

**relapse** The tendency to return to the addictive behavior after a period of abstinence.

**religion** A system of beliefs, practices, rituals, and symbols designed to facilitate closeness to the sacred or transcendent.

**REM sleep** A period of sleep characterized by brain-wave activity similar to that seen in wakefulness; rapid eye movement and dreaming occur during REM sleep.

**repetitive motion disorder (RMD)** An injury to soft tissues, tendons, muscles, nerves, or joints due to the physical stress of repeated motions.

**resting metabolic rate (RMR)** The energy expenditure of the body under BMR conditions plus other daily sedentary activities.

**restless legs syndrome (RLS)** A neurological disorder characterized by an overwhelming urge to move the legs when they are at rest.

**Rh factor** A blood protein related to the production of antibodies; if an Rh-negative mother is pregnant with an Rh-positive fetus, the mother may manufacture antibodies that can kill the fetus, causing miscarriage.

**rheumatic heart disease** A heart disease caused by untreated streptococcal infection of the throat.

**rheumatoid arthritis** An autoimmune inflammatory joint disease.

**RICE** Acronym for the standard first aid treatment for virtually all traumatic and overuse injuries: rest, ice, compression, and elevation.

**rickettsia** A small form of bacteria that live inside other living cells.

**risk behaviors** Actions that increase susceptibility to negative health outcomes.

**RLS** *See* restless legs syndrome.

**RMD** *See* repetitive motion disorder.

**RMR** *See* resting metabolic rate.

**rubella (German measles)** A milder form of measles that causes a rash and mild fever in children and may damage a fetus or a newborn baby.

**SAD** *See* seasonal affective disorder.

**SA node** *See* sinoatrial node.

**satiety** The feeling of fullness or satisfaction at the end of a meal.

**saturated fats** Fats that are unable to hold any more hydrogen in their chemical structure; derived mostly from animal sources; solid at room temperature.

**SBS** *See* sick building syndrome.

**schizophrenia** A mental illness with biological origins that is characterized by irrational behavior, severe alterations of the senses, and often an inability to function in society.

**scrotum** External sac of tissue that encloses the testes.

**seasonal affective disorder (SAD)** A type of depression that occurs in the winter months, when sunlight levels are low.

**secondary sex characteristics** Characteristics associated with sex but not directly related to reproduction, such as vocal pitch, degree of body hair, and location of fat deposits.

**secondhand smoke** *See* environmental tobacco smoke.

**self-disclosure** Sharing personal feelings or information with others.

**self-efficacy** Belief in one's ability to perform a task successfully.

**self-injury** Intentionally causing injury to one's own body in an attempt to cope with overwhelming negative emotions; also called self-mutilation, self-harm, or non-suicidal self-injury (NSSI).

**self-nurturance** Developing individual potential through a balanced and realistic appreciation of self-worth and ability.

**self-talk** The customary manner of thinking and talking to yourself, which can affect your self-image.

**semen** Fluid containing sperm and nutrients that increase sperm viability and neutralize vaginal acid.

**seminal vesicles** Glandular ducts that secrete nutrients for the semen.

**serial monogamy** A series of monogamous sexual relationships.

**set point theory** Theory that a form of internal thermostat controls our weight and fights to maintain this weight around a narrowly set range.

**sexual abuse of children** Sexual interaction between a child and an adult or older child.

**sexual addiction** Compulsive involvement in sexual activity.

**sexual assault** Any act in which one person is sexually intimate with another without that person's consent.

**sexual aversion disorder** Desire dysfunction characterized by sexual phobias and anxiety about sexual contact.

**sexual dysfunction** Problems associated with achieving sexual satisfaction.

**sexual fantasies** Sexually arousing thoughts and dreams.

**sexual harassment** Any form of unwanted sexual attention related to any condition of employment or performance evaluation.

**sexual identity** Recognition of oneself as a sexual being; a composite of biological sex characteristics, gender identity, gender roles, and sexual orientation.

**sexual orientation** A person's enduring emotional, romantic, sexual, or affectionate attraction to other persons.

**sexual performance anxiety** A condition of sexual difficulties caused by anticipating some sort of problem with the sex act.

**sexual prejudice** Negative attitudes and hostile actions directed at sexually identified social groups; also referred to as sexual bias.

**sexuality** All the thoughts, feelings, and behaviors associated with being male or female, experiencing attraction, being in love, and being in relationships that include sexual intimacy and activity.

**sexually transmitted infections (STIs)** Infectious diseases caused by pathogens transmitted through some form of intimate, usually sexual, contact.

**shaping** Using a series of small steps to gradually achieve a particular goal.

**shingles** A disease characterized by a painful rash that occurs when the chickenpox virus is reactivated.

**SI** *See* spiritual intelligence.

**sick building syndrome (SBS)** Problem that exists when 80 percent of a building's occupants report maladies that tend to lessen or vanish when they leave the building.

**sidestream smoke** The cigarette, pipe, or cigar smoke breathed by nonsmokers.

**SIDS** *See* sudden infant death syndrome.

**simple carbohydrates** A major type of carbohydrate, which provides short-term energy; also called simple sugars.

**simple rape** Rape by one person, usually known to the victim, that does not involve physical beating or use of a weapon.

**simple sugars** *See* simple carbohydrates.

**single-gene disorder** A disorder characterized by structural and/or functional impairments resulting from a defect involving only one gene.

**sinoatrial node (SA node)** Cluster of electric pulse-generating cells that serves as a natural pacemaker for the heart.

**situational inducement** Attempt to influence a behavior through situations and occasions that are structured to exert control over that behavior.

**sleep** A readily reversible state of reduced responsiveness to, and interaction with, the environment.

**sleep apnea** A disorder in which breathing is briefly and repeatedly interrupted during sleep.

**sleep debt** The difference between the number of hours of sleep an individual needed in a given time period and the number of hours he or she actually slept.

**sleep inertia** A state characterized by cognitive impairment, grogginess, and disorientation that is experienced upon rising from short sleep or an overly long nap.

**sleep study** A clinical assessment of sleep in which the patient is monitored while spending the night in a sleep disorders center.

**snuff** A powdered form of tobacco that is sniffed or absorbed through the mucous membranes in the nose or placed inside the cheek and sucked.

**social anxiety disorder** *See* social phobia.

**social bonds** Degree and nature of interpersonal contacts.

**social cognitive model** Model of behavior change emphasizing the role of social factors and thought processes (cognition) in behavior change.

**social death** A seemingly irreversible situation in which a person is not treated like an active member of society.

**social health** Aspect of psychosocial health that includes interactions with others, ability to use social supports, and ability to adapt to various situations.

**social learning theory** Theory that people learn behaviors by watching role models— parents, caregivers, and significant others.

**social phobia** A phobia characterized by fear and avoidance of social situations; also called social anxiety disorder.

**social physique anxiety (SPA)** A desire to look good that has a destructive effect on a person's ability to function well in social interactions and relationships.

**social support** Network of people and services with whom you share ties and from whom you get support.

**socialization** Process by which a society communicates behavioral expectations to its individual members.

**SPA** *See* social physique anxiety.

**spermatogenesis** The development of sperm.

**spermicide** Substance designed to kill sperm.

**spiritual health** The aspect of psychosocial health that relates to having a sense of meaning and purpose to one's life, as well as a feeling of connection with others and with nature.

**spiritual intelligence (SI)** The intelligence of the deep self; a capacity to live in alignment with our inner wisdom, values, and vision.

**spirituality** An individual's sense of purpose and meaning in life, beyond material values.

**spontaneous abortion** *See* miscarriage.

**stages of change model** *See* transtheoretical model.

**stalking** The willful, repeated, and malicious following, harassing, or threatening of another person.

**standard drink** The amount of any beverage that contains about 14 grams of pure alcohol (about 0.6 fluid ounce or 1.2 tablespoons).

**staphylococci** A group of round bacteria, usually found in clusters, that cause a variety of diseases in humans and other animals.

**starch** Polysaccharide that is the storage form of glucose in plants.

**static stretching** Stretching techniques that slowly and gradually lengthen a muscle or group of muscles and their tendons.

**stent** A stainless steel, meshlike tube that is inserted to prop open the artery.

**sterilization** Permanent fertility control achieved through surgical procedures.

**stigmas** Negative stereotypes about groups of people.

**stillbirth** The birth of a dead baby.

**stimulants** Drugs that increase activity of the central nervous system.

**STIs** *See* sexually transmitted infections.

**Streptococcus** A round bacterium, usually found in chain formation.

**stress** A series of physiological responses and adaptations in response to a real or imagined threat to one's well-being.

**stress inoculation** Stress-management technique in which a person consciously tries to prepare ahead of time for potential stressors.

**stressor** A physical, social, or psychological event or condition that upsets homeostasis and produces a stress response.

**stroke** A condition occurring when the brain is damaged by disrupted blood supply; also called cerebrovascular accident.

**subjective well-being** An uplifting feeling of inner peace.

**suction curettage** An abortion technique that uses gentle suction to remove fetal tissue from the uterus.

**sudden cardiac death** Death that occurs as a result of abrupt, profound loss of heart function.

**sudden infant death syndrome (SIDS)** The sudden death of an infant under 1 year of age for no apparent reason.

**suicidal ideation** A desire to die and thoughts about suicide.

**Superfund** Fund established under the Comprehensive Environmental Response, Compensation, and Liability Act to be used for cleaning up toxic waste dumps.

**suppositories** Mixtures of drugs and a waxy medium (designed to melt at body temperature) that are inserted into the anus or vagina.

**survivorship** Physical, psychological, emotional, and economic issues of cancer from diagnosis until the end of life.

**sympathetic nervous system** Branch of the autonomic nervous system responsible for stress arousal.

**sympathomimetics** Food substances that can produce stresslike physiological responses.

**synergism** The interaction of two or more drugs that produces more profound effects than would be expected if the drugs were taken separately; also called potentiation.

**syphilis** One of the most widespread bacterial sexually transmitted infections; characterized by distinct phases and potentially serious results.

**systolic pressure** The upper number in the fraction that measures blood pressure, indicating pressure on arterial walls when the heart contracts.

**tar** A thick, brownish substance condensed from particulate matter in smoked tobacco.

**target heart rate** The heart rate range of aerobic exercise that leads to improved cardiorespiratory fitness (i.e., 70% to 90% of maximal heart rate).

**TB** *See* tuberculosis.

**TCM** *See* traditional Chinese medicine.

**temperature inversion** A weather condition occurring when a layer of cool air is trapped under a layer of warmer air.

**teratogenic** Causing birth defects; may refer to drugs, environmental chemicals, X rays, or diseases.

**terrorism** The unlawful use of force or violence against persons or property to intimidate or coerce a government, the civilian population, or any segment thereof in furtherance of political or social objectives.

**testator** A person who leaves a will or testament at death.

**testes** Male sex organs that manufacture sperm and produce hormones.

**testosterone** The male sex hormone manufactured in the testes.

**tetrahydrocannabinol (THC)** The chemical name for the active ingredient in marijuana.

**thanatology** The study of death and dying.

**THC** *See* tetrahydrocannabinol.

**thrombolysis** Injection of an agent to dissolve clots and restore some blood flow, thereby reducing the amount of tissue that dies from ischemia.

**thrombus** Blood clot attached to a blood vessel's wall.

**TIA** *See* transient ischemic attack.

**time** As part of the FITT prescription, refers to how long a person needs to exercise each time to improve a parameter of physical fitness.

**tinctures** Herbal extracts usually combined with grain alcohol to prevent spoilage.

**TMS** *See* triple marker screen.

**Today sponge** A contraceptive device, made of polyurethane foam and containing nonoxynol-9, that fits over the cervix to create a barrier against sperm.

**tolerance** Phenomenon in which progressively larger doses of a drug or more intense involvement in a behavior is needed to produce the desired effects.

**total fertility rate** The hypothetical average number of children born to women during their lifetime, given prevailing fertility and mortality rates.

**toxic shock syndrome (TSS)** A potentially life-threatening disease that occurs when specific bacterial toxins multiply and spread to the bloodstream, most commonly through improper use of tampons, diaphragms, or cervical caps.

**toxins** Poisonous substances produced by certain microorganisms that cause various diseases.

**toxoplasmosis** A disease caused by an organism found in cat feces that, when contracted by a pregnant woman, may result in stillbirth or an infant with mental retardation or birth defects.

**trace minerals** Minerals that the body needs in only very small amounts.

**traditional Chinese medicine (TCM)** Ancient comprehensive system of healing that uses herbs, acupuncture, and massage to bring the body into balance and to re-

move blockages of vital energy flow that lead to disease.

***trans* fats (*trans* fatty acids)** Fatty acids that are produced when polyunsaturated oils are hydrogenated to make them more solid.

**transdermal** The introduction of drugs through the skin.

**transgendered** Having a gender identity that does not match one's biological sex.

**transient ischemic attack (TIA)** Brief interruption of the blood supply to the brain that causes only temporary impairment; often an indicator of impending major stroke.

**transsexual** A person who is psychologically of one sex but physically of the other.

**transtheoretical model** Model of behavior change that identifies six distinct stages people go through in altering behavior patterns; also called the *stages of change model.*

**traumatic injuries** Injuries that are accidental and occur suddenly and violently.

**trichomoniasis** Protozoan sexually transmitted infection characterized by foamy, yellowish discharge and unpleasant odor.

**triglycerides** The most common form of fat in the body; excess calories consumed are converted into triglycerides and stored as body fat.

**triglycerides** The most common form of lipid in the body; excess calories are converted into triglycerides and stored as body fat.

**trimester** A 3-month segment of pregnancy; used to describe specific developmental changes that occur in the embryo or fetus.

**triple marker screen (TMS)** A maternal blood test that can be used to help identify fetuses with certain birth defects and genetic abnormalities.

**TSS** *See* toxic shock syndrome.

**tubal ligation** Sterilization of the woman that involves the cutting and tying off or cauterizing of the fallopian tubes.

**tuberculosis (TB)** A disease caused by bacterial infiltration of the respiratory system.

**tumor** A neoplasmic mass that grows more rapidly than surrounding tissue.

**type** As part of the FITT prescription, refers to what kind of exercises a person needs to do to improve a parameter of physical fitness.

**type 1 diabetes** Form of diabetes mellitus in which the pancreas is not able to make insulin and therefore blood glucose cannot enter the cells to be used for energy.

**type 2 diabetes** Form of diabetes mellitus in which the pancreas does not make enough insulin or the body is unable to use insulin correctly.

**typical-use failure rate** The number of pregnancies (per 100 users) that are likely to occur in the first year of use of a particular birth control method if the method's use is not consistent or always correct.

**UC** *See* ulcerative colitis.

**ulcerative colitis (UC)** An inflammatory disorder that affects the mucous membranes of the large intestine, producing bloody diarrhea.

**ultrasonography (ultrasound)** A common prenatal test that uses high-frequency sound waves to create a visual image of the fetus.

**ultrasound** *See* ultrasonography.

**underweight** Having a body weight more than 10 percent below healthy recommended levels; in an adult, having a BMI below 18.5.

**unintentional injury** Any injury committed or sustained without intent of harm.

**unsaturated fats** Fats that do have room for more hydrogen in their chemical structure; derived mostly from plants; liquid at room temperature.

**urethral opening** The opening through which urine is expelled.

**urinary incontinence** Inability to control urination.

**uterus (womb)** Hollow, pear-shaped muscular organ whose function is to contain the developing fetus.

**vaccination** Inoculation with killed or weakened pathogens or similar, less dangerous antigens in order to prevent or lessen the effects of some disease.

**vagina** The passage in females leading from the vulva into the uterus.

**vaginal intercourse** The insertion of the penis into the vagina.

**vaginismus** A state in which the vaginal muscles contract so forcefully that penetration cannot occur.

**values** Principles that influence our thoughts and emotions, and guide the choices we make in our lives.

**variant sexual behavior** A sexual behavior that is not practiced by most people.

**vas deferens** Tube that transports sperm from the epididymis to the ejaculatory duct.

**vasectomy** Sterilization of the man that involves the cutting and tying off of both vasa deferentia.

**vasocongestion** The engorgement of the genital organs with blood.

**vegetarian** A person who follows a diet that excludes some or all animal products.

**veins** Vessels that transport waste and carry blood back to the heart from other regions of the body.

**ventricles** The heart's two lower chambers, which pump blood through the blood vessels.

**venules** Branches of the veins.

**very low-calorie diets (VLCDs)** Diets with a daily caloric value of 400 to 700 calories.

**violence** A set of behaviors that produces injuries, as well as the outcomes of these behaviors (the injuries themselves).

**virulent** Strong enough to overcome host resistance and cause disease.

**viruses** Minute microbes consisting of DNA or RNA that invade a host cell and use the cell's resources to reproduce themselves.

**visualization** The creation of mental images to promote relaxation.

**vitamins** Essential organic compounds that promote growth and reproduction and help maintain life and health.

**VLCDs** *See* very low-calorie diets.

**vulva** Collective term for the external female genitalia.

**waist-to-hip ratio** Waist circumference divided by hip circumference; a high ratio indicates increased health risks due to unhealthy fat distribution.

**water intoxication** *See* hyponatremia.

**wellness** The achievement of the highest level of health possible in each of several dimensions.

**whole grains** Grains that are milled in their complete form, and so include the bran, germ, and endosperm, with only the husk removed.

**whole medical systems** *See* alternative medical systems.

**withdrawal 1** A method of contraception that involves withdrawing the penis from the vagina before ejaculation; also called coitus interruptus.

**withdrawal 2** A series of temporary physical and biopsychosocial symptoms that occurs when an addict abruptly abstains from an addictive chemical or behavior.

**womb** *See* uterus.

**work addiction** The compulsive use of work and the work persona to fulfill needs for intimacy, power, and success.

**XDR-TB** *See* extensively drug resistant TB.

**X-linked dominant disorder** Single-gene disorder that occurs in individuals who have inherited at least one copy of an X chromosome with the affected dominant allele.

**X-linked recessive disorder** Single-gene disorder that occurs in individuals who have inherited only one copy of an X chromosome with the affected recessive allele.

**yeast infection** *See* candidiasis.

**yoga** A system of physical and mental training involving controlled breathing, physical postures (asanas), meditation, chanting, and other practices that are believed to cultivate unity with the Atman, or Absolute.

**yo-yo diets** Cycles in which people diet and regain weight.

# Photo Credits

**Chapter 1** Opener: Laura Doss/Corbis; p. 2 left to right: AP Wide World Photos; Shutterstock; Mitchel Gray/Jupiter Images; p. 3 left to right: Randy Faris/Corbis; Christina Kennedy/Alamy; fig. 1.1: Ale Ventura/PhotoAlto/Jupiter Images; p. 4: sumnersgraphicsinc/iStockphoto; p. 5: AP Wide World Photos; p. 6: Shutterstock; p. 7: Digital Stock/Corbis; fig. 1.2: IT Stock Free/AGE Fotostock; fig. 1.5 top left: iStockphoto; fig. 1.5 top right: Shutterstock; fig. 1.5 bottom right: Grantly Lynch/Alamy; fig. 1.5 bottom left: iStockphoto; p. 11: Shutterstock; p. 12: David R. Frazier Photolibrary, Inc./Photo Researchers, Inc.; p. 14 top: Suzy Allman/Getty Images; p. 14 bottom: Liz Van Steenburgh/iStockphoto; p. 17: iStockphoto/ThinkStock; p. 18: Mitchel Gray/SuperStock/Jupiter Images; p. 20: Liz Van Steenburgh/iStockphoto; p. 21: Randy Faris/Corbis; p. 22: Christina Kennedy/Alamy; p. 24: Jacob Wackerhausen/iStockphoto; p. 25: Lisa F. Young/iStockphoto; p. 26: iStockphoto.

**Chapter 2** Opener: Noel Hendrickson/Getty Images; p. 30 left to right: Pascal Broze/AGE Fotostock; Randy Faris/Corbis; Comstock/Jupiter Images; p. 31 left to right: David H. Seymour/Shutterstock; endostock/fotolia; p. 33: Ed Bock/Corbis; fig. 2.3 left: Thinkstock/Jupiter Images; fig. 2.3 right: Terry Vine/Blend Images/Getty Images; p. 35: Pascal Broze/AGE Fotostock; p. 37 top: Randy Faris/Corbis; p. 37 bottom: Image Source; p. 38: George Doyle/Getty Images; p. 39: Sharon Dominick/iStockphoto; p. 41: Photolibrary; p. 42: Shutterstock; p. 43: Comstock Images/Jupiter Unlimited; p. 44: Peter Hvizdak/The Image Works; p. 45 top: John Bell/iStockphoto; p. 45 bottom: Losevsky Pavel/Shutterstock; p. 47: Bubbles Photolibrary/Alamy; p. 48: Hank Morgan/Photo Researchers; p. 49: Simon Rawley/Alamy; p. 51: Shutterstock; p. 52: David H. Seymour/Shutterstock; p. 54: endostock/fotolia; p. 55: Jon Helgason/iStockphoto; p. 56: iStockphoto.

**FOCUS ON Cultivating Your Spiritual Health** Opener: Stephen Shepherd/Alamy; p. 60 left to right: Ari Joseph/Middlebury College; Jochem D Wijnands/Getty Images; George Doyle/Getty Images; Image Source; p. 61: Jim West/Alamy; p. 62 Jochem D Wijnands/Getty Images; p. 64: K-King Media Co. Ltd /Getty Images; p. 65: Blend Images/Alamy; p. 66 top: mvp64/iStockphoto; p. 66 bottom: Slobo Mitic/iStockphoto; p. 67 top: PhotoAlto/Alamy; p. 67 bottom: DAJ/Getty Images; p. 68 left: Sharon Dominick/iStockphoto; p. 68 right: Blend Images/Alamy; p. 69: Jumpstart; p. 70 top: Alex Slobodkin/iStockphoto; p. 70 bottom: Aldo Ottaviani/iStockphoto.

**Chapter 3** Opener: Comstock Images/Getty Images; p. 72 left to right: Aliosha Marquez/AP World Wide Photo; Alamy; Workbook Stock/Jupiter Images/Getty Images; Ryan McVay/Photodisc/Getty Images; p. 73 left to right: Sam Chrysanthou/Photolibrary; Alamy; p. 74 left: Aliosha Marquez/AP World Wide Photo; p. 74 right: Alamy; fig. 3.2: Sam Diephuis/CORBIS; fig. 3.3: Michael Krinke/iStockphoto; p. 77: Masterfile; p. 78 top: Murat Giray Kaya/iStockphoto; p. 78 bottom left: Workbook Stock/Jupiter Images/Getty Images; p. 79 top: Shutterstock; p. 79 bottom: David De Lossy/Photodisc/Getty Images; fig. 3.4 Radius Images/Corbis; p. 81: Marili Forastieri/Getty Images; p. 82 top: iStockphoto; p. 82 bottom: Ryan McVay/ Photodisc/Getty Images; p. 83: Bridget Montgomery/AP Wide World Photos; p. 84: iStockphoto; p. 85: Sam Chrysanthou/Photolibrary; p. 87: Chuck Savage/Corbis; p. 88: Jamie Grill/Getty Images; p. 89: DEX IMAGE/Jupiter Images; p. 90: Tetra Images/Alamy; p. 93 top: Richard Rodvold/iStockphoto; p. 93 bottom: Creatas Images/Jupiter Images; p. 94: Andy Crawford/Dorling Kindersley; fig. 3.7: John Dowland/Photolibrary; p. 96: iStockphoto; p. 97 top: Sharon Dominick/iStockphoto; p. 97 bottom: iStockphoto.

**FOCUS ON Improving Your Sleep** Opener: Rubberball/Getty Images; p. 102 left to right: Patrick Keen/iStockphoto; Brooklyn Production/Corbis; GoGo Images/Jupiter Images; Radius Images/Jupiter Images; p. 104 top: Ryan McVay/Getty Images; p.104 bottom: Patrick Keen/iStockphoto; p. 106: SuperStock/Alamy; p. 108 left: Brooklyn Production/Corbis; p. 108 right: GoGo Images/Jupiter Images; p. 109: Stockxpert/Jupiter Images; p. 110: Radius Images/Jupiter Images; p. 111: sumnersgraphicsinc/iStockphoto; fig. 3: Inga Spence/Photo Researchers, Inc.; p. 113: Mark Douet/Getty Images; p. 114 top: stephanie phillips/iStockphoto; p. 114 bottom: Emrah Turudu/iStockphoto.

**Chapter 4** Opener: JGI/Jamie Grill/Getty Images; p. 116 left to right: Jose Luis Pelaez/Corbis; Somos Images/Alamy; Masterfile; p.117 left to right: David Young-Wolff/PhotoEdit; PhotoAlto/John Dowland/Getty Images; p. 118: Jose Luis Pelaez./Corbis; p. 119: Laura Doss/Fancy/PhotoLibrary; p. 121: Somos Images/Alamy; p. 124 top: Masterfile; p. 124 bottom: Marina Krasnorutskaya/Shutterstock; p. 125 left: Marina Krasnorutskaya/Shutterstock; p. 125 right: Masterfile; p. 126: David Nagel/Getty Images; p. 128 top: David Young-Wolff/PhotoEdit; p. 128 bottom: Sharon Dominick/iStockphoto; p. 130: Purestock/Getty Images; p. 131: Purestock/Jupiter Images; p. 132: Ryan McVay/Getty Images; p. 133: Jaroslaw Grudzinski/Shutterstock; p. 134 left: Corbis/SuperStock; p. 134 right: iStockphoto; p. 136: Martyn Vickery/Alamy; p. 138: Yanik Chauvin/iStockphoto.com.

**Chapter 5** Opener: Buena Vista Images/Getty Images; p. 142 left to right: David J. Green/Alamy; DK Stock/Veronique Krieger/Getty Images; Kevin Dodge/Masterfile; p. 143 left to right: Orenstein/Photodisc/Getty Images; PhotoAlto/Alamy; p. 144: Sharon Dominick/iStockphoto; p. 147: David J. Green - lifestyle themes/Alamy; p. 149: Matthias Clamer/Getty Images; p. 150: DK Stock/Veronique Krieger/Getty Images; p. 152: Kevin Dodge/Masterfile; p. 153: Gallo Images/Getty Images; p. 154: Getty Images; p. 155: Allison Michael Orenstein/Photodisc/Getty Images; p. 156: Huntstock/Getty Images; p. 157: Ranald Mackechnie/Getty Images; p. 158: Sieto Verver/iStockphoto; p. 159: PhotoAlto/Alamy; p. 160: sumnersgraphicsinc/iStockphoto; p. 161 top: Banana Stock/Jupiter Images; p. 161 bottom: Getty Images; p. 162: shoo_arts/Shutterstock; p. 163: iStockphoto.

**Chapter 6** Opener: Gary John Norman/Getty Images; p. 168 left to right: Adam Hart-Davis/Photo Researchers; Maureen Spuhler/seelevel.com; Fancy/Alamy; p. 169 left to right: Newscom; Stockbrokerxtra Images/PhotoLibrary; p. 170: Michael Keller/Corbis; p. 171: Corbis; p. 173: Murat Giray Kaya/iStockphoto; fig. 6.2: Dorling Kindersley; p. 175: Creative Digital Visions; fig. 6.3: Jules Selmes and Debi Treolar/Dorling Kindersley; p. 176 left: Reproduced with permission from FemCap, Inc. and Alfred Shihata, MD; p. 176 right: Allendale Pharmaceuticals, Inc.; p. 177: Adam Hart-Davis/Photo Researchers, Inc.; p. 179: Johnson & Johnson Pharmaceutical Services, LLC; p. 180 top: NuvaRing, Inc., Organon USA, Inc.; p. 180 bottom: Phanie/Photo Researchers, Inc.; p. 181: Saturn Stills/Photo Researchers, Inc.; p. 182: Teva North America; p. 183: Maureen Spuhler/seelevel.com; p. 186 Fancy/Alamy; p. 188: Imagesource/PhotoLibrary; p. 189: Newscom; p. 192: Stockbrokerxtra Images/PhotoLibrary; fig. 6.11: Lisa Spindler Photography, Inc./Getty Images; fig. 6.12a: Claude Edelman/ Photo Researchers; fig. 6.12b: Petit Format/Nestle/Photo Researchers, Inc.; fig. 6.12c: Petit Format/Nestle/Photo Researchers, Inc.; p. 197: Leland Bobbe/Getty Images; p. 199: Golden Pixels LLC/Alamy; p. 202: Plush Studios/Getty Images; p. 203: Donna Coleman/iStockphoto; p. 205 left: Christoph Achenbach/iStockphoto; p. 205 right: Marc Dietrich/iStockphoto.

**Chapter 7** Opener: Radius Images/Getty Images; p. 210 left to right: Mohr Images/StockFood Creative/Getty Images; Noel Hendrickson/Getty Images; Imagesource/PhotoLibrary; p. 211 left to right: Brian Hagiwara/Jupiter Images; Reg Charity/Corbis; fig. 7.1: webphotographeer/iStockphoto; p. 214: design56/Shutterstock; fig. 7.2: PLG/Pearson Science; p. 216: Mohr Images - Stockfood Munich/Stockfood; p. 217: HO/Reuters/Corbis; p. 218: Sharon Dominick/iStockphoto; p. 219: Brian Leatart/FoodPix/Jupiter Images; p. 220: Noel Hendrickson/Getty Images; table 7.2 top to bottom: Brand Pictures/AGE Fotostock; Brand Pictures/AGE Fotostock; Corbis; Photodisc/Getty Images; Corbis; Corbis; table 7.3 top to bottom: BrandPictures/AGE Fotostock; Corbis; Corbis; Brand Pictures/AGE Fotostock; p. 224: Fresh Food Images/PhotoLibrary; p. 225 top: Monika Adamczyk/iStockphoto; p. 225 bottom: Suzannah Skelton/iStockphoto; table 7.4 top to bottom: Brand Pictures/AGE Fotostock; Brand Pictures/AGE Fotostock; Corbis; Brand Pictures/AGE Fotostock; Corbis; table 7.5: Corbis; p. 228: Imagesource/PhotoLibrary; fig. 7.5 top to bottom: Flashon Studio/iStockphoto; Chris Bence/Shutterstock; Westmacott Photography/iStockphoto; JR Trice/Shutterstock; Stargazer/Shutterstock; Morgan Lane Photography/Shutterstock; p. 230 left to right: PLG/Pearson Science; Flashon Studio/

iStockphoto; Corbis; Brand Pictures/AGE Fotostock; Corbis; Brand Pictures/AGE Fotostock; Corbis BrandPictures/AGE Fotostock; Brand Pictures/AGE Fotostock; JR Trice/Shutterstock; Corbis; Corbis; Corbis; Corbis; Corbis; p. 232: Brian Hagiwara/Jupiter Images; p. 233: Suzannah Skelton/iStockphoto; p. 235: Reg Charity/Corbis; p. 239: Eric Gevaert/iStockphoto; p. 240 top: USDA; p. 240 bottom: rtyree1/iStockphoto; p. 241: MorePixels/iStockphoto; p. 242: Joel Nito/AFP/Getty Images; p. 244: Denise Kappa/iStockphoto.com; p. 245 top: iStockphoto; p. 245 bottom: Jaimie Duplass/iStockphoto.

**Chapter 8** Opener: Erik Isakson/age footstock; p. 250 left to right: Alex Mares-Manton/Getty Images; UPI/Newscom; Custom Medical Stock/Alamy; p. 251 left to right: UpperCut Images/Alamy; Evan Vucci/AP Wide World Photos; fig. 8.2: Big Cheese Photo LLC/Alamy; p. 253: Ariel Skelley/Corbis; p. 255: UPI/Brian Kersey/Newscom; p. 256: Anton J. Geisser/AGE Fotostock; p. 257: Brand X Pictures/Getty Images; p. 258: Jose Luis Pelaez, Inc./Getty Images; p. 259: Image Source/Alamy; p. 260: Russell Underwood/Getty Images; p. 262 Jim Esposito Photography LLC/Getty Images; p. 264 top to bottom: PhotoEdit; Custom Medical Stock Photo; May/Photo Researchers, Inc.; Phanie/Photo Researchers, Inc.; Life Measurement, Inc.; fig. 8.6 left: Girl Ray/Stone/Getty Images; fig. 8.6 right: Image Source Pink/Getty Images; p. 267: Murat Giray Kaya/iStockphoto; p. 268: UpperCut Images/Alamy; p. 270 top: Evan Vucci/AP Photo; p. 270 bottom: Aleksei Potov/Shutterstock; p. 271: Kevin Winter/American Idol 2009/Getty Images for FOX; p. 272: Dennis MacDonald/PhotoEdit; p. 273 LIU Jin/Agence France Presse/Getty Images; p. 274 top: Catherine Lane/iStockphoto; p. 274 bottom: Sharon Dominick/iStockphoto; p. 275: iStockphoto; p. 276: iStockphoto.

**FOCUS ON Enhancing Your Body Image** Opener: Stockbyte/Getty Images; p. 280 left to right: CBS Photo/Getty Images; Bettmann/Corbis; Travel Ink/Alamy; Simona Ghizzoni/Redux Pictures; Pascal Broze/Getty Images; fig. 1 left: Custom Medical Stock Photo/Alamy; fig. 1 right: Sakala /Shutterstock; p. 283 top left: CBS Photo Archive/Getty Images; p. 283 top right: Bettmann/Corbis; p. 283 bottom: Jupiter Images; p. 284 Travel Ink/Alamy; fig. 2 left: Brand X Pictures/Jupiter Unlimited; fig. 2 right: gollykim/iStockphoto; p. 286: Chistopher LaMarca/Redux Pictures; fig. 4: Simona Ghizzoni/Redux Pictures; fig. 5: Corbis; p. 288: WireImage/Getty Images; p. 289: Pascal Broze/Getty Images; p. 290 left: Loretta Hostettler/iStockphoto; p. 290 right: Sharon Dominick/iStockphoto; p. 291 top: Lucas Allen White/Shutterstock; p. 291 bottom: Photodisc/Thinkstock; p. 292: Gustavo Andrade/Getty Images.

**Chapter 9** Opener: Stockbyte/Getty Images; p. 294 left to right: Stockbyte/Getty Images; David Sacks/Getty Images; Jupiter Images; p. 295 left to right: Thomas Smith Photography/Alamy; AGE Fotostock; p. 296 top: Neo Vision/Getty Images; p. 296 bottom: Kazuhiro Nogi/AFP/Getty Images; fig. 9.1 left to right: Teo Lannie/Getty Images; Pearson Education; Photodisc/Getty Images; Superstock; JLP/Jose Luis Pelaez/Corbis; p. 298: Sharon Dominick/iStockphoto; fig. 9.2: Pete Saloutos/Corbis; p. 300: Stockbyte/Getty Images; p. 301: Stockbyte/Getty Images; p. 302: David Sacks/Getty Images; p. 303: James Whitaker/Alamy; table 9.3 top left to right: Walter Cruz/Dallas Morning News/MCT/Newscom; Craig Veltri/iStockphoto; Tatuasha/shutterstock; Paul Maguire/iStockphoto; Melvin Levine/Time & Life Pictures/Getty Images; Graca Victoria/Shutterstock; Sandra Caldwell/Shutterstock; Masterfile; table 9.3 bottom left to right: K. J. Pargeter Images/iStockphoto; enderbirer/iStockphoto; Bob Jacobson/Corbis; Ali Ender Birer/shutterstock; Dandanian/iStockphoto; p. 305: Masterfile; p. 306 left to right: Dan Dalton/Getty Images; MIXA/Getty Images; Image Source Pink/Getty Images; fig. 9.6a: Creative Digital Visions; fig. 9.6b: Karl Weatherly/Getty Images; p. 308: Abelimages/Getty Images; p. 309 OSU Office of News & Communication; p. 310: Masterfile; table 9.4 left to right: Jac Mat Communication Marketing; Pearson Education; Pearson Education; HOGGAN Health Industries, Inc.; fig. 9.7c–d: Elena Dorfman; p. 313: Jupiter Images; p. 314: Sheer Photo, Inc/Getty Images; p. 316: Thomas Smith Photography/Alamy; p. 317 top: Kristin Piljay, Pearson Science; p. 317 bottom: iStockphoto; fig. 9.8: Thomas Northcut/Getty Images; p. 318: AGE Fotostock; p. 319: Radius Images/PhotoLibrary; p. 320: Ingram Publishing/PhotoLibrary; p. 321 top: Aleksandr Lobanov/iStockphoto; p. 321 bottom: Elena Dorfman, Pearson Science; p. 322: Creative Digital Visions; p. 323: Pearson Canada; p. 324 top: Eliza Snow/iStockphoto; p. 324 bottom: Jacqueline Perez/iStockphoto.

**Chapter 10** Opener: Eric Bean/Getty Images; p. 328 left to right: Hill Creek Pictures/Alamy; Steve Cole/Getty Images; Cassiede Alain/Shutterstock; p. 329 left to right: UpperCut Images/Alamy; Kristy-Anne Glubish/Jupiter Images; p. 330 left: Philip & Karen Smith/Getty Images; p. 330 right: Hill Creek Pictures/Alamy; p. 331: Steve Cole/Getty Images; p. 332: sumnersgraphicsinc/iStockphoto; p. 333: Cassiede Alain/Shutterstock; p. 334: RubberBall/Alamy; p. 335: John Howard/Getty Images; p. 336: Ike Van de Velde/Digital Vision/Alamy; p. 337: Denis Pepin/iStockphoto; p. 338: Antonio Mo/Getty Images;

fig. 10.3: Corbis Super RF/Alamy; p. 339: UpperCut Images/Alamy; p. 340: Kristy-Anne Glubish/Jupiter Images; p. 341: Blend Images/Alamy; p. 342: Catchlight Visual Services/Alamy; p. 343: Oleg Prikhodko/iStockphoto; p. 344 top: Kasia Biel/iStockphoto; p. 344 bottom: afhunta/iStockphoto; p. 345: Chris Bernart/iStockphoto.

**Chapter 11** Opener: Andersen Ross/Getty Images; p. 348 left to right: Getty Images; Goodshoot/Jupiter Images; Image Source/Getty Images; p. 349 left to right: Roger Lee/SuperStock/PhotoLibrary; vario images GmbH & Co. KG/Alamy; p. 350: Stockbyte/Getty Images; p. 351: Fuse/Getty Images; p. 352: Rafael Laguillo/iStockphoto; p. 355: Goodshoot/Jupiter Images; p. 356: INSADCO Photography/Alamy; fig. fig. 11.6: I Love Images/PhotoLibrary; p. 359 top: Benjamin Brandt/iStockphoto; p. 359 bottom left: Image Source/Getty Images; p. 359 bottom right: Murat Giray Kaya/iStockphoto; fig. 11.7a CNRI/SPL/Photo Researchers, Inc.; fig. 11.7b: Martin M. Rotker/Photo Researchers, Inc.; p. 362 Ellen B. Senisi/The Image Works; p. 363: Roger Lee/SuperStock/PhotoLibrary; p. 364: Thinkstock/Getty Images; p. 365: Sharon Dominick/iStockphoto; p. 367: vario images GmbH & Co. KG/Alamy; p. 368: Mark Peterson/Corbis; p. 370: Superstock; p. 371: Stanislav Fadyukhin/iStockphoto.com.

**Chapter 12** Opener: Radius Images/Alamy; p. 376 left to right: Kristin Piljay, Pearson Science; Rayman/Getty Images; Image courtesy of Romano & Associates, Inc./Oral Health America; p. 377 left to right: Image Source/Alamy; Comstock Images/Getty Images; p. 378: Steve Wanke/Taxi /Getty Images; p. 379: Kristin Piljay, Pearson Science; p. 380: Tony Cenicola/The New York Times/Redux; p. 382: Stringer/Getty Images; fig. 12.2: Elizabeth Weinberg/PhotoLibrary; p. 383: Rayman/Digital Vision/Getty Images; p. 384: Elvele Images Ltd/Alamy; fig. 12.3 James Stevenson/Photo Researchers, Inc.; p. 387 left: image100/Alamy; p. 387 right: Image courtesy of Romano & Associates, Inc./Oral Health America; fig. 12.4: TPH/allOver photography/Alamy; p. 389: Sharon Dominick/iStockphoto; p. 390: Getty Images; p. 392: John Howard/Digital Vision/Getty Images; p. 393 left: Image Source/Alamy; p. 395: Comstock Images/Getty Images; table 12.4 top to bottom: Josh Sher/Photo Researchers, Inc.; Bloombeg/Getty Images; Michael Newman/PhotoEdit; Gustoimages/Photo Researchers, Inc.; Jane Stockman/Dorling Kindersley; Custom Medical Stock Photo; ICP/Alamy; p. 398: fStop/Alamy; p. 400: Milos Luzanin/iStockphoto.com.

**Chapter 13** Opener: Falko Updarp/Corbis; p. 404 left to right: Arnd Wiegmann/Reuters/Corbis; David Hoffman Photo Library/Alamy; Luc Beziat/Getty Images; p. 405 left to right: Jon Bradley/Getty Images; Jupiterimages/Getty Images; fig. 13.1: Image Source/Getty Images; p. 407: Craig Wactor/Shutterstock; fig. 13.2: Science Photo Library/Alamy; p. 408: sumnersgraphicsinc/iStockphoto; p. 409 left: Lori Sparkla/Shutterstock; p. 409 right: Arnd Wiegmann/Reuters/Corbis; p. 411: Chris Haston/Fox/Everett Collection; p. 412: Jeff Greenberg/Alamy; fig. 13.4: Image Source/Getty Images; p. 415: Banana Stock/PhotoLibrary; p. 417: Charles Tatlock; p. 419 top: iStockphoto; p. 419 bottom: Jamie Grill/Iconica/Getty Images; p. 420: Park Street/PhotoEdit; p. 421: Gregor Buir/Shutterstock; p. 422: David Hoffman Photo Library/Alamy; p. 423: Luc Beziat/Getty Images; p. 424 top: Martyn Vickery/Alamy; p. 424 bottom: Bob Cheung/Shutterstock; p. 426: Janine Wiedel Photolibrary/Alamy; p. 426: Hiroko Masuike/Getty Images News; p. 427: Jon Bradley/Getty Images; p. 428: Jupiterimages/Getty Images; p. 429: Cappy Thompson/Arresting Images; p. 430: iStockphoto.

**Chapter 14** Opener: Image Source/Getty Images; p. 434 left to right: Tschilar Marco/PhotoLibrary; age fotostock/SuperStock; Peter Llewellyn/Alamy; p. 435 left to right: Steve Mercer/Getty Images; Gideon Mendel/Corbis; fig. 14.2: John Howard/Getty Images; p. 440: Michael Krinke/iStockphoto; p. 441: Murat Giray Kaya/iStockphoto; p. 442: Tschilar Marco/PhotoLibrary; fig. 14.5a: Gary Gaugler/Photo Researchers, Inc.; fig. 14.5b: Dr. Linda Stannard, UCT/Photo Researchers, Inc.; fig. 14.5c: Steve Gschmeissner/Photo Researchers, Inc.; fig. 14.5d: Eye of Science/Photo Researchers, Inc.; fig. 14.5e: David Scharf/Image Source/Getty Images; p. 444: Science Photo Library/PhotoLibrary; p. 445: Kelly Mooney Photography/Corbis; p. 446: iStockphoto; p. 447: age fotostock/SuperStock; p. 448: Dai Kurokawa/epa/Corbis; fig. 14.7: Sidea Revuz/Photo Researchers, Inc.; p. 450: iStockphoto; p. 451: Peter Llewellyn/Alamy; p. 452: Reuters/Corbis; p. 455: Steve Mercer/Getty Images; p. 456: Jupiterimages/Getty Images; fig. 14.10: Western Ophthalmic Hospital/Photo Researchers, Inc.; fig. 14.11: Centers for Disease Control and Prevention; fig. 14.12a–c: Photo Researchers, Inc.; p. 458: Sharon Dominick/iStockphoto; fig. 14.13a: Wellcome Trust Library/Custom Medical Stock Photo; fig. 14.13b: CDC Public Health Image Library; fig. 14.14 left: Photo Researchers, Inc.; fig. 14.14 right: Centers for Disease Control and Prevention; p.461: John Amis/AP Wide World Photos; fig. 14.15: Eye of Science/Photo Researchers, Inc.; p. 462: Gideon Mendel/Corbis; p. 464: Stonehill/zefa/Corbis; p. 465: Das Fotoarchiv/PhotoLibrary;

p. 466: Nick Ut/AP Wide World Photos; p. 467 top: Tomaz Levstek/iStockphoto; p. 467 bottom: iStockphoto; p. 468: Simon Valentine/iStockphoto.

**FOCUS ON Understanding Your Health Inheritance** Opener: Blend Images/SuperStock; p. 472 left to right: Scott Bauer/Photo Researchers, Inc.; Adam Hart-Davis/Photo Researchers, Inc.; Ryan McVay/Getty Images; Leila Cutler/Alamy; p. 473: sumnersgraphicsinc/iStockphoto; p. 474: Ingram Publishing/PhotoLibrary; p. 475: Scott Bauer/Photo Researchers, Inc.; fig. 2 Addenbrookes Hospital/Photo Researchers, Inc.; p. 476: Stefanie Sudek/Getty Images; p. 477 top: Adam Hart-Davis/Photo Researchers, Inc.; p. 477 bottom: Friedrich Stark/Alamy; fig 5: Exactostock/SuperStock; p. 479 top: Ryan McVay/Getty Images; p. 479 bottom: Bridge/PhotoLibrary; p. 481: Leila Cutler/Alamy; p. 482: NLshop/iStockphoto; p. 483: Sharon Dominick/iStockphoto.

**Chapter 15** Opener: Jack Hollingsworth/PhotoLibrary; p. 486 left to right: John Shearer/WireImage/Getty Images; Ian Hooton/SPL/Getty Images; Fotokia/Getty Images; p. 487 left to right: Thinkstock/Getty Images; Purestock/Alamy; p. 490: John Shearer/WireImage/Getty Images; p. 493: Paul Conklin/PhotoEdit; p. 494: Sharon Dominick/iStockphoto; p. 495: iStockphoto; p. 497: Ian Hooton/SPL/Getty Images; fig. 15.7: Radius Images/Alamy; p. 499: Fotokia/Getty Images; p. 500: Julien Bastide/Shutterstock; p. 501: Cusp/PhotoLibrary; p. 502: Koki lino/Getty Images; fig. 15.9: Moodboard/PhotoLibrary; p. 504: Thinkstock/Getty Images; p. 505 top: Stefan Ataman/iStockphoto; p. 505 bottom: Michael Ventura/Alamy; p. 506: Purestock/Alamy; p. 507: Tetra Images/Getty Images; p. 508: Red Images, LLC/Alamy; p. 509: Ioana Davies/iStockphoto; p. 510 top: iStockphoto; p. 510 bottom center: Max Delson Martins Santos/iStockphoto; p. 510 bottom right: Mark Stay/iStockphoto.

**FOCUS ON Minimizing Your Risk for Diabetes** Opener: Ismael Lopez/PhotoLibrary; p. 514 left to right: John Giustina/Getty Images; Terry Vine/Blend Images/Corbis; Stockxpert/Jupiter Unlimited; Jerilee Bennet/Colorado Springs Gazette/Newscom; p. 516: Rob Hoffman/JBE/Getty Images; p. 517: Donna Day/Getty Images; p. 518: John Giustina/Getty Images; p. 519: Elfina Photo Art/iStockphoto; p. 520: Terry Vine/Blend Images/Corbis; fig. 3a: Medicimage/PhotoLibrary; fig. 3b: Paul Parker/Photo Researchers, Inc.; p. 521: Murat Giray Kaya/iStockphoto; p. 522: Stockxpert/Jupiter Unlimited; p. 523: Jerilee Bennet/Colorado Springs Gazette/Newscom; p. 524: Andrew Gentry/Shutterstock.

**Chapter 16** Opener: Purestock/Getty Images; p. 526 left to right: Philippe Psaila/SPL/Photo Researchers, Inc.; Blend Images/Alamy; BSIP SA/Alamy; p. 527 left to right: Rick Gomez/Masterfile; Kevin Winter/Getty Images; p. 529: Philippe Psaila/SPL/Photo Researchers, Inc.; p. 530: PhotoLibrary; p. 531 top: Sharon Dominick/iStockphoto; p. 531 bottom: iStockphoto; p. 532: Allen Russell/PhotoLibrary; p. 533: iStockphoto; p. 534 top: Blend Images/Alamy; p. 534 bottom: ERproductions Ltd/Getty Images; p. 536: BSIP SA/Alamy; p. 537: Garo/Photo Researchers, Inc.; p. 539: Sharon Dominick/iStockphoto; p. 540: Rick Gomez/Masterfile; fig. 16.3a: James Stevenson/SPL/Photo Researchers, Inc.; fig. 16.3b: Dr. P. Marazzi/SPL/Photo Researchers, Inc.; fig. 16.3c: Dr. P. Marazzi/SPL/Photo Researchers, Inc.; p. 541: David Sacks/Getty Images; p. 542: FilmMagic/Getty Images; p. 543: Joel Saget/Agence France Presse/Getty Images; p. 547 top: Science Photo Library, Photo Researchers, Inc.; p. 547 bottom: Kevin Winter/Getty Images; p. 548 Steve Prezant/Corbis; p. 550 mark wragg/iStockphoto.

**Chapter 17** Opener: Agencja FREE/Alamy; p. 554 left to right: Custom Medical Stock Photo/Alamy; Science Photo Library/Alamy; Gladskikh Tatiana/Shutterstock; p. 555: JLP/Jose L. Pelaez/Corbis; Chassenet/BSIP SA/Alamy; fig. 17.1: allOver photography/Alamy; p. 557: Reinhard Krause/Reuters/Landov; p. 558: Adam Gault/Getty Images; fig. 17.2: PhotoAlto/Alamy; p. 559: Custom Medical Stock Photo/Alamy; p. 561: Science Photo Library/Alamy; p. 562: Vanja Gavric/Alamy; p. 563: Corbis Premium RF/Alamy; p. 565: Alexander Tsiaras/Photo Researchers, Inc.; p. 566: Gladskikh Tatiana/Shutterstock; p. 569: JLP/Jose L. Pelaez/Corbis; p.570: sumnersgraphicsinc/iStockphoto; p. 571 left: Jack Sullivan/Alamy; p. 571 right: BSIP SA/Alamy; p. 572: Ken Kaminesky/Getty Images; p. 573 left: Gilmanshin/Shutterstock; p. 573 right: Slyadnyev Oleksandr/Shutterstock; p. 574 top: Jim Jurica/iStockphoto; p. 574 bottom: Stefano Lunardi/iStockphoto; p. 575: claudiobaba/iStockphoto.

**Chapter 18** Opener: Darren Kemper/Corbis; p.578 left to right: Jiang Jin/Superstock; Luca Tettoni/Corbis; Willie Hill, Jr./The Image Works; p.579 left to right: Michael Newman/PhotoEdit; Bruce Laurance/Getty Images; p. 580: Peter Scholey/Getty Images; p. 581: Jiang Jin/Superstock; p. 583: Tatiana Popova/shutterstock; p. 584: Ilene MacDonald/Alamy; p. 587: Luca Tettoni/Corbis; p. 589: Bananastock/Jupiter Images; p. 590: Willie Hill, Jr./The Image Works; p. 591 Murat Giray Kaya/iStockphoto; p. 592: Steve Snowden/Shutterstock; p. 595: Michael Newman/PhotoEdit; table 8.2 top to bottom: Elena Elisseeva/Shutterstock; WILDLIFE GmbH/Alamy; Shapiso/shutterstock; Joanna Wnuk/Shutterstock; WEKWEK/iStockphoto; eAlisa/shutterstock; bildagentur-online.com/th-foto/Alamy; Richard Griffin/Shutterstock; WILDLIFE GmbH/Alamy; fig. 18.6: U.S. Pharmacopeia; p. 598: Jochen Tack/Alamy; p. 599: Bruce Laurance/Getty Images; p. 602: Comstock Images/Jupiter Unlimited; p. 603: Pixland/PhotoLibrary; p. 604: Viviane Moos/Corbis; p. 605: Fabio Cardoso/Corbis; p. 606 top: iStockphoto; p. 606 bottom: jo unruh/iStockphoto.

**Chapter 19** Opener: Chris Rout/Alamy; p. 610 left to right: Catherine Ursillo/Photo Researchers, Inc.; D. Hurst/Alamy; Paula Bronstein/Getty Images; p. 611 left to right: Bill Aron/PhotoEdit; William Thomas Cain/Getty Images; fig. 19.1: Jochen Tack/Alamy; p. 613: Alamy; p. 614: Catherine Ursillo/Photo Researchers, Inc.; p. 615 top: Alamy; p. 615 bottom: Sharon Dominick/iStockphoto; p. 616: D. Hurst/Alamy; p. 617: iStockphoto; fig. 19.3: Thinkstock; p. 619: Paula Bronstein/Getty Images; p. 620 top: Hill Creek Pictures/Getty Images; p. 620 bottom: Sharon Dominick/iStockphoto; p. 622: Bill Aron/PhotoEdit; p. 623: Peter M. Fisher/Corbis; p. 624: iStockphoto; p. 626 top: Patti Sapone/Star Ledger/Corbis; p. 626 bottom: William Thomas Cain/Getty Images; p. 628: Justin Sullivan/Getty Images; p. 630 top: Gerville Hall/iStockphoto; p. 630 bottom: iQoncept/Shutterstock; pl 631 top: Felix Mizioznikov/Shutterstock; p. 630 bottom left: Eric Ferguson/iStockphoto; p. 631 right: Daniel Deitschel/iStockphoto.

**FOCUS ON Reducing Your Risk of Unintentional Injury** Opener: INSADCO Photography/Alamy; p. 636 left to right: Radius Images/Alamy; Martin Heitner/PhotoLibrary; Laurel Scherer/PhotoLibrary; Jeff Greenberg/PhotoEdit; p. 637: Radius Images/Alamy; p. 638 top: Martin Heitner/PhotoLibrary; p. 638 bottom: PhotoEdit; p. 640: Laurel Scherer/PhotoLibrary; fig. 1: Kristin Piljay, Pearson Science; p. 641: PNC/Getty Images; p. 643: Jeff Greenberg/PhotoEdit; p. 644: sumnersgraphicsinc/iStockphoto; p. 645: Caterina Bernardi/Getty Images; fig. 3: Alamy; p. 648 top: Dmitry Melnikov/ shutterstock; p. 648 bottom: Cosmonaut Creative Media, LLC/iStockphoto.

**Chapter 20** Opener: Alix Minde/Getty Images; p. 650 left to right: Lonely Planet Images/Getty Images; Masterfile; Real World People/Alamy; p. 651 left to right: David McNew/Getty Images; qaphotos.com/Alamy; p. 653: Murat Giray Kaya/iStockphoto; p. 654: Lonely Planet Images/Getty Images; p. 655: Masterfile; p. 657: Will and Demi McIntyre/Photo Researchers, Inc.; p. 660: Real World People/Alamy; p. 662: Ari Joseph/Middlebury College; p. 663: David McNew/Getty Images; p. 664: qaphotos.com/Alamy; p. 666: Raphael Van Butsele/Getty Images; p. 667: Philip James Corwin/Corbis; p. 668: Blend Images/Alamy; p. 670: p.imagebroker.net/PhotoLibrary; p. 671: iStockphoto; p. 672 top: iStockphoto; p. 672 bottom left: iStockphoto; p. 672 bottom right: Jupiter Images.

**Chapter 21** Opener: Jim Naughton/Getty Images; p. 676 left to right: Avik Gilboa/WireImage/Getty Images; Dan Bosler/Stone/Getty Images; Thinkstock/Getty Images; p. 677 left to right: DreamPictures/Blend Images/Corbis; Bodenham, LTH NHS Trust/Photo Researchers, Inc.; p. 678 top: Ronnie Kaufman/Blend Images/Getty Images; p. 678 bottom: Avik Gilboa/WireImage/Getty Images; p. 680: Markos Dolopikos/Alamy; p. 681: Klaus Guldbrandsen/Photo Researchers, Inc.; fig. 21.3: moodboard/Corbis; p. 682: Sharon Dominick/iStockphoto; p. 683: Ariel Skelley/Corbis; p. 684 top: Karen Massler/iStockphoto; p. 684 bottom: Dan Bosler/Stone/Getty Images; p. 686: John Henley/Corbis; p. 687: Thinkstock/Getty Images; p. 689: DreamPictures/Blend Images/Corbis; p. 691: Matthew Plexman/Masterfile; p. 692: Bodenham, LTH NHS Trust/Photo Researchers, Inc.; p. 694: Pascal Broze/Reporters/Photo Researchers, Inc.; p. 695: Richard Hutchings/PhotoEdit; p. 696: Apex News and Pictures Agency/Alamy; p. 698: Daniel Cardiff/iStockphoto.

# Index

# O

Oat fiber, 591
Obama, Michelle, 251
Obesity. *See* Overweight/obesity
Obesogenic, 251
Objectification of women, 625
Object meditation, 68
Obsession, sign of addiction, 330
Obsessive-compulsive disorder (OCD), 45
Obstetrician/gynecologist, 197t
Obstructive sleep apnea, 111–112
OCD. *See* Obsessive-compulsive disorder
OGTT. *See* Oral glucose tolerance test
Older adults
ethical and moral considerations, 680–681
exercise and, 309
growing number of, 678–679, 679fig
health care costs, 679, 679p
housing and living arrangements, 679–680, 679fig
sexual response and, 150–151
*See also* Aging
Omega-3 fatty acids, 218, 503
Omega-6 fatty acids, 218
*Omnivore's Dilemma, The* (Pollan), 238
Oncogenes, 531
*On Death and Dying* (Kübler–Ross), 688
One hundred-mile diet, 238
One repetition maximum (1 RM), 298, 309–310
Online medications, 592, 592p
Open relationships, 130
Ophthalmologists, 585
Opioids, 421–422, 421p, 422p
*See also* Drug misuse/abuse; Drugs; Narcotics
Opium, 421, 421p
Opium poppy seedpod, 421, 421p
Opportunistic infections, 438, 463–464
Optometrists, 585
Oral contraceptives, 171t, 172t, 177–178, 177p, 178fig
Oral–genital stimulation, 157
Oral glucose tolerance test (OGTT), 521, 521fig
Oral herpes, 458, 459fig
Oral ingestion, of drugs, 407, 407fig
Organ donation, 697, 697fig
Organelles, 358
Organic foods, 235–236, 236p
Orgasmic disorders, 159–160
Orgasmic phase, 150, 151fig
Orgasmic standard of sex, 155
Ornish, Dean, 211
Ortho Evra (contraceptive patch), 172t, 179, 179p
Osteoarthritis, 570–571, 682
Osteopaths, 583, 585
Osteoporosis, 300, 682, 683, 683p
OTC. *See* Over-the-counter (OTC) drugs
"Outercourse," 184
Outpatient behavioral treatment, 426
Ovarian cancer, 528t, 542–543
Ovarian follicles, 145, 146fig
Ovaries, 144–146, 145fig, 146fig, 152

Overload
in resistance exercise program, 309, 310
stress, 82
Overpopulation, 13
growth rates by nation, 653–654
measuring, 652, 652fig
total fertility rates, 653, 653t
zero population growth, 654
Over-the-counter (OTC) drugs, 406, 563, 593–594, 593t, 594fig
misuse/abuse of, 408–409
sleeping aids, 108–109
supplements as, 234
*See also* Drug misuse/abuse; Drugs; Medications
Overuse injuries, 316–317
Overweight/obesity
as a disability, 272, 272p
body fat measures, 263–264, 264fig
body fat percentage recommendations, 261t
body mass index (BMI), 251, 262, 263fig
body type and genes, 252–254, 253p
cancer and, 531
cardiovascular disease and, 500–501, 501p
children and, 257–258, 258p
costs of, 6–7, 252
defining, 261
diabetes and, 517–518
environmental factors, 256–258
exercise and, 308
fat cells and predisposition to fatness, 256
fat cells at various stages of weight loss, 256fig
fiber and, 219
health risks associated with, 251–252, 253fig
hormones: ghrelin and leptin, 255–256
lifestyle factors, 258, 260–261
metabolic rates and, 254–255
obesity stigma, 260, 260p
pregnancy and, 197
psychosocial and economic factors, 258
puberty and, 145
by race/ethnicity, 251
sitting and, 260, 260p
sleep and, 103–104, 104p
stress and, 77
trends, 252fig
waist circumference and ratio measurements, 262–263
*See also* Weight management
Oviducts (fallopian tubes), 144, 145fig
Ovulation, 146, 146fig
Ovum, 145
Oxidative stress, 224–225
OxyContin, 411, 411p, 416t
Oxytocin, 120
Ozone, 655, 656t
Ozone layer depletion, 660

# P

PAD. *See* Peripheral artery disease
Pain, 11, 441, 507, 563, 563p
Palliative care, 447, 693, 694
Pancreas, 516

Pancreatic cancer, 389, 528t, 531
Pandemic flu, 452, 452p
Pandemics, defined, 435
Panic attacks, 45
Panic disorders, 45, 45p
Pap test, 459, 543
ParaGard, 181, 182, 182p
Paranoid personality disorder, 46
Parasitic worms, 443fig, 451
Parasomnias, 112–113
Parasympathetic nervous system, 75
Parental influence, violence and, 612–613
Parenting choices, 134–135, 134p, 135t
Parenting styles, 135t
Parkinson's disease, 567t
Partial birth abortion (intact dilation and extraction), 190
Partially hydrogenated oils, 220
PAs. *See* Physician assistants
Passionate love, 120, 120fig
Passive (attentive) listening, 127
Passive euthanasia, 693
Passive smokers, 391
Paternal health, 192–193
Pathogens
animalborne, 436
bacteria, 442–446, 443fig, 445p, 446p
body's defenses against, 438–439, 439fig
cardiovascular disease and, 504
defined, 435
foodborne illnesses, 239t
fungi, 443fig, 450–451
parasitic worms, 443fig, 451
prions, 451
protozoans, 443fig, 451
routes of transmission, 436, 436t
viruses, 443fig, 447–450, 447p, 448fig, 448p, 450p
*See also* Bacteria; Diseases/disorders; Viruses
PCBs. *See* Polychlorinated biphenyls
PCOS. *See* Polycystic ovary syndrome
PCP. *See* Phencyclidine
PCP. *See* Primary care practitioner
PDAs. *See* Personal digital assistants
Pedophilia, 158
Pelvic inflammatory disease (PID), 203, 455–456, 456p
Penicillin, 443
Penile cancer, 148
Penis, 148, 148fig
Peptic ulcers, 446
Percocet, 411
Perfectionism, 86
Perfect use failure rate, 170
Performance, physical activity for, 298
Performance-enhancing drugs, 315, 315t
Perineum, 144, 145fig
Periods of communicability, 454
Peripheral artery disease (PAD), 491–492
Permissive parenting style, 135t
Personal digital assistants (PDAs), 81
Personal flotation device, 641
Personality
genetics and, 481
well-being and, 36–37

Personality disorders, 46
Personality types (A, B, C, D), 84
Pessimism, 86
Pesticides, 665
PET scan. *See* Positron emission tomography (PET) scan
Peyote, 416t, 424, 424p
Pharmaceutical waste, 602
Phencyclidine (PCP), 406, 416t, 424
Phenylethylamine, 121
Phobic disorders, 45, 45p
Photochemical smog, 655–656, 656t
Physical activity
body composition and, 297fig, 298
cancer and, 531
cardiorespiratory fitness, 296, 297fig, 298–299
defined, 296
for fitness, 296–298, 297fig, 297t
flexibility, 297fig, 298
guidelines for, 297t, 687t
for health, 296
for improved bone mass and reduced risk of osteoporosis, 300, 683
for improved immunity, 301
incidence of, 295
lack of, 10
for longer life span, 301
for mental health, 301
muscular strength and endurance, 297fig, 298
overcoming obstacles to, 301–302, 302p, 302t
for performance, 298
for reduced cancer risk, 299–300
for reduced risk of cardiovascular diseases, 298, 501
for reduced risk of metabolic syndrome and type 2 diabetes, 299, 522
sleep and, 107
for special populations, 308–309, 308p
for stress management, 301
for weight management, 268, 300–301
*See also* Exercise; Physical fitness; Physical fitness programs
Physical attraction, 123
Physical checkups, 50
Physical environment, health effects and, 12
Physical fitness
assessing yourself, 321–324
benefits of, 298–301, 299fig
components of, 297fig
defined, 296
diabetes and, 522
fitness-related injuries, 316–320, 317p, 318fig, 320p
FITT principle (frequency, intensity, time, type), 306–312, 306fig
gadgets and equipment for, 304t
goals for, 301
incorporating into your life, 302–303
motivation and commitment to, 298–301
older adults, 686–687, 687t, 687p
overcoming obstacles to, 301–302, 302t
websites for, 326

Psychosocial health
    cancer and, 531
    overweight/obesity, 258
    sleep and, 104
    spirituality and, 64
    stress and, 79–83, 82*p*, 83*p*
    *See also* Psychological health
PTSD. *See* Post-traumatic stress
    disorder
Puberty, 144–145, 152
    *See also* Menstrual cycle
Pubic lice, 460–461, 462*fig*
Public health achievements, of the
    20th century, 8*fig*
Public health model, 7–8
    *See also* Ecological model of
      health
Public policies, 12
Purpose, spirituality and, 63, 63*fig*

## Q

*Qi*, 93, 590
Qigong, 93, 314, 587, 590
Quality of life, 5
    spirituality and, 64

## R

*Rabbi Ben Ezra* (Browning), 678
Rabies, 450, 450*p*
Race/ethnicity
    alcohol use and, 366, 366*t*
    cardiovascular disease, 489, 503,
      504*fig*
    depression, 42
    genetic disorders and, 479–480
    health disparities and, 14
    health insurance, 598
    illicit drug use, 412, 412*t*, 412*p*
    obesity, 251, 257
    sleep disorders, 110*t*
    smoking, 377–378, 378*t*, 380–381
Radiation
    cancer and, 533–534
    ionizing, 669
    nonionizing, 667–669, 668*p*
    nuclear power plants, 669–670,
      670*p*
    *See also* Food irradiation
Radiation absorbed doses (rads),
    669
Radionuclides, 505
Radiotherapy, 546
Radon, 659
Rads. *See* Radiation absorbed doses
RAM. *See* Remote Area Medical
    (RAM) clinics
Ramstad Act (Campus Sexual
    Assault Victim's Bill of Rights),
    622
Rape
    acquaintance (date) rape, 353,
      622, 622*p*
    date rape drugs, 161
    defined, 621
    marital rape, 622
    on U.S. campuses, 422, 612, 613,
      622, 622*p*
    what to do if rape occurs, 627
    *See also* Sexual victimization
Rating of perceived exertion scale,
    307
Rational suicide, 693
Raynaud's syndrome, 567*t*
RBD. *See* REM sleep behavior
    disorder

RDAs. *See* Recommended Dietary
    Allowances
RDIs. *See* Daily Reference Intakes
Reactive aggression, 615
Realistic expectations, 38
Rebound relationships, 137
Receptor sites, 408
Recessive genes, 476–478, 478*fig*,
    479*p*
Reciprocity, 123
Recommended Dietary Allowances
    (RDAs), 233
Recovery
    from cardiovascular disease, 508
    from drug addiction, 426–427,
      427*p*
Recreational drugs, 406–407
    *See also* Alcohol; Caffeine; Drug
      misuse/abuse; Drugs;
      Tobacco use
Recreational safety, 639–642,
    640*fig*, 640*p*, 641*p*
Rectal cancer, 539, 545*t*
Recycling, 666, 666*fig*, 667*p*
Red wine, 503
Registered nurses (RNs), 585
Rehabilitation, from cardiovascular
    disease, 508
Relapse from recovery, 341–342,
    370
Relationships
    choosing romantic partners,
      122–123
    cohabitation, 132
    communication and, 125–130,
      125*p*, 126*fig*, 128*p*
    Defense of Marriage Act
      (DOMA), 133, 133*p*
    ending, 135–137, 136*p*, 137*p*
    expectations and, 124–125
    family, 118
    friendships, 119, 119*p*
    gay/lesbian partnerships,
      132–134, 132*p*
    gender roles, 124
    healthy vs. unhealthy, 121–122,
      122*fig*
    intimate, 117–121, 118*p*, 119*p*,
      120*fig*
    jealousy in, 123–124, 124*p*
    marriage, 130–132, 130*fig*, 130*p*,
      131*p*
    meeting people online, 123
    older adults, 686
    parenting choices, 134–135,
      134*p*, 135*t*
    power in, 124
    romantic, 119–121, 120*fig*
    with self, 118–119
    singles, 134
    spirituality and, 62–63
    stress and, 80–82
    *See also* Communication;
      Intimate relationships
Relaxation techniques, 89–90
    biofeedback, 95
    diaphragmatic or deep
      breathing, 94, 94*p*
    hypnosis, 95
    meditation, 94
    massage therapy, 95
    progressive muscle relaxation,
      95, 95*fig*
    qigong, 93
    tai chi, 93–94

    visualization, 94
    yoga, 92–93, 93*p*
Religion
    contraception and, 187
    violence and, 613
    vs. spirituality, 62, 62*p*, 62*fig*
Remote Area Medical (RAM)
    clinics, 14*p*
REM sleep, 105–106, 105*fig*
REM sleep behavior disorder
    (RBD), 113
Repetitive motion disorders
    (RMDs, repetitive stress
    injuries), 81, 646–647, 647*fig*
Reproduction, 143
    female hormones, 144–146
    male hormones, 148–150
    *See also* Childbirth; Contracep-
      tion (birth control);
      Pregnancy; Sexual
      anatomy/physiology
Residential treatment programs,
    426
Resiliency, 37
Resistance phase of general adap-
    tation syndrome, 75, 75*fig*
Resistance training, 305–306,
    306*fig*, 309–310, 310*p*, 311*t*
Resolution phase, 150, 151*fig*
Respiratory disorders
    coping with, 555–560
    smoking and, 390
    *See also* Asthma; Chronic
      obstructive pulmonary
      disease (COPD)
Resting metabolic rate (RMR),
    254–255
Restless legs syndrome (RLS), 112
Restrictive surgeries, for weight
    loss, 271
Reverse transcriptase, 465
Rewards, 23
Reye's syndrome, 447
Rheumatic heart disease, 497
Rheumatoid arthritis, 571
Rh factor, pregnancy and, 201
RhoGAM, 201
RICE: rest, ice, compression, eleva-
    tion, 317–318, 317*p*
Rickettsia, 446
Right to die, 692–693
Risk behaviors
    body piercing and tattooing, 464,
      464*p*
    defined, 8
    HIV/AIDS, 463
    sexually transmitted infections
      (STIs), 453–454, 454*fig*
Risk factors
    addiction, 333–334, 333*fig*, 333*p*,
      334*p*
    alcohol abuse, 365
    breast cancer, 539
    cancer, 528–535
    cardiovascular disease, 497–505
    colon and rectal cancers, 539
    eating disorders, 286, 286*fig*
    HIV transmission, 462–463,
      463*fig*
    infectious diseases, 436–438,
      437*fig*
    mental illness, 39
    metabolic syndrome, 497–498,
      498*fig*
    modern maladies, 567–568*t*

    lung cancer, 536
    osteoporosis, 682, 683
    ovarian cancer, 543
    overweight/obesity, 252–261
    prostate cancer, 541–542, 541*p*
    sexually transmitted infections,
      453–454, 454*fig*
    skin cancer, 540–541
    suicide, 48
    type 2 diabetes, 516–517
    *See also* Health determinants
Risk reduction
    cancer, 299–300, 533, 536*p*, 538,
      538*fig*, 541, 544, 544*fig*, 545*t*
    cardiovascular disease, 298–299,
      497–505
    dating violence, 627
    driving, 639
    home injuries, 642–645, 643*p*,
      644*fig*, 645*p*
    infectious diseases, 436–437
    metabolic syndrome, 299
    motor vehicle accidents,
      637–639, 637*p*, 638*p*
    obesity, 300–301
    osteoporosis, 300, 683, 683*p*
    rape and assault, 626–627
    recreational activities, 639–642,
      640*fig*, 640*p*, 641*p*
    type 2 diabetes, 299, 519
    work injuries, 645–647, 646*fig*,
      647*fig*
    *See also* Prevention
Risks
    for cancer, 529–535
    foodborne illnesses, 240, 240*p*,
      241
    of obesity, 252
R. J. Reynolds, 379
RLS. *See* Restless legs syndrome
RMDs. *See* Repetitive motion
    disorders
RMR. *See* Resting metabolic rate
RNs. *See* Registered nurses
Road rage, 615, 615*p*
Rocky Mountain spotted fever
    (RMSF), 446
Roetgens, 669
*Roe v. Wade* (1973), 187
Rogers, Carl, 125
Rohypnol (date rape drug), 161,
    416*t*, 422, 423, 622
'Roid rage, 425
Role models, 20–21
Rolfing, 589
Romantic relationships, 119–121,
    120*fig*, 122–123
Romantic standard of sex, 155
Roosevelt, Teddy, 281
Rosacea, 568*t*
Rosen, Larry, 81
Rosenman, Ray, 84
Rosenstock, I., 15
RTFQ (Read the Full Question), 85
RU-486 (early abortion pill), 183
Rubella (German measles), 198, 450
Runner's knee, 316–317
Running shoes, 318, 318*fig*
Runoff, 664, 664*fig*
Russert, Tim, 491

## S

SAD. *See* Seasonal affective disorder
Sadomasochism, 158
Safe Drinking Water Act (SDWA), 664